LEGAL MEDICINE

American College of Legal Medicine Textbook Committee

S. Sandy Sanbar, M.D., Ph.D., J.D., F.C.L.M.
Chairman and Project Director (1994-1995)
Past President, ACLM (1989-1990)

Allan Gibofsky, M.D., J.D., F.A.C.P., F.C.L.M.
President, The American College of Legal Medicine (1994-1995)

Marvin H. Firestone, M.D., J.D., F.C.L.M.
Immediate Past President, ACLM (1993-1994)

Theodore R. LeBlang, J.D., F.C.L.M.
Publications Committee Chairman, ACLM (1994-1995)

Third Edition

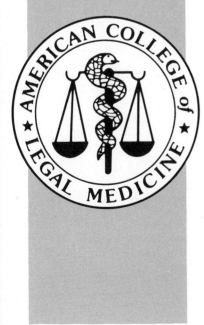

AMERICAN
COLLEGE
OF
LEGAL
MEDICINE

M Mosby

St. Louis Baltimore Boston Carlsbad Chicago Naples New York Philadelphia Portland
London Madrid Mexico City Singapore Sydney Tokyo Toronto Wiesbaden

Ⅳ Mosby

Dedicated to Publishing Excellence

**A Times Mirror
Company**

Editor: Susie H. Baxter
Developmental Editor: Ellen Baker Geisel
Project Manager: Karen Edwards
Senior Book Designer: Gail Morey Hudson
Editing and Production: Spectrum Publisher Services
Manufacturing Supervisor: Tim Stringham

THIRD EDITION

Printed in the United States of America
Composition by Graphic World, Inc.
Printing/binding by Maple-Vail Book Mfg. Group

Mosby–Year Book, Inc.
11830 Westline Industrial Drive
St. Louis, Missouri 63146

Library of Congress Cataloging in Publication Data

Legal medicine / American College of Legal Medicine. —3rd ed.
    p. cm.
   Includes bibliographical references and index.
   ISBN 0-8151-0131-7
   1. Medical laws and legislation—United States. 2. Medical
jurisprudence—United States. I. American College of Legal
Medicine.
   KF3821.L44 1995
   344.73′041—dc20
   [347.30441]   94-43455
                                        CIP

95 96 97 98 99 / 9 8 7 6 5 4 3 2 1

Contributors

JOHN A. ANDERSON, M.D., J.D., F.C.L.M.

VP Medical Care
West Paces Medical Center
Atlanta, Georgia
Chapter 29: The Process of Dying

RICHARD R. BALSAMO, M.D., J.D., F.C.L.M.

Vice President and Medical Director
CIGNA HealthCare of Illinois
Des Plaines, Illinois
Chapter 20: Risk Management

EMIDIO A. BIANCO, M.D., J.D., F.A.C.P., F.C.L.M.

Clinical Associate Professor of Family Medicine
University of Maryland, School of Medicine
Baltimore, Maryland
Medical Officer Case Analyst
Consultation Case Review Branch
Office of the Army Surgeon General
Walter Reed Army Medical Center
Washington, D.C.
Chapter 22: Consent to and Refusal of Medical Treatment

GARLAND L. BIGLEY, R.N., J.D.

Assistant Attorney General
Office of the Attorney General
Richmond, Virginia
Chapter 32: Children as Patients

STEVEN B. BISBING, Psy.D., J.D.

Clinical Assistant Professor of Psychology
Drexel University
Philadelphia, Pennsylvania
Chapter 4: Competency, Capacity, and Immunity

BARRY H. BLOCH, J.D.

Hollowell & Associates, P.A.
Raleigh, North Carolina
Chapter 45: Coproviders and Institutional Practice

MAX DOUGLAS BROWN, J.D.

Vice President and General Counsel
Office of Legal Affairs
Rush-Presbyterian-St. Luke's Medical Center
Associate Professor, Department of Health Systems
Management
College of Health Sciences
Associate Professor (Conjoint Appointment)
Rush University College of Medicine
Chicago, Illinois
Adjunct Assistant Professor
Business School of Rosary College
River Forest, Illinois
Chapter 20: Risk Management

JOHN T. BURROUGHS, M.D., J.D., F.C.L.M.

San Diego, California
Chapter 10: Peer Review, Disciplining, Hearings, and Appeals

MICHAEL S. CARDWELL, M.D., J.D., M.P.H., F.C.L.M.

Director, Maternal-Fetal Medicine
Department of Obstetrics and Gynecology
St. Vincent Medical Center
Toledo, Ohio
Chapter 31: Reproduction Patients

DAVID P. CLUCHEY, M.A., J.D.

Professor of Law
University of Maine School of Law
Portland, Maine
Chapter 16: Antitrust

ARTHUR J. COHEN, M.D., J.D., F.C.L.M.

Private Law Practice
Sarasota, Florida
Private Medical Practice
Bradenton, Florida
Chapter 44: Practice Organizations and Joint Ventures

EDWARD DAVID, M.D., J.D., F.C.L.M.

Neurology Associates of Eastern Maine, P.A.
Bangor, Maine
Chapter 16: Antitrust

JOHN R. FEEGEL, M.D., J.D., M.P.H., F.C.L.M.

Adjunct Professor
College of Public Health
University of South Florida
Tampa, Florida
Chapter 14: Liability of Health Care Entities for Negligent Care

BERNARD J. FICARRA, M.D., Sc.D., LL.D., F.C.L.M.

President, The Catholic Academy of Sciences
Washington, D.C.
Chapter 26: Ethics and Bioethics

MARVIN H. FIRESTONE, M.D., J.D., F.C.L.M.

Neuropsychiatric Consultant
Brain Injury Rehabilitation Unit
Division of Mental Health and Rehabilitation
Palo Alto VA Medical Center
Stanford University School of Medicine
Stanford, California
Former Professor
Schools of Medicine, Law, and Health Services
Administration
George Washington University
Washington, D.C.
Chapter 43: Psychiatric Patients and Forensic Psychiatry

MARTIN B. FLAMM, M.D., J.D., F.C.L.M.

Associate Clinical Professor
Department of Radiology
Louisiana State University Medical Center
Assistant Clinical Professor
Department of Radiology
Tulane University Medical Center
New Orleans, Louisiana
Chapter 11: Health Care Provider as a Defendant

DANIEL J. GAMINO, J.D.

Oklahoma City, Oklahoma
Chapter 9: Education and Licensure

RICHARD F. GIBBS, M.D., J.D., LL.D., F.C.L.M.

Vice Chairman, Board of Directors, Medical Malpractice
Joint Underwriting Association of Massachusetts
Assistant Professor of Anesthesia
Harvard Medical School at the Brigham and Women's
Hospital
Cambridge, Massachusetts
Chapter 19: Medical Liability Insurance

ALLAN GIBOFSKY, M.D., J.D., F.A.C.P., F.C.L.M.

Professor of Medicine
Cornell University Medical College
Adjunct Professor of Law
Fordham University
Attending Physician
Department of Medicine
The Hospital for Special Surgery
New York, New York
Chapter 37: Impaired and Disabled Patients

RICHARD S. GOODMAN, M.D., J.D., F.A.A.O.S., F.C.L.M.

Private Practice in Orthopedics
Orthopedic Consultant
Smithtown, New York
Chapter 40: Sports Medicine

RICHARD L. GRANVILLE, M.D., J.D., F.C.L.M.

Department of Legal Medicine
Armed Forces Institute of Pathology
Washington, D.C.
Chapter 4: Competency, Capacity, and Immunity

KENNETH D. HANSEN, M.D., J.D., F.C.L.M.

Clinical Assistant Professor of Ophthalmology
University of Maryland, School of Medicine
Baltimore, Maryland
President, International Health Foundation
McLean, Virginia
Arlington Eye Associates, Ltd.
Arlington, Virginia
Chapter 2: American Legal System
Chapter 3: Judicial System

C. GORDON HECKEL, M.D., J.D., F.C.L.M.

Consultant in Legal Medicine
Armed Forces Institute of Pathology
Staff Anesthesiologist
Walter Reed Army Medical Center
Washington, D.C.
Chapter 48: Medical Technology

CHARLES G. HESS, M.S., M.D.

Clinical Instructor of Pediatrics
Baylor College of Medicine
Former Chairman of Pediatric Sections
Heights Hospital
Memorial Hospital Northwest
Houston, Texas
Chapter 47: Physician as an Employer

HUGH F. HILL III, M.D., J.D., F.C.L.M.

President, Medical Claims Control
Medical Director of Risk Management
Emergency Medical Services Associates
Consultant in the Professions
Bethesda, Maryland
Chapter 5: Contracts, Agency, and Partnership

HAROLD L. HIRSH, M.D., J.D., F.C.L.M.

Distinguished Visiting Professor
Health Services Management and Policy
George Washington University
Washington, D.C.
Chapter 22: Consent to and Refusal of Medical Treatment
Chapter 23: Medical Records
Chapter 24: Disclosure about Patients
Chapter 37: Impaired and Disabled Patients
Chapter 46: Cost Containment and Reimbursement

WAYNE HODGES, M.D., Psy. D., F.A.A.P.M.

Medical Director
Department of Pain Medicine
Coastal Pain Center
Savannah, Georgia
Chapter 38: Pain Management

ALAN C. HOFFMAN, J.D., F.C.L.M.

Partner, Alan C. Hoffman & Associates
Chicago, Illinois
Chapter 6: Civil Trials
Chapter 12: Medical Malpractice

EDWARD E. HOLLOWELL, J.D., F.C.L.M.

Adjunct Professor of Medical Jurisprudence
School of Medicine
East Carolina University
Greenville, North Carolina
Hollowell & Associates, P.A.
Raleigh, North Carolina
Chapter 45: Coproviders and Institutional Practice

MATTHEW L. HOWARD, M.D., J.D., F.C.L.M.

Associate Physician
Department of Head and Neck Surgery
Kaiser Permanente Medical Group
Santa Rosa, California
Associate Clinical Professor
Department of Otolaryngology
University of San Francisco
Attending Staff, Department of Otolaryngology
San Francisco General Hospital
San Francisco, California
Chapter 21: Physician-Patient Relationship

MARSHALL B. KAPP, J.D., M.P.H.

Professor, Department of Community Health
Wright State University School of Medicine
Dayton, Ohio
Chapter 33: Geriatric Patients

HARVEY KATZ, M.D.

Chapter 25: Telephone Contacts and Counseling

EDWIN KELLERMAN, M.D., J.D., F.C.L.M.

Wynnewood, Pennsylvania
Chapter 28: Organ Donation and Transplantation

IRVING LADIMER, J.D., S.J.D., F.C.L.M.

Adjunct Associate Professor
Department of Community Medicine
Mt. Sinai School of Medicine
New York, New York
Chapter 7: Alternative Dispute Resolution in Health Care

CAROLYN S. LANGER, M.D., J.D., M.P.H.

Instructor in Occupational Medicine
Lecturer in Occupational Health Law
Harvard School of Public Health
Boston, Massachusetts
Chapter 39: Occupational Health Law

BRADFORD H. LEE, M.D., J.D., M.B.A., F.A.C.E.P., F.C.L.M.

Corporate Counsel
Lee, Lee, & Lee, Inc.
Oakland, California
Chapter 18: Countersuits by Health Care Providers

ARTHUR H. LESTER, M.D., J.D., F.A.C.O.G., F.C.L.M.

Attending Physician
Department of Obstetrics and Gynecology
White Wilson Medical Center
Fort Walton Beach, Florida
Chapter 30: Physician-Assisted Suicide

MARTIN J. MacNEILL, D.O., J.D., F.C.L.M.

Brigham Young University
Provo, Utah
Chapter 15: Pharmaceutical Product Liability

JOSEPH P. McMENAMIN, M.D., J.D., F.C.L.M.

Associate, McGuire, Woods, Battle & Boothe
Richmond, Virginia
Chapter 4: Competency, Capacity, and Immunity
Chapter 32: Children as Patients

RICHARD W. MOORE, Jr., J.D., C.P.C.U.

President, Medical Malpractice
Joint Underwriting Association of Massachusetts
Boston, Massachusetts
Chapter 19: Medical Liability Insurance

DONALD L. NEWMAN, M.D.

Detroit Institute of Physical Medicine & Rehabilitation
Southfield, Michigan
Chapter 48: Medical Technology

MAX KARL NEWMAN, A.B., M.D., F.A.C.P.

Biomechanics (Physical Medicine and Rehabilitation)
Michigan State University
East Lansing, Michigan
Retired, Chairman, PMR
Mt. Sinai Hospital
Detroit, Michigan
Detroit Institute of Physical Medicine & Rehabilitation
Southfield, Michigan
Chapter 48: Medical Technology

STEVEN E. NEWMAN, M.D.

Active Staff
Department of Internal Medicine, Section of Neurology
Mt. Sinai Hospital
Detroit, Michigan
Attending Staff
Department of Internal Medicine, Section of Neurology
William Beaumont Hospital
Royal Oak, Michigan
Detroit Institute of Physical Medicine & Rehabilitation
Southfield, Michigan
Chapter 48: Medical Technology

FREDERICK ADOLF PAOLA, M.D., J.D., F.C.L.M.

Assistant Professor
Department of Medicine
S.U.N.Y. at Stony Brook
Stony Brook, New York
Attending Physician
Division of General Medicine
Nassau County Medical Center
East Meadow, New York
Chapter 27: Fetal Interests
Chapter 29: The Process of Dying

JOSEPH D. PIORKOWSKI, Jr., D.O., J.D., M.P.H., F.C.L.M.

Associate, Williams & Connolly
Adjunct Professor
Georgetown University Law Center
Washington, D.C.
Chapter 13: Medical Testimony and the Expert Witness

MIKE A. ROYAL, M.D., J.D., F.C.L.M.

Assistant Professor of Anesthesiology and Critical Care Medicine
University of Pittsburgh School of Medicine
Director, Acute Pain Service
University of Pittsburgh Medical Center
Pittsburgh, Pennsylvania
Chapter 36: Patients with Human Immunodeficiency Virus (HIV) Infection and Acquired Immunodeficiency Syndrome (AIDS)

S. SANDY SANBAR, M.D., Ph.D., J.D., F.C.L.M.

Clinical Assistant Professor
Department of Medicine
Oklahoma University School of Medicine
President, Royal Oaks Cardiovascular Clinic
Law of Medicine
Sanbar Law Firm
Oklahoma City, Oklahoma
Chapter 1: Legal Medicine, Medical Ethics, and Legal Medicine Education in America
Chapter 8: Selected Health Care Statutory Provisions
Chapter 9: Education and Licensure
Chapter 17: Crimes Against and by Health Care Providers and Criminal Procedures

MELVIN A. SHIFFMAN, M.D., J.D., F.C.L.M.

Private Medical Practice
Medicolegal Consultant
Tustin, California
Chapter 34: Oncology Patients

MELINDA THOMPSON, M.D., J.D., F.C.L.M.

Consultant, Legal Medicine
Huntsville, Alabama
Chapter 1: Legal Medicine, Medical Ethics, and Legal Medicine Education in America

STAN TWARDY, J.D., LL.M., A.C.L.M.

Private Legal Practice
Oklahoma City, Oklahoma
Chapter 17: Crimes Against and by Health Care Providers and Criminal Procedures

LOUIS B. VOGT, M.D., J.D., F.C.L.M.

Consultant in Legal Medicine
Department of Legal Medicine
Armed Forces Institute of Pathology
Washington, D.C.
Chapter 21: Physician-Patient Relationship

JAMES E. WARNER, J.D.

Law of Medicine
Sanbar Law Firm
Oklahoma City, Oklahoma
Chapter 8: Selected Health Care Statutory Provisions
Chapter 9: Education and Licensure

CLARK WATTS, M.D., J.D.

Professor, Department of Neurosurgery
University of Texas Health Sciences Center
San Antonio, Texas
Special Counsel
Ford & Ferraro
Austin, Texas
Chapter 35: Brain-Injured Patients

CYRIL H. WECHT, M.D., J.D., F.C.L.M.

Clinical Adjunct Associate Professor
Department of Pathology
University of Pittsburgh School of Medicine
Adjunct Professor of Law
Duquesne University School of Law
Chairman and Chief Pathologist
Department of Pathology
St. Francis Central Hospital
Pittsburgh, Pennsylvania
Chapter 41: Forensic Use of Medical Information
Chapter 42: Forensic Pathology
Chapter 49: Research and Experimentation

VICTOR WALTER WEEDN, M.D., J.D., F.C.L.M.

Lieutenant Colonel, U.S. Army
Chief Deputy Medical Examiner
Program Manager, DOD DNA Registry
Office of the Armed Forces Medical Examiner
Armed Forces Institute of Pathology
Washington, D.C.
Chapter 28: Organ Donation and Transplantation

WILLIAM R. WICK, J.D.

Nash, Spindler, Dean & Grimstad
Manitowoc, Wisconsin
Chapter 25: Telephone Contacts and Counseling

Preface

Since its founding in 1955, the American College of Legal Medicine (ACLM) has been devoted to addressing problems that exist at the interface of the law and medicine. As the foremost established organization in the United States concerned with medical jurisprudence and forensic medicine, the college serves as a natural focal point for those professionals interested in the study and advancement of legal medicine.

The membership of the college includes not only dual-degreed physician-attorneys, but also many health science professionals and attorneys who specialize in health law. Accordingly, central to the mission of the college is education in legal medicine, and this text has been prepared with the hope and expectation that the more knowledge that is available concerning the relevant legal concepts, principles, and rules, the more effective an individual can become as a medical or legal practitioner.

The nature and frequency of legal problems confronting physicians continue to expand in modern-day society and will undoubtedly multiply in future years. It simply is not possible to practice medicine with wisdom, sensitivity, and total concern for patients' welfare and safety, unless the physician is cognizant of basic legal rules and generally accepted mandates. There is no logical or justifiable reason to remain ignorant of and hospital to the legal system, which is an integral and essential part of our government. Physicians, like all other citizens, are obliged to function within the parameters of civil and criminal law, and they should feel comfortable and safe in doing so as they pursue their medical careers.

This text attempts to highlight those areas of professional endeavor in a health care institution that constitute potential pitfalls and problems of a legal nature. The field of legal medicine is extremely broad and far reaching, with new developments of a significant nature occurring constantly.

The text explores and illustrates the legal implications of medical practice and the special legal issues attendant to organized health and medical care. Although originally conceived as a book for physicians and physicians-in-training, it should also prove useful for other health care organizations and law students with an interest in medical and health care issues. For those beginning the study of legal medicine, it may serve well as a comprehensive survey of the discipline.

On behalf of the ACLM, I extend my deepest appreciation to all the authors and contributors of the chapters and to the editorial committee and its director, Dr. S. Sandy Sanbar, who edited the textbook. Their contributions represent the true labors of love to the college and a monumental work in the field of legal medicine.

Finally, I wish to express my thanks to Mosby–Year Book, especially Susie Baxter, Medical Editor; Ellen Baker Geisel, Developmental Editor; and Karen Edwards, Project Manager, as well as to Kristin Miller, Editorial Manager, and Kelly Ricci, Production Manager, of Spectrum Publisher Services.

Allan Gibofsky, M.D., J.D., F.A.C.P., F.C.L.M.

American College of Legal Medicine Textbook Committee:

S. Sandy Sanbar, M.D., Ph.D., J.D., F.C.L.M.
Chairman and Project Director (1994–1995)
Past President, ACLM (1989–1990)

Allan Gibofsky, M.D., J.D., F.A.C.P., F.C.L.M.
President, The American College of Legal Medicine (1994–1995)

Marvin H. Firestone, M.D., J.D., F.C.L.M.
Immediate Past President, ACLM (1993–1994)

Theodore R. LeBlang, J.D., F.C.L.M.
Publications Committee Chairman, ACLM (1994–1995)

Contents

PART ONE LEGAL MEDICINE AND MEDICAL ETHICS

1 Legal Medicine, Medical Ethics, and Legal Medicine Education in America, 3

S. SANDY SANBAR
MELINDA THOMPSON

PART TWO LEGAL ASPECTS OF HEALTH CARE

SECTION I Legal process and precepts

2 American Legal System, 17

KENNETH D. HANSEN

3 Judicial System, 24

KENNETH D. HANSEN

4 Competency, Capacity, and Immunity, 27

STEVEN B. BISBING
JOSEPH P. McMENAMIN
RICHARD L. GRANVILLE

APPENDIX 4-1 Some areas of law in which competency is an issue, 44

APPENDIX 4-2 Some general tests of competency, 45

5 Contracts, Agency, and Partnership, 46

HUGH F. HILL III
JOSEPH P. McMENAMIN

6 Civil Trials, 70

ALAN C. HOFFMAN

7 Alternative Dispute Resolution in Health Care, 78

IRVING LADIMER

APPENDIX 7-1 Checklist and guidelines for ADR programs for health care, 78

SECTION II Regulation of medical practice

8 Selected Health Care Statutory Provisions, 87

JAMES E. WARNER
S. SANDY SANBAR

APPENDIX 8-1 Advanced health care directive statutes, by state, 90

APPENDIX 8-2 Controlled substances statutes, by state, 91

APPENDIX 8-3 Medical licensure statutes, by state (statutes annotated), 91

APPENDIX 8-4 Medical malpractice claims statutes, by state, 92

9 Education and Licensure, 93

S. SANDY SANBAR
DANIEL J. GAMINO
JAMES E. WARNER

10 Peer Review, Disciplining, Hearings, and Appeals, 105

JOHN T. BURROUGHS

SECTION III Professional medical liability

11 Health Care Provider as a Defendant, 118

MARTIN B. FLAMM

12 Medical Malpractice, 129

ALAN C. HOFFMAN

13 Medical Testimony and the Expert Witness, 141

JOSEPH D. PIORKOWSKI, Jr.

14 Liability of Health Care Entities for Negligent Care, 156

JOHN R. FEEGEL

15 Pharmaceutical Product Liability, 168

MARTIN J. MacNEILL

16 Antitrust, 180

DAVID P. CLUCHEY
EDWARD DAVID

17 Crimes Against and by Health Care Providers and Criminal Procedures, 196

STAN TWARDY
S. SANDY SANBAR

18 Countersuits by Health Care Providers, 213

BRADFORD H. LEE

19 Medical Liability Insurance, 220

RICHARD F. GIBBS
RICHARD W. MOORE, Jr.

APPENDIX 19-1   **Insurance glossary,** 235

20 Risk Management, 237

RICHARD R. BALSAMO
MAX DOUGLAS BROWN

APPENDIX 20-1   **Top malpractice allegations by frequency and cost, PIAA data,** 260

APPENDIX 20-2   **Malpractice allegations with the highest indemnity, PIAA data,** 260

APPENDIX 20-3   **Top ten malpractice allegations by average cost,** 260

APPENDIX 20-4   **Top ten malpractice allegations by frequency,** 261

APPENDIX 20-5   **All malpractice allegations by location,** 261

APPENDIX 20-6   **Major malpractice allegation issues,** 261

APPENDIX 20-7   **Unusual incident report,** 262

PART THREE   MEDICAL AND ETHICAL ENCOUNTERS

SECTION I   *Physicians and patients*

21 Physician-Patient Relationship, 265

MATTHEW L. HOWARD
LOUIS B. VOGT

22 Consent to and Refusal of Medical Treatment, 274

EMIDIO A. BIANCO
HAROLD L. HIRSH

23 Medical Records, 297

HAROLD L. HIRSH

24 Disclosure about Patients, 312

HAROLD L. HIRSH

25 Telephone Contacts and Counseling, 343

WILLIAM R. WICK
HARVEY KATZ

SECTION II   *Ethical-legal issues in medicine*

26 Ethics and Bioethics, 351

BERNARD J. FICARRA

27 Fetal Interests, 364

FREDERICK ADOLF PAOLA

28 Organ Donation and Transplantation, 372

VICTOR WALTER WEEDN
EDWIN KELLERMAN

APPENDIX 28-1   **Organs used in transplantation,** 392

APPENDIX 28-2   **Amended Uniform Anatomical Gift Act (1987),** 393

APPENDIX 28-3   **National Organ Transplant Act,** 397

29 The Process of Dying, 404

FREDERICK ADOLF PAOLA
JOHN A. ANDERSON

APPENDIX 29-1   **Current opinions of the Council on Ethical and Judicial Affairs of the American Medical Association, 1992,** 419

APPENDIX 29-2   **ACP Ethics Manual,** 420

APPENDIX 29-3   **"Proportionality/disproportionality" of proposed treatment,** 421

APPENDIX 29-4   **New York's Do-Not-Resuscitate Law,** 422

APPENDIX 29-5   **New York's Health Care Agents and Proxies Law,** 423

30 Physician-Assisted Suicide, 424

ARTHUR H. LESTER

SECTION III *Care of special patients*

31 **Reproduction Patients,** 432
MICHAEL S. CARDWELL

32 **Children as Patients,** 456
JOSEPH P. McMENAMIN
GARLAND L. BIGLEY

33 **Geriatric Patients,** 488
MARSHALL B. KAPP

34 **Oncology Patients,** 494
MELVIN A. SHIFFMAN

35 **Brain-Injured Patients,** 509
CLARK WATTS

36 **Patients with Human Immunodeficiency Virus (HIV) Infection and Acquired Immunodeficiency Syndrome (AIDS),** 516
MIKE A. ROYAL

APPENDIX 36-1 **Sources of HIV information,** 522

APPENDIX 36-2 **1993 Revised Classification System for HIV infection and expanded surveillance case definition for AIDS among adolescents and adults,** 523

APPENDIX 36-3 **Guidelines on evaluation and management of early HIV infection,** 529

APPENDIX 36-4 **Reporting requirements for HIV infection,** 530

37 **Impaired and Disabled Patients,** 531
ALLAN GIBOFSKY
HAROLD L. HIRSH

38 **Pain Management,** 534
WAYNE HODGES

39 **Occupational Health Law,** 545
CAROLYN S. LANGER

40 **Sports Medicine,** 554
RICHARD S. GOODMAN

SECTION IV *Forensic science and medicine*

41 **Forensic Use of Medical Information,** 558
CYRIL H. WECHT

42 **Forensic Pathology,** 567
CYRIL H. WECHT

43 **Psychiatric Patients and Forensic Psychiatry,** 585
MARVIN H. FIRESTONE

PART FOUR **LEGISLATIVE AND BUSINESS ASPECTS OF MEDICINE**

SECTION I *Medical practice finance and management*

44 **Practice Organizations and Joint Ventures,** 617
ARTHUR J. COHEN

45 **Coproviders and Institutional Practice,** 635
EDWARD E. HOLLOWELL
BARRY H. BLOCH

46 **Cost Containment and Reimbursement,** 662
HAROLD L. HIRSH

47 **Physician as an Employer,** 683
CHARLES G. HESS

SECTION II *Health care industry*

48 **Medical Technology,** 691
C. GORDON HECKEL
MAX KARL NEWMAN
DONALD L. NEWMAN
STEVEN E. NEWMAN

49 **Research and Experimentation,** 711
CYRIL H. WECHT

APPENDIX 49-1 **The Nuremberg Code,** 727

APPENDIX 49-2 **The Declaration of Helsinki,** 727

PART ONE

Legal medicine and medical ethics

Legal medicine, medical ethics, and legal medicine education in America

S. SANDY SANBAR, M.D., Ph.D., J.D., F.C.L.M.

MELINDA THOMPSON, M.D., J.D., F.C.L.M.

DEFINITION OF LEGAL MEDICINE
DEFINITION OF OTHER MEDICOLEGAL TERMS
MEDICAL JURISPRUDENCE
NINETEENTH-CENTURY AMERICAN SCHOLARS IN LEGAL MEDICINE
THE AMERICAN COLLEGE OF LEGAL MEDICINE
LEGAL MEDICINE JOURNALS
MEDICAL ETHICS
LEGAL MEDICINE EDUCATION IN LAW SCHOOLS
LEGAL MEDICINE EDUCATION IN MEDICAL SCHOOLS
MD/JD DEGREES
MEDICAL AND LAW SCHOOL CLINICS
HEALTH LAW STUDY
ETHICS AND LEGAL MEDICINE IN THE 1990s
CONCLUSION

Legal medicine is currently recognized in America as an organized specialty within academic medicine and, as such, is viewed as a clinical specialty in medicine. Legal medicine in America is not a new concept. Its roots can be traced back to sixteenth-century Italy, and to British legal medicine, which began in the late eighteenth century. Published treatises generated from Italy and Britain guided the development of legal medicine in Germany, France, and the United States.

DEFINITION OF LEGAL MEDICINE

"Medicine legale," or legal medicine, is a French term that first appeared during the late eighteenth and early nineteenth centuries.[1] The French legal medicine subject was broad and included not only medical evidentiary matters, but also medical areas of legal significance, for example, the criminally insane and rehabilitation of criminals, among other subjects.

In 1877, Harvard University established a separate professorship in legal medicine. In 1942, Dr. Alan R. Moritz, who was then the occupant of the Harvard professorship in legal medicine, defined legal medicine as follows:

Legal medicine is ordinarily defined as the application of medical knowledge to the needs of justice. Although by definition this would appear to be a broad and scientifically heterogeneous field, the practice of legal medicine is concerned chiefly with what might be most adequately described as forensic pathology.[2]

As recently as 1955, Dr. Moritz suggested that the model course in legal medicine in American medical schools should focus on death-case investigations and concentrate on the fields of pathology and allied sciences, such as toxicology.[3]

Interestingly enough, the most recent definition of legal medicine was suggested in 1975 by another prominent Harvard professor of legal medicine, William J. Curran, an attorney and a scholar, who has published extensively in the field of legal medicine. In 1975, Professor Curran published an article on "Titles in the Medicolegal Field: A Proposal for Reform," which offered an analysis of the historical roots of the terminology that has been applied in the medicolegal field and also a proposal for reform. Professor Curran, who is an Honorary Fellow of the American College of Legal Medicine, defined the term *legal medicine* as follows:

Legal medicine: the specialty areas of medicine concerned with relations with substantive law and with legal institutions. Clinical medical areas—such as the treatment of offenders and trauma medicine related to law would be included herein.[1]

DEFINITION OF OTHER MEDICOLEGAL TERMS

In addition to the definition of legal medicine *supra*, Professor Curran proposed in 1975 that the following set of defined terms be utilized with respect to interdisciplinary discourse in the broad field of medicolegal relations. The terms have consistency and specificity for the medicolegal field.

Environmental law: a specialty area of law, not related to *medical law*, but concerned with all the legal aspects of the regulation of environmental safety and health programs.

Forensic medicine: the specialty areas of medicine, medical science and technology, concerned with investigation, preparation, preservation, and presentation of evidence and medical opinion in courts and other legal, correctional, and other law-enforcement settings.

Forensic pathology: a sub-specialty of pathology concerned with medicolegal autopsies and with primary emphasis on investigation, preparation, preservation and presentation of death-case evidence in law and law-enforcement settings. The forensic pathologist may also be the operational head of a public health investigational program including other forensic medical specialists and forensic scientists.

Forensic toxicology, forensic biochemistry, forensic orthopedic surgery, etc.: other sub-specialties of medical practice fields concerned, as defined under *forensic medicine*, with producing evidence for the legal system.

Health law: a specialty area of law and law practice related to the medical and other health fields—such as dentistry, nursing, hospital administration, and environmental law.

Hospital law: a sub-specialty of *medical law* related to legal aspects of hospital administration and hospital legal liability.

Legal psychiatry: a sub-specialty of psychiatry concerned with both the clinical and the forensic aspects of psychiatry in relation to law, law enforcement, and corrections.

Medical evidence law and procedure: a sub-specialty area of *medical law* related to the utilization of medical evidence and admissibility and competency questions concerning medical fact evidence and expert medical opinion testimony and reports.

Medical law: a specialty area of law and law practice related to legal regulation of medicine and medical practice and other legal aspects of medicine.

Medicolegal relations: the broad interrelationship of the fields of medicine and law, both in regard to subject matter and professional activities of a cooperative nature.

Programs of public (medicolegal) death investigation: organized medical examiner's offices or coroner's office programs, usually headed by a forensic pathologist, including a forensic scientific laboratory, and a faculty and staff of forensic scientists and technicians.

Public health law: a specialty area of law and law practice related to legal regulation and legal administration of public health programs."[1]

MEDICAL JURISPRUDENCE

The introduction of the term *medical jurisprudence* in America was the result of developments in Great Britain. In 1788, Dr. Samuel Farr of Britain published the *Elements of Medical Jurisprudence*. Until that time, Great Britain neither systematically studied nor taught legal or forensic medicine, and no comprehensive British work on the subject was available.[4]

In 1789, Dr. Andrew Duncan (1744-1828) was appointed professor of the Institutes of Medicine at the University of Edinburgh, and he began forthwith to give lectures in medical jurisprudence and public hygiene.[4] Indeed, Dr. Duncan was the first in Britain to provide systemic instruction in legal medicine. He used the term *medical jurisprudence* to encompass both "medical police and juridical medicine." In 1798, Dr. Duncan presented a *Memorial to the Patrons of the University of Edinburgh* in which he delivered what he called "A short view of the Extent and Importance of Medical Jurisprudence, considered as a Branch of Education."[4]

Interestingly, Dr. Andrew Duncan, Jr., followed his father as professor of the institutes of medicine at the University of Edinburgh; he occupied that chair until 1819. In 1807, Dr. Duncan, Jr., was also appointed professor of medical jurisprudence at one of the universities. This appointment triggered a public debate in the English House of Commons questioning Dr. Duncan's understanding of the duties of such a professor and what was meant by the science which he professed. Subsequently, Dr. Duncan, Jr., went on to give a course of instructions on medical jurisprudence, and he wrote essays and reviews about the subject in the *Edinburgh Medical and Surgical Journal*, of which he was editor.[4]

As noted later, Dr. James S. Stringham of New York was at Edinburgh earning his MD in 1799. He was undoubtedly influenced by the teaching of the Duncans, and he brought with him to America the term *medical jurisprudence*. In 1804, Dr. Stringham defined

> Medical Jurisprudence as that science which applies the principles and practice of the different branches of medicine to the elucidation of doubtful questions in courts of justice.[5]

Dr. Benjamin Rush was also influenced by the Duncans' lectures and used the term *medical jurisprudence* in his lecture on the subject in 1810. In a letter to his son, James Rush, Dr. Rush made references to Dr. Duncan's lecture and his own lecture on medical jurisprudence in 1810. Dr. Rush wrote:

> I regret that I did not request you obtain a copy of young Dr. Duncan's lectures upon medical jurisprudence while you were in Edinburgh. At a future date that science I hope will be taught in the University of Pennsylvania. I propose making the state of mind which is proper to legalize testimony, wills and crimes, the subject of my next introductory lecture.[4]

In the United States, the term *legal medicine* is currently preferred over *medical jurisprudence*. In fact, the latter term is not favored. In 1975, Harvard Professor William Curran noted:

The unfortunate title of "medical jurisprudence" should at long last be relegated to the lexicographer's scrap heap. It was incorrectly applied to the **medical** side of the field in the first place. It is now either inappropriate or too pretentious a term for the legal aspects of the subject.[1]

NINETEENTH-CENTURY AMERICAN SCHOLARS IN LEGAL MEDICINE

Numerous excellent articles on the history of legal medicine have been published in the medical and legal professional journals, some of which are referred to in this chapter. Four extensive and authoritative references of articles on the general history of legal medicine are those by Gilbert H. Stewart in 1910,[5] Sir Sydney Smith in 1954,[4] Chester R. Burns in 1977,[6] and James C. Mohr in 1993 as well as William Curran in 1980.[7] Some of these publications also include discussions of the history of medical ethics. The following focuses on the history of legal medicine and the early legal medicine scholars in America.

In the United States, legal medicine started to develop at the beginning of the nineteenth century. Dr. James Sackett Stringham studied medicine first in his native city of New York, and subsequently at Edinburgh, in Great Britain, where he graduated with the degree of MD in 1799. In 1804, Dr. Stringham instituted a course of lectures in legal medicine at Columbia College of Physicians and Surgeons in New York. He was the first to use the title "Medical Jurisprudence" in American lectures, and also has the distinction of being the first systematic teacher of legal medicine in America. In 1813, he was appointed professor of medical jurisprudence at the College of Physicians and Surgeons in New York, a post he held until his death in 1817. In 1814, Dr. Stringham published the *American Medical and Philosophical Register,* which dealt with sundry topics in legal medicine.

In 1810, Dr. Benjamin Rush is credited with emphasizing the significance of the relationship between law and medicine. As the nation's first surgeon general and a signatory of the Declaration of Independence, Dr. Rush established American legal medicine with his published lecture "On the Study of Medical Jurisprudence," which he delivered to medical students at the University of Pennsylvania, Philadelphia, in 1811.[8] The lecture dealt with homicide, mental disease, and capital punishment.

The work of Dr. Stringham and Dr. Rush inspired the teaching of medical jurisprudence in other American medical schools. Among the early teachers were Dr. Charles Caldwell in Philadelphia and Dr. Walter Channing at Harvard.

In 1819, Dr. Thomas Cooper, who was a legal officer of distinction and also president of the College of South Carolina, published *Tracts on Medical Jurisprudence.* This volume contained almost all available recent literature in English on legal medicine, evidencing an increasing interest in the field.

In 1815, Dr. T. Romeyn Beck was appointed lecturer on medical jurisprudence at Western Medical College, New York State. In 1823, Dr. Beck first published the *Elements of Medical Jurisprudence,* which defined the field of legal medicine for about half a century of American medical practitioners. Beck's two volumes included impressive topics such as rape, impotence and sterility, pregnancy, delivery, infanticide and abortion, legitimacy, presumption of survivorship, identity, mental alienation, wounds, poisons, persons found dead, and feigned and disqualifying diseases.

In 1838, Isaac Ray published a "Treatise on Medical Jurisprudence of Insanity." In 1855, the year when Dr. Beck died, Francis Wharton, a lawyer, and Dr. Moreton Stille, a physician, collaborated to publish "A Treatise on Medical Jurisprudence."

In 1860, physician/attorney John J. Elwell published a book entitled *A Medico-Legal Treatise on Malpractice, Medical Evidence, and Insanity, Comprising the Elements of Medical Jurisprudence,* which highlighted the issue of malpractice in the medical jurisprudence literature. Elwell's book presented excerpts from contemporary cases for the purpose of teaching physicians what to expect from malpractice litigation.

Another physician/attorney, John Odronaux, published *Jurisprudence of Medicine* in 1867 and *Judicial Aspects of Insanity* in 1878. In 1894, Randolph A. Witthaus and Tracy C. Becker published *Medical Jurisprudence, Forensic Medicine and Toxicology.*

Throughout most of the 1800s, medical jurisprudence for medical students and physicians assumed the position of central importance in schools of medicine in the United States. During the course of the nineteenth century, the institutions, laws and judicial decisions in America showed the increasing influence of sound medicolegal principles, especially those pertaining to mental disease and criminal lunatics.

By 1876, however, things had changed drastically; legal medicine became temporarily dormant. American Professor and Dean Stanford Emerson Chaille expressed his view of the deplorable condition of medical jurisprudence in the United States. He demonstrated how the teaching of medical jurisprudence had deteriorated by noting that in some medical colleges the course had been dropped altogether, in others it had been attached to some other subject, and in many colleges the teaching of medical students was entrusted to a lawyer with no formal teaching in the medical field.[4]

Even in the early part of the twentieth century, the teaching of medical jurisprudence was relegated to a position as an occasional subject taught outside the mainstream. However, by the middle of the twentieth century, legal medicine underwent a renaissance, as evidenced by the establishment of the American College of Legal Medicine and the rekindling of contemporary interest in a vast array of legal medicine, medical ethics, physician and patient rights, and the business and professional aspects of medical practice.

THE AMERICAN COLLEGE OF LEGAL MEDICINE

Recognizing the growing impact of legislation, regulations, and court decisions on patient care and the general effect of litigation and legal medicine on modern society, in 1955 a group of physicians and surgeons, some of whom were learned in the law, organized what was later to become the American College of Legal Medicine. The college was incorporated on September 23, 1960, by nine doctors of medicine, three of whom were lawyers. Of the 36 physicians who were designated "founding fellows," 10 had earned law degrees.

The American College of Legal Medicine is the oldest and most prestigious organization in the United States devoted to problems at the interface of medicine and law. Its membership is made up of professionals in medicine, osteopathy, and allied sciences including dentistry, nursing, pharmacy, podiatry, psychology, and law.

The American College of Legal Medicine has published a scholarly journal, the *Journal of Legal Medicine,* since 1973. In 1988, the College also published it first edition of this textbook, *Legal Medicine;* the second edition was published in 1991.

LEGAL MEDICINE JOURNALS

A list of some of the legal medicine journals published in the nineteenth and twentieth centuries follows:

1867-1876	*Quarterly Journal of Psychological Medicine and Medical Jurisprudence*
1874-1924	*Medicolegal Journal*
1900-	Medico-Legal column of the *Journal of the American Medical Association*
1948-	*Journal of Forensic Sciences*
1973-	*Journal of Legal Medicine* of the American College of Legal Medicine
1975-	*American Journal of Law and Medicine*
1976-	*Journal of Health Politics, Policy and the Law*
1978-	*American Journal of Forensic Psychiatry*
1980-	*American Journal of Forensic Medicine and Pathology.*

This list is by no means an all-inclusive list of publications and journals dealing with legal medicine. Numerous publications and journals are published currently that deal more specifically with the topic of medical ethics, and also include legal medicine topics.

MEDICAL ETHICS

Medical ethics, conduct, morality, and philosophy have evolved gradually over the past 4500 years, beginning with the Babylonian and Egyptian societies who promulgated rules and sanctions to control the activities of physicians and surgeons.

Babylonians: Code of Hammurabi

Conceived by the Babylonians around 2500 BC, the Code of Hammurabi was the earliest written code of ethical principles and conduct for medical practice. The code detailed the nature of the conduct required of physicians at that time.

Egyptian: Papyri

Egyptian papyri from the sixteenth century BC represent the first documented descriptions of the priest-physician, as well as methods of establishing diagnoses and appropriate treatment decisions. Innovative or unconventional treatments on a patient that caused the death of the patient could also result in loss of the treating physician's life.

Greek: Hippocratic oath

During the fifth century BC, the Greeks conceived the Oath of Hippocrates. The oath represented a statement of principles and ideals to be cherished by the physician. Greek (Hellenic) medicine carried forward the Hippocratic tradition and intermingled it with the ethical teachings of Plato, Aristotle, and the Stoics. The original Oath of Hippocrates made reference to pagan gods. Around the tenth century AD, the Oath of Hippocrates was christianized and reference to pagan gods was eliminated. To date, some 2400 years since its conception, the Hippocratic oath has survived as an expression of the ideal conduct of the physician in our modern civilization.

The Hippocratic ethic is indeed the touchstone of modern medical ethics. The Hippocratic Ethic, particularly the oath, was incorporated into the teaching of Moslem, Jewish, and Christian physicians, thereby spreading throughout the Middle East and Europe. However, it permitted holding the truth from patient and family if it served the patient's good, and it tolerated different standards of care for the rich and the poor.

Greek God: Aesculapius

Around the fourth century BC, Greek medicine had formally separated itself from religion. However, the Greeks deified Aesculapius, who was believed to have ministered, with his sons, to the Greek army at the siege of Troy. The priests of Aesculapius healed through art and magic and had little science. They stressed equality of care for rich and poor. To date, the staff and snake of

Aesculapius remain the symbol of healing of the medical physicians.

Roman: Galan

Roman medical ethics was influenced by Stoic philosophy emphasizing virtue and duty. Galan (130-201 AD), a Greek, worked in Rome and advanced the ethical stance that combined Hippocratic and Stoic Hellenic ethics.

Chinese and Hindu medical ethics

Chinese medicine established ethical precepts and a canon that were in accord with the Aesculapian ethics. Hindu medical mores, on the other hand, were akin to those of the Babylonians and the Greeks.

Arab and Persian medical ethics

During the Middle Ages, medical science and philosophy were sustained and transmitted to the West by the Arabs and their allies as they moved along the Mediterranean littoral and into Spain. Two Persians, Avicenna (980-1036 AD) and Rhazes (865-925 AD), were renowned physicians, philosophers, and clinicians who wrote extensively about medicine.

Jewish medical ethics

Moses Maimonides (1135-1204 AD) was one of the greatest physician-philosophers who compiled a canon of Jewish law and medicine.

Christian medical ethics

St. Thomas Aquinas (1224-1274 AD) integrated the philosophy and ethics of Aristotle with Christian theology in his "Summa Theologica" and developed the classical doctrine of virtue ethics to a high sophistication.

Sicily: Frederick II, father of quality assurance of medical care

Around 1200 AD, Frederick II of Sicily involved the state and the government with medicine. He established rules for the education of future physicians, methods of practice, charges for medical services, and mechanisms for ensuring the purity of drugs. Frederick II can probably be considered the father of quality assurance of medical care and possibly health care reform.

English medical ethics

In 1520, the Royal College of Physicians of London drew up a penal code for physicians. In 1543, the word "penal" was changed to "ethical" to avoid the implication of criminology.

In 1769, Samuel Bard published "A Discourse Upon the Duties of a Physician." In 1803, Thomas Percival, an English physician and philosopher, published "Medical Ethics: A Code of Institutes and Precepts Adapted to the Professional Conduct of Physicians and Surgeons." In 1858, the British Medical Association published its Code of Ethics.

World medical association

In 1948, the World Medical Association adopted the Declaration of Geneva, which represented a revision of the Hippocratic oath. Also, the Nuremberg Code and the Declaration of Helsinki of 1964 were conceived. These documents emphasized the concept of voluntary consent for human research subjects and expressed significant characteristics of modern medicine.

Code of medical ethics of the American Medical Association (Chicago, 1994)

The American Medical Association (AMA), at its first real meeting in Philadelphia in 1847, adopted a Code of Ethics that was based partly on Percival's code, Bard's publication, and the code of the Royal College of Physicians of London.

In June 1957, the AMA House of Delegates adopted the short version of the AMA Principles of Medical Ethics, which states:

The medical profession has long subscribed to a body of ethical statements developed primarily for the benefit of the patient. The following Principles adopted by the American Medical Association are not laws but standards of conduct which define the essentials of honorable behavior by the physician.

  I. A physician shall be dedicated to provide competent medical service with compassion and respect for human dignity.
 II. A physician shall deal honestly with patients and colleagues and strive to expose those physicians deficient in character or competence, or who engage in fraud or deception.
III. A physician shall respect the law and also recognize a responsibility to seek changes in those requirements which are contrary to the best interests of the patient.
 IV. A physician shall respect the rights of patients, of colleagues, and of other health professionals and shall safeguard patient confidences within the constraints of the law.
  V. A physician shall continue to study, apply and advance scientific knowledge, make relevant information available to patients, colleagues and the public, obtain consultation, and use the talents of other health professionals when indicated.
 VI. A physician shall, in the provision of appropriate patient care except in emergencies, be free to choose whom to serve, with whom to associate, and the environment in which to provide medical services.
VII. A physician shall recognize a responsibility to participate in activities contributing to an improved community.

LEGAL MEDICINE EDUCATION IN LAW SCHOOLS

In 1867, the Medico-Legal Society was organized in New York. It was the first society in the world to be organized for the purpose of carrying out the principle that a lawyer could not be fully equipped either for the prosecution or for the defense of an individual indicted for the crime of homicide without some knowledge of anatomy or pathology, and that no physician or surgeon could give absolute satisfaction as an expert witness without some knowledge of the law.[5]

The existing tension between the medical and legal professions has been traced to many possible sources. At the core of this tension, however, is the intellectual process that each profession takes in seeking the ultimate truth. The legal profession pursues the truth through the conflicting forces of an adversarial confrontation. By partisan assertion of a legal position in a given setting against a competing assertion of different principles, the adversary process pursues a full statement of issues and evidence from two sides' opposing efforts. The physician, on the other hand, proceeds in terms of insightful scientific analyses, moving from hypothesis to data to working hypothesis to conclusion. A medical diagnosis is made by objective evaluation of neutral subjective facts, often in consultation with colleagues. When one realizes how different this teamwork approach is compared to the adversarial contests over valuation of rights and powers that take place in courtrooms, it becomes easier to comprehend how a lack of understanding developed between the two disciplines. For those involved in medicolegal education the problem is one of finding the most effective way to harmonize these differences and to exchange valued information from profession to profession.

The law student's training is primarily derived from the Socratic method, which employs a continuous dialogue between professor and student, exploring all possible avenues as potential solutions to a legal problem. The medical student begins with didactic lectures, followed by clinical experience. Therefore, although it would not be a shock for the law student to be exposed to medicine through a series of didactic lectures, a number of questions are raised when electing to add medicine, or medically oriented courses, to the law school curriculum. The medical content, the educational method, and the point in time in the curriculum at which to offer legal medicine are all matters of conjecture when the medical course is considered.

When no medical courses are offered in law school, self-education is the method used by lawyers involved in legal medicine cases. Aside from the lack of time to prepare for medical case issues and to acquire a medical-legal background, the foremost obstacle for a lawyer is the move from the inductive reasoning of law to the deductive logic of the basic sciences. An additional problem is the diversity of medical knowledge required. A legal case may involve questions of anatomy, embryology, physiology, biochemistry, pharmacology, and pathology in a myriad of medical specialties and subspecialties. Lawyers, however desirous they may be of acquiring some medical training, lack the underlying basic science courses to support effective self-education.

Formal education is essential if the lawyer is to be effective in evaluating medical evidence, both friendly and adversarial. A lawyer who specializes in legal medicine must possess a specific knowledge of pertinent medical services and specialties required in any particular case situation. To undertake a medical issues case with a lack of such knowledge could constitute legal malpractice.

In an effort to bridge the gap between law and medicine, some lawyers are enrolling in medical school, or in dual-degree MD/JD programs. The number of medical school courses extraneous to a legal practice with medical specialization also discourages lawyers from a formal medical education.

A well-developed legal medicine program designed to fit into the law school curriculum can prepare an attorney to work competently with medical issues. Existing programs are unfortunately few in number and often lack formal structure. An ideal program would cover clinical sciences including diagnosis, treatment, and laboratory work, and working with a coroner, including participation in autopsies, histology, and toxicology.

While a combined MD/JD program would appear to be the most effective way of teaching medical concepts to law students, it is doubtful whether enough students are willing to pursue such a long period of training, or whether they would actually need to practice in both fields to function appropriately in one, with contributions from the other.

Alternatively, a team approach has been suggested, employing doctors and lawyers together, in order to convey to the students the problems unique to each discipline. Such training gives the law student a greater understanding of the problems present in the physician's medical practice. Regardless of the instructor, however, the consensus of legal medicine educators is that the material should be presented during the third year of law school, after the student has obtained an adequate background in the basic major fields of the law. It is even possible that a law school could develop a mini-curriculum for students interested in legal medicine, incorporating both classroom and clinical work during the third year.

LEGAL MEDICINE EDUCATION IN MEDICAL SCHOOLS

The major problem caused by the differences in basic intellectual approach and teaching methods between law and medical schools is exacerbated by the belief of both doctors and lawyers that they can effectively practice their professions without being trained in legal medicine. Physicians uniformly assert that if the lawyers would just depart, medicine could be practiced effectively and beneficially for patient and physician.

Nevertheless, most medical school curriculum committees now recognize the need for some form of instruction in legal medicine. The legal aspects of medical practice have appeared in various treatises, culminating in 1931 with a full course in legal medicine being taught at the University of Illinois Medical School. A 1958 survey of medical school catalogs showed 58% offering some form of instruction in legal medicine.

Progress in medicolegal education has not proceeded at great speed, however. Although a 1973 survey showed that 60.3% of the medical schools responding offered some type of formal instruction in law and medicine, a 1978 survey showed that only 39.6% of the reporting colleges actually required the students to take such course offerings, and another 27.8% indicated they had no such offerings at all. The surveys seem to indicate that not only are formal course offerings in legal medicine absent from many medical schools, but, even when offered, a student is not necessarily exposed to this important subject matter.

Such a low priority of legal medicine is reflected in the methods used to teach law to medical students. By often refusing to use the Socratic method, and instead resorting to didactic techniques, the medical student not only loses a feeling for the law, but is also denied the critical insight into legal reasoning so essential for a basic understanding of the law. Finally, while the medical schools emphasize core curricula by requiring additional clinical work, no clinical programs exist for legal medicine.

It will be the role of both law and medical schools to increase the level of understanding between the professions in years to come. For the physician, this will require a change in the medical school curriculum. The requisite educational materials must not be a cursory review course, consisting of a recitation of general law, which is slipped into the curriculum at a convenient and minimal slot. The ideally structured course would provide an overview of the legal system with the emphasis placed on the legal decision-making and dispute resolution process and the values derived from the process. The student should be exposed to those substantive and procedural areas that have a direct bearing on medical practice.

Most importantly, the restructuring of medical education must start with making course offerings in legal medicine mandatory, to guarantee that all students will be exposed to this crucial information. For maximum benefit these courses should be offered in the third and fourth years, to allow integration of medical clinical experience.

In 1952, the Committee on Medicolegal Problems of the American Medical Association published its report of a survey of the teaching of law in 72 schools of medicine.[9] The report noted that 15 medical schools had departments of legal medicine, and 16 offered required courses in legal medicine that were judged on the basis of the committee's standards as "satisfactory." Instruction in legal medicine alone was described by 23 other medical schools. The AMA Committee on Medicolegal Problems recommended that every medical school in the United States create a department or division of legal medicine and offer a 20-hour course in legal medicine focusing on basic material of general interest and importance to medical doctors, such as forensic medicine, legal duties of physicians, patient rights, malpractice, expert testimony, and the physician's responsibility to third parties. The committee also recommended specialized elective forensic training in residency programs and appropriate continuing education.

In 1968, the AMA Committee on Medicolegal Problems published a suggested curriculum for the study of law and medicine in American medical schools.[10] The Committee updated the 1952 curriculum and noted that the purpose of the course was to provide physicians the legal knowledge regarding the professional as well as the *business* aspects of medical practice, thereby permitting the physician to function effectively in society.

In 1971, Beresford assessed the teaching of legal medicine by surveying the 96 existing American medical schools.[11] Of the 79 schools responding, 11 reported separate divisions of legal medicine, 42 reported formal course work for medical students, and 1 reported a combined MD/JD program. Malpractice or professional liability, physician testimony, informed consent, and forensic pathology were the subjects most frequently covered, in that order.

In 1977, the American College of Legal Medicine Task Force on Medical-Legal Education published a recommended medical-legal curriculum in its *Journal of Legal Medicine*.[12] The task force recommended a medical legal curriculum for all American medical schools. The curriculum consists of two parts. The first is a mandatory 14 to 15 hours of lecture or discussions that are essential in a basic legal medicine course for undergraduate medical students. The second part consists of optional topics to be included if there is available curriculum time.

MD/JD DEGREES

In 1993, Jonas, Etzel and Barzansky, reporting on the educational programs in U.S. medical schools, noted that students can earn a combined doctor of medicine and doctor of jurisprudence degree (MD/JD) in only 9 out of 125 degree-granting, U.S. medical schools, fully accredited by the Liaison Committee on Medical Education (LCME).[13] In contrast, students can earn a combined doctor of medicine and doctor of philosophy (MD/PhD) in 113 out of the 125 U.S. medical schools. The majority of individuals who currently have dual-degree MD/JDs, however, earned their doctorate degrees separately, with most of them earning the MD first.

In 1985, Schneller and Weiner[14] published their findings regarding dual-degree MD/JD individuals, and noted that cross-professional education in law and medicine remains a relatively rare phenomenon in the United States. They concluded that "Without the development of institutionalized career lines and the acceptance of cross-disciplinary approaches to problem solving, MD/JDs must negotiate their jobs and job descriptions within an occupational structure that rewards disciplinary efforts. The marginal status of the interprofessional specialist persists in the decade of the 1980s."[14]

MEDICAL AND LAW SCHOOL CLINICS

One proposal for meeting the needs for legal-medical course work for both the medical and law school settings has been the concept of jointly sponsored clinics operated by both schools. In such a setting, law students, under the supervision of faculty or appropriately trained attorneys, would be available for consultation to the medical students and interns at the medical school. The law student, working as a legal intern, could actually represent medical students, or physicians, as they perform in their roles as health care providers. They would have regular office hours, be available to prepare memoranda on particular questions, assist in negotiations, prepare physicians as witnesses in pending litigation, or perhaps even represent a health care provider in actual litigation, under the practicing attorney's supervision.

There are numerous advantages to such a system as opposed to the present modes of teaching legal medicine. A joint clinic would give lawyers and physicians an opportunity to interact with each other in real-life settings. Both parties would be exposed to the particular vulnerabilities of each profession in medicolegal matters. It is this type of interaction, more than any other factor, that should lead to greater understanding between the professions.

One example of an attempt to bridge the chasm between physicians and lawyers is a joint effort occurring between the University of Wisconsin Medical School and Marquette University Law School. This project was conceived by the deans of the respective professional schools, with the following objectives:

1. To create an atmosphere of interaction between law and medicine concerning ethical, moral, societal, and legal issues surrounding health care.
2. To provide an opportunity for medical students to experience firsthand the various legislative and legal restrictions placed on medical practice.
3. To endow law students with an understanding of the foibles of medical practice, the difficulties in the decision-making process in medicine, and the practicing of defensive medicine.
4. For both groups to pool their knowledge in relation to the serious ethical problems of the 1980s, including attempting a satisfactory definition of death, establishing proper standards for informed consent, and other timely issues.

When the representatives of the two schools convened at the first organizational meeting, several projects were proposed. The first conferences in 1981 were in a seminar format. Each seminar was attended by a liaison committee from each school, both deans, and core members of each profession. Early topics included brain death, problems of psychiatric commitment, and expert witness testimony. An average of 15 to 20 faculty members attended each session, with no students or outside audience in attendance.

During the second year of the program, faculty members were added to the medical side of the joint committee. Additionally, a Bioethics Center was established in the medical school. The center set up public lectures and published newsletters that discussed ethical issues confronting doctors and lawyers. In December 1982, another year of faculty seminars was approved. Three possible formats were proposed:

1. Weekend retreats, uniting both faculties, in which previously discussed topics could be examined in greater detail
2. Future development of continuing education programs for alumni of both schools
3. Joint research programs involving faculty from both schools.

Future interfaculty seminar programs were planned on the subjects of liability for medical innovations and unapproved use of drugs, controlling the cost of litigation in today's economy, orphan drugs, and the right to die. An undergraduate curriculum at the medical school is also being developed. This would be approximately 15 to 20 hours in length and would concentrate on the role of the physician in the medical community.

The joint committee proposed that two distinct courses be offered at the start. The first would be taught by the medical school faculty to law students interested in practicing personal injury litigation. It would contain an introduction to forensic medicine, medical jurisprudence, an overview of the basic sciences, and an evaluation of medical diagnosis and treatment. It would also cover principles of medical training, hospital organization, and medical literature.

The second course offering would be aimed at both medical and law students. It would address policy questions facing attorneys and physicians, using the team teaching method by faculty members from both schools. The topics covered would include such items as psychosurgery and psychoactive drugs in behavior control, genetic engineering, and regulating human experimentation.

HEALTH LAW STUDY

With the rapidly changing face of health care delivery, and the increasing need for lawyers to sort through the myriad rules and regulations that control health care dispensing, health law, as well as the more specialized field of legal medicine, is becoming more and more attractive to law students. Unfortunately, such students often find the normal law school curriculum unsatisfactory, particularly if they intend to pursue more specialized areas of health law.

To meet the needs of such students, some law schools, such as St. Louis University, are offering specific electives that address health law issues. Among such course offerings are health law and the special legal problems of the elderly. In addition to electives, however, law schools such as St. Louis University are offering more highly structured attempts to educate future lawyers for the health care field. Two of these proposals are the dual-degree program and the health law center.

The dual-degree program is common in law schools, but the additional degree is more often a master's of business, or a master's of public administration. In rare situations, a school may offer an MD/JD program. Although such programs may offer degrees in a shorter period than if they were taken sequentially, many times they are simply a matter of the school's going out of its way to ease scheduling for the student.

An alternative to the dual-degree program is the Center for Health Care Studies. In such a situation, the center provides those courses not found in the usual law school curriculum, without requiring the student to register for the second degree program. To effectively create such a center, a university must provide several key factors, including faculty, multidisciplinary relationships, curriculum, students, and a specialized library.

The very nature of the health care law makes a multidisciplinary approach necessary, and the faculty should include members from the law school who possess training and experience in health care law. The cooperation of all disciplines is essential in order to provide the highest quality degree program. The curriculum and libraries require specialization to a degree, but not to the exclusion of all other materials. Note that a good health law library can be an expensive proposition. Thus a health law center will require the continuing support of the university and alumni.

The physician and the lawyer, however, are not the only individuals affected by the interface of law and medicine. Numerous groups, including health care administrators, risk management professionals, prepaid care operators, and others, have a vested interest in this evolution of health care law. In the past, the health care administrator was viewed as extraneous to the physician-patient relationship. However, with the increasing responsibility of the hospital administrator for the care of the patient, and for the overall activities of the hospital, this is no longer the case. Not only must the administrator be familiar with the law as it affects the hospital, he or she must also have some knowledge of the legal issues involved in the physician-patient relationship.

To expect the nonattorney health care manager to have an attorney's knowledge of the law would be too much to expect. Therefore, any attempt at training hospital administrators in the law should be oriented toward giving the administrator an overview of the legal issues involved in health care, when to obtain legal counsel, and how to use that counsel effectively.

ETHICS AND LEGAL MEDICINE IN THE 1990s

In today's increasingly complex society, the American College of Legal Medicine is providing greater insight into the field of legal medicine—or health care law—especially as it touches on such thorny issues as the economics of health care, patients' rights, conflicts of interest, and professional ethics.

Economics of health care

During the past decade, medical practice has changed radically through the combined impact of competition, prospective payment, managed care, and the evolving role of peer review. However, the farthest reaching change is yet to be realized. Today, more than 40 million Americans are disenfranchised from receiving adequate health care as a result of inadequate or nonexistent insurance. Nearly 90% of Americans believe that health care should be a universal right, and this change may come in the 1990s. The cost of health care has soared from $50 billion in 1969 to more than $600 billion today—nearly 13% of our gross national product.

Why have health care costs risen so dramatically? Some have suggested a prevalence of unnecessary, inappropriate, and costly medical procedures.

In the field of cardiology, for example, there exists a

broad spectrum of diagnostic tests ranging from exercise testing, including exercise echocardiography, to nuclear medicine techniques and angiography. The costs of these tests vary widely, as do the accuracy of the results. A $240 treadmill test can spiral to more than $1000 or $2000 in additional cardiac testing.

The initial capital investment by physicians for testing equipment requires a certain patient volume to justify the expenditure, so that totally asymptomatic high-risk patients are encouraged to undergo "screening" for a variety of cardiac risk factors and for silent ischemia. Typically, when exercise stress tests do reveal myocardial silent ischemia, the patient may be subjected to angiography and possibly angioplasty without differentiation of relative risk for cardiac event.

In today's medicine, conservative medical treatment is viewed frequently as antiquated and suboptimal, and yet many patients are likely to exhibit an excellent outcome when treated noninvasively and nonsurgically.

Conflict of interest

Ethical, legal, and economic concerns arise in which a number of nonclinical factors might be compelling a management approach that is not necessarily in the patient's best interest. Public obsession with cardiac health—as documented by the extraordinary market in aspirin, oat bran, antioxidants, and aerobics—predisposes an individual to seek risk factor screening. This is indeed a bed of roses for many.

In addition, pharmaceutical and device-manufacturing companies deliver insistent messages through advertising, symposia, and clinical research designed to evaluate their products' effectiveness. Concerns about conflict of interest have been voiced when physicians themselves become investors in such companies or in separate business ventures that provide screening services.

The free enterprise system in our country has generated increasing commercial interest in health care. Because physicians do control the type and volume of health delivery, they are the focus of marketing for commercial interests. As competition increases, so do the marketing efforts. Company-sponsored symposia, clinical research, and investment portfolio opportunities cloud the question of whether the subsequent use of these products and services so marketed was the result of fair and objective assessment and consideration.

Ethical and legal standards

Few standards exist to guide physicians through this morass. Clearly, physicians have the same rights as anyone else to engage in profit-making activities. But should they profit directly from the treatments they prescribe for their patients without restraint of disclo-

sure? While we must assess in the next decade appropriate ethical and legal standards by which to measure our changing world, we must also be concerned with the appearance of conflict of interest and its potentially damaging impact.

Ethical and legal standards have positive implications for reinforcing patient trust and public regard. Furthermore, such standards would address the basic issues of tort liability and quality assurance, and they would also provide much-needed guidance to physicians on how to conduct their practice of medicine.

In the 1990s, some physicians are being required to rethink their ethics and priorities. A recent survey published in the *Journal of the American Medical Association* revealed that the majority of physicians felt that telling the truth had a lower priority than the impact of the truth on the patient.[15] Most physicians were willing to deceive insurance companies intentionally to help patients receive maximum coverage. Few physicians, however, would be willing to withhold information about a teen's pregnancy and abortion from her parents.

These fairly simple ethical issues represent only the tip of the iceberg. As medical horizons expand, we begin to confront widening dichotomies—between our perceptions of the origin and meaning of human life and our degree of dominion over it, between moral and legal sanctions, and the conflict between theological and utilitarian ethical systems. Current questions about voluntary euthanasia for the terminally ill, on surrogate motherhood, and on the use of fetal tissue in medical research for afflictions such as Parkinson's disease, Alzheimer's, Huntington's chorea, and diabetes illustrate all too vividly how important this issue has become.

Hospital ethics committees

More and more frequently, physicians find themselves addressing moral questions in the hospital setting. Guidance is often sought from ethics committees and ethics consultants.

Ethics committees are concerned with the nonclinical evaluation of policy. Medical ethicists or ethics consultants identify the moral aspects of patient care, gathering data, identifying arguments, and restoring focus to the moral dilemma. Some medical ethicists are nonclinicians; others are medical practitioners. Those ethicists trained as clinicians seem to have an advantage in that they also bring to the table hands-on knowledge of patient care skills and an ability to distinguish among complex medical indices.

Legal medicine consultant

In a world where people are more likely than ever before to sue their physicians, many ethical questions carry legal implications. The legal medicine consultant or the specialist in health care law is uniquely qualified to analyze the application of laws and regulations in the clinical setting and help physicians ensure better quality health care.

The ethical, legal, and economic constraints of medicine in the 1990s could have a greater potential to modify the course of medical practice than do advances in technology. The requirements for increased funds to implement new medical technologies, the necessity for reduced health care spending, the rights of health care providers, and patients' rights are all on a collision course. In our litigious society, that collision course will in all likelihood be adjudicated in courts of law, far from the clinical setting.

CONCLUSION

Legal medicine is a field uniquely poised to benefit physicians and the public interest through its capacity to reconcile the adversarial relationship that often exists between the medical community and legal community. With one foot in either world, legal medicine consultants and specialists in health care law have a leadership responsibility to help build unified standards of ethical conduct and safety precautions so as to ensure the highest quality of care and with it the advancement of medical potential. Medicine is truly a bed of roses but they are expensive flowers and unfortunately have many sharp and painful thorns.

END NOTES

1. William J. Curran, *Titles in the Medicolegal Field: A Proposal for Reform,* 1 Am. J.L. Med. 1-11 (1975).
2. Alan R. Moritz, *The Need of Forensic Pathology for Academic Sponsorship,* 33 Arch. Pathology 382-386 (1942).
3. Alan R. Moritz, *Scientific Medicolegal Investigation in the Undergraduate Medical Curriculum,* 158 JAMA 243-244 (1955).
4. Sir Sidney Smith, *The History and Development of Legal Medicine,* in *Legal Medicine,* 1-19, (R. B. H. Gradwohl ed., C. V. Mosby Co. 1954).
5. Gilbert H. Stewart, *Legal Medicine* 1-6 (Bobbs-Merrill Co. 1910).
6. Chester R. Burns, *Legacies in Law and Medicine* (Science History Publications, 1977).
7. James C. Mohr, *Doctors & the Law: Medical Jurisprudence in the Nineteenth Century America* (Oxford University Press 1993). *Also see* William J. Curran, *History and Development,* in *Modern Legal Medicine, Psychiatry, and Forensic Science,* 1-26 (William J. Curran et al. eds., F. A. Davis Co. 1980).
8. B. Rush, Introductory Lectures upon the Institutes and Practices of Medicine 363 (Philadelphia 1811). See Curran *supra,* Ref. 1.
9. Regan, *Report of Committee on Medicolegal Problems,* 150 JAMA 716 (1952).
10. Fischer, *Teaching Medical Law,* 205 JAMA 245 (1968).
11. Beresford, *The Teaching of Legal Medicine in Medical Schools in the United States,* 46 J. Med. Educ. 401 (1971).
12. The Task Force on Medico-Legal Curriculum, *A Recommended Medico-Legal Curriculum,* 5 J. Legal Med. 8EE (1977).
13. Harry S. Jonas, Sylvia I. Etzel & Barbara Barzansky, *Educational Programs in U.S. Medical Schools,* 270 JAMA 1061-1068 (1993).
14. Eugene S. Schneller & Terry S. Weiner, *The M.D.-J.D. Revisited—A Sociological Analysis of Cross-Educated Professionals in the Decade of the 1980s,* 6 J. Legal Med. 337-359 (1985).
15. D. H. Novack, B. J. Detering & R. Arnold, *Physicians' Attitudes Toward Using Deception to Resolve Difficult Ethical Problems,* 261 JAMA 2980-2985 (1989).

PART TWO Legal aspects of health care

CHAPTER 2   American legal system

KENNETH D. HANSEN, M.D., J.D., F.C.L.M.

CONSTITUTIONS
STATUTES
ADMINISTRATIVE LAW
COMMON LAW
FULL FAITH AND CREDIT TO OUT-OF-STATE JUDGMENTS
CONFLICT OF LAWS
CASE AND CONTROVERSY
RIGHT TO SUE AND APPEAL

In common with the legal systems of most other countries, American jurisprudence was developed to bring civility to the settlement of individual disputes. Thus "trial by combat" gave way to "trial by law." The "law" settles differences by having the parties to a dispute present their legal and factual arguments to a judge and jury. The judge, as the legal expert, decides the legal issues, whereas the jury—peers of the parties—decides the factual issues. The courtroom was established as the forum for the controversy, and lawyers, as officers of the court, serve as the "champions" of the opposing parties. The outcome of a civil trial usually involves the awarding of monetary damages, although the court may also order other remedies such as requiring a party to refrain from doing certain acts (an *injunction*). Law is a system of conduct that is derived from competent authority and is capable of being enforced. All laws derive from the power inherent in an authority, whether the authority is that of a country, state, county, city, or town. The power may be exercised in the form of a democracy, republic, monarchy, dictatorship, or totalitarian state.

Most individuals recognize that certain general rules of conduct provide order in everyday commerce. To secure person and property, individuals collectively transfer certain rights to authority so that such authority can apply laws to govern all. Government, the result of this transfer of rights, is based on the principle that the benefits derived from stability are worth the rights surrendered to create the government.

In the United States, individuals are governed and laws are established under a dual form of government.

Each of these two governments—federal and state—derives power from enabling documents called *constitutions*. Such constitutions not only embody the rights transferred by the citizens but also contain restraints that limit the power of the government.

CONSTITUTIONS

The U.S. Constitution was adopted and ratified as a part of the founding of the nation. Each of the states has its own constitution, adopted at the time of statehood or prior to entry into statehood while still a territory. All constitutions describe generally the powers of the government and allocate these powers to executive, legislative, and judicial branches. Thus, a framework is provided on which to build a functioning government.

The U.S. Constitution restricts the powers of the states in certain areas of national importance. For example, the federal government has exclusive powers in matters relating to the postal system, citizenship, immigration, naturalization, interstate commerce, national taxation and spending, maintaining an army, and waging war. All powers not specifically delegated to the federal government are reserved to the states.

Although the Constitution is an amazingly enduring document, it was not intended to be static, and provisions were made in Article V to amend it from time to time. All amendments to the Constitution become incorporated into the Constitution and as such become part of the supreme law of the land.

The process of amendment was deliberately intended to be cumbersome. Amendments may be proposed either by a two-thirds vote of both houses of Congress or by a national convention called by Congress on application of two-thirds of the legislatures of the states. A constitutional amendment becomes effective as of the date on which a sufficient number of states (three-fourths) ratify a proposed amendment. On the effective date, the amendment applies to all states regardless of whether any particular state rejected ratification. To date, the U.S. Constitution has been amended 26 times. With the exception of the Eighteenth Amendment (alcohol prohibition), which was repealed by the Twenty-first Amendment, all are operative.

United States constitutional supremacy clause

Article VI, Section 2, of the U.S. Constitution states that the Constitution, its amendments, and all laws passed by Congress in conformity with the Constitution constitute the absolute and unqualified law of the land. It is binding on all officers and judges of both federal and state governments. No governmental unit—agency, city, county, court, department, legislature, state, or town—can take any action that is inconsistent with the U.S. Constitution. Any provision of any state or federal law found to be inconsistent with the Constitution is void and cannot be enforced.

Bill of Rights and subsequent amendments

The first 10 amendments are known as the *Bill of Rights.* These 10 amendments guarantee that certain rights of individual citizens may not be infringed on by the federal government (i.e., freedom of speech, freedom of the press, freedom of religion, the right to bear arms, and the right to petition the government).

Before the Civil War, the U.S. Supreme Court[1] held that the protections contained in the Bill of Rights regarding the power of government over the citizen were intended to restrict the power of the federal government but not the individual states. For example, President Lincoln's famous Emancipation Proclamation freeing the slaves became effective on January 1, 1863. However, it was clearly a war measure and had no effect in those states that had remained in the Union (Delaware, Maryland, Missouri and Kentucky) and had no effect on the seceding Southern states after their readmission into the Union on conclusion of the Civil War. The Thirteenth Amendment, which abolished slavery, was adopted in 1865 to address this problem. This amendment not only prohibited the federal government from engaging in slavery activities but, by virtue of its Section 2, gave the federal government the power to enforce the abolition of slavery in all the states.

This set the stage for what may be the most important and certainly the most debated amendment to our Constitution—the Fourteenth Amendment. Not only did this amendment clearly define citizenship for the first time, it also made the distinction between U.S. citizenship and state citizenship.

But the most important and far-reaching effect of the Fourteenth Amendment is that it prohibits the *states* from abridging the privileges and immunities of citizens, from depriving any person of life, liberty, or property without due process of law, and from denying any person the equal protection of the laws.

Fourteenth amendment

Privileges and immunities clause. The federal courts have had some difficulty interpreting the scope of the privileges and immunities clause of the Fourteenth Amendment. At first it appeared that the amendment gave the federal government complete power to regulate all business and civil rights of citizens and made the first 10 amendments (the Bill of Rights) enforceable against the individual states. However, in a victory for those espousing states' rights, the U.S. Supreme Court in the famous "Slaughter House" cases gave a restrictive interpretation to the privileges and immunities clause.[2] It held that when a citizen's rights were derived either from the U.S. Constitution and laws promulgated thereunder or from the citizen's state constitution and laws that the state controlled. Most fundamental personal rights were deemed to flow from the consequence or incidence of state citizenship, therefore remaining beyond the reach of the privileges and immunities clause. This led to situations in which a state could be prohibited from discriminating against freed slaves but that individuals, such as hotel operators, were free to discriminate.

Privileges of national citizenship were protected. These included, but were not limited to, the right to travel freely among the various states, to petition the Congress, to vote for national offices, and to inform federal authorities of violations of federal law.[3]

Although the "Slaughter House" cases still have some validity today, a relentless pressure to protect individual citizen rights from not only federal infringement but also state infringement has slowly led to extension of most of the Bill of Rights to the individual states and their citizens.

The U.S. Supreme Court has adopted an approach that uses the Fourteenth Amendment selectively to enforce the Bill of Rights against the states. Thus the Court has held that the states are bound by the First, Fourth, Fifth, Sixth, and Eighth Amendments. Whereas the Second Amendment aims to prevent the Congress from interfering with the right of the states to maintain armed bodies of militia and from banning citizen ownership of weapons, the states themselves have significant latitude in regulating possession and use of firearms. The Third Amendment, which prohibits quartering of soldiers in private houses, has never been violated and thus has never been litigated. The Seventh Amendment, which guarantees a trial by jury in cases wherein the controversy exceeds $20 in value, has not been applied to the states, which are free to set their own limits in civil cases. The Ninth and Tenth Amendments reiterate that power not specifically delegated to the federal government is reserved to the states or to the people. These last two amendments have been liberally construed by the Court to expand rather than constrict the power of the federal government.

Substantive due process. Fundamental to American values and noted in both the Declaration of Independence and the U.S. Constitution is that all persons are endowed by their creator with certain basic natural rights that are immune from governmental interference. This philosophy of "natural law" requires that some constitutional basis be found if these natural rights are to remain secure. Initially when the Court found such natural rights, it employed what is called *substantive due process.* Essentially, the due process clause of the Fourteenth Amendment provided the process by which the Court confers constitutional protection to several unenumerated individual rights. The Court did not begin to employ this process with vigor until the nineteenth century. In the famous case of *Lochner v. New York,* the U.S. Supreme Court decided that the New York state legislature had violated the natural rights of bakery employees (according to the due process clause of the Fourteenth Amendment) when it passed a statute limiting bakery working hours.[4] Thus the U.S. Supreme Court substituted its judgment for that of the entire New York legislature. Following this decision lower federal courts began to also freely substitute their own subjective judgments as to the advisability of state legislative actions, especially in matters deemed to deal with the public interest.

Advocates of states rights were outraged by this action and somewhat rightfully exclaimed that the Court's substantive due process cases had trampled on the protections granted by the Tenth Amendment. In the absence of any meaningful standard by which the courts could determine which human interests could rise to the level of constitutional protection, predictably an inconsistent and irreconcilable line of court decisions developed. It was not until the Depression years that the Court suddenly reversed itself and began to find that previously prohibited governmental acts were now quite permissible. The Court adopted a new rule that regulatory schemes that neither impinged on the Bill of Rights nor improperly restricted political process must be

upheld, unless, under any reasonably conceivable facts, the law was "of such a character as to preclude the assumption that it rests upon some rational basis."[5]

Thus the U.S. Supreme Court provided the constitutional basis for the political movement referred to as the "New Deal" and it was during this time and decades after that the concept of "natural law" with its protections of unenumerated rights lay in repose. Meanwhile the power of the federal government expanded relatively unimpeded by judicial action.

Substantive due process II. The 1960s and 1970s were a time of considerable political change in the United States and this change began to have a profound impact on the U.S. Supreme Court. In 1965, a new form of substantive due process began to evolve.

The Court recognized its predicament. If it revived the substantive due process method of *Lochner,* consistency would require that the Court invalidate much of the federal social and economic schemes that had enabled the massive expansion of federal power during the previous three decades. On the other hand, failure to act to provide for individual rights could result in not only social injustice but also social unrest.

The Court acted in the only way it knew how: it created another legal fiction. In what should be called *substantive due process II,* the Court found that the Constitution included "a zone of privacy created by several fundamental guarantees" found within the first eight amendments and in the "penumbrae" of the entire constitution. Using this reasoning and carefully declaring that it was not resurrecting *Lochner,* the Court struck down a Connecticut criminal statute prohibiting use of contraceptive devices by married couples.[6] In 1973, the "penumbrae" of rights theory was extended "to encompass a woman's decision whether or not to terminate her pregnancy" in *Roe v. Wade.*[7] The Court held that only a compelling interest could justify state regulation of abortion.

How far the "zone of privacy" will be extended remains to be seen.

Procedural due process. Whereas substantive due process required a review of the judgments of the legislative branches of government, *procedural due process* deals with an individual's opportunity to be heard in a timely manner and in a meaningful way in matters of controversy. Underlying procedural due process is the recognition that procedural safeguards are necessary to assure fundamental fairness and reliability of results.[8]

The threshold problem for the courts is the determination of when procedural due process is required. The Fifth and Fourteenth Amendments tell us that deprivation of life, liberty, or property activates due process guarantees. But these issues are themselves somewhat elastic and the Court has provided further guidance that these "core" liberty interests include "not merely freedom from bodily restraint, but also the right of the individual to contract, to engage in any of the common occupations of life, to acquire useful knowledge, to marry, to establish a home, and bring up children [and] to worship God according to the dictates of...conscience."[9]

In dealing with the application of procedural due process to property interests, the Court has adopted the *entitlement doctrine,* which requires a person to have "a legitimate claim of entitlement" to a benefit, as opposed to a need or expectation.[10] A claim of entitlement may emanate from explicit state law or official custom and practice. A license to practice medicine is a form of property that receives procedure due process protection. The entitlement doctrine helps explain why due process requirements are different when a physician first makes application for admission to the hospital staff and when a physician finds himself the subject of a staff revocation proceeding. In the first the physician has only an "expectation" of receiving staff privileges and in the second the physician, having already been granted staff membership, has a "legitimate claim of entitlement."

Once it is determined that an interest is entitled to the protections of procedural due process, it is somewhat unclear as to the extent or formality of the due process required. The current rule is actually a flexible guideline which states that due process "calls for such procedural protections as the particular situation demands" and the type of hearing required (formal or informal) is determined by the careful balancing of respective interests.[11]

Equal protection. Although it is a fundamental principle of our constitution, equal protection under the law does not mean that everyone must be treated the same: "Equal protection does not require that all persons be dealt with identically, but it does require that a distinction made have some relevance to the purpose for which the classification [which results in unequal treatment] is made."[12]

The traditional equal protection standard requires that the classifications that could result in unequal treatment (or benefits) be reasonably related to a permissible governmental purpose. The courts will apply close judicial scrutiny to classifications that result in unequal treatment of persons by race. Other "suspect areas" have been created by statute and include sex, color, national origin, religion, and age.

Physicians do not belong to any of the suspect classifications, and laws providing special taxation of physicians to pay for care of the indigent have been upheld as aiding a permissible governmental purpose. In addition, several federal appeals courts have ruled that price controls dealing with Medicare recipients can be imposed on physicians without violating constitutional protections.

STATUTES

All constitutions invest one body of the government with the power to make laws. The federal body so empowered is the Congress. The state bodies are called assemblies or legislatures. Laws enacted by a legislative body are referred to as *statutes*. Statutes may deal with a wide range of subjects limited only by the U.S. Constitution and, in the case of state statutes, by the additional limitation of the state constitution.

Following enactment by a legislative body, statutes are published in chronological order, usually on an annual basis (e.g., *United States Statutes at Large*). The statutes are then codified so that statutes dealing with similar subject matter can be found in one volume. For example, all federal laws dealing with veterans and their benefits are found in Volume 38 (referred to as Title 38) of the *United States Code*. State laws are similarly codified. All of the states' legislatures delegate certain law-making powers to the state's political subdivisions (i.e., counties, cities, and towns). These political subdivisions operate under the provisions of charters (similar to a constitution) and may enact laws of a local nature. Such laws are usually called *ordinances* and have effect only within the boundaries of the political subdivision.

Preemption clause

Federal laws promulgated in conformity with the Constitution and its amendments are supreme to any state or lesser political subdivision's statutes. Indeed, under the federal preemption doctrine, Congress has the power, by legislating on a particular subject, to preclude the states from legislating on that subject. For example, Congress has preempted the subject of aviation and established the Federal Aviation Administration and the Civil Aeronautics Board to administer the country's aviation.

As stated earlier, the final arbiter of whether a governmental action or law conforms to the requirements of the Constitution rests with the courts. State courts generally make determinations regarding state laws and constitutions but also will frequently strike down state laws on U.S. constitutional grounds.

State court actions on purely state matters (state statutes, regulations, ordinances, or constitutions) are not subject to review by federal courts. The federal courts may hear appeals from state court actions when such actions are based on a U.S. constitutional issue or when the appealing party alleges that the state court action violates certain U.S. constitutional guarantees of rights.

ADMINISTRATIVE LAW

Congress or state legislatures often enact statutes that provide for the performance of certain ongoing tasks (e.g., the licensing of health care personnel). Such legislation establishes an administrative agency (licensing board) and charges the agency with the task of carrying out the legislative intent contained within the broad wording of the enabling statute. In a sense, the enabling statute is the "constitution" of an administrative agency that, within the confines of the statute, performs the "legislative" task of promulgating rules and regulations governing the subject matter within the agency's authority. These rules not only regulate the day-to-day operations of the agency but also serve to fine-tune the broader mandate of the enabling legislation.

When an administrative agency's rules have been properly promulgated (i.e., issued in conformity with a valid statute), such rules will have the force of law as if enacted by the legislature. These rules often confer judicial-like powers that allow an agency to decide individual complaints, to issue or deny licenses, and, in certain instances, to grant monetary awards or levy fines. Administrative bodies exercise their judicial functions at hearings. Although these hearings are not as formal as court trials, evidence may be presented and witnesses called. In addition, legal counsel may represent parties challenging agency action. After it is established that an agency has acted within the lawful scope of its powers and has not acted arbitrarily as concerns any individual, courts are generally foreclosed from reviewing the merits of the agency's decision. The courts recognize that Congress or state legislatures have entrusted certain decisions involving expert knowledge to the agency, and the courts generally do not judge the merits of agency decisions, according to the principle of separation of powers between the legislature and the judiciary.

Challenges to the regulatory system are frequent, but courts have generally upheld administrative agencies' exercises of power. In a typical case, an employer challenged the legality of action by the Occupational Safety and Health Administration (OSHA). The employer claimed that the imposition of civil penalties by the OSHA Review Board in the absence of a jury trial violated the Seventh Amendment of the U.S. Constitution. In upholding the administrative agency, the U.S. Supreme Court stated[13]:

Congress found the common law and other existing remedies for work injuries resulting from unsafe working conditions to be inadequate.... It created a new cause of action, and remedies theretofore unknown to the common law, and placed their enforcement in a tribunal supplying speedy and expert resolution of the issues involved. The 7th amendment is no bar to the creation of new rights or to their enforcement outside the regular courts of law.

During the past 30 years, statutes have established administrative agencies that control a wide range of human endeavors. Administrative rules and regulations are issued by agencies at all levels of government—federal, state, and local. The impact of these rules and regulations in the health care field is substantial, and rules issued by the Department of Health and Human Services (DHHS), Health Care Financing Administration (HCFA), Peer Standards Review Organizations (PSROs), and others are myriad and likely to proliferate even further.

COMMON LAW

The "common law" in the United States is based on a system of law that arose in England during the Middle Ages. During this time, all executive, legislative, and judicial power was centralized in the monarchy. As the burden of adjudicating individual conflicts increased, the king delegated almost autonomous judicial power to the various lords and barons, who in turn appointed judges under their control. Subsequently, the power to appoint judges was regained by the king, and the lords and barons were restricted to executive functions. The first adjudications by English judges were based on prior rulings of the king (or lord) and, when no such ruling existed, on common custom. The laws made by the judges were not broad in application but were restricted to the resolution of the particular conflict at hand. The court's pronouncement was absolutely binding on the parties to the conflict (subject only to appeal to the king), but other parties having similar conflicts could escape applicability of an unfavorable decision by citing factual differences.

The decisions of the English courts were recorded in permanent form for the first time during the reign of Henry II in the year 1195. These case books were known as *plea rolls*. With the introduction of written decisions, a large body of common law accumulated over the centuries. Fairness required that the court abide by and adhere to previously decided cases whenever the facts were the same. Thus, one of the most important principles of the common law was born—*stare decisis*.

Stare decisis literally translates to "let the decision stand." The stability derived from such a principle is apparent. Citizens could expect comparable treatment in similar circumstances. When the facts of a given controversy did not substantially resemble any prior case, the English courts had the flexibility to apply judicially derived principles to fit the new fact pattern. The courts rarely overruled prior rulings, and then only when strong justification existed. It was this ability of the

English courts to maintain both stability and flexibility in light of changing circumstances that gave the system of common law its strength. At the time of the founding of the American colonies, the English common law system was firmly in place and well developed. Original colonial decisions were based on English decisions; however, different circumstances and changing customs eventually diminished reliance on English pronouncements.

After the American Revolution, the states feared that the federal government would institute a national common law with potential for abuse by the central power. To reserve the common law for the states, a movement to establish a national statutory code was undertaken during the late eighteenth and early nineteenth centuries. This movement was successful in limiting the jurisdiction and powers of the newly established federal courts. Federal judges were not allowed to make law (as were the English judges); they were restricted to merely applying existing federal laws. If no federal law existed to cover the issue, the federal court had no jurisdiction to hear the case. However, the exception to this principle is found in diversity of citizenship cases, in which the citizens of different states can ask the federal court to resolve their controversy. If the federal court finds it has jurisdiction over the controversy, it may hear and decide the case. However, the federal judge must render a decision in conformity with state common law and state statutory law.

FULL FAITH AND CREDIT TO OUT-OF-STATE JUDGMENTS

The framers of the U.S. Constitution recognized that the diverse and often competing interests of the various states would lead to conflict in the application of laws and individual judgments. To minimize this conflict, Article IV, Section 1, requires that the states give "full faith and credit" to the court judgments of the other individual states. In general, this clause requires that a court in another state give the first state's judgment the same effect it would have had if the defendant were still in the jurisdiction of the first.

The rationale for full faith and credit is the prevention of inconsistent judgments in neighboring jurisdictions and the more efficient use of both the court system and individual resources required for litigation. Because of the potential for abuse on the part of litigants attempting to enforce "foreign" judgments, the doctrine is subject to various limitations. In order for full faith and credit to be given to a *foreign* or out-of-state judgment, that judgment must have been obtained under proper jurisdiction. In other words, did the foreign court have the right to try the parties in the first place? Was proper notice given to all interested parties, and were they afforded an adequate opportunity to defend?

Second, the judgment must be *final.* Many jurisdictions take the position that whenever a lower court decision is being appealed, there is no final judgment that can be enforced. Third, the judgment must have been *on the merits.* In certain cases a plaintiff may sue a defendant in the wrong court (*improper venue*) and the defendant may succeed in having the case dismissed. If the defendant were to attempt to use the dismissal as a bar to suit by the plaintiff in another state, the dismissal would not merit full faith and credit because the issue at controversy had not been decided *on the merits* but rather had been dismissed on a technicality.

CONFLICT OF LAWS

In a modern and mobile society, controversies between citizens of different states are bound to occur. A system of legal rules to deal with these conflicts has evolved to bring order and reasonable predictability to such conflicts. The full faith and credit clause of the Constitution does not require the states to abide by the often varying laws of neighboring states. To do so would allow one state to legislate for another. The U.S. Supreme Court in *Klaxon Co. v. Stentor Electric Mfg. Co.* stated: "Nothing in the Federal Constitution insures unlimited extraterritorial recognition of all (state) statutes or of any statute under all circumstances."[14] It has been said that absent the full faith and credit rules in regard to enforcement of foreign court judgments, the states are free to adopt their own rules to resolve controversies involving the laws of various jurisdictions.

For any court to have power to render a judgment it must first have jurisdiction over the parties to the controversy. If both parties to the lawsuit are citizens of state *X,* then there exists no jurisdictional problem. However, if the defendant is a citizen of state *Y,* it may be difficult for the court to obtain "personal" jurisdiction over said defendant, and where none can be obtained there can be no lawsuit.

Several methods to obtain jurisdiction over *foreign* citizens have been devised, one of which is called the *long arm statute.* These statutes utilize the fiction of *implied consent* whereby certain acts imply consent to submit to the jurisdiction of the courts of the state in which the acts occur. For example, persons driving on the roads of state *X* imply consent to the jurisdiction of state *X* courts for controversies arising out of use of the highways or a vehicle in state *X.*

Likewise, courts are able to obtain jurisdiction over *foreign* citizens who *do business* in state *X.* A physician who has an office in Arlington, Virginia, and who sees patients from the District of Columbia and Maryland may be subject to the jurisdiction of the D.C. and Maryland courts if the physician's contact with those jurisdictions is considered to be significant. It has been held that merely providing a telephone diagnosis and treatment plan across state lines is sufficient to establish jurisdiction for the purposes of a malpractice lawsuit.

In general, the court asked to entertain the lawsuit will determine the presence or absence of jurisdiction according to state court guidelines and, if jurisdiction is found, the court will also usually apply its own court procedures in the conduct of the case at controversy.

CASE AND CONTROVERSY

The terms *case* and *controversy,* as used in the U.S. Constitution, embrace claims or contentions of litigants brought before the court for adjudication by regular proceedings established for the protection or enforcement of rights, or the prevention, redress, or punishment of wrongs; and whenever the claim or contention of a party takes such a form that the judicial power is capable of acting on, it has become a case or controversy.[15] These two terms are to be distinguished because there may be a "separable controversy" within a case, which may be removed from a state court to a federal court,[16] although the case as a whole is not removable. The term *controversy,* if distinguishable from *case,* is so in that it is less comprehensive than the term *cases* and includes only suits of a civil nature.[17]

RIGHT TO SUE AND APPEAL

Under the Sixth Amendment to the Constitution, a person has a right to sue provided the plaintiff can demonstrate an iota or scintilla of evidence indicating that he or she has been wronged and entitled to redress. There is no concomitant right of appeal upon loss in the lower court; it is at the discretion of the appellate court.

END NOTES

1. *Barron v. Baltimore,* 32 U.S. 243 (1833) ("The Constitution was ordained and established by the people of the United States for themselves; for their own government; and not for the government of individual states").
2. 83 U.S.36 (1883).
3. *Twining v. New Jersey,* 211 U.S. 78 (1908).
4. *Lochner v. New York,* 198 U.S. 45 (1905).
5. *United States v. Carolene Products Co.,* 304 U.S. 144 (1938).
6. *Griswold v. Connecticut,* 381 U.S. 479 (1965).
7. *Roe v. Wade,* 410 U.S. 113 (1973).
8. *Fuentes v. Shevin,* 407 U.S. 67 (1972).
9. *Meyer v. Nebraska,* 262 U.S. 390, 399 (1923).
10. *Board of Regents v. Roth,* 408 U.S. 564 (1972).
11. See *Goss v. Lopez,* 419 U.S.565 (1975) (required only a rudimentary hearing for a public school student suspended for 10 days). *Also see Goldberg v. Kelly,* 397 U.S. 254 (1970) (held that a welfare recipient was entitled to a full evidentiary hearing before benefits could be terminated).
12. *Baxstrom v. Herold,* 383 U.S. 107 (1966).
13. *Atlas Roofing Co. v. OSHA Review Board,* 430 U.S. 442 at 461 (1976).
14. 313 U.S. 487, 85 L. Ed. 477, 61 Sup. Ct. 1020 (1940).
15. *Interstate Commerce Comm'n v. Brimson,* 154 U.S. 447, 14 Sup. Ct. 1125, 38 L. Ed. 1047 (1894).
16. *Snow v. Smith,* C.C.Va., 88 Fed. 658 (1882).
17. *Smith v. Blackwell,* C.C.A.S.C., 115 F2d 186, 188 (1940).

CHAPTER 3

Judicial system

KENNETH D. HANSEN, M.D., J.D., F.C.L.M.

THE FEDERAL COURT SYSTEM
STATE COURTS

Our judicial system is rooted in the common law and has two distinct characteristics: (1) an adversary system, modified by the use of "discovery" (ability of each side to acquire essential factual information from the other), and (2) consistency and continuity based on appellate decisions resulting in precedents or stare decisis. Our judicial system not only resolves legal disputes in the courts, it also creates law when there is a public need and the other two branches—executive and legislative—do not act. The system is predicated on the theory that for every wrong there should be a remedy. To that end, disputes between people, between people and the government, and between governments—federal and state—are resolved by the judiciary.

All court systems, whether federal, state, or local, have trial and appellate levels. The trial court "hears" the case first, taking oral testimony and considering other evidence. Its decisions are usually reached by a judge and jury or by a single judge sitting without a jury. When a jury is involved, it weighs the evidence presented and determines the true facts of the case. The judge interprets the applicable law and states it for the jury to apply to the facts. When the judge sits without a jury, the courts act as both fact finder and interpreter of the law.

In contrast to the trial court, the appellate court does not take evidence, but instead relies on the facts as determined at trial. The appellate court hears legal arguments, which are directed to either support the law as applied by the trial judge or to show how the trial judge erred in his or her application of the law. Appellate courts consist of three to nine judges, and rulings are based on majority vote. If a tie vote occurs, the trial court's ruling is upheld. Appellate court decisions usually appear as written opinions and are published in chronological order in books of cases called *reporters*. The lines of cases set forth in these reporters comprise the body of law and legal principles currently referred to as the American common law. The U.S.

Supreme Court resolves the questions of supremacy, preemption, and the full faith and credit clause inherent in the Constitution.

THE FEDERAL COURT SYSTEM

The federal courts are courts of limited jurisdiction. Courts of limited jurisdiction have the power to render decisions only in those cases dealing with specific subject matter. Federal courts can exercise jurisdiction only over those types of cases specified in the U.S. Constitution or specified by an act of the Congress. This limited jurisdiction of the federal courts grew out of the fear of a too-powerful national court system, such as that found in Great Britain.

As the U.S. Constitution states[1]:

The judicial power shall extend to all cases, in law and equity, arising under this Constitution, the laws of the United States, and treaties made, or which shall be made, under their authority; to all cases affecting ambassadors, other public ministers and counsels; to all cases of admiralty and maritime jurisdiction; to controversies to which the United States shall be a party; to controversies between two or more states; between a state and citizens of another state; between citizens of different states, between citizens of the same state claiming lands under grants of different states, and between a state, or the citizens thereof, and foreign states, citizens or subjects.

This clause was restricted by the Eleventh Amendment to the Constitution ratified January 8, 1798. The Eleventh Amendment guaranteed the individual states immunity from suit. The effect of such "sovereign immunity" is that an individual state may be sued only with its permission.

The Constitutional Convention in 1787 originally made provision only for a Supreme Court that would be a final arbiter of federal controversies. Many state delegations, wanting to keep the great bulk of judicial power within their own boundaries, were against the establishment of inferior, or lower, federal courts. A compromise resolution left the establishment of lower federal courts to the discretion of the Congress[2]:

The judicial power of the United States shall be vested in one Supreme Court, and in such inferior courts as the Congress may from time to time ordain and establish . . ."

The U.S. Constitution became effective March 4, 1789. It did not take long for Congress to exercise its discretion in the establishment of lower federal courts; by September 24, 1789, the Judiciary Act of 1789 was passed. This act established two lower federal court systems, provided for one federal district court to be established in each state, and provided for three circuit courts of appeals to act as intermediate courts.

Being a federal court justice in those days was not a lucrative profession; federal judges often had to literally "ride the circuit" in order to hear federal cases. When circuit judges were unavailable, district judges acted on occasion as circuit courts of appeals judges, and in many instances heard appeals from their own decisions. It was not until 1891, with the adoption of the Evarts Act of 1891, that a judge was prohibited from hearing an appeal from a case over which that same judge had previously presided.[3]

District courts

The United States (including the District of Columbia and Puerto Rico) is divided into 91 federal judicial districts. Each federal district has its own district court and, with only one exception, federal judicial districts do not extend across state lines. (The District Court for Wyoming includes Wyoming and those parts of Yellowstone National Park extending across the Wyoming border into Montana and Idaho.) Several states have more than one judicial district and thus more than one district court. These include California, New York, and Texas, each of which has four judicial districts.[4] With few exceptions, all cases dealing with federal issues must be brought to the federal district courts. This is termed *original jurisdiction,* that is, no controversy or appeal may be heard in any federal appellate court unless it has been first brought to and decided by the district court. The jurisdiction of the federal district courts has been greatly expanded in the last 20 years due to the great number of federal statutes that confer federal jurisdiction (e.g., consumer and environmental protection laws, labor rights statutes, etc.).

Federal courts of appeals

Although the Judiciary Act of 1789 had created circuit courts of appeals, there had been considerable confusion as to the jurisdiction of such courts. In many cases there was concurrent jurisdiction between the courts of appeals and the district courts. The Evarts Act of 1891 clarified the jurisdiction and powers of the circuit courts of appeals and provided for a system that is very similar to the current system. Renamed the United States Court of Appeals by the 1948 Judicial Code, the system consists of 11 courts of appeals — one for the District of Columbia and 10 others. Each court has jurisdiction over between 3 and 10 state judicial districts. The great bulk of the work of the courts of appeals is appellate: hearing appeals of cases tried in the lower courts. The courts of appeals do retain some original jurisdiction, the most notable being review of decisions made by many federal administrative agencies.

The Supreme Court

The U.S. Supreme Court was created by the U.S. Constitution. Its size has varied from six to ten members, and the current number (nine) was set in 1869.

As with the courts of appeals, the jurisdiction of the Supreme Court is primarily appellate. There are special cases, however, in which the Supreme Court may sit as the court of original jurisdiction. As the Constitution states[5]:

[I]n all cases affecting ambassadors, other public ministers and counsels, and those in which a state shall be a party, the Supreme Court shall have original jurisdiction. In all the other cases before mentioned the Supreme Court shall have appellate jurisdiction, both as to law and fact, with such exceptions, and under such regulations as the Congress shall make.

During the nineteenth and twentieth centuries, the Supreme Court had little power to refuse to hear appeals from lower courts, and the Court became increasingly over-burdened with appellate cases. In the early 1920s, a committee of Court justices drafted a bill (later called the Judge's Bill) that reduced the burden on the Supreme Court.[6] In this law, the Supreme Court was given the right of discretionary review of cases it felt to be of particular importance and urgency. This bill greatly expanded the use of the writ of certiorari, which was first allowed under the Evarts Act of 1891. This writ is essentially a request that the Supreme Court hear a particular case; again, the Court exercises discretionary power over whether or not to accept the case. An example of the magnitude of the discretion to refuse to hear cases is found in Supreme Court statistics from 1974: the Court addressed 3,876 cases, 3,349 of which were denials or dismissals of appeals or petitions for review. Only 527 of the cases were actually decided on their merits.

There is no appeal from a decision of the Supreme Court, although the Court may agree to rehear a case. In those instances in which the Court interprets a statute or a law in a manner at odds with a congressional interpretation, the only remedy afforded Congress is to rewrite the statute; this was the case with the snail darter decision in which the Court decided that the Endangered Species Act prohibited the completion of the Tellico Dam.[7] The congressional response was to amend the law. In four instances, the Constitution has been amended to overcome Supreme Court decisions.[8]

Other federal courts

Several other federal courts not within the system are outlined here. The Court of Claims was established in 1855 and is the oldest of the special courts. This court has jurisdiction to hear claims against the United States.[9] The Court of Customs and Patent Appeals was established in 1909 and deals with patent issues as well as questions of customs laws and policy.[10] The newest of the special courts of the United States is the Tax Court, which was established in 1969 to hear issues arising under the Internal Revenue Code.[11]

Judicial tenure

The judges of the federal courts, including the Supreme and lower courts, enjoy lifetime tenure, assuming they refrain from criminal activities and are able to perform their tasks. There have been very few instances of judges being impeached or removed from their judicial office.

STATE COURTS

Like the federal court system, state courts are generally established by statute or by constitutional provisions. Unlike the federal courts, however, state courts have general jurisdiction to hear cases arising under their laws and to hear the complaints of their citizens. For example, the state of Michigan provides in its constitution[12]:

The judicial power of the state is vested exclusively in one court of justice, which shall be divided into one Supreme Court, one Court of Appeals, one trial court of general jurisdiction known as the circuit court, one probate court, and courts of limited jurisdiction created by the legislature.

Similar provisions exist in all other states, establishing a multilevel system of courts. The Michigan system is typical of many state court systems.

- The Supreme Court of Michigan has jurisdiction over any matter brought to it by "any appropriate writ" from any inferior court; any question of law or request for review under rules written by the court. The court has the power to refuse to hear any case and, in this way, is somewhat unique in having totally discretionary jurisdiction.[13]
- The Michigan Court of Appeals has jurisdiction over appeals from decisions of all the lower courts of the

state. In many instances this is the court of last resort for most litigants, given the discretionary nature of the state supreme court jurisdiction. The state supreme court also has the power to order the state court of appeals to hear any question it determines should be reviewed by a higher court.[14]

- The Michigan circuit courts are general trial courts, empowered to hear all matters of law and equity and appeals concerning state administrative agency actions.
- The Michigan district courts, established by the Michigan legislature, are also general jurisdiction courts, but with some limitations: the amount in controversy must be less than $10,000 and traditional equity matters, such as divorce or suits for injunctive relief, are barred. The creation of these courts was simply a response to the clogged dockets of the circuit courts.
- The Michigan Small Claims Court, a division of the district courts, hears claims under $600 and is a much less formal setting for the resolution of small disputes.[15]
- The Michigan Probate Court is a specialized court, having jurisdiction over matters concerning trusts, wills, and estates, juvenile problems, adoption proceedings, and other areas of family law.
- The Michigan Court of Claims, similar to the federal claims court, was established to hear claims against the state and its agents.

Unlike federal judges who enjoy lifetime tenure, most state judges are elected officials who serve for a fixed term of office. The rationale for election of state judges rests with the notion that elected judges are more in tune with the wants and needs of the electorate. Many commentators, however, criticize the practice of electing judges, citing dangers inherent to the politicization of the court system and the pressures of conducting a political campaign and soliciting contributions.

END NOTES

1. U.S. Const. art. III, §2.
2. *Id.* at §1.
3. Evarts Act of March 3, 1891, 26 Stat. 826 (1891).
4. 28 U.S.C.A. §§81-131.
5. U.S. Const., *supra,* at §2.
6. Act of February 13, 1925, 43 Stat. 936 (1925).
7. *TVA v. Hill,* 437 U.S. 153, 98 S. Ct. 2279, 57 L. Ed. 2d 117 (April 18, 1978).
8. 9 Wright and Miller, *Federal Practice and Procedure,* §3507, note 14.
9. 28 U.S.C.A. §§171-175.
10. *Id.* at §§251-255.
11. 26 U.S.C.A. §744i.
12. Mich. Const. art. 6.
13. Mich. Comp. Laws Ann. §600.215.
14. *Id.* at §600.308.
15. *Id.* at §600.8401.

CHAPTER 4

Competency, capacity, and immunity

STEVEN B. BISBING, Psy.D., J.D.
JOSEPH P. McMENAMIN, M.D., J.D., F.C.L.M.
RICHARD L. GRANVILLE, M.D., J.D., F.C.L.M.

COMPETENCY AND CAPACITY
IMMUNITY

COMPETENCY AND CAPACITY
Introduction to the law

Definition. Nearly every area of human endeavor is affected by the law and, as a fundamental condition, the law requires that a person be mentally competent. Essentially, *to be considered legally competent* can be defined as "having sufficient ability . . . possessing the requisite natural or legal qualifications. . . ."[1] This definition is deliberately vague and ambiguous because the term *competency* is a broad concept that encompasses many different legal issues and contexts. As a result, the definition, requirements, and application of the term can vary greatly, depending on the nature of the legal issue.

In general, competency refers to some minimal mental, cognitive, or behavioral ability, trait, or capability required to perform a particular jural act or to assume some legal role. Appendix 4-1 outlines a sample of the various contexts in which competency may be an issue. The term *capacity*, which is often interchanged with the word *competency*, refers to an individual's actual ability to understand or form an intention with regard to some act. Appendix 4-2 summarizes several areas in which capacity is defined in order for a person's actions to be legally recognized as being competent. As a distinction, *incompetent* is applied to an individual who fails one of the tests of capacity and is therefore considered by *law* not to be mentally capable of performing a particular act or assuming a particular role.

It is important to realize that the adjudication of incompetence is *subject*- or *issue*-specific. For example, the fact that a person is adjudicated incompetent to execute a will does not automatically render him or her incompetent to do other things, such as consent to treatment or testify as a witness.

The law in general. Generally, the law recognizes only those decisions or choices that have been made by a competent individual. The reason for this is because the law seeks to protect the incompetent from the effects of their acts and from being taken advantage of because of their lack of capacity. Persons over the age of majority, which is now considered to be 18,[2] are presumed to be competent.[3] However, this presumption is *rebuttable* by evidence of an individual's incapacity.[4]

The issue of competency, in either a civil or a criminal context, is commonly raised in two situations: with a person who is a minor or one who is mentally disabled. In many situations, minors are not considered legally competent and therefore require the consent of a parent or designated guardian. Exceptions to this general rule include minors who are considered emancipated[5] or mature[6] and, in some cases, those in medical need[7] or in an emergency.[8]

The mentally disabled present a slightly different problem in terms of competency. Lack of capacity or competency cannot be presumed because of either treatment for mental illness[9] or because a person is institutionalized.[10] Moreover, mental disability or illness does not, in and of itself, render a person incompetent or incompetent in all areas of functioning. Instead, scrutiny should be given to determining whether certain specific functional incapacities render a person incapable of making a particular kind of decision or performing a particular type of task. Respect for individual autonomy[11] demands that individuals be allowed to make decisions of which they are capable, even if they are seriously mentally impaired. As a rule, therefore, a patient or person with a history of mental illness generally must be judicially declared incompetent before he or she loses the legal power to do what normal adult persons have the right or power to do. A person's current or past history of mental illness is but one factor to be weighed in terms of determining whether a particular test of competency is met.

Scope of this section. Appendix 4-1 outlines a number of the areas of the law in which competency is required. This is by no means an exhaustive list, but it should provide an adequate overview of the persuasiveness and importance of this element. This chapter addresses a sample of that list, concentrating on some of the more common issues raised in civil law. Appendix 4-2 provides a summary of some of the general tests for competency depending on the act to be committed. Of course, the specific language of these and other tests is typically defined by state or federal statute, and their interpretation and practical usage are outlined in the case law in which competency was an issue. As a general rule, it is important to keep in mind the distinction between mental illness or disability and competency. One commentator has pointed out that where competency is concerned, the issue raises two questions[12]:

1. Is there evidence of mental illness or deficiency (as in alcohol-induced, advanced age, organically related illness, and so on)?
2. If so, does this condition prevent the person from satisfying the relevant legal test or criterion for competency?

Thus although it is not always obvious from the legal tests themselves (see Appendix 4-2), there is often a threshold condition of mental illness, defect, or deficiency that serves as a qualifying consideration.

Competency areas

Capacity to contract. The law recognizes that to execute any business transaction between two parties, each must have sufficient *capacity* to give a free and relatively knowing consent to enter into an agreement or contract. Minors and the mentally incompetent historically have been recognized as being incapable of executing a legally recognized transaction owing to their presumed lack of requisite cognitive capacity.

This presumption goes back as far as Roman law, which held that "an insane person cannot contract any business whatever, because he does not know what he is doing." Similarly, the common law of contracts in England required that two persons wishing to enter into a business agreement must reach a "meeting of the minds." If one of the parties lacked the necessary mental capability to reach such a meeting, the law would not recognize the contract. In *Dexter v. Hall,* the U.S. Supreme Court articulated the effects of mental illness on the legality of a contract by holding

[T]he fundamental idea of a contract is that it requires the assent of two minds. But a lunatic, or person *non compos mentis*

("not of sound mind") has nothing which the law recognizes as a mind, and it would seem, therefore, upon principle, that he cannot make a contract which may have efficacy as such.[13]

As noted, unsoundness of mind incorporates not only mental infirmities but also any condition that impairs a person's capacity to reason. For example, narcotics,[14] organic brain disease[15] or disorder, mental retardation,[16] alcoholism,[17] aging,[18] and other conditions all would be relevant contributing factors of incompetence.

It is important to note that the lack of capacity to contract may be total or partial. In cases of total incapacity, a person is unable to enter into any contractual obligation, and any indication of an intent to do so would be considered void. For instance, a person whose property is under the supervision of a legal guardian as a result of a legal adjudication of incompetence is considered "totally lacking contractual capacity." Capacity to contract may also be partial, as is generally the case with minors, the mentally ill, and those whose cognitive faculties have been impaired by drugs, alcohol, or medication.[19] The extent of their ability to legally contract depends on the nature of the transaction and the surrounding circumstances.

For instance, in *United Pacific Insurance Co. v. Buchanan,*[20] a Washington State court of appeals held that an incompetent individual could enter a binding contract, despite evidence of memory loss and dementia caused by chronic alcoholism, where his guardians failed to enforce the guardianship or carry out their duties. The defendant was adjudicated to be incompetent in 1981, and his son and daughter were appointed guardians. For seven years they neither evaluated his estate nor maintained any of his business interests. Following completion of an alcohol treatment program, the defendant returned to the community and set up residence on his own. He resumed work with a general contracting company, a firm in which he had one-third interest with his son/guardian and another party. Buchanan and some partners in the contracting firm, in their individual capacities, entered into a construction contract that they eventually defaulted on. A bonding company sued Buchanan to recover payments it had made as a result of the default. Buchanan's children, in their role as guardians, sought to have the suit dismissed, claiming that his contractual obligation was void because he was incompetent and had executed the original construction contract without their (guardians') representation. In reversing a trial court's granting of the guardians' motion, the court of appeals noted that, among other things, there was a triable question concerning whether Mr. Buchanan was incompetent. Moreover, it noted that because of the children's inactivity as guardians, their role had been constructively abandoned and thus the defendant did not necessarily require their representation to sign corporate documents.

UNDERLYING BASIS OF THE LAW AND LEGAL APPLICATION. The interests of commerce underlie the basic values associated with requirement of competency and contracts. When a contract is affected by the incapacity or mental unsoundness of one of the parties, two contrary public policies come into play. From a business perspective, there is a fundamental view that the security of the transaction should be upheld in order to promote the development of commerce and to ensure the fulfillment of the reasonable expectations of the parties. However, a countervailing public policy, grounded in notions of morality and fairness, states that persons unable to appreciate the consequences of their actions should not be held accountable for them.

At one time, the law regarding contracts entered into by persons lacking capacity was that such contracts were void[21]; however, the overwhelming weight of modern authority is that they are merely *voidable* at the incompetent person's option.[22] An exception to this rule is when a party is so mentally disabled that he or she has been adjudicated mentally incompetent and a guardian of the property has been appointed prior to entering into the transaction; in many states this contract will be considered void.[23]

Generally, insanity that rises to the level of incompetency to contract is said to exist where a "party does not understand the nature and consequences of his acts at the time of the transaction."[24] This rather broad and flexible test often leads to the implicit conclusion that if the contract is fair and beneficial to the alleged incompetent there is a great tendency to conclude that he was "sane"; otherwise, the tendency is to find him incompetent.[25] The more contemporary view uses both a cognitive test ("ability to understand") and the contention that the contract is voidable if the party "by reason of mental illness or defect . . . is unable to act in a reasonable manner in relation to the transaction and the other party has reason to know of this condition."[26] This approach allows for the incompetent person to disaffirm an agreement or contract that he or she might be capable of understanding if the incompetent cannot control his or her behavior in a rational manner.[27]

Cases involving challenges to a party's competency typically involve one of two scenarios. In one, there is evidence of a mental condition that impairs a person's *cognitive ability* — the ability to understand the nature and consequences of the proposed transaction. In the other, the evidence indicates that there are mental conditions that impair a party's *motivation* or ability to act rationally. Where a party to a contract lacks cognitive capacity, the contract is voidable without regard to whether the other person knew or had reason to know of the mental impairment. However, when one party has an impaired motivational control, the contract is usually held to be voidable only if the other party knew or had reason to know of the mental condition (e.g., alcohol or narcotics intoxication[28]).

Finally, two situations exist in which the incompetency of a party may not necessarily void the provisions of an agreement: restitution and necessities. Sometimes a contract may be executed and its conditions performed before the issue of competency is ever raised. A person seeking to avoid a contract has the burden of proof of the requisite facts.

Generally, if one of the parties is incompetent and the contract is still to be executed[29] or if the contract is based on grossly inadequate provisions,[30] rescission will be granted. If, however, the other party had no reason to know of the mental infirmity and the contract is not otherwise unfair, the right to void the agreement may be lost to the extent that the contract has already been executed.[31] At the very least in this latter situation, the incompetent would have the responsibility of placing the other party in the *status quo ante* (place he was before the contract).

In the second situation, mental incompetents, like minors, cannot void a contract in which "necessities of life" have been provided.[32] Whether a good or service is considered a necessity is a matter for the jury, but certainly food, shelter, and clothing would qualify. Other provisions such as medical assistance, legal services, transportation, and others are evaluated based on a party's situation at the time of the contract.

Wills/testamentary capacity. Another form of competency that contains significant legal implications is whether a person was competent at the time of executing a will. This form of competency, like that concerning contracts, does not refer to general competency, but rather to the capacity to meet the legal threshold required to perform a particular act. In this situation, the act is the writing of a will. If the person writing the will, or the *testator,* is judged to be without the requisite competency *(testamentary capacity)* at the time of writing the will, the will is not admitted to probate and judged legally valid. As a result, its provisions have no legal effect. If this occurs, the distribution of the testator's estate will be guided by any valid will that does exist, or if no other will is available, the estate will be distributed under the rules of *intestate secession* (favoring the immediate family and/or relatives). If no immediate family is available, the estate can *escheat* (revert) to the state.

The conveyance of property through some form of testamentary process has a long and colorful history. Prior to the sixteenth century, no law recognized the written conveyance of real property to third parties. What typically took place was that property rights were passed from one person to another or one family member (e.g., father) to another (e.g., eldest son) in the form of an oral agreement or understanding. Public declaration or formal representation in writing of this change of ownership was uncommon and generally had no legal effect even if instituted. The basic integrity and good faith of the two parties involved provided the basis for any exchange of property. If a person died without settling his estate, personal or real, his personal possessions were considered to be "up for grabs" and his real property typically was seized by the local authorities in the name of the King or the Crown.

In 1540, the first English Statute of Wills was passed.[33] This statute, and its later amendments, authorized wills of land, provided that they were in writing, but required no other formality.

LEGAL REQUIREMENTS. Today, the law recognizes that a person may dispose of his or her property in any way he or she sees fit, as long as it does not violate state law. However, in order for a will to be considered valid, it must, like a contract, be executed knowingly and voluntarily. Challenges to the validity of a will frequently revolve around whether the testator had sufficient testamentary capacity (knowingly made) when making the will or was free from any undue influences (voluntarily made).

Any person wishing to execute a legally binding will has to possess, among other things, testamentary capacity. Analogous to the fundamental criminal law concept of mental competency, testamentary capacity involves having a certain level of understanding of what he or she is doing in terms of disposing of his or her property. There are no hard-and-fast rules or requisite elements that define what constitutes testamentary capacity. However, the majority of jurisdictions in the United States require some variations of the elements articulated in the classic case, *Banks v. Goodfellow*.[34] In *Banks*, the court fashioned the following five-part test:

To make a valid will one must be of sound mind though he need not possess superior or even average mentality. One is of sound mind for testamentary purposes only when he can understand and carry in his mind in a general way:

(1) The nature and extent of his property;
(2) The persons who are the natural objects of his bounty, and
(3) The disposition which he is making of his property.

He must also be capable of:

(4) Appreciating these elements in relation to each other, and
(5) Forming an orderly desire as to the disposition of his property

If a will is challenged on the basis that the testator lacked the requisite capacity, a probate judge generally inquires: Was the testator aware that he or she was making a will? Was he or she able to assess and appraise the amount and value of the property? Was he or she aware of legal heirs? Finally, was there some organized or rational scheme to the distribution of the property?

In assessing each of these or similar criteria, a probate judge entertains any evidence by the challengers that indicates a contrary finding of fitness. A testator, as with all questions involving adults and issue of competency, is presumed to possess the requisite capacity. Therefore, the burden is on the challenger to prove that at the time of the making of the will the testator lacked the requisite capacity.

In determining whether testamentary capacity exists under the standards just articulated, the law does not require *perfect capacity* or knowledge. As with many tests of competency, only a minimum level of functioning is required. For example, in *In re Estate of Fish*,[35] a New York appellate court held that a testator "did not need to know the precise size of estate" in order to be considered competent. Also, a testator is not automatically considered to lack testamentary capacity simply because of the existence of mental illness, alcoholism, or drug addiction.[36] Although these conditions may obviously cloud or impair a person's competency, if the will is written during a "lucid interval," it will be deemed valid.[37] Similarly, mere personality quirks, abnormalities in perception, and idiosyncracies in and of themselves are not sufficient to support a claim of testamentary incapacity.

UNDUE INFLUENCE. A similar ground for challenging the provisions of a will occurs when there is sufficient proof that the will was not executed voluntarily or was not the result of the testator's free will. This issue is commonly framed in terms of the presence of undue influence being applied by one party, usually a nonbeneficiary, to the testator. Persons who are in a vulnerable mental state because of old age or physical or mental infirmity are particularly susceptible to the overreaching influence of others.

No specific rules exist concerning what constitutes undue influence. This is generally a matter for the courts to decide, using common law precedent to guide it. *Neil v. Brackett*[38] neatly summarizes a common interpretation of what undue influence is and how it invalidates a will:

Fraud and undue influence in this connection mean whatever destroys free agency and constrains the person whose act is under review to do what is contrary to his own untrammeled desire. It may be caused by physical force, by duress, by threats, or by the establishment and maintenance of conditions intolerable to the particular individual. It may result from more subtle conduct designed to create an irresistible ascendancy by imperceptible means. It may be exerted either by deceptive devices or by material compulsion without actual fraud. Any species of coercion, whether physical, mental or moral, which subverts their sound judgment and genuine desire of the individual, is enough to constitute undue influence. . . . Fraud or undue influence, such as is found to have been exercised, invalidates a will, and may be manifested in diverse ways. It is not practicable or desirable to attempt to lay down any hard and fast rule. Whatever may be the particular form, however, in all cases of this character three factors are implied:

(1) A person who can be influenced;
(2) The fact of the deception or improper influence existed;
(3) Submission to the overmastering effect of the unlawful conduct.

Undue influence incorporates the concept of coveted result, which includes obtaining for oneself or another a benefit that one could normally not receive and that disadvantages a deserving party (e.g., a rightful beneficiary). For example, bequests to attorneys, physicians,[39] and clergy who attend to the testator during the remaining phase of terminal illness or failing health are generally considered suspect. Any person who assumes a fiduciary role in the execution of the testator's will and who is also named a beneficiary assumes a legally recognized duty to demonstrate that he or she has not applied undue influence on the testator.[40]

Competency to testify

GENERAL LEGAL TEST. *Black's Law Dictionary* defines competency as "[I]n the law of evidence, the presence of those characteristics, or the absence of those disabilities, which render a witness legally fit and qualified to give testimony in a court of justice."[41] The determination of whether a witness is competent to provide testimony[42] rests solely within the sound discretion of the trial court.[43] The standard in which such a determination is made typically is composed of four separate inquiries:

(1) Whether, at the time of the event in question, the witness had the capacity "to observe intelligently";
(2) Whether at the time of the trial the witness possesses the capacity to recollect that event;
(3) Whether the witness has the "capacity mentally to understand the nature of the questions put and to form and communicate intelligent answers"; and
(4) Whether the witness has "a sense of moral responsibility, of the duty to make the narration correspond to the recollection and knowledge (i.e., to speak the truth as he sees it)."[44]

District of Columbia law provides a good illustration of how the issue of competency of witnesses to testify is treated by the courts. For instance, one general section of the local statutes regarding court testimony states that

No person is incompetent to testify, in either civil or criminal proceedings, by reason of his having been convicted of a criminal matter.[45]

The Criminal Rules of the Superior Court of the District of Columbia, further provides that

The admissibility of evidence and the *competency* and privileges of witnesses shall be governed, except when an act of Congress or these rules otherwise provide, by the principles of the common law as they may be interpreted by the courts in the light of reason and experience.[46]

In other words, no statutorily defined definitions or standards typically exist for evaluating the competency of a witness to provide testimony. Instead, the courts (judges) apply traditional common law principles in making this determination.[47] It is important to note that there is no single, fixed standard of competency to be applied "across the board" to all witnesses. For example, in *United States v. Crosby*,[48] the court acknowledged that

The competency of a defendant to stand trial is, of course, crucial to fairness, and is governed by a somewhat stricter standard *than is* the competency of a witness to testify. Likewise, the competency standard for witnesses *may vary* depending upon the importance of the witness in the case. Where, as here, the witness is the *key* witness for the prosecution, justice demands a strict standard of competency [emphasis added].[49]

A good example of the need for flexibility in assessing the competency of witness to testify is in the case of a child witness[50] and persons suspected of being mentally disabled.

Consent to medical treatment

INFORMED CONSENT. Under the doctrine of informed consent, health care providers have a legal duty to abide by the treatment decisions made by their patients unless a compelling state interest exists. The term *informed consent* is a legal principle in medical jurisprudence which generally holds that a physician must disclose to a patient sufficient information that will enable the patient to make an informed decision about a proposed treatment or procedure.[51]

If a patient's consent is to be considered informed, it must adequately address three essential elements: information, competency, and voluntariness. In general, the patient must be given adequate information in which to make a truly knowing decision, and that decision (consent) must be made voluntarily by a person who is legally competent. Each of these elements must be adequately met or any consent given will not be considered informed and legally valid.

Only a *competent* person is legally recognized as being able to give informed consent. For health care providers working with patients who may be of questionable competence because of mental illness, narcotic abuse, or alcoholism, this can be a particularly important issue. The law presumes that a person *is* competent unless judicially determined to be incompetent or unless the person has been incapacitated by a medical condition or emergency. The mere fact that a person is being treated for a mental illness[52] or institutionalized[53] does not automatically render him or her incompetent. Accordingly, physicians have a duty to make a reasonably complete and fair disclosure of the risks of treatment and to obtain, in most situations, a psychiatric patient's informed consent prior to the initiation of treatment.[54]

From a legal perspective, the term *competency* is narrowly defined in terms of *cognitive capacity*. No established set of criteria exists for determining a patient's competence. In fact, some authors have noted that "the search for a single test of competency is a search for a holy grail."[55] Physicians and psychiatrists should, however, ensure that at a minimum the patient is capable of the following:

1. Understanding the particular treatment being offered[56]
2. Making a discernible decision, one way or another, regarding the treatment that has been offered[57]
3. Communicating, verbally or nonverbally, that decision.[58]

Mental patients who have been determined to be lacking the requisite competency to make a treatment decision, except typically in cases of emergency,[59] will have an authorized representative or guardian appointed to make medical decisions on their behalf.[60]

Competency and consent to die. The majority of case laws addressing the issue of a patient's "right to die" deal with individuals who are incompetent at the time that removal of life-support systems is sought.[61] A small, but growing body of cases is emerging that involves competent patients—usually suffering from excruciating pain and terminal diseases—who seek the termination of further medical treatment.

The single most significant influence in the development of this body of law is the doctrine of informed consent, which developed out of medical malpractice litigation. Beginning with the fundamental tenet that "no right is held more sacred . . . than the right of every individual to the possession and control of his own person,"[62] the courts have fashioned the present-day "informed consent" doctrine.

Notwithstanding these principles, the right to decline life-sustaining medical intervention—even for a competent person—is not absolute. As noted in *In re Conroy,* four countervailing state interests may limit the exercise of that right: preservation of life, prevention of suicide, safeguarding the integrity of the medical profession, and the protection of innocent third parties.[63] In each of these situations and depending on the surrounding circumstances, the trend in cases thus far has been to support a competent patient's right to have artificial life-support systems discontinued.[64]

In cases involving incompetent persons, courts are often faced with the situation of trying to *figure out* what the patient most likely would have wanted, since many incompetent patients have never articulated their desires. The New Jersey Supreme Court decision in *In re Conroy* fashioned a "limited-objective" and "pure-objective" best-interest test to determine the incompetent person's best interests, which is likely to be followed or adapted by other courts.[65]

Under the "limited-objective" test, life-sustaining treatment may be withheld or withdrawn when there is "some trustworthy evidence" that the patient would have refused the treatment, and the decision-maker is satisfied that the burdens of the patient's continued life with the treatment outweigh the benefits of that life for the patient. In the absence of such trustworthy evidence, a "pure-objective" test will be employed. If the "net burdens of the patient's life with treatment should clearly and markedly outweigh the benefits that the patient derives from life," *and* if "the recurring unavoidable and severe pain of the patient's life with the treatment should be such that the effect of administering life-sustaining treatment would be inhumane," then, life-sustaining treatment may still be withheld or withdrawn from such an incompetent person.[66]

Guardianship

Definition. Guardianship can be defined as the delegation by the state of the authority over an individual's person or estate to another party. Historically, the state or sovereign possessed the power and authority to safeguard the estate of incompetent persons.[67] This traditional role still reflects the purpose of guardianship today. In some states, there are separate provisions for the appointment of a guardian of one's *person* (e.g., for health care decision-making) and another guardian of one's *estate* (e.g., with authority for making contracts to sell one's property).[68] This latter guardian is frequently referred to as a *conservator,* although this designation is not uniformly used throughout the United States. A further distinction, also found in some jurisdictions, is *general* (plenary) and *specific* guardianship.[69] As the name implies, the latter guardian is restricted to exercising decisions about particular subject areas. For instance, the specific guardian may be authorized to make decisions about major or emergency medical procedures, and the disabled person retains the freedom to make decisions about all other medical matters. General guardians, in contrast, have total control over the disabled individual's person, estate, or both.[70]

Determination of need for guardian. A guardian is needed only when there is some question as to whether the individual is *de facto* (or actually) incompetent. An interesting aspect of the guardianship proceeding is its relatively flexible and relaxed atmosphere. In most states any interested person can petition to have someone declared incompetent and subject to guardianship.[71]

Often no specific allegation is required in the petition, and notice to the respondent is limited to the fact that a hearing will be held.[72] At the hearing itself, the respondent frequently has no right to counsel[73] or trial by jury.[74] In some jurisdictions the respondent is rarely present.[75] If counsel is appointed, he or she is often designated as a *guardian ad litem,* who is free to act in what he or she believes is in the respondent's best interest.[76] Moreover, if the respondent is determined to be in need of a guardian, the incompetent person usually bears the burden of raising the issue at a later time if he or she believes that a guardian is no longer needed.[77] At a later hearing, such a person is placed in the awkward position of persuading the court that the situation has changed and that he or she is now competent. This is required even though the respondent has had no opportunity to manage his or her own affairs, which would be compelling evidence that competency has been restored and a guardian is no longer needed!

The informality and procedural permissiveness that define a guardianship proceeding are equally matched by the vagueness of the standards by which the need for a guardian is determined. For a *general guardianship,* most jurisdictions simply require evidence of deficient mental status (e.g., mental illness, senility) and incapacity to "care for oneself or one's estate."[78] Standards for *specific guardianship* are not much better in terms of providing concrete requirements or descriptions. Despite this lack of rigor in definition, some state courts require considerable evidence of incompetency and incapacity before they will order guardianship.[79] Other courts are less stringent in the extent of their analysis of the facts.[80]

Selection of guardian. Anyone can petition the court to become a guardian over the person or estate of another. A diversity of parties may be appointed, ranging from family members and relatives to government agencies and law enforcement authorities.[81] As a rule, the selection of one guardian over another is more likely than not a matter of policy or law.

Role of the guardian. Guardians are generally charged with the responsibility of safeguarding an incompetent person's interests pursuant to one of two decision-making models. In one model an *objective test* is employed. This test guides the guardian by framing his or her responsibilities in terms of the question: What action will most effectively serve and protect the incompetent individual's best interests? The second model, relying on a *subjective model,* utilizes a form of "substituted judgment." With this model the guardian is asked to assume the role of the ward and to "act as he or she thinks the ward would have acted, if the ward had been competent."[82] In situations in which there is no relevant history or reliable information to hypothesize

how a ward might have acted if competent, a guardian is usually left with no alternative but to employ a form of best-interest test.[83] What is likely to occur, under these circumstances, is that the guardian will objectively evaluate as much relevant information as is available and then determine a course of action that best serves the ward's interests.

IMMUNITY

Whenever the legal process thought it necessary to accomplish a purpose, it gave the actor protection, or immunity. Although some other reasons were advanced, the law developed the doctrine of governmental immunity, also called sovereign immunity, to protect the financial integrity of the government. In the same manner, the doctrine of charitable immunity developed to protect the financial integrity of the charitable and nonprofit hospital. These doctrines have been all but abandoned because the needs they served are no longer viable.

Physicians have also been objects of grants of immunity. In an effort to encourage physicians to help people in an emergency, Good Samaritan statutes have been enacted to protect the physician who may be negligent while offering volunteered medical services. This doctrine has now been extended to sometimes include other health care providers and even other lay persons. To have an open and free discussion about the questioned competence of a physician, immunity for peer review members has been established. Federal physicians and other health care providers are given immunity from their possible negligence; the government stands in their places if liability is ever in question.

Abuse of children, spouses, and the elderly has become a serious problem. Its prevention and control may be accomplished by prompt reporting of the situation. Thus the various state legislatures have given immunity from liability for defamation to the reporter, who need only suspect the abuse. Mandatory reporting, with civil and criminal penalties, exists in most jurisdictions.

Physician immunity

Immunity was traditionally defined as freedom from suit or liability. Immunity was justified as an important social value or policy. For instance, in recent years society has encouraged citizens to help victims at the scene of an accident. As a result, Good Samaritan statutes, which intended to foster such aid, were eventually passed in all states. Such statutes immunize the health care provider from liability for negligence.

How does an immunity statute help the individual defendant, such as the physician? An individual notified of a complaint filed against him or her may oppose the suit by asserting immunity. For example, in the federal system, the defendant may move to dismiss the complaint. More specifically, the defendant may state that the complaint "fails to state a claim upon which relief can be granted" under the *Federal Rules of Civil Procedure.*[84] The basis for this motion is that the defendant is immune from being sued because of an immunity statute. The immunity statute does not protect the defendant from the initiation of suit. It does, however, furnish the defendant with an affirmative defense that can be raised in response to the plaintiff's complaint.

In addition to immunity from suit for certain persons, the defense of immunity may also apply to freedom from discovery during litigation. Some states have statutes that protect certain hospital and peer review committee records from discovery.

Before discussing several specific areas of immunity, it is important to recognize that immunity statutes vary from state to state. Each physician should consult the applicable state statute to determine the immunity provisions governing medical practice.

Areas in which physicians and other health care providers, such as nurses or emergency medical technicians, are likely to encounter immunity provisions include Good Samaritan laws, child abuse statutes, medical staff committee immunity, and the immunity of government-employed physicians.

Charitable immunity

The doctrine of charitable immunity had its origin in English common law.[85] It relieved charitable institutions, including charitable hospitals, from liability. American courts adopted this doctrine of charitable immunity during the nineteenth century. The doctrine was first declared in this country in 1876 in the landmark decision *McDonald v. Massachusetts General Hospital.*[86] In that case, a charity patient suffered a fractured leg, which was treated in a negligent fashion. The court stated that the hospital could not be held liable and was immune from suit. The rationale for such a holding was similar to that of the earlier English cases. Public and private donations that supported charitable hospitals constituted a trust fund and could not be diverted. This "charitable trust" theory of immunity was widely relied on in suits against charitable hospitals. Courts did not want to deplete a hospital's trust funds and defeat the intent of the benefactor. If suits were allowed, prospective donors would be less likely to make gifts to hospitals. Another reason for upholding such immunity was that individuals receiving benefits directly from the charitable institutions assumed the risk of receiving treatment. There was tremendous public interest in maintaining charitable hospitals and fostering their charitable immunity.

The next major decision concerning charitable immunity, *Schloendorff v. Society of New York Hospital,* was heard in 1914.[87] In that case, the plaintiff was admitted with a fibroid tumor, which was removed at surgery. Subsequent to the operation, the plaintiff developed gangrene in her left arm, which resulted in significant pain and required the subsequent amputation of several fingers. The court of appeals affirmed the trial court's decision in favor of the hospital. The court used a theory of implied waiver by the patient. One who had accepted the services of a charitable organization could not complain if these services happened to be negligently administered.

Another major trend established by *Schloendorff* was the refusal of the courts to apply the doctrine of *respondeat superior* to hospitals. The court reasoned that physicians were not servants or employees of the hospitals, but rather independent contractors because of their unique skill. They practiced their profession to the best of their abilities and were in no way under the control of the hospitals. Because they were described as independent contractors, they were liable for their own torts, and the hospital was thus insulated from the physicians' tortious conduct. The court also expanded the role of charitable immunity to cover paying patients in a private, or profit-making, hospital.

The *Schloendorff* decision underwent many amendments and qualifications in subsequent years and demonstrated a great deal of incongruity. In *Bing v. Thunig,*[88] a 1957 New York case, the plaintiff received a burn during surgery. Tincture of Zephiran, an alcoholic antiseptic, was used to prepare the patient's back for spinal anesthesia. The nurses had been instructed to remove the inflammable antiseptic, but some drops remained on the sheets underneath the patient. The nurses failed to change the sheets. The physician then used a heated electric cautery, which ignited the soiled linen. He extinguished the fire with water and proceeded with the operation, but a later examination of the patient revealed severe burns on her body. The defendant hospital distinguished between medical and administrative acts and argued that the nurse's action was a "medical" act; therefore, the hospital was not liable.

The court pointed out that hospitals' liability should not be based on such distinctions. Rather, the court stated that there was no reason to exclude hospitals from the doctrine of *respondeat superior*. It was noted that hospitals did more than furnish facilities for treatment; they employed physicians and nurses, and they also charged patients. The test to be used in applying the doctrine of *respondeat superior* was whether the individual was an employee and was acting within the scope of his or her employment. The court, in deciding to reject the doctrine of charitable immunity, held that hospitals operate in a businesslike fashion. Even charitable organizations, the court reasoned, must be just before they are generous. They should operate so that they do not injure anyone through carelessness. The *Bing* court expressed rather definite disapproval of the doctrine of charitable immunity.

Not until the past 20 years has the doctrine of charitable immunity clearly declined; a majority of courts now reject it. This is significant, because our legal system is generally based on the idea that once a particular issue has been decided in the courts of a given state, the same result should occur in subsequent cases on the same issue in that jurisdiction. This is known as the doctrine of *stare decisis*. Old precedents, if obsolete, may be overturned if new circumstances arise or the doctrine becomes unfair. If justice and reason require that a change be made, judges may choose not to follow a precedent.

Recent courts have moved away from protecting institutions and toward allowing recovery for wrongful conduct. Although economics and social benefits were the rationales advanced in favor of protecting charitable hospitals in the past, there are a number of reasons for rejecting charitable immunity.

First, adequate redress for various torts, including compensation for injuries negligently inflicted by medical personnel, has become a more important public policy. Second, most individual health care providers and hospitals have obtained liability insurance. The insurance company, and not the hospital, provides the compensation. Third, the immunization of the hospital and health care providers could adversely affect medical competence. Medical personnel might not exercise the same degree of care and diligence if they were guaranteed immunity. Fourth, the heavy burden of injury without compensation would be unjust to the charity hospital patient, especially because patients at other hospitals might be compensated for similar injuries. For these reasons, most courts have rejected the doctrine of charitable immunity.

In *Colby v. Carney Hospital,* the Massachusetts Supreme Court upheld the doctrine, but stated that it would abolish it when next confronted with it as a defense.[89] Some courts have applied the doctrine of *respondeat superior* in finding hospitals liable. For instance, in *Bilonoha v. Zubritzsky,* a 1975 Pennsylvania case, a surgeon left a hemostat in the patient's abdomen.[90] The patient was having intraabdominal surgery and an umbilical hernia repair. The Superior Court of Pennsylvania found that the surgeon's assistants were paid by the hospital; the hospital had control of the operating room and instruments used by the surgeon and charged the plaintiff. Since the surgeon's assistants were paid employees of the hospital, the

court found the hospital liable for the negligence of its personnel.

A few states have maintained a remnant of charitable immunity through statute. Otherwise, however, the doctrine has been all but abolished.

Medical staff committee immunity

The responsibility for the quality of medical care lies with the medical staff. The physicians who serve on various hospital committees, such as the credentials committee, the tenure committee, and the the executive committee, review the medical care provided by the institution and thereby ensure the quality of its practitioners. The Joint Commission on Accreditation of Hospitals, in its accreditation manual for hospitals, mandates, in Standard MS. 6, "As part of the hospital's quality assurance program, the medical staff strives to assure the provision of quality patient care through the monitoring and evaluation of the quality and appropriateness of patient care."[91] To maintain appropriate accreditation, a hospital must have an adequate system of peer review through various committees.

A great deal of litigation has involved the confidentiality of these meetings and the immunity of the members. To guarantee total candor at such meetings, individual participants are immunized from liability, and the information discussed is protected from discovery in civil proceedings.

Many states have enacted statutes that effectively give immunity to members of peer review committees. The statutes differ concerning which individuals receive protection. In some states, only members of the particular committee are protected. In many states, not only members of the committee are protected, but also persons reporting problems to the peer review committee. One example is the Maryland statute, which states that "A person who acts in good faith and within the scope of jurisdiction of a medical review committee is not civilly liable for any action as a member of the medical review committee or for giving information to, participating in, or contributing to the function of the medical review committee."[92] The Maryland legislature chose to protect both committee members and those individuals who report information to such committees.

The Florida statute states "There shall be no monetary liability on the part of, and no cause of action for damages shall arise against, any member of a duly appointed medical review committee or any health care provider furnishing any information . . . . to such committee, for any act or proceeding undertaken or performed within the scope of the functions of any such committee if the committee member or health care provider acts without malice or fraud."[93] Florida, like Maryland, has chosen to protect both committee members and those health care providers who furnish information to such committees.

The California statute states[94]:

There shall be no monetary liability on the part of, and no cause of action for damages shall arise against, any . . . duly appointed member of a committee of a professional staff of a licensed hospital (provided the professional staff operates pursuant to written bylaws that have been approved by the governing board of the hospital), for any act or proceeding undertaken or performed within the scope of the functions of any such committee which is formed to maintain the professional standard of the society established by its bylaws or any member of any peer review committee whose purpose is to review the quality of medical or dental services rendered by physicians and surgeons, dentists or dental hygienists, for any act or proceeding undertaken or performed in reviewing the quality of medical or dental services rendered by physicians and surgeons, dentists, or dental hygienists in reviewing the quality of medical services rendered by members of the staff if such committee or board member acts without malice, has made a reasonable effort to obtain the facts of the matter as to which he or she acts, and acts in reasonable belief that the action taken by him or her is warranted by the facts known to him or her after such reasonable effort to obtain facts.

The California code, in a separate section, also provides immunity for those individuals who report information to such a committee.[95]

Most state statutes granting immunity to members of peer review committees require the good faith of the members and the person reporting information. There must be no malice. The statements of individuals involved must be based on a reasonable belief that the allegations are true, and must properly relate to the function of the committee.

Several general issues arise in establishing immunity from liability for members of peer review committees. First, each member of a peer review committee should be familiar with the state statute granting immunity. The statutes differ somewhat concerning who is covered, which committees are covered, and good faith requirements. Adverse statements concerning a health care professional should be made only at a formal proceeding of the committee. Proceedings of committee meetings should not be revealed to nonmembers. Finally, individuals who make statements at committee meetings should act with a reasonable belief that those statements are true. The statements should be made without malice.[96]

A related issue concerns the privilege of confidentiality. State statutes, as well as judicial decisions, provide protection from discovery, the process by which evidence is shared between plaintiff and defendant before a civil trial.

For example, the Florida statute provides[97]:

The proceedings and records of committees as described in the preceding subsection shall not be subject to discovery or introduction into evidence in any civil action against a provider of professional health services arising out of the matter which are the subject of evaluation and review by such committee, and no person who was in attendance at a meeting of such committee shall be permitted or required to testify in any such civil action as to any evidence or other matter produced or presented during the proceedings of such committee or as to any findings, recommendations, evaluations, opinions or other actions of such committee or any member thereof.

Even in the absence of a statute, many judicial decisions have supported the protection of statements made in peer review committee meetings. There is a strong public interest in the improvement of patient care and treatment through self-evaluation and criticism by members of the hospital staff. In *Mayfield v. Gleichert,* the plaintiff, Dr. Mayfield, sued the defendant, Dr. Gleichert, Chief of Obstetrics and Gynecology at Methodist Hospital in Dallas.[98] She alleged that the defendant had spoken and published slanderous and libelous statements against her to the executive committee of the medical staff, in conjunction with a peer review proceeding that resulted in her discharge, removal, and expulsion from the staff of the hospital. The court held that a qualified privilege existed, requiring a showing of actual malice or falsity for the plaintiff to recover. A qualified privilege exists if a communication is made in good faith on a subject in which the speaker has an interest, right, or duty to another with a similar interest, in a manner fairly warranted by the occasion and interests of the parties. The court stated that, in this case, there was no malice on the part of the defendant. The failure to investigate the accuracy of an allegation was not, by itself, enough to constitute malice. The defendant physician believed his statement to be true. A common law privilege existed in this case, and it proved to be a successful defense for the defendant in this defamation suit.

The essential elements of qualified or conditionally privileged communications include good faith, an interest to be upheld, a proper occasion (such as a peer review meeting), and publication to only proper parties. This privilege promotes full and unrestricted communication for medical staff committees.

The most important recent case regarding physician immunity involving medical staff committee immunity is the case of *Patrick v. Burget.*[99] The filing of this suit was actually one basis for the creation of the Health Care Quality Improvement Act of 1986,[100] which provides immunity for peer review committee members acting in good faith. The immunity provisions of this act are described later.

The *Patrick* case creates a dilemma for many physicians who are asked to serve on peer review committees in their hospitals. Any physician who does serve on such a committee takes a risk of being sued in the future. The Health Care Quality Improvement Act of 1986 certainly should help to minimize some of this concern. However, if proper due process is not given to a defendant physician or if the actions are undertaken in bad faith, a successful suit against the medical staff peer review committee members is possible. It would be important for all physicians to be familiar with the Health Care Quality Improvement Act as well as its standards for peer review and due process requirements.

In *Patrick,* Dr. Timothy Patrick, a vascular surgeon in Astoria, Oregon, became an employee of the Astoria Clinic and a member of the Columbia Memorial Hospital medical staff in 1972. A year later, he ended his association with the clinic physicians and established an independent practice in competition with the surgical practice of that clinic. The physicians associated with the Astoria Clinic consistently refused to have professional dealings with him after that time. He received no referrals and patients were referred to surgeons as far away as 50 miles from Astoria. The physicians employed by the clinic often declined to give consultation to Dr. Patrick or to provide him with backup coverage. He was criticized by the clinic physicians for failing to obtain outside consultation or to have adequate backup coverage. In 1979 Dr. Patrick left a patient in the care of a recently hired associate who in turn left the patient in the hands of a general practitioner. The patient deteriorated, and later a complaint about this case was forwarded to the State Board of Medical Examiners from the executive committee of the Columbia Memorial Hospital. Information about other cases handled by Dr. Patrick also were forwarded to the Board of Medical Examiners. A letter of reprimand was drafted but retracted two years later after judicial review of these proceedings was obtained.

Two years later Dr. Richard Harris, an Astoria Clinic surgeon, asked the executive committee of the Columbia Memorial Hospital medical staff to review Dr. Patrick's hospital privileges. The committee voted to terminate his privileges because of substandard care. Before a final decision was rendered, he resigned from the hospital staff rather than risk termination.

During the hospital peer review proceedings, Dr. Patrick filed suit in U.S. District Court. He alleged that the clinic partners had participated in hospital peer review proceedings to reduce competition rather than to improve patient care. A verdict against clinic physicians

was awarded to Dr. Patrick in the amount of $650,000 on the two antitrust claims with treble antitrust damages.

This case was appealed to the United States Court of Appeals 9th Circuit on March 4, 1986, and decided on September 30, 1986. The court of appeals held that because the action of the physicians engaged in peer review fell under the doctrine of state action, the action of the physicians was exempted from federal antitrust liability. The court argued that supervision by the Board of Medical Examiners, a state agency, was equivalent to supervision by the state. Also the hospital's decision to terminate or restrict privileges also was judicially reviewable. The fact that the legislature contemplated the kind of activity complained of was sufficient to demonstrate a clear articulation of state policy. This was necessary to acquire immunity from federal antitrust laws. The court concluded that the physician's activities on the peer review committee were extensions of state action and immune from federal antitrust immunity. Whether the physicians acted in bad faith was a question for state courts. The case was also remanded for the purposes of reviewing any state law claim based on bad faith.

The Supreme Court of the United States decided this case on May 16, 1988. It held that the state action doctrine did not protect Oregon physicians from federal antitrust liability for their activities on hospital peer review committees. Sufficient state supervision by the state officials with the power to review the acts of the peer review committees was not present in this case. There was no showing that the state health division, the State Board of Medical Examiners, or the state judiciary reviewed or could review private decisions regarding hospital privileges. Therefore, the Supreme Court held that the state action doctrine did not protect the peer review activities from the application of federal antitrust laws. The Court, therefore, reversed the judgment of the court of appeals. The Court did note that the Health Care Quality Improvement Act of 1986 was not in effect at the time of this case. This act immunizes peer review committee members from liability if the committee members act in good faith and in the reasonable belief that they were furthering quality health care.

On November 14, 1986, President Reagan signed into law the Health Care Quality Improvement Act of 1986.[100] The act was introduced because of the increasing occurrence of medical malpractice suits and the national need to restrict the ability of incompetent physicians to move from state to state. Professional peer review was one means through which incompetent physicians could be precluded from practicing medicine. Antitrust cases have indicated that the threat of liability unreasonably discourages physicians from participating in effective peer review. Therefore a national peer review act has been created. Part A of the Health Care Quality Improvement Act involves the promotion of professional review activity. Section 411 of the Act involving the immunity provision is stated as follows:

(a) In general
  (1) Limitation on damages for professional review actions—If a professional review action (as defined in section 431(9)) of a professional review body meets all the standards specified in section 412(a), except as provided in subsection (b)—
    (A) the professional review body,
    (B) any person acting as a member or staff to the body,
    (C) any person under a contract or other formal agreement with the body, and
    (D) any person who participates with or assists the body with respect to the action, shall not be liable in damages under any law of the United States or of any State (or political subdivision thereof) with respect to the action. The preceding sentence shall not apply to damages under any law of the United States or any State relating to the civil rights of any person or persons, including the Civil Rights Act of 1964, 42 U.S.C. 2000e, et seq. and the Civil Rights Acts, 42 U.S.C. 1981, et seq. Nothing in this paragraph shall prevent the United States or any Attorney General of a State from bringing an action, including an action under section 4C of the Clayton Act, 15 U.S.C. 15C, where such an action is otherwise authorized.
  (2) Protection for those providing information to professional review bodies—Notwithstanding any other provision of law, no person (whether as a witness or otherwise) providing information to a professional review body regarding the competence or professional conduct of a physician shall be held, by reason of having provided such information, to be liable in damages under any law of the United States or of any State (or political subdivision thereof) unless such information is false and the person providing it knew that such information was false.
(b) Exception—If the Secretary has reason to believe that a health care entity has failed to report information in accordance with section 423(a), the Secretary shall conduct an investigation. If, after providing notice of noncompliance, an opportunity to correct the noncompliance, and an opportunity for a hearing, the Secretary determines that a health care entity has failed substantially to report information in accordance with section 423(a), the Secretary shall publish the name of the entity in the Federal Register. The protections of subsection (a)(1) shall not apply to an entity the name of which is published in the Federal Register under the previous sentence with respect to professional review

actions of the entity commenced during the 3-year period beginning 30 days after the date of publication of the name.

It can be seen that significant immunity is provided for physicians who take part in professional review activities as well as those who provide information to the review body. The immunity is contingent on two conditions, however. First, the professional review action must meet certain standards. The action must be in the reasonable belief that it was furthering quality health care and that it was undertaken after a reasonable effort to obtain the facts of the matter. Adequate notice and hearing procedures must be afforded to the physician involved. The action must be in the reasonable belief that it was warranted by the facts known after such reasonable effort to obtain facts. The requirements for adequate notice and hearing are outlined in the act as well. Secondly, to ensure immunity, the health care entity must report information to a central data bank concerning all adverse actions. This is necessary under Part B of the act whereby a central data bank of adverse professional review actions by boards of medical examiners and health care entities as well as malpractice payments made by insurance companies and other entities are reported. If a health care entity fails to report adverse professional review actions that it undertakes against a given physician, then it suffers the loss of its immunity.

This national legislation has received tremendous support from various specialty societies and hospital associations. It is intended to help hospitals, HMOs, and so on, to screen their applicants in order to prevent that very small segment of the medical profession that may practice substandard care from continuing their practices.

It is recommended that each peer review committee member review the Health Care Quality Improvement Act and be aware of the various provisions stated in the act in order to ensure that immunity is not forfeited for failure to follow a specific provision of the act.

Good Samaritan statutes

Good Samaritan statutes are another area of medicolegal interface in which significant statutory law has provided immunity for health care providers. Since 1959, every state has adopted some form of Good Samaritan legislation, which provides immunity from civil liability to physicians and others for negligent acts committed in the treatment of an injured party at the scene of an accident. The rationale is that health care providers would be much less willing to render emergency aid if threatened with a possible malpractice suit by doing so; immunity is granted in the interest of public health.

The laws of the various states differ as to the degree of

immunity provided. They may confer immunity on only physicians, may include other medical personnel, or may even extend immunity to anyone who renders aid. The Pennsylvania statute is a good example, and contains several elements found in many state statutes[101]:

Section 8331. Medical good Samaritan civil immunity: (a) General rule. Any physician or any other practitioner of the healing arts or any registered nurse, licensed by any state, who happens by chance upon the scene of an emergency by reason of serving on an emergency call panel or similar committee of a county medical society or who is called to the scene of an emergency by the police or other duly constituted officers of a government unit or who is present when an emergency occurs and who, in good faith, renders emergency care at the scene of the emergency shall not be liable for any civil damages as a result of any acts or omissions by such physician or practitioner or registered nurse in rendering the emergency care, except any acts or omissions intentionally designed to harm or any grossly negligent acts or omissions which result in harm to the person receiving emergency care.

(b) Definition. As used in this section "good faith" shall include, but is not limited to, a reasonable opinion that the immediacy of the situation is such that the rendering of care should not be postponed until the patient is hospitalized.

Section 8332. Nonmedical good Samaritan civil immunity: (a) General rule. Any person who renders emergency care, first aid or rescue at the scene of an emergency, or moves the person receiving such care, first aid and rescue to a hospital or other place of medical care, shall not be liable to such person for any civil damages as a result of any acts or omissions in rendering the emergency care, first aid or rescue, or moving the person receiving the same to a hospital or other place of medical care, except any acts or omissions intentionally designed to harm or any grossly negligent acts or omissions which result in harm to the person receiving the emergency care, first aid or rescue or being moved to a hospital or other place of medical care.

The Pennsylvania legislature chose to protect both medical and nonmedical rescuers. A majority of states, in fact, grant immunity to any rescuer, and not merely medical professionals. Some states protect only physicians, or perhaps only resident physicians. Others may protect only physicians, other medical personnel, policemen, and firemen.

The Good Samaritan statutes in some states require good faith on the part of the health care provider. In general, it is an evaluation of the state of mind of the person who renders aid. The Pennsylvania legislature, as seen previously, determines good faith based on a reasonable opinion that the immediacy of the situation warrants the rendering of care.

The extent of protection afforded may be stated in the statute. The issue is whether immunity extends beyond the scene of the emergency and includes the period during which the patient is transferred to the hospital. Some state statutes, including the Pennsylvania statute,

specifically immunize the physician or other allied health personnel during transport of the patient to the hospital. Other statutes are silent in this regard. Again, the health care professional should review the statute to determine his or her protection.

The standard of care required of the health care personnel is outlined in the Pennsylvania statute. This provision varies widely among states. Most state statutes, including Pennsylvania's, require that the rescuer not commit gross negligence, recklessness, or willful or wanton misconduct. A few states do not provide immunity, even for ordinary negligence, whereas some states allow immunity for gross misconduct.

Some states also require that there be no expectation of payment on the part of the health care provider for emergency treatment. The Pennsylvania statute is silent in this regard. This obviously creates some confusion in certain situations; for example, emergency medical technicians and paramedics may receive a salary for their duties. However, many states specifically provide immunity for ambulance personnel.

Extended applications of the Good Samaritan laws occurred in more recent cases. For instance, in Illinois case *Johnson v. Matviuw,*[102] a patient had a cardiac arrest in the hospital. A physician, not that patient's doctor, was in another room and was called to assist in beginning cardiopulmonary resuscitation. The patient died. The physician was sued and he alleged that he was immune under the Good Samaritan statute. The appellate court ruled that the Good Samaritan statute does apply to physicians who are acting in good faith with no prior notice of the illness and who are providing emergency medical treatment without charge to a patient. The fact that this occurred in the hospital did not alter application of the Good Samaritan statute in this case. The physician was therefore immune from liability.

In addition, some states such as California have passed laws that grant immunity to individuals from civil liability when they provide cardiopulmonary resuscitation (CPR).[103] Again good faith is required. A gross negligence standard is used if the individual is not a member of a rescue team. Those who train individuals to perform CPR are also covered in the statute.

In a recent case, *Lowry v. Henry Mayo Newhall Memorial Hospital,*[104] the leader of the hospital code blue team was sued after unsuccessfully treating a patient in cardiac arrest. The court relied on specific legislation other than the Good Samaritan statute, which provided immunity to all members of the hospital rescue team. The physician was therefore granted immunity from liability.

Governmental (sovereign) immunity

Under the English common law, the sovereign was immune from suit. This immunity was continued under

American common law; governmental immunity prevented lawsuits against the federal and state governments. In 1946, Congress abandoned governmental immunity by enacting the Federal Tort Claims Act.

The states have generally followed the federal government in abrogating their immunity. Some have retained partial immunity by limiting the amount of recoverable damages; others have not included their political subdivisions. Local jurisdictions may thus have governmental immunity. Employees performing their duties are also immune. There is no governmental immunity for breach of contract.

Federal physicians' immunity

Another significant immunity is that granted to federal physicians. In 1946, the U.S. government waived sovereign immunity with regard to the negligence of its employees acting within the scope of their duties. Prior to 1946, the government could not be sued. The Federal Tort Claims Act enabled plaintiffs to sue the government in United States District Court.[105] If a patient was injured in a military or other federal hospital, the patient could sue the United States government. The Federal Tort Claims Act provides that a suit against the United States shall be exclusive of any other civil action or proceeding against the federal employee. Recent case law that resulted in erosion of federal employee immunity gave rise to the recent passage of the Federal Employees Liability Reform and Tort Compensation Act of 1988.[106] This act upholds the exclusiveness of the remedy against the United States. It thus reestablishes the immunity of federal officials from common law tort liability for actions taken within the scope of their employment.

In 1974, the Gonzales Act was passed (it was amended in 1976).[107] The Gonzales Act states, in part[108]:

(a) The remedy against the *United States* [emphasis added] provided by sections 1346 (b) and 2672 of Title 28 for damages for personal injury, including death, caused by the negligent or wrongful act or omission of a physician, dentist, nurse, pharmacist, or paramedical or other supporting personnel (including medical and dental technicians, nursing assistants and therapists) of the armed forces . . . while acting within the scope of his duties or employment therein shall hereafter be exclusive of any other *civil action* or *proceeding* [emphasis added] by reason that the same subject matter against such physician, dentist, nurse, pharmacist or paramedical or other supporting personnel (or the estates of such person) whose act or omission gave rise to such action or proceeding.

By this act, if a military doctor, nurse, or other support personnel is negligent, the U.S. government may be sued under section 1346, but the doctor himself is immune from suit.

This particular statute provides protection for members of the armed forces. Similar statutes provide protection for other federal physicians, such as Department of State personnel,[109] NASA personnel,[110] and Public Health Service personnel.[111]

A number of judicial decisions have addressed immunity statutes in determining physicians' liability. In *Baker v. Barber and Talmage,* a federal civilian employee was injured on the job and taken to Breland Army Hospital, Fort Knox, Kentucky, where he received treatment by the two defendant army doctors.[112] The government moved to dismiss his later malpractice action on grounds that it was barred by the Gonzales Act, which provided that the Federal Tort Claims Act is the exclusive remedy for a claimant in cases of malpractice suits against military medical personnel. The district court concluded that Congress intended to provide immunity to individual military doctors in such situations and dismissed the suit. On appeal, the court affirmed the dismissal, holding that Congress, by enacting the Gonzales Act, felt a special need to protect military doctors against the threat of malpractice suits because armed services medical personnel, unlike their civilian counterparts, must respond to military orders in providing medical services. In addition, the lower pay of defense medical personnel, relative to private medical practice, makes it especially difficult for them to afford malpractice insurance.

In another case, *Apple v. Jewish Hospital and Medical Center,*[113] the defendant physician, an employee of the National Health Service Corps, had performed an allegedly negligent cesarean section. The government moved to dismiss the action against the doctor and substitute the United States as defendant instead. The doctor's membership in the Corps made him immune from suit pursuant to statutory authority. The government argued that the exclusive remedy for damage allegedly resulting from performance of medical functions by an officer or employee of the Public Health Service, acting within the scope of his or her employment, was that provided by the Federal Tort Claims Act.[114] The court granted the motion to dismiss. The United States was found to be the sole defendant; the physician was immune from suit.

Recently, the immunity of federal physicians has been questioned in cases in which a military physician is performing duties at a civilian institution. In *Anderson v. O'Donoghue,* the plaintiff's popliteal artery was severed during a surgical procedure on the left knee.[115] Gangrene eventually developed and the left leg was amputated above the knee. One of the surgeons was an employee of the U.S. Navy, working on a civilian assignment. The court in this case held that the military physician was not immune from suit. The fact that the defendant was at a civilian institution created a situation in which the United States was not a party to the action.

This case has important implications for physicians who are in the armed services and assume that the immunity statute will protect them from personal liability. This problem is being addressed through training agreements between the military and the civilian institution to ensure malpractice coverage for the individual trainee by the facility. Additionally, these residents are considered to be employees of the United States acting within the scope of their federal duties. The United States would therefore be substituted as the defendant.

In addition to federal statutory law, immunity exists for state employees as well. For example, in *Hudson v. Rausa,* the Mississippi Supreme Court ruled that a physician and nurse supervisor employed by the State Board of Health were immune from a wrongful death action.[116] The physician had prescribed isoniazid for a patient with tuberculosis. The patient died several months later secondary to hepatic failure. The court stated that the discretion given to the physician and nurse to prevent the spread of tuberculosis applies only to their decisions regarding tuberculosis and to treatment administered according to the policies of the State Board of Health. They were therefore immune from suit. State public officials may have a qualified immunity from a civil action when acting in the performance of official functions. They lose that immunity only when they exceed their authority or commit willful or malicious acts.

Child abuse reporting

Every year, more than a million children in the United States are abused by their parents or other adults; 2000 to 5000 die as a result of such abuse. The Council on Scientific Affairs, Division of Drugs and Technology, of the American Medical Association has formulated and published diagnostic and treatment guidelines.[117]

Every state legislature has passed a statute concerning the reporting of child abuse. In many instances, immunity for civil and criminal action has been provided for physicians and other health care providers who report in good faith suspected instances of child abuse.

Every health care practitioner should be aware of the specific requirements of the appropriate state statute. Emergency room personnel are especially likely to confront cases of child abuse and should be familiar with the appropriate state statute.

For example, the California Penal Code provides, in part[118]:

... any child care custodian, medical practitioner, nonmedical practitioner, or employee of a child protective agency who has knowledge of or observes a child in his or her professional capacity or within the scope of his or her employment whom he or she knows or reasonably suspects has been the victim of child abuse shall report the known or suspected instance of child abuse to a child protective agency immediately or as soon as practically possible by telephone and shall prepare and send a written report thereof within 36 hours of receiving the information concerning the incident.

This statute demonstrates several important characteristics of the reporting statutes. First, the categories of personnel may include nonmedical individuals, as well as physicians and nurses. Second, a reasonable suspicion of child abuse is necessary. Third, the timing and method of reporting may be outlined. In addition to mandatory reporting of child abuse, such statutes also provide for some form of immunity for physicians and other health care personnel if they are sued for reporting a case of suspected child abuse.

The California Penal Code further states[119]:

No child care custodian, medical practitioner, nonmedical practitioner, or employee of a child protective agency who reports a known or suspected instance of child abuse shall be civilly or criminally liable for any report required or authorized by this article. Any other person reporting a known or suspected instance of child abuse shall not incur civil or criminal liability as a result of any report authorized by this article unless it can be proven that a false report was made and that the person knew that it was false.

The Michigan legislature has provided the following immunity[120]:

The identity of a reporting person shall be confidential subject to disclosure only with the consent of that person or by judicial process. A person acting in good faith who makes a report or assists in any other requirement of this act shall be immune from civil or criminal liability which might otherwise be incurred thereby. A person making a report or assisting in any other requirement of this act shall be presumed to have acted in good faith. This immunity from civil or criminal liability extends only to acts pursuant to this act and does not extend to a negligent act which causes personal injury or death or to the malpractice of a physician which results in personal injury or death.

The use of the immunity statute was reviewed in *Ackerman v. TriCounty Orthopedic Group, P.O.,* a Michigan case.[121] A five-year-old boy had a history of five bone fractures during a four-month period in 1979. A diagnosis of osteogenesis imperfecta was suspected but ruled out. A report of suspected child abuse was soon after filed. The child was removed from the custody of the parents and placed with an uncle. While in his foster placement, the boy sustained another fracture by dropping a toy on his toe. Another physician then made the diagnosis of osteogenesis imperfecta. The charges of child abuse were dismissed and after four months of foster care the child was returned to the parents. The parents sued the doctors for negligence in failing to diagnose osteogenesis imperfecta; they alleged that the misdiagnosis had resulted in an erroneous report of child abuse, causing them shame and humiliation.

The appellate court affirmed judgment for the physicians and interpreted the Michigan statute as providing immunity for the erroneous reporting of child abuse in good faith. The immunity did not, however, extend to negligence in the treatment of the patient if the injury resulted directly from the negligent act.

It is evident that physicians and other health care personnel have some degree of protection from liability for reporting child abuse in good faith. However, angry or guilt-ridden parents may sue the health care provider for negligence in the care of the child, if that negligence causes an injury.

Although every state has a reporting statute for child abuse and a growing number of states have elder abuse reporting statutes, very few states have reporting and immunity provisions for physicians regarding spousal abuse. Nearly all states have recognized the alarming incidence of spousal abuse and have enacted some form of domestic violence or protection from abuse statute. In general, they do not contain reporting and immunity provisions for physicians, in contrast to child abuse and elder abuse statutes. Rather, spousal abuse statutes define domestic violence, establish domestic violence centers, and outline the procedures that an abused person must take to seek a legal remedy.

One state that explicitly grants immunity to physicians and others who make a report concerning spousal abuse is Mississippi. The statute provides the following[122]:

Reports of abuse: Confidentiality of reports. A written report of any known or suspected abuse may be made to the state department of public welfare as soon as possible by any person having knowledge of such abuse. Reports of abuse made under the provisions of this chapter and the identity of those persons making the reports shall be confidential.

Participants in reports or proceedings presumed acting in good faith; Immunity from liability. Any licensed doctor of medicine, licensed doctor of dentistry, intern, resident or registered nurse, psychologist, social worker, preacher, teacher, attorney, law enforcement officer, or any other person or institution participating in the making of a report pursuant to this chapter or participating in judicial proceedings resulting therefrom shall be presumed to be acting in good faith, and if found to have acted in good faith shall be immune from any liability, civil or criminal, that might otherwise be incurred or imposed. The reporting of an abused person shall not constitute a breach of confidentiality.

This immunity statute is similar to the child abuse statutes in that any person can report abuse and the reporting must be done in good faith. The statute differs from standard child abuse statutes, however, in that reporting is not mandatory but may be done at the discretion of the reporting individual.

With greater awareness and concern about spousal abuse, we can expect more state legislatures to enact provisions concerning the reporting of spousal abuse and the accompanying immunity of the health care provider.

Miscellaneous immunity statutes

Besides child abuse, other reportable conditions include injuries due to firearms. The Pennsylvania legislature has passed a statute requiring a physician who treats a person injured by a deadly weapon to report the injury and the name of the injured person to the police. The statute also provides that no physician or other person will be subject to civil or criminal liability because such a report was filed.[123] Other examples of statutory immunity for physicians include mass immunization projects[124] and emergency medical services training programs.[125]

Concerning emergency medical services, some states such as California provide immunity for those who train individuals to provide emergency medical services, that is, those who actually provide emergency care including those at the site of the emergency and the physicians who direct those individuals. Again, there must be no gross negligence and good faith is required.

END NOTES

1. *Black's Law Dictionary* 257 (5th ed. 1979).
2. *See, e.g., The Legal Status of Adolescents 1980,* U.S. Dept. of Health & Human Services, 41 (1981).
3. *See, e.g., Meek v. City of Loveland,* 85 Colo. 346, 276 P. 30 (1929).
4. *See, e.g., Scaria v. St. Paul Fire & Marine Insurance,* 68 Wis. 2d 1, 227 N.W. 2d 647 (1975).
5. Smith, J.T., *Medical Malpractice: Psychiatric Care* 178-179 (1986).
6. *See, e.g., Gulf Southern Railroad Co. v. Sullivan,* 155 Miss. 1, 119 So. 501 (1929).
7. *See, e.g., Planned Parenthood v. Danforth,* 428 US 52, 74 (1975) (abortion); Ill. Rev. Stat. ch. 91 1/2, para 3-501(a) (1983) (mental health counseling).
8. *See, e.g., Jehovah's Witnesses v. King County Hospital,* 278 F.Supp. 488 (WD Wash 1967).
9. *See, e.g., Wilson v. Lehmann,* 379 S.W.2d 478, 479 (Ky. Ct. App. 1964).
10. *See, e.g., Rennie v. Klein,* 462 F.Supp. 1131 (D N.J. 1978).
11. *See, e.g., Schloendorff v. New York Hospital,* 211 N.Y. 125, 105 N.E. 92 (1914).
12. H. Weihofen, *The Definition of Mental Illness,* 21 Ohio St. L.J. 1 (1960).
13. *Dexter v. Hall,* 82 U.S. 15 (1872).
14. *See, e.g., Michigan v. Leighty,* 411 N.W. 2d 778 (Mich. Ct. App. 1987) (effects of cocaine free-basing several days preceding arrest considered but ruled not sufficient to invalidate defendant's waiver of right to silence).
15. *See, e.g., Hess v. Arbogast,* 376 S.E. 2d 333 (W.Va. 1988) (diagnosed evidence of arteriosclerosis and organic brain syndrome raises jury questions regarding decedent's capacity to convey property and execute a will).
16. *See, e.g., Edmunds v. Chandler,* 203 Va. 772, 127 S.E. 2d 73 (1962).
17. *See, e.g., In re Estate of Villwok,* 413 N.W. 2d 921 (Neb. 1987).
18. *See, e.g., Daughton v. Parson,* 423 N.W. 2d 894 (Iowa Ct. App. 1988) (transfer of property set aside where the grantor did not have sufficient mental capacity to execute the deed because of "senile psychosis").
19. *See, e.g., Sharpe, Medication as a Threat to Testamentary Capacity,* 35 N.C.L. Rev. 380 (1957).
20. *United Pacific Insurance Co. v. Buchanan,* 765 P.2d 23 (Wash. Ct. App. 1988).

21. *See, e.g., Hovey v. Hobson,* 53 Me. 451 (1866).

22. *See* 2 Williston, *Contracts* §§249-252.

23. Restatement Second, *Contracts,* §13.

24. *See, e.g., Cundick v. Broadbent,* 383 F.2d 157 (10th Cir. 1967), *cert. den.* 390 U.S. 948 (1968). *See also* Guttmacher & Weihofen, *Mental Incompetency,* 36 Minn. L. Rev. 179 (1952).

25. *See, e.g.,* Green, *Proof of Mental Incompetency and the Unexpressed Major Premise,* 53 Yale L. J. 271 (1944); Green, *The Operative Effect of Mental Incompetency on Agreements and Wills,* 21 Tex. L. Rev. 554 (1943).

26. Restatement Second, *Contracts* §15.

27. *See, e.g.,* Danzig, *The Capability Problem in Contract Law,* 148-204 (1978); *but see* Hardisty, *Mental Illness: A Legal Fiction,* 48 Wash. L. Rev. 735 (1975).

28. *See generally* McCoid, *Intoxication and Its Effect upon Civil Responsibility,* 42 Iowa L. Rev. 38 (1956); 2 Williston, *Contracts* §§258-263.

29. *See, e.g., Cundell v. Haswell,* 23 R.I. 508, 51 A 426 (1902).

30. *See, e.g., Alexander v. Haskins,* 68 Iowa 73, 25 N.W. 935 (1885).

31. *See, e.g.,* Restatement Second, *Contracts* §15(2).

32. *See, e.g., Coffee v. Owens' Admiralty,* 216 Ky. 142 (1926).

33. E. Clark, L. Lusky & A. Murphy, *Gratuitous Transfers,* 372 (3d ed. 1985).

34. *Banks v. Goodfellow,* 5 Q.B. 549 (1870).

35. *In re Estate of Fish,* 522 N.Y.S. 2d 970 (App. Div. 1987).

36. 79 Am. Jur. 2d *Wills* §§77-101.

37. *See generally* 18 Am. Jur. POF.2d *Mentally Disordered Testator's Execution of Will during Lucid Interval* §1 (1979).

38. *Neil v. Brackett,* 234 Mass. 367, 126 N.E. 93, 94 (1920).

39. *See, e.g., Estate of McRae,* 522 So.2d 731 (Miss. 1988).

40. *See, e.g., Succession of Hamiter,* 519 So.2d 341 (La. Ct. App. 1988); *but see Succession of Cahn,* 522 So.2d 1160 (La. Ct. App. 1988).

41. *Black's Law Dictionary* 257 (5th ed. 1979).

42. Competency issues are frequently raised about a number of aspects of witnesses' or defendants' conduct or litigation procedures (e.g., waive right to silence, counsel, or jury; to stand trial; to be sentenced; to serve a sentence and be executed).

43. *See generally Wheeler v. United States,* 159 U.S. 523, 524-25 (1895); *United States v. Benn,* 155 U.S. App. D.C. 180, 476 F.2d 1201 (1972); *In re B.D.T.,* 435 A.2d 378, 379 (D.C. 1981).

44. II Wigmore, *Evidence,* §493 (3d ed. 1940).

45. D.C. Code §14-305(a).

46. D.C. Super. Ct. (Crim.) R. 26.

47. The four-part test enunciated by Professor Wigmore would be a typical example of a common-law rule or guiding principle.

48. 149 U.S. App. D.C. 306, 462 F.2d 1201 (1972).

49. 149 U.S. App. D.C. at 308, 462 F.2d at 1203.

50. There is no precise age that determines the question of competency. *Wheeler v. United States,* 159 U.S. 523, 524 (1895) (five-year-old boy determined to be competent to testify).

51. *Black's Law Dictionary* 701 (5th ed. 1979).

52. *See, e.g., Wilson v. Lehmann,* 379 S.W.2d 478 (Ky. Ct. App. 1964).

53. *See, e.g., Rennie v. Klein,* 462 F.Supp. 1131 (D.N.J. 1978).

54. *See, e.g., Rivers v. Katz,* 504 N.Y.S.2d 74 (App. Ct. 1986) [psychopharmacotherapy]; *Pickle v. Curns,* 435 N.E.2d 877 (Ill. App. 1982) [ECT].

55. Meisel, Roth & Lidz, *Tests of Competency to Consent to Treatment,* 134 Am. J. Psychiatry 279, 283 (1977).

56. Meisel, Roth & Lidz, *Toward a Model of the Legal Doctrine of Informed Consent,* 134 Am J. Psychiatry 285, (1977).

57. M. Perlin, *Mental Disability Law — Civil and Criminal,* vol. 3, 1989, Charlottesville, Va., Michie, p. 80.

58. Meisel, Roth & Lidz, *Toward a Model of the Legal Doctrine of Informed Consent,* 134 Am. J. Psychiatry 285, 287 (1977) *citing* 139

Am. Law. Reports 1370 (1942); *but see Lipscomb v. Memorial Hospital,* 733 F.2d 332, 335-36 (4th Cir. 1984).

59. *See, e.g., Frasier v. Department of Health and Human Resources,* 500 So.2d 858, 864 (La. Ct. App. 1986).

60. *See, e.g., Aponte v. United States,* 582 F.Supp. 555, 566-69 (D.P.R. 1984).

61. *See, e.g., In re Quinlin,* 355 A.2d 647 (N.J.), *cert. denied sub nom Garger v. New Jersey,* 429 U.S. 922 (1976); *In re Conroy,* 486 A.2d 1209 (N.J. 1985).

62. *Union Pacific Railroad Co. v. Botsford,* 141 U.S. 250, 251 (1891); *also see Schloendorff v. New York Hospital,* 211 N.Y. 125, 105 N.E. 92 (1914) ("Every human being of adult years and sound mind has a right to determine what shall be done with his own body. . .").

63. *In re Conroy,* 486 A.2d 1209, 1222-23 (N.J. 1985).

64. *See, e.g., Tune v. Walter Reed Army Medical Hospital,* 602 F.Supp. 1452 (D.D.C. 1985); *Bartling v. Superior Court,* 163 Cal.App.3d 186, 209 Cal. Rptr. 220 (1984); *Bouvia v. Superior Court,* 225 Cal. Rptr. 297 (1986); *In re Farrell,* 529 A.2d 404 (N.J. 1987); *In re Peter,* 529 A.2d 419 (N.J. 1987); *In re Jobes,* 529 A.2d 434 (N.J. 1987).

65. *In re Conroy,* 486 A.2d at 1230-31.

66. *Id* at 1232 (footnotes omitted).

67. *See generally* Regan. *Protective Services for the Elderly: Commitment, Guardianship, and Alternatives,* 13 Wm. & Mary L. Rev. 569, 570-73 (1972).

68. B. Sales, D.M. Powell & R. Van Duizend, *Disabled Persons and the Law: State Legislative Issues* 461 (1982).

69. *Id.* at 462.

70. *Id.* at 461-62.

71. *Id.* at 463.

72. Regan, *supra* note 67, at 605.

73. Sales, Powell & Van Duizend, *supra* note 68 at 463 (as of 1988, 10 states provide no statutory right to counsel).

74. *Id.* (as of 1988, 22 states provide the respondent with the right to jury).

75. *Id.* (as of 1988, the right to be present is guaranteed in only 38 states, and that right is often waivable with only a doctor's certificate that the respondent is unable to attend).

76. Sales, Powell & Van Duizend, *supra* note 68, at 463.

77. *Id.* at 464.

78. *Id.* at 469-474.

79. *See, e.g., Plummer v. Early,* 190 Cal. Rptr. 578 (Ct. App. 1983) (evidence that schizophrenic respondent was dirty, disheveled, and incontinent, and spent the majority of his time in the backyard of his home was insufficient to warrant conservatorship or guardianship of person).

80. *See, e.g., In re Oltmer,* 336 N.W.2d 560 (Neb. 1983).

81. *See generally* Hodgson, *Guardianship of Mentally Retarded Persons: Three Approaches to a Long Neglected Problem,* 37 Alb. L. Rev. 407 (1973).

82. *See, e.g., In re Roe III,* 383 Mass. 415, 421 N.E.2d 40 (1981); *Rogers v. Commissioner of Mental Health,* 390 Mass. 489, 458 N.E.2d 308 (1983).

83. *See generally* Melton & Scott, *Evaluations of Mentally Retarded Persons for Sterilization: Contributions and Limits of Psychological Consultation,* 15 Prof Psychol: Research, Practice 34, 35-36 (1984).

84. Fed. R. Civ. P. 12 (b)(6).

85. *Feoffees of Heriot's Hospital v. Ross,* 8 Eng. Rpt. 1508 (1846).

86. *McDonald v. Massachusetts General Hospital,* 120 Mass. 432 (1876).

87. *Schloendorff v. Society of New York Hospital,* 211 N.Y. 125, 105 N.E. 92 (1914).

88. *Bing v. Thunig,* 2 N.Y.2d, 163 N.Y.S.2d 3, 145 N.E.2d 351 (1957).

89. *Colby v. Carney Hospital,* 254 N.E.2d 407 (1969).

90. *Bilonoha v. Zubritzky,* 233 Pa. Super. 339, 336, A.2d 351 (1975).

91. Joint Commission on Accreditation of Hospitals, Accreditation Manual for Hospitals 117 (1989 ed.).
92. Md. Health Occ. Code Ann. §§14-601F (1981).
93. Fla. Stat. Ann. § 768.40(2) (West 1986).
94. Cal. Civ. Code § 43.7 (West 1982).
95. Cal. Civ. Code § 43.8 (West 1982).
96. Norman, *So-called Physician "Whistle Blowers" Protested: Immunity of Peer Review Committee Members from Suit,* Legal Aspects Med. Pract., Feb. 1983, at 3.
97. Fla. Stat. Ann. § 768.40(4) (West 1986).
98. *Mayfield v. Gleichert,* 484 S.W. 2d 619 (C.A. Tex. 1972).
99. *Patrick v. Burget,* No 85-1145, slip op. (S. Ct. May 16, 1988).
100. The Health Care Quality Improvement Act of 1986, Pub. L. No. 99-660, sec. 401-432, 100 Stat. 3784 (1986).
101. 42 Pa. Cons. Stat. Ann. §§ 8331,8332 (Purdon 1982).
102. *Johnson v. Matviuw,* 531 N.E. 2d 970 (Ill. App. Ct. 1988).
103. Cal. Health and Safety Code § 1799,100. Cal. Civ. Code § 1714 2 (c)-(d).
104. *Lowry v. Henry Mayo Newhall Memorial Hospital,* 229 Cal. Rptr. 620 (Cal. Ct. App. 1986).
105. 28 U.S.C.A. § 1346 (West 1976).
106. The Federal Employees Liability Reform and Tort Compensation Act of 1988, Pub. L. 100-694 (1988).
107. 10 U.S.C.A. § 1089 (West 1983).
108. *Id.*
109. 22 U.S.C. § 817 (West 1979).
110. 42 U.S.C. § 2458(a) (West 1983).
111. 42 U.S.C. § 233 (West 1983).
112. *Baker v. Barber and Talmage,* 673 F. 2d 147 (6th Cir. 1982).
113. *Apple v. Jewish Hospital and Medical Center,* 570 F. Supp. 1320 (D.N.Y. 1983).
114. 42 U.S.C. § 233 (West 1983).
115. *Anderson v. O'Donaghue,* 677 P. 2d (Okla. 1983).
116. *Hudson v. Rausa,* 462 So. 2d 689 (Miss. Sup. Ct. 1984).
117. *AMA Diagnostic and Treatment Guidelines Concerning Child Abuse and Neglect,* 254 J.A.M.A. 796-800 (1985).
118. Cal. Penal Code § 11166 (West 1982).
119. Cal. Penal Code § 11172 (West 1982).
120. Mich. Comp. Laws Ann. § 722.625 (West 1987).
121. *Ackerman v. TriCounty Orthopedic Group,* 373 N.W. 2d 204 (1985) (Mich. Ct. of App., 1985).
122. Miss. Code Ann. 93-21-25 (1987).
123. 42 Pa. Cons. Stat. Ann. § 8334 (Purdon 1982).
124. 18 Pa. Cons. Stat. Ann. § 5106 (Purdon 1982).
125. Cal. Health & Safety Code § 1799.100 (West 1987).
126. *See, e.g., In re Guardianship of Pamela,* 519 N.E.2d 1335 (Mass. Sup. Jud. Ct. 1988).
127. *See, e.g., McAlister v. Deatheridge,* 523 So.2d 387 (Ala. 1988).
128. *See, e.g., Daughton v. Parson,* 423 N.W.2d 894 (Iowa Ct. App. 1988) (transfer of property set aside where the grantor did not have sufficient mental capacity to execute the deed).
129. *See, e.g., Annas & Densburger, Competence to Refuse Medical Treatment: Autonomy vs. Paternalism,* 15 U. Tol. L. Rev. 561 (1984).
130. *See, e.g., Weldon v. Long Island College Hospital,* 535 N.Y.S.2d 949 (N.Y. Sup. Ct. 1988).
131. *See, e.g., Pace v. Pace,* 513 N.E.2d 1357 (Ohio Ct. App. 1986).
132. *See, e.g., Manhattan State Citizen's Group, Inc. v. Bass,* 524 F.Supp. 1270 (S.D. N.Y. 1981).
133. *In re Conservatorship Estate of Moehlenpah,* 763 S.W.2d 249 (Mo. Ct. App. 1988).
134. *See, e.g.,* D.C. Code §16-904 (d) (1)-(5) (grounds for annulment of marriage including "insanity" at the time of marriage).
135. *See, e.g., In re Marriage of Steffan,* 423 N.W.2d 729 (Minn. Ct. App. 1988) (divorce decree binding where the wife's mental condition did not interfere with her comprehension).
136. *See, e.g., In re Jason Y,* 744 P.2d 181 (N.M. Ct. App. 1987).
137. *See, e.g., In re J.O.L.II.* 409 A.2d 1073 (D.C. 1979) (Defining factors used in the District of Columbia that delineate whether an adoption by a petitioning party is in the "best interests of the child." Among those factors is the *mental state* of the petitioning party. Clearly, if the petitioner was incompetent, placement would not be in a child's best interests).
138. *See, e.g., Dusky v. United States,* 362 U.S. 402 (1960).
139. A defendant who has been found "competent" is not necessarily capable of making intelligent decisions on all issues, *e.g.,* the decision to waive an insanity defense. *Frendak v. United States,* 408 A.2d 364, 379 (D.C. 1979).
140. *See, e.g., Nebraska v. Tully,* 413 N.W.2d 910 (Neb. 1987) (defendant's confession and guilty plea held to be "knowingly, intelligently, and voluntarily made despite IQ of 81 and diagnosis of mild mental retardation).
141. *See, e.g., Ex parte Ford,* 515 So.2d 48 (Ala. 1987).
142. *See, e.g.,* Note, *Mental Aberration and Post Conviction Sanctions,* 15 Suffolk Univ. L. Rev. 1219 (1981); *State v. Hehman,* 520 P.2d 507 (Ariz. 1974); *Commonwealth v. Robinson,* 431 A.2d 901 (Pa. 1981).
143. *See, e.g., In re Hews,* 741 P.2d 983 (Wash. 1987).
144. *See, e.g., Jurney v. Arkansas,* 766 S.W.2d 1 (Ark. 1989).
145. *See, e.g., Ford v. Wainwright,* 477 U.S. 399 (1986); Note, *The Eighth Amendment and the Execution of the Presently Incompetent,* 32 Stan. L. Rev. 765 (1980).
146. *See, e.g., United States v. Thornton,* 498 F.2d 749, 162 App. D.C. 207 (1974); *Bethea v. United States,* 365 A.2d 64 (App. D.C. 1976).
147. *See, e.g., Fuller v. Texas,* 737 S.W.2d 113 (Tex. Ct. App. 1987).

APPENDIX 4-1   Some areas of law in which competency is an issue

CIVIL

- Guardianship—care for one's self and property[126]
- Enter into a contract[127]
- Make a will[128]
- Consent to treatment[129]
- Authorize disclosure of medical records
- Sue[130] or be sued[131]
- Testify in court
- Vote[132]
- Obtain a driver's license
- Act in public or professional capacity
- Receive benefits (e.g., Social Security)
- Retain private counsel[133]

FAMILY LAW

- Marry[134]
- Divorce[135]

- Terminate parental relations with a child[136]
- Adopt[137]

CRIMINAL LAW

- Stand trial[138]
- Assume responsibility for a criminal act
- Waive the insanity defense[139]
- Make a confession[140]

- Waive the right to counsel[141]
- Undergo sentencing[142]
- Make a plea[143]
- Provide testimony in court[144]
- Be executed[145]
- Entertain premeditation or "specific intent" of a crime[146]
- Consent to sexual intercourse[147]

APPENDIX 4-2 Some general tests of competency

Relevant act	General legal test regarding competency
Make a will	Understand the nature and object of the will, one's holdings, natural objects of one's bounty
Make a contract	Understand the nature and effect of the proposed agreement or transaction
Marry	Understand the nature of the marital relationship and the rights, duties, and obligations it creates
Drive	Understand the pertinent laws of the state with regard to licensure; not drive in a dangerous manner
Testify in court	Be capable of observing, remembering, and communicating about events in question; understand the nature of an oath
Responsibility for a criminal act	Possess sufficient capacity (cognitive) to understand and appreciate the criminality of one's acts and conform one's conduct to the requirements of the law
Stand trial	Possess sufficient capacity to rationally and factually understand the nature of the proceedings and be able to assist and consult with legal counsel
Make a confession	Possess sufficient capacity to make a knowing and intelligent waiver of certain constitutional rights and a knowing and voluntary confession
Be executed for a criminal act	Possess sufficient capacity to rationally and factually understand the nature of the trial proceedings and purpose of punishment
Consent to treatment	Possess sufficient mental capacity to understand the particular treatment choice being proposed and any relevant adverse effects associated with it

CHAPTER 5 Contracts, agency, and partnership

HUGH F. HILL III, M.D., J.D., F.C.L.M.
JOSEPH P. McMENAMIN, J.D., F.C.L.M.

THE LAW OF CONTRACTS FOCUSES ON ENFORCEABILITY
BACKGROUND AND RATIONALE OF CONTRACT LAW
ELEMENTS OF AN ENFORCEABLE CONTRACT
DEFENSES—GENERAL REASONS WHY OTHERWISE VALID CONTRACTS MAY
  BE UNENFORCEABLE
HOW ARE CONTRACTS ENFORCED?
RULES OF INTERPRETING CONTRACT LANGUAGE
EFFECT OF STATUTES ON CONTRACTS AND CONTRACT LITIGATION
REMEDIES—THE RELIEF GRANTED BY THE COURT
NEGOTIATING AND MAKING A CONTRACT
HOW TO READ A CONTRACT; SPECIFIC CLAUSES
TYPES OF CONTRACTS
CONTRACTUAL LIABILITY OF MINORS

Contracts are agreements. In popular context, a contract is a formal agreement that evidences a serious commitment and carries the possibility of legal action if the promises are not kept.

THE LAW OF CONTRACTS FOCUSES ON ENFORCEABILITY

Contract law is an area of the law about which common understanding, though deficient in detail, is correct in spirit. Many think of their contractual commitment in a unilateral, personal way. The contract is thought of as an obligation that individuals bear to the party with whom they have contracted. Although there may be an intellectual awareness that the contract results from an exchange of commitments, the focus is on the individual's own obligations. This is, at least in part, because an individual is aware that failure to meet these obligations gives the other party the opportunity to threaten or use legal action.

The law of contracts, like the man or woman involved in a contract, is concerned with whether (and what parts of) an agreement will be enforced by the law. The forms and details of contractual agreements reflect the infinite variety of human relationships and interactions. The question "What is a contract?" is moot. The functional question for anyone thinking about

contracting is "What agreements will be enforced by a court of law?"

BACKGROUND AND RATIONALE OF CONTRACT LAW
Historical development of contract law

Development of contract law is a feature of a commercial society. Precommercial societies, even if relatively advanced in other ways, do not have laws addressing mutual promises that are to be carried out at a later date. Among tribal peoples, commitments involving behavior not otherwise required by custom, or whose fulfillment was not ensured by the potential application of force, were guaranteed by some exchange of security. Alliances were forged with marriages, not treaties. Kings and chiefs exchanged sons and daughters.

In a society without law or custom governing contracts, promises could not be enforced on an individual level, but complaints regarding unfulfilled promises could at least be taken to the sovereign. As European civilization progressed out of the Dark Ages, church courts began to enforce agreements on grounds of fairness. Governments also found it increasingly expedient to utilize consistent, reliable rules of contract enforcement.

Contract law developed later than other areas of the law. In the thirteenth century, European merchants created their own "courts" and were using them in a procedure akin to modern commercial arbitration. This was necessary because businessmen could not rely on the law courts to enforce agreements. As mercantile interests expanded beyond simple dealings with a known, local group of individuals, the need for consistency and reliability increased. To members of a political unit, especially when dealing with those outside the unit, the advantages of a dependable method of enforcement of contractual agreements were apparent.

Roman law influences

Part of the reason for the late development of contract law is the profound influence on Western civilization of Roman jurisprudential thinking and codification. Roman law treated disputes regarding contractual obligations as problems of property. In other words, someone who had broken a promise to give some item was said to be in unlawful possession of the item. Thus, a contract made up of promises to act at a later time (an *executory contract*) was not enforceable by law in Rome until very late in that culture's history. As the Dark Ages descended on Europe and its once lively commercial society regressed to a more isolated and agrarian one, this late development of Roman law diminished in importance and was lost.

Beginning of modern contract law systems

The Roman foundations of contract law were rediscovered in the Renaissance that percolated out of northern Italy starting as early as the tenth century. Driven by the needs and actual practices of the merchant class, which became more important as the middle of the second millennium approached, contract law grew and contracts became enforceable everywhere. In the continental, civil law countries of Europe, codifications of contract law principles were influenced by scholars, theorists, and academicians. The results were similar to the law that developed in England as judges decided real disputes between real people. These English judges of the common law applied and distinguished decisions and rules enunciated in previous cases. This practice of following precedent resulted in fairly consistent and, for the most part, cohesive principles of contract interpretation and rules of enforcement. Considering the differences in approach, the similarities between the English common law and the continental civil law systems are remarkable. This is in part because civil law codifications included an attempt to write common custom into statute.

Where the common law and civil law approaches to contracts differ, it is usually a minor difference of technique or procedure, with both designed to achieve the same end result. For example, civil law holds offers open to a response, unless the offer states otherwise. Common law offers can be revoked, but acceptance is effective when mailed. Both rules respond to the need of the person receiving the offer to be able to rely on the agreement once accepted; both rules balance this need with fairness to the person making the offer. Differences in approach persist to this day, but so do the similarities in policy aspirations, which are the goals of the contract law of both systems.

Reasons for enforcing contracts

The history just summarized suggests why societies promulgate and maintain a system of contract law. The juxtaposed, sequential appearance of commerce and contract law betrays the latter's economic policy basis. As the legal system becomes a reliable source of contract enforcement, the reliability and attraction of contractual agreements is enhanced. Business activity is thereby advanced. It is rare for a government not to be interested in increased commercial development.

Reliable contract enforcement was and is especially important to outside business interests. Roman law recognized different law applicable to different people—the *lex barbarosum* versus the *lex Romanum*. This was not usually a means of favoring Roman citizens, but rather a more subtle technique of subjugation. The local or barbarian customs were incorporated into the applied Roman law, encouraging order and acceptance. After the reception of Roman jurisprudence into the law of the Western Renaissance, nations applied one law to all people within their borders. Where distinctions of application were wanted, they were specifically stated as such. Thus, outside traders could contract and rely on that society's courts to enforce contracts in accord with their law.

The advantages of policies encouraging executory contracts are apparent. Consider the situation of a society without reliable contract enforcement. Agreements involving promises to perform in the future are a gamble. Secure transactions are limited to immediate exchanges. Commercial situations in which immediate exchange is impractical or economically inefficient require the parties to take risks, to depend on extrajudicial enforcement (force), or to act inefficiently. This inhibits both the society and the individual.

Contract law policy, in addition to general societal interests, is also the result of special group interests. Intuitively, the result is proportional to the political influence and power of the group. Commercial interest groups are aided by contract enforcement. Business people can enter into agreements confident that a remedy is available if the other party violates the contract.

But does this mean that contract law protects only the

stronger business interest against the weaker? The commercial policy-maker who sees at all beyond his or her immediate interests realizes the benefits of encouraging weaker players to stay in the game. A Marxist might say that all capitalist law protects the haves from the have-nots by giving the weak the illusion that a fair court system protects them. Thus, goes the argument, contract law encourages the weak to enter and keep contractual agreements. The strong have less need of legal protection; they can protect themselves.

Contract enforcement creates a mechanism for the society to influence an otherwise private process. For example, by refusing to enforce abusive or illegal agreements, the law distinguishes disfavored arrangements from those that will be supported and encouraged. Common understandings can be codified by the legislature if the pattern of judicial decisions is not acceptable, even though individual cases cannot be so affected. If a pattern of contractual business practices arises with potential harm to a segment of society or the society in general, the means exist to limit the damage and make necessary changes by statute.

Court enforcement of contracts provides a forum for dispute resolution. As with tort disputes, society has a clear interest in a peaceful end to disagreements. Methods outside the law used to enforce commitments by organizations and businesses are disruptive and sometimes dangerous, even to nonparticipants.

But no society blindly enforces all contracts. After the means of enforcement through the courts is established, two principal groupings of issues arise. The first has to do with the individual contract before the decision-maker. What did the parties to the contract intend when they entered the agreement? A second major grouping of issues addresses, in more general terms, what contracts the courts should and will enforce. These concerns have, over centuries of judicial decisions in contract cases, resulted in a pattern of principles. These principles reflect the history of contract development and the policies behind contract law. These principles determine whether a contract will be enforced.

ELEMENTS OF AN ENFORCEABLE CONTRACT

The person considering a contract faces concerns, some of which are common to all types of agreements. Will the other party fulfill his or her end of the bargain? What if disputes arise as to whether the agreement was fulfilled or as to what the agreement requires? If someone goes to court to sue on the basis of this contract, what will be the result? A preliminary consideration is whether the agreement contains the basics that will cause a court to recognize the agreement as a contract and then as an enforceable contract.

Through the historical development of the common law, judicial decisions and reasoning have come to consistently require three principal elements in a contract before enforcement will be possible: offer, acceptance, and consideration. If the party requesting the aid of the law in enforcing the contract can prove that these elements were included, then a court-ordered remedy will be possible. Without them, the court will declare the agreement, if there was one, to be something other than a contract and therefore not enforceable.

Offer

The origin of a contractual commitment is the initial suggestion of willingness to enter a contract. An offer is a communication that creates the possibility of a contract; if it is accepted, a contract can exist. Disputes will arise over whether there was an offer. Does the physician who states at a medical meeting that he or she is looking for a partner state an offer? If so, then a physician at the meeting who accepts has bound both self and the first physician. The first physician might argue, however, that he or she was merely offering to negotiate or indicating a willingness to entertain offers and would probably win in court.

The determination of whether an offer was made is, in the law, a practical one. The terms of the offer must be sufficiently firm to allow court enforcement. In the previous example, the terms and conditions of the partnership "offer" are so unclear that a court would not be able to determine whether or how to enforce the agreement; therefore, there was no offer and thus no contract. This legal principle also explains why advertising does not create a contract when the target of the marketing effort accepts and expresses willingness to purchase. The terms are too indefinite; conditions such as number of items and times of delivery are not stated. Therefore, an advertisement is simply a price quote or an invitation for offers, not a true offer.

An offer is considered to be open for the time stated or for a reasonable time. The common law allows the offer to be withdrawn or revoked by the party making the offer at any time prior to acceptance. Again, the specific terms of the offer can express different conditions; like many other contract law principles, the presumption of revocability at will functions in the absence of a statement on the subject by the parties. The party making the offer can, for whatever reason or for no reasons at all, withdraw or change the offer if the other party has not yet accepted. The law also presumes the offer closed on the death of the person making the offer or on the destruction of some essential to the offer. A prospective tenant cannot accept the offer of the lease after the building has burned to the ground and then expect the court to enforce that contract. An essential to the agreement, the building, the continued existence of which was a presumed condition to the agreement, has been destroyed, and the law closes the offer at the time of the destruction. An offer also is closed by the rejection of that offer.

The principle that an offer is closed on rejection creates a common misunderstanding. In negotiating the purchase of one year's worth of medical supplies, the prospective purchaser might counterpropose a lower price. This counterproposal functions as a rejection and is a counteroffer. The counteroffer is not a form of acceptance of the original offer; it is a rejection and a new beginning of the process. If the seller rejects the counteroffer, the purchaser may not then bind the seller by accepting the original offer. If the purchaser wants to keep the original offer open and make a parallel, but separate, counteroffer, then he or she must state this clearly. A respondent might have to write back, "I have received, am interested in, and am keeping under consideration your offer to work in your hospital. Would you consider the following proposed change in schedule and vacation allowance?" Here again, the legal principle operates only when the parties have not addressed the issue.

Acceptance

Before a court will enforce a contract, the court must find that an offer was accepted. There must be some act manifesting assent and willingness to be bound by the terms of the contract. The acceptance must be made in response to, or at least with knowledge of, the offer. Consider a physician who writes to a colleague, "I will buy your practice on the terms we discussed if you will fire your receptionist." If the owner of the practice terminates the receptionist before this letter is received, no contract is created; there must be some other manifestation of acceptance. A coincidental act, although specified in the offer, is not enough.

The common law rule was that the acceptance had to be in the terms set by the offer and had to be unequivocal. This strict rule is being modified by time and subsequent decisions into a rule requiring that the offer be definite enough. For example, where an offer states "Reply by wire," a letter may be sufficient to make a binding contract. Silence constitutes acceptance only when custom demands it and a continuing relationship exists that makes such an assumption fair.

In addition to the statement "I accept," or its equivalent, acceptance is manifested in a variety of ways. One common method is to communicate a promise in return. If the offer does not clearly require performance as acceptance, then the return promise makes a contract. A physician writes, "I will stay in town and continue to do surgery at your hospital if you will buy that operating microscope I've wanted." The physician has left unclear whether immediate purchase of the equipment is required. A contract may be created by the return promise of "We will buy the damn thing, since you insist," even though no one has specified a time limit within which the purchase will take place. Acceptance is also shown by doing the required act (e.g., buying the microscope in the previous example). Taking control of and using offered goods can also constitute acceptance, although some jurisdictions protect the user of unsolicited goods.

Agreements to make a contract in the future are problematic. At times, professionals make commitments to contract or to reduce an agreement to a written document. The reviewing court must determine whether this was an acceptance, a promise to bargain in good faith, or a rejection—that is, an expression that the party was not yet willing to be bound but wished to continue the discussion. The old common law rule was simply that agreements to make an agreement were not enforceable contracts.

A response to an offer that proposes new terms is a new offer, not an acceptance. But a carefully worded acceptance can make a binding contract while proposing changes for consideration. If the acceptance is in any way conditional on the new terms, then it is a new offer. If the acceptance is clearly unconditional, new terms may be proposed without voiding the acceptance. Thus the following response makes a binding contract: "I accept your offer to fill the open slot in your residency program. Would you consider letting me start August 1, instead of July 1?" The program director cannot take this as a rejection by counteroffer and hire someone else. However, the cautious recipient of such an acceptance will take additional steps to ensure clear mutual understanding.

How does the party considering acceptance know the offer is still open? Many offers are made for a limited, stated time. When the parties fail to specify, the rule of law states that an offer is revocable until accepted, within a reasonable period of time. But another rule makes the contract binding on acceptance. For example, the manager of a housekeeping service organization has in hand a hospital's recent letter offering her a three-year contract on set terms. The manager can mail an acceptance and begin hiring personnel to fulfill the contract, without fear that the hospital has revoked its offer. The manager's acceptance was effective when mailed, and a contract has been created.

Offer and acceptance alone do not make an enforceable contract. Because of our common law heritage, a court also requires proof of the formality of consideration before finding an enforceable contract.

Consideration—mutuality of obligation

Taken together, offer and acceptance mark a threshold—from negotiations to commitment. But this is not enough to prove an enforceable contract. The law requires another essential element. Something of value must have been exchanged. Consideration is the *quid pro quo* that cements the deal.

Historically, the law could have taken the direction of enforcing commitments without consideration, but the common law did not. Consideration not only helps to show a bargained exchange, it also justifies enforcement. A promise of a gift might be accepted, but a naked promise will not be enforced by a court. Something must flow back in return for the promise. An expression of acceptance such as "Thanks," following the statement "I will pay your medical school tuition," does not make an enforceable contract. However, "I will pay your tuition if you will go to medical school" may allow a contract to be created. The relative value or the nature of the consideration is not ordinarily examined by the court. Even a promise in return for a promise constitutes valid consideration.

Because a promise can fulfill the requirement for consideration, an exchange of promises can make a contract. Therefore, questions about consideration will not be a concern in many contracts. But one common situation in which the lack of consideration defeats an assertion of contract arises in modifications of existing contracts. Consider Dr. T, the contracted medical director of a hospice. Dr. T already serves gratuitously but is concerned about malpractice insurance. He secures a promise from the hospice to include his professional activities under their institutional policy. This promise is not enforceable; there is no new consideration flowing from Dr. T to the hospice in return for the contract modification. Had Dr. T offered to refrain from resigning, in return for the insurance coverage, consideration could be found and the arrangement enforced. Dr. T cannot rely on an unstated threat to resign to show consideration.

Some promises can be implied, if necessary to validate consideration and to effectuate the parties' obvious intent. Thus, where the buyer and seller of a medical practice failed to include in their agreement language committing the buyer to pursue the practice and work it, but did provide that the purchase price was to come from practice proceeds, the court may imply a promise to service and maintain the practice. But where a stated promise is not of any real value, a court will not rewrite the promise. For example, if in response to an offer to sell custom-made splints, the practitioner promises to buy ". . . as many as I like," there is no consideration. The practitioner may purchase none. To imply consideration, the court would have to change the agreement, which it will not do.

Many contract documents contain recitations about consideration, but in fact nothing described changes hands (e.g., "For and in consideration of $1.00 and other good and valuable consideration, receipt of which is hereby acknowledged . . ."). These statements are an attempt to prove that consideration changed hands, that the agreement was a bargained exchange, and that the contract is enforceable. In a few jurisdictions, evidence to show that the consideration clause was a sham may be allowed by the court.

A party acting on another party's promise can be protected in another fashion. The concept of reliance, or acts in reliance, at one time functioned as a substitute for consideration. If B substantially changes his position because of and depending on A's promise, such that B would suffer a significant detriment if A does not fulfill the promise, then B may argue that there is an enforceable agreement between the two. In modern theory, the detrimental reliance forms an independent basis for enforcing the agreement. The party who relied on a promise and who seeks enforcement must show that injustice would result otherwise.

These three basic elements—offer, acceptance, and consideration—must be proven by a disappointed party to a contract who seeks court-ordered enforcement of that contract. However, the defendant has an opportunity to defend on grounds other than the lack of a crucial element. A contract with the required elements may still be unenforceable for other reasons.

DEFENSES—GENERAL REASONS WHY OTHERWISE VALID CONTRACTS MAY BE UNENFORCEABLE

Some contracts meet the definitional requirements—they may show that offer, acceptance, and consideration were exchanged—but will not be enforced by a court. The defenses in this section are generally available and they are not necessarily dependent on the specific language in the document. Disputes often arise about the interpretation and intent of contract wording, but defenses based on interpretation are discussed later in this chapter in the section on enforcement of contracts. The defendant may also claim that the terms of the contract were fulfilled and thus there was no breach. Defenses based on adequate performance are also addressed later.

Illegal terms and public policy

The rationale for court enforcement of contracts dissipates in the face of contracts and clauses that are damaging to society. The defendant can argue that although he entered the agreement, the court should not enforce it against him because of general policy considerations.

Courts will not enforce a contractual obligation to do something illegal. This is obvious in extreme cases such as murder for hire and gambling debts. But laws with less social opprobrium can invalidate contract commitments and trip the unwary. For example, a physician might agree to serve an institution's patients on a fee-for-service basis but may be unable to enforce the institution's promise to pay because the agreed-upon fees are in technical violation of a freeze.

Courts will also not enforce contract commitments that violate public policy; they are not unlawful because of statute or regulation but because of a general understanding about the policies underlying our laws. Defendants may assert that a clause should not be enforced because it restrains trade. Every contract restrains trade at least to some degree. Every commitment limits the ability to make other commitments, so the court considers the relative seriousness of the restraint or other policy violation.

Noncompetition clauses frequently confront contracting physicians. This is the classic dispute regarding policy and restraint of trade. Many court cases result from an attempt by the nonbreaching party to the contract to enforce an agreement not to compete. A clause might say, "If this partnership is dissolved, then the junior partner won't practice for two years within 25 miles of the current office." These clauses are disfavored because they restrain trade and limit the person's ability to earn a living; they must be carefully drawn to ensure enforcement. The clause must not be unreasonably restrictive in time or place. "Unreasonable" depends on the circumstances: how much time and distance is required to protect the interests of the party seeking enforcement? In physician practice cases, time restraints of up to three years have been held acceptable, although two years is more common. Geographical limits can depend on speciality. Thus, a metropolitan areawide restriction might be valid for a subspecialist but not for a primary care practitioner. If the clause is unenforceable because it unreasonably restrains trade and violates public policy, the breaching party is not bound and can compete wherever and whenever he chooses. In some few cases, the court has rewritten the clause to meet reasonable restrictions. This acts as a powerful inducement not to *overreach*. The senior partner who attempts to bind the junior to a long or far-flung noncompetition clause risks defeat and unenforceability.

Another common clause confronting health professionals is the *liquidated damages* provision. The contract includes a sum of money payable if some other provision is not met. Insofar as this amount is an estimate of the value of the damages resulting from violation, it can be enforced. But if the amount is out of proportion and is in fact a penalty, a court will not order it paid.

Contract provisions that attempt to relieve one party of responsibility for negligent acts may be unenforceable because of public policy. This is one of the reasons why contracts between patients and physicians or hospitals

that prohibit the patient from suing for medical malpractice are not enforced. Other policy considerations in this setting include the presumed unequal bargaining power of the parties and unequal control once treatment begins.

Duress and undue influence

Contracts may be unenforceable because of great disparity in the positions of the two parties. However, if the results of the enforcement are purely economical, this defense is not likely to succeed.

The party defending against enforcement of a contract because of duress must show that he acted under the threat of something wrongful or unlawful. Don Corleone's "offer he can't refuse" is duress, but Snidely Whiplash's threat to foreclose on the mortgage is not. In addition to illegality, the threat must have been so serious as to cause the defendant to accept the contract when otherwise he would have not accepted. A contracting party who threatens to refuse to fulfill the contract, and thereby wins new concessions, may find the new agreement unenforceable. Employers in terminable-at-will contracts can be caught by this restriction as well. The doctor who threatens an employee nurse with termination if the nurse will not agree to a wage cut may lose when the nurse later sues for the original wage.

The defense of undue influence addresses mental capacity, at the time of the contract, of the party asserting this defense. It is more limited in scope and application than the defense of duress. The focus here is on whether the assent to the contract was real and knowing. If the plaintiff in the contract suit took unfair advantage of a trusting relationship with the defendant, or of a mental infirmity in the defendant at the time the contract was entered, then this defense may be applicable. The defense of undue influence is akin to an inquiry into the mental state of the person making out a will. Fraud and duress focus on behavior.

Both undue influence and duress are difficult to prove and are applied by the courts in a spotty fashion. Therefore, they are unreliable. A party planning to breach a contract and then claim that the agreement is unenforceable because of duress or undue influence is taking a considerable risk.

Not all contracts in which there is a great disparity of terms will be unenforceable. Many normal business agreements are "take it or leave it" and are obviously stacked in favor of the party authoring the contract. Contracts that are, on their face, strongly biased against the other party or are standard forms without opportunity for negotiation are called *contracts of adhesion*. Even contracts of adhesion will be enforced by courts, but they are subject to more intense judicial scrutiny than other contracts. The authors of the *Restatement of the Laws*, a learned commentary thought authoritative by most courts, have suggested that where the party offering such a standard contract had reason to believe that the other party would not have agreed if that other party had known of a particular term, then that term should not be an enforceable part of the agreement.

Fraud and misrepresentation

To make a successful defense against enforcement of a contract based on fraud, the defendant must show that the plaintiff's assertions were made with knowledge of their falsity and with intent. If the inducement was truly fraudulent, like the classic land sales of worthless properties, relief in the form of a suit in tort for fraudulent misrepresentation is available as well as a defense to the contract.

Misrepresentation, however, can be an honest mistake, so the misrepresentation must be something that induced the defendant to agree to the contract. The court reviewing such a case will consider whether the defendant acted reasonably in relying on the mistaken statements. For example, the purchaser of a software system who wishes to void the contract and obtain a refund by showing that the salesperson misrepresented the system as likely to improve income by 20% has a stronger case than the purchaser who relied on the assertion that the system would triple income.

Capacity and mistake

Lack of capacity is the legal principle that makes minors' contracts void and unenforceable. Unlike the more vague defense of undue influence, capacity refers to an absolute inability to commit meaningfully to a contract. Insane persons, retarded persons, and others may be incompetent to enter contracts. The defendant is required to show that, as a result of a certain mental state or infirmity, he or she was incompetent at the time the contract was made.

Intoxication as a basis for a defense of incapacity depends on whether the intoxication was voluntary. Drugs, including alcohol, taken involuntarily, can be a basis for relief from the contract's obligation only if there is an additional showing that the other party to the contract knew (or should have known) that the defendant was incapacitated at the time. Prescription drugs may be considered to result in an involuntarily intoxicated state, thus voiding a contractual commitment.

Lack of capacity, like the other defenses, is much more likely to be successful where the plaintiff was at fault, such as knowledge of the defendant's incapacity and an attempt to take advantage of the situation. In clear cases of incapacity, however, the contract may be found unenforceable even though this works a hardship on the innocent party suing on the agreement. The remedy or relief granted may be adjusted accordingly under these circumstances.

Mistake is another defense that is bolstered considerably by the misdeeds of the nonmistaken party. If the plaintiff knew that the other party was mistaken about the terms or intended differently from the final agreement, then that nonmistaken party appears to be taking unfair advantage.

Relief from a contract entered into mistakenly will not be granted if the mistaken party acted unreasonably. In other words, there is a general understanding that parties to a contract must act responsibly, with reasonable caution to investigate where necessary and understand the agreement they are entering. An assertion of mistake is possible whenever one party or the other is disappointed in a contract; therefore, courts are not likely to grant relief easily on this basis. Failure to read a contract is not grounds for claiming that there was a mistake.

Successful defenses of mistake are particularly susceptible to reform of the contract by the reviewing court, as opposed to simply voiding all obligations. Although refusing to enforce any part of the contract may be the proper remedy if nothing has been done yet in fulfillment of the terms or in reliance on them, in many situations it may be appropriate for the court to rewrite the contract to meet the parties' intentions.

Impossibility and acts of God

Relief from enforcement of contracts for these reasons is only very rarely granted if economic hardships create the difficulties. Performance of the contract's terms must be impossible, not merely more difficult or expensive than a party would prefer. The impracticality must be objective, not subjective according to the defendant, and is almost always the result of some change in conditions on which the parties relied. Where the impossibility or an act of God affects the consideration and makes it valueless, the contract can be found to have failed for lack of consideration. Where consideration was good and changed hands, the defense of impossibility is still available.

Examples of how this defense operates can be seen in the situation of a middle-man contracting group, which purchases and supplies services. If a contracting group has an arrangement to provide emergency care at a hospital, the group will then contract with individual physicians, as subcontractors or employees. If the master contract with the hospital is terminated, then the group may assert the defense of impossibility against a physician suing to enforce his contract with the group. If the group's contract with the hospital was terminated because of a violation by the group, then the defense of impossibility may not be available to the group. If the hospital burns or is condemned, then all parties may be relieved by asserting this defense.

HOW ARE CONTRACTS ENFORCED?

Participants in a contract who believe they have been wronged may seek relief through the courts. The procedure followed is generally similar to other civil lawsuits. The standards applied, the elements that must be proven, the defenses and the remedies available all follow from the nature of the suit. It is a suit *in contract*.

Procedure of the suit in contract

As in other civil suits, the party seeking court-ordered relief files a demand in the court of proper jurisdiction. The filing asserts that there was a contract and that it was breached. This initial *pleading* gives notice to the defendant and states the basis on which the requested relief can be granted. The relief, or desired response by the court, is stated, either in money or other specific relief. After a period of discovery (an opportunity for both sides to learn about the other's theories and evidence), the trial commences. Each side offers evidence and argues the case, hoping for a favorable decision by the judge or jury. The written document itself, if there is one, is usually the most important piece of evidence.

The parole evidence rule can prevent the use of prior agreements to explain the contract

Many written contracts contain a clause indicating that the document is the full and final expression of the parties' intent, or words to that effect. Such clauses attempt to make use of the *parole evidence rule*. This rule prevents both parties from introducing at trial other agreements made before or at the same time as the one in question, in an effort to modify or add to that contract. These prohibited agreements may be written. "Parole" once meant verbal, but the rule now refers to extrinsic evidence.

The parole evidence rule comes up when one party attempts to claim that words exchanged at or before the time of contracting indicate a different intent from that expressed in the written document. The holder of a medical malpractice insurance contract may assert that even though the policy states one thing, the agent assured her of another. She may be prevented from introducing evidence about the agent's assurances because of the rule.

The parole evidence rule has limited application and does not prevent the use of extrinsic agreements offered to prove certain defenses, such as fraud or mistake. For the rule to apply at all, there must have been a writing, and the court must find that the writing was the final and complete expression of the parties' intent.

Court review of contracts

A court may enforce a valid contract and order that the party to the contract receive that to which he or she is entitled. Interpretation of the language of the contract and determination of the adequacy of performance, as well as the basic finding of the existence of a valid contract, affect the relief ordered by the court. For example, it is possible to enforce an invalid contract where one of the parties has performed and the other alleges there was no contract in order to avoid performance. The court may stop the nonperforming party from asserting there was no contract in the interests of fairness. This is called *equitable estoppel*.

Was there a breach of contract?

Following (sometimes as part of) a determination that there was a valid contract and that no defenses apply, the court then considers the allegation with breach. Were the contract obligations met or not?

In determining whether there was a breach of contract, a court decides whether the breached commitment was conditional, and if it was conditional, whether that condition was met. The obligation to pay on a mortgage loan is not conditional; the monthly payment is due regardless. A sale contract providing for payment on delivery makes that obligation to pay conditional on the delivery. A contract plaintiff attempting to prove breach of a conditional promise must show that the condition was met, in addition to proving the breach. In the sale of goods example above, the purchaser need not offer payment prior to instituting suit for the nondelivery of the goods. Only where both obligations are to be met simultaneously, where each could wait for the other and no absolute duty would then arise, must the contract plaintiff perform or tender an offer of performance before instituting suit.

Did performance take place?

Performance refers to compliance with the contract obligations, both the performance that fulfills—and defeats—an allegation of breach as well as the performance required of the party who sues. For example, an employee who has worked as required has performed, but an employer who has not paid the employee has not performed.

Performance is not an absolute concept in the law of contracts. Partial, especially substantial, performance can still be enough to allow that party to sue on the contract if the other side has not kept its promise. The concept of substantial performance also concerns conditions that must be met before the other parties' obligations are triggered.

Picture a physician who has hastily entered a contract for interior decoration of his office. Following the signing of the agreement, the physician has reconsidered and wishes to be relieved of the agreement, but the interior decorating firm is adamant. Imagine the numerous ways in which the decorator might fail to meet various details of the contract, from the extremely minor to the very important. The physician cannot safely repudiate the contract and refuse to pay because of an insubstantial breach, without language in the agreement indicating the essential nature of all details. If the decorator supplies waiting room chairs of a different brand name than that called for in the contract, but of substantially similar quality and appearance, the physician can not rely on the substitution to excuse him from his obligations under the agreement. A reviewing court might find that there was substantial performance and that the condition that had to be met before the doctor's obligation was triggered (completion of the interior decorating work) had been substantially met and that the doctor's obligation to pay had become absolute. Contract law is not like contributory negligence law in torts; without bad faith, a minor mistake by one party to the contract does not relieve the other of liability on the agreement.

Fairness and common sense in determining performance also appear in the *doctrine of severability*. This rule means that noninterdependent subparts of the contract that can be separated may be enforced separately. Partial performance may trigger an obligation for partial payment. The physician who has contracted to work for one year and who leaves after 11 months can be sued by the employer for breach of contract because of the early departure. However, the departing physician can still demand, and sue for, if necessary, the periodic wage or salary called for in the contract and earned during the 11 months of work.

Because of the law's general approach to performance determinations in contract litigation and the doctrines of fairness, substantial performance, and severability, even a party who performs perfectly under the agreement cannot take unfair advantage of the other party's imperfect performance. It is not safe for one party to pounce on the other party's minor performance failures.

Occasionally, a party to a contract announces or otherwise indicates an intention to violate the agreement. This repudiation of a contractual obligation occurs before the performance is finally due, and this breach occurs in anticipation of the due date of the obligation. The other party is not then required to perform, knowing that the repudiating party will not perform. This form of breach, called *anticipatory repudiation,* may occur when a party realizes that he or she will be unable to fulfill the contract and so advises the other party in an effort to reduce the damages or injury that will result. In most situations, the other party then has a right to go to court and sue for breach, but occasionally the time of performance must pass and the anticipated breach actually take place before suit can be filed.

RULES OF INTERPRETING CONTRACT LANGUAGE

"Ordinary meaning prevails" is the oft-quoted rule. However, once a contract dispute arises, meanings that seemed ordinary and obvious become subject to disagreement about intent and effect under the circumstances. Each party may have had entirely different assumptions when the agreement was made. There can be powerful incentives to discover areas of disagreement as the dispute evolves. Common law principles of interpreting contract language are used by courts in resolving disputes.

The court will take an overall view of the document and the circumstances, within limits. It is generally said that the contract writing is to be viewed as a whole and that all the facts and circumstances are to be taken into account. Put simply, contract clauses are not analyzed in a vacuum. In reviewing a disputed word or phrase, the court looks at the rest of the document and the facts of the case. However, the parole evidence rule just explained prevents simultaneous or prior agreements from being presented to the court if the contract in dispute is a complete and final expression of the parties' intent. For example, the physician in court over a contract with his residency program might wish to introduce evidence of a conversation he had with the residency director prior to signing the agreement. The physician will argue that this conversation is part of the surrounding facts and circumstances that should be considered by the court, but the director may respond that the parole evidence rule prevents this information from coming out at trial.

The rule favoring interpretation as a whole is also affected by severability clauses. These purport to make the remainder of the document good if one part is declared invalid. Another rule of interpretation that affects the general construction rule states that specific, separately negotiated clauses have more weight than standard clauses. For example, a court reviewing a contract on a preprinted standard form with handwritten alterations or typed-in additional clauses will consider those special writings as determinative if there is a conflict between them and the printed form.

In interpreting the language of a contract, the court also considers evidence of accepted trade or business dealings and the past dealings of the parties. Trade practices may, of course, be overridden by specific language in the contract, but in the absence of such statements and where there is dispute as to the meaning of contract language, generally accepted business practices will influence the outcome. In situations in which the contract is fulfilled in separate, sequential steps, then past practices and what the parties have found acceptable previously will be considered in determining what the parties expected.

Consider a physician whose contract arrangement with a laboratory service contains language indicating that specimens will be picked up at a reasonable time. After months of the laboratory picking up specimens from the previous day on the following morning, the physician now demands daily evening pick-ups and argues that the contract language requires this. The laboratory company can be confident of success if the physician takes them to court on the contract, because the pattern of performance established what the parties meant by "reasonable time." This also suggests that silently tolerating an unacceptable situation may interfere with later opportunities to demand correction. To preserve her rights to sue later, the doctor need not have brought immediate legal action on the day of the first unacceptable pick-up. But by writing and protesting expeditiously, she would have preserved her ability to indicate that the pick-up times were a matter of dispute from the outset.

The reviewing court attempts to take the subjective expectations of the parties into account. The court is attempting to effectuate the results intended by the parties at the time of signing. It is generally said that good faith is required in performance and enforcement of contract obligations, but not in the negotiations as to their terms. However, a disputed contract term will be interpreted in accordance with the subjective understanding of one of the parties if the other party knew of the different meaning attached to the language by the first party. Thus, a contract to install a chart rack in a physician's office may be rescinded if the physician intended it for a certain space where it does not now fit and if the salesperson knew it wouldn't fit, but interpreted the contract language "right for your office" as meaning a compatible color scheme. Providing the salesperson's knowledge will, of course, be difficult.

Where the intended result to be derived from fulfillment of the contract is apparent, the court will interpret the language to prevent an unintended result. If, for example, one interpretation of the wording makes an agreed-upon project possible and another interpretation of the wording makes completion impossible, a court tends to favor the former interpretation.

An important rule of contract interpretation requires

that ambiguities be resolved *against* the interests of the author of the document. This is especially true in the "take-it-or-leave-it" standard form contracts, in which no real negotiation or bargaining took place. This is a major reason why form contracts have so many specific details. The authors of the contract know that any lack of clarity in the language can result in an interpretation against their interests. This rule is justified by the assumption of superior bargaining power in the hands of the author of the contract, plus an assumption that the contract writer will have taken care of himself in the language. The nonauthor signator to the agreement may not have had an opportunity to affect the language.

EFFECT OF STATUTES ON CONTRACTS AND CONTRACT LITIGATION

Common law principles are subject to statutory revision. The legislature may pass laws that guide the courts in settling contract disputes and supercede common law principles derived from previous cases. However, these new statutes must also be interpreted by courts. Although many statutes codify common law principles, sometimes with only minor changes, other statutes dramatically alter the results that would have been obtained without them.

In the United States, commercial dealings are affected by the Uniform Commercial Code (UCC). Despite the term "Uniform," the states made various modifications to the code when they adopted it. Some sections of the code are made applicable by their language only to certain people in certain situations, such as merchants engaged in the sale of goods. Like other uniform laws, such as the Uniform Partnership Act, the UCC was the result of the consensus of a group of legal scholars. It was then presented to the state legislatures for their consideration and adoption, at least in part in an attempt to achieve better consistency in the law and interpretation of the laws among the jurisdictions within the United States. The UCC is the most important statute controlling contract enforcement by the courts, but for the most part, it follows previously understood common law contract principles.

The Statute of Frauds is an example of legislation adopted to alter common law contract rules. The English Parliament adopted the statute first in 1677. It was a response to perceived contract law abuses that the common man was powerless to prevent. The statute required that a writing be shown as proof of certain contracts before they could be enforced. Adoption of the statute on this side of the Atlantic varies among the states, such that the list of contracts that must be in writing varies, depending on the jurisdiction.

The evidentiary requirement of a written document has several effects. Parties are protected against claims based on oral agreements. People are put on notice that a serious commitment is involved when a written document is required and are, to some degree, protected against hasty decisions. These statutes also encourage discussions without fear that a binding contract will be made before a written document is signed. Generally, the trend of the law in the United States has been toward more requirements for written evidence of contracts, while in England the opposite trend has developed.

The kinds of agreements that require a document before they can be enforced, depending on the jurisdiction, are listed as follows:

1. Contracts that cannot be performed within a year. Thus, in states that have adopted this part of the Statute of Frauds, an employment contract extending more than one year must be in writing to be enforced.
2. Contracts in consideration of marriage. The abuse potential in this area was probably greater in the seventeenth century than today; however, prenuptial agreements may reawaken interest in this old rule.
3. Real property transactions. Historically, this portion of the Statute of Frauds addressed the worst problem facing the English peasantry. The wealthy could claim an oral agreement for the transfer of land and because of the difference in resources, could sue the common man to exhaustion. The requirement of a written document to effectuate the transfer of an interest in real property is generally understood and accepted today.
4. Commitments to answer for the debt of another (*suretyship*) is another area in which there is significant abuse potential. Specious claims of these obligations might be commonplace if it were not for the requirements of the statute.
5. Commitments to make a will.
6. Sales of goods of more than $500 or personal property of more than $5000. The adoption of restrictions in these areas is especially varied among the states.

The variation in application of statutory as well as common law principles makes the choice of which state's law will apply a critically important factor. Many contracts include a clause identifying the applicable law. Consider two parties in a contract dispute regarding the provision of billing services for a three-year period. The physician, relying on the laws of her state, which provide that such an agreement must be in writing to be enforced, claims that there was no contract. She believes she only has to pay the billing company its percentage of income actually generated by its services for the few months it served her. The billing company, relying on the laws of another state, which allow such contracts to be enforced without a written document, claims that there was a valid verbal commitment to a three-year arrangement and sues for a percentage of the physician's income for the entire three-year period. The importance of determining which jurisdiction's law will apply is apparent.

In the absence of a statement by the parties, the court determines the applicable law based on several principles, including where the contract was signed. The court also looks at, as another example, where the performance on the contract was to take place.

Two important cautions can be derived from this example. First, statement of the applicable law in the agreement is usually wise. Second, one should use caution in dealing with parties from jurisdictions in which contract law rules differ from those of his or her native jurisdiction.

REMEDIES — THE RELIEF GRANTED BY THE COURT

A court will grant a successful contract litigant the relief necessary and fair under the circumstances. Contract law is not criminal law and does not seek to punish the person who commits a breach of contract. While a wrong-doer or party acting in bad faith may be unable to enforce unfair dealings or may have contract language interpreted against his or her interest, the court will not award more than what was due under the contract against the breaching party. At least in concept, tort law also is intended to grant only the measure of relief required to make the injured person whole again. But tort law has developed the anomalous notion of punitive damage awards, clearly intended to punish the tort-feasor. Contract law has no such anomalous principle. The innocent party to a contract cannot obtain more than he or she would have been entitled to under the agreement itself, regardless of outrageous behavior on the part of the party breaching the contract.

This principle has obvious advantages of fairness and simplicity. However, one potentially negative aspect is that the principle allows a party to a contract to cold-heartedly calculate what he or she might lose if he or she was to breach the contract. He or she then decides whether that breach could be economically advantageous. Scholars who analyze the law in economic terms, on the other hand, argue that this policy encourages economic efficiency, because it allows the most economically efficient choice to be made by the party to a contract.

Measure of damages

The result of a successful contract suit is the court award of money to the victorious party. It is unusual for the court to order actual performance on the contract.

Prohibitions against involuntary servitude and the difficulty of supervising enforcement are the two most important reasons for this tendency. Legal systems of some other countries do provide for enforcement by requirement of specific performance and thus they avoid the difficulties of determining the proper amount of monetary damages required to put the matter right.

In general, the amount awarded by the court is that required to put the party where he or she would have been if the contract had been performed. Consider the physician who has contracted with a stenography service to handle overflow typing of charts and correspondence for a certain period at $1.00 per page. If the service breaches the contract, then the physician must purchase the typing elsewhere, at say $1.50 per page, for the duration of the contract period. The proper measure of damages is not the $1.50 per page that the physician now must pay, but the 50 cents per page differential. The physician would have had to pay $1.00 per page under the terms of the contract, so only the difference is required to give the physician the benefit of the former bargain.

Damages are also sometimes calculated by the amount necessary to put the nonbreaching party back to where it was before performance started. This measure may be appropriate when one party has acted in reliance on the contract and materially changed its position.

A third measure of damages is a calculation of the costs of *restitution,* or what is required to pay back the offended party for what it had already given to the party violating the contract. The plaintiff in a contract suit litigation usually asserts the most favorable measure of damages and offers proof of same. The defendant can then argue that this measure is inappropriate and claim that a different calculation should be used.

The consequences of a breach of contract can extend beyond that contract itself. A researcher who has a commitment from a supplier to provide a certain number of a strain of rats by a certain date, to be used in an ongoing experiment, may find that a delay in delivery ruins the entire procedure and it must be restarted. The costs of this result far exceed the purchase price of the rats, but the supplier would be liable for these consequential damages only if it were foreseeable that this harm might result from delay. The fairness of this restriction on consequential damages may be demonstrated. If the supplier knows of the possible outcome of delay or breach of contract, the supplier has a better sense of how much difficulty and expense he should undertake to assure proper performance. The researcher who wishes to make certain that the risk of a consequential loss is placed on the supplier will specify the possible results of delayed delivery in the contract document.

Fairness considerations also function when the court is reviewing the innocent party's conduct following notification of the breach. In the previous example, if the wronged researcher could have purchased the necessary rats on the day of delivery from a nearby supply house at a slightly higher price (and if he had the knowledge and the ability to do so), then the court won't award the damages that could have been avoided by this purchase. This is the result of a failure to *mitigate,* or act reasonably to reduce the injury resulting from a contract breach. This is another situation in which a party to a contract is not permitted to take unfair advantage of a breach by the other party.

Relief for third parties — those affected by but not parties to the contract

Failure to perform a contract's obligation can reach beyond its effects on the parties to the contract. Persons or business entities other than those signing the agreement are termed *third parties.* Enforcement of contracts *intended* to benefit third parties is handled differently from contracts that affect third parties incidentally.

Someone who is not a party to a contract can enforce that contract in court, if, and only if, the original parties intended to benefit that third party. The third party need not be named in the contract document, but need only be identifiable. Third-party beneficiary contracts arise most frequently in situations involving a promise to pay a debt owed to another. If Dr. B contracts to purchase the office building owned by Dr. S and to assume the loan, then the mortgage holder of the note is a third-party beneficiary of Drs. B and S's contract. The mortgage holder has enforceable rights and can sue either the original debtor (Dr. S) or the buyer of the property (Dr. B). The suit against Dr. B is based on the promise made to Dr. S — the promise to pay the mortgage holder.

Collection — enforcement of the judgment

The contract litigant victorious in court often faces the beginning of another arduous process: losing contract defendants do not always simply shrug their shoulders and write a check. Some successful contract litigants expend thousands of dollars pursuing their rights, win a substantial judgment in court, and never collect a penny.

If the losing defendant refuses to pay, the plaintiff must go through additional procedures to collect the money. Assets of the losing defendant must be found and attached. Legal procedures are used whereby the sheriff, or other official, is paid a fee to identify, take into possession, and then sell the loser's assets. The court can also order that a portion of the defendant's wages be paid to the victorious plaintiff. This garnishment procedure is valuable only if there is an employer making regular wage or salary payments to the defendant. If the party ordered to pay the award by the court does not have the necessary assets or the prospect of obtaining them, then there is little the plaintiff can do but hold the judgment and hope that some asset will appear.

Two methods are commonly employed to avoid this problem. One is refusal to contract with parties who are or may become *judgment-proof,* that is, parties with an impoverished state that renders them immune to any court's money judgment. The second is to demand a performance bond at the time of entering the contract. This is a form of insurance that is an added guarantee that compensation will be available if the contract is breached.

NEGOTIATING AND MAKING A CONTRACT

When most people think of a contract, they envision a paper, with or without negotiation. It is not difficult to recognize that one will be bound by a contract when presented with a document to sign. This is the usual method and, for some subject matters, is the only way to make a binding agreement that will be enforced by a court of law (see the previous section on the Statute of Frauds). It is still possible, though, to find oneself bound by contractual commitments without signing a written document.

Verbal contracts are possible

The majority of exchanges in daily life are immediate and not contractual. The goods are taken to the counter, money is tendered to the clerk, change and a receipt may be proffered, and the sale is complete. Verbal contracts arise when some part of the exchange is to happen in the future and the exchange is not thought to be of such importance or value that the parties require a written documentation of their understanding. The difficulty for reviewing courts in verbal contract situations is obviously one of proof. One party asserts that there was a verbal contract; the other party denies this. How is the court to determine which side is correct?

Proof of a verbal contract is offered in the usual and generally understood ways. Witnesses to the agreement might be produced; cancelled checks may be offered to the court as evidence. It was probably the difficulty of proof that Samuel Goldwyn had in mind when he quipped, "A verbal contract isn't worth the paper it's written on."

Acts in reliance can become especially important in proving a verbal contract. The act in reliance is a change in position undertaken by a party to a contract, which depends on that contract for its success. In other words, if the contract was breached, the party acting in reliance would be harmed, as compared with not changing positions, or not acting in reliance. Following a verbal contract, the act in reliance may be the best proof that

the nonbreaching party has of the existence of that verbal agreement. If the innocent party prepares for or undergoes expenses associated with the anticipated performance of the contract by the other party, then there has been an act in reliance, which may show there was a verbal contract.

Quasi contract

The theory of quasi contract allows enforcement of a contractual commitment, although there has been no explicit commitment. It is based on a theory of *unjust enrichment;* if the court were not to enforce the obligation, the breaching party would be unfairly benefited. Older contract theory based quasi-contract enforcement on the idea of an assumed promise.

Quasi-contract obligations are a common part of daily life. After ordering a meal in a restaurant, the diner has assumed the obligation to pay on the theory of quasi contract. This theory is the basis for upholding the obligation of the patient to pay the physician's reasonable fee. There was no written or verbal contract between physician and patient, but treatment was rendered and professional time expended. If the patient does not pay, the patient will have received a benefit without paying for it and be unjustly enriched.

For a quasi contract to be enforced, the plaintiff must have actually expected compensation at the time. Thus, the Good Samaritan who renders aid in an emergency may not be able to use this theory if he or she attempts to bill for the services.

Quasi-contract obligations can be triggered by an honest mistake. Consider the example of a copier company that misdelivers a copier to a physician's office, rather than to the neighboring physician down the hall. If that lucky physician uses the copier for a time, the company is entitled to recover something in quasi contract for the use. This example shows why the theory has changed. The older notion of assumed promise did not fit or justify this kind of situation, but unjust enrichment explains the court's enforcement of the obligation to pay the copier company.

The amount due under quasi contract is a customary measure. It is set by trade practices in the market and is determined by the value of what the defendant received. This is why the physician whose patient fails to pay the bill cannot be assured of recovering in quasi contract every penny of the amount charged, but rather only the usual fee or value of the service in the community.

Contracting – a process

Except for take-it-or-leave-it contracts, such as those offered by insurance companies, banks, and some sellers of goods, the natural sequence of a contract process involves discussions or negotiations toward the desired end, a meeting of the minds, and then an attempt to put down in writing the understanding of the parties.

Consider the example of Drs. S and J, which will be used throughout this discussion of negotiation. After 15 years of successful solo practice, Dr. S is thinking about taking on a partner. Dr. J has completed a residency and a fellowship and has worked for 2 years in another state. Both S and J have previously experienced problems with partnerships. Dr. J worked 2 years with a physician with whom he anticipated partnership and feels that he was treated unfairly. After 10 years of practice, Dr. S had a partner for a brief period, but their styles were so different that they had an acrimonious parting of the ways. Each of the two physicians is thinking about raising the idea of partnership to the other.

Prenegotiation considerations

Parties who might potentially enter a contract do not always have the time and foresight to consider their future needs. Frequently, someone suggests a contractual relationship and discussions immediately follow. The discussions are a form of negotiation, and sometimes the parties are thinking about their own needs and interests for the first time while the discussions are under way. On other occasions, potential contracting parties have an opportunity to consider as individuals, or with their own advisors, what they need and what they hope to achieve. This preliminary strategic work enhances chances for long-term success. More important in some situations, as with Drs. S and J, it gives the parties a chance to clarify, in their own minds, their needs and expectations.

Each party to a potential contract should take an opportunity for reflection prior to discussions with the other party. For example, Dr. J should think about what he really wants. He must ask himself why he is changing practice locations and what he seeks in a location that this particular community has or lacks. If his personal cost/benefit analysis favors moving to Dr. S's city, a similar analysis must take place regarding potential practice with Dr. S. Dr. J must ask himself what alternatives there are, such as establishing solo practice or joining another group in that city. Then the relative advantages or disadvantages of contracting with Dr. S may be weighed against realistic alternatives. The questions asked should focus on what is realistic, not some idiosyncratic notion of what is fair. Often, the result of such prenegotiation ruminations is the realization of the need for additional information. Dr. J may find he must investigate the community, the alternatives, and even Dr. S before entering into discussions.

Dr. S must also ask himself what he really wants. Does he want someone to round out his practice and provide a different facet for marketing purposes, or does he

simply want someone to share the load and the call schedule? Dr. S, too, must consider the alternatives: continuing to practice alone, recruiting for a different potential partner, or perhaps some more creative solution. Often, the result of these prenegotiation considerations is the realization of possible new answers to old problems. For example, Dr. S might realize that he could organize a call group among similarly situated practitioners in his area, if that is his only reason for seeking a partner. Dr. S may also want to contact his accountant or attorney regarding the relative advisability of taking on a partner. A necessity for both Drs. S and J, and anyone considering entering a contract discussion, is to understand his or her own needs, so as not to be operating from a vague, ill-informed, and potentially ill-advised feeling that something should be done.

This is also an opportunity for parties to make realistic projections of what may be achieved. Both Drs. S and J need to imagine themselves in the other's shoes and consider what is reasonable and right under the circumstances. Dr. J would be happy to have $100,000 a year guaranteed and an immediate full partnership to avoid the problems that he faced in his previous partnership, but he may be unlikely to win such concessions from anyone with whom he would want to practice. Realistic expectations of the other party also involve market considerations. What are the other party's reasonable alternatives? Is it a buyer's or a seller's market for what the individual is offering? Dr. J must ask himself whether there is a paucity or plethora of newly certified, well-trained physicians in his field looking for work in Dr. S's city. Dr. S must ask himself whether there are other senior physicians looking for junior partners in his area and he must also consider the relative difficulty Dr. J will face in establishing a new solo practice.

Negotiations

The discussions that lead to a signed document are important beyond the efforts of both parties to get what they want into the agreement—the discussions must also lead to a true meeting of the minds. Contracting parties who are bright, aggressive, and inexperienced in business dealings (some physicians), are apt to make one common error in negotiating long-term commitments. In the midst of the attempt to achieve short-term goals in the negotiation, physicians sometimes forget about the long-term need for both parties to be satisfied.

Much has been written on negotiations. Some of it is surprisingly useful because it stimulates thinking about the process. The best printed work on the subject has come from the Harvard negotiating group, which has conceived and articulated the Best Alternative To a Negotiated Agreement (BATNA). Considering what one will do if no agreement is reached in the negotiations helps keep the entire process in perspective and helps the negotiator deal with bottom-line concerns. The concept of a BATNA can also be applied to specific problems that are subfeatures of a negotiation. If Dr. S cannot win a certain concession from Dr. J, is it important enough to keep him from contracting with Dr. J? What is his BATNA on this particular issue?

Answers to problems in negotiations may often be found by inquiring into the real concerns of the participants. This is especially useful when a comfortable, long-term relationship is desired. For example, Dr. S absolutely refuses to take call more than one night out of four and Dr. J absolutely refuses to take call more often than every other night. Is a compromise possible? If the negotiations are a confrontation, then success is unlikely. For example: Dr. S: "I want you to take call three-fourths of the time." Dr. J: "That's unfair. I will not take call more than half of the time." If Dr. S is forthright and Dr. J learns that the senior physician's true wish is to reduce his own call load and not to force the junior man into an excessive call situation, then an alternative solution may be possible. In this scenario, Dr. J may then suggest sharing call with another nearby group. Although it may be necessary to keep some background information to oneself, it must be realized that chances of a true meeting of the minds and a true meeting of needs are enhanced by a clear understanding of each other's concerns. For example, Dr. J might not wish Dr. S to know that J is very concerned about immediate cash flow because Dr. J is in financial trouble. On the other hand, it may be important and productive for both parties to know of each other's past difficulties with other partnership arrangements. The parties are then more likely to find acceptable solutions to their respective concerns.

If a continued, cordial, and long-term relationship is a desired outcome, then the parties must keep this uppermost in mind. A short-term negotiating victory can be a Pyrrhic one. Drs. S and J may negotiate a 50% division of the income of the practice. Dr. J may see the solution as advantageous because he realizes that the older man moves faster and sees more patients than he ever will. Dr. S may not realize this and will be exceedingly disappointed later in the arrangement if income is disproportionate to work. A potentially mutually beneficial partnership will fail because of short-sightedness.

Use of counsel

Although many parties may wish to bring in their lawyers before the written document is prepared, review by counsel of a writing should certainly be considered. Usually, the parties think they have an agreement and seek counsel to record their understandings. Questions by counsel then cause the parties to realize that there are possible unintended results and potential problems that have not been discussed.

The proper role of counsel may be a difficult determination in many situations. Sometimes contracts are not signed and agreements are called off after the lawyers get involved. In many cases, this is because the interests of one or the other party require this result. Sometimes, however, counsel's involvement is inappropriately disruptive and destroys what might have been a satisfactory arrangement.

A brief reflection on the training and focus of lawyers reveals the reason for their seemingly negative bias. In contract law, attorneys are trained as legal pathologists: They dissect the wording of judicial decisions in court cases in which something has gone wrong. The attorney's job is to protect the client from bad results. It is not normally the attorney's job to tell the client wonderful things that will happen as the result of an agreement, but rather to point out the negatives, that is, what will happen if something goes wrong or one party is disappointed.

Purchasers of legal services should remember that they are in control. The client who wishes to reach an agreement must insist that the attorney apply his or her skills to find a creative solution to problems raised. Although creative solutions do not carry the same security as tried-and-tested language, novel solutions may be the only way that the parties in some situations can achieve an enforceable agreement—a contract.

HOW TO READ A CONTRACT; SPECIFIC CLAUSES

The nonlawyer can and should read his or her own contracts. Assistance of legal counsel will be required in some situations, but the layperson can understand most contract language. Slow reading and perhaps rereading can make the contract comprehensible. Reading speed studies have shown that only legal textual reading is slower than medical technical reading.

Standard sections

Most contracts are organized in a consistent fashion, permitting analysis by the layperson. Look for the caption, recitals, commitments, restrictions, and signatures.

At the beginning of most agreements, a heading identifies the type of contract. Sometimes this appears in the first line. The agreement may contain atypical features, but the caption indicates for a reviewing court the general category of contract intended by both parties.

Introductory statements usually follow. They often

begin with the term "whereas." The reasons for the agreement are recited here. This is not superfluity. As explained earlier, the intention of the parties is very important when the contract is reviewed in court.

The commitments are the heart of the agreement. The promises that are exchanged are the statements as to what each party will or will not do. These commitments can be in the form of multiple paragraphs, sometimes over many pages, but they are usually set off and identifiable as such.

Immediately after the promises, and sometimes included in them, are the restrictions or conditions. The parties list conditions in an effort to meet "what-if" concerns. They may be stated in definitive terms, but a careful reading will reveal that they are, in fact, restrictions on, or triggers of, the promises made elsewhere in the document.

Finally, the signature section should not be ignored. All the important parties must sign. In general, the document may be enforced in court only against a party who has signed it. The formality of the seal is being eliminated by many states, but some still require it. Grandiose wax impressions are a thing of the past, but the simple word "seal" following the signature is still needed in some jurisdictions.

Liquidated damages

Many contracts provide specified amounts of money to be paid in the event of a violation of the contract. These agreed amounts are "liquidated" damages because the parties to the contract have determined the monetary value of the breach or violation. Like liquid assets, they are reduced to a dollar value.

Starting with the most general rule that people are free to make whatever contracts they wish, liquidated damages clauses seem permissible and enforceable by courts. An important policy consideration countervails, however, that penalties in contracts are not enforced.

The rule against penalties developed as the equity courts struggled with grossly unfair contracts.[1] From a great discrepancy in bargaining positions came liquidated damages clauses that punish a party for breaching a contract and deter that breach. Traditionally, the difference between a penalty and a liquidated damages clause was determined by (1) the intent of the parties, (2) the difficulty or ease with which the court could quantify damages for the breach, and (3) whether or not the amount specified was a reasonable *ex ante* estimate of the losses associated with the breach. The first and last of these criteria depend on the amount, and the second is infrequently applied.[2]

Difficulty in determining damages has been used to justify a liquidated damages clause in a noncompetition agreement. An Indiana court enforced the required payment of $25,000 liquidated damages against an orthopedist who had violated his covenant not to practice in the same area for two years.[3]

The trend in the law is to look at the amount of the liquidated damages and question its reasonableness.[4] This does not imply a passive acceptance but rather a different analytical viewpoint. Courts still strongly disfavor and refuse to enforce agreements that suggest penalty, not appraisal.[5] The reasonableness of the amount can be assessed as of the time the contract was made or as of the time of the actual loss caused by the breach.[6]

Economic analysis, the current vogue in legal thinking, supports the use of these clauses, perhaps at a cost to morality and custom. It makes good commercial sense to allow parties to a contract to buy their way out of deals that have become bad. Holding a party to an agreement that is more costly than anticipated, simply to fulfill the other party's expectations and because there is a contract, is economically inefficient.

Restrictive covenants not to compete (noncompetition clauses)

Noncompetition clauses are common in health care contracts. An important public policy disfavoring restrictions on trade or the practice of a profession clashes with the general freedom to contract. Courts will not enforce restrictions on competition that are unreasonable, even if freely entered originally. Suits seeking enforcement of noncompetition clauses can demand that the court order the breaching party to stop or pay money damages or both. General distaste for ordering specific performance, especially where personal service is involved, moves the deliberations quickly to the money alternative.[7] What is considered "reasonable" does not vary as much as one might expect, as the cases discussed later suggest. The trend appears to favor the restriction if carefully drawn.[8] One particular area of difficulty is agreements not to compete made after the employment has commenced. It is recognized that without some enforceable means of securing business secrets, promotion and new phases of employment will bypass some worthy employees.[9]

Restrictions must be reasonable both in time and geographical area.[10] The area is generally wider for a specialist, and time limits vary. There may be reciprocal balancing—where one (e.g., time) is especially narrow, more restraint may be allowed in the other (e.g., geographical area). A contract clause preventing a chiropractor from practicing for five years within 10 miles was upheld as "eminently reasonable."[11] The court in that case noted, with approval, contract language allowing any reviewing court to revise restrictions as necessary to make them lawful.[12]

Traditional rationales for allowing restrictive covenants involved trade secrets or customer contacts.[13] A third, uniqueness of services, has come under attack.[14] None of these would seem to justify preventing the average physician from setting up shop down the street, if no patient lists are taken or announcements made to current patients. Still, these covenants are allowed and enforced against health care professionals. The party seeking enforcement may have to show that it is protecting a legitimate interest,[15] but this standard is far too loose and will lead to insecurity and litigation unless broadly defined. "Legitimate interest" may depend on the courts' perception of public need and good, not individual rights. In a suit involving a radiologist, an Ohio court refused to enforce a two-year noncompetition clause.[16] It was "unreasonable" in view of the local citizens' need for radiological services.

Noncompetition clauses are often accompanied by liquidated damages estimates (see previous discussion under "Liquidated damages"). A $30,000 liquidated damages clause was allowed in a suit against a physician for violation of his noncompetition agreement.[17] In a Wisconsin case, the unenforceability of a liquidated damages subsection did not render the entire noncompetition feature of the contract unenforceable.[18] The amount must be an estimate of cost with violation, not a penalty.

Indemnification

To *indemnify* is to promise to pay. An insurance contract is an indemnification agreement. A liability insurance policy is a promise to pay in the event of liability to a third party. The health care professional or institution that contracts to indemnify is insuring against the other party's losses.

Indemnification clauses are appearing in health care–related contracts with increasing frequency. They are dangerous, sometimes open-ended, and should generally be avoided.

Arbitration

Arbitration is an alternative means of dispute resolution that is justifiably becoming increasingly popular. Parties to a contract may agree to submit any disputes to arbitration, and may specify the form of the arbitration. Even without such a contract clause, once the dispute arises, the parties may then both agree to submit their problem to binding arbitration. Usually, however, one of the parties sees an advantage in taking the case to a traditional law court.

Binding arbitration agreements have long been used by major commercial interests. It is especially advantageous when the parties wish to continue their relationship following resolution of the dispute. In the typical arbitration, each of the parties appoints an individual and those two individuals select a third. An arbitration panel (or sometimes a single arbitrator) hears evidence and reviews documents. The procedure is much less formal than court, and the parties can sometimes represent themselves. Because it is less formal, restrictions on evidence that apply in court cases are not used. The inquiry can be more broad and more general than in a traditional lawsuit. Following the decision by the arbitration panel, the victorious party may seek to have the judgment enforced through a court of law, if necessary. Argument will then ensue over the validity of the commitment to submit to arbitration and the arbitration itself, but in the current crises of overwork facing today's courts, judges are not usually interested in rehearing the case.

The advantages of arbitration of contract disputes include time and money. The costs of pursuing an arbitration award are considerably less than the lawsuit, with its attendant pleadings, legal maneuvering, and formalities. Arbitration decisions can be had on a much more timely basis, which can be an advantage to both parties, not just one. Arbitration can also be conducted in private. Arbitration is especially useful in technical contracts. Arbitrators with expertise in the area can be appointed; they can bring to bear a knowledge base not shared by lay jurors or even judges. The possible need for and advisability of an arbitration clause should be considered in every contract.

Disappointingly, use of arbitration agreements in avoiding malpractice lawsuits has not spread beyond Michigan and Hawaii.[19] It should still be a consideration, especially where HMO or other prepaid contracts are in use.

TYPES OF CONTRACTS
Physician-patient contract

Although general contracting principles apply to all forms of agreements, different kinds of contracts have differing considerations, nuances, and points of emphasis.

The physician-patient relationship is based on a contract that creates a fiduciary relationship between the parties, and in which the physician impliedly promises the patient that he or she will exercise that degree of skill ordinarily possessed by his or her colleagues and practice according to accepted standards.

Most courts insist that negligence is the only type of lawsuit applicable to the physician-patient contract, since malpractice constitutes a breach of duty to the patient by the physician. They are unwilling to recognize breach of contract lawsuits premised on the theory of an implied promise by the physician.

Courts generally frown on implied contracts and are reluctant to enforce them, but those courts that apply the breach of contract laws do so on the theory that when a patient obtains a physician's services, there exists an implied contract in which the physician warrants that he or she will treat the patient with the degree of skill ordinarily possessed by members of the medical profession. These courts also hold that there is an implied promise to render care according to accepted practices. To confuse matters further, there are numerous reported cases espousing both legal philosophies.

Although a lawsuit for medical negligence and breach of contract may arise out of the same professional relationship, each one is distinct as to theory, proof, and damages. A few courts do allow the patient suing for malpractice to claim either negligence or breach of contract. These courts apply contract law on the theory that when a patient engages a physician's services, a contract ensues and failure to treat properly is a breach of contractual duty rather than breach of professional duty.

In the past, almost all malpractice lawsuits for breach of contract against physicians were based on an expressed promise by the physician to perform a specific procedure, cure the patient within a specific time, or achieve a certain result. Although a physician is free to do so, normally he or she would not ensure a result or guarantee improvement or a cure. A physician would be foolish to be more than optimistic or encouraging.

The relationship of the health care professional to the patient is not usually a contractual one. The patient has a quasi-contractual obligation to pay for the services rendered, but there are no implied warranties (as there are in the sale of goods) or contract commitments.[20] The parties to this relationship can enter a true contract, however, and can do so inadvertently.

Health care professionals can find themselves subject to a contract if specific promises are made. A general commitment to a good result, albeit inadvisable, is not enough to trigger contract liability.[21] An expressed guarantee of a stated result can create a contract.[22] These claims arise after plastic surgery (and may increase given the number of plastic surgeons using advertisements, pictures, and computer-generated depictions). More recently, the problem comes up in failed sterilization cases.

The physician should be aware that another source of malpractice involving breach of contract suits is for alleged abandonment of patients. Abandonment is usually claimed when the physician unilaterally discontinues the care of a patient without proper notice and opportunity for the patient to reasonably secure other medical care. Breach of contract actions have also been instituted when invasion of privacy and breach of confidentiality have been alleged, and for indiscretions on the part of the physician in regard to the patient's personal rights.

From a practical viewpoint in negligence suits, as compared with breach of contract actions, proof and procedural rules are much more formidable for the patient, and actually run in favor of the physician. In negligence the patient must establish the standard of care and the physician's failure to meet it. Expert testimony from another physician is usually required.

Despite these legal barriers, lawyers almost always sue for negligence because of the potential for large general damages for pain, suffering, and mental anguish. In breach of contract actions, only out-of-pocket losses, so-called special damages, are available. Several states allow general damages in breach of contract malpractice suits.

Contract suits are pressed where the statute of limitations has run and prevents civil lawsuit. The time during which a contract suit may be brought, i.e., the statutory limitations period, is usually longer than a tort suit. Although pain and suffering damages cannot be won in contract, at least some claim can be brought where the first deadline is passed. Insurance coverage may also be an issue. Lack of consideration is raised in defense of these cases, but if the promise was made before treatment, no separate consideration is required to make a contract.[23]

The potential dangers to physicians for more breach of contract lawsuits are on two fronts. As a result of the reactions to the malpractice crises, states are imposing significant restrictions on negligence suits. This may make breach of contract actions more attractive despite the limitations in damages. The more formidable potential danger lies in the development of HMOs. These are predicated on written, express contracts between provider and patient. Courts will have difficulty accepting breach of contract suits when the physician deviates from accepted standards of care since there is a written contract. Some HMO or other PPO literature allows the implication of a "superstandard" for health providers. Brochures or material that promise "the best," "the highest," or similar lofty ideals of care can reappear to haunt the organization in a contract suit.

Insurance contracts

Courts apply contract law principles when insureds attempt to enforce insurance policies against the issuing company. When an insurance company and policyholder disagree about coverage for a particular act or mischance, the court looks to the contract of insurance. Ordinary meaning prevails, with ambiguities interpreted against the author of the document—the company. Disputes often focus on exclusionary clauses and claims that the insurer acted in bad faith. Courts read exclusionary clauses (and the whole contract) in light of public policy considerations, which may void contracted coverage.

Exclusionary clauses and public policy. Exclusionary clauses and public policy become especially important in health care contracts for malpractice insurance. A contract of insurance often states what is not covered, for example, damages resulting from willful acts. There are also important reasons for society not to allow insurance coverage of such acts. Insurance payment of civil money penalties defeats whatever deterrent effect exists in tort awards. Intentional torts, punitive damages, and antitrust claims do arise in the health care setting, raising the question of insurance coverage.

Intentional torts. The general rule is that intentional torts cannot be covered by insurance. Confronted with an injured party and a choice of who will pay, an individual or an insurance company, courts appear to favor assessing the solvent (or impersonal) source. When interpreting the rule against coverage and when interpreting contract exclusionary clauses, the law can attempt to discriminate between an intended *act* and an intended *injury.* Some courts say that an unplanned magnification of the degree of harm or injury is not enough to escape the rule and maintain insurance coverage, if the eventual damage could have been foreseen.[24] Other courts require specific intent to do the harm caused before the insurance coverage is voided.[25] The lay public reads reports of court cases disputing contract language in such cases and is bemused. "Distinctions without a difference," they say. But fights like these over contract language are not mere lawyers' sophistry. The results are very important to the parties, great sums of money can be involved, and the precedential effects can be far-reaching.

Consider the physician sued for assault and battery by his patient. Will his malpractice contract of insurance provide coverage? The claim is based on an "intentional tort." After many suits and judicial decision, it is fairly well established that intentional tort claims arising in the setting of routine patient care are covered. Insurance contracts are written to cover these claims and public policies do not usually prohibit coverage, but other public policies can have an impact. Cases of sexual misconduct can defeat coverage.[26] However, courts read language in the contract broadly and maintain coverage, especially in the medical professional setting.[27] Public policy allows insurance coverage for the intentional wrongs of an employee and for other vicarious liability situations.

Punitive damages. Courts use a similar analytical process when the question is coverage for punitive damages: Did the contract provide for coverage of these extraordinary awards, and what are the public policy considerations? Punitive damages awards punish the

defendant and deter others from similar behavior. This penalty is more like a criminal law result, but may be applied in cases of outrageous misconduct in civil litigation. Even if the contract of insurance fails to exclude coverage for punitive damages, courts can disallow the coverage because the purpose of the award would be defeated.[28] Judges who allow insurance coverage of punitives point to a lack of deterrent effect[29] and the importance of freedom of contract.[30] When the plaintiff in a malpractice case threatens or demands a punitive damage award, the contracts of insurance and public policy become critically important.

Antitrust claims. Lawsuits for restraint of trade and antitrust violations also stimulate insurance coverage disputes. If there is an insurance contract that might cover such claims, it will be associated with the business of practice, rather than the practice itself. Activities as part of a medical staff or group practice, or as a trustee or officer, can lead to antitrust risk. Again, the contractual analysis is: Does the language of the policy cover this risk? Does the public interest allow coverage? Courts deciding whether coverage will be allowed focus on the punitive or compensatory nature of the treble damages awarded in antitrust suits.[31] This is true in any situation in which a statute allows multiples of damages.[32]

Duty to defend. Many court cases have supported the idea that the insurance company has a broader duty to defend than to indemnify.[33] That is, the company may be able to refuse to pay for the damages, but still may be required to provide a defense. The company will notify the insured of the possibility of no coverage, but then hire counsel and proceed with the defense of the case as if there were coverage. It is in the company's interest to defend; a court may later rule against the company's claim of exclusion. The insurer may be required to defend, even when public policy prohibits coverage,[34] by the contract of insurance[35] or by specific statute.[36] This is an important part of the insurance contract; legal expenses in defense of cases of even questionable merit can exceed $50,000.

Bad faith. Liability insurers seem powerful and implacable, but policyholders often succeed in suits on the contract of insurance. A growing area of litigation is against insurance companies in "bad faith." The insured asserts that the company has not acted in its policyholder's best interest, usually after a disastrous outcome in a malpractice case. In contracts of insurance for medical expenses, companies are vulnerable to claims that they unreasonably refused to pay.[37] Similarly, liability insurers are vulnerable to claims that they unreasonably refused to offer sufficient settlement. Policyholders usually bring these claims after a judgment exceeding policy limits, but they are sometimes brought by the patient-plaintiff in the original case.[38] State funds, created by statute, are not as susceptible to claims of bad faith, if those funds act in accord with their legislated responsibilities.[39] Although "bad faith" by the insurer may cause extended liability, the policyholder cannot get punitive damages and damages for emotional distress because of the company's refusal to settle.[40]

Although as yet unreported, contract claims of bad faith may arise under employment or subcontracting arrangements that promised to provide malpractice coverage. If the language in the agreement doesn't specify, the employer or group may not buy occurrence insurance, leaving questions of tail coverage for physicians leaving.

Claims-made coverage. As claims-made policies have become the dominant (and often only) form of malpractice coverage available, litigation over these contracts of insurance has become more common. In an Illinois case, Mr. and Mrs. Freeman sued Dr. A. At the time the suit was filed, Dr. A was covered by a St. Paul's Hospital claims-made policy, but he was not served (and did not notify St. Paul's) until after the policy cancellation. The trial court let St. Paul's out of the case, but on appeal, the contract language was held to be sufficiently ambiguous to require further proceedings.[41]

Dr. H was accused of leaving a needle in the knee of his arthroscopy patient. The patient's lawyer wrote Dr. H and then filed with the state's arbitration panel, all within the policy coverage term. Dr. H did not formally notify the company, as required in the policy, until three months later, 43 days after the expiration of claims made coverage period. The company attempted to deny coverage, but the court said that the company would have to show that it was prejudiced by the delay to avoid responsibility.[42] Although these cases exemplify the lengths to which the law favors an insured over an insurer, coverage over no coverage, it is foolish to rely on this attitude. Strict compliance with the contract's reporting requirements is fundamental.

Control with health plans. Health professionals confront increasing opportunities/demands to contract with HMOs, IPAs, and PPOs, as employees and as independent practitioners in a relationship with the organization. These entanglements must be regarded seriously, with a cautious eye to any effects on liability produced by the contract. The adage about marriage applies: Contract in haste – spend at leisure.

Vicarious liability. It should be apparent that the contracting organization assumes risk for the professional negligence of its employees and subcontractors. Hospital-employed[43] and independent contractor[44] physicians have triggered vicarious liability for the institution. PPOs are exposed to similar risks.[45] Less clear is the independent liability of the PPO. Hospitals are increasingly held to an independent duty of care.[46]

It is less apparent that contracts with PPOs create liability risks for the practitioners, risks that may be acceptable, but still must be considered. Consider the case of Dr. S. She has signed up with a PPO and that organization's patients are being referred to her. Dr. S usually sends the biopsy specimens taken in her office to a lab of her choosing, well known to her but expensive. The PPO has cut costs by making an arrangement with a discount lab service. The PPO's lab reports as benign a specimen Dr. S felt certain was malignant. Her own reading of the slide confirms her suspicion. Although the arrangement is otherwise satisfactory, Dr. S drops the PPO because of concern for her patients. Additional risks attend PPO contracts because of the inherent conflict between the physician's traditional broad, deep responsibilities and the surrender of control required in these contracts.

Getting in and out of the arrangement. The physician considering contracting with a PPO should read the entire document carefully, asking, "What happens if I want out?" Is the plan providing liability coverage not otherwise in place? If so, what happens on termination of the relationship? Will the PPO provide tail coverage or an extended endorsement? Circumstances of departure should be anticipated. Are there due process protections for the panel physicians? What are the limitations on the plan's use of the physician's name? The answer is, plan for the worst and hope for the best.

Disappointment is common among physicians entering PPO contracts. An easy exit on short notice probably offers the best protection. Although contracts for terms of years are the rule elsewhere in health care, a 60-day notice should be bargained for in the PPO contract with an individual physician. The master plan, the contract between the group of providers and the IPA or HMO, will be for a longer term and for more notice on termination.

Beware of "evergreen" clauses. Contracts often provide for automatic renewal, that is, if the party doesn't notify the other, the term of the contract extends for another stated period. Thus, the physician who assumes that she may by inactivity resign from the plan can be disappointed.

Payment provisions. The major source of disappointment for physicians contracting with PPOs is compensation. These organizations save money and offer reduced costs to insurance companies, employers, and the public. PPOs often advertise enhanced quality, concern, and convenience. Furthermore, the plan must take overhead out for the promotion and operations. Where does this money come from? The theoretical advantage of bulk purchasing power and utilization efficiencies are rarely sufficient. Providers must be paid less, and usually later.

Examine the contract for compensation provisions. A controlled fee schedule is easily recognized, but typically the plan will hold back a percentage against losses (and promise a bonus if there is a surplus). How will these amounts be calculated? What expenses are costed against the withheld pool? Are the books open to individual physicians or the physician group's representatives? Are rights to earned compensation lost on withdrawal? In some parts of the United States where HMOs and PPOs are ubiquitous, brokers invite providers to sign agreements, obtaining access to multiple plans. These may be in the form of "power of attorney," giving extensive authority to the broker. Unlimited powers of attorney can enmesh the physician in multiple and varied commitments, without even the rudimentary notice provisions of responsible plans. Capitated physicians, usually the primary care providers, should ask about what happens if there is an unexpectedly high utilization. Can the plan obtain catastrophic reinsurance?

Unjust dismissal and employment contracts. Suits over hiring and firing practices are burgeoning, affecting physicians as employees and employers. In most reported cases involving physicians as plaintiffs, physicians base employment or staff privileges claims on civil or statutory rights.[47] More often, physicians find themselves the target of these lawsuits, brought by disgruntled or dismissed employees. This risk can be minimized or eliminated.

Problems most often arise over the dismissal of "at will" employees. At will employment can be ended at any time by either party for any reason; the verbal or written contract provides for no fixed term and no procedures for termination. Statutes and recent court cases limit at will discharges. State and federal legislation contains multiple specific reasons that cannot be the basis for terminating an employee; the legislation creates a right to sue for the employee fired for one of the impermissible reasons.[48] Judges have allowed suits against firing employers in three areas: public policy,[49] good faith and fair dealing, and violations of employee handbook provisions.[50] Other courts have found that employee manual provisions do not give the employee the right to sue.[51]

To avoid or win suits brought by fired or dissatisfied employees, common sense will help, and knowledge and documentation will succeed. Take, for example, sexual harrassment. Foreknowledge may have saved Dr. F. After she fired Nurse M, he sued Dr. F, claiming he'd been sexually harrassed and sexually discriminated against. According to federal law, sexual harrassment is "unwelcome sexual advances, requests for sexual favors, and other verbal or physical conduct of a sexual nature. . . ."[52] Dr. F defended the case on three bases: (1) M had willingly participated; (2) the cartoons, jokes,

pinches, and so on, were not harrassment; and (3) she treated all her employees that way. Even without being aware of all the details of sex discrimination law, Dr. F could have done much to prevent the problem. A thought-out program of assessment and documentation is now necessary for every employee, and these efforts should be coordinated with the basic contract of employment.

Physicians should adopt a few of the procedures used by bigger businesses. Regular recorded performance reviews should include opportunities for the employees to express any dissatisfactions. Poor work habits, absenteeism, and especially any patient care problems will be rational bases for termination. The extent of documentation should be balanced between the need to protect against employment claims and the need to protect against claims of negligence in maintaining a dangerous employee. Respondeat superior hiring and liability for the employee cannot be avoided by this balancing, however. Violation of statutory prohibitions are avoided by concentrating on the requirements of the job. Group practices with 15 or more empoloyees are subject to Title VII restrictions. A group with a large Hispanic practice may not refuse to hire or retain anyone who is not Hispanic, but may require that the staff speak Spanish. The orthopedist in the group may not fire her technician because he has reached the age of 70, but may fire the technician because he can no longer perform the physical requirements of the job. Contract terms and employment manuals can help, but there must be awareness of legal requirements beyond the employment agreement to avoid these problems.

CONTRACTUAL LIABILITY OF MINORS

In general, without a statute to the contrary, a minor has the capacity to incur only voidable contractual duties.[53] Loosely stated, this means that although a minor may bind an adult in contract, the adult may not bind the minor.[54] The infant's right to avoid his or her contract is not defeated merely because he or she is nearly of age.[55] Nor may another person purporting to act for the minor bind the minor in contract unless the actor is authorized by a court to do so.[56]

Necessaries

In common law under the doctrine of necessaries, one who sells goods to a minor can charge the minor's father if the goods are necessary for the maintenance or support of the child. Depending on the jurisdiction and the circumstances, the minor may be liable for the value of the necessaries furnished.[57] This is particularly true where the necessaries were provided to the minor on his or her own credit.[58] However, if the minor makes a bad bargain, enforcement of a minor's contract for necessaries is limited to the reasonable market value of the necessaries furnished.[59]

The meaning of the term "necessaries" varies from case to case and jurisdiction to jurisdiction.[60] It may include not only those services required to sustain life but also those suitable for the individual according to his or her circumstances and condition in life.[61] Whether articles furnished to a minor are necessaries may depend on the minor's financial situation, his or her social position as well as the family's, their requirements and needs, the nature and quality of the articles furnished, the adaptability of such articles to the needs of the minor and the family, and what alternative sources may exist to obtain those articles.[62] An article may not be necessary if the minor already has a sufficient supply of it[63] or if a parent or guardian is able and willing to supply it.[64]

In some jurisdictions, whether goods furnished to a minor are necessaries is a question for the court.[65] In others, the judge defines the class and character of articles that may be held as necessaries, and the jury then decides whether the articles at issue fall within the class.[66]

Health care

Medical, dental, or hospital services reasonably required by a minor are usually classified as necessaries.[67] Thus, the minor may be held liable for such services,[68] particularly if the services were furnished on his or her own credit.[69] However, a minor may not be liable for even necessary health care services when living with or supported by a parent or guardian,[70] unless the parent or guardian refuses to provide those services to the infant[71] or is unable to do so.[72] In at least one case, the court ruled that a minor was liable for the value of necessary medical services even though the minor lived with or was supported by a parent or guardian.[73] An emancipated minor is generally liable for necessary health services,[74] as may be the case with one whose parents are deceased.[75]

Legal services

Legal services may also be necessaries in some circumstances[76]; hence, an infant may be liable for the value of such services.[77] Whereas prosecution of a personal injury claim may be necessary,[78] protection of an infant's rights to or interest in an estate may not be.[79] Some courts have held minors liable for attorneys' fees whether or not the associated legal services were necessaries.[80]

END NOTES

1. J. Calamari & J. Perillo, *The Law of Contracts* 639-40 (1987).
2. *Id.* at 641.
3. *Raymundo v. Hammond Clinic Ass'n.* 449 N.E.2d 65 (Ind. 1983). The court was impressed by the figures quoted. The clinic made more than $8 million in 1974, the year before Dr. Raymundo's breach of contract. The orthopedic department brought in $384,595 and Dr. Raymundo $103,262 of that. The contract provided for a 2-year limit in a 25-mile radius and liquidated damages at $25,000 in the event of competition in the first year after breach, $15,000 in the second. The clinic surely spent more than $25,000 in pursuing the case, as did Dr. Raymundo in defending it.
4. Restatement Second, *Contracts* §356(1). Damages for breach by either party may be liquidated in the agreement but only at an amount that is reasonable in light of the anticipated or actual loss caused by the breach and difficulties of proof of loss. A term fixing unreasonably large liquidated damages as a penalty unenforceable on grounds of public policy. See especially Illustration no. 2.
5. *Vernitron Corp. v. CF48 Ass'ns,* 104 A.D.2d 409, 478 N.Y.S.2d 933 (1984).
6. Restatement, *supra,* note 3.
7. Impossibility of enforcement and the taint of involuntary servitude are involved.
8. The cost of litigating these clauses is recognized. Note *Post-Employment Restraint Agreements: A Reassessment,* 53 U. Chic. L. Rev. 703, 705 (1985).
9. Leibman and Nathan, *The Enforceability of Post-Employment Non-competition Agreements Formed After At-Will Employment Has Commenced: The "Afterthought" Agreement,* 60 So. Cal. L. Rev. 1465 (1987).
10. "Covenants not to compete are unreasonable restraints unless they are tightly limited as to both time and area." *Pathology Consultants v. Gratton,* 343 N.W.2d 428, 434 (Iowa 1984).
11. *Wyatt v. Dishong,* 127 Ill. App. 3d 716, 469 N.E.2d 608 (1984).
12. *Id.* at N.E.2d 610. More often, courts reject these reformation opportunities.
13. Applicability of these principles to a specific situation may justify broad restraints. *Sigma Chems. v. Harris,* 586 F. Supp. 704 (1986). The former employee was held to worldwide restrictions with no fixed time limits.
14. J. Calamari & J. Perillo, *Contracts* 686 (3d ed. 1987).
15. *Reddy v. Community Health Found. of Man.,* 298 S.E.2d 287 (W. Va. 1982). Allowed a 3-year and 30-mile limit.
16. *Williams v. Hobb,* 9 Ohio App. 3d 331, 460 N.E.2d 287 (1983).
17. *Webb v. West Side District Hospital,* 193 Cal. Rptr. 80 (2d Dist. 1983).
18. *Fields Found. Ltd. v. Christensen,* 103 Wis. 2d 465, 309 N.W.2d 125 (1981).
19. Saunders, *The Quest for Balance: Public Policy and Due Process in Medical Malpractice Arbitration Agreements,* 23 Harv. J. Leg. 267 (1986). The author states that there is no conclusory evidence that contracts to arbitrate disputes have reduced costs in Michigan.
20. *Dorney v. Harris,* 482 F. Supp. 323 (D. Colo. 1980).
21. *Depenbroh v. Kaiser Found. Health Plan,* 144 Cal. Rptr. 724, 70 Cal. App. 3d 170 (2d Dist. 1978).
22. *Murray v. University of Penn. Hospital,* 490 A.2d 839 (Penn. Super. 1985).
23. *Sard v. Hardy,* 379 A.2d 1014 (Md. 1977).
24. It is "[i]rrelevant [that the injury was] different in character or magnitude from the harm . . . subjectively intended." *Farmer in the Dell Enterprises, Inc. v. Farmers Mutual Ins. Co.,* 514 A.2d 1097 (1986). In this case, setting a fire to trash outside a building resulted in a foreseeable destruction of the entire structure.
25. *Brown v. St. Paul Fire & Marine Ins. Co.,* 177 Ga.App 215, 338 S.E.2d 721 (1985). The unintended result of an intentional act did not trigger the exclusion clause when the insured's gunfire killed a bystander.
26. *Illinois Farmers Insurance Co. v. Judith G.,* 379 N.W.2d 638 (Minn. App 1986).

27. *St. Paul Fire & Marine Insurance v. Asbury,* 149 Ariz. 565, 720 P.2d 540 (1986). The contract's words "providing or withholding of professional services" were held to cover the claimed improper manipulations during a gynecological exam.

28. *See, e.g., Northwestern Casualty Company v. McNulty,* 307 F.2d 432 (5th Cir. 1962).

29. *See, e.g., Lazenby v. Universal Underwriters Ins. Co.,* 214 Tenn. 639, 383 S.W.2d 1 (1964).

30. *Koehring Co. v. American Mutual Liability Ins. Co.,* 564 F.Supp. 303 (E.D. Wis. 1983).

31. *See California Shoppers Inc. v. Royal Globe Ins. Co.,* 175 Cal.App.3d 1, 221 Cal.Rptr. 171 (1985).

32. For example, a Wisconsin case addressed triple damages allowed by statute for dog bites in *Cieslewicz v. Mutual Service Casualty Ins. Co.,* 84 Wis.2d 91, 267 N.W.2d 595 (1978).

33. *See, e.g., National Grange Mutual Ins. v. Continental Casualty Ins.,* 650 F.Supp. 1404 (S.D. N.Y. 1986).

34. *Burnham Shoes, Inc. v. West American Ins. Co.,* 813 F.2d 328 (11 CA 1987). Many insurance policies will, as in this case, expressly commit the company to providing a defense.

35. Sharpe and Shaffer, *The Parameters of an Insurer's Duty to Defend,* 19 Forum 555 (1984).

36. *Cf. Jaffe v. Cranford Ins. Co.,* 168 Cal.App.3d 930, 214 Cal.Rptr. 567 (1985), where the court, as an aside, said: "[A]n insured may be entitled to legal defense against a cause of action even though the insurer is ultimately prohibited from paying losses therefrom." In *Jaffe,* a psychiatrist asserted that his insurance company should have defended him against criminal charges of fraud and theft arising from his practice.

37. In a Mississippi court, Crenshaw won the $20,000 he had demanded from his insurance company *and* won $1.6 million in punitive damages based on the company's bad faith refusal to pay. *Bankers Life and Casualty Co. v. Crenshaw,* #85-1765, USSC, May 16, 1988. Aetna denied Ms. Armstrong's post-CVA home care coverage and the home care agency sued Ms. Armstrong. She sued Aetna. The jury awarded $35,000 compensation (on a $25,000 home care bill), $50,000 for Aetna's breach of duty to act in good faith, and $125,000 in punitive damages. Aetna had asserted that the care was custodial, Ms. Armstrong said that it was blended. On appeal, the court dropped the punitive damages for lack of malicious intent by Aetna. *Staff Builders, Inc. v. Armstrong,* #87-196, 37 Ohio St.3d 298, Ohio SC, July 6, 1988.

38. *Phillips v. Southern California Physicians Ins. Exchange,* #B016723, Calif. Ct. App. 2d App.Div., Aug. 27, 1986. Conclusive establishment of the liability of the insured is a prerequisite. *Synch v. Ins. Co. of North America,* #B-003996, Calif. Ct. App., Oct. 15, 1985.

39. *Isaacson v. California Ins. Guarantee Ass'n,* #LA 32116, Calif.SC, March 7, 1988. *Finkbinder v. Medical Professional Liability Catastrophe Loss Fund,* #381 C.D. 1988, Pa. Commonwealth Ct., Sept. 1, 1988.

40. *Benkert v. Medical Protective Co.,* #86-1177 & -1587, 6th Cir., March 16, 1988.

41. *St. Paul Ins. Co. of Illinois v. Armas,* #87-3017, Ill.App.Ct., 1st Dist., Aug. 2, 1988.

42. *St. Paul Fire and Marine Ins. Co. v. House,* # 322, Md.Ct.Special App., Nov. 12, 1987.

43. *Bing v. Thunig,* 2 N.Y.2d 656, 143 N.E.2d 3 (1957).

44. *Adamski v. Tacoma General Hospital,* 20 Wash.App. 98, 597 P.2d 970 (1978).

45. *Boyd v. Albert Einstein Medical Center,* 3133 Philadelphia 1987. Pa. Sup.Ct., Sept. 22, 1988.

46. *Darling v. Charleston Community Memorial Hospital,* 33 Ill.2d 326, 211 N.E.2d 253 (1965), *cert. denied,* 383 U.S. 946 (1966).

47. *See, e.g., Zaklama v. Mt. Sinai Medical Center,* #87-5428 & -6554, 11th Cir., April 12, 1988.

48. Examples include the Civil Rights Act, the Age Discrimination in Employment Act, and veterans' protections. State statutes may include service in the national guard or jury duty; even local jurisdictions may have such laws.

49. For example, if the employee claims he was fired for refusing to obey an illegal or otherwise impermissible order. Whistle-blowers' suits are under this category.

50. *Duldulao v. Saint Mary of Nazareth Hospital,* 505 N.E.2d 314 (Ill. 1987).

51. Discharge procedures in manual asserted to have been violated. *Garmon v. Health Group of Atlanta, Inc.,* 359 S.E.2d 450 (Ga. App. 1987).

52. 23 U.S.C. Sect. 703, Sect. 1604.11 of the E.E.O.C. Guidelines. The harrassment must adversely affect the employment as well.

53. Restatement, *Contracts* 2d § 14 (1979), 42 Am. Jur. 2d, Infants, § 58. For a criticism of this principle, *see* Note, *A Reevaluation of the Contractual Rights of Minors,* 57 UMKC L. Rev. 145 (1988). For an analysis of analogous concepts under civil law, *see* Note, *The Contractual Capacity of Minors: A Survey of the Prior Law and the New Articles,* 62 Tul. L. Rev. 745 (1981). Some states have codified the voidability of minors' contracts. *See, e.g., Ehrsan v. Borgen,* 185 Kan. 776, 347 P.2d 260 (1959). *Paulson v. McMillen,* 8 Wash.2d 295, 111 P.2d 983 (1941). Others have legislatively permitted minors to contract. *See, e.g., Valley National Bank v. Glover,* 62 Ariz. 538, 159 P.2d 292 (1945).

54. *Williston on Contracts,* § 223 (W. Jaeger ed., 3d ed. 1967); *Hersh v. Lopez,* 70 Ariz. 201, 218 P.2d 727 (1950); *Cain v. Garner,* 169 Ky. 638, 185 S.W. 122 (1916); *but see Porter v. Wilson,* 106 N.H. 270, 209 A.2d 730 (1965), *Kelly v. Furlong,* 194 Minn. 465, 261 N.W. 460 (1935), and *Valencia v. White,* 134 Ariz. 139, 654 P.2d 287 (Ariz. App. 1982) for the minority, contrary view. *See also, Parks v. Lyons,* 219 S.C. 40, 64 S.E.2d 123 (1951) (an infant who asserts contractual rights is bound by reciprocal obligations). An infant's contracts are also voidable when both contracting parties are infants. *Hurwitz v. Barr,* 193 A.2d 360 (D.C. App. 1963), *Drude v. Curtis,* 183 Mass. 317, 67 N.E. 317 (1913).

55. *Ex parte McFerren,* 184 Ala. 223, 63 So. 159 (1913).

56. 42 Am. Jur. 2d Infants § 58.

57. *Mutual Life Ins. Co. v. Schiavone,* 63 App. D.C. 257, 71 F.2d 980 (1934), *In re O'Leary's Estate,* 352 Pa. 254, 42 A.2d 624 (1945), *Foster v. Adcock,* 161 Tenn. 217, 30 S.W. 2d 239, (1930), *Russell v. Buck,* 116 Vt. 40, 68 A.2d 691 (1949). In some states, minors are bound by statute on their contracts for necessaries. *Ehrsam v. Borgen, supra,* note 1, 185 Kan. 776, *Paulson v. McMillen, supra,* note 1, 8 Wash. 2d 295.

58. *Burnand v. Irigoyen,* 30 Cal.2d 861, 186 P.2d 417 (1947). Conversely, the minor may not be liable for necessaries furnished him or her on the credit of another. *In re Johnstone's Estate,* 64 Ill. App.2d 447, 212 N.E.2d 143 (1965).

59. *Merrick v. Stephens,* 337 S.W. 713 (Mo. App. 1960).

60. *Id., Smitti v. Roth Cadillac Co.,* 145 Pa. Super. 292, 21 A.2d 127 (1941).

61. *Trask v. Davis,* 297 S.W.2d 792 (Mo. App. 1957).

62. *Spaulding v. New England Furniture Co.,* 154 Me. 330, 147 A.2d 916 (1959).

63. *Mitchell v. Campbell & Fetter Bank,* 135 Ind. App. 523, 195 N.E.2d 489 (1964).

64. *Bensinger's Coexecutors v. West,* 255 S.W.2d 27 (Ky. 1953).

65. *Publishers Agency, Inc. v. Brooks,* 14 Mich. App. 634, 166 N.W.2d 26 (1968).

66. *Wiggins Estate Co. v. Jeffrey,* 246 Ala. 183, 19 So.2d 769 (1944).

67. *Santasiero v. Briggs,* 278 A.D. 15, 103 N.Y. S.2d 1 (1951). *See generally* Annotation, *Infant's Liability for Medical, Dental, or Hospital Services,* 53 ALR 4th 1249.

68. *Hagerman v. Mutual Hospital Ins., Inc.,* 175 Ind. App. 293, 371

N.E.2d 394 (1978), *Reed Bros. v. Giberson,* 143 Me. 4, 54 A.2d 535 (1947), *Rehg v. Giancola,* 391 S.W.2d 934 (Mo. App. 1965), *Przestrzelski v. Board of Ed.,* 71 A.D.2d 743, 419 N.Y. S.2d 256 (1979). *See also Madison General Hospital v. Haack,* 124 Wis. 2d 398, 369 N.W.2d 663 (1985) (limited to express or implied-in-fact contracts to pay for necessaries; "necessaries doctrine not applicable to sick, indigent 16-year-old in labor, as she was in no condition to agree to anything").

69. *Estate of Hammond v. Aetna Casualty,* 141 Ill. App. 3d 963, 491 N.E.2d 84 (1986), *Mackey v. Schreckengaust,* 27 S.W.2d 752 (Mo. App. 1930). *See* note 6, *supra,* and accompanying text.

70. *Estate of Hammond, supra,* note 17, 141 Ill. App. 3d 963, *Gaspard v. Breaux,* 413 So.2d 288 (La. App. 1982), *Blue Cross/Blue Shield of New Hampshire-Vermont v. St. Cyr,* 123 N.H. 137, 459 A.2d 226 (1983), *Albany Medical Center Hospital v. Johnston,* 102 A.D.2d 915, 477 N.Y. S.2d 499 (1984), *Lane v. Aetna Casaulty & Surety Co.,* 48 N.C. App. 634, 269 S.E.2d 711 (1980), *petition denied,* 302 N.C. 219, 276 S.E.2d 916 (1981).

71. *Charles S. Wilson Memorial Hospital v. Puskar,* 26 Misc.2d 281, 208 N.Y. S.2d 229 (1960), *Gardner v. Flowers,* 529 S.W.2d 708 (Tenn. 1975).

72. *Przestrzelski v. Board of Ed., supra,* note 16, 71 A.D.2d 743, *Greenville Hospital System v. Smith,* 269 S.C. 653, 239 S.E.2d 657 (1977), *Gardner v. Flowers, supra,* note 19, 529 S.W.2d 708.

73. *Scott County School Dist. Iv. Asher,* 263 Ind. 47, 324 N.E.2d 496 (1975) (parent also held liable).

74. *Cidis v. White,* 71 Misc.2d 481, 336 N.Y. S.2d 362 (1972), *Daubert v. Mosley,* 487 P.2d 353, 56 A.L.R. 3d 1328 (Okla. 1971), *Chappell v. Smith,* 208 Va. 272, 156 S.E.2d 572 (1967).

75. *Nugen v. Hildebrand,* 145 W.Va. 420, 114 S.E.2d 896 (1960).

76. *Fanelli v. Barclay,* 100 Misc.2d 471, 419 N.Y. S.2d 813 (1979). *See generally* Annotation, *Infant's Liability for Services Rendered by Attorney at Law Under Contract with Him,* 13 A.L.R. 3d 1251.

77. *Leonard v. Alexander,* 50 Cal. App.2d 385, 122 P.2d 984 (1942), *Yellen v. Bloom,* 326 Ill. App. 134, 61 N.E.2d 269 (1945).

78. *Goldberg v. Perlmutter,* 308 Ill. App. 84, 31 N.E.2d 333 (1941).

79. *Watts v. Houston,* 65 Okla. 151, 165 P.128 (1917).

80. *Porter v. Wilson,* 106 N.H. 270, 209 A.2d 730, 13 A.L.R. 3d 1247 (1965), *Sneed v. Sneed,* 681 P.2d 754 (Okla. 1984).

CHAPTER 6

Civil trials

ALAN C. HOFFMAN, J.D., F.C.L.M.

COMMENCEMENT OF ACTION AND SERVICE OF PROCESS
PLEADINGS AND MOTIONS
DISCOVERY
TRIAL PRACTICE
THE TRIAL ITSELF
POST-TRIAL PROCEEDINGS

American law, like its predecessor, English common law, has evolved to facilitate the resolution of disputes among parties. To implement this legal philosophy and public policy, the legislatures have developed procedural rules—in other words, the game plan that will be followed in the pursuit of justice.

It is well known that victory or defeat at trial may depend purely on the lawyer's knowledge of and skill in applying the rules of procedure. We are a country of laws and, even though victory or defeat at trial is not predicated only by justice and who is right, but also on who is best in the courtroom, the outcome is supported by procedural rules and how they are employed.

The procedural aspects of a medical malpractice action are governed by the rules of civil procedure in effect in the jurisdiction in which the action is commenced. To litigate successfully (either as a plaintiff or as a defendant) in a medical malpractice action, it is necessary to understand the applicable procedural rules and act accordingly. Although each of the 50 states has different civil rules, an increasing number of states model their rules after the Federal Rules of Civil Procedure. Because an evaluation of the rules of each jurisdiction is beyond the scope of this textbook, we discuss the procedural aspects of medical malpractice litigation using the Federal Rules of Civil Procedure as an example. The Federal Rules of Civil Procedure govern the procedure in U.S. district courts in all suits of a civil nature whether they are cases at law in equity, or in admiralty, with the exceptions set forth in Rule 81. Recent changes, which are discussed later, state that the rules are to be construed and administered to secure the just, speedy, and inexpensive determination of every action.

COMMENCEMENT OF ACTION AND SERVICE OF PROCESS

Malpractice actions do not appear out of nowhere; someone must first decide to sue someone else. Even if the plaintiff, the one who brings the action, concludes that the action is one for which the courts will grant relief, a litigant must consider the probability of winning a lawsuit. The plaintiff must ask whether the defendant, the person who has caused the injury, can be found and brought into court; whether witnesses and documents will be available to support the claims being sued on; whether this proof will be believed; whether the potential adversary can justify its conduct or establish any defenses to the action; and whether an accurate assessment of the law can be made ahead of time.

A plaintiff must consider whether what is won will be worth the time, the effort, and the expense it will cost, and must weigh against this the alternatives to suit, among them settlement or arbitration. The potential litigant must decide whether the injury is one for which a monetary payment will be satisfactory; for instance, does the defendant have insurance?

Initially the plaintiff must determine in which court to bring action. The plaintiff may have some choice, but it will be a limited one, because the court selected must have jurisdiction over the subject matter (that is, the constitution and statutes under which the court operates must have conferred on it the power to decide this type of case) and must also have jurisdiction over the person.

The subject-matter jurisdiction of the federal courts is severely limited.

The courts of original jurisdiction are the courts on which cases are brought and tried, and one court of appellate jurisdiction sits only to review the decisions of lower courts. The courts of general jurisdiction are organized into districts comprising for the most part several counties, although the largest or most populous counties each may constitute single districts. These district courts hear cases of many kinds and are competent to grant every kind of relief, but in order to bring a case in one of them a plaintiff must have a claim for more than a specific amount. The federal government of course also operates a system of courts. The principal federal courts are the U.S. district courts, courts of original jurisdiction of which there is at least one in every state; the 13 U.S. courts of appeals, each of which reviews the decisions of federal district courts in several states within its circuit (with the exception of the courts of appeals for the District of Columbia Circuit and Federal Circuit); and the Supreme Court of the United States, which not only reviews the decisions of federal courts but also reviews decisions of state courts that turn on an issue of federal law. The jurisdiction over subject matter of the U.S. district courts extends to many cases involving federal law, and also to many cases that do not involve federal law; the latter are cases in which there is diversity of citizenship and the required amount in controversy is at stake. Not every court that has jurisdiction over the subject matter and jurisdiction over the defendant will hear a case. It also is necessary that an action be brought in a court having proper venue.

A medical malpractice action is initiated by filing a complaint with the court.[1] When the complaint is filed, the appropriate informational forms are filled out for the clerk of courts and the filing fee is paid. Thereafter, the summons (which is issued by the clerk) and the complaint are served on the defendant.[2] Service can be made in any number of ways. For instance, a defendant may be served by regular or certified mail (initiated by either the plaintiff or the clerk) or in person by a U.S. marshall, sheriff, or process server. Depending on the rules in effect in the jurisdiction, the defendant may be served in person, at his or her residence, at his or her workplace, or by publication of a notice in a newspaper of general circulation.

PLEADINGS AND MOTIONS

After the defendant has been served, he or she must, through an attorney, file with the court and serve a response on the plaintiff's counsel. Failure to do so will result in the entry of a default judgment. Rules 7 through 16 of the Federal Rules of Civil Procedure deal with pleadings and motion practice.

Pleadings

Rule 7 deals with the forms of pleadings allowed, including a complaint, an answer, a counterclaim (a claim against the person making the complaint), or a third-party claim (a claim against yet another individual). Rule 7 is specific in that no other pleading shall be allowed other than as set forth. Rule 7 also states that all motions when an individual seeks to have something done shall be according to a written motion, except at hearing and shall be in the form prescribed by the local jurisdiction or in the court as heard. In addition, Rule 7 abolishes the ancient forms of demurrers and pleas. Rule 8 requires that a pleading set forth a claim for relief as well as a short and plain statement of the grounds on which the court's jurisdiction depends, a short and plain statement of the claim showing that the pleader is entitled to relief, and a demand for judgment for the relief to which the plaintiff deems he or she is entitled. Relief in the alternative may be demanded. A party may state in short and plain terms defenses to each claim and shall admit or deny the averments on which the adverse party relies. A party may allege affirmative defenses in the pleadings. Under federal rules, if there is an averment in a pleading to which a responsive pleading is required, other than the *ad damnum,* then it is admitted when not denied in responsive pleadings. In earlier federal rules, it was required that the plaintiff plead facts setting forth the cause of action. Under the new federal rules, only noticed pleading is required, which requires the barest necessity of pleadings.

Motions in general

It has been said that an excess of 200 motions can be made prior to, during, and subsequent to trial. Some of the motions are motion to dismiss, motion to amend a complaint, motion to suggest or spread death of record, motion to amend pleadings, motion to add parties, motion to disqualify, motion for a mistrial, motion for a physical examination inspection, motion to exclude, motion for relief from the final judgment, and so on. When motions are made, they must be noticed up in accordance with the local rules, and motions will be argued accordingly. Depending on the nature and the type of motion, the motion itself may be briefed.

Generally speaking, the defendant files an answer to the complaint, setting forth in short and simple terms his or her defenses to each claim, as well as any affirmative defenses that exist.[3] In the answer, the health care defendant may assert any counterclaim against the plaintiff. For instance, if a defendant physician remains unpaid for services rendered to the plaintiff, a claim for the unpaid balance should be set forth in the counterclaim.[4] Failure to assert this claim as a counterclaim may constitute a waiver to assert it later. The initial complaint is usually couched in general terms. Frequently, the answer attempts to obtain specifics and details from the plaintiff. As a result, several exchanges of supplemental complaints and answers can occur.

In some instances the health care professional may file a third-party complaint against a person, not a party to the original action, who is or may be liable to the professional for all or part of the plaintiff's claim.[5] Although it is rather unusual to find third-party complaints filed in medical malpractice actions, there have been instances in which a physician was sued for an untoward effect that resulted from use of a prescription medication, and the physician initiated a third-party action against the pharmaceutical company.

Sometimes a motion, instead of an answer, is filed in response to the complaint. In fact, Rule 12(b) specifically provides that certain defenses may, at the option of the defendant, be made by motion. These include the following:

1. Lack of jurisdiction over the subject matter
2. Lack of jurisdiction over the person
3. Improper venue
4. Insufficiency of process
5. Insufficiency of service of process
6. Failure to state a claim on which relief may be granted
7. Failure to join a party under Rule 19.

The number of motions that may be made in response to the complaint is practically endless. The law of the jurisdiction and the specific facts of the situation must always be carefully considered to determine whether dispositive motions should be filed in response to the complaint. Alternatively, motions to strike certain portions of the complaint may be successful, leaving a limited number of allegations to which an answer must be filed.

After all the preliminary filings have been completed, the defendant may appear before a judge who has reviewed the pleading on a motion for summary judgment or judgment on the pleading. The judge then decides whether there are sufficient facts for the case to go forward and, if so, sets a preliminary trial date. Dismissal of the case may be appealed by the plaintiff.

DISCOVERY

After the identities of the parties have been determined, service has been completed, and preliminary motions have been decided, the litigation enters its so-called "discovery" phase. In the federal court system, discovery is governed by Section V of the Federal Rules of Civil Procedure (Depositions and Discovery). To investigate thoroughly the merits of the allegations and defenses, parties may discover by one or more of the following methods: (1) depositions upon oral interroga-

tories or written questions[6]; (2) written interrogatories[7]; (3) production of documents[8]; (4) physical and mental examinations of the plaintiff[9]; and (5) requests for admission.[10] Federal Rule 26 was amended effective December 1993 and the result was substantial changes on several procedures including disclosure of witnesses and subject matter of testimony; in addition, all relevant documents must be identified and damage calculations must be presented.

The Federal Rules of Civil Procedure do not dictate the order of discovery. Usually, all parties proceed by initially filing interrogatories and requests for production of documents. The defendant health care practitioner may, for example, file written interrogatories requesting that the plaintiff provide certain background information relevant to the issues. For instance, the plaintiff may be required to identify all health care received as a result of the alleged negligence that is the subject matter of the lawsuit, the costs of that health care, an outline of the damages sought in the litigation, and the identity of expert witnesses who will be testifying on the plaintiff's behalf. After the plaintiff has provided the answers to the interrogatories, the defendant may then file a request for production of the report from an expert witness for the plaintiff. The plaintiff proceeds in a similar fashion against the defendant.

After the interrogatories have been answered and the documents produced, the litigants proceed to the deposition phase of discovery. Although it is possible to conduct written depositions on written interrogatories (i.e., where the court reporter reads questions prepared by counsel and records the answers), this is generally limited to mundane matters such as obtaining medical records from the offices of health care practitioners and hospitals. Generally, depositions are conducted orally. It is conventional for the defendant's counsel first to take the plaintiff's deposition to develop the factual basis of the plaintiff's case and obtain information helpful to the defense.

The counsel for the plaintiff will depose the defendant health care practitioner to obtain information that will assist in the prosecution of the lawsuit. Prior to taking the deposition, the counsel for the plaintiff will have received and reviewed interrogatory answers, minutely dissected the appropriate and relevant medical records, and perhaps consulted with an expert of his or her own to conduct the deposition intelligently. The depositions of the parties and their expert witnesses are the most important aspects of a medical malpractice case. After the depositions have been taken, the counsel may evaluate their respective positions and, if appropriate, make efforts to settle the litigation.

Discovery includes a request for admission of facts, which is a request to the opposing party to admit that a given set of facts or statement is true. If the request is not denied, it is deemed admitted and can be taken as an admitted fact at trial.

During the course of discovery, a party has to cooperate with the opposing party to see that discovery is fulfilled. Various state rules as well as federal rules require the working together of counsel to facilitate discovery. Before bringing a motion for sanctions or a motion to compel discovery, the parties are usually required to confer among themselves. If they are unable to resolve their differences, they can then apply to the courts for relief.

Failure to give information or to respond to discovery requests, provide answers to interrogatories, or supply witnesses for depositions can result in sanctions that include but are not limited to one or more of the following:

1. Assess attorney's fees and other costs against the guilty party.
2. Bar a witness from trial in the proceedings for failure to comply with the request for discovery.
3. Hold parties or witnesses in contempt of court.
4. Stay all proceedings until the discovery requested has been fulfilled.
5. Strike the defendant's pleadings and enter a default judgment against him or her.
6. Dismiss the cause of action.

When a discovery deposition is taken, the only limitation of the scope of a deposition is that it must be confined to matters that are relevant to the subject of the lawsuit or what may lead to evidence or further issues so long as it does not invade the areas of privilege.

There are numerous reasons to take oral depositions, including the following:

1. To preserve evidence.
2. To use portions of the deposition for possible impeachment at a later date.
3. To obtain admissions.
4. To acquire unknown facts.
5. To use in support of a motion for summary judgment.
6. To expedite settlement.
7. To lock the deponent into a definite version of the facts.

After discovery has been completed and the case reviewed by a judge, the parties again appear before the judge. Again, a dismissal may be requested and granted, with the right of appeal by the plaintiff. It is not unusual for the judge to recommend settlement, including suggested terms. If not, a new trial date is set in accordance with the court schedule.

TRIAL PRACTICE

Rule 16 of the Federal Rules of Civil Procedure sets forth the criteria for a pretrial conference. If the litigation cannot be settled out of court, the parties then undertake the appropriate preparation for trial. In an effort to simplify the trial of the action, the parties may serve requests for admission pursuant to Rule 36 of the Federal Rules of Civil Procedure. Many parties use this rule to obtain concessions or admissions concerning statements or opinions of fact, the application of laws to facts, or the genuineness of certain documents. Any matter admitted is established conclusively for the purpose of that case and requires no further proof at trial.

Motions in limine

A motion in limine is a motion made prior to the selection of the jury wherein the movant moves the court to instruct the defendant's counsel that any reference to the testimony or to the immaterial issue of whether the plaintiff acted in a certain way should be barred, because it could highly prejudice the jury.

THE TRIAL ITSELF

The procedural aspects of trials are governed by Rules 38 through 53 of the Federal Rules of Civil Procedure. Although the parties may waive a jury and try a case to the court, malpractice actions are seldom tried without a jury. Many members of the defense bar believe juries in malpractice actions do not objectively evaluate the evidence and are willing to award large verdicts out of sympathy for the plaintiff. Although many defense counselors are willing to waive a jury trial and proceed before the court alone, this seldom occurs, because counsel for the plaintiffs often prefer to take their chances with a lay jury.

Jury selection

The selection of jurors, or voir dire, is governed by the provisions of Rule 47 of the Federal Rules of Civil Procedure. The number of jurors varies from jurisdiction to jurisdiction. In fact, in federal courts throughout the United States, it is not uncommon to find 6, 8, or 12 jurors, plus a number of alternates.

The extent of the voir dire examination of prospective jurors also varies. In many state courts, the counsel conducts the examination, whereas in federal court, the court itself often selects the jurors. In those situations in which the court conducts the examination, it is required by Rule 47(a) to permit the parties or their attorneys to supplement the examination by further inquiry as it "deems proper" or to submit to the prospective jurors additional questions of the parties or their counsel as it "deems appropriate and proper."

In all cases, the court or counsel determines first who may be unqualified for or exempt from jury service. For instance, an individual is not qualified to serve on a jury unless he or she is a citizen of the United States, is 21 years of age, and has resided within the judicial district for one year. Depending on the jurisdiction, the preliminary questions may be posed by the court, the clerk, or counsel.

Next, the voir dire process ascertains whether the jurors can act in an impartial manner. Those who exhibit prejudice or bias may be challenged for cause. Although the bases for challenges for cause vary, the following list is representative:

1. Lack of comprehension of the English language
2. Suspicion of prejudice against or partiality for either party
3. Conviction of a crime
4. An interest in the case
5. A party to an action pending against either party
6. Prior jury service in the same action
7. The employer, employee, or the spouse, parent, son, or daughter of the employer or employee, counselor, agent, steward, or attorney of either party
8. Related by consanguinity or affinity within the fourth degree to either party or to the attorney of either party
9. Defendant or his or her spouse, parent, son, or daughter is a party to another action then pending in any court in which an attorney in the case then on trial is an attorney, either for or against the defendant
10. Prior jury service in the county within the preceding 12 months
11. Inability to follow the court's instructions on the law
12. Inability to be a fair and impartial juror.[11]

The number of challenges for cause that a party can make is not limited, but the burden of demonstrating bias and prejudice is on the party making the challenge. By statute, each party is entitled to three preemptory challenges. A preemptory challenge to a given juror may be made without showing any cause or reason. In a medical malpractice action involving several defendants, the court may consider the defendants as a single party for the purposes of making challenges. In other words, the several defendants have the collective right to exercise only three preemptory challenges. However, the court may allow additional preemptory challenges for both sides.

Following the selection of the jury, counsel customarily makes an opening statement to acquaint the jury with the facts they expect to prove. In some jurisdictions, however, it is possible for counsel for the defendant to reserve the opening statement until the plaintiff has rested and the defendant presents his or her case.

Because the plaintiff has the burden of proving the elements of his or her case by a preponderance of the evidence, he or she proceeds first with the presentation of evidence. The admissibility of evidence in the federal courts is governed by the Federal Rules of Evidence.

Although many states have adopted evidentiary rules that are similar to the Federal Rules of Evidence, in many states the admissibility of evidence is governed by the common law. Evidence may be in the form of oral testimony, deposition testimony, exhibits, stipulations by the parties, or matters of which judicial notice is taken by the court.

Most evidence is in the form of personal, direct testimony. Invariably there will be fact witnesses—the plaintiff, if alive, and other persons who have some knowledge of the case. The plaintiff meets the burden of proof by employing expert witnesses to advise the jury and/or judge, one of whom must ultimately decide whether the plaintiff has met the burden of proof. All witnesses are subject to cross-examination. To extract more information from the experts, additional or redirect examination may be necessary.

Opening statement

The case begins with an opening statement. Generally, an opening statement is made to a jury to familiarize them with the facts to be presented during the case in trial. The purpose of an opening statement is to develop a road map that the jurors can use during the course of litigation. An opening statement is especially helpful if witnesses, especially experts, are called out of sequence. A study from the University of Chicago Law School established that 65% of juries ultimately decided the case consistent with their first impressions immediately following opening statements. In certain situations, an opening statement may be waived until prior to the presentation of the case in chief.

In making an opening statement, the facts should not be overstated, but counsel should clearly and concisely state what the party intends to prove. It is necessary to make sure that the facts that are alleged will be admissible. If inconsistencies are expected, they should also be pointed out. In opening statements the pleadings should be summarized. During an opening statement, visual aids may be used, such as charts, diagrams, and other aids, to help the jury to become familiar with the facts. This is especially valuable in medical malpractice cases to familiarize jurors with various parts of the anatomy.

Direct examination

The plaintiff's case in chief is presented next and consists of direct examination by the plaintiff and then cross-examination by the defendant. It is extremely important that the witness be well prepared. During direct examination evidence can be objected to as being irrelevant and immaterial. The order in which witnesses appear can also be very important in terms of continuity with the case.

When a witness is called to the stand in a case in chief, it is called direct examination. During direct examination the attorney cannot ask leading questions of his or her own witness. It is therefore important that the witnesses be well prepared and familiar with the style of the attorney and know what to expect.

There are certain areas in which a lay witness can give opinions, such as the speed of a moving vehicle; however, in many cases, such as medicolegal cases, an opinion can be offered only by an expert. For an individual to be qualified as an expert, one would have to get his or her name; address; information as to college, medical school, residency, board certification, and state licensures; any books, treatises, or publications written; professional associations or affiliations; hospital staffs on which the neutral witness serves; and other similar types of questions. Experts often include physicians, but there may be other health care providers who have the requisite knowledge, training, and experience.

Attorneys vary in terms of their opinion as to whether or not to elicit all the background of an expert witness or to stipulate it. Many attorneys who have well-credentialed experts like to list all of the credentials because it impresses the jury.

After a witness has testified on direct examination, visual and graphic aids are distinguished from exhibits. An exhibit is an item that is marked by the court and is later offered into evidence. A visual or graphic aid is something that merely assists the witness or the jury to better understand what the witness is testifying about. Therefore, an anatomical chart would be a visual aid, whereas a death certificate would be an exhibit. Invariably demonstrative data are used, including photographs, models, tables, x-rays, and other laboratory depictions. Testimony has also been presented by videotapes obtained prior to the trial under trial-like circumstances.

The direct examination procedure rests on the premise that the defendant's lawyer attempts to refute or discredit the plaintiff's evidence through an adversarial system. Each side may object to the other side's presentation of evidence.

Cross-examination

When the plaintiff concludes examination of a witness, the defendant is entitled to cross-examine that particular witness. The objectives of cross-examination are: (1) to establish that the witness is lying on one or more material points; (2) to show that the witness is prejudiced; (3) to show that testimony of the witness is improbable; (4) to force the witness to admit to certain facts; (5) to supplement testimony that the witness has already given; (6) to weaken the testimony of the witness by showing that his or her opinion is questionable because of inability to observe, to hear conversation, or to see because of poor lighting conditions, or by showing other facts to reduce the value of the witness's opinion; (7) to show that an expert witness or lay witness who has testified to an opinion is not competent or qualified because of a lack of necessary training or experience (to negate or reduce the probative value of the expert's opinion); (8) to impeach the witness by showing that he or she has given a contrary statement at other times; (9) to show that the witness has been convicted of an infamous crime in order to cast doubt on credibility; and (10) to obtain necessary evidence to establish the case through examination of an adverse witness during the case in chief.

After cross-examination is concluded and new issues are brought out, the plaintiff's attorney has the right to re-direct examination and subsequent to that the defense attorney has the right to conduct re-cross-examination if additional information was brought out on the re-direct examination.

At the conclusion of the plaintiff's case, the defendant may move for a directed verdict, pursuant to the provisions of Rule 50(a) of the Federal Rules of Civil Procedure, or the equivalent state rule. Such a motion tests the legal sufficiency of the evidence presented by the plaintiff. For the defendant to obtain a directed verdict, the evidence must be such that, without weighing the credibility of the witnesses, or otherwise considering the weight of the evidence, reasonable persons could conclude only in favor of the defendant. The court is obligated to view the evidence most favorably to the party against whom the motion is directed, that is, the plaintiff. In most instances, the motion for a directed verdict is overruled, although a motion may be sustained for a portion of the plaintiff's case. For instance, if the plaintiff asserted liability on the basis of lack of informed consent and negligence, the court could direct a verdict in favor of the defendant on one of these theories but leave the other intact.

If the motion for a directed verdict is denied, the defendant then has the opportunity to present evidence in his or her favor. Since the defendant is not obliged to prove anything (unless he or she has asserted a counterclaim), it is theoretically unnecessary for him or her to present any evidence at all. However, conventional thinking asserts that the defendant must present substantial evidence in favor of his or her position, or run the risk of conveying the impression that the position is meritless. The defendant uses most of the tactics used by the plaintiff.

At the close of the defendant's case (or rebuttal, if there was any), all parties frequently move for directed verdicts. Because the evidence must be construed in favor of the party against whom the motion is made, generally motions are again overruled. There are, however, certain circumstances in which an affirmative defense may be established with sufficient clarity that a motion for a directed verdict in favor of the defendant is granted.

Closing arguments

Following the presentation of evidence, the counselors for both sides have the right to argue their cases to the jury (or to the court, in a nonjury case). Because the plaintiff has the burden of proof, he or she has the right of opening and closing the argument. The court has broad discretion in controlling the closing arguments. The arguments of counsel must be limited to the issues in the case and the evidence presented, as well as any fair and reasonable inferences and deductions from that evidence. Although the practice varies from jurisdiction to jurisdiction, charts and drawings used during the course of the trial may be referred to in the closing argument. In addition, the counsel may outline the obligations of the jurors. It is inappropriate (and a potentially reversible error) for the counsel for the plaintiff to excite the prejudice of the jury or appeal to their sympathies.

Instructions

Following the closing arguments, the jury is given its instructions on the applicable law. These instructions are generally referred to as the *jury charge*. In a typical malpractice case, the jury is instructed in the law of negligence, burden of proof, proximate cause, and damages. The jury is instructed that it is to determine or resolve the factual issues in the case in accord with the law, as given by the court.

The verdict forms are discussed with the jury, which is instructed as to the manner in which it will deliberate. The form of the verdict varies; in some instances, there will be a general verdict in which the jury indicates simply whether it finds for the plaintiff or the defendant and, if it finds for the plaintiff, the amount of damages. Under Rule 49(a) of the Federal Rules of Civil Procedure, the court may require the jury to answer certain questions that are referred to as special verdicts. Under Rule 49(b), the court may submit a general verdict to the jury with written interrogatories on one or more issues of fact—a decision on which is necessary to a verdict.

The percentage of jurors required to render a verdict also varies. In the federal system, a unanimous verdict is required, unless the parties, pursuant to Rule 48 of the Federal Rules of Civil Procedure, stipulate otherwise. In various states, a three-quarters or five-sixths majority is necessary.

Judgments

Following the jury verdict, the clerk prepares, signs, and enters the judgment. The judgment is the final determination of the lawsuit, absent an appeal. Judgment may be rendered on default when the defendant does not appear; or following the granting of demurrer, a motion to dismiss, or a motion for summary judgment; or upon the jury's verdict, or the finding of fact and conclusions of law of the trial judge in a nonjury case.

POST-TRIAL PROCEEDINGS

Every judicial system provides for review by an appellate court of the decisions of the trial court. Generally a party has the right to appeal any judgment to at least one higher court. In the federal courts, district court decisions are reviewed by the courts of appeals, but review in the U.S. Supreme Court must be sought in most cases by a petition for a writ of certiorari, which that Court may deny as a matter of discretion without reaching any conclusion as to the merits of the case. The record on appeal will contain the pleadings, at least a portion of the transcript of the trial. The parties present their contentions to the appellate court by written briefs and in addition, in most cases by oral argument. When the judge has sat without a jury, an appellate court will rarely reexamine a question of fact. The appellate court has the power to affirm, reverse, or modify the judgment of the trial court. It may order that judgment be entered or it may remand the case to trial court for a new trial or other proceedings not inconsistent with its decision. The decision of an appellate court is usually accompanied by a written opinion.

In the federal court system, the losing party may file a motion for a new trial no later than 10 days after the entry of a judgment.[12] In this motion the nonprevailing party sets forth the alleged trial errors that entitle it to a new trial.

The nonprevailing party may also file a motion for a judgment notwithstanding the verdict (JNOV), in which the losing party asserts that the evidence is such that reasonable persons could only have reached a conclusion against the prevailing party.

Most states have procedures that are similar to the motion for a new trial or motion for JNOV. Although these motions are frequently filed, they are rarely granted. In any event, the judge may reject the jury's verdict, just as he or she may avoid jury deliberation with a directed verdict during or at the conclusion of the trial.

Following the post-trial proceedings, a limited number of alternatives are available. A judgment in favor of the plaintiff may be satisfied and the litigation terminated. A judgment in favor of the defendant may be accepted by the plaintiff and no further action taken. Alternatively, either side may appeal the case to the appropriate court of appeals.

END NOTES

1. Fed. R. Civ. P. 3.
2. Fed. R. Civ. P. 4.
3. Fed. R. Civ. P. 8.
4. Fed. R. Civ. P. 13.
5. Fed. R. Civ. P. 14.
6. Fed. R. Civ. P. 8.
7. Fed. R. Civ. P. 30, 31, 32.
8. Fed. R. Civ. P. 33.
9. Fed. R. Civ. P. 33.
10. Fed. R. Civ. P. 35.
11. Fed. R. Civ. P. 36.
12. Ohio Rev. Code §§2313.42, 2313.43.
13. Fed. R. Civ. P. 59(b).

CHAPTER 7

Alternative dispute resolution in health care

IRVING LADIMER, J.D., S.J.D., F.C.L.M.

CURRENT INTEREST IN ALTERNATIVE DISPUTE RESOLUTION
ALTERNATIVE DISPUTE RESOLUTION METHODS
ARBITRATION IN PRACTICE
DESIGNING AN ARBITRAL SYSTEM
ADR PRACTICE TIPS
CONCLUSION

The complexity of a national health program and allied state systems will inevitably generate conflict.[1] The sheer magnitude of a combination of plans with public/private authorities as monitors and regulators will create disagreements and disputes. Differences will occur at several levels and stages and will involve managers and providers, engaged and independent professionals, contractors and consultants, and, certainly, consumers—patients, subscribers, applicants, dependents—and the insurers and employers offering and administering health plans. Issues will range from the basic obligations to provide service, coverage, and control to the familiar claims of eligibility, entitlement, and payment. In addition, disputes will arise concerning practice liability, institutional and hospital care, admission and discharge, and other aspects of patient service. In sum, although there may be no essential change in the character of conflict, there will be an exponential rise in number of conflicts and in participants.

All programs have recognized the need for expeditious disposition of complaints and claims.[2] The litigation burden and cost of conventional settlement, especially for the expected volume of similar requests of members and subscribers, cannot reasonably be imposed on a new and expanding mix of health services. Thus, almost all concerned with the delivery of care and professional practice have proposed alternatives to resolve conflicts of all types.

A comparison of proposed health reform legislation shows that, despite differences on other issues, the major bills, including the president's Health Security Act (H.R. 3600/S. 1770), would require the approved health plans to establish alternative dispute mechanisms for malpractice and other claims. No definitions are provided but these mechanisms might include rapid settlement offers, mediation, and arbitration.

Major medicolegal organizations have endorsed alternative dispute resolution (ADR), including the American College of Legal Medicine, which "supports the premise that ADR should play a larger role than now assigned to it."[3] This is based on the realization that multiple legal issues inherent in health care reform "including but not limited to contractual equities, appropriate physician management status, protection of physician and patient rights and their attendant risks, raise many considerations for resolution."

In a straightforward op-ed editorial, presaging the current call for arbitration, Senator Pete Domenici of New Mexico, then ranking Republican member of the Senate Budget Committee, and former Surgeon General Everett Koop endorse an administration (Bush) proposal: "We want to overhaul the system by removing virtually all malpractice claims from courts and resolving them in binding arbitration."[4] They would require participants in all entitlement health programs and tax-break employer plans to arbitrate such claims. The main thrust is the provision for "more consistent, more expert, more reasonable and more timely decisions at lower cost and with better results."

Under this proposal, states would be encouraged to enact legislation with guidelines on procedure, compensation, and collateral sources. Also, the bill (which later would have to be reintroduced) would stimulate provision of medical standards.

CURRENT INTEREST IN ALTERNATIVE DISPUTE RESOLUTION

Use of arbitration, the best known and most popular alternative, is not new. Medical malpractice arbitration was provided as early as 1929 in the subscriber contracts of the Ross-Loos Medical Group in California, a prepaid group practice plan. The Kaiser program adopted a similar approach some 40 years later and set the pattern for use by health maintenance organizations (HMOs). In 1969, a project involving Southern California hospitals demonstrated that voluntary, binding arbitration served to reduce time and cost and provide fair resolution. Subsequently, the reform movement resulting from the malpractice crisis of the 1970s and the landmark report of the Secretary's Commission on Medical Malpractice, which recommended trial study of this option, stimulated statutory and voluntary action.

Federal action

The most recent expression of federal interest is the enactment of the Administrative Dispute Resolution Act (ADRA) of 1990 (Public Law No. 101-552,104 Stat. 2736, 1990), which establishes a statutory framework for federal use of alternative dispute methods for contract issues.[5] In 1925, Congress passed the Federal Arbitration Act, which permitted enforcement of arbitration agreements in federal courts. Now, noting that ADR modes have been "used increasingly by States, courts and private entities within the past decade," these are made available for government contracts. The law adopts recommendations of the Administrative Conference of the United States and refers specifically to prior statutes covering administrative arbitration, ALJ authority, contract disputes, FMCS authority, tort claims, and other government claims. ADRA thus puts to rest the long-standing doctrine that the government cannot submit to arbitration.

ADRA was followed by the Negotiated Rule-making Act to resolve issues under proposed regulations. In addition, Executive Order 12866 directs agencies "to explore, and where appropriate, use continual mechanisms for developing regulations." The American Bar Association's new Section of Dispute Resolution has joined with many organizations and the Administrative Conference to "promote use of consensus based resolution methods for disputes involving the federal government."[6]

ADRA is a five-year experiment in the use of arbitration and mediation to settle disputes with the government, chiefly contract claims. Any appropriate method can be used—conciliation, mediation, minitrials, and arbitration, to name the most prominent. Parties may submit all or selected issues for consideration. Agencies are encouraged to train staff to utilize these methods. The burgeoning health field should benefit from this opportunity.[7]

Statutory malpractice arbitration. In the wake of the malpractice crisis, all states enacted some type of reform, usually stressing procedural changes such as shortened statutes of limitation, indemnity limits, prior notice, insurance obligations and review prior to litigation by a screening panel, and incorporating mediation and arbitration. As of 1994, the American Arbitration Association (AAA) lists 15 states with laws providing for voluntary arbitration of medical malpractice claims.[8] Some statutes, passed in the first reform wave, were repealed or have expired. Others remain as originally drawn. Only Michigan required hospitals to notify patients of the availability of arbitration, and it maintained a program, under its Insurance Department, for administering claims. From 1975 to 1991, there were 20,000 litigated cases, and about 1000 arbitrations, mostly managed by the AAA. Because of the relatively small number, the ambitious legislation was repealed. In explanation of the demise, a representative of the U.S. General Accounting Office, which studied arbitration for Congress, noted that when voluntary arbitration is offered in parallel to litigation, which is familiar to lawyers and reputedly favors higher awards, the alternative tends not to be selected. But "when mandatory arbitration is linked to the provision of health care, as is done by some health maintenance organizations, experience suggests that it is an acceptable alternative to litigation."

Although the several state statutes for medical malpractice are not widely used, except by group practices and similar organizations, their features may be significant under health care reforms.

The typical statute provides for voluntary or elective use on the basis of an offer by a hospital, physician, or other provider. Most permit arbitration of future as well as present claims. For this form, the parties have to agree in advance that any dispute subject to the arbitration clause or contract would be available on demand of either party. The customary way of effecting such a future-dispute compact is by presignifying or authorization by the provider, such as an HMO, and signing of a form or statement by the patient, usually on entry to a hospital, clinic, or office. Some statutes specify the elements of such an agreement to ensure understanding and enforceability.[9] Also, because of differences in interpretation or comprehension, the validity of such agreements has often been questioned when the patient elects to sue rather than arbitrate.

ALTERNATIVE DISPUTE RESOLUTION METHODS

Alternatives to conventional litigation have in common three purposes: conservation of time, expense, and procedural steps; expert or experienced adjudicators; equitable and rational disposition.[10] These objectives may be found in (1) arbitration, (2) mediation and screening, and (3) fact-finding and variations of these methods, utilized independently or annexed to court processes. Also, usually included as an alternative is a *no-fault* option, applied in general or in part to specific issues.[11]

Arbitration is a process of dispute settlement, pursuant to law, whereby the parties agree to submit specified present or future controversies to a neutral third party for final determination. Binding arbitration is essentially a voluntary, contractual process that seeks final resolution; some forms are nonbinding, permitting appeal or review for specific reasons. Binding arbitration is not subject to court reconsideration or appeal except for procedural flaws, bias, or fraud. It is enforceable in every jurisdiction today under contract law or statute providing for general or specific arbitration, including malpractice or health claims.

Mediation is a process intended to encourage the parties to settle through the use of an expert facilitator (mediator) to arrive at their own terms of resolution. A form of mediation, used for malpractice by statutory authority or option, is the *pretrial screening panel,* available in the majority of states enacting tort reforms. These methods do not bind the parties who, under certain conditions, maintain recourse to the court, without reference to panel recommendations.

Fact-finding is a party-agreed process of investigation, including a review of the case by one or more experts who are expected to recommend a settlement or course of negotiation leading to settlement. Unlike arbitration, it is not binding and generally not subject to any special legislation. It is an informal method used by professionals, akin to peer review. Fact-finding serves to clarify the issues and provide a basis for agreement.

No-fault plans would provide a system of compensation for medical or hospital injury without regard to fault or negligence as the basis of liability. Various plans, generally limited to specific or designated injuries, incidents or events, have been proposed as alternatives to the common fault-centered tort system. The oldest effective model is workers' compensation. A federal program for vaccine-related injuries and two state systems for neurologically impaired infants are in operation.

Arbitration-mediation in health care

A program illustrating use of mediation and arbitration was jointly developed in 1992 by the American Arbitration Association and the health care service units of Duke University. Under the Health Care Claim Settlement Procedures of the AAA, patients may, on their own or on a dependent's behalf voluntarily submit any claim, dispute, or demand, first to mediation and, if inconclusive, to arbitration. Entry into the system waives litigation; for example, "By signing this Agreement, you are voluntarily selecting alternative dispute resolution as an exclusive alternative to exercising your right to trial by jury."[12]

The explanation to patients notes that experience has shown that 80% of disputes are acceptably resolved by mediation, the process of settlement by the parties through guided discussion. It closes by restating the voluntary aspect: "Your participation is voluntary. If you do not choose to participate, you will still receive the same high level of professional care for which Duke University is so well known."

In this system, as in the 10-year Michigan program, the Kaiser plans, and the New York State Medical Society and Hospital Association project (1975-1979), patient education and verifiable understanding are essential to cooperation and enforcement. As noted in the checklist of Appendix 7-1, early attention must be given to proper consent, notice, and forms of agreement.

No-fault compensation option

The radical alternative, the "no-fault" plan, is not one of process, but purpose. Thus, instead of expediting resolution through mediation or arbitration within the negligence-tort system, some type of compensation would be provided without consideration of negligence as the determinant of liability and payment.[13] Although "no-fault" was proposed as a legislative option as early as 1976 in the influential Report of the New York Special Advisory Panel on Medical Malpractice, following numerous studies and references to workers' compensation in the United States and foreign compensation systems, there has been no significant movement.[14] Again, in New York, the 1988-1990 review of hospital records by the Harvard University team strongly suggested this alternative to overcome the inefficiencies and inequities of the tort system.[15]

As of late 1994, limited no-fault systems for medical malpractice are found only in Virginia (1987) and Florida (1988) solely for birth defect cases, based on the workers' compensation principle.[16] In 1986, federal legislation was enacted to cover medical liability for DPT vaccination injury or damage, and similar state legislation was passed by North Carolina in the latter part of the same year with provision to avoid duplication.[17] Under the vaccination statutes, liability is administratively determined by a panel of experts, based on cause-and-effect criteria without regard to medical or provider negligence.

A special form of no-fault "economic damage guarantee" seeks to induce defendants to foreclose a claim by a timely offer to compensate for net economic loss with collateral offset plus fees.[18] If no offer is made within the time specified, the claimant may proceed to litigate. Advantages to the claimant are speed and certainty of payment even though the payment would likely be for a lesser amount. The lower payment and time costs are the advantages to the defendant.[19]

This approach is under evaluation though a program adopted in 1982 by the national Federation of High School Associations to cover serious athletic injuries. The 1985 Federal Medical Offer and Recovery bill included such a proposal but no congressional action was taken. In 1986, "offer and recovery" was made part of the New York malpractice reform legislation, but this option has not been used.

Enforcing arbitration

In general, an arbitration award is accepted without further review or appeal since the grounds for court reconsideration are few and limited.[20] However, problems arise not merely from the actions of arbitrators or procedural flaws, claimed by either party, but from the scope or application of the initial agreement.[21]

Two 1993 Michigan cases illustrate this issue and thus underscore the importance of party comprehension and clarity of contract. In *Grazia v. Sanchez*, 502 N.W. 2d 751 (Mich. Ct. App. 1993) the appellate court affirmed a lower court's enforcement of arbitration for later-date surgery and hospitalization as well as for preoperative tests. The patient entered for an elective laparotomy and signed the usual consent form and arbitration agreement on the day of testing. She maintained that the agreement referring to "this hospital stay" limited the arbitration. The court ruled that there was no evidence that her visit for testing constituted a "stay" and, in fact, the parties' conduct in light of all circumstances showed an intent to relate to the upcoming operation. This interpretation accorded with an earlier appellate court ruling that an arbitration accord signed after care was rendered reasonably related back to date of service [*Harte v. Sinai Hospital of Detroit* 144 Mich. Ap. 659, 375 N.W. 2d 782 (1985)].

Place rather than time was at issue in *Villarreal v. Chun*, 501 N.W. 2d 227 (Mich. Ct. App. 1993). At trial, medical care, the activity subject to arbitration, was extended to out-of-hospital treatment as well as in-hospital surgery. At each hospital visit, the patient signed an arbitration agreement applying only to care in the hospital. The trial court found that the majority of the alleged malpractice occurred in the hospital but held that arbitration applied to both aspects of care since they were related. In a reversal, the appellate court decided that, although the entire claim must be arbitrated when damages are inextricably related, this agreement was "unambiguously limited to in-house" care. Thus, the malpractice could be tried in respect to out-of-hospital treatment but arbitration applied to in-hospital care.

Objections to arbitration are often framed by lawyers in cases expected to succeed in court or result in higher compensation.[22] This view tends to restrict the proper use of a method initially and fairly chosen by the parties and just as likely to provide a fair review and outcome.

ARBITRATION IN PRACTICE

Use of arbitration for providers, consumers, and others involved in health service disputes will depend on the perception of success of this method in actual practice. Although appealing in concept, arbitration for this field must also be accessible, practical or feasible, and enforceable if it is to be willingly and widely accepted.[23]

Accessibility

Arbitration is a private, party-designed or accepted system employed for a specific set of problems or issues. In its most familiar and appropriate form, it is voluntary; that is, parties may agree in advance or at the time or occasion of dispute to submit the matter to a chosen or preselected arbitration panel or individual for final determination. To utilize arbitration, generally, some formal plan must be in place. In the health context, three customary approaches have made or caused arbitration to be available and accessible:

1. Provision in a health care or delivery program such as an HMO, group practice, or special service agency stipulating that subscribers, members, or others eligible or entitled to benefits may or shall use arbitration for resolution of disputes. These may be broadly defined to include issues of practice, entitlement, eligibility, availability, payment, and ancillary service or may be restricted to practice and service, for example, medical malpractice and hospital referral and care. It is usually linked to the internal grievance or complaint program that must first be utilized.

   The system may call for a single arbitrator or a panel and may include medical, legal, or other members. The procedure requires notice, definition of scope and application, conditions for use (time, forms, complaint), and nature of remedy (compensation, service, referral). The binding or final nature of the process must be clear. Court review is limited to procedural error, bias, or misapplication to a claim or party not within intended coverage.

2. Some states permitting arbitration of malpractice disputes specify the information to be given, the limits of the arbitral process, and requirements for

judicial review. Programs for arbitration must conform. Some that have challenged the imposition of arbitration have alleged failure to notify or to explain, for example, that arbitration, once selected or entered, is the exclusive remedy without recourse to trial by judge or jury.[24]

3. Where the system is administered by an outside professional agency, these matters are usually routinely managed. The hearings are conducted under prescribed rules for the parties, attorneys, or other advocates and for the arbitrators, including schedules, fees, awards, and documentation for enforcement.

Practicality

The singular advantage of arbitration is informality, including adaptability to the needs of the parties, expertise of adjudicators, and economy with due respect for fair process. Generally, arbitration is undertaken within the provisions of a contract, which may be the health insurance policy, statement of program, or an agreement specifically fashioned for the issues, such as a disciplinary proceeding for a professional or administrator.

Although informal relative to a court proceeding, arbitration works within statutory, regulatory, or agency rules and the contract conditions. The court rules of evidence, discovery, presence of witnesses, and introduction of relevant material need not be followed.

Generally, the experts who serve as arbitrators are capable of evaluating evidence without reliance on rules of admission and exclusion. Parties may stipulate what can or cannot be covered and have considerable influence as to conduct of a case, subject to the agreement and arbitration control. (This strength is often seen as a weakness by litigation attorneys who maintain that only the court and statutory prescriptions can assure a fair hearing and just result). Arbitrators have substantial leeway to set awards and remedies and are not restricted to legal confines.

Such procedural efficiency, time savings, and avoidance of docket delays should result in economy to all parties. When there is acceptance of the process and effective administration, the outcomes are generally satisfactory.

Enforceability

Enforcement is the critical question. In the court system, a verdict is enforced by power of the law as interpreted by the judge. Courts have authority to command. But lower court actions are subject to appeal on a variety of grounds, thus often relegating finality to a long, expensive appellate process.

Arbitral awards are rendered as final, with only a highly limited basis for review. But arbitration is a legally constituted system and its awards may be submitted to the court of proper jurisdiction for enforcement. It is customary to conclude many an arbitration by application for confirmation. As such, the award becomes a court order, with all due sanctions for enforcement.

Objections to the use of arbitration reside in the frequency and nature of court review, thus negating the speed, economy, and finality claimed for this alternative. The body of case law suggests that arbitration has been frustrated in two major respects: challenges to the process and coverage and challenges to the awards and application.

Analyses of the use of arbitration have established first and foremost that the process is valid and constitutional and not an improper or unlawful substitute for the right to trial [*Doyle v. Giulicci* (62 Cal. 2d 606, 401 P.1 (1965)], upholding the validity of arbitration in a group practice agreement (Ross-Loos), which goes back to its early use in the 1960s. Subsequent cases involving Kaiser plan contracts for subscribers similarly supported the legality of arbitration when properly introduced and explained.[25] The Michigan arbitration law, which required hospitals to offer arbitration, was likewise upheld as a proper forum and process.

Cases that confounded the issue have dealt with technical aspects: scope of coverage; clarity of terms; application to nonsigners, such as dependents or executors; multiple parties; issues of timeliness; and procedure for enrollment. As these were resolved, arbitration when used in Michigan, for example, became more efficient, faster, and less expensive.

Evaluation

Several studies sought to assess the value or influence of arbitration on claims frequency and disposition either directly or inferentially compared with litigation.

The first case study, based on a single program—that of the Ross-Loos Medical Group of California—was performed by physician attorney David Rubsamen in 1972. He reviewed 35 closed claims subject to arbitration of which three were arbitrated and the rest closed within the arbitration context. He concluded that for physicians "arbitration had a calming effect and was seen as an unqualified success because it stimulated settlement rather than continued controversy. For the defense, it proved economical. Lawyers were satisfied with a qualified neutral arbitrator. Moreover, the ease of review did not generate more cases.[26]

In 1975, Duane Heintz compared cases closed by eight Southern California hospitals in a project using arbitration and a control group of earlier cases and those of similar hospitals during 1970-1973, and later, until 1975.

Although, as in Ross-Loos, few proceeded to hearing, all were influenced by the choice of method. Recognizing the small size and the selective character of the study, Heintz nonetheless concluded that objectively the demonstration hospitals had fewer claims, they were settled faster, and both average payouts and defense costs were markedly lower.[27]

Ladimer, Solomon, and Mulvihill in 1980-81, conducted the most extensive study. They compared data on 205 cases closed between 1967 and 1979 administered by the American Arbitration Association with similar information on litigated cases relating to frequency, severity, disposition, time, defense costs, and procedural steps. The control cases were drawn from the National Association of Insurance Commissioners (NAIC) database of malpractice cases closed during 1975-1978, adjusted for the period covered. This study also reviewed contemporary legislative case law and detailed descriptions of the arbitral process to illustrate the realities of practice.[28]

The Ladimer study concluded that (1) arbitration can be effectively used for malpractice cases; (2) arbitration formats for current and future controversies can be appropriately applied in different situations; (3) even with challenges, the use of this mode is faster, less expensive, and procedurally acceptable to the parties; and (4) arbitration offers the dimension of equity and responsiveness by virtue of its expert, private, and informal character.

DESIGNING AN ARBITRAL SYSTEM

Although state and federal statutes may prescribe general outlines for alternative resolution of disputes involving medical practice, health service, commercial aspects, or special programs, the design and establishment of a system for particular purposes will be the responsibility of the administrator. First consideration, of course, will be compliance or conformance with statutes and regulations. For the agency, however, the policy and local practice or environment must be determined.

An arbitral plan for an HMO, for instance, would mesh with the internal grievance procedure and would necessarily involve consumer or member understanding and participation regarding coverage, entitlement, eligibility, payment and notice issues, and medical and ancillary health services. A hospital plan would encompass physician, staff, and managerial interests as well as patient concerns.[29]

The versatility of alternatives, as the name ADR implies, provides ample opportunity to create and develop a truly responsive system, which could include elements of less and more formal structures—mediation and arbitration—acceptable and fair to all concerned.[30]

Experience in the use of alternatives, still relatively spare and even untried by many lawyers and managers, suggests that the following features are essential:

1. *Application:* Must provide a clear statement as to parties, issues, and availability.
2. *Use:* Its use is optional or mandatory [arbitration is customarily optional or voluntary (one or both) at entry and binding or final at conclusion].
3. *Fair:* Process must be and appear to be just to all concerned with respect to access, inclusion, and representation as well as determination by qualified adjudicators.
4. *Simple:* Rules, internal appeals, and time/cost delays frustrate the system. Preset guidelines, suitable to the problem and parties, should be employed to avoid procedural technicalities.
5. *Cost:* Fees should be appropriately shared to permit consumer use.
6. *Information:* Most important, parties should be provided with sufficient information, by appropriate media, to comprehend the purpose and scope of the system and the advantage of alternative methods for resolutions.

To assist in developing a viable system, avoiding the obstacles of objection and enforcement (although appeal is limited, issues of application, understanding, due process, and scope of award, among others, may require court review and judgment), and benefiting from the support of statute and case law, a checklist for guidance is provided in Appendix 7-1.

ADR PRACTICE TIPS

In the last two decades, the ADR movement has generated a dynamic and, for many law firms, significant practice area. The creation of a full-fledged ADR Section by the American Bar Association, inclusion of courses in most law schools, use of annexed arbitration by courts, and, mainly, the development of ADR agencies, companies, and programs have all given ADR an identity and purpose. Litigation has been recognized as too expensive, time consuming, and ridden with technicalities.[31]

The consequence has been a turn to alternatives, out of need and, admittedly, out of frustration with courts, juries, and unpredictable outcomes. Many attorneys and others have seized the opportunity to engage in some aspect of ADR service chiefly as mediator or arbitrator but also as consultant, system designer, and administrator. An attractive feature is the novelty of private adjudication (previously regarded as a drawback), the potential for change, and, frankly, the chance for additional income. Civic-minded practitioners will also find pro bono or equivalent activity in neighborhood dispute resolution, mediation projects covering domestic relations, representation of the indigent, or arbitration of assigned civil or minor criminal cases.

A variety of training courses and more formal education is now available through professional societies at the national and local level. The well-established organizations, such as the American Arbitration Association, and the specialty agencies for health care, insurance, labor, and commercial areas are also within easy reach. Directories of practitioners in this field; books, periodicals, and services for training and case reports; and focus programs are among the resources.[32]

The growing health industry, encompassing all manner of public and private service and the financial component, clearly stands out as a major ADR arena. Federal and state governments have for some time utilized and encouraged arbitration and mediation and have increasingly extended these modes for entitlement, business, technical, and contractual programs.[33]

Arbitration of physician discipline by hospitals is now fairly common and accepted as an independent means of resolution. Arbitral processes have also been introduced by federal legislation to monitor physician practices. The Health Care Quality Improvement Act of 1986 and the Medicare and Medicaid Protection Act of 1987 provide for identification and reporting of substandard practitioners.[34] The National Practitioner Data Bank, established under the 1987 statute, contains specified information on disciplinary actions and reports of malpractice claims and would exclude disciplined practitioners from federal programs. A hearing program was therefore included for review of any proposed action (Ch. 117, Sec. 11111-11115). It authorizes determination "before an arbitrator mutually acceptable to the physician and the health care entity" or a neutral hearing officer approved by the entity or a panel. In cases of disputed accuracy, the government must provide procedures for review and correction.

ADR is now a familiar feature, easily adapted to resolution of health issues under various sponsorships.

CONCLUSION

Assessment of alternatives to the current system suggests that in the health field, these methods — as for labor contract and employment issues — may become primary. They can constructively respond to recognized deficiencies in litigation and court processes.

Even though questions of introduction, explanation, and application will arise, as for any specially defined system, the advantages of access, practicality, and enforceability should prevail. Legislation may be required to encourage use and adaptation to different issues and to assure the validity of such approaches. The

law can be used creatively. With good will, education, and the options available, there are favorable opportunities for all concerned.

END NOTES

1. Healthcare Reform will Include ADR Dispute Resolution Journal p3 (Dec. 1993).
2. Kaiser Commission on the Future of Medicaid, *Health Reform Legislation: A Comparison of Major Proposals* (Jan. 1994).
3. American College of Legal Medicare, *Health Care Reform Paper. A Position Statement* (1994).
4. P. V. Domenici and C. E. Koop, *Sue the Doctor? There's a Better Way (Take the Case to Binding Arbitration),* N.Y. Times, June 6, 1991, Op Ed.
5. Administrative Dispute Resolution Act, Pub. L. No. 101-552, 104 Stat. 2736, 5 U.S.C. 5581-593 (1990); J. Babbin and G. Cox, *Saving Time and Money — Arbitration and Mediation of Government Dispute Under the ADRA* Contract Management 20-25 (Jan. 1992).
6. R. D. Raven, *The Future of Court-Annexed ADR (From the Chair)* 1 Dispute Resolution Magazine (ABA Section of Dispute Resolution) 2 (Spring 1994).
7. *U.S. Health Plan will include ADR,* Dispute Resolution Times (ADR News from the American Arbitration Association), 1, 7 (Winter 1993/94).
8. States enacting or amending statutes were Alabama, Alaska, California, Colorado, Florida, Georgia, Illinois, Louisiana, Michigan, New York, North Dakota, Ohio, South Dakota, Vermont, and Virginia. Of the 15 states with malpractice arbitration laws, 10 also had pretrial screening panels. Some statutes were repealed or were time limited.
9. J. Zaremski and L. Goldstein, *Medical and Hospital Negligence, in* 4 Alternative Dispute Resolution (Ladimer ed., Callaghan and Co., 1988).
10. U.S. (DHEW) Secretary's Commission on Medical Malpractice DHEW, DHEW Pub. No. (os) 73-88 Report (Jan. 16, 1973).
11. U.S. General Accounting Office, *Medical Malpractice: No Agreement on the Problems or Solutions,* HRD-86-50 (1986); U.S. General Accounting Office, *Medical Malpractice: A Framework for Action,* HRD 87-73 (1987).
12. American Arbitration Association, *Letter and Form for Duke University Hospital Arbitration Project* (1992).
13. R. Latz, *No-Fault Liability and Medical Malpractice — A Viability Analysis* 10 J. Legal Med. 479-525 (1989); Havighurst and Tarcredi, *Medical Adversity Insurance: A No-Fault Approach to Medical Malpractice and Quality Assurance,* 51 Milbank Memorial Fund Q 125 (1973) and 613 Insurance Law J. 69 (1974); Havighurst, *Medical Adversity Insurance — Has Its Time Come?* 2975 Duke L.J. 1233. Kenneth Jost, *Fault-Free Malpractice: Two More States (New York and Utah) Propose Testing Waters in a Controversial Approach to Medical Injury Claims.* 80 ABA Jnl. 46-49 (Jan. 1994).
14. New York Special Advisory Panel on Medical Malpractice, Report (Jan. 1976).
15. Harvard Medical Practice Study, *Patients, Doctors and Lawyers: Medical Injury, Malpractice Litigation and Patient Compensation in New York,* a report (Feb. 1990).
16. Virginia Code Ann 38.2-5000 to 5021 (Supp. 1989) passed 1987; Florida Stat. Ann. 766.301 to 316 (West Supp. 1989) passed 1988. Few cases were brought under these programs.
17. National Childhood Vaccine Injury Act of 1986 (and amendments) Pub. L. 99-660; 42 U.S.C.A. §300 aa-1 (1986); N.C. Sess. L. 1985 (Reg. Sess. 1986) c. 1008 S.J. later made effective Oct. 1, 1986 (the same effective date as federal law) L. 1987 c. 215 5.8; Lenchek, *A*

Shot in the Arm: The National Vaccine Injury Act of 1986, 3 Wash. Lawyer 24-28, 58 (Mar-Apr. 1989).

18. Moore and O'Connell, *Foreclosing Medical Malpractice Claims by Prompt Tender of Economic Loss* 44 La. L. Rev. 1267 (1984).
19. Medical Offer and Recovery Act, H.R. 3084, 99th Cong. (July 25, 1985).
20. G. Friedman, Note, *Medical Malpractice Arbitration: Time for a Model Act* 33 Rutgers L. Rev. 454 (1981).
21. I. Ladimer, *The Case for Arbitration: Hospital Physician Disputes,* Hospital Trustee 33-35 (Feb. 1981); *Ciacco v. Cazayoux,* 519 So. 2d799 (La App. 1st Cir. 1987) typifies the problem of application and enforceability. In a wrongful death case, court held arbitration agreement valid and binding on patient who signed but not on husband minor deceased children who did not sign.
22. Powsner and Hamermesh, *Medical Malpractice Crisis the Second Time Around* 8 J. Legal Med. 283-291 (1987).
23. Kaiser Permanente Letter to James Clyne Deputy Superintendent New York State Insurance Department, describing nature, experience on program in Kaiser health benefits contracts (Sep. 23, 1985).
24. Maine law requires health insurers to provide nonbinding arbitration of disputes over benefit claims (Me. Rev. Stat. Ann tit 24, 2747, 2816) (1989).
25. *Madden v. Kaiser Foundation Hospitals,* 131 Cal. Rptr. 882, 552 P. 2d 1178 (1976). Golann, *Making Alternative Dispute Resolution Mandatory: The Constitutional Issues,* 68 Or. L. Rev. 487-568 (1989) (these issues were widely discussed by the House Ways and Means Committee consultations on mandating arbitration for Medicare and Medicaid claims).
26. D. Rubsamen, *The Experience of Binding Arbitration in the Ross-Loos Medical Group,* prepared for Secretary's Commission on Medical Malpractice, DHEW Contract No. HEW-OS 72-122, Report No. SCMM-DR-AS (1973).
27. D. Heintz, *An Analysis of the Southern California Arbitration Project National Center for Health Service Research* DHEW Publ. No. HRA 77-3159 (Mar. 1975).
28. Ladimer, Solomon, and Mulvihill, *Experience in Medical Malpractice Arbitration,* Legal Med. 433-463 (1981).
29. Ladimer, *Malpractice Arbitration of Medical and Hospital Claims,* 2 Health Care Man. Rev. 29 (Winter 1988).
30. I. Ladimer, *Versatility of Arbitration,* New York L.J. 1 (Mar. 8, 1979).
31. Eric R. Galton, *Building an ADR Practice (Practice Tips)* 23 The Brief (Amer. Bar Assoc.) 56-60 (Fall 1993) [referring also to Alan Aldehaff, *A Preparation Guide to Mediation,* 20 The Brief 53 (Summer 1991)].
32. American Bar Association 1993 Dispute Resolution Directory (1993). Reference to more than 400 programs and services.
33. Allison and Stahlhat, *Arbitration and the ADA: A Budding Partnership,* 48 Arbitration J. 53-60 (Sep. 1993).
34. *Promotion of Professional Review Activities,* 42 USC 11049, 1986, amended by Pub. L. 100-177 (1987) 101 Stat. 1007. (Medicaid Patient and Protection Act).

APPENDIX 7-1 Checklist and guidelines for ADR programs for health care

Note: This outline for an administrator or attorney suggests only issues to be considered, not solutions. It may apply to malpractice and other health/medical issues.

A. Jurisdiction and application
   1. Type of case or claim to be covered
   2. Mandatory (within a contract or program) or optional application by one or both parties
   3. Disputes: present, future, or both
   4. Parties directly or indirectly affected (minors, survivors, third parties)
   5. Conditions or regulations of local law or public agency
   6. Possible conflict with litigation

B. Acceptance and agreement
   1. Avoidance of adhesion; proper consent
   2. Legal and administrative conditions: notice, form of agreement, contract terms; time periods
   3. Coverage of single and multiple providers; staff, consultants, contractors (hospital, pharmacy, laboratory, suppliers)
   4. Marketing, education, and information; renewal agreements; relationship to other contract or health plan elements
   5. Recording of individual acceptances; modifications and cancellations

C. Arbitration or mediation in relation to prior complaint processes
   1. Use and exhaustion of internal remedies
   2. Single or dual paths for different types of claims (e.g., service, entitlement, medical practice)
   3. Joint review of multiple or related claims
   4. Decision points in system
   5. Financial implications of dual system with respect to insurance or organizational budget

D. Operation of ADR system — entry or access
   1. Conditions for starting process
      a. Under administered system (e.g., American Arbitration Association; state or federal program regulation)
      b. Under contract or party-developed system
   2. Time limits for initiation and later steps
   3. Problems of compliance or remand by court: motions affecting entry (see part I, "Enforcement and follow-up")

E. Administration — rules, procedures, consumer and attorney information
   1. Availability of general rules (e.g., use of AAA or other rules)
   2. Development of special rules: models; clearance, approval, and interpretation
   3. Prehearing processes

    a. Discovery procedures

    b. Informal settlement: mediation, use of ombudsmen

    c. Role of insurers, administrator, representatives of interested parties

    d. Closure or termination of case without hearing

  4. Representation: attorneys or others; witnesses; costs and fees

F. Arbitration tribunals or panels

  1. Number and type of fact finders, arbitrators, or mediators (specialty, qualifications and disqualifications)

  2. Selection under administered and party-appointed systems

  3. Development of rosters: local, national

  4. Payment of arbitrators

    a. Amount and source (parties, special fund, from award)

    b. Fees for neutral expert and demonstrations

G. Financial support of system and individual cases

  1. Fund for administration; for payment of filing and other fees; for education; for evaluation

    a. Supported by percentage of capitation

    b. Supported as an operational expense

    c. Supported by portion of awards

  2. Case fees

    a. Amount; contributions by parties

    b. Free consumer or indigent filing (and other expense; special fund)

H. Awards and remedies

  1. Limits on compensation or indemnity (noneconomic; collateral source; other limitations or requirements based on state law)

  2. Composite award: monetary compensation, medical care rehabilitation, other costs

    a. Position of insurance carrier

    b. Collateral support from government sources; health plan (e.g., medical care or other aid)

    c. Use of neutral agencies for medical supervision

  3. Written opinions accompanying awards

  4. Use of opinion and disposition data, if any, for:

    a. Improvement of health care and medical practice

    b. Guidelines (not precedents) for future cases

    c. Training: staff, arbitrators, attorneys, others

    d. Participation in data collection (research)

    e. Requirements of local law or public agency (e.g., state insurance, health department)

I. Enforcement and follow-up

  1. Action to compel arbitration per agreement (parties, terms, issues)

  2. Entry of judgment and enforcement by court

  3. Compliance through noncourt process (e.g., guarantee fund)

  4. Supervision of parties subject to award and remedy

  5. Reports to tribunal or agency

J. Evaluation

  1. Review of claims processing and disposition: time, awards, administrative costs; court involvement

  2. Use of system: types of cases, frequency, parties, essential issues, disposition, and follow-up

  3. Comparisons with prior experience or experience of others

  4. Effects on insurance premiums

  5. Consumer, attorney, and staff satisfaction

  6. Proposals for modification and improvement

Note: This outline may be more extensive than necessary, especially in jurisdictions or programs governed by state or lay agency regulations specifying arbitration, mediation, or other forms of conflict settlements. It is designed mainly for managed care systems such as HMO plans (in which arbitration is most likely to be used) and provider arrangements with professionals as well as consumers. Thus, it emphasizes the relationship between the arbitral process and the end stage of prior complaint and grievance systems.

CHAPTER 8   Selected health care statutory provisions

JAMES E. WARNER, J.D.
S. SANDY SANBAR, M.D., Ph.D., J.D., F.C.L.M.

ANTITRUST
THE FEDERAL FOOD, DRUG, AND COSMETIC ACT
MEDICAL DEVICES
LABORATORY REQUIREMENTS
HOSPITALS
HEALTH MAINTENANCE ORGANIZATIONS AND OTHER ORGANIZATIONAL STRUCTURES
THE SOCIAL SECURITY ACT
AREAS OF STATE JURISDICTION
QUESTIONS OF FRAUD
MILITARY PHYSICIANS
NATIONAL HEALTH SERVICE CORPS
THE PRISON SYSTEM
SPECIAL TYPES OF PATIENT EMPLOYMENT
ALTERNATIVE MEDICINE THERAPIES
RESEARCH AND MULTIDISCIPLINARY APPROACHES
PEER REVIEW
PHYSICIAN PAYMENT REVIEW COMMISSION
MISCELLANEOUS

There was a time when the legal aspects of the practice of medicine were defined in terms of the common law. The chief areas of concern were negligence, breech of contractual agreements, and breeches in the confidentiality of the doctor-patient relationship. Those times are now gone.

In their place exists a complicated regulatory web, woven of laws at all levels of government. The statutory scheme touches on such diverse aspects as environmental concerns, antitrust law, product liability, and civil rights. Health care regulation is an ocean both broad in scope and deep in complexity. A Westlaw search of "physicians" and "health care," for example, provided citations to more than 9900 separate federal statutes and regulations. Health care law is increasingly constitutional, statutory, and administrative law, rather than common law doctrines.

This chapter provides a reference to certain types of federal and state statutes, so that health care practitioners have a starting point for research into their specific concerns. Case law interpreting the statutes has been omitted. So too has material touching on a number of overly broad or overly specialized topics.

ANTITRUST

The major statutes in the area of antitrust are the Sherman Act, 15 U.S.C. Section 21 *et seq.,* and Section 7 of the Clayton Act, 15 U.S.C. Section 18. Guidance on allowable types of mergers for business entities in general, including health care institutions, can be found in the 1992 Merger Guidelines, 4 Trade Reg. Rep. (CCH) Para. 13,104, at 20,571. Guidelines for the health care field can be found in the Safe Harbor Regulations of the Medicare Anti-Kickback Provisions, 42 CFR 1001 *et seq.,* specifically at 1001.952 (1991).

Restrictions on the ability of physicians to diversify the business aspects of their practice can be found in the Self-Referral Provisions, 42 U.S.C. Section 1395nn, Section 1877 of the Social Security Act.

THE FEDERAL FOOD, DRUG, AND COSMETIC ACT

A major section of the regulatory structure related to health care is provided by the Federal Food and Drug Administration. Of primary interest to the practicing physician is the Federal Controlled Substances Act, 21 U.S.C. Section 801 *et seq.,* which details the allowable usages and requirements for the possession, use, and recording of controlled substances, including narcotics. Information regarding the Substance Abuse and Mental Health Services Administration is codified at 42 U.S.C.A. Section 290aa, *et seq.* Approval of new drugs is handled under 21 U.S.C.A. Section 355.

Cancer control programs under the National Cancer Institute are set forth at 42 U.S.C.A. Section 284 *et seq.*

The Department of Health and Human Services is responsible for creating a board for the development of drugs and devices for rare diseases or conditions. This board is known as the Orphan Products Board (42 U.S.C.A. Section 236).

Payment for covered outpatient drugs under the Social Security Act is covered at 42 U.S.C.A. Section 1396r-8. Significant recent amendments to the Act include the following:

Pub. L. 103-80, Section 1, 107 Stat. 773 (Aug. 13, 1993), the Nutrition Labeling and Education Act Amendments of 1993.

Pub. L. 102-571, Title I, Section 101(a), 106 Stat. 4491 (Oct. 29, 1992), the Prescription Drug User Fee Act of 1992.

Pub. L. 102-571, Title II, Section 201, 106 Stat. 4500 (Oct. 29, 1992), the Dietary Supplement Act of 1992.

Pub. L. 102-353, Section 1(a), 106 Stat. 941 (Aug. 26, 1992), the Prescription Drug Amendments of 1992.

MEDICAL DEVICES

The general provisions respecting control of devices intended for human use are found at 21 U.S.C.A. Section 360j. The practitioner should also note that significant questions regarding implantable medical devices also arise in the area of patent law.

42 U.S.C.A. Section 1395m sets out special payment rules under the Social Security Act for durable medical equipment.

LABORATORY REQUIREMENTS

Laboratory requirements for all types of medical laboratories, including those in a physician's office, are set under the Clinical Laboratories Improvement Amendments of 1988 (CLIA) at Pub. L. 100-587, 102 Stat. 2903, 42 U.S.C. Section 263a. The Stark law specifically prohibits physicians from sending lab work to a laboratory in which they retain an economic interest under virtually all circumstances (42 U.S.C.A. Section 1395nn).

Hazardous substances releases, liability, and compensation are covered at 42 U.S.C.A. Section 9604.

Patient radiation health and safety is discussed at 42 U.S.C.A. Section 10003 *et seq.*

HOSPITALS

Regulation of hospitals has progressed to the point where it is proper to speak in terms of a hospital being a theoretically private, but government-structured, institution. Pertinent statutes are as follows:

The Hospital and Medical Facilities Act of 1964 can be found at 42 U.S.C. Sections 201 nt, 247c, 291 *et seq.*

The Hospital and Medical Facilities Construction and Modernization Assistance Act of 1968 can be found at 42 U.S.C. Sections 201 nt, 291a, 291b.

Definitions on ambulatory and outpatient facilities are found at 42 U.S.C. Section 291o.

Special rules exist for rural areas, including grant funding to facilitate increased health care service in rural areas (42 U.S.C.A. Section 294p). Establishment of programs for improving trauma care in rural areas is covered by 42 U.S.C.A. Section 300d-3.

Requirements for, and assurance of quality of care in, skilled nursing facilities are set forth at 42 U.S.C.A. Section 1395i-3 and Section 1396r.

Note: The Safe Harbor Regulations of the Medicare Anti-Kickback Provisions also apply to hospitals (42 CFR 1001 *et seq.*).

HEALTH MAINTENANCE ORGANIZATIONS AND OTHER ORGANIZATIONAL STRUCTURES

The Health Maintenance Organization Act of 1973, Pub. L. 93-222, Pub. L. 95-626, codified at 12 U.S.C. Section 1721, 42 U.S.C. Sections 201 nt, 280c, 300e to 300e-14a, 2001, as amended, established the existence of health maintenance organizations (HMOs) and mandates their structure.

Payments to health maintenance organizations and competitive medical plans under the Social Security Act are at 42 U.S.C.A. Section 1395mm.

Federal mortgage insurance for group practice facilities and medical practice facilities is covered at 12 U.S.C.A. Section 1749aaa-5.

THE SOCIAL SECURITY ACT

The Social Security Act can be found at 42 U.S.C.A. Section 405 *et seq.,* and 42 U.S.C. 1395c *et seq.*

Rules for the exclusion of certain individuals and entities from participation in Medicare and state health care programs can be found at 42 U.S.C.A. Section 1320a-7. Exclusion for filing invalid claims can result in civil monetary penalties and, in cases of persons knowingly and willfully making a false statement or representation of a material fact in any application for repayment, criminal prosecution.

The federal anti-Kickback law has been specifically held applicable to Medicare and Medicaid claims (42 U.S.C. Section 1320a-7b). The provisions of this act have also been applied by the Internal Revenue Service (26 U.S.C. Section 162) and the Securities and Exchange Commission to cases in their respective areas of responsibility (*HLH*, 26-7).

The specific rules for determining disability and blindness under the act are found at 20 CFR Section 404.1512 *et seq.*

AREAS OF STATE JURISDICTION

In a number of cases, the federal statutes act to extend areas of traditional state law to actions taking place on federal lands. 42 U.S.C. Section 13031, for example, requires reporting of child abuse taking place on federal land or in federal facilities. Another example is trauma care modifications to state plans for emergency medical services, found at 42 U.S.C.A. Section 300d-13, which affects formula grants from the federal governments to the states.

State plans for medical assistance are included in the Social Security Act at 42 U.S.C.A. Section 1396a *et seq.*

QUESTIONS OF FRAUD

Large sections of federal law, including specifically provisions under the Social Security Act, provide for the imposition of penalties for noncompliance with, or attempts to defraud, the federal government as part of a medical reimbursement effort. A number of such statutes are cited elsewhere in the chapter. Other applicable statutes include:

The False Claims and Civil Actions for False Claims, 31 U.S.C. Sections 3729-3733.

The Program Fraud Civil Remedies Act of 1986, Pub. L. 99-509, 31 U.S.C. Sections 3801-3812.

The Major Fraud Act of 1988, Pub. L. 100-700.

MILITARY PHYSICIANS

A detailed discussion of federal law relating to military duty by physicians has been omitted. General rules are found at 10 U.S.C.A. Section 1087. The standard for defense of medical malpractice suits is found at 10 U.S.C.A. Section 1089. Basic relevant statutes on licensure, appointment, retention, etc., can be found at 10 U.S.C. 1094, 50 Ap Sections 454, 456.

Treatment of veterans and their medical benefits are covered at 38 U.S.C.A. Section 7316 (defense of malpractice and negligence suits) and 38 U.S.C.A. Section 7462 (major adverse actions involving professional conduct or competence).

NATIONAL HEALTH SERVICE CORPS

The provisions of the National Health Service Corps program can be found at 42 U.S.C.A. Section 254h *et seq.*

THE PRISON SYSTEM

A number of federal statutes involve medical care provided to persons being detained or incarcerated. 18 U.S.C.A. Section 4244, for example, covers hospitalization of a convicted person suffering from mental disease or defect.

Claims under 42 U.S.C.A. Sections 1981 and 1983 often result out of an incarceration context. Specifics on Section 1983 claims by prisoners can be found in 42 U.S.C.A. Section 1983, at heading XII, Medical Care of Prisoners, 841-890.

Civil commitment of persons not charged with any criminal offense is covered at 42 U.S.C.A. Section 3412.

SPECIAL TYPES OF PATIENT EMPLOYMENT

Statutes providing special treatment for certain types of employment are given in the following list:

5 U.S.C.A. Section 7901, services to government employees

5 U.S.C.A. Section 8103, compensation for work injuries

5 U.S.C.A. Section 8904, government employees' health insurance

22 U.S.C.A. Section 4084, health care program for foreign service

33 U.S.C.A. Section 907, medical services and supplies to longshore and harbor workers

26 U.S.C.A. Section 9712, coal industry health benefits

50 U.S.C.A. Section 2051, Central Intelligence Agency retirement and disability system, retirement for disability or incapacity.

46 U.S.C.A. Section 11102 of the Merchant Seamen Protection and Relief Act provides for the maintenance of medicine chests on board vessels.

ALTERNATIVE MEDICINE THERAPIES

Information about grants for chiropractic demonstration projects is available at 42 U.S.C.A. Section 295a.

Provisions for the establishment of an Office of Alternative Medicine, to evaluate alternative medical treatment modalities, including acupuncture and Oriental medicine, homeopathic medicine, and physical manipulation therapies, can be found at 42 U.S.C.A. Section 283g.

RESEARCH AND MULTIDISCIPLINARY APPROACHES

A number of advisory boards on specific disease types exist, including the National Heart, Lung, and Blood Institute, the National Diabetes Advisory Board, the National Digestive Diseases Advisory Board, the Office of Research on Women's Health, and the National Kidney and Urologic Diseases Advisory Board (42 U.S.C.A. Section 285b-2 *et seq.*).

Restrictions on fetal research are codified at 42 U.S.C.A. Section 289g.

Research grants for genetic diseases are provided at 42 U.S.C.A. Section 300b-1.

42 U.S.C.A. Section 300cc-3 *et seq.* covers research for acquired immune deficiency syndrome (AIDS).

PEER REVIEW

The peer review process is mandated at 42 U.S.C.A. Section 299b-1, under the Forum for Quality and Effectiveness in Health Care. The administrator is authorized to enter into contracts with public and nonprofit private entities for the purpose of developing and periodically reviewing and updating guidelines for medical care.

The general provisions for peer review are contained at 42 U.S.C.A. Section 1320b-12.

The obligations of health care practitioners and providers of health care services are set forth at 42 U.S.C.A. Section 1320c-5.

42 U.S.C.A. Section 11111 *et seq.* covers promotion of professional review activities.

PHYSICIAN PAYMENT REVIEW COMMISSION

42 U.S.C.A. Section 1395w-1 creates the Physician Payment Review Commission, which makes recommendations to Congress regarding adjustments to the rea-

sonable levels at which physicians should charge for services. The actual provision for payment fee schedules is at 42 U.S.C.A. Section 1395w-4. Determination of entitlement, and provisions for appeal of a negative determination, are at 42 U.S.C.A. Section 1395ff *et seq.*

Establishment of the Provider Reimbursement Review Board is at 42 U.S.C.A. Section 1395oo.

MISCELLANEOUS

Subrogation of third-party claims by the United States is covered at 42 U.S.C.A. Section 2651.

It is important that the physician and his or her office manager be aware of the requirements of the Equal Employment Opportunities Act, at 42 U.S.C.A. Section 2000e *et seq.* Note also that 42 U.S.C.A. Section 2000d imposes a prohibition against exclusion from participation in, denial of benefits of, and discrimination under federally assisted programs on the grounds of race, color, or national origin.

Child abuse prevention and treatment and adoption reform is covered at 42 U.S.C.A. Section 5106g *et seq.* and 42 U.S.C.A. Section 13001b *et seq.* There is a specific reporting requirement for health care personnel, which is contained at Section 13031.

APPENDIX 8-1   Advanced health care directive statutes, by state

Alabama	§22-8A-1 to §22-8A-10	Nebraska	—
Alaska	§18.12.010 to §18.12.100	Nevada	§449.535 *et seq.*
Arizona	§36-3201 to 3262	New Hampshire	§177.H.1 *et seq.*
Arkansas	§20-17-201 *et seq.*, §20-13-901 to 908	New Jersey	—
California	Health and S. §7185 *et seq.*	New Mexico	§24-7-1 *et seq.*
Colorado	§15-18-101 *et seq.*	New York	Pub. HE §2980 *et seq.*
Connecticut	§19A-570 *et seq.*	North Carolina	§32A.15 to §32A.26, §90.320 to §90.323
Delaware	Title 16, §2501 *et seq.*	North Dakota	§23-06-5-1, §23-06-4 *et seq.*
Florida	§744.3115	Ohio	§2133.01, Durable Power §1337.11 *et seq.*
Georgia	§88.4101 *et seq.*	Oklahoma	Title 63, §3-101 *et seq.*
Hawaii	§327F.2 *et seq.*, §327D.2 *et seq.*	Oregon	—
Idaho	§39-4501 *et seq.*	Pennsylvania	20 PS 5401 *et seq.*
Illinois	755 ILCS 35/1 *et seq.*, 210 ILCS 50/10.3	Puerto Rico	—
Indiana	§16-36-4-1 *et seq.*	Rhode Island	Gen. Laws 23-4-11-1 *et seq.*
Iowa	§144A.1 *et seq.*	S. Carolina	§44-66-10, §44-77-10, §44-66-110 *et seq.*
Kansas	§65-28-101 *et seq.*	S. Dakota	§34-12D-1 *et seq.*, §34-12C-1 *et seq.*, §39-7-2 *et seq.*
Kentucky	§311.622 *et seq.*		
Louisiana	§40:1299 *et seq.*, §58.1	Tennessee	§32-11-101 *et seq.*, §34-6-101 *et seq.*
Maine	Title 18A, §5701 *et seq.*	Texas	H + S 672.001 *et seq.*
Maryland	HG §5-601 *et seq.*	Utah	§75-2-1101 *et seq.*
Massachusetts	Chap. 201D-1 *et seq.*	Vermont	Title 18, §5252 *et seq.*
Michigan	§700.496 *et seq.*	Virginia	§54-1-2981 *et seq.*
Minnesota	§145B.01 *et seq.*	Washington	§70.122.010 *et seq.*
Mississippi	§41-14-101, §41-41-151 *et seq.*	W. Virginia	§16-30-1 *et seq.*, §16-30B-1 *et seq.*, §16-30C-1 *et seq.*
Missouri	§459.010 *et seq.*		
Montana	§50-9-102 *et seq.*, §50-10-101 *et seq.*	Wisconsin	§154.01 *et seq.*, §155.01 *et seq.*
		Wyoming	§35-22-101 *et seq.*

APPENDIX 8-2   Controlled substances statutes, by state

Alabama	§20-2-1 to §20-2-144	Montana	§50, Chap. 32 *et seq.*
Alaska	§11.30 generally, §11.71, §11.73	Nebraska	§28-401 *et seq.*
Arizona	§36-2501 *et seq.*, §32-1901 *et seq.*	Nevada	§453.021 *et seq.*
Arkansas	§5-64-101 *et seq.*	New Hampshire	§172.1, §318.B.1 *et seq.*
California	Health and S. §11000 *et seq.*	New Jersey	§24:21-1 *et seq.*
Colorado	§18-5-601 *et seq.*, §18-18-419	New Mexico	§30-31-1 *et seq.*
Connecticut	§21A-240 *et seq.*	New York	Pub. HE §3302 *et seq.*
Delaware	Title 16, §4701 *et seq.*	North Carolina	§90.86 to §90.113.8
Florida	§893.01 *et seq.*	North Dakota	§19-03-1-1 *et seq.*
Georgia	§79a.803 *et seq.*	Ohio	§3719.01 *et seq.*
Hawaii	§329-1 *et seq.*	Oklahoma	Title 63, §2-101 *et seq.*
Idaho	§37-2701 *et seq.*	Oregon	§167.203, §475.005, §475.035 *et seq.*
Illinois	720 ILCS 570/1001 *et seq.*, 720 ILCS 570/40	Pennsylvania	35 PS 780.101 *et seq.*
Indiana	§35-48-1 *et seq.*	Puerto Rico	—
Iowa	§124.101 *et seq.*	Rhode Island	Gen. Laws 21-28-2-01 *et seq.*
Kansas	§65-655g *et seq.*, §65-4101 *et seq.*	S. Carolina	§44-53-10 *et seq.*
Kentucky	§218A.010 *et seq.*	S. Dakota	§34-20B-11 *et seq.*
Louisiana	§40:961 *et seq.*	Tennessee	§39-17-401 *et seq.*
Maine	Title 17A, §1101 *et seq.*, Title 32, §1081 *et seq.*	Texas	H + S 481.001 *et seq.*
		Utah	§58-37-2 *et seq.*
Maryland	HO §27-277 *et seq.*	Vermont	Title 18, §4201 *et seq.*
Massachusetts	Chap. 94c-1 *et seq.*	Virginia	§54-1-3401 *et seq.*
Michigan	§333.7101 *et seq.*	Washington	§69.50.101 *et seq.*
Minnesota	§151.01 *et seq.*, §152.01 *et seq.*	W. Virginia	§60A-1-101 to §60A-7-707
Mississippi	§14-29-101 *et seq.*	Wisconsin	§161.001 *et seq.*
Missouri	§195.010, §196.010 *et seq.*	Wyoming	§33-24-201 *et seq.*

APPENDIX 8-3   Medical licensure statutes, by state (statutes annotated)

Alabama	§34-24-50 to 84, -310-406	Missouri	§334.031 *et seq.*
Alaska	§08.64.107-360,	Montana	Chap. 3, P. 3 (§301) *et seq.*
Arizona	§32-1421 *et seq.*	Nebraska	§71-1.102 *et seq.*
Arkansas	§17-93-400 to 500	Nevada	§630.160 *et seq.*
California	Bus. & P. §2030 *et seq.*	New Hampshire	§329.10 *et seq.*
Colorado	§12-36-101 to 137	New Jersey	§45:9-12 *et seq.*
Connecticut	§20-8a, -10 *et seq.*	New Mexico	§61-6-11 *et seq.*
Delaware	Title 24, §1701 *et seq.*	New York	Educ. Law §6524 *et seq.*
District of Columbia	§2-3505 *et seq.*	North Carolina	§90-6 *et seq.*
		North Dakota	§43-17-17 *et seq.*
Florida	§455.01, Licensure and Sanctions 458.301 *et seq.*	Ohio	§4731.08 *et seq.*
		Oklahoma	Title 59, §481 *et seq.*
Georgia	§84.906 *et seq.*	Oregon	§677-100 *et seq.*
Hawaii	§453-4 *et seq.*	Pennsylvania	Title 63, §422.22, 422.25 *et seq.*
Idaho	§54-1801 to 1841	Puerto Rico	Title 20, §30 *et seq.*
Illinois	225 ILCS 60/1 *et seq.*	Rhode Island	Gen. Laws 5-37-2 *et seq.*
Indiana	§25-22.5-1-1.1 *et seq.*	S. Carolina	§40-47-140 *et seq.*
Iowa	§148.1 *et seq.*	S. Dakota	§36-4-10 *et seq.*
Kansas	§65-2802 *et seq.*	Tennessee	§63-6-201 *et seq.*
Kentucky	§311.550 *et seq.*	Texas	Civil Stat., Art. 4495b, 3.01 *et seq.*
Louisiana	§37:1271 *et seq.*	Utah	§58-12-30 *et seq.*
Maine	Title 32, §3269 *et seq.*	Vermont	Title 26, §1391 *et seq.*
Maryland	HO §14-101 *et seq.*	Virginia	§54.1-2930 *et seq.*
Massachusetts	Chap. 112, §2 *et seq.*	Washington	§18.71.021 *et seq.*, §18.120.010
Michigan	§333.17011 *et seq.*	W. Virginia	§30-3-10 *et seq.*
Minnesota	§147.02 *et seq.*	Wisconsin	§448.01 *et seq.*
Mississippi	§73-43-1 *et seq.*, 73-25-1 *et seq.*	Wyoming	§33-26-303 *et seq.*

APPENDIX 8-4   Medical malpractice claims statutes, by state

Alabama	Medical Liability Act of 1987, §6-5-480 *et seq.*
Alaska	§09.55.530-560
Arizona	§32-1854, §12-563 *et seq.*
Arkansas	§16-114-201 to 209
California	Bus. & P. §3527 *et seq.*, 801, 802; CC 3333.1 to 2
Colorado	§13-64-401 *et seq.*
Connecticut	§52-184c
Delaware	Title 18, §6801 *et seq.*
Florida	§461.013 *et seq.*, 766.101 *et seq.*
Georgia	§81a.1089 *et seq.*
Hawaii	§671-3 *et seq.*
Idaho	§6-1001 *et seq.*
Illinois	735 ILCS 5/2 *et seq.*
Indiana	§27-12-1-1 to §27-12-18-1,
Iowa	§147.135 *et seq.*
Kansas	§60-3401, §65-4901 *et seq.*
Kentucky	§413.140 *et seq.*
Louisiana	§40:1299.39 *et seq.*
Maine	Title 24, §2501 *et seq.*
Maryland	HO §14-101 *et seq.*
Massachusetts	CJ, §3-2A-01 *et seq.*
Michigan	§600.1483 *et seq.*, §500.2477 *et seq.*
Minnesota	§145.682, §573.02 *et seq.*
Mississippi	§11-1-59 *et seq.*, 15-1-36
Missouri	§484.190 *et seq.*
Montana	§27-6-103 *et seq.*
Nebraska	§44-2801 *et seq.*
Nevada	§41A.003 *et seq.*
New Hampshire	§507C.1, §507E.1 *et seq.*
New Jersey	§17:30D-1 *et seq.* (Liability Insurance Act)
New Mexico	§41-5-1 *et seq.*
New York	CPLR §3017 *et seq.*
North Carolina	§90.21.11 to .14
North Dakota	§28-01-18, §28-01-46, §43-17.1 *et seq.*
Ohio	§2305, §2307, §2317 *et seq.*
Oklahoma	Title 76, §17 *et seq.*
Oregon	§18-470 *et seq.*, §30-080 *et seq.*
Pennsylvania	40 PS 1301.301 *et seq.*
Puerto Rico	Title 20, §52a, Title 31, §2991, *et seq.*
Rhode Island	Gen. Laws 9-19-32 *et seq.*
S. Carolina	§40-47-60, §40-47-190, §40-47-260
S. Dakota	Arbitration §21-25-1 *et seq.*
Tennessee	§29-26-115 *et seq.*
Texas	Civil Stat., Art. 4591i *et seq.*
Utah	§78-14-1 *et seq.*
Vermont	Title 12, §700 *et seq.*, §1908, §1909
Virginia	§55-7B-1 *et seq.*
Washington	§655.001 *et seq.*
W. Virginia	§9-2-1501 *et seq.*
Wisconsin	§448.01 *et seq.*
Wyoming	§33-26-303 *et seq.*

CHAPTER 9 **Education and licensure**

S. SANDY SANBAR, M.D., Ph.D., J.D., F.C.L.M.
DANIEL J. GAMINO, J.D.
JAMES E. WARNER, J.D.

THE "RIGHT" TO BE A PHYSICIAN
MEDICAL SCHOOL ADMISSION CRITERIA
MEDICAL SCHOOL RETENTION AND GRADUATION
MEDICAL LICENSURE: THEORY AND REQUIREMENTS
MEDICAL LICENSURE: SUPERVISION AND DISCIPLINARY SANCTIONS
CONCLUSION

This chapter covers pivotal, threshold issues. Medical education, from admission to medical school to completion of postgraduate training, occurs in a definite legal framework. Both the student and the state enjoy certain legal rights and duties.

State licensure to practice medicine and surgery is also basic. The requirements for licensure and the ways in which that medical licensure may be lost or curtailed are many.

More than 400 years ago Shakespeare observed, "Oh, how full of briers is this working-day world."[1] That is still true for medicine today. This chapter points out these briers.

THE "RIGHT" TO BE A PHYSICIAN

There is no vested property or constitutional right to attend medical school. However, selection to a medical school class may not be based on any violation of the applicant's general civil rights, nor may requirements be arbitrary or capricious. A medical school may not employ quotas, but may employ some affirmative action in selecting students. The relationship of the medical student and the school is an enforceable contractual relationship. Some courts have held a student admitted to medical school to have a "liberty right or interest," mandating procedural due process necessary for administrative problems and substantive due process for disciplinary situations. The general rule is one of fair play in making rules regarding information, discipline, and punishment.

MEDICAL SCHOOL ADMISSION CRITERIA

Each medical school, public or private, can establish its own admission standards. The admission criteria must be uniformly applied to each candidate. The primary area of legal interest in medical school admissions is that of affirmative action admissions programs, which make race, gender, or ethnic origin a factor of greater or lesser degree in the acceptance decision.

Early medical school admission cases focused on a variety of legal theories. The courts have allowed the return of entrance application fees under a theory of false pretenses when the standards used for admission were not in keeping with those advertised in the medical school's bulletin.[2] Professional schools have been ordered to award degrees to students when they were denied admission or retention on an arbitrary or unreasonable basis.[3]

Judicial review

Judicial review of the medical school admissions process on constitutional equal protection grounds requires the existence of "state action" sufficient to trigger the provisions of the applicable constitutional provision or federal statute. In *Cannon v. University of Chicago,*[4] a female student's suit under the federal sex and age discrimination statutes was deemed as failing to state a cause of action because of a failure to prove the existence of state action.

In a decision foreshadowing the *Bakke* decision, the Court of Appeals of New York held that a strict scrutiny standard of review applied to racial reverse discrimination in medical school admissions. The New York court did not discuss less restrictive alternatives available to the university, because the cessation of the minority admissions program would still not have entitled the plaintiff to a place in the incoming class.[5]

The Bakke decision

The seminal legal decision involving medical school admission requirements is that of *University of California Regents v. Bakke.*[6] In that case Mr. Bakke was denied admission to the University of California–Davis Medical School because his credentials failed to meet the standards required for admission as a nonminority applicant. School policy established a quota-based affirmative action program setting aside 16% of the available places in the entering medical class for minority applicants, defined as Blacks, Chicanos, and Asian-Americans. Bakke's entrance scores were higher than those of certain persons accepted under the minority entry program. Thus, but for Mr. Bakke's race and ethnic origin, he most likely would have been accepted for entry into medical school.

Bakke sued, claiming a violation of the Equal Protection Clause of the U.S. Constitution and Title VI of the 1964 Civil Rights Act. No clear majority opinion developed from the U.S. Supreme Court's review of the case. Six separate opinions were written, with no more than four justices agreeing on any one chain of reasoning behind their decision. Evaluation of the *Bakke* decisions is thus somewhat difficult.

Four justices of the Court held that the Davis plan was completely constitutional. Four held the quota plan in violation of Title VI and failed to reach the constitutional equal protection issue.

The swing vote was cast by Justice Powell. He considered that Title VI was primarily a codification of the constitutional equal protection standard, and thus the applicable standard of review was identical under either a constitutional or statutory evaluation.

Justice Powell, applying a strict scrutiny standard of review, considered the use of race to be a valid factor in the evaluation of potential medical candidates, but stressed that the quota system was not necessary to achieve the university's desired goal and thus was not permissible.

The four-justice group led by Justice Brennan agreed with Justice Powell's approach (allowing the use of race as a factor in the admissions process), but considered the applicable standard of review to be an intermediate level of scrutiny, as is applied in sex discrimination cases such as *Craig v. Boren.*[7] The *Bakke* decision did not answer all questions. The decision established that affirmative action programs in a medical school admissions process could be structured to avoid constitutional legal protection violations, and further that certain types of affirmative admissions programs, such as quota-based systems, were a violation of equal protection rights. The difficulty of *Bakke* was that the Court failed to articulate a definitive standard of review for affirmative action admissions programs.

Reaction to Bakke

Reaction to the *Bakke* decision was mixed both during and after the decision was rendered. The National Conference of Black Lawyers and the National Lawyers Guild, for example, urged that the Supreme Court refuse to hear the case at all on the grounds of inadequate records regarding possible past racial discrimination by the University.[8]

In a similar case, the U.S. Supreme Court had previously refused to decide a similar case on the merits at all, declaring the matter moot, since the student in question was about to complete his legal education.[9] On remand the Supreme Court of Washington upheld its earlier decision holding the minority admissions policy of the university to be valid.[10]

General rule

Generally, affirmative action minority placement programs for medical schools are permissible, as long as race is not used as the sole determining factor in the evaluation process. It is important to remember that state action requirements must be established before a standard of review is applicable.

Americans with Disabilities Act

The 1990 Americans with Disabilities Act (ADA) provides that "no qualified individual with a disability shall by reason of such disability be excluded from participating in or be denied the benefits of the services, programs, or activities of a public entity...."[11] This mandate requires medical schools, both public and private,[12] to make "reasonable accommodations" in evaluating applicants. Case law on ADA is nearly nonexistent. Requirements for accommodation may include granting additional time to candidates to take entrance examinations, providing a reader to the sight-impaired or dyslexic candidate, and perhaps instituting a different standard of review of a disabled candidate's undergraduate transcript and grades.

MEDICAL SCHOOL RETENTION AND GRADUATION

The primary concern of most medical students is successful graduation. Numerous suits have occurred as a result of student dismissals, either on academic or disciplinary grounds. The nature of legal challenges raised in an attempt to prevent academic dismissals is quite varied.

Academic dismissals

Once accepted into the medical school program at a public institution, students are deemed to have a liberty or property interest in the continuation of their medical school education and in eventually receiving their medical degrees. Private medical schools, while not subject to Fourteenth Amendment due process itself, are subject to the standards set by accreditation requirements, and any standard or procedures that have been internally adopted.

Attention to the due process requirement during an academic dismissal proceeding is essential on the part of the medical school administration. Strict adherence to due process protects the rights of the student and helps reduce the risk of future litigation by the student.

Academic dismissals (i.e., those that are based on poor academic performance or failure to complete the requirements for graduation) are evaluated differently from disciplinary dismissals. Notice of the potential dismissal must be given by the institution to the student, but traditional legal procedures for fact-finding, such as for a hearing, are not legally required. Academic dismissals may arise from either strict academic performance or from clinical performance.

A key case on academic dismissals is *Board of Curators of the University of Missouri v. Horowitz.*[13] Therein, the U.S. Supreme Court ruled that in the case of academic dismissals notice of the impending dismissal was required to be given to the student, but a formal hearing was not mandatory. The Supreme Court based its decision on the long tradition of judicial deference to academic discretion, and that the academic evaluation of a student is more properly placed in the academic setting rather than the judicial courtroom.

Post-*Horowitz* decisions have tended to uphold medical schools' decisions for academic dismissal over procedural due process challenges of medical school students. In most cases, medical schools have provided procedural protections far beyond the scope required by *Horowitz,* including multiple forms of notice and multiple opportunities for academic hearings and inquiry prior to final dismissal on academic grounds. In *Sanders v. Ajir,*[14] for example, the Court held that a student going through the dismissal process on two separate occasions, with two levels of hearing on each occasion, had been afforded a level of procedural protection in excess of the requirements set by the *Horowitz* case.

Where academic hearings have been offered to a student prior to academic dismissal, court decisions have not required the same degree of formal procedural protection that has been required in other Fourteenth Amendment property or liberty settings. Most academic procedures do not provide for the presence of an attorney during hearings or for a formal transcript of the proceedings. Records consisting of the initial notice of dismissal and a summary of the final decision of the academic hearing committee are sufficient. Witnesses, including faculty members, are often questioned by the dismissal panel outside the presence of the student.

Hearings are thus informal and nonadversarial in nature. The hearings normally consist of the student making a statement to the appeals board and then answering questions.

Even in the post-*Horowitz* cases that have required a hearing, the Court has required only that the student be given the opportunity to explain his or her poor scholarship, and to provide any additional information that might lead to an expectation of future satisfactory performance.[15]

Disciplinary dismissal

In contrast to dismissal for academic grounds, disciplinary dismissal entitles the student to a greater standard of procedural protection.

Disciplinary dismissal of students occurs on the basis of nonacademic considerations, usually specified in a formal academic code of conduct by the medical school. Reasons for disciplinary dismissal include plagiarism, cheating, and disruptive behavior. The legal requirements for due process in disciplinary dismissal cases include notice to the student of the intended dismissal, an opportunity to be heard, and an opportunity to rebut the school's grounds for dismissal. Disciplinary dismissal due process directly parallels protection afforded individuals prior to the deprivation of a liberty or a property interest. An example is *Goss v. Lopez.*[16] There, the U.S. Supreme Court held that a high school student could not be suspended for improper behavior without notice of the charges against him, an explanation of the evidence, and an opportunity to present his side. The standard for procedural process is the *Matthews v. Eldridge*[17] test, which weighs the strength of the private interest, the strength of the state interest, the risk of error under the current procedures used, and the probable value of additional or substitute procedural safeguards.

Substantive due process claims

Substantive due process consists of the concept that the individual is entitled to a decision that is not arbitrary or capricious, when a liberty or property interest exists. Educational institutions cannot act in an arbitrary way or in a capricious manner. In a dismissal case the burden of proof is on the student to demonstrate an arbitrary or capricious decision, that is, no real basis for dismissal existed or that malice, bad faith, or ill-will existed on the part of the medical school or its acting employees.

Exercise of discretion by the medical school in terms of retention based on academic failure has not been considered to be arbitrary or capricious action by the courts.

In contrast, a student mandatorily dismissed for first-year academic failure, when three other students with an equal or greater number of failures were allowed to repeat the first year, was judged arbitrary by a New York court at the trial level, but was reversed on an appeal.[18] In Michigan, a decision resulted against the medical school when a student was singled out on the basis of his initial score on the NBNE examination, and was deprived of his opportunity to retake the test along with 40 other students from the same school who had failed the same part of the examination.

Mere general allegations by a student that a particular grade or dismissal was improper usually fails to meet the requirements of proof to establish arbitrary, capricious action by the medical school. In contrast, if the student can demonstrate by objective evidence how he was singled out for disparate treatment from fellow students, his chances of proving arbitrary and capricious behavior on the part of the medical school are considerably enhanced.

Contractual relations between medical school and student

Related to the concept of substantive due process is the use of contractual claims by the student to establish procedural or substantive legal rights. The trend of the courts has been to construe liberally the terms of the contract in favor of the medical school. This approach is typical in educational contract cases. But it is at variance from the more traditional contract viewpoint that a contract should be construed strictly with respect to the person drafting the contract, in this case the medical school.[19]

Handicapped students

The Americans with Disabilities Act, originally enacted by Congress in 1990, is changing how medical schools and all other schools approach handicapped students.[20] This act requires medical schools to make "reasonable accommodations" toward students with certain physical and mental disabilities. Dyslexia, narcolepsy, drug and alcohol abuse, and mental disorders all fall within the scope of disabilities and certain protections of the law, along with the more traditional physical handicaps.[21] Little case law has yet developed today.

Substance of content of medical school education

Increasingly, the demands to include new information in the medical school curriculum, for example, courses on AIDS, have produced a problem of serious dimensions in medical school class scheduling. The phenomenon can be seen both within the medical school educational process and the process of health care law instruction within the legal community.[22]

The AIDS crisis exemplifies the difficulty of providing education and medical ethics within the medical school process. The medical student is presented with the dilemma when assigned to a rotation that requires treatment of AIDS patients. AIDS demonstrates the potential for new requirements of specific substantive courses within medical school education by state law, a step that would be historically unique within the medical school process.[23]

Substance of content requirements has also been increasingly dictated in a variety of other areas, on both a voluntary and involuntary basis.[24] These trends point to the potential tendency toward further standardization of the medical school education process.

House officers

A medical school graduate is required to complete at least one year of postgraduate training in an internship, usually in a hospital. Many then go on to advanced training programs, residencies, and fellowships certified by a variety of organizations.

In the past, house officers were considered to be employees and subject to the whim of the hospital administration. A recent California court decision,[25] noting the impact of the arbitrary cancellation of a house officer contract on his career, imposed the requirement of a due process hearing, with all its protection. In light of the increasing scrutiny of courts over actions of hospital boards of trustees in dealing with their professional staffs, this case is a harbinger of increasing legal scrutiny.

Clinical training programs present a serious potential for questions in the area of medical malpractice. There is considerable divergence among jurisdictions on the standard of care for residents in the academic medical context. Although *Rusk v. Akron General Hospital*[26] represents the position that a special standard of care is applicable for interns and residents within the medical school and clinical context, more recent cases suggest that the standard of care to be applied will either be the standard of a general physician[27] or the standard of the specialty to which the resident is being trained.[28] Although there appear to be no reported cases covering the standard of care for medical students,[29] it is important for the medical student, intern, or resident to be aware of the potential for being held to the standard of care applicable to the attending physician supervising his or her education and clinical process. Also, the team-teaching approach presents additional informed consent issues. It is important to recognize that the consent is specific for the individual physician. Thus, consent by the patient for one attending physician to engage in a procedure does not automatically grant consent for the procedure to be performed by proxy (e.g., by a resident or intern), even though the procedure is done at the attending physician's or senior resident's request.[30] Thus, in the academic medical context several possibilities for liability arise that do not normally occur within the private practice setting. The attending physician and student must be aware of the potential for liability, take steps to ensure proper consent on the part of the patients, and maintain the highest possible standards of care.[31]

MEDICAL LICENSURE: THEORY AND REQUIREMENTS
Power of the state

The state may require the professional to obtain a license to carry out the practice of medicine and surgery in order to exclude any incompetent practitioners. The state has a right to continue to evaluate a physician's professional practice. "The right of a physician to toil in his profession . . . with all its sanctity and safeguards is not absolute. It must yield to the paramount right of government to protect the public health by any rational means."[32]

Licensing statutes are justified under a state's sovereign power to protect the health and welfare of its citizens. Medical practice acts create and define the composition of a state medical board, define the requirements for licensure, and vest the board with the authority to license candidates. The state medical board is mandated to regulate the practice of medicine in the public interest and for the advancement of the medical profession. Establishing and vigilantly enforcing standards of conduct to ensure the competence and the scruples of physicians is the responsibility of the board. This stewardship is viewed by courts as an entrustment by the state, and is subject to judicial review.

Licensure statutes were originally designed to exclude the untutored, unskilled, and incompetent from the practice of medicine by certifying a minimally acceptable qualification of training, knowledge, and competence after evaluating and certifying submitted credentials. In a landmark case in 1898, the U.S. Supreme Court stated that licensure powers could be extended beyond credentialing to include standards of behavior and ethics. The case held that, in a doctor, "character is as important a qualification as knowledge."[33]

Sanctions may include denial of license, revocation, suspension, probation, oral or written reprimands, imposition of monetary fines, and censuring.

The authority of the courts to oversee the licensing of physicians is also mandated by statute. The courts, however, seldom intercede until the physician has completely exhausted his administrative remedies, unless the licensing board has acted wholly outside of its jurisdiction. At the conclusion of the administrative proceedings, the courts typically intervene only when the physician successfully argues that the licensing board violated the physician's constitutional rights, that it acted outside of its jurisdiction, or that it failed to follow its own rules and regulations.

Types of licensure

Virtually all state medical licenses are unlimited, that is, unrestricted to any branch of medicine or surgery. Thus, the holder of a medical license may perform routine histories and physicals or specialized neurosurgery under the same license.

Some states have a restricted license for postgraduate training, such as residency. In some cases, the credentialing process is delegated *de facto* to the supervising institution. Physicians in state hospitals or correctional facilities sometimes hold licenses restricted to such institutional use. Again, the respective state legislature and/or medical board will set forth the specific types of licensure available in that state.

As a sanction, some physicians may be restricted to institutional practice as a result of disciplinary proceedings in which supervision of practice is deemed appropriate. Such licensure curtailment is sometimes supplanted by other restrictive techniques, such as probation.

Some states allow temporary licensure, to allow *locum tenens* work or to allow a visiting expert to a medical school to engage in clinical activities.

Obtaining a license

As a necessary function of its duty to protect the public interest, a state board may require physicians and related practitioners to demonstrate a certain degree of skill and learning. It may also include conditions of licensure bearing a direct, substantial, and reasonable relationship to the practice of medicine, such as a statutorily specified amount of malpractice insurance coverage before the licensee may practice medicine. In exercising its licensing authority, the state has the inherent power to determine precisely the qualifications the applicant must possess. It may investigate educational credentials, professional competence, and moral character. The applicant bears the burden to prove his fulfillment of all requirements for licensure.

U.S. citizenship was once required for medical licensure, but that requirement was struck down by the U.S. Supreme Court in 1973 as unconstitutional discrimination. Another barrier to licensure was a residency requirement of a specific number of months. That requirement, too, was struck down as discrimination that only furthered the parochial interest of state physicians. Closely related to residency restrictions is reciprocity licensure. A state is not required to license a physician based merely on his holding a license from another state; otherwise the state would be obligated to automatically grant a license to everyone who held a license in another state. Thus, reciprocity is neither constitutionally discriminatory nor an infringement on one's rights and privilege of practice. Most states have also established a minimum age of 21 for licensure.

Invariably, "good moral character" is required for licensure. A typical reason for denying a license on that ground is a prior criminal conviction, even if the crime on which the conviction was based has no obvious connection with the practice of medicine. Such candidates must be prepared to demonstrate total rehabilitation. The nature of the offense is a material consideration. For example, a licensing board should be prepared to differentiate between a trespass conviction arising out of a 1970s antiwar demonstration and the offense of grand larceny.

State requirements of educational achievement for licensure vary, but have generally been upheld. Educational requirements cannot be arbitrary and must be rationally related to competence. Requirements of preprofessional education and professional education from "accredited" schools has been held reasonable and valid.[34] Experience requirements of postgraduate education are likewise considered to be rational, reasonable, and valid. If experience provided comparable or superior education but licensure required a diploma, it has been held that the diploma requirement was not capricious or arbitrary, and did not deprive one of a constitutional right of due process or equal protection.[35]

Requiring malpractice insurance, a recent mandate in at least one state (Idaho), was upheld as reasonable because it bears a rational relationship to the welfare of citizens.

MEDICAL LICENSURE: SUPERVISION AND DISCIPLINARY SANCTIONS
Grounds for discipline

Until a few years ago, licensure sanctions against physicians because of their inadequate care of patients were few and far between. In large part, this was due to the reluctance of physicians to report or take action against colleagues. In particular, physicians feared that their colleagues who were reported would sue them for libel, slander, or restraint of trade. Additionally, the boards were nearly impotent, having more restricted investigative ability and less sanctioning authority.

This situation has now changed. Courts have held not only hospitals but also physicians liable for failure to ferret out bad physicians. Legislatures have given administrative agencies new power and have granted immunity to honorable informants and their authorized listeners. Licensing boards no longer wait for a formal report or complaint; they may now begin an inquiry and proceedings on their own initiative. Some courts have even allowed licensing board proceedings while a criminal proceeding is still pending.

Grounds for discipline of the medical licensee are generally set forth in statute as "unprofessional conduct." These may include the following:
1. Alcohol or drug dependency
2. Fraudulent procurement of a license
3. Failure to cooperate with a medical board investigation
4. Participation or involvement in a criminal abortion
5. Sexual advances toward or involvement with patients
6. Sales of medical licenses
7. False and/or inaccurate patient records
8. Misrepresentation of hospital status to patients
9. Revocation or curtailment of hospital privileges
10. Fraud involving reimbursement of patients' expenses by third parties
11. Improperly prescribing, administering, or dispensing controlled substances
12. Diverting or giving away controlled substances
13. Transmission of disease by improper sterilization procedures
14. Weight control therapy abuse
15. Patient neglect—abandonment, real or constructive
16. Unprofessional or dishonorable conduct, or gross misconduct
17. Malpractice
18. Communication of confidential patient information
19. Failure to comply with legal requirements, such as reporting of venereal disease, birth registration, and suspicious death or injury
20. Permitting, aiding, or abetting unlicensed personnel to perform medical procedures normally restricted to a physician (If a physician's practice policies were challenged by the licensing board, the courts have held the practices must be harmful or misleading and not merely generally unacceptable to the medical community.)
21. Conviction of a crime, if the crime in question has been made a basis for a license revocation by statute
22. Criminal activities that have been the basis for licensing board action include fraud involving Medicare, Medicaid, the state insurance companies and patient reimbursement; improperly prescribing, administering, or dispensing controlled dangerous substances; and conviction of a felony or misdemeanor—sexual assault, possession of an unlicensed firearm, accepting a bribe, in violation of either a state or federal law.

The least precise ground for disciplinary action is the allegation of unprofessional,[36] immoral,[37-39] dishonorable, or gross misconduct.[40] Such concepts are difficult to define. It is manifestly impossible to categorize all of the acts subject to discipline. Such unspecific and vague standards are enforceable because there is a common professional understanding of what the public interest requires. Precise definitions made by the state medical boards are usually left intact, but there are occasions when courts have sometimes reversed them and imposed their own definitions. As long as a board bases its finding of unprofessional conduct or gross misconduct on expert testimony, in the record, as to the proper standard of care, the board should be upheld.

Discipline on grounds of incompetence, negligence, or malpractice is also somewhat vague and difficult to define. Incompetence is not established by rare and isolated instances of inadequate performance; rather, repeated defects in the exercise of everyday skills are the gist of such complaints. In rare cases, a single act of gross negligence is so wanton that it sufficiently demonstrates incompetence.

Fraud and deceit in the practice of medicine are grounds for discipline; most often this is alleged when a physician bills a third party (Medicare or insurance company) for work he did not perform. Fraud or deceit in nonprofessional activities are offenses more in the nature of moral turpitude or immoral conduct.

A felony conviction[41] empowers the board in most states to revoke a license. In some states, revocation cannot occur until all appeals have been exhausted. Misconduct in another state may also be grounds for revocation. Fraudulently obtaining a license and aiding and assisting an unlicensed practitioner in the practice of medicine are also grounds for revocation.

Discipline for failure to complete training and educational requirements, if mandated by a state statute, has been upheld as constitutional. Discipline for violation of medical board regulations is typically upheld, particularly if the legislative intent was to delegate to the state medical board the power to set standards of competence and conduct. Such regulations must be in the public interest and, although generally viewed favorably, are nevertheless subject to judicial review.

Medical boards have become increasingly active in dealing with physicians impaired by alcohol or controlled substances. Some states track these physicians through the traditional disciplinary route. Other states have formally established recovery programs that give physicians an opportunity to avoid formal disciplinary proceedings if they quickly agree to comprehensive treatment, supervision of their medical practice, and random monitoring of their bodily fluids.

Defenses to disciplinary charges

One of the most common practitioner defenses is that due process of law was denied by the board's commingling of investigative and adjudicatory functions within the same administrative agency. Courts have generally rejected this argument, stating that, absent a showing of bias, there was not sufficient risk of prejudice to taint the decision.[42]

A number of specific defenses may be raised by the practitioner at the initiation of disciplinary procedures. The defenses include the statute of limitations, entrapment, unlawful search and seizure, double jeopardy, recovery from impairment (with or without impaired physician committee monitoring), and jurisdictional challenges to a medical board proceeding after voluntary surrender of a license.

Occasionally, disciplinary proceedings are brought years after the alleged conduct of the physician. This occurs most often because of the initial unwillingness of witnesses to come forward or lengthy processes in state and federal courts. Generally, a defense of inordinate delay in prosecution for an alleged offense from the too distant past, though valid in criminal and civil judicial proceedings, has been held as an invalid defense in administrative disciplinary proceedings.[43] However, some states specifically include a statute of limitations. Whether or not the physician practices in one of the few states with a statute of limitations on medical board disciplinary proceedings, the physician can defend by asserting the "equitable doctrine of laches." This doctrine protects defendants in cases of an unexcused delay in bringing a disciplinary procedure that is inequitably prejudicial to the defendant.

Entrapment is a defense that asserts that the defendant physician was coerced, tricked, induced, or persuaded to commit an offense by law enforcement agents, an offense that would not have been committed without the agent's conduct. Entrapment may be a valid defense but a few cases have rejected the defense as limited to criminal proceedings.[44]

Evidence gained by unlawful search and seizure may sometimes be suppressed and constitutes a successful defense. Courts typically explore the policies underlying the exclusionary rule before automatically applying it to professional licensure proceedings.[45] However, this evidence is not always subject to the usual prohibition because of the necessity of strict supervision in certain highly regulated business activities (firearms, narcotics).[46]

Double jeopardy (the risk of double punishment for a single offense), alleged in instances of multiple license revocations, has been held an invalid defense. In addition, a board may impose discipline even when the physician has prevailed in a related criminal proceeding and the principle of double jeopardy does not apply.[47]

A defense of recovery from an impairment (with or without monitoring from an impaired physician committee) or assertion of the right to resumption of practice after voluntary surrender of license, is not of itself a defense in sanction proceedings. Typical board considerations when recovery is alleged include establishing that the impairment was the cause of misconduct, that the subject has indeed recovered, that the recovery has arrested the threat to public health and safety, and that relapse is not likely to occur.

Presentation by a convicted felon of "certificate of rehabilitation" under a "rehabilitated convicted offenders act" is not a dispositive defense; proof of a degree of rehabilitation does not preclude a license authority from disqualifying . . . applicants.[48]

A jurisdictional challenge based on voluntary surrender of (or failure to renew) a license depends on whether the physician retains any remaining rights to revive the license. Furthermore, the state can assert an interest in going forward with its proof at a time when evidence and witnesses' memories are fresh.[49]

R. P. Reeves describes the defense of winning by "intimidation."[50] Such defenses include "tying up" board members or assistant attorney generals and staff with repeated requests for continuance, voluminous discovery requests, subpoenas for spurious documents or witnesses, floods of character witnesses, applications for stays, and collateral attacks in federal court.

Finally, physicians brought on disciplinary charges have tried to bring federal civil rights actions under 42 U.S.C. Section 1983. Because boards are sitting in both their prosecutorial and quasijudicial capacities when carrying out disciplinary functions, board members and their staffs are usually granted absolute immunity from such suits.[51] Physicians who bring such suits may also be ordered to pay the attorney fees of their successful opponents.

Commingling investigative and judicial functions

It is a common objection to disciplinary action that a fair hearing was denied when matters are judged by a board that is also investigating the charges. Commingling sometimes occurs because of practical limits of funds and personnel. Commingling has been recognized as prejudicial only when there was an actual showing of bias.[52] Thus, a court found no denial of due process in a situation wherein the physician asserted

. . . That the member of the Board who moved that the order to show cause be served upon him was thereafter appointed hearing officer and conducted the hearing, that complainant counsel was employed by the Board, and that before the hearing all the Board members, including the hearing officer, had access to the investigatory materials collected in the...complaint file. In addition, he (appeared) to assert that one or more of the Board members who participated in the decision to issue the order to show cause also participated in the ultimate decision to revoke his license.[53]

Contrast a court finding of necessary bias in which two

board members commenced an unauthorized investigation. One posed as a patient; they then filed formal charges and appeared as investigators and witnesses before their fellow board members, who voted to suspend an optometrist's license.[54]

Disciplinary proceedings before formal charges are filed

A physician can be brought to the board's attention by a variety of sources: professional colleagues, nurses and other health care professionals, anonymous written or oral communications, overheard conversations by board employees, news exposés, etc. Frivolous complaints are not pursued. Granting of public access to dismissed complaints varies from state to state. States must balance the danger of unjustified notoriety against the value of keeping boards accountable by allowing the public to scrutinize dismissed complaints. Formal complaints or reports filed by patients, hospitals, other physicians, insurance companies, clerks in the courthouse, state or federal agencies, and the Federation of State Medical Boards constitute major informational sources of disciplinary procedures.

Although it is usually not required, the board may notify the physician that a complaint has been received, thus providing the physician an opportunity to respond. Many complaints, however, can be dismissed without prior notice to the physician.

The investigative powers of boards vary. All, by statute, have subpoena powers. However, successful challenges limiting subpoena powers have been made. Some state and federal laws, to protect confidentiality, limit discovery of records from mental health or alcohol and drug treatment centers.

The accused physician does not have the right to subpoena board witnesses for deposition or to subpoena the board's investigative files. Civil trials typically have a wide-open discovery process that seeks to uncover all the opposition's facts. However, professional disciplinary discovery proceedings are much more limited, especially prior to the filing of formal charges.

Disciplinary proceedings after formal charges are filed

The license to practice medicine and surgery is a right substantive enough to want compliance with all the requirements of due process, that is, proper notice of charges, notice of the hearing before a properly constituted tribunal, the right to cross-examine and produce witnesses, and a right to a full consideration and fair determination based on the facts.

Proper notice need not be exact and formal, but it must be sufficient to permit a full opportunity to prepare an adequate defense.[55] Hearings, usually required by statute to be public, are typically before a hearing officer or, due to financial constraints, the board *en banc* without a hearing officer. The structure of the hearings is controlled by statute or by agency rules. Some boards employ a hearing officer who reviews the records of the investigative officers, makes findings of fact, conclusions of law, and recommendations. Other boards employ the hearing officer to sit only as a judge who rules on motions and admissibility of evidentiary documents while the board sits as a jury. Other board cases are tried by a subcommittee of the entire board and the subcommittee then reports its findings and recommendations to the Board *en banc.*

In whatever process is devised under state law, full opportunity must be given to challenge the testimony of adverse witnesses and other evidence in a proceeding before the full board.[56] The right to appear with counsel is uniform. During the pendency of the formal adjudicatory hearing, the board, as the decisionmaker, must be sufficiently separated from its own investigative agents so that it may be free from bias and prejudice.[57]

The rules of evidence in a board hearing are not identical to courthouse rules of evidence. Hearsay testimony, both written and oral, is commonly admissible, as long as it goes to prove an issue and sustain a finding. The evidence must be substantive. Whether the evidence must be sufficient to establish a "preponderance" or a "clear preponderance" or "clear and satisfactory proof" or "clear and convincing proof" varies by state.

The final decision, rendered by a hearing officer or a board *en banc,* must adopt specific findings of fact, which is a concise and explicit statement of the events supporting the decision. It must also contain conclusions of law in a form that permits judicial review. Appeals to the judicial process are generally limited to reviews, not retrials. Stays pending further appeal are within the discretion of the court. Courts are sometimes prohibited by statute from granting such stays, but even then a court can intervene with a stay if the physician successfully asserts that he is likely to prevail on a procedural due process claim.

When a board has determined its sanction, courts are generally reluctant to interfere unless persuaded there has been a clear abuse of discretion.

Discovery

Efforts to find out the nature and extent of witnesses against a defendant physician prior to the time of hearing are termed *discovery.* The administrative law process normally offers opportunity for full use of normal pretrial discovery. Depositions, interrogatories, requests to produce, requests for admission, and inspection of site, can all be used to determine the strength and intensity of the state board's case.

Because the administrative context is sometimes more informal, legal counsel or a defendant physician may in some jurisdictions merely request copies of evidentiary documents in an informal manner to shortcut the normal formal discovery process. Diligent legal counsel should inquire with the board attorney about specific board rules or procedures related to expediting the pretrial discovery process.

Recusal of board members

Generally, state administrative law will provide a mechanism to request the recusal of any board member who "cannot accord a fair and impartial hearing or consideration."[58] Generally, that request must be accompanied by affidavit and promptly filed on discovery of the alleged disqualification, stating with particularity the grounds on which it is claimed that a fair and impartial hearing cannot be accorded. This threshold issue must be determined promptly by the board.

This pretrial remedy must be exercised with care. An unsuccessful or frivolous attempt to disqualify a board member may ignite other board members' passions against the defendant physician. Historically this remedy is not often sought in the administrative law process and is not often granted. There is a strong presumption that the administrative tribunal is unbiased.[59] However, if evaluation of the case and the board's process indicates substantial grounds that make this necessary, then it should be strongly considered.

Attorney fees

Some states' statutes provide that when an administrative proceeding is brought without reasonable basis or is frivolous, the board may become liable for the licensee's attorney fees.[60] This is a powerful statute where it occurs. Under the proper circumstances it can be an "equalizer" to help the defendant physician retain his rights. Aggressive demands for attorney fees and putting the agency on notice may give a defendant physician leverage in settlement negotiations or may result in dismissal of charges.

Sanctions

All state boards have laws authorizing sanctions, some more detailed than others.

License revocation is the most severe sanction available because its term is indefinite, usually "forever placing the offender beyond the pale."[61] Other sanctions include suspension, probation, written or oral reprimand, censure, curtailment of professional activities, and monetary fines.

Restoration of a revoked license requires a petition and review process that could take years to complete. If the cause was physician impairment and if a board so chooses, a surrendered license may be restored without protracted and formalized procedures if and when demonstrated recovery can be established. Suspension of a license is like a revocation, except that it is for a limited period of time.

Probation is a formalized sanction in which a formal surveillance procedure, most typically for mental illness and including alcohol and drug impairment, is initiated. Terms and conditions of probation must be set forth in the board order. Systematic and periodic reviews are implemented, typically for years, because relapse years later is a valid concern.[62]

Reprimand (a formal and sharp rebuke) and censure (a judgment of fault and blame) are intended to induce a mending of ways. They are lenient sanctions, granted when probation is deemed too severe. In practice, such actions are more effective as a means of defining minimal acceptable levels of conduct than as a means of disciplinary enforcement. Licenses may be restricted to prohibit writing of any prescriptions, to prohibit Schedule II controlled dangerous substance prescriptions, or to limit hospital practice or all practice except supervised positions in state hospitals or teaching centers. In the past, restricted licensure has been used to provide supervision of the wayward, but that has fallen from favor because of an insufficient emphasis on the rehabilitation of restricted physicians.

Sanctions are generally imposed only after the physician has received notice and an opportunity to be heard in the adversary proceeding, with witnesses, cross-examination, etc., as set forth earlier. However, if a board determines there is an imminent and material danger to patients or public health, safety, and welfare, a summary suspension, with later hearing, can be imposed. However, the physician is entitled to a prompt, postsuspension hearing that concludes without appreciable delay.[63] Summary suspension is the single exception to the rule that sanctions are imposed only after full hearing.

Sanctions to protect the public are the primary responsibility of the medical board. Public opinion has become increasingly critical of the paucity of revocations, inadequate supervision, and investigative impotence.[64] A perception persists that professional compassion for a colleague sacrificed public protection and that some sanctions were inconsistent, lenient, and seemingly ineffective. Contributing factors to the inadequacy of the boards include court-issued stay orders, injunctions, appeals, new trials granted on technical grounds, inadequate financing, and resistance by defense attorneys, hospital administrators and district attorneys.

National collectors of disciplinary data

Two national clearinghouses currently collect disciplinary data on physicians. These data are retained and made available to other state boards where a physician may hold a license, principally in response to reports of physicians "jumping jurisdictions" after disciplinary action is taken in one state where they hold a license.

The Federation of State Medical Boards in Ft. Worth, Texas, has maintained a national clearinghouse on physician discipline for several years.[65] The federation collects information about disciplinary actions taken by the 65 member jurisdictions and then transmits a summary of those actions to each of the other jurisdictions on a monthly basis. This allows state medical boards to contact a sister state to obtain details of disciplinary action taken on a physician who is also licensed in their state.

A part of the 1986 Health Care Quality Improvement Act (Pub. L. 99-660) established the National Practitioner Data Bank.[66] Like many federal projects, the data bank was initially slow to receive adequate funding and slow to get under way. The legislation included a requirement that hospitals must query the data bank at least every two years on all physicians on their staff. Medical boards and certain others may also query the data bank. Federal law requires medical boards and hospital staffs that impose a curtailment on a license of more than 30 days to report that incident to the data bank.

Open meeting act and open record act

The traditional perception exists in the medical profession that the medical boards should regulate and discipline in private. This has aroused suspicion of conspiracies of silence. Exposés by the media and the increasing publicity of malpractice claims have created legislative pressure to revamp the traditional regulatory process of a medical board.

Most states have enacted "sunshine" laws that include an Opening Meetings Act and an Open Records Act.[67] States have also enacted "sunset" laws, which require an administrative board to reprove periodically its reason for existence to a legislative body. The purpose of those laws is to require all government agencies, including medical boards, to give advance public notice of all activities and further to carry them out in public view and open to the press. However, most do not require that frivolous complaints become public matters, and most do not allow public inspection of board investigative records before they are made public at a hearing.[68] Some boards distribute periodic newsletters listing regulations and specific sanctions imposed on physicians, including the practitioner's name, address, and listed infractions. Such measures are made to assure the public that regulation is active and vigorous.

Appeals

Judicial review of an administrative decision is normally limited to determining whether the administrative agency acted arbitrarily, capriciously, or fraudulently; whether the order was substantially supported by the evidence presented; or whether the administrative agency's actions were within the scope of its legal authority as created by the statute. Although courts do review a decision of law by the administrative agency, decisions regarding the credibility of evidence and witnesses are normally a matter for the administrative agency itself and are overturned only if they are clearly contrary to the overwhelming weight of the evidence. Courts seldom intervene to substitute their judgment in determining a sanction or an assessment of mitigating circumstances.

Although there is no fundamental right of appeal of an administrative decision, virtually all jurisdictions grant appeal by state statute. Licensees have fought any limitation of the appeals process by arguing that such limits would compromise access to the judicial process and limit board accountability.

Typically, courts restrict appeals to the appeals process specified by statute. This could mean denying judicial access until the board has had a rehearing or the petitioner has exhausted all other administrative remedies. Some statutes typically limit judicial appeals to those approved by the board, known as "by leave" appeals as opposed to those "by right." Courts typically limit their scope of review to the issues of law. Rarely, however, courts have granted a new trial as part of the appeals process, as if no administrative proceeding had occurred.

As a practical matter, some state courts may choose to review cases however they like, accepting limits that suit their convenience or needs. On the one hand, they may choose to protect a licensee from administrative arbitrariness with strict scrutiny.[69] On the other hand, they may choose to accept virtually all board findings with routine affirmance.

Restoration of a license

Restoration of a license following revocation or suspension is a matter of serious concern for the public, the profession, and the physician. The odds of restoration are against the physician. And the physician clearly bears the burden of proof to demonstrate that there has been a substantial change of conditions in his qualifications and/or practice methods since the discipline was originally imposed. The process of reinstatement has no due process entitlements, supposedly because reinstate-

ment rights are not a substantive enough property right to warrant such protection.[70]

A surrendered license cannot be used to avoid a restoration process and consequent hearing and sanction. Licenses so surrendered are deemed final. In suspension, as compared with revocation, resumption of practice is automatic. There is also an early automatic reinstatement for a licensee who has failed to pay a routine renewal fee.

In the restoration process, a petition must be submitted (normally after at least one year) to initiate a preliminary investigative process. The investigation might involve an interview of the petitioner, review of character references, and contacts with other law enforcement agencies. The board might take steps to ensure that those providing character references are fully familiar with the facts the board found that led to the initial loss of license. Board concern focuses on rehabilitation and maintenance of skills, and it always keeps the public interest in mind. If a restoration petition is denied, reconsideration, future resubmission, or court challenges are available as alternative appeals. A court appeal of a denied reinstatement petition has virtually no chance of success because the decision is left to the board's exercise of its discretion. A board may require a minimum waiting period before resubmission of a reinstatement petition.

CONCLUSION

Physicians and the medical services they provide greatly affect public health, safety, and welfare. Because of that impact, and the historically high-profile nature of the medical profession, state government has the authority to regulate both medical education and to erect a medical licensure process. The state also exercises a continuing jurisdiction over the professional activities of licensed and practicing physicians and may impose sanctions thereon.

Currently, the pendulum of public opinion is swinging to favoring more oversight and accountability of physicians, rather than less.

END NOTES

1. Shakespeare, *As You Like It,* Act 1, Scene 3.
2. *Steinberg v. Chicago Medical School,* 354 N.E.2d 586 (Ill. App. 1976).
3. *DeMarco v. Chicago Medical School,* 352 N.E.2d 356 (Ill. App. 1976); *In re Florida Board of Bar Examiners,* 339 So.2d 637 (Fla. 1970).
4. *Cannon v. University of Chicago,* 559 F.2d 1063 (7th Cir. 1977).
5. *Alevy v. Down State Medical Center,* 384 N.Y.S.2d 82 (1976).
6. *University of California Regents v. Bakke,* 438 U.S. 265 (1978).
7. *Craig v. Boren,* 429 U.S. 190 (1976).
8. Smith, *A Third Rate Case Shouldn't Make Hard Law,* Jurisdoctor 31 (Feb. 1978).
9. *BeFunls v. Odegoard,* 416 U.S. 312, 94 S.Ct. 1704, 40 L.Ed.2d 164 (1974).

10. *BeFunls v. Odegoard,* 529 P.2d 438 (Wash. 1974).
11. Pub. Law 101-336, 104 Stat. 327 (codified at 42 U.S.C. Sec. 12101 *et seq.*). An excellent discussion of the ADA is found at Jones, *Overview and Essential Requirements of the Americans With Disabilities Act,* 64 Temple L.R. 471 (Summer 1991).
12. 42 U.S.C. § 12181.
13. *Board of Curators of the University of Missouri v. Horowitz,* 96 S.Ct. 948 (1978).
14. *Sanders v. Ajir,* 555 F.Supp. 240 (W.D. Wis. 1983).
15. *Ross v. Pennsylvania State University,* 445 F.Supp. 147 (M.D. Penn. 1978).
16. *Goss v. Lopez,* 95 S.Ct. 729 (1975).
17. *Matthews v. Eldridge,* 424 U.S. 319 (1976).
18. *Ewing v. Board of Regents University of Michigan,* 742 F.2d 913 (6th Cir. 1984), *cert. granted* 53 U.S.L.W. 3687 (U.S. Mar. 25, 1985).
19. *Lions v. Salva Regina College,* 568 F.2d 200 (1st Cir. 1977).
20. 42 U.S.C. § 12101 *et seq.*
21. S. Rep. No. 116, 101st Cong., 1st Sess. 22 (1989); H.R. Rep. No. 485, 101st Cong., 2nd Sess. 56 (1990).
22. *Teaching Health Law, A Symposium,* 38 J. Legal Educ. 489-497, 505-509, 545-554, 567-576 (Dec. 1988).
23. J. W. Burnside, *AIDS and Medical Education,* 10 J. Legal Med. 19 (Nov. 1, 1989).
24. Allen R. Felhous and Robert D. Miller, *Health Law and Mental Health Law Courses in U.S. Medical Schools,* 15 Bull. Am. Acad. Psychiatric Law 319 (Dec. 1987).
25. *Eneklal v. Winkler,* 20 Cal.3d 267, 142 Cal. Rptr. 418, 572 P.2d 32 (1977).
26. *Rusk v. Akron General Hospital,* 84 Ohio App. 2d 292, 171 N.E.2d 378 (1987).
27. *McBride v. United States,* 462 F.2d 72 (9th Cir. 1972).
28. *Pratt v. Stein,* 298 Pa. Super 92, 444 A.2d 674 (1982).
29. Ben A. Rich, *Malpractice Issues in the Academic Medical Center,* 36 Del. Law J. 641-646 (Dec. 1987).
30. *Id.* at 652.
31. Harold I. Hirsch, *The Evils of Admitting Private Patients to Hospitals with Teaching Programs; A View From Outside the Ivory Tower,* 16 Legal Aspects Med. Prac. (Nov. 1988).
32. *Lawrence v. Board of Registration in Medicine,* 239 Mass. 424, 428, 132 N.E. 174 (1921).
33. *Hawke v. New York,* 170 U.S. 189, 194 (1898).
34. *Dent v. West Virginia,* 129 U.S. 114, 123 (1888).
35. *In re Hansen,* 275 N.W.2d 700 (Minn. 1978).
36. This includes false or deceptive advertising. Many states have specific statutes and regulations providing for discipline on this ground.
37. *Brun v. Lazzell,* 172 Md. 314, 191 A. 240 (1937) (revocation of license to practice dentistry based upon guilty plea to criminal charges of indecent exposure).
38. *Raymond v. Board of Registration in Medicine,* 387 Mass. 708, 443 N.E.2d 391-394 (1982) (where the board disciplined a physician upon his conviction for possession of unregistered submachine guns the court held that ". . . lack of good moral character and conduct that undermines public confidence in the integrity of the medical profession are grounds for discipline.").
39. *Urick v. Comm. Board of Osteopath Examination,* 43 Pa. Commw. 348, 402 A.2d 290 (1979) (court upheld licensure revocation for committing a crime of "moral turpitude" where the physician was convicted of conspiracy to use the mails to defraud and conspiracy to unlawfully distribute and possess Schedule II controlled substances).
40. *Lawrence v. Board of Registration in Medicine,* 239 Mass. 424, 428, 430, 132 N.E. 174 (1921) (gross misconduct in the practice of medicine is not too indefinite as a ground for discipline).
41. Includes felonies clearly unrelated to the practice of medicine, such as income tax evasion.
42. *Withrow v. Larkin,* 421 U.S. 35 (1975).
43. Note that a statute of limitations defense was not valid to block admission into evidence in a licensure proceeding, a felony conviction more than three years old, even where that state required that legal actions be commenced within three years. *Colorado State Board of Medical Examiners v. Jorganson,* 198 Colo. 275, 599 P.2d 869 (1979).
44. *See generally* R. P. Reaves, *The Law of Professional Licensing and Certification* 255-57 (1st ed. 1984).
45. *See, e.g., Emslie v. State Bar of California,* 11 Cal. 3d 210, 520 P.2d 991, 1000 (1974) (rule not applied to attorney disciplinary action); *Elder v. Board of Medical Examiners,* 241 Cal. App. 2d 246, 50 Cal. Rptr. 304 (1966), *cert. denied* 385 U.S. 1001 (1967) (rule applied in disciplinary action against physician).
46. *United States v. Biswell,* 406 U.S. 311 (1972).
47. *Arthurs v. Board of Registration in Medicine,* 383 Mass. 299, 418 N.E.2d 1236 (1981).
48. *Hyland v. Kehayas,* 157 N.J. Super. 258, 384 A.2d 902 (1978).
49. *See Cross v. Colo. State Bar of Dental Examiners,* 37 Colo. App. 504, 508, 552 P.2d 38 (1976) ("It is logical and sensible that where such grave charges of . . . unprofessional or dishonorable conduct are alleged, the Board has the right to preserve (any) evidence . . . of these charges otherwise witnesses may disappear and the passage of time itself may well dim or even eradicate the memory of the witnesses and thus preclude the construction of an adequate record.").
50. R. P. Reeves, *The Law of Professional Licensing and Certification* 258 (1st ed. 1984).
51. *See, e.g., Horowitz v. State Board of Medical Examiners of Colorado,* 822 F.2d 1508 (10th Cir.) (members of state medical board absolutely immune for actions in connection with suspension of podiatrist's licensure), *cert. denied* 484 U.S. 964 (1987); *Vakas v. Rodriquez,* P.2d 1293 (10th Cir.), *cert. denied* 469 U.S. 981 (1984); *see Batz v. Economou,* 438 U.S. 478, 508-517 (1978).
52. *See Withrow v. Larkin,* 421 U.S. 35 (1975).
53. *Raymond v. Board of Registration in Medicine,* 387 Mass. 708 (1982).
54. *3600 I. Rogers v. Texas Optometry Board,* 609 S.W.2d 248 (Tex.) (1980).
55. *Bloch v. Ambach,* 528 N.Y.S.2d 204 (N.Y. App. Div. 1988).
56. *Physicians and Surgeons,* 61 AmJur 2d. § 105 (1981).
57. *Morrissey v. Brewer,* 408 U.S. 471, 92 S.Ct. 2593, 33 L.Ed.2d 484 (1972).
58. *See, e.g.,* 75 O.S. 1991, § 316.
59. *Schneider v. McClure,* 456 U.S. 188, 102 S.Ct. 1665, 72 L.Ed.2d 1 (1982); *National Labor Relations Board v. Ohio New & Rebuilt Parts, Inc.,* 760 F.2d 1443 (6th Cir.), *cert. denied* 474 U.S. 1020 (1980).
60. *See, e.g.,* 12 O.S. 1991, § 941B.
61. Derbyshire, *Offenders and Offenses,* 19 Hosp. Prac. 981 (1984).
62. Shore, *The Impaired Physician, Four Years After,* JAMA 248:3127 (1982).
63. *See Barry v. Barchi,* 443 U.S. 55, 66 (1979); *Ampueto v. Department of Professional Regulation,* 410 So.2d 213 (Fla. D.C. App. 1982) (six-month delay in postsuspension hearing found unreasonable).
64. *See* Vol. 18, *Hosp. Prac.,* 251 (1983) (ten-year saga of a license revocation).
65. Federation of State Medical Boards, 2630 West Freeway, Suite 138, Ft. Worth, TX 76102-7199.
66. Codified at 42 U.S.C. § 11101 *et seq.*
67. *See, e.g.,* 25 O.S. 1991, § 301 *et seq.,* and 51 O.S. 1991, § 24A.1 *et seq.*
68. *See, e.g.,* 51 O.S. 1991, § 24A.12 *et seq.*
69. R. P. Reeves, *supra* note 50, at 276.
70. *Hicks v. Georgia State Board of Pharmacy,* 553 F.Supp. 314 (Ga. 1982), *citing Meachum v. Fano,* 427 U.S. 215, 228 (1976).

CHAPTER 10

Peer review, disciplining, hearings, and appeals

JOHN T. BURROUGHS, M.D., J.D., F.C.L.M.

PEER REVIEW
ECONOMIC CREDENTIALING
JUDICIAL REVIEW
CONCLUSION

The present state of peer review evolved from the long-standing process initiated by physicians to maintain appropriate care of the hospitalized patient by the medical staff. Standing committees within the medical staff organization, such as surgical review, tissue review, medical records review, credentials, utilization review, and other such committees, represent this earlier approach to maintaining the quality of care rendered in the hospital. Physicians traditionally approached this task as professional peers, fulfilling their responsibilities on a collegial level.

The current process of peer review within the medical profession sharply contrasts the "user-friendly" approach formerly in place. Today, adversarial dynamics are intrinsic to all legal actions, whether they are transactional, quasijudicial, or judicial proceedings. The adversarial approach has become the standard applied to peer review as a result of the profession being ruled by "standard business practices" and managed by lay people, administrative personnel, and organizations, including but not limited to the HMO (Health Maintenance Organization), PPO (Preferred Provider Organization), IPA (Independent Practice Association), PHO (Physician-Hospital Organization), MSO (Medical Service Organization), GPWW (Group Practice Without Walls) structures. Explosive expansion of integrated health care entities has accelerated this transformation.

The former, collegial method of peer review was subject to abuse by physicians being overprotective of their brethren, thereby allowing physicians whose care was substandard to "slip through the cracks." This was the "good old boy" mind-set, which led to accusations and improper and inadequate peer review by physicians alone standing in judgment of their comrades.

Changes were bound to occur and did. Such cases as *Johnson v. Misericordia Community Hospital*[1] and *Elam v. College Park Hospital*[2] decreed that hospitals have a responsibility to govern peer review processes to assure that doctors are competent and deserve staff privileges. These cases and their progeny place liability on the hospital if there is negligence in overseeing the peer review process.

Nevertheless, the courts recognize that the physician has the right to pursue his livelihood without arbitrary and capricious exclusionary practices, although those rights require balance against the interests of the general public to receive quality medical care and against the duty of the hospital to provide competent staff physicians.[3] The courts have taken the view that "a hospital may not deprive a physician of staff privileges without granting him minimal due process of law protection."[4]

Further changes have occurred. Medicine has become a business, run by business practice rules and for-profit motives. This has placed a different emphasis on the practice of medicine. Contractual relationships between entities and physicians, even physicians and physicians, have taken on a different atmosphere. Competition at all levels has brought about more strident relationships. Formal disciplinary procedures are now in place, adversarial in their very nature, presenting a different and frightening arena to the practicing physician. The pendulum has swung to the other end of the spectrum, and the physician is not familiar enough with the applicable rules to protect or defend himself adequately in many instances. The adversarial process, the traditional trend of attorneys, has permeated the relationships between physicians, their colleagues, and the very organizations they are being beleaguered to join. The

105

hospital/organization attorney is business oriented and many have little or no insight into the tremendous impact on the physician of losing his or her staff privileges. The physician is becoming a medium-level supervisor, or in many organizations an employee-at-will. The credentialing process has become, in many instances, an economically controlling hammer, which can devastate the physician's livelihood and career.

However, one must not lose sight of the fact that incompetent physicians do indeed exist as a result of lack of training, not staying abreast of the rapid changes in medicine, lack of skill, impairment from drugs or alcohol, and psychological problems. Until recently, because of the confidentiality of state medical board proceedings, these physicians often disappeared from one environment only to reappear in another, reopening a practice because there was no mechanism to obtain information about previous problems. Only *minimum* standards need be met for licensure. The National Practitioner Data Bank was formed under the Health Care Quality Improvement Act of 1986, Title 4 (hereinafter HCQIA),[5] in an attempt to mollify the problem.

The purpose of this brief overview is to address some of the salient features and issues in the peer review process. It is not meant to be a comprehensive law review of the entire subject; included citations refer to relevant jurisdictional statutes, case law, and Supreme Court decisions. California law was used for many examples because it is a leader in this developing area of the law.

We discuss the subject under three broad headings:
1. Peer review
2. Economic credentialing
3. Judicial review

PEER REVIEW
Legal representation

The right to representation. Physicians are vulnerable to adversarial confrontations that may suddenly jeopardize their professional activity. Even so, there is no unanimity as to whether or not the physician even has the right to legal counsel at a peer review hearing. For example, in California, the applicable code, the California Business and Professions Code (hereinafter Cal. Bus. & Prof.), provides only that "The peer review body shall adopt written provisions governing whether a licentiate shall have the option of being represented by an attorney at the licentiate's expense. No peer review body shall be represented by an attorney if the licentiate is not so represented."[6] In contradistinction, The California Medical Association Model Staff Bylaws, section 7.4-2, widely used as an exemplar throughout the United States, recommend that "The member shall be entitled to representation by legal counsel in any phase of the

hearing, should he/she so choose." Further, the statute not only allows for an option by the peer review body to decide whether counsel shall be permitted, but the standards differ for medicine vis-à-vis dentistry, the result of conflicting decisions by the two professions. Cal. Bus. & Prof. § 809.3(c) has been modified by adding to the section:

No peer review body shall be represented by an attorney if the licentiate is not so represented, *except dental professional society peer review bodies may be represented by an attorney provided that the peer review body grants each licentiate the option of being represented by an attorney at the licentiate's expense, even if the licentiate declines to be represented by an attorney.*

Conflict of interest. The number of attorneys who appreciate the position of the physician and who can equitably and properly represent him with in-depth knowledge and compassion for the nature of the intimate and trusting doctor-patient relationship, who understand the physician's need of facilities where his patients can be served, and who appreciate what it means to dislodge a physician from his base of practice are in the minority.

Most attorneys who practice health care law primarily represent hospital administration, governing boards of organizations (HMO, IPA, PHO, etc), or the hospital medical staff as a whole. Yet they will hold themselves out as qualified to represent the *individual* physician when he or she comes under attack from one or more of these entities. The conflict of interest, when viewed from the physician's point of view, seems obvious. But the practice is all too common and, until recently, was not challenged by the courts. As a matter of fact, in 1988, a court stated "[w]e are aware of no rule requiring hospitals to hire separate counsel to represent the medical staff and the board in these proceedings."[7]

However, the innate conflict of interest of attorneys when they, or other members of their firm, represent more than one party in a controversy has been recognized in California. This is particularly true when the situation is made more acute by the appointment of a supposedly independent and disinterested judicial review committee (JRC) for peer review, which does not have an independent investigative arm. Rather, the JRC relies on the adversarial presentations of the accused versus the medical entity, where each has the right to present evidence, cross-examine witnesses, and advocate his position in the formal hearing process.

A recent case has addressed the issue. In *Howitt v. Superior Court of Imperial County,*[8] attorneys from the same firm, the county counsel office, were the advocates for the county department opposing the employee and at the same time were advising the decision-making board. The court found that "to allow an advocate for one party to also act as counsel to the decision-maker creates the substantial risk that the advice given to the decision maker, . . . 'perhaps unconsciously,' will be skewed" (citation omitted).[9] In the absence of screening from any inappropriate contact, such a relationship was deemed probably to violate due process.

Due process

Definition and interpretation. The fundamental access to due process lies in the finding that the rights at issue constitute either protected interests in "liberty" or "property" deserving of appropriate due process before those rights are removed.[10] The right to practice medicine without undue interference is recognized as a protected property right, not liberty protection per se,[11] although liberty protection may attach. The pivotal question then becomes one of determining what type of hearing process will satisfy due process requirements. The Supreme Court delineated the factors to be balanced in determining the process that is appropriate to protect a property interest in *Mathew v. Eldridge,*[12] holding that "[d]ue process is flexible and calls for such procedural protections as the particular situation demands." Such a determination:

[G]enerally requires consideration of three distinct factors: first, the private interest that will be affected by the official action; second, the risk of an erroneous deprivation of [a property] interest through the procedures used, and the probable value, if any, of additional or substitute procedural safeguards; and finally, the government's interest, including the function involved and the fiscal and administrative burdens that the additional or substitute procedural requirement would entail.[13]

But the type of hearing is not always the same and may vary from case to case. Due process merely requires that the person be given *"some kind of hearing"*[12] (emphasis added).

Several basic tenets in the fabric of due process are relevant to the issues involved in peer review. First, there is no constitutional requirement that the decision-maker be an uninvolved person when a property interest protected by due process is at stake.[14] Secondly, it is generally accepted that "in a highly technical occupation, the members of the profession should have the power to set their own standards. Due process requires that the evaluations of whether one gets along and meets the standards not be made in bad faith or arbitrarily and capriciously." It does not always require a full and formal adversarial hearing.[15]

These basic premises must be taken into account when interpreting the law of due process particularly as applied by HCQIA, 42 U.S.C. § 11112. The following questions, raised by the formulation of the due process requirements in HCQIA, are cited as examples of

ambiguity and issues arising therefrom, but are not meant to be a complete listing of all the deficiencies. Two examples are:

1. Under § 11112 (b)(1)(ii), concerning notice of the proposed action, the physician must be provided with "reasons for the proposed action." The particularity with which the reasons must be articulated is not addressed.
2. Under § 11112 (b)(3)(A), "the hearing shall be held (as determined by the health care entity) — (iii) before a panel of individuals who are appointed by the entity and are not in direct economic competition with the physician involved." This provision would make it possible for the board of directors, who ordinarily must follow the recommendations of their "independent medical staff," to sit as the decision-maker JRC. There is no limitation as to the qualifications of panel members, so that it is possible that a health care entity could appoint a JRC of nonphysician members to sit in judgment, including members of the governing board.

Further, the final sentence of § 11112(b)(3)(D) states "A professional review body's failure to meet the conditions described in this subsection shall not, in itself, constitute failure to meet the standards of subsection (a)(3) of this section." The broad interpretation of what minimal due process is, combined with the exceptions inferred herein, may virtually preclude successful judicial review challenge of unfair JRC proceedings under this statute (see the section on Judicial Review *infra*).

Modification and expansion of HCQIA peer review

California law overview. The ground rules of peer review must be precisely delineated in the hospital bylaws and followed by all parties so as to protect their interests when disputes arise, including the governing body, administration, the hospital medical staff as a whole, and the individual physician. Self-governance by the medical staff is paramount. Neither the governing body nor the medical staff may unilaterally amend the medical staff bylaws. Because of the importance of the concepts, the Joint Commission on Accreditation of Healthcare Organizations (JCAHO) has promulgated provisions for self-governance, accountability, fundamental fair-hearing, and appellate review mechanisms in the Medical Staff section of its manual, section MS.3.[16]

With appropriately written bylaws, a "level playing field" for all concerned can be established. The rules promulgated by JCAHO and the provisions of HCQIA are minimal and inadequate. Because of the deficiencies, California, as provided in the act, opted out of the professional review aspects of HCQIA because it had developed proceedings equal to or exceeding the requirements of the statute. The California law represents the most equitable and fair procedure rules of any jurisdiction, achieving better protection of and equity for the parties. The sections of the California codes relevant to this discussion are Business and Professions Code, sections 805 *et seq.,* 809 *et seq.,* and Government Code, section 11503.

The law was enacted under California Senate Bill 1211 (SB1211) which became the law of California on January 1, 1990, the legislature enacted the pertinent legislature, now codified as cited *supra.* Before SB1211 became the California law of due process, the general rule was that "a hospital may not deprive a physician of staff privileges without granting him minimal due process of law protection."[4] The inadequacies and scarcity of elements satisfying minimal due process were enunciated by the definition supplied in *Pinsker v. Pacific Coast Society of Orthodontists,*[17] where the court stated:

The common law requirement of a fair procedure does not compel formal proceedings with all the embellishment of a court trial, nor adherence to a single mode of process. It may be satisfied by any one of a variety of procedures which afford a fair opportunity for an applicant to present his position. As such, this court should not attempt to fix a rigid procedure that must invariably be observed. Instead, the [entities] themselves should retain the initial and primary responsibility for devising a method which provides an applicant *adequate notice of the 'charges' against him and a reasonable opportunity to respond.* . . . [T]he organization should consider the nature of the tendered issue and should fashion its procedure to insure a *fair* opportunity for an applicant to present his position.[18] (first emphasis added)

The laws apply to a medical or professional staff of a hospital, licensed health facility, or ambulatory surgical center certified by Medicare, a health care service plan or a nonprofit hospital service plan, any physician, conducting or the subject of peer review *organized* by any facility, such as an HMO, PHO, IPA, PPO, hospital or other health entity with 25 or more licentiates, and to any medical, psychological, dental, or podiatric professional society having as members at least 25% of the eligible licentiates in the area in which it functions and which includes at least one county. (Cal. Bus. & Prof., section 809(a)) The code also states, *inter alia:*

(2) Because of deficiencies in the federal act and the possible adverse interpretations by the courts of the federal act, it is preferable for California to "opt out" of the federal act and design its own peer review system.

(3) Peer review, fairly conducted, is essential to preserving the highest standards of medical practice.

(4) Peer review which is not conducted fairly results in harm both to patients and healing arts practitioners by limiting access to care.

(7) It is the intent of the Legislature that peer review of

professional health care services be done efficiently . . . with an *emphasis on early detection of potential quality problems and resolutions through informal educational interventions.* (emphasis added)

(8) . . . It is the intent of the Legislature that written provisions implementing Sections 809 to 809.8, inclusive, in the acute care hospital setting, shall be included in medical staff bylaws which shall be adopted by a vote of the members of the organized medical staff and which shall be subject to governing body approval, which approval shall not be withheld unreasonably.

Preliminary investigation. Included in these sections is the most important policy that the peer review be performed by *licentiates.* Also, the *initiation* of the process should be performed at a *collegial* level by a duly appointed and designated investigative committee having no bias or financial interest in the outcome, as intended by the legislature and enunciated in subsection 7 of Cal. Bus. & Prof. Code, section 809(a) *supra.* The committee must be organized by a recognized medical entity to which the provisions of Cal. Bus. & Prof. Code, section 805 attach (see *infra*). The investigational committee shall conduct a fair, unbiased investigation and is charged with arriving at a "final proposed action." This preliminary, informal procedural process, absent legal interference, provides the parties the opportunity to resolve the issues on a collegial level. The final proposed action may well be of such a nature that no further action need be taken.

Obviously, such provisions must be established in the bylaws of the entity involved. All too often, even with such provisions incorporated into the intent of the law, as in California, the appropriate steps for protection have not been taken by the members of the medical staff. This is a critical step in the process, because the "final proposed action" can be remedial education, alteration of behavior, or other alternatives with none of the reportable sanctions included. The process is at an end, with agreement and correction confidentially attained.

Where this preliminary, informal procedure is properly spelled out, the physician has the opportunity to approach the entity, offer cooperation, and develop his defenses through marshalling his friendly colleagues, obtaining appropriate formal review by a disinterested expert or experts, and preparing a detailed and thorough legal defense, necessary not only to informally end the process, if possible, but also to be adequately prepared for potential future actions. To do this effectively, the physician needs expert legal counsel *at the onset.*[19] The truth of the matter is that most physicians do not seek help until this opportunity to stop the process at a nonreportable level may have passed. The available data indicate that most physicians do not seek help until the process has been under way for six months or more. The expenses become exponentially greater and the chances of success exponentially less.

Reportable sanctions. Under both HCQIA and the California statutes, the latter found in Cal. Bus. & Prof. Code, section 805, the following findings constitute a reportable disciplinary action:

1. Any denial, reduction, suspension, revocation, restriction, denying or failure of renewing of any staff privileges or membership of more than 30 days cumulatively in any 12-month period
2. Termination or revocation of any staff privileges, employment, or membership
3. Acceptance of the surrender or restriction of clinical privileges while the physician or dentist is under investigation or in return for not conducting an investigation.

Voluntary relinquishment is not a shield from reporting.

Bias by the Judicial Review Committee. Another problem area concerns bias on the part of a member of the JRC. An attempt to protect the accused physician was made in the California law, by providing that the licentiate will have the right:

to a reasonable opportunity to voir dire the panel members and any hearing officer, and the right to challenge the impartiality of any member or hearing officer. Challenges to the impartiality of any member or hearing officer shall be ruled on by the presiding officer. . . .[20]

Unfortunately, this provision did not elucidate what would be interpreted as "a reasonable opportunity to voir dire the panel members." Severely limiting rulings by hearing officers have eroded the intent of this provision in many instances. The need for explicit and detailed bylaws to ensure proper procedural description is mandatory. Also, the hearing transcript, recorded by a court stenographer, is the record relied on by the courts for judicial review. It is critical to make and preserve an appropriate record during the JRC hearing, to obtain successful judicial review (see *infra*).

Notice requirements. There is no definition of the particularity required for stating the "reasons for the proposed action" (*supra*). The peer review statutes of California, sections 805 *et seq.* and 809 *et seq.*, do not contain this information. Fortunately, however, California Government Code, section 11503, does delineate what must be elucidated in an administrative adjudication where the purpose of the hearing is "to determine whether a right, authority, license or privilege should be revoked, suspended, limited, or conditioned:

The accusation shall be a written statement of charges which shall set forth in ordinary and *concise* language the acts or omissions with which the respondent is charged, to the end that

the respondent will be able to prepare his defense. (emphasis added)

To give an example of how important this language is, the notice of hearing in a particular case, among other vague and ambiguous accusations, alleged that the physician had ordered "excessive chemistries." The named patient had terminal, metastatic carcinoma to bone. His calcium levels were extremely high, with resulting cognitive disruption virtually to the state of coma. His calcium, creatinine, and BUN, along with other lesser but significant electrolyte abnormalities, were very high. In the course of several days with careful, repetitive blood chemistry monitoring of the abnormalities, the treating physician was able to bring the CA++ levels down to reasonable levels, the chemistries relevant to renal function returned toward normal, and the patient left the hospital. He lived nearly another year, during which time he enjoyed his family. How, from the accusation, was one to determine, with any specificity, which or how many of the chemistries ordered were supposed to be excessive under the circumstances of this case? Without this information, there could be no effective cross-examination of the accusers, or ability to find out if all of them agreed on certain lab tests as excessive, etc. Unfortunately, this kind of broad, vague accusation appears all too frequently and must be challenged before the hearing occurs. Since the law is unclear concerning the specificity of allegations in many jurisdictions, and is not assisted by HCQIA, the fairness of a peer review hearing may depend on the rulings of the hearing officer. Preserving the record carefully and thoroughly may permit challenge on appeal (see section on Judicial Review *infra*).

Rights of discovery of evidence. The Health Care Quality Improvement Act is also silent concerning what documents and evidence the physician may obtain in discovery. California law mandates that the physician has the right "to inspect and copy at the licentiate's expense *any* documentary information relevant to the charges which the peer review body has in its possession or under its control." (The JRC has the same right to discovery of relevant evidence in the possession of the physician.) (emphasis added)[21]

Immunities. Both HCQIA and jurisdictional laws provide for immunities from liability to those involved in peer review. Once again, however, California law serves as a beacon for defining the extent of immunities for all parties. There is immunity only so long as the review functions are conducted in a fair and unbiased manner. HCQIA provides for only one exception to immunity, in addition to antitrust actions, namely, a participant providing false information knowing the information to be false.[22] (42 U.S.C. §111101 *et seq.,* §§11111(a)(2); §11112)

California law, on the other hand, provides absolute immunity to any participant in the proceedings, including preliminary actions. But the immunity does not apply to "communications made to individuals not properly concerned with credentialing or disciplinary functions."[23] Absolute immunity also applies to anyone communicating relevant information to the medical or podiatric boards and the Department of Justice. Also there is provision of legal counsel to anyone under contract with the medical boards who may be sued for defamation concerning opinions rendered, statements made or testimony given, either in any disciplinary action or any report concerning an impaired physician under the diversion program of California.[24]

Overlap of investigatory, prosecutorial, and adjudicatory functions. This issue was considered by the Supreme Court in *Withrow v. Larkin,*[25] concerning the suspension of a physician's license by a state examining board. The physician challenged the proceedings as violative of due process, because the board first undertook an "investigative hearing" where the physician could not fully participate, followed by the same board conducting a "contested hearing." His challenge, that the combination of investigative and adjudicatory functions deprived him of an impartial hearing, was granted certiori because the challenge constituted a "substantial issue." The Court found that "No specific foundation has been presented for suspecting that the Board has been prejudiced by its investigation or would be disabled from hearing and deciding on the basis of the evidence to be presented at the contested hearing. The mere exposure to evidence presented in nonadversary investigative procedures is insufficient in itself to impugn the fairness of the Board members at a later adversary hearing."[26]

Confidentiality. Any information furnished to an organized peer review proceeding is confidential and nondiscoverable. But the confidentiality may not attach to any group or committee that is not formally "organized" (under bylaws and state law), to statements made outside of formally convened peer review meetings, or to statements or documents voluntarily divulged to a party to the action.[27]

There is an innate conflict between confidentiality of information in peer review and information sought in a medical malpractice action. This issue has recently been addressed in *Alexander v. The Superior Court of Los Angeles County.*[28] The issue was whether there was a difference between documents and evidence "generated" by the peer review committee and documents or evidence "submitted" to such a review entity. The court decided that the intent of the evidence code was not to "draw the 'generated versus submitted' distinction . . ."

(citation omitted).[29] The court specifically addressed the issue at hand by stating, "It evinces a legislative judgment that the quality of in-hospital medical practice will be elevated by armoring staff inquiries with a measure of confidentiality".[30] Further the court reiterated the impact of the conclusion by restating its effect from *Matchett v. Superior Court*[31]:

> This confidentiality exacts a social cost because it impairs malpractice plaintiffs' access to evidence. In a damage suit for in-hospital malpractice against doctor or hospital or both, unavailability of recorded evidence of incompetence might seriously jeopardize or even prevent the plaintiff's recovery. Section 1157 represents a legislative choice between competing public concerns. It embraces the goal of medical staff candor at the cost of impairing plaintiff's access to evidence.

The strong public policy position of protecting confidentiality demonstrated by this case has been followed in other jurisdictions,[32] and addressed in the legal literature.[33]

Peer review appeal. Peer review *may* include an appellate procedure, which is adequately described in the Model Medical Staff Bylaws of the California Medical Association.[34] However, administrative appeal is not mandated, at least not in California or in the provisions of the HCQIA. Most medical staff bylaws provide rules for an appellate process. In essence the hearing shall be an appellate format, based on the record of the JRC proceedings. Acceptance of additional evidence is recommended and legally permissible, subject to a foundational showing that such evidence could not have been made available to the JRC in the exercise of reasonable diligence and that the evidence would materially have affected the decisions of the JRC. Also such evidence would be subject to the same rights of confronting and cross-examining the party presenting the evidence.

There shall be the right to legal counsel at this level of hearing, if appeal is provided for. The appeal shall include the information to which the appellant has rightful access, including (1) the written decision of the JRC, including findings of fact and a conclusion articulating the connection between the evidence produced at the hearing and the decision reached; (2) a written explanation of the procedure for appealing the decision, if any appellate mechanism exists; (3) the right to receive the written decision of the appellate body.[35]

When the peer review process may not attach. No contract with an organized medical entity, recognized under the bylaws or state statutes may waive peer review rights, as established under California law or in other jurisdictions with similar provisions. The California provisions, however, specifically limit application to entities with 25 or more licentiates. Suppose that a physician is a shareholder in a corporate entity of 15 members. Assume that one or more of the other shareholders decide, for whatever reason, that the physician is no longer wanted in the group. Under business law, if they can persuade a majority of the shareholders (in this case eight of them), the one shareholder may be disenfranchised by the majority vote. Absent specialized exceptions, resort to the courts will not, as a general rule, aid the aggrieved party; corporate law will prevail.

ECONOMIC CREDENTIALING

There may be no redress for loss of privileges under what is termed as *economic credentialing*, because peer review does not apply without statutory or bylaw provision. The term *economic credentialing* is broad and somewhat vague. It includes the use of economic factors to decide whether a physician will be granted membership and/or certain privileges, employment by a health care entity, revocation of privileges or dismissal from employment. It also includes evaluation of the economic impact of a physician's practice on an organization, particularly playing a major role in the hiring and firing of the "gatekeeper" in HMOs, PHOs, etc.

One of the seminal cases in this arena is that of *Rosenblum v. Tallahassee Memorial Regional Medical Center, Inc.*[36] The case involved a cardiothoracic surgeon who had contracted to direct the heart surgery program at Tallahassee Community Hospital (TCH), to develop a referral market into the program, and to market the system. He was very successful at accomplishing this task and, thereby, caused TCH to become a major competitor of the other program in Tallahassee, at Tallahassee Memorial Regional Hospital (TMRH). Then Dr. Rosenblum applied for staff privileges at TMRH. He was denied and appealed to the court. The court found:

1. The bylaws relevant to peer review did not apply, since the bylaws constitute a contract and Dr. Rosenblum, as an applicant, was not privy to contract at TMRH.
2. Under a Florida statute, section 395.011(5) Fla. Stat., permitting the governing board of a hospital to consider "such other elements" when deciding to accept an applicant, the court found that "economic credentialing" was such an element, so long as such factors were not arbitrary or capricious. Since Dr. Rosenblum was the director of fierce competition and his presence on the staff of TMRH might serve to further his primary goal of marketing the program at TMRH, the court found that the decision to deny privileges was based on considerations that were economically valid. The decision was limited to an applicant, not a staff member.

Overutilization or improper and excessive utilization have become bases for economic credentialing. As noted, this has become of particular moment in regard to the "gatekeeper." The usual economic basis of an HMO or other medical entity is capitation, with or without some discounted fee-for-service for certain limited-use specialists. Ordinarily, anywhere from 15% to as much as 25% of the earned income of the primary physician will be a "withhold," in order to compensate for unanticipated losses. If the primary physician is "conservative" in his referral to other specialists, he will probably acquire part of the withhold, now really a "bonus" in effect. Thus, there is a personal economic incentive to restrict referral. Also, he will be a "satisfactory" employee of his health care organization, not producing economic drain. But if he refers on an increased level, he not only will not have reserved the "bonus" fund, but the organization may determine that he is an economic burden. Almost all these contracts contain a "terminate without cause" clause. The physician may find himself or herself dismissed purely on economic grounds. Because this can be construed as a "business necessity," and because there is a basis for termination without peer review considerations, there seems little chance of redress legally. (Again, business law prevails; i.e., employment/labor law.) Parenthetically, the other side of the coin is possible medical negligence action against the primary physician for failure to properly refer, leading to consequent injury to or death of a patient—and the very HMO, PHO, etc., producing the problem will probably cross-claim against him for indemnification.

A case in point is that of *Knapp v. Palos Community Hospital.*[37] In this case, three physicians who were practicing pulmonary medicine were accused of excessive use of respiratory equipment and procedures, which was having an economic effect on the hospital. Consequently, on review of the use of ventilatory facilities and after a duly appointed ad hoc committee review, the privileges of the three to use the respiratory facilities of the hospital were terminated. The court upheld the decision of the JRC and the appellate review by the hospital, based on no violation of the hospital bylaws.

More directly inferring "pure" economic credentialing is the case of *Maltz v. New York University Medical Center.*[38] This case involved an application from a gastroenterologist, a clinical instructor with the university. He was denied privileges on the grounds that there were bed limitations and adequate staffing in oncological gastroenterology. He filed the complaint first with the New York Public Health Council, based on New York law, which stated that it was improper for the governing body of a hospital to refuse to act on a staff application or to deny or withhold such without stating the reason, or *if the reasons therefore were unrelated to patient care, welfare, objectives of the institution, or character or competency of the applicant.* The Public Health Council held that the action taken was related to its "business objectives." The appellate court affirmed on the grounds that there were no issues of not acting in good faith. This decision demonstrates the propensy of courts to uphold decisions based on "business reasons," that is, economic credentialing.

"Pure" economic credentialing was reflected in the decision in *Bhogaonker v. Metropolitan Hospital.*[39] Here, the physician employment at the institution was cut due to budget cuts. The court upheld the hospital decision, stating in part "[T]o hold otherwise would impose an unworkable economic burden upon employers to stay in business to satisfy employment contracts and related agreements terminable only for good or sufficient cause. . . ."

Upholding the validity of an exclusive contract, the court in *Belmar v. Cipolla*[40] affirmed termination of anesthesiology services, with an exclusive contract being given to another group. The hospital contended that by doing so, there was more efficient use of operating rooms, reduction in administrative problems, ability to process more operative procedures, avoidance of fee splitting between surgeons and anesthesiologists, and better 24-hour coverage. The Supreme Court of New Jersey upheld the hospital action on the grounds that the exclusive contract was a reasonable business decision, did not violate public policy, and did not demonstrate antitrust violations.

One of the more significant cases in this area, is that of *Redding v. St. Francis Medical Center.*[41] Drs. Redding and Lawrence, on staff for 11 or more years, brought an action against the hospital as a result of the decision by St. Francis to form an exclusive contract with a cardiac surgeon who was to be brought to the facility to direct the cardiac surgery program. It was conceded that both Dr. Redding and Dr. Lawrence had a very low mortality rate. However, there were several other independent cardiac surgeons working at St. Francis, and all of these surgeons were working at other hospitals. The hospital contended several identified problems were the result of the spread of activity over a wide geographical area, including a high *overall* mortality rate of 8.4%, failure of cardiac surgeons to conduct peer review, inability to schedule needed surgeries, and unavailability of cardiac surgeons for needed backup, for handling emergencies, and for giving follow-up care. The hospital contended that the team approach, fostered by a "closed" program, would be a 24-hour-a-day arrangement and would foster teamwork, uniformity of high standards, dedication to this program, and *lower mortality rates.* When notification was served that none of the existing staff members would be able to

perform independent bypass surgery in 38 days, the complaint was filed, alleging (1) breach of contract; (2) breach of the covenant of good faith and fair dealing; (3) negligence; (4) negligent interference with prospective economic advantage; (5) interference with present and prospective contractual rights and professional relationships; and (6) unfair competition. An application for a temporary restraining order was granted, but upon the hearing, all of the allegations were dismissed, declaring that there was no basis for intervention in the internal affairs of St. Francis. An appeal was filed.

Grounds to grant or deny a preliminary injunction, a TRO, rest within the discretion of the trial court and cannot be interfered with on appeal unless abuse of discretion occurs. The grounds for finding such abuse sound in a finding that the trial court "exceeded the bounds of reason or contravened the uncontradicted evidence."[42] The probability of such findings in the context of case law concerning credentialing and when bylaws are reasonably followed are very unlikely and were not found here.

Additionally, the court individually addressed each of the six allegations in the complaint and found none of them valid. One of the basic premises of common law on hospital-physician relationships is an established principle that an action will lie where the right to pursue a lawful business, calling, trade, or occupation is *intentionally interfered with either by unlawful means or by means otherwise lawful when there is lack of sufficient justification.* In view of the decisions concerning staff privilege vis-à-vis "reasonable business action," "business necessity," and now definitive application of economic considerations, justification probably will be found. "It will not be set aside by the court unless it is substantively irrational, unlawful, contrary to established public policy, or procedurally unfair."[43] The law is based on a balancing, with due consideration of all the circumstances, of the respective importance to society and the parties of protecting the activities interfered with on one hand and permitting the interference on the other. Further, the common law generally holds that a physician, otherwise qualified, cannot be unreasonably or arbitrarily excluded from membership on the medical staff. Further, the greater number of cases in which appeal, by one means or another, has been brought deal with fair and equitable procedure. Further, the courts have recognized that a physician or surgeon, deprived of staff membership, has been denied the right to fully practice his profession.

But the common law also recognizes that there is a distinction between *intentional actions of a medical entity directed specifically toward exclusion of a particular physician or group of physicians, and the actions of a medical facility which, as a practical matter, may result in exclusion but which actions were undertaken for less personally directed reasons.* In the first instance, physicians will be protected. In the latter, the case law favors, in nearly all cases, the medical entity, especially in the present milieu where the case law upholds the right of medical entities to make rational management decisions.

Based on the law herein discussed, the court found that none of the six allegations in the complaint were valid in *Redding*.[41]

There is one aspect of this case that might have made a difference. As pointed out earlier, Cal. Bus. & Prof. Code, section 809.6(c), precludes any waiver in any instrument of hearing rights provided in the hearing statute, Cal. Bus. & Prof. Code, sections 809.1 to 809.4. But there was originally a phrase that hearing rights could not be waived "for any other reason." The latter was expunged from the enacted law.

In *Redding*,[41] it was stated by the court that Drs. Redding and Lawrence had "very low mortality rates." The high rate of 8.4% was recognized as due to other surgeons who were not evaluated. Further, the surgeon who took over the exclusive contract, and his group, did not do well and developed a mortality rate 50% to 75% higher, in the 13% to 14% range. Consequently that surgeon was dismissed from St. Francis. It is possible that the outcome would have been different if peer review had been required in the procedural functions to be followed by St. Francis. Under the law, and with disregard for peer review in evaluating business relations, the good surgeons left the hospital and those in both the first and second group with high mortality rates went elsewhere in medicine to continue a less than satisfactory operative expertise.

One final note concerning economic credentialing is the possibility of antitrust considerations. Exclusive contracts have been upheld by the Supreme Court.[44] However, a spokesman for the Department of Justice has stated a concern that economic credentialing decisions could be used to lock out physicians willing to work for lower prices by denying them a place to practice, resulting in higher consumer prices.

JUDICIAL REVIEW

Administrative judicial review for certain actions, such as those against physicians, may be treated in a specialized manner. For example, in California Code of Civil Procedure, section 1094.5, those characteristics are specifically delineated. The writ is issued for the purpose of inquiring into the validity of any final administrative order or decision made as the result of a proceeding in which, *by law:*

1. a hearing is required to be given;
2. evidence is required to be taken; and
3. discretion in the determination of facts is vested in the hearing panel, be it a formal tribunal, corporation, board or officer.

A final administrative order or decision is predicated on completion of all administrative hearings, thereby satisfying "exhaustion" of administrative procedures before the court may accept the case. Exceptions to this rule exist: where administrative review will serve no purpose because there is no need for the hearing officer to either decide disputed factual issues or furnish expertise essential for judicial review, or where, even though there is an administrative remedy to exhaust, the exhaustion requirement is excused where its pursuit would be futile, idle, or useless. The latter is very narrow and apparently can only be applied where the petitioner can positively state the administrative agency has declared what its ruling will be in a particular case.[45] The record below may be filed in part or in full at the discretion of the parties. The fundamental questions to be addressed by judicial review are (1) whether there was a fair trial and (2) whether there was any *prejudicial* abuse of discretion.

The basis for determination of whether or not there was any abuse of discretion in the administrative procedure will be predicated on the issues of due process, discussed in the previous section of this chapter. The measure of appropriate due process depends on the furnishing of *minimally* acceptable due process. As delineated *supra,* there is no "litmus test" of what encompasses minimum due process in the context of this type of quasijudicial hearing concerning disciplinary action in a medical setting; it is obvious that the requirement is low, unless modified by statute, as in California. Included in the determination is a fundamental policy issue embraced by the courts that the rights of the physician must be balanced against the public peril of overlooking lack of medical competence.

An enunciation of this standard was well expressed in *Rhee,*[7] where the court stated that "[t]he appropriate standard to bring to bear on judicial review of hospital disciplinary procedures is therefore this: courts must not interfere to set aside decisions regarding hospital staff privileges unless it can be shown that a procedure is 'substantively irrational or otherwise unreasonably susceptible of arbitrary or discriminatory application . . .'" (citations omitted).

But the standard of review may be greatly influenced by the scope of review to be applied. There are two, very different premises on which review at the trial court level may be based. The first is the independent judgment rule; the second is the substantial evidence rule. The difference between the two can and does result in opposite conclusions by the court of first impression.

The two alternative review methods require review of the entire record from the tribunal below, the JRC and the appeal board decision, if any. There the two methods part company. Under the independent judgment rule, the court may find abuse of discretion if it determines that the findings are not supported by the *weight* of the evidence, that is, whether or not the evidence fairly and reasonably supports the decision. In essence, the proceeding becomes a mini-trial *de novo* similar to civil appeal. Only errors of law are subject to its cognizance. Factual findings can be overturned only if evidence received by the trial court, including the record of the administrative proceeding(s), is insufficient as a matter of law to sustain the findings.[46]

Under the substantial evidence rule, however, the trial court may not reexamine the weight of the evidence; it may only determine if there is substantial evidence to support the conclusion in light of the entire record.[47]

The entry question as to whether the independent evidence rule shall be applied is whether or not the subject decision substantially affects a "a fundamental vested right."[48,49] In *Anton,* the court pointed out that the scope of judicial review to be afforded administrative decisions of an adjudicatory nature "is the importance of the affected right to the individual who stands in jeopardy of losing it".[50] The basis was stated in *Bixby,* where the Supreme Court of California explained: "[i]f . . . the right has been acquired by the individual, and if the right is fundamental, the courts have held the loss of it is sufficiently vital to the individual to compel a full and independent review. The abrogation of the right is too important to the individual to relegate it to exclusive administrative extinction."[51]

After the first *Anton* case,[47] the California legislature decided that the rule should not apply, even though a physician has such a vested interest, when the case involves a private hospital. Thus, by statute, California added to their Code of Civil Procedure 1094.5 a new section (d), which states:

Notwithstanding the provisions of subdivision (c), in cases arising from *private* hospital boards, abuse of discretion is established if the court determines that the findings are not supported by substantial evidence in the light of the whole record. . . .[52]

But in *Kimble v. Los Angeles City Board of Education,*[53] the court stated that "Substantial evidence means evidence which is of ponderable legal significance. Obviously, the word cannot be deemed synonymous with "any" evidence. It must be reasonable in nature, credible, and of solid value; it must actually be "substantial" proof of the essentials which the law requires in a particular case".[54] The court pointed out that hearsay evidence, for example, though admissible in an administrative proceeding, cannot be considered on appeal as substantial evidence in support of the findings.[55]

Further, in *Miller v. Eisenhower Medical Center,* the Supreme Court of California also stated:

It is well settled, of course, that in cases involving imposition of a penalty or other disciplinary action by an administrative body, when it appears that some of the charges are not sustained by the evidence, the matter will be returned to the administrative body in all cases where there is 'real doubt' as to whether the same action would have been taken upon *a proper assessment of the evidence.* (emphasis added) (citations omitted)[56]

[T]he existence of 'real doubt' as to the probable determination of the administrative body upon a *proper view* of the evidence will necessitate a redetermination.[57] (emphasis added) (citations omitted)

Thus in evaluating the scope of review in any given jurisdiction, this most important distinction must be carefully appraised. One might also consider examining the constitutional issue of discrimination where the substantial evidence rule has been imposed by such a limitation.

If the writ is appealed, the scope of appellate review is essentially the substantial evidence standard. Thus, when the substantial evidence rule is applicable, the trial court and appellate level perform essentially identical functions. However, "the conclusions of the trial court are not conclusive on appeal."[58]

Bias

The administrative hearing must be conducted by an unbiased panel. The defendant, therefore, must have the right to voir dire the members, including the hearing officer, if there is one. If there is curtailment of reasonable voir dire, it is imperative that an appropriate record be made so that the court can adequately evaluate any charge to that effect brought before it in judicial review.

In that regard, there is the issue of "overlapping" of investigatory, prosecutorial, and adjudicatory functions at the administrative level, but it has been clearly enunciated by the Supreme Court that some overlapping may have occurred, but that ordinarily will not be of sufficient merit so as to rise to the level of denial of due process.[25]

As an example of the elements that will be considered by the court, another California case will serve for demonstrating the tenets, *Applebaum v. Board of Directors of Barton Memorial Hospital.*[59] An obstetrician, and competitor of Dr. Applebaum, was given a complaint by the head nurse, questioning Dr. Applebaum's delivery techniques. In accord with the bylaws, a letter was written to the chief of staff requesting an investigation, with a listing of various charges. The hospital's Medical Executive Committee (MEC) reviewed the problem and appointed an ad hoc committee to investigate it. The same competing obstetrician and another competing obstetrician were members of the MEC; and both were appointed to the ad hoc committee. The ad hoc committee recommended suspension of Dr. Applebaum's privileges. The MEC, in turn, reviewed the recommendation and affirmed it. Five of the six members of the ad hoc committee attended that meeting of the MEC, including both of the competing obstetricians.

Dr. Applebaum, in accord with the hospital bylaws, filed an appeal. An appellate review panel consisting of three physicians who had not been involved in the previous proceedings was appointed. While the appeals process was under way, before any decision was reached, two of these physicians were appointed to the MEC. They attended an MEC meeting at which the events surrounding Dr. Applebaum were deliberated. The suspension of privileges was sustained.

Upon judicial review, at both the trial and appellate court level, the judges determined that this scenario presented a "practical probability of unfairness." The decision was predicated on the fact that the instigator of the investigation also conducted the investigation. Additionally, there was overlapping membership in the committee that reviewed both the initial and final decisions. Also, a majority of the adjudicators belonged to this same committee. The court found that "the risk of prejudgment or bias was too high to maintain the guarantee of fair procedure."[60] Keep in mind, also, that the concept of overlapping usually applies to ascending levels of adjudication that would allow a trier of fact to review his own previous decisions and/or judge a physician whom he had charged or investigated.

In *Rhee*,[7] as mentioned previously, the court found no case law as to overlapping roles of counsel, where there were two members from the same firm involved, representing the medical staff and the board of directors. As discussed above, however, the *Howitt*[8] decision has offered correction of that obstacle to fair due process.

Of importance in *Rhee*[7] is the fact that Dr. Rhee charged that the panel members were biased against him, that they used a prosecutorial approach by questioning of witnesses; that they gave credibility to hospital witnesses while criticizing the witnesses for Dr. Rhee. However, the court could find no evidence in the record to support this claim and dismissed it. The importance of demanding a complete record, and making a complete record is most certainly underlined by these findings in the case.

Categories have been identified where the probability of actual bias by a panel member will be found unacceptable. These fall into four categories:

1. A member has a direct pecuniary interest in the outcome.

2. A member has been the target of personal abuse or criticism from the person before him.
3. A member is enmeshed in other matters involving the person whose rights he is determining.
4. A member may have prejudged the case because of prior participation as accuser, investigator, factfinder, or initial decisionmaker.[61]

Violation of hospital bylaws

The concept of due process does not require strict adherence to any particular set of rules. In the deliberations of any effect of bylaws violations, the courts have interwoven the balance of a physician's rights vis-à-vis the rights and safety of patients. Thus, substantial departures from the procedures delineated in the bylaws may occur, but still the substantive effect may be outweighed by the balancing of these considerations. A difficult question thereby arises as to whether or not the violation resulted in definitive unfairness, which also deprived the physician of a basic right to due process, such as notice, opportunity to be heard, or trial by a demonstrably partial JRC.

Sufficiency of evidence

The substantial evidence rule provides that where a finding of fact is attacked on the ground that it is not sustained by the evidence, the power of an appellate court begins and ends with a determination of whether there is substantial evidence, contradicted or uncontradicted, supporting the finding. The court will consider the evidence in the light most favorable to the prevailing party, giving him the benefit of every reasonable inference and resolving conflicts in support of the judgment. The court is without power to judge the effect or value of the evidence, weigh the evidence, consider the credibility of witnesses, or resolve conflicts in the evidence or in the reasonable inferences that may be drawn from it. Unless a finding, viewed in light of the entire record, is so lacking in evidentiary support as to render it unreasonable, it may not be set aside.[62] Abuse of discretion is established if the court determines that the findings are not supported by substantial evidence in light of the whole record.

In considering the totality of the administrative procedures, the judicial review may consider prejudicial violations of bylaws. For example in *Huang v. Board of Directors*,[63] the accusations of a nurse that she had been threatened were discounted and charges against Dr. Huang dropped at the JRC. The decision was appealed by the hospital. The hospital appellate review panel reopened inquiry into the evidence, found against Dr. Huang, and reversed the decision.

Upon judicial review, the staff bylaws were demonstrated to have stated that "The proceeding by the

Appeal Board shall be in the nature of an appellate review based upon the record of the hearing before the Judicial Review Committee." The rule that the appellate panel could accept additional oral or written evidence only upon a showing that such evidence could have materially affected the decisions of the JRC in the exercise of reasonable diligence was included in the deliberations (see discussion of additional evidence on appeal *supra*).

The court found that the appellate panel had impermissibly reweighed the evidence, that the JRC finding was dispositive, and reversed the final decision by the MEC based on the appellate panel's error.

Finally, it should not be overlooked that some violations of procedure, from the onset, may cause immediate and irreparable harm to a physician. For example, a board of directors, against the hospital bylaws, may try to wrest from the hands of the MEC its designated duty to investigate and adjudicate disciplinary actions. By so doing and planning to render a reportable disciplinary action, thereby going to both the state board of medical examiners and the National Practitioner Data Bank, established by HCQIA, there may be immediate, severe, irreparable harm to the livelihood and reputation of a physician. Under circumstances such as these, it is possible to obtain an *ex parte* TRO, preventing such action, so long as the medical staff is prepared to undertake and carry out timely its duties.

CONCLUSION

Peer review is an expanding area in the law. The shift of health care to a business orientation, with its development of both horizontal and vertical integration, is having a profound and permanent effect. An attempt has been made in this chapter to focus on major issues. Physicians and attorneys alike must pay more attention to the medical staff bylaws, statutes, and other sources of law, including contractual relationships between physicians and medical entities, which govern health care organizations. We must take a more active role in assuring that the precise wording and clear interpretation of those governing rules are equitable, justifiable, and give all parties the opportunity to participate on a level playing field. We have the best system of health care in the world. The parties involved in the delivery of that care cannot afford to take economic and personal advantage of one another.

END NOTES

1. *Johnson v. Misericordia Community Hospital,* 99 Wis.2d 708; 301 N.W.2d 156 (1981).
2. *Elam v. College Park Hospital,* 132 Cal. App. 3d 332, 183 Cal. Rptr. 156 (1982).
3. *Id.* 321 Cal. App. 3d 332, at 337-341.
4. *Cipriotti v. Board of Directors,* 147 Cal. App. 3d 144, 157, 196 Cal. Rptr. 367 (1983).
5. Health Quality Improvement Act, 42 U.S.C. §§ 11101 *et seq.*
6. California Business & Professions Code, § 809.3(c).
7. *Rhee v. El Camino Hospital District,* 247 Cal. Rptr. 244, 201 Cal. App. 3d 477, 493. (1988).
8. *Howitt v. Superior Court of Imperial County,* 5 Cal. Rptr. 2d 196; 3 Cal. App. 1575 (1992).
9. *Id.* (Cal. Rptr.) at 204.
10. *Board of Regents v. Roth,* 408 U.S. 564, 92 S.Ct. 2701, 33 L.Ed.2d 548 (1972).
11. *Anton v. San Antonio Community Hospital,* 19 Cal. 3d 802, 823, 140 Cal. Rptr. 442, 567, 567 P.2d 1162 (1977).
12. *Mathews v. Eldridge,* 424 U.S. 319, 335, 96 S.Ct. 893, 903, 47 L.Ed.2d 18.
13. *Id.* L.Ed.2d, at 33.
14. *Arnett v. Kennedy,* 416 U.S. 134, 94 S.Ct. 1633, 40 L.Ed.2d 15 (1974).
15. *Stretton v. Wadsworth Veterans Hospital,* 537 F.2d 361, 369, note 18.
16. *Joint Commission Accreditation Manual for Health Care Organizations,* § MS.3 (1993).
17. *Pinsker v. Pacific Coast Society of Orthodontists,* 12 Cal. 3d 541, 116 Cal. Rptr. 245, 526 P.2d 253 (1974).
18. *Id.* Cal. 3d, at 555-556.
19. Bond, Charles, Esq., Representing Physicians in Disciplinary Peer Review Proceedings, Address at National Health Lawyers Association Seminar on The Medical Staff: Legal Issues in a Changing Delivery System (November 12-13, 1992).
20. California Business and Professions Code, § 809.2(c).
21. *Id.* at 809.2(d).
22. 42 U.S.C. § 111101 *et seq.,* § 11111(2)(2), § 11112.
23. *California Civil Code,* §§ 43.8, 47.
24. *California Business and Professions Code,* §§ 2317, 2318.
25. *Withrow v. Larkin,* 421 U.S. 35; 95 S.Ct. 1456; 43 L.Ed.2d 712 (1975).
26. *Id.* 421 U.S., at 55; 95 S.Ct. at 1468.
27. *California Evidence Code,* § 1157 *et seq.*
28. *Alexander v. The Superior Court of Los Angeles County,* 226 Cal. Rptr. 2d 397; 859 P.2d 96, 62 USLW 2296 (1993).
29. *Id.* 226 Cal. Rptr. 2d 397, at 401.
30. *Id,* at 402.
31. *Matchett v. Superior Court,* 40 Cal. App. 3d 623, 629, 115 Cal. Rptr. 317 (1974).
32. *Cruger v. Love,* 599 So.2d 111 (Fla. 1992).
33. *Anatomy of the Conflict Between Hospital Medical Staff Peer Review Confidentiality and Medical Malpractice Plaintiff Recovery: A Case for Legislative Amendment,* 24 Santa Clara L.Rev. 661 (1984).
34. California Medical Association, *Model Medical Staff Bylaws,* §§ 7.5-5, 7.5-6 (1992).
35. California Business and Professions Code, § 809.4.
36. *Rosenblum v. Tallahassee Memorial Community Hospital,* Case no. 91-589, (June 18, 1992).
37. *Knapp v. Palos Community Hospital,* 125 Ill. App. 3d 244; 80 Ill. Dec. 442 (1984).
38. *Maltz v. New York University Medical Center,* 121 A.2d 323; 503 N.Y.S.2d 570 (1986).
39. *Bhogaonker v. Metropolitan Hospital,* 164 Mich. App. 563; 417 N.W.2d 501 (1987).
40. *Belmar v. Cipolla,* 96 N.J. 199, 475 A.2d 533 (1984).
41. *Redding v. St. Francis Medical Center,* 208 Cal. App. 3d 98; 255 Cal. Rptr. 806 (1989).
42. *IT Corp. v. County of Imperial,* 35 Cal. 3d 63, 69; 196 Cal. Rptr. 715, 715, 672 P.2d 121.
43. *Centeno v. Roseville Community Hospital,* 107 Cal. App. 3d 62, 63; 167 Cal. Rptr. 183 (1979).

44. *Jefferson Parish Hospital, Dist. No. 2 v. Hyde,* 466 U.S. 2 (1984); *Coastal Neuro-Psychiatric Assoc., P.A. v. Onslow Memorial Hospital,* 795 F.2d 340 (4th Cir. 1986); *Burnham Hospital,* 101 F.T.C. 991 (1983) (FTC advisory opinion).

45. *Bollengier v. Doctors Medical Center,* 222 Cal. App. 3d 1115, 1126; 272 Cal. Rptr. 273 (1990).

46. *Merrill v. Department of Motor Vehicles,* 80 Cal. Rptr. 89, 458 P.2d 33, 71 Cal. 2d 907 (1969).

47. *Anton v. San Antonio Community Hospital,* 9 Cal. 3d 802; 140 Cal. Rptr. 442; 567 P.2d 1162 (1977).

48. *Id.* 9 Cal. 3d 802, at 821; *see also Bixby v. Pierno,* 4 Cal. 3d 130, 93 Cal. Rptr. 234, 481 P.2d 242 (1971).

49. *Strumsky v. San Diego County Employees Retirement Assn.,* 11 Cal. 3d 28, 112 Cal. Rptr. 805, 520 P.2d 29 (1974).

50. *Merrill, supra* note 46, at 821.

51. *Bixby, supra* note 48, Cal. 3d 130, at 144.

52. *Anton v. San Antonio Community Hospital,* 132 Cal. App. 3d 638, 183 Cal. Rptr. 423 (1982).

53. *Kimble v. Los Angeles City Board of Education,* 192 Cal. App. 3d 1423, 238 Cal. Rptr. 160 (Cal. App 3rd Dist. 1987).

54. *Id.* at 162.

55. *Id.* at 164.

56. *Miller v. Eisenhower Medical Center,* 27 Cal. 3d 614, 166 Cal. Rptr. 826, 614 P.2d 258 (1980).

57. *Id.* at 635.

58. *Lewin v. St. Joseph Hospital of Orange,* 82 Cal. App. 3d 368, 387, 146 Cal. Rptr. 892 (1978).

59. *Applebaum v. Board of Directors of Barton Memorial Hospital,* 104 Cal. App. 3d 648, 163 Cal. Rptr. 831 (1980).

60. *Id.* 104 Cal. App. 3d 648, at 660.

61. *Hackethal v. California Medical Assn.,* 138 Cal. App. 3d 435, 443, 187 Cal. Rptr 811 (Dec. 1982); *see also Applebaum, supra* note 59; *Crampton v. Michigan Dept. of State,* 395 Mich. 347, 235 N.W.2d 352 (1975); Prygoski, *Due Process and Designated Members of Administrative Tribunals,* 33 Admin. L. Rev. 441.

62. See 9 Witkin, Cal. Procedure (3d ed. 1985) Appeal §§ 281-282.

63. *Huang v. Board of Directors,* 220 Cal. App. 3d 1286, 270 Cal. Rptr. 41 (1990).

CHAPTER 11 # Health care provider as a defendant

MARTIN B. FLAMM, M.D., J.D., F.C.L.M.

HISTORY OF PHYSICIAN AS DEFENDANT IN MALPRACTICE SUITS
PLAINTIFF THEORIES AGAINST PHYSICIANS
PHYSICIANS' DEFENSE THEORIES AGAINST PLAINTIFFS' CLAIMS
NEGOTIATION AND SETTLEMENT OF MALPRACTICE CLAIMS

Medical "malpractice" does not imply general lack of competence. However, it is more than a mere mistake or a bad outcome. The term *malpractice* refers to any professional misconduct that encompasses an unreasonable lack of skill or unfaithfulness in carrying out professional or fiduciary duties. Although the term *medical negligence* may be preferable to *medical malpractice,* which is heavily charged with emotional baggage, *medical malpractice* will be used in this chapter because of the common and traditional usage of this term.

HISTORY OF PHYSICIAN AS DEFENDANT IN MALPRACTICE SUITS

It may comfort the modern physician to know that holding physicians accountable for an acceptable standard of care is not a recent phenomenon. The history of liability of health care providers for improper practice of medicine is surprisingly lengthy.

Malpractice laws can be traced back at least two millennia. Hammurabi, the King of Babylonia from 2025-2067 B.C., delivered to the courts of his empire great laws from the sun god Shamash. According to the Code of Hammurabi, if a physician unsuccessfully treated a gentleman with a lancet of bronze and caused the patient's death, the physician was penalized by the loss of his hand. If the patient were a slave, the penalty was replacement with another slave. Ancient Egyptian law also provided for sanctions against the physician who committed malpractice, providing for the healer's banishment or death, depending on circumstances. Roman civil law also punished medical practitioners who committed malpractice with exceedingly severe penalties, and medieval law was equally hard on barbers and surgeons.

In 1533, Holy Roman Emperor Charles I established an important concept in medical malpractice law—that medical malpractice must be judged by medical practitioners. Under the American legal system, patients have always been entitled to sue their physicians for medical malpractice. Until the 1950s, however, lawsuits alleging malpractice were relatively uncommon in the United States. From 1950 until the mid-1960s, such lawsuits increased gradually, and by the mid-1960's, the rate of increase accelerated. Despite a trend to "tort reform," which may have led to a recent decrease of such suits, physicians are frequently defendants in medical negligence suits.

Medical malpractice law has evolved continuously in this country to its current state. The law of medical malpractice is continually evolving, however, and it is likely that some interesting historical developments will occur in medical malpractice law within the reader's lifetime.

PLAINTIFF THEORIES AGAINST PHYSICIANS

Currently, there are a number of legal theories or causes of action by which a patient as plaintiff may bring a lawsuit against a health care provider. Although negligence is the most common basis of medical malpractice actions for imposing liabilities on physicians, physicians may also find themselves involved in legal actions brought on other legal theories. For purposes of completeness, alternative plaintiff theories against physicians are considered after a discussion of the basic principles of medical negligence suits. The physician must be aware that suits often will be brought under several theories in one legal action. If the patient as plaintiff wins under any of these theories, recovery of a monetary award from defendant physicians and their professional liability insurance carriers may result.

Negligence

Most medical malpractice suits are based on the legal theory of negligence. Briefly, negligence is a breach of the duty of the physician to behave reasonably and prudently under the circumstances, causing foreseeable harm to another. For a successful suit under a theory of negligence or, in legal terms, to present a cause of action for negligence, a patient as plaintiff must prove each of the following four elements of negligence.

Duty. The first element of the negligence theory of liability is that of duty, recognized by law as created by a physician-patient relationship. This duty requires that a physician possess and bring to bear on the patient's behalf that degree of knowledge, skill, and care usually exercised by a reasonable and prudent physician under similar circumstances, given the prevailing state of medical knowledge and available resources. In other words, physicians owe their patients a duty to act in accordance with the specific norms or standards established by their profession, commonly referred to as "standards of care" to protect their patients against unreasonable risk.

This legal fiction requires every physician to possess the requisite skill, care, and diligence that a particular case demands. A patient may show that his or her physician failed to exercise the required care by either the commission or omission of an act — in other words, by doing something that shouldn't have been done or by failing to do something that should have been done. It may not matter that the physician has performed at full potential and in complete good faith. Instead, the physician must have conformed to the standard of a "reasonable physician" under similar circumstances.

Unfortunately, such statements do not provide a definition of the duty of a particular physician in a particular case. Because most medical malpractice cases are highly technical, it is necessary that witnesses with special medical qualifications provide guidance to the judge or jury by giving them the knowledge necessary to render a fair and just verdict. As a result, the standard of medical care must be determined from expert testimony in nearly all cases. In the case of a specialist, the standard of care generally is the care and skill commonly possessed and exercised by similar specialists under similar circumstances. The specialty standard of care may often be higher than that required of general practitioners.

Although courts recognize that medical facts and medical practices are usually not within the realm of common knowledge, and require expert testimony, it should be clear that physicians themselves or bodies of physicians or professional societies do not set the "standard of care." The standard of care is an objective standard against which the conduct of a physician sued for malpractice may be measured. Because it must be objective, this standard does not depend on any individual physician's own knowledge.

The law does not equate the mental ability of various individuals. By attempting to fix a uniform standard by which a jury or judge may determine whether or not a physician has properly performed his or her duties toward the patient, expert medical testimony from both plaintiff and defense experts is required. The judge or jury, however, ultimately determines the standard of care, after listening to the testimony of the medical experts. Of course, there are exceptions to every rule, and expert testimony may not be required where a patient presents evidence showing that his or her physician's lack of care is so obvious as to be within the comprehension of a layperson. For example, an instrument left within the abdomen during surgery may qualify under a legal doctrine called *res ipsa loquitur.*

Breach of duty. The second element of medical negligence is that a physician did not comply with his or her duty toward a patient, by failing to act in accordance with norms or standards of care by his or her commission or omission of a certain act. Of course, the standard of care and duty must first be proven before the plaintiff can prove that the health care provider breached such duty.

In most cases, testimony of plaintiff and defense expert witnesses will address the question of breach of duty during the same testimony elicited to describe the standard of care owed. The plaintiff must prove that the defendant health care provider failed to comply with the standard of care by the greater weight or preponderance of the evidence.

Causation. The third element of medical malpractice or negligence is that of causation. The plaintiff must show that a reasonable close and "causal" connection exists between the act or omission and the resulting injury. In legal terms, this is commonly noted as "legal cause" or "proximate cause."

Particular note should be made that this legal concept of causation differs markedly from medical causation in that it refers to a single cause and not necessarily the only cause or even the most immediate cause of the injury, as is the case with medical causation. Although the requirement that the patient as plaintiff prove that the defending physician's breach of duty caused his or her damages may seem simple on the surface, causation is sometimes the most complex and elusive concept in a medical malpractice negligence case.

Legal causation consists of two principal branches: causation in fact and foreseeability. Causation in fact may be stated as follows: An Event A is the cause of another Event B, if and only if Event B would not have occurred when and as it did but for Event A. This definition is often called the "but for" test.

This test is easily met in some cases but not in others. Contrasting examples would be an intestinal perforation from an instrument left by a surgeon in the abdominal cavity, so that a subsequent abdominal abscess, surgery, or death of the patient would be due to a breach of the standard of care, in that but for the retained instrument such complication would not have occurred, whereas a delay in the diagnosis and treatment of a highly aggressive malignant neoplasm might not necessarily affect the patient's chance of cure or survival.

Foreseeability is the second breach of the causation element. In other words, a patient's damages must be the foreseeable result of a defendant health care provider's substandard practice. Generally, the patient must prove only that his or her injuries were of a type that would have been foreseen by a reasonable physician as likely resulting from the breach of the medical standard of care. The patient's damages are included within that zone.

The law of causation varies widely from jurisdiction to jurisdiction and is an area currently in flux. For example, in *Daubert v. Merrell Dow Pharmaceuticals,*[1] the U.S. Supreme Court recently addressed the question of admissibility of scientific evidence in a case involving expert testimony concerning causation. The ultimate effect of this recent decision, which directly applies to federal courts (and the states that adopt or follow the Federal Rules of Evidence) cannot be accurately predicted. In general, this decision allows judges greater discretion in deciding which scientific evidence is or is not admissible.

Damages. The fourth element of the medical negligence suit is proof of damages. In general, the concept of damages encompasses the actual loss or damage to the interests of the patient by the physician's breach of the standard of care. If the patient is not harmed, there can be no recovery.

Damages of several kinds may be recovered in the malpractice suit, but almost always these are expressed in terms of a monetary award. Damages may encompass a wide range of financial, physical, or emotional injury to the patient. The law has identified various injuries and recognizes certain categories of damages, but categorization is often imprecise and inconsistent because some of these categories will overlap and are not strictly adhered to by courts of all jurisdictions.

The most common categories of damages include general damages, without any reference to any special circumstances of the particular patient, such as generalized pain and suffering. Special damages are those that are the actual but not necessarily the inevitable result of

the injury complained of and that follow the injury as a natural and proximate cause in that particular case. Typical items of special damages that are compensable by a monetary judgment include past and future medical, surgical, hospital, and other related costs; past and future loss of income; funeral expenses in a death case; and unusual physical or medical consequences of the alleged injury, such as an aggravation of a preexisting condition.

Punitive or exemplary damages may be given above the patient's actual losses where a wrong done was aggravated by special circumstances of fraud, malice, violence, or intentional conduct on the part of the health care provider. Punitive damages, which are quite unusual in medical negligence cases, are intended to make an example of the defendant or to punish negative behavior.

Battery

This cause of action for medical injury is really not a negligence action, but an intentional tort. The law in general recognizes the principle that an individual is to be free from unwarranted and unwanted intrusion. In legal terms, the touching of another without that person's express consent is a battery. The attempt to touch another without express consent is an assault. Assault can be considered as an attempt at battery.

The law in all jurisdictions places considerable importance on the principle of this personal autonomy, and traditionally this has been reinforced in legislation dealing with patients' rights. In the medical setting, battery is most often seen in the context of undesired medical treatment or unconsented sexual contact. To successfully prove a claim for medical assault or battery, a patient as plaintiff must show that he or she was subjected to an examination or treatment for which there was no express or implied consent. The treatment provided must be a substantially different form of care than that which was agreed to by the patient and physician. There must also be proof that the departure from the agreed-to form of care was intentional on the part of the physician.

Unlike claims made under the negligence theory of consent, which is discussed later, there is no need to prove actual harm in battery cases, although harm may have occurred. The amount of damages, of course, will relate directly to the amount of harm in most cases. For example, an unconsented-to operation that saves a patient's life will likely not result in damages, except in rare cases. However, where damages are due to a physician who operates without consent and the patient suffers painful, crippling, or lingering effects, damages may be awarded.

Specific examples of medical battery cases historically include sexual "therapy" by a psychiatrist or other mental health care professional in the name of treatment, unauthorized extension of a surgery to nonconsented matters different and unjustified by the original procedure, and the unconsented treatment of Jehovah's Witnesses or others whose religious convictions limit their therapeutic alternatives.

Although there are still some jurisdictions where recovery may be based on assault-and-battery theories, most jurisdictions have removed by legislation (sometimes as part of reform measures) the right to bring such an action. This change, however, has come about because of the now nearly universal acceptance of the negligence theory of consent.

Failure of informed consent

A physician may be negligent if he or she proceeds to diagnose or treat a patient by failing to obtain informed consent or failing to obtain an adequate informed consent for such diagnosis or treatment.

Patients must be capable of giving consent and must possess adequate information through which to reach a decision regarding treatment, and must be given ample opportunity to discuss proposed diagnosis and treatment methods and alternatives with the physician. A failure to meet the requirements for an appropriate and adequate informed consent may be a departure from the recognized standard of care and may result in an action for negligence in obtaining proper consent against a health care provider.

It is wise to remember that consent is actually a process, not a form. Physicians may, for this reason, fail in their duty to patients when they rely on a form or document for achieving "informed consent." Such a form can never replace the exchange of information between a patient and health care provider, which is necessary to fulfill the requirements of an adequate informed consent.

Although some physicians are paternalistic and cannot believe that their patients want to make or are capable of making their own medical decisions, the law generally respects a competent individual's right to determine what happens to his or her own body. Most patients are quite concerned about the risks, benefits, and reasonable alternatives to a recommended procedure and want to know what possible impact a specific course of medical care or surgical treatment will have on their health. For a physician to presume otherwise may subject him or her to a successful cause of action based on negligence of informed consent. Additionally, patients are generally now more aware and conscious health care consumers, and knowledgeable of their individual liberties. They are more likely now than in the past to question the need for or the cost of a specific procedure, for example, when presented with alternatives.

Generally, any physician who undertakes to treat or diagnose a patient has a duty to advise that patient or that patient's responsible party about:

1. The problem to be treated or symptom to be diagnosed
2. The proposed test or prescription
3. The risks, consequences, complications, or side effects of the test or treatment
4. The indications for the choice
5. The expected results or goal to be achieved by the test or treatment
6. Reasonable available alternative methods and costs of diagnosis and treatment
7. The consequences of doing nothing

A practical problem is not in obtaining consent, but in obtaining an adequate and informed consent. As with other aspects of medical practice, adequacy of informed consent must be measured against a legal standard. Standards of informed consent that are currently used by courts in various states include:

1. What a reasonably prudent physician would tell a patient, under the same or similar circumstances.
2. What a reasonably prudent patient would wish to know in order to decide among several alternatives, under the same or similar circumstances. The patient, as the plaintiff, must show that an ordinary reasonably prudent patient under the same circumstances would have declined diagnosis or treatment when informed about the possible risks and alternatives under this commonly used reasonable patient standard. It is not legally adequate to contend that he or she would not have consented having been fully informed, if a reasonable patient would have done so.
3. Reasonably common complications and sequelae that a panel of physicians and attorneys has determined that patients need to be warned about for each medical and surgical procedure.
4. A statutory list of the elements necessary for the presumption of informed consent.

The practicing physician must know which standard is applicable in his or her state and stay abreast of current developments in this field, which is in a state of flux.

Suits involving failure to obtain adequate informed consent are decided by applying general legal principles. A patient as plaintiff who persuades the judge or jury that he or she was not adequately informed according to the applicable legal standard is also required to prove causation and damages to prevail.

Abandonment

Generally, a physician has no duty to treat any person who is not already a patient. However, a physician who consents to diagnose, advise, or treat a patient accepts the duty to provide continuity of care. Legal recognition of this duty follows from the reality that a sick or injured person is at risk until cured or stabilized. If abandonment is alleged, it is not tried as a tort in and of itself, but such cases are judged according to a negligence standard.

No physician can be available at all times and in all circumstances. Prudent physicians must provide an adequate surrogate when they are out of town, ill, enjoying recreational pastimes, or attending another patient. Many physicians meet this obligation by making arrangements with a partner or nearby colleague in the same or similar field of practice. Backup may be provided by residents in a teaching hospital or by directing ambulatory patients to a nearby, physician-staffed emergency room. Brief lapses of coverage are generally reasonable. For example, doctors would unlikely be successfully sued for failure to attend simultaneous cardiac arrests, for which no other physician was available. They are sued at times when the unavailability of coverage for several hours harms a hospitalized patient.

This duty to provide care is extinguished when the physician dies, when the patient no longer requires treatment for the illness under consideration, or when the physician notifies the patient of his or her intention to withdraw. In the latter case, however, the physician must give the patient a reasonable time to arrange for care from another qualified physician or must arrange for a substitute physician who is acceptable to the patient. The original physician must also provide emergency care for the patient's same or related medical problems, until the patient has established a relationship with the new doctor.

An acceleration of growth of managed health care plans has resulted in many physicians becoming members of various health care networks. In some cases, physicians may opt to leave a network to join others. Such an action, per se, does not necessarily end a physician-patient relationship, particularly because patients may opt to continue the relationship outside of the network payment scheme. Any physician wishing to discontinue seeing patients previously seen in such a system may wish to notify those patients of a change in managed care participation, and arrange for appropriate transfer of care to a successor physician.

Breach of confidentiality

Physicians have a duty to respect the privacy interests of their patients. Generally, everything said by a patient or family member to a physician in the context of medical diagnosis and treatment is confidential and may be revealed only under certain circumstances. In many states, a physician-patient relationship is recognized by a statute that sets forth exceptions to the general rule of confidentiality. Some states rely on common law in this

area. Every practitioner needs to know the rules that apply in his or her state and to establish procedures for his or her employees to act accordingly.

In general, health care providers can safely release medical information to other treating physicians or consultants. In life-threatening emergencies, certain information necessary to treat the patient may also be revealed to other medical personnel, even if the patient is unaware.

Generally, a health care provider can safely release medical information to other third parties, including insurance companies, if the patient consents. As a precaution, however, memorialization of consent in writing is advisable. A consent to release selected information is not a consent to release other information, however. For example, if a physician is asked to release information concerning a back injury, this is not necessarily permission to release other medical information, such as psychiatric history, that may not be relevant. A health care provider may release information to his or her own attorney if a patient sues for malpractice, or if the physician is suing a patient for payment of fees.

When a patient sues a physician, the patient's statements to his or her attorney are privileged. This testimonial privilege, in other words, allows a client to talk with the attorney or the attorney's employees in confidence, and such matters discussed may not be inquired into by the court during the negligence suit.

No such privilege exists for nonmedical confidences between a physician and patient, however. A physician called on to testify in a criminal or civil matter can therefore be required by the court to testify concerning the patient's conduct, habits, condition, or utterances at the court's discretion. A difficult situation arises when the public interest outweighs patient confidentiality. This can occur, for example, when a physician learns that a patient is about to commit a crime. In this situation, courts have held that a physician has a duty to warn the potential victim, police authorities, or both. This has been held in common law, and some states have statutes setting forth this duty. In the event that a patient carries out the threatened crime, the timeliness and adequacy of the physician's warnings may be evaluated to determine whether a physician is liable for negligence.

Breach of contract or warranty to cure

When a physician promises to effect a cure or to achieve a particular result and the patient submits himself or herself for treatments, the physician is generally liable if the treatments fail to achieve the promised result. The unhappy patient in such a situation can sue the physician in contract, rather than in tort. This form of medical malpractice suit has become less common in recent decades. The major advantage for the plaintiff in a contract suit is that a medical standard of care need not be shown. The plaintiff need prove only that a promise was made and relied on and that the promise was not kept, and that damages resulted due to the broken promise.

The plaintiff in such suits must prove how he or she was damaged by the physician's breach of promise. A successful plaintiff generally recovers an amount of money that would place him or her in a position comparable to not having agreed to be treated. In many cases, that amounts to a return of the surgeon's fees, plus a small sum for related expenses. Damages may be exceedingly high in some instances, however, such as when a professional performer is scarred or killed. Professional medical negligence liability policies often exclude payment of damages in this form of legal action.

Most physicians at one time or another prognosticate for their patients. Courts understand that aspect of medical practice. Breach of contract/warranty actions usually arise when a physician sells a patient on a particular operation. The statement, "Mr. Jones, after your nose job, your friends won't know you from Robert Redford," is far more likely to produce a lawsuit than, "Mrs. Smith, removing your gallbladder may reduce your indigestion and cause vomiting after consumption of fatty foods." Obviously, many medical predictions fall somewhere between such outright hucksterism and bland assertions. In order to prevent a plethora of unwarranted suits, many states provide that no legal action may be taken for breach of a contract to cure, unless the physician's promise is in writing.

Strict liability for drugs and medical devices

Strict liability (i.e., not negligence based) is imposed on manufacturers/sellers of unreasonably dangerous and defective products for injuries resulting from their use. Such liability is independent of negligence law, and a manufacturer's/seller's degree of care is irrelevant in lawsuits based on the concept of strict liability. However, the law recognizes that every drug and device used in medical practice is potentially hazardous. Therefore, manufacturers/sellers of such products are not liable for damages if they give adequate warnings that make their products as safe as possible. These warnings must be given clearly, prominently, and in a timely manner, and they must be given to the proper person. Overpromotion of a product can negate the effect of otherwise adequate warnings.

Strict liability applies to manufacturers, wholesalers, and retailers of all products, not just medical products. The nature of the required warning, the question of who must be warned, the seller's duty to investigate and learn of all known hazards, and the matter of indemnification among sellers in the distribution chain are treated elsewhere in this book. Strict liability is mentioned here because many medical malpractice suits include claims for harm caused by inadequate warnings of product hazards.

Because it may be impractical or impossible for a manufacturer of medical products to notify each patient who has been treated, warnings are often given from the manufacturer to the physician, who acted as a "learned intermediary." In this event, the health care provider may have the duty to inform and adequately warn the patient of a defective product.

One reason for strict liability suits is to reduce the plaintiff's burden of proof. It is much easier to prove that a product warning was not given or was inadequate than to show that a physician violated the standard of care. It is also easier to prove causation in a strict liability suit. The plaintiff need show only either that the product was defective or that the warning of its nondefective hazards was faulty and that the deficiency of product or warning was a producing cause of the injury. Foreseeability is not required to make a case against a strict liability defendant.

Another setting for bringing in a strict liability defendant is when a defendant physician is uninsured or underinsured and a solvent pharmaceutical house or device manufacturer may be found liable to pay a share of any judgment. Sometimes, a defendant physician will bring the drug manufacturer or device company into the suit, as a "third-party defendant," to require it to pay part or all of plaintiff's damages. A similar situation may arise when the defendant-treating physician is also the seller of the drug or device.

Physician liability for other health care providers

Physicians usually supervise other health team members. Physicians therefore owe their patients the duty to supervise nurses, technicians, and other subordinates properly. That duty creates vicarious liability, whereby one person may be liable for the wrongful acts and omissions of another. There are several legal doctrines that must be discussed in this context.

The simplest such doctrine is known as *respondeat superior*: An employer is liable for the negligence of his or her employees. If a physician's office nurse injects a drug into a patient's sciatic nerve, causing injury, that patient may sue the nurse or the physician or both. Should the patient recover damages from the physician, the physician may be entitled to reimbursement from the nurse, at least in theory. The physician's employee is judged by the standard of care for a person of the same profession or occupation, not by the same standard as the physician performing the same service. In the example stated, the trier of fact would determine whether the nurse violated the nursing standard of care for administering an injection. If they find that he or she did, the judge can rule that his or her employer-physician must pay.

One physician may be employed by another physician or by a hospital or other institution. In that case, the acts of the treating physician are judged against the applicable standard of care for physicians. Therefore, when an emergency room physician is found to be negligent, he or she is liable for damages as is the hospital or physician group that employed this individual. For this reason, many physicians and other health professionals adopt an independent contractor format in their practices. An independent contractor is one who is paid to do a particular job and who controls the manner in which it is performed. Obviously, many sticky "gray areas" arise in malpractice suits, when the issue is whether or not one party is an employee or an independent contractor. Physicians may wish to consult their own legal counsel for advice on ways to avoid such potential liability for others.

Another example of vicarious liability is that physicians may be liable for the negligence of certain hospital employees they supervise. For example, surgeons are sometimes sued for errors and omissions by operating room personnel, under the "captain of the ship" doctrine. This doctrine is a poor legal fiction, which holds that a surgeon is like the captain of a ship at sea and is therefore responsible for all the wrongs perpetrated by the crew. It was intended to offer a remedy for the many persons injured over the years by careless employees of charitable hospitals. For many years, such hospitals were immune from suit, and injured patients were not compensated for damages sustained at their hands. Many courts created a "captain of the ship" doctrine and held surgeons liable for all operating room negligence, in order to afford patients a measure of compensation for their injuries.

Obviously, a surgeon is not a captain and lacks a captain's enormous power over the crew, and an operating room is not a ship. As the doctrine of charitable immunity was overturned, patients could sue and recover from charity hospitals (or the organizations/governments that operated them) for injuries caused by operating room personnel and other staff/employees. The "captain of the ship" doctrine has been largely replaced by the "borrowed servant" doctrine in such situations. This latter doctrine holds surgeons responsible for hospital employees' negligence that is committed under their direct supervision and control.

Physicians today frequently request consultations from other physicians, especially regarding hospitalized patients. The consulting physician may be either a general practitioner or a specialist. The consulted physician visits with the patient, examines him or her, writes or dictates a report, shares diagnostic impressions, and recommends treatment. Sometimes, the consulted practitioner does not prescribe or administer treatment. To assume part or all of the consulting physician's responsibilities for ongoing care, a consulted physician must receive a referral of the patient.

A referring physician usually is not liable for the negligence or other misdeeds of the specialist. However, the referring physician may be liable for the referred-to physician's misdeeds, if each physician assumes the other will provide certain care that is omitted by both, or if they neglect a common duty (e.g., postoperative care). When the standard of care requires consultation or referral, failure to request one would be negligent and would make the treating physician liable for the resulting injury. Of course, a referring or consulting physician may also be required to answer for the negligence of a partner.

Physicians cannot attend or be available to all patients at all times. They have the duty to provide another physician to care for their patients when they cannot. Just as physicians are generally not liable for consultants' malpractice, they need not answer for care provided by other physicians who cover their practice. Exceptions include covering physicians who are also partners, or negligently selecting covering physicians.

Physicians may also be liable for their own negligence in hiring, training, assigning, supervising, or retaining employees who harm their patient or others. Failure to check credentials and references, failing to test skills, and failing to maintain surveillance over a practice can make physicians liable for their employees' acts and omissions, even when they are not themselves negligent. Worse yet, physicians' neglect in these areas can make them liable for injuries intentionally inflicted by employees.

PHYSICIANS' DEFENSE THEORIES AGAINST PLAINTIFFS' CLAIMS
Negligence

A defendant physician can defeat a negligence claim by showing the absence of one or more of the requisite elements for the patient to prove medical negligence.

Absence of duty. The first defense in a negligence case would be an attempt to show that there is no duty owed to the patient by the physician. If a physician can show that no physician-patient relationship exists, this "no duty" defense may suffice to defeat the plaintiff's action.

Physicians generally have no duty to treat new patients or even patients of years past, with some exceptions. In some cases, even though a physician treats or diagnoses a condition, a duty is sometimes seen only between the physician and the patient's employer, as in certain occupational settings such as a plant physician.

In general, courts rarely hold that the "no duty" defense applies and have even held that a simple telephone consultation between a physician and emergency room personnel may be sufficient to create a professional relationship between the physician and that patient with the attendant requirements to comply with such duty.

A physician wishing to withdraw from taking care of certain patients, planning to relocate his or her practice, or simply retiring, must notify his or her patients who will be affected in the manner of an ordinary and reasonably prudent physician in the same circumstances. Such notice is best made in writing, and mailed postpaid to the patient's last known address. All patients who are receiving ongoing care for potentially serious ailments should be notified by certified mail, return receipt requested, at the last known address. Such patients should be informed that their physician will continue to see them for emergencies during a certain fixed and reasonable period of time. A successor physician or list of physicians can be recommended or given, but if not, an offer to forward records or copies of records, at a reasonable or no cost, to other successor physicians of the patient's own choice may be made.

In practice, if a physician retires, or moves and sells the practice to a succeeding health care provider, patients' records are often sold as part of the transaction. However, physicians should be warned that many states have medical record retention acts, and that these acts usually do not provide an exception for record-keeping requirements in such transfer. In such jurisdictions, physicians had best comply with statutory law and provide copies, and/or keep copies, of all pertinent records for the required statutory period.

Although such medical retention statutes typically do not provide penalties for violation of the record-keeping act, physicians should follow such act or, at an absolute minimum, protect themselves by keeping such records for the minimum period of time for which they can personally be sued for medical negligence. In many states, this period is actually shorter than the period of time required by the medical retention act statutes.

Absent fraud, once the statutory period of limitations for filing a medical malpractice suit has passed or prescribed, physicians still may wish to check with their medical malpractice insurers concerning disposal of old records in order to avoid lack of protection under the insurance policy carrier's rules.

No breach of duty (compliance with the standard of care). A physician may also controvert the second requirement of the plaintiff's negligence case: That there was a breach of the standard of care owed by the

physician to the plaintiff. If the physician can convince the judge or jury by evidence and argument that he or she complied with the requisite standard of care, the plaintiff will lose the case. Because the plaintiff has the burden of proving the case, if testimony and evidence are equally balanced, the physician will prevail in this respect.

Because rules of evidence generally prevent nonphysicians from testifying about the standard of care in most medical cases, the physician will best attempt to prove compliance with the standard of care with appropriate medical testimony. Such testimony may be given on his or her behalf, but more often by expert witnesses, who may be other treating physicians or experts hired to serve in this capacity. Both the plaintiff and the defendant physician may use a nondefendant treating physician as an expert with respect to any possible deviation of the standard of care.

In practice, especially in past years, nondefendant treating physicians were often reluctant to appear, especially if they received regular referrals from defendant physicians or were otherwise socially or professionally connected with them, except in the defense of their physician cohorts. For this reason, physicians engaged to testify for the plaintiff have often been nontreating physicians who may have had no personal connection with the case. Defendant physicians, however, may also employ nontreating physicians at will. In cases involving potentially substantial damages, paid expert witnesses who were not treating physicians will often testify for both sides with respect to deviation of the standard of care issue.

Because physicians are not held to be insurers against harm nor guarantors of a favorable result, an applicable defense would be to bring experts to testify at trial that the physician in the case used the skill and knowledge common to other physicians in that specialty and applied such skills appropriately under the circumstances. Such physicians will attempt to show that although there may have been a bad result, the bad result occurred without deviation from the standard of care.

Such testimony may state that if a physician is available to a patient, interviews and examines him or her appropriately, forms a reasonable differential diagnosis, performs the indicated tests to establish a diagnosis and to rule out potentially more serious conditions, refers for consultation when appropriate, forms a reasonable diagnosis, treats, follows up, and nevertheless makes an error, such a physician has *not* violated the standard of care owed by the defendant physician to the patient, even though the patient may have suffered harm by the error.

Another source to demonstrate that there has been no deviation from the standard of care is the use of medical textbooks or other published medical data. However, the admissibility of such evidence as proof of the standard of care varies markedly among jurisdictions.

A traditional rule is that medical texts may be used in medical negligence lawsuits only to cross-examine a medical expert, such cross-examination accomplished by framing a proposition in the exact language used by the author of the medical text and asking if the witness agrees or disagrees. In such a situation an expert witness cross-examined need not initially agree that the text is standard or authoritative. Medical negligence cases tried in federal court, under the federal rules of evidence, allow statements from texts or medical journals to be read directly into evidence.

A defendant physician is not necessarily bound by a standard of care shown by the patient's medical experts. If a choice can be made among various methods of medical diagnosis or treatment, and a substantial minority of physicians agree with such methods, a physician may not be negligent for using such a method. This may be true even though other methods are thought to be good medical practice by the majority of physicians. In other words, employing a different method of diagnosis or treatment from that commonly used is not by itself evidence of the violation of the standard of care, especially if a "substantial minority" of physicians would have acted similarly under similar circumstances.

Defense physicians' experts sometimes refer to this as a "mere error in judgment." In fact, that is a misstatement because an error in judgment may or may not be negligent. Unsuccessful use of a minority approach to diagnosis or treatment is not negligence per se.

Lack of causation. A plaintiff cannot recover from a physician for damages unless the physician's malpractice caused the plaintiff's injuries. Under negligence and most other theories of recovery, a plaintiff is required to prove that such negligence was the actual cause-in-fact of injuries and that those damages were reasonably foreseeable. This area occasionally affords an adequate defense for the physician.

For example, delay in diagnosis and treatment is generally not compensable if any delay did not materially affect the ultimate treatment and outcome of the disease. For example, a delay in the diagnosis of a fatal high-grade malignancy when the delay is short likely would not have made a difference in the patient's outcome and would not be compensable. The damages, in other words, would have ensued even without delay in diagnosis and treatment. Many jurisdictions hold that in such a situation, a plaintiff cannot recover any damages unless he or she can prove that there was a greater than 50% chance of survival if diagnosis had been made earlier and treatment more timely made.

Recently, a growing trend has been to go beyond traditional causation principles to allow for recovery for loss of a chance of a cure. Some jurisdictions no longer require plaintiffs to show that they have already suffered an actual loss because of a delay in diagnosis and treatment, but only some potential loss. In such a case, there may be a reduction in the amount of damages in proportion to the reduction in the odds of the plaintiff surviving. Complications may arise when a plaintiff in such cases has been treated and is apparently well at trial, but there is a sizable chance of recurrence later. Recovery for the possibility of such recurrence may be allowed in some jurisdictions.

Harm suffered by a plaintiff may have several causes. Most biological effects are known by medical science to have many causes. A plaintiff can generally recover for malpractice, even if it is only one of many actual causes, as long as the effect was foreseeable. However, a defendant physician can win on causation if he or she can prove later that an intervening or independent event was the proximate cause of the patient's injury, and not the complained of negligent act of the physician.

No damages. The ability to disprove or reduce legal damages is often a defendant physician's best defense in a medical malpractice suit. To recover a monetary award, a plaintiff must introduce testimony and other evidence of damages, which often in practice is a difficult burden. In some cases, a patient may get insurance or government benefits to cover expenses. In states not having a collateral source rule, evidence of such payment may obviate a showing of damage or at least mitigate the amount of damages owed for negligence.

Other defenses. Even if the plaintiff can prove all four elements of negligence, the physician may employ other defenses.

CONTRIBUTORY NEGLIGENCE, COMPARATIVE NEGLIGENCE, AND COMPARATIVE FAULT. At common law, a patient's contributory negligence acted as a complete bar to any recovery for the negligent act of the defendant physician, no matter how slight the patient's negligence was compared to the physician's. This doctrine of contributory negligence was created to avoid "rewarding" persons for their own folly and to reduce the likelihood of collusion in suits between parties.

To avoid many harsh results, however, contributory negligence as a concept has been largely replaced by the doctrine of comparative negligence. This innovation lets the trier of fact determine the relative negligence of each party to a lawsuit and requires the judge or jury to assess any monetary awards accordingly. Some states only permit a plaintiff to recover if he or she is less negligent than the defendants.

A physician's duty to protect his or her patient from harm is often greater than the patient's duty to protect himself or herself. Only in limited circumstances can a physician reduce or escape liability because of a patient's negligence. An example might be where an inadequately treated diabetic patient, who resists treatment, continues a hazardous sport and, despite a physician's clearly documented directions and warnings, passes out as a complication of the diabetes and is injured as a result. However, defendant physicians have great difficulty in proving legally sufficient negligence on the part of the plaintiff. Even such socially destructive acts as smoking and drinking alcohol while pregnant are not in most cases considered negligence by courts.

Comparative fault is a more recent legal doctrine, designed by courts to allow apportionment of damages among negligent defendants. Some jurisdictions have experimented with various tests, including allocating damages based on a comparison of causation among all parties. In this case, previous rules on contribution and indemnification among defendants have been rewritten. This is an area of expected change.

SOVEREIGN GOVERNMENT IMMUNITY. In medieval times, the concept that "the king can do no wrong" allowed the state to escape liability. As a consequence, if the state could do no wrong, its physicians and hospitals could not be sued for malpractice. This was the law until relatively recently, when both federal and state governments passed tort claims acts, which allow suits against the sovereign and its representatives.

These acts permit persons negligently injured by government workers, including its employed physicians, to sue and recover from the government. These acts often impose limitations on suits against the respective government authorities, such as statutory limits of liability.

STATUTE OF LIMITATIONS. That misdeeds must be punished within a reasonable time is the basis for the statute of limitations. Actually, each state has many statutes of limitations that apply in various legal situations: felonies, breach of contract, torts, disputes over land ownership, and so on.

The statute of limitations for medical negligence is generally the same as for other torts: assault, automobile accidents, and product liability. If an injured patient sues a doctor after the time set forth in the applicable statute of limitations has passed, the defendant may be entitled to dismissal. Plaintiffs are held to a duty to bring suit before time makes defense an unreasonable burden.

The time allowed for filing suit is said to run from the date the negligent act occurred. That may present a special problem when the negligence was an omission. Most states stop or "toll" the running of time set forth in the statute, during periods when the plaintiff would not be able to commence the lawsuit without great difficulty. Some examples are while plaintiff is a minor or mentally incompetent, while the defendant is out of state, or before the plaintiff has a chance to learn about the defendant's negligence or its effects. Examples of the latter include cases when the physician fraudulently conceals the misdeed and those where neither physician nor patient learns of the problem for years.

EXCULPATORY AGREEMENTS AND INDEMNIFICATION CONTRACTS. These two types of written agreements have more differences than similarities. Exculpatory agreements are those between physicians and patients that appear to relieve the physician of liability for negligence. Although such contracts are occasionally upheld in other settings, they are consistently struck down in the medical malpractice context. The basis is simply that they are contracts of adhesion. An ill patient is not in a position to negotiate terms or to reach a fair meeting of the minds that is essential for a binding contract.

Contracts of indemnification usually arise between physicians and other persons or institutions. For example, a hospital may agree to indemnify the president of its medical staff for any legal damages he or she sustains for carrying out the duties of that office. Conversely, the chief of anesthesiology may agree to indemnify the hospital for any malpractice damages arising from the operation of the department, when no hospital employee is found to be negligent. Both types of contracts are generally upheld and are effective to transfer enormous financial burdens from one entity to another. Although such agreements are often misrepresented as standard terms in an employment contract, they must be studied carefully by qualified counsel.

NEGOTIATION AND SETTLEMENT OF MALPRACTICE CLAIMS

Practical aspects of defending any particular malpractice claim against a physician are best handled by proper consultation of that physician with his or her attorney and malpractice insurer. In most cases, a malpractice insurer will provide counsel under the policy to defend the claim. Although a physician may believe that the best time to settle a malpractice claim, from his or her point of view, is at the time such claim occurs, procedural matters as well as substantive matters must be considered, and the physician's legal counsel may be able to give the best advice on this point.

In particular, and in practice, the physician should contact his or her professional liability carrier as soon as there is even a suggestion of a possible claim, and ask for a representative to handle the matter. The physician should always insist that the matter be handled by an attorney rather than a claims adjuster, even if the physician is willing to admit fault. If a physician has no insurance, private counsel should be retained to negotiate and reach a settlement in the course of the litigation.

A physician may wish, at his or her own additional

expense, to retain private counsel in addition to any counsel assigned or allocated by the insurance company under a malpractice insurance policy. This is particularly important, because the Health Care Quality Improvement Act of 1986[2] requires reporting the settlement of any medical malpractice claim, with few exceptions, to the National Practitioner Data Bank.

In practice, negotiation and settlement of a malpractice claim rarely occur before discovery, which is a set of pretrial procedures that go on during the weeks or months between the filing of the suit and the scheduled trial. Discovery measures include interrogatories, requests for admissions, requests for production of documents or other items such as X rays or fetal monitoring strips and such, depositions, subpoenas, and motions for summary judgment. All these measures are useful for ferreting out different information; the same methods are used both by plaintiff and defense counsel to determine the nature of the opposing party's case.

END NOTES

1. *Daubert v. Merrell Dow Pharmaceuticals*, 61 U.S. 6W 4805 (1993).
2. Health Care Quality Improvement Act, 42 U.S.C. §11101 *et seq.* (1986).

CHAPTER 12 Medical malpractice

ALAN C. HOFFMAN, J.D., F.C.L.M.*

HISTORICAL BACKGROUND
INTENTIONAL TORTS
FALSE IMPRISONMENT
NEGLIGENCE
STRICT LIABILITY
RES IPSA LOQUITUR — THE THING SPEAKS FOR ITSELF
ABANDONMENT
DEFAMATION
NEGLIGENT INFLICTION OF EMOTIONAL DISTRESS
COMPENSATION FOR LOSS OF A CHANCE
DUTY TO WARN AND CONTROL
JOINT AND SUCCESSIVE TORTFEASORS
REPORTING STATUTES
LOSS OF CONSORTIUM
WRONGFUL DEATH — SURVIVAL ACTS
STATUTES OF LIMITATIONS
DAMAGES

Torts are private civil wrongs, in contrast to crimes, which are public wrongs. A tort arises from the breach of a legal duty one person owes another to act reasonably in a way that will not harm another's person or property. In contrast, a contract is an agreement between parties with a breach occurring when one or both parties do not abide by the terms. Health care providers incur both legal and contractual duties incident to their professional roles. The law does not consider the professional and patient to be on equal terms; greater legal duties, or burdens, are imposed on the health care provider.

Historically, the duties and responsibilities of health care providers to patients were limited, and a breach of a duty resulting in a tort was narrowly defined and invoked. That is no longer true. The courts have increasingly broadened the duties of health care providers and the bases on which they may be held liable in tort.

The law now declares that health care providers not only have duties to their patients, but may also owe a duty to third parties, who may be strangers to the physician-patient relationship.[1] Privity, the requirement of direct dealing or an immediate relationship, has been abandoned as a necessary basis for a duty owed. The health care facility has a duty to control or to warn the proper persons when their patients are dangerous to themselves or others, even when it breaches the patients' confidentiality. The courts have ruled that when a patient's confidentiality confronts the public's need to know or the public's safety and welfare, the patient's confidentiality must yield to the public good.

Health care providers are responsible for both the safety and efficacy of the medication, materials, and devices that are employed in the facility. Defective physician orders must be corrected before they are implemented. There is a "duty to recall" or warn when a treated individual is discovered to be vulnerable to danger, even when the person would, under ordinary circumstances, no longer be considered a patient. Patients have a right not only to informed consent, but also to informed refusal — a discrete warning as to the potential harm of not taking treatment.

HISTORICAL BACKGROUND

To understand fully the law of torts, we must understand the historical objectives and theories of tort liability. In an effort to understand torts, one must distinguish between tort law and criminal law. Prosser and Keaton, in the handbook *The Law of Torts,* fourth

*The author gratefully acknowledges work from previous contributors: Joseph P. McMenamin, M.D., J.D., F.C.L.M.; Janet B. Seifert, J.D.; and James G. Zimmerly, M.D., J.D., F.C.L.M.

edition, state that a "really satisfactory definition of torts has yet to be found."[2] Generally stated, a tort is a breach of a duty (other than a contractual or quasi-contractual duty) that gives rise to an action for damages. To put it briefly, the English law of torts is merely a list of actual omissions, which in certain conditions have been found actionable.

Tortious conduct generally arises from the breach of a duty. It is a civil wrong for which the remedy is a common law action for damages. It does not include the breach of a contract or the breach of a trust or other merely equitable obligation. By contrast, a crime is an offense against the state or the public at large for which the state is the representative of the people—it is the "people" who bring proceedings to prosecute the crime. The purpose of the criminal proceeding is to protect and vindicate the interest of the public by punishing the offender. A criminal prosecution is generally not concerned in any way with compensation of the individual against whom the crime was committed. In recent years, some courts have seen fit to require, as part of the sentence, restitution to the victim by the offender. That restitution is still considered part of the penal action and is not a civil action for tort. In early English common law, an act could be both a tort and a crime. If the crime was a felony, the tort was "merged" into the crime and the civil action was stayed until the criminal action was completed. While very early American cases adopted this rule, numerous American courts have discarded it. Originally, tort damages were at first applied to the injured individual, incident to a criminal prosecution, when the two remedies were administered by the same court. Because of the common origin, both a tort and a crime could have the same names, such as assault, battery, trespass, or libel. Although such terms refer to similar conduct, the theory of tort law and criminal law and the rights and remedies attendant to each have developed along totally different lines.

One must go back to the very earliest of times to examine tort law. Long before the development of English common law, peoples' rights and duties and the penalties for failure to perform as required were regulated by codes of conduct. Even before that, the earliest tribal or communal law depended on local practice and custom for controlling the actions of members. Probably one of the oldest known codes is the Code of Hammurabi, which was developed by Babylon's kings some 20 centuries before the Christian era. This code required that the doctor's hand be cut off if he treated a man with a metal knife and the man died. In the ancient Mosaic law, the Israelites, barely eight centuries later, perpetuated further the concept of "Lex Talionis" or "Law of the Talion" by demanding "an eye for an eye, a tooth for a tooth."

Development of the form and principles of the laws we use today in America can probably be traced no further back than the thirteenth century, or nearly two centuries after the Norman conquest of the British Isles in 1066. During the course of many hundreds of years, we subsequently developed today's court system from the common pleas courts and the royal courts (or bench). During this developmental period, these courts established a variety of procedural rules, which required that the offense charge should be in the form of a specific court writ before the plaintiff could be heard by the court. Frequently, there was no appropriate writ for the complaining party; consequently, considerable innovation or the creation of "legal fictions" was necessary before the court would administer justice.

However, more important than the development of the system of courts with their rules of procedures was the accumulation of a vast body of decisions from both criminal and civil cases beginning during the reign of Edward I in the fourteenth century. It was during this period that the first "year book" was published, which consisted simply of a compilation of informal notes of cases and comments made by lawyers and students. It was this body of decisions, and the custom of applying those prior decisions of the royal court cases, that became known as the "common law." It was subsequently brought to this country by the early colonists from England. In the United States, the state of Louisiana is unique in that it does not follow the English common law, but still bases its legal system on the Napoleonic Code. The Napoleonic Code came to this country from France when France controlled what is now Louisiana.

Since its early beginning more than 600 years ago, tort law has been evolving in the United States. The object of the law has always been the determination of legally protected rights of the individual's person, property, and reputation, which must not be interfered with or invaded. Therefore, it is within the basic precepts of tort law that the components of medical legal liability are found. The most important types of these are intentional interference, negligence, and strict liability.

INTENTIONAL TORTS

The tort of intentional interference, sometimes more simply referred to as an *intentional tort,* is a direct outgrowth of the ancient writ of trespass. A variety of terms originally associated with trespass have been continued into a modern classification of intentional torts (e.g., assault, common battery, false imprisonment, defamation, deceit, or fraud).

In general, the law deals much more harshly with those accused of intentional tort than other torts. In many cases of intentional torts, it is unnecessary for the plaintiff to prove an injury resultant from a tortious act to obtain a judgment for damages. The burden of proving the defendant's intent is often one of the greatest obstacles for the plaintiff. It is frequently sufficient to show only that the act was a "practical joke" that misfired or that the act was directed toward someone else but nevertheless caused an injury to the plaintiff. The distinction here is that the defendant intended to perform the act but did not intend the result.

An important distinction between an intentional tort and one that is not intentional is that it is necessary in professional negligence cases to show that there was a departure by the defendant from the usual and customary standards of practice. This is done through the use of expert witnesses. Such evidence is not required in the case alleging an intentional tort. The fact that the surgeon removes an organ during surgery, without the informed consent of the patient, constitutes the intentional tort of "battery." The patient-plaintiff is not required to introduce testimony by an expert witness that the removal of the organ did not comport with the reasonable medical standards. A battery is described by Prosser and Keaton[3]:

The interest in freedom from intentional, unpermitted contact with the plaintiff's person is protected by an action for the tort called battery. This protection extends to any part of the body or anything which is attached to it. A battery is the intentional, harmful or offensive contact of another, either directly or indirectly through an object (such as a club). A battery takes place when there is actual physical contact to which the plaintiff has not consented. Battery requires the intent to strike another, as does assault. A battery can occur even if an individual is not aware of it at the time it occurs, and intent may be "transferred" when an intended contact occurs with an unintended victim.

Assault is distinguished from battery. No actual contact is necessary for an assault to occur; all that is necessary to constitute the tort of assault is that the plaintiff be placed in reasonable apprehension of receiving a harmful or offensive contact. Therefore, if a psychiatrist makes certain sexual advances toward a patient, which places the patient in fear of receiving an offensive or harmful contact—a battery—the threat is an assault. Parenthetically, malpractice insurance policies cover actions alleging negligence but do not consider or insure for intentional acts. Therefore, one would most likely not have insurance for assault, battery, or other similar intentional acts.

Assault can be found as an actionable wrong in tort in civil law and also in criminal law. In civil law, assault is the placing of an individual in apprehension of receiving a battery or otherwise harmful or offensive contact. Assault should be distinguished from battery in that in an assault, no actual contact is necessary and the plaintiff may only suffer a mental trauma in order to substantiate a recovery. When an individual apprehends a battery, the degree of apprehension that would be applied would be

that applied to a reasonable person. Further, unless there is apprehension at the immediate time, no assault takes place. Therefore, if an individual was not aware until some time after the incident that someone was pointing a loaded gun at him or her, no assault would take place. For there to be an apprehension, there must be some overt act. Words and acts taken together may create an assault. In order that a defendant be liable in tort for assault there must be specific intent to interfere with the plaintiff's person. Even if the defendant were to cease and desist from the act, once the plaintiff has suffered the physical apprehension of receiving a battery, that is sufficient for him or her to maintain the cause of action.

The intentional tort of "deceit" is quite often referred to today as either fraud or misrepresentation. Although many authorities distinguish between these two, their common features are sufficient to treat them collectively in this discussion.

A showing of deceit requires the following:
1. The defendant knowingly made a false representation.
2. The false representation was made in order to benefit the person making the representation or to cause harm to another person.
3. The plaintiff relied on the misrepresentation as true.
4. The plaintiff was injured as a result of his or her reliance.

This intentional tort can be applied to the practice of medicine. Suppose a physician left a foreign body in a patient during an earlier procedure, but fails to tell the patient the real cause of the resultant complications or symptoms. The patient's consent for the second surgical procedure is obtained on a false basis. This constitutes the intentional tort of deceit (as well as a battery, because informed consent was not given). In such a case, the testimony of an expert may not be required. Additionally, a professional liability insurance carrier may not provide a defense to an action for damages against a physician in this situation, except under a reservation of the right to deny coverage should an intentional tort be proved.

Finally, there are certain areas in which intentional interference with a person is permitted. Most notably are the areas of self-defense of the person and protection of property. However, those areas are specifically limited to very strict circumstances.

FALSE IMPRISONMENT

False imprisonment and false arrest are similar torts. False imprisonment is a tort that protects an individual from restraint from movement. False imprisonment may occur if an individual is restrained against his or her will in any confined space, whether it be an elevator, a home, or even a city. Note also that false imprisonment may occur where there may be access or egress to a given area, but the plaintiff is not aware of same. In order for there to be false imprisonment, the plaintiff must be aware of it at the time (although there is some case law to the contrary). In an action for false imprisonment, nominal damages may be awarded even if no actual damages are proven, and punitive damages may then be awarded in addition.

The plaintiff is entitled to compensation for loss of time, for any inconvenience suffered, for physical or emotional harm, and for related expenses, sometimes including attorneys' fees. The restraint of an individual's freedom imposed by a legal authority constitutes an arrest, and if it is an improper arrest, it constitutes false arrest. The defendant does not have to have a warrant, or even be a police officer, to be liable for false arrest. If an individual is under legal duty to release one from confinement and fails to do so, that constitutes false imprisonment. A physician or staff member of a hospital, holding a patient against his or her will, without court order, could be held liable for false imprisonment. Such situations arise in cases involving mental illness, where a patient is held without compliance with laws governing civil commitments.

NEGLIGENCE

Negligence is a separate and distinct tort, relatively new to the law. Negligence may be considered as "conduct which involves an unreasonable risk of causing damage," or perhaps better, "conduct which falls below the standard established by law for the protection of others." Medical negligence is medical care that falls below the established standard of care expected of physicians. Four distinct elements are necessary to prove negligence as a cause of action:

1. A duty owed, or standard of conduct required to be met by the alleged "tortfeasor," or wrongdoer, in relation to the injured party
2. Failure to conform to that duty or standard of conduct
3. A link showing that the failure was a "proximate" or direct cause of injury to the complaining party
4. Actual loss or injury that can be measured for compensation in money damages.

The first recorded action brought for medical negligence occurred in England in 1374. The first American case occurred more than 400 years later, in 1794, in Connecticut. Numerous American cases were recorded during the eighteenth and nineteenth centuries in which patients sought to recover damages for injuries alleged to be the proximate result of medical negligence. Probably the most frequently quoted early case dealing with medical negligence in America is the 1898 case of *Pike*

v. Honsinger.[4] In that case, the Court of Appeals of New York stated four principles of law that continue, to some extent, to affect the daily practice of medicine in the United States, nearly nine decades later. In that case, Pike sought damages against Dr. Honsinger for the negligent treatment of his injured knee. The court of appeals, in reversing the decision of the lower court and ordering a new trial, stated that: "A physician . . . impliedly represents that he possesses . . . that reasonable degree of learning and skill . . . ordinarily possessed by physicians in the locality. . . ." Furthermore, the court held, "it becomes his duty to use reasonable care and diligence in the exercise of his skill and his learning . . ." and added, "he is bound to keep abreast of the times, and . . . departure from approved methods and general use, if it injures the patient, will render him liable." Finally, the court required the physician to give "proper instructions to his patient in relation to conduct, exercise, and use of an injured limb."

Statutes of limitations have been passed in all states to limit the time in which an action may be brought following the injury. The limitations period may be shorter for medical negligence than other kinds of negligence. The statute of limitations does not begin to run against the plaintiff until the damage has occurred. It may be tolled (stopped) if the plaintiff is incompetent by reason of age or incapacity. There has been some real difficulty in the area of medical malpractice in cases in which the statute of limitations has run out before the plaintiff has discovered any injury. Under many court decisions and statutes, the plaintiff's cause of action does not accrue, and the statute does not run, until plaintiff discovers (or, in the exercise of reasonable diligence, should have discovered) that there has been an injury occasioned by negligence. Courts have also attempted to ameliorate the statute of limitations by saying that the defendant's duty is continued until the relation of physician and patient has ended. Fraudulent concealment of the damage also tolls the running of the statute. The courts also have found "constructive," or implied, fraud in the physician's silence when he knows of the failure to discover, such as when he has failed to remove a sponge or other foreign object left in the plaintiff's body. It is sometimes held to be a "continuing negligence" as long as the defendant remains silent.

The court, in tort law, looks to establish a standard of care to measure negligence. Courts have dealt with the standard of care by creating a fiction called "the reasonable man." In medical negligence, the standard is to possess and exercise that degree of skill and knowledge that would be expected of a reasonable physician under similar circumstances.

Some time ago, the "locality" standard of care was

instituted; it was held that the standard of care in the "same locality" or "similar locality" would be the standard of care to be imposed. Because of improved medical facilities and board certification, the locality rule for medical negligence has been abandoned in many jurisdictions. Now one would look to a national standard, such as the skills and knowledge necessary for board certification, to define the standard of care.

Under some circumstances, a statute may be interpreted as setting a community standard, such that deviation from the standard constitutes negligence. This is referred to as negligence per se. The statute may be one of civil or criminal law. It must have been intended to protect a class of persons, of which the plaintiff is a member, against harm. When the court finds that there is a violation of the statute, the effect is to find that the defendant's conduct is necessarily negligent. For example, a statute requiring a landowner to clear ice and snow from sidewalks adjacent to his property is intended to protect pedestrians, and failure to do so which results in a slip-and-fall injury to plaintiff will be negligence per se. Various defenses, such as contributory fault of the plaintiff, may still be raised as in other forms of negligence.

STRICT LIABILITY

Today's concept of "strict liability" is probably the purest survivor of the early forms of action, having grown out of the tort of trespass. Early tort law was much more concerned with providing an appropriate remedy, and thereby to keep peace among the citizens, than with determining responsibility based on "fault."

During the last 200 years, we find the inexorable movement of the law toward the identification and recognition of fault to form the basis of legal liability for damages. Although the theory of negligence was developing rapidly, many continued to argue that a finding of liability without fault provided a more equitable basis for assessing damages than did the determination of fault. Even today, legal scholars continue this debate, with some indications that negligence is losing to the "no-fault" concept as a more equitable basis for determining damages in certain types of cases (such as automobile accidents).

During the past century, a growing social policy has developed that seeks to impose liability on the party who can best bear the loss. Those who engage in dangerous activities (e.g., blasting), those who keep animals (e.g., zoos, refuges, and private persons), and those who operate dangerous equipment (e.g., heavy construction) are subjected to liability arising from their creation of an unusual risk of harm to other members of the community. Where an expected harm materializes—broken windows, personal injury, or property destruction—the activity need not have been conducted negligently in order for an injured plaintiff to recover.

The legal doctrine of strict liability has not been directly applied by American courts in any action brought by a patient-plaintiff against a physician-defendant. Nevertheless, it has been applied to the pharmaceutical and medical appliance industries.

Other tort actions that may be predicated on the physician-patient relationship and accepted standards of care include actual or constructive abandonment, invasion of privacy, breach of confidentiality, defamation (e.g., libel or slander), battery, lack of informed consent and refusal, and false commitment or imprisonment.

RES IPSA LOQUITUR—THE THING SPEAKS FOR ITSELF

In a malpractice action for negligence, the plaintiff has the burden of proving the following:

1. That there is a standard (or are standards) of care for the treatment of the medical (in its generic sense) problem or conditions—creating a duty for the health care provider.
2. That the health care provider breached this duty; that is, failed to conform or abide by the standard(s), in fact, deviated or departed from the standard(s).
3. That this breach was the proximate or direct cause of the patient's injury.
4. That damages were incurred.

Medical malpractice defendants have long had the benefit of special rules established by the courts, most notably the doctrine that the degree of skill and standard of care required of physicians or any health care provider may be evaluated solely by other doctors or appropriate health care providers. A patient can only prove a case against one health care provider through the mouth of another. This means that the patient must find an expert willing to testify. For many years, physicians were reluctant to fill that role. Plaintiff's attorneys called this a "conspiracy of silence." Most physicians and other health care providers hesitate to become involved in legal matters of any kind, particularly those that require a negative characterization of a colleague or facility. Thus, it is not surprising that plaintiffs have had difficulty obtaining appropriate expert testimony.

A long-accepted substitute for the medical expert has been the use of *res ipsa loquitur,* which literally means "the thing speaks for itself." Under *res ipsa loquitur,* the plaintiff need not prove negligence if the injury is one that could not occur in the absence of negligence, and the defendant was in control of the instrumentality that caused the injury. Causation and damages must still be proven. *Res ipsa loquitur* is not uniformly accepted and implemented in the various states. Where applied, the doctrine may relieve the plaintiff from the requirement of proving fault through an expert witness and, thus, the plaintiff's lack of an expert is removed as a shield for the defendant health care provider. Of course, the invocation of *res ipsa loquitur* may necessarily impress a jury as much as a live expert, whose credibility can be tested and demeanor observed. All the rule means is that in certain cases, the defense can no longer rely on the natural reluctance of physicians and other health care providers to get involved in litigation, because negligence may be proved without expert testimony. In other words, negligence is presumed unless the defendant proves otherwise. This doctrine applies to nonmedical torts as well. If a piano falls onto a pedestrian from a warehouse's second floor loading door, the plaintiff need not name names and describe and prove events leading to the fall. *Res ipsa loquitur* requires the plaintiff only to show that the outcome was caused by an object or instrumentality in the exclusive control of the defendant; that the plaintiff did not voluntarily contribute to the result; and that the injury was the type not normally occurring in the absence of negligence. After the plaintiff shows these conditions, the burden of proof shifts to the defendant to show how no negligent act on his or her part was responsible for the damage or injury.

ABANDONMENT

Courts have recently come to recognize a cause of action in tort for abandonment. This is more specifically directed against medical professionals than any other field. Abandonment may also be considered a breach of contract. Damages will be awarded as in any other form of negligence or contract action.

DEFAMATION

Courts throughout various jurisdictions have provided for legal redress for injury to reputation through the tort of defamation. A statement is defamatory if it impeaches a person's integrity, virtue, human decency, respect for others, or reputation, and lowers that person in the esteem of the community or deters third parties from dealing with that person. A defamatory statement can either be in writing, which is libel, or verbal, which is slander. In some states, truth is an absolute defense to defamation. Some states have adopted a rule which states that, in actions for defamation, the truth, when published with good motives and justifiable ends, shall be a sufficient defense. A statement cannot amount to defamation in many states if it is substantially true, even though it may not be literally true. Therefore, nothing is defamatory about a newspaper report that a nursing home has 37 retired residents when in fact it has only 7 such residents.

In one notable case, Dr. Nagiv sued the *News-Sun* for libel.[5] In its morning edition the newspaper had reported that a hospital's credentialing committee dismissed Dr. Nagiv for 54 instances of professional irregularities. The evening edition said that the committee had considered only 3 such instances. The court found that there were in fact 190 such instances. The Illinois Appellate Court affirmed a dismissal of Dr. Nagiv's case. The court noted, however, that if the paper had stated that there were in excess of 190 instances, then there might have been a question of fact presented on which the trier of fact could have found defamation.

NEGLIGENT INFLICTION OF EMOTIONAL DISTRESS

The *Restatement (Second) of Torts* recognizes the tort of outrageous conduct, or negligent infliction of emotional injury. Negligent infliction of emotional distress has been applied in cases of indecent, immoral, unethical, or improper disposition of bodies or parts thereof, as well as for countersuits by physicians against plaintiffs.

Courts have begun to recognize liability based on the tort of "outrage"—that is, negligent infliction of emotional distress by extreme and outrageous conduct. Physical injury, or at least contact, has traditionally been required, but in some jurisdictions the tort of outrage is applicable when there is deliberate or reckless infliction of mental suffering on another, even without physical injury. The aggrieved party may be either the direct victim or a third party affected only indirectly. There are four elements of outrage.

1. The wrongdoer's conduct must be intentional or reckless. This is satisfied when the wrongdoer either acted with the specific purpose of causing emotional distress, or when the behavior was intentional and the wrongdoer knew, or should have known, that emotional distress would be likely to occur.
2. The conduct must be outrageous and intolerable in offense of generally accepted standards of decency and morality. This requirement is aimed at limiting frivolous suits for "outrage" and preventing litigation in situations in which only bad manners, unpleasantness, or hurt feelings are involved.
3. There must be a causal connection between the wrongdoer's action and the emotional distress.
4. The emotional distress must be severe.

COMPENSATION FOR LOSS OF A CHANCE

Loss of a chance involves negligence that causes a decrease in the injured plaintiff's prospects of recovering from a serious illness or injury. The question of whether, or how, to weigh diminished prospects for a plaintiff whose future expectations are already severely impaired has caused many courts to reexamine the traditional analysis of causation. The issue is this: Should liability be imposed for negligence that merely increased the probability of an already probable negative outcome?

The majority of U.S. jurisdictions retain the "but for" test of causation, or "actual cause," in addition to proximate, or direct, cause in tort actions. Therefore, many courts require that a negligently injured patient must prove that his chance for recovery or survival was "probable," "more likely than not," or "better than even." The rationale for this approach is that less-than-probable losses are speculative. The position of the majority of courts having considered the issue is that negligence that "might have caused" the loss of a chance of recovery is an insufficient quantum of cause, even if proximate.

In a minority of jurisdictions, courts have said that recovery is allowed so long as the negligence was a "substantial factor" in causing the death or injury of the plaintiff. The acceptance of the "substantial factor" measure reflects the courts' desire to compensate plaintiffs whose prospects of recovery or survival were less than even, but more than zero.

A leading, majority-view medical malpractice case involving loss of a chance is *Cooper v. Sisters of Charity of Cincinnati.*[6] In *Cooper,* the plaintiff's 16-year-old son arrived in the defendant's emergency room after a truck hit his bicycle. He complained that he had hit his head, hurt his back, and had a headache. Several hours had passed since the accident, and the boy had vomited before coming to the emergency room. While waiting, he again vomited. The physician examined the patient and ordered X rays. The boy's mother testified she called the doctor's attention to the fact that the back of the boy's head was injured, and recalled that she had seen a red spot there at home. The physician did not examine the back of the head, nor did he test the patient's gait or use an ophthalmoscope. He ordered the patient to be released to his home, with the usual directions on a "head injury sheet." The boy returned home with his mother, and he died soon after.

The cause of the boy's death was a basal skull fracture. The parents sued the hospital for medical malpractice. The trial court granted the defendant's motion for a directed verdict. On appeal, the judgment for defendant was affirmed. The Supreme Court of Ohio held that when medical malpractice is alleged as the cause of death, and the plaintiff's evidence indicates that a failure to diagnose injury prevented the patient from an opportunity to be operated on, the failure of which eliminated any chance of the patient's survival, the issue of proximate cause can be submitted to a jury only if there is sufficient evidence showing that with proper diagnosis, treatment, and surgery, the patient probably would have survived. The court cited a 1938 case, stating

"Loss of chance of recovery, standing alone, is not an injury from which damages will flow." Rejecting cases in which judgment was based on causation not proven to a standard of probability, the court held "we consider the better rule to be that, in order to comport with the standard of proof of proximate cause, plaintiff in a malpractice case must prove that the defendant's negligence, in probability, proximately caused the death."

Similarly, in the Florida case of *Gooding v. University Hospital Building, Inc.,*[7] the court held that even though a hospital emergency room staff was negligent in treating the plaintiff's husband, no liability could be imposed on the hospital because the evidence did not prove plaintiff's having a greater-than-even chance of survival. In this wrongful death action, the plaintiff's expert testified that the inaction of the hospital staff in failing to prevent a ruptured abdominal aortic aneurysm was negligence; however, he did not testify that immediate diagnosis and surgery, more likely than not, would have enabled the patient to survive. The trial court instructed the jury that they could find liability if the hospital destroyed the patient's chance to survive. The jury found the hospital liable and awarded $300,000 to the estate. On appeal, the court examined cases allowing recovery of damages for a less-than-even chance of survival. It expressly rejected the cases holding that a negligent diagnosis that destroys even the smallest chance to prolong life, or reduce suffering, may be actionable.

Two cases from Arizona reflect the current trend toward relaxing the probability requirement for causation, and moving toward recognition of loss of a chance as the compensable injury. In the 1980 case of *Hizer v. Randolph,*[8] the Arizona court found that the plaintiff was required to show that the defendant's delay in treating the plaintiff's wife, who came to the hospital suffering from acute hypoglycemia, was the probable cause of her death. The court stated that the mere loss of "an unspecified increment of chance for survival is . . . insufficient to meet the standard of probability."

In the 1986 case of *Thompson v. Sun City Community Hospital,*[9] the plaintiff brought action against the hospital and emergency room physicians for injury to her son from negligent transfer. The 13-year-old boy was injured in a traffic accident and taken by ambulance to the Sun City Community Hospital. Among his injuries was a transected femoral artery. The child was examined at the hospital and diagnosed as needing surgery. At some point, the decision to transfer the boy to a county hospital was made, based on economic considerations. His medical condition was considered stabilized, so he was certified as medically transferable. Testimony indicated that transfer was instituted if the patient was judged by a physician to be medically safe to transport. At the county hospital, the boy's condition worsened. He underwent abdominal surgery and then surgery to repair his femoral artery, and incurred a residual impairment in one leg.

The Supreme Court of Arizona found the hospital negligent in deciding to transfer the patient. The defendant argued that the residual injury is the kind that occurs in injuries of this type and requested the court to instruct the jury that recovery could be allowed only if proof established that the negligence probably caused the injury. The plaintiff asked that the instruction include discussion of negligence, which increased the risk of harm to the plaintiff, as provided by the *Restatement (Second) of Torts,* section 323.13. The court in *Thompson* expressly overruled the *Hizer* case, stating:

There is much to be said against the Hizer rule. . . . It puts a premium on each party's search for the willing witness. Human nature being what it is, and the difference between scientific and legal tests for "probability" often creating confusion, for every expert witness who evaluates the lost chance of 49%, there is another who estimates it at closer to 51%.

In the *Thompson* case, defense experts testified that even if the failure to admit caused a delay in vascular surgery, the chances were only 5% to 10% that the plaintiff would have achieved complete recovery with prompt surgery. Though unwilling or unable to quantify the chance of complete recovery with prompt surgery, the plaintiff's experts testified that there could have been a "substantially better chance" of full recovery if surgery had been performed at once. They testified that the longer the delay, "the greater the risk of residual injury."

In *Thompson,* the court held that the protection of the chance interest was within the range of the duty breached by the defendant and the harm that followed was the type from which the defendant was to have protected the plaintiff. The jury was allowed to consider the increase in the chance of harm, on the issue of causation. Under this rationale, if the jury finds that the defendant's failure increased the risk of harm, from this fact, the jury may find a "probability" that the negligence caused the harm. The court ruled that the issue of causation may go to the jury on proof of increase in the risk of harm. The jury is left to decide the defendant's share of responsibility for the risk's materializing.

The leading case of *Hicks v. United States*[10] similarly rejected the defendant physician's argument that the success of surgery for bowel obstruction was speculative. The physician had misdiagnosed the patient's condition, and death resulted. The court found that where the defendant's negligence terminates any chance of survival, the defendant may not raise conjectures of what

has been made impossible. It further stated, "If there was any substantial possibility of survival and the defendant has destroyed it, he is answerable."

Another landmark case is *Hamil v. Bashline.*[11] In that case, the patient presented with severe chest pain to the defendant hospital emergency room. Lacking necessary equipment for diagnosis, the hospital did not treat the patient. The patient's wife took him to a physician's private office, where he died of a myocardial infarction. Although the hospital's negligence could not be proved to have caused the death, evidence showed that the negligence increased the risk of the death of the patient. The court allowed the jury to weigh whether the increased risk was a substantial factor in producing the injury.

Health care providers argue that under the substantial factor rationale, they may find themselves defending lawsuits involving merely a bad outcome, rather than actual negligence. However, compensating the loss of chance recognizes the realities inherent in medical negligence. People who seek medical treatment are diseased or injured. Failure to diagnose or properly treat them denies some opportunity to recover. Including this lost opportunity within causality gives recognition to a real consequence of medical negligence. Under the majority, or *Cooper,* rationale, health care providers are free of liability for even the grossest malpractice if the patient had only a 50-50 chance of surviving the disease or injury with proper treatment.

DUTY TO WARN AND CONTROL

A physician's duty of care includes the duty to identify reasonably foreseeable harm from treatment and, if possible, to prevent it. It is increasingly recognized that a health care provider has the responsibility to warn patients of dangers involved in their care. Failure to advise the patient of known, reasonably foreseeable dangers leaves the physician open to liability not only for harm the patient suffers, but also for injuries that patient may cause to third parties.

The failure of the physician to warn the patient or third party of a foreseeable risk is a separate and distinct negligent act. The courts have imposed the duty to warn upon a health care provider when medications with potentially dangerous side effects are administered. If a drug is administered that might affect a patient's functional ability (such as in ambulating), the health care provider is obliged to explain the hazard to the patient and/or to someone who can control the patient's movements (e.g., the family members or others who can reasonably be expected to come in contact with the patient). The same duty is owed to patients engaged in any activity that may be hazardous, such as operating a car or machinery.

Similarly, when a health care provider ascertains a medical condition with dangerous propensities that may impair the patient's control of his or her activities, the health care provider has a duty to warn proper persons—patient, family, or others in contact with the patient. This may be true whether the condition is completely diagnosed or still under study.

There are a number of cases in which health care providers have been held liable to injured third parties for failure to warn of the potentially dangerous mental condition of the patient. Similarly, next of kin have successfully sued after a patient's suicide that could have been foreseen and potentially prevented.

Every jurisdiction has a list of diseases that must be reported to the authorities. The health care provider's failure to conform to the statutory requirement has made the provider liable to criminal penalties. It has also been held to be negligence per se (not requiring proof of negligence) in civil suits brought by the injured patients and/or third parties.

The doctrine of *informed consent* is one reflection of this duty to warn the patient. The purpose of the doctrine, implicit in its name, is to require the health care provider to give the patient sufficient information so that he or she has the opportunity to make a knowledgeable and informed decision about the course of his or her treatment. In the absence of adequate information concerning the risks and alternatives to a procedure or medication, a patient's consent is invalid, and the physician's treatment may then constitute a battery.

Depending on the circumstances, the warning should be made to the patient, to third parties known to be in proximity to the patient where the risk of harm may extend to them, and/or to the proper authorities. This provides an opportunity for measures to be taken to obviate the potential dangers.

Expanding the doctrine of strict product liabilities, the courts have established a precedent that health care providers and drug or device manufacturers have a duty to notify present and past patients of any hazards incident to the use of a defective treatment or therapy when such risks become known. This is the "duty to recall."

Other duties of the physician may run to persons who are not the patient. The duty to third parties is an outgrowth of the law's abandonment of the doctrine of privity and to the trend toward enforcement of the public health responsibilities of health care providers. The law has recognized, for example, the duty of a health care provider to warn the public of the communicability of contagious diseases, such as scarlet fever, smallpox, syphilis, or tuberculosis.

As to the question of confidentiality, when the patient's privacy conflicts with the public's health and safety and need to know, the patient's right must yield to that of the public.

The physician-patient relationship gives rise to a host of duties on the part of the physician that go beyond health care. Physicians have also been required to aid patients in litigation and to testify on behalf of patients. Treating physicians have also been required to fill out insurance forms promptly, adequately, and accurately.

Recent court decisions also indicate that a physician has the duty to divulge results to a patient who is examined at the behest of an employer.

JOINT AND SUCCESSIVE TORTFEASORS

The term *joint tortfeasor* means that where a tort is committed by more than one person, all persons who were involved in committing the tortious act are jointly liable. Because all could be joined as defendants and each was liable for all, the jury would normally not be required to apportion damages among the defendants. Today, where there is a common plan or design among the tortfeasors, all are equally liable unless joint liability has been modified by statute.

The law in the United States is quite clear that where the separate tortious acts of two or more wrongdoers join to produce an indivisible injury, and where the injury cannot be apportioned with reasonable certainty to the individual wrongdoers, all the wrongdoers will be held jointly and severally to be liable for the entire damages. If, however, the incidents of wrongdoing can be separated, and the successive wrongdoer commits a second act, the successive wrongdoer would be responsible for his own act. If the jury finds that the plaintiff's injuries and damages from the accidents are separable or divisible, it must be determined which portion resulted from the first accident and which from the subsequent accidents. If the first accident merely created the risk of harm, which then resulted from the second, independent accident, then the question is one of causation rather than apportionment.

REPORTING STATUTES

Statutes in many states require a health care provider to report certain matters, including communicable diseases and battered children, to the proper authorities. The physician is generally exempted from any civil or criminal liability for making a report pursuant to the terms of the statute. If the physician fails to report that which is required to be reported, he may be held liable to an individual who is damaged by the failure.

LOSS OF CONSORTIUM

The law is expanding a physician's liability to third parties where the physician negligently treats a patient. There is increasing recognition on the part of the courts that people can sustain emotional injuries and damages as an isolated phenomenon, not only as a consequence of a physical injury. This recognition has come about as a result of the evolution of psychiatry, particularly in the comprehension of emotional problems.

Consortium is that conjugal fellowship of husband and wife, and the right of each to the company, cooperation, affection, and aid of the other in every conjugal relation. Traditionally, only husbands were entitled to recover for the loss of their wives' "services." Damages for loss of consortium are now being awarded to wives, parents, children, and even unmarried partners. This development is due to the legal recognition of the fact that all family members suffer emotional injury when one is injured. Until recently, parents were not compensated for grief on the loss of a child, because the law did not recognize that the loss was more than merely a loss of services. In reality, one may lose companionship, security, society, aid, comfort, love, affection, solace, and guidance. It is no more difficult to determine the worth of the loss of such emotional intangibles than it is to determine intangible damages in general, such as pain and suffering from a physical injury. As a result, courts may be willing to compensate such losses.

WRONGFUL DEATH—SURVIVAL ACTS

Under English common law, when a person was killed by another's fault, the right of a cause of action against the wrongdoer died with the individual. Thus, it was more advantageous for the defendant to kill than to severely injure an individual. To remedy the situation, every jurisdiction in the United States, as well as England, passed what is known as a wrongful death act. The wrongful death act is a statute that allows the survivors to seek compensation for the death of another. Under wrongful death acts, the statutes define who the survivors are and who may recover. Many statutes have been enlarged on recently with the addition of parents, siblings, and even cousins to the list of potential plaintiffs. The theory of a wrongful death act is to compensate the decedent's survivors for the loss of economic benefit that might have been received from the decedent in the form of services, contributions, or support. Although strict construction of the law requires that damages for a minor child or for an aged individual be nominal (since there is usually little proof of an economic loss), many courts have put aside strict construction of the law and have allowed substantial recoveries in those cases. Recovery for the wrongful death of a child is often limited by statute, as well.

A survival action is one that had accrued to the decedent at or before the time of his death and that, by statute, "survives" the death and may be brought by an heir, estate, or other successor in interest. Even where death is not the proximate result of negligence, other damages occasioned by negligence may be recovered after the death of the injured patient. Usually, noneconomic damages, particularly those for pain and suffering, are not recoverable in a survival action.

In addition to wrongful death and survival actions, due to the great advances in the area of human reproduction, physicians now face the specter of claims of preconception negligence, negligent genetic counseling, wrongful conception or pregnancy, wrongful birth, or even wrongful life.

STATUTES OF LIMITATIONS

No wrongdoer, whether he or she committed a tort, a crime, or a mere breach of contract, should be held in legal jeopardy in perpetuity. The plaintiff must bring the complaint against the defendant within a legislatively prescribed period of time, contained in the applicable statute of limitations. Each jurisdiction has its own statutes of limitations for various offenses and torts. Except for the crime of murder, statutes of limitations have been established for most crimes and civil causes of action.

Statutes of limitations for tort actions are generally shorter than those for crimes or breaches of contract. In most jurisdictions, the statute of limitations for medical malpractice in negligence is three years or less. Recently, some jurisdictions have even reduced their statutes of limitations for medical malpractice actions to a minimal period of one year.

Frequently the crucial question in a malpractice action concerns when the statute began to run. Originally, it was universally held that the statute began to run when the injury occurred. However, it became apparent that in some situations, this was unfair to the patient. Many times the patient continued under the care of the physician, and was unable to discover the occurrence or cause of the injury while remaining in that care. The courts thus developed the "continuous treatment" rule, which held that the statute did not begin to run until the last date of treatment. Subsequently, almost all jurisdictions have adopted another test known as the "discovery" rule. Under this principle, the statute will not begin to run until the patient discovers the harm or, in the exercise of reasonable diligence, ought to have discovered it.

The plaintiff may also assert that the onset of the statute of limitations should be tolled when he or she can demonstrate that the failure to discover the injury was due to willful fraud, deceit, or concealment by the defendant.

DAMAGES

Under the common law, the purpose of tort law was to ensure that a person harmed by a tort is made "whole" again, or returned to the position or condition that existed prior to the injury. Since it is often impossible to alleviate the effects of an injury, public policy demands redress through the award of monetary damages to the victim. To prove entitlement to receive damages, the victim must substantiate the amount of loss incurred, within reasonable limits.

Occasionally, a person has been injured in principle but has essentially no actual loss. Under these circumstances, the jury or judge may award the plaintiff *nominal damages,* or a token sum—one cent or one dollar. What is the value of such a judgment? Although it is economically worthless, there is some virtue to such an award. The plaintiff, who has had his or her honesty, integrity, or virtue challenged, has the satisfaction of having his or her claim vindicated. Also, the defendant must pay court costs, which are often not insignificant, and sometimes the plaintiff's attorney's fees. Finally, the award of nominal damages may serve as a prerequisite to the award of a significant sum in punitive damages, as discussed later.

When the injury has resulted in a loss, the claimant is awarded *compensatory damages.* There are two types of compensatory damages—special and general damages. *Special damages* are reimbursement for actual economic loss, that is, out-of-pocket damages. These include payment for medical care and related expenses incurred in recovering from the injury, plus lost wages, future losses, and disability. These must be shown to be causal and foreseeable. *General damages* are awarded for the noneconomic injuries, including pain and suffering, mental anguish, grief, and other related symptoms or complaints. Because these cannot be measured exactly in monetary terms, our legal system allows the trier of fact to determine the monetary value of such injuries based on their own knowledge and experience, and depending on the proof that the plaintiff can establish. Injuries that are merely speculative are not compensable in damages.

It has been suggested that juries cannot value complex and convoluted economic interests. To the contrary, juries can and do find values in complex and technical litigation. Even when a specific defendant cannot be identified, the law has devised equitable theories, such as market share liability, on which to base valuation of damages. Under market share liability, damages may be apportioned among a number of defendants even when it cannot be shown with certainty that any of them actually caused the injury of the plaintiff. This has been limited to product liability actions such as the cases brought for injuries caused by use of the drug DES during pregnancy, leading to birth defects. In *Sindell v. Abbott Laboratories,*[12] market share liability was imposed on several manufacturers of the drug even though the plaintiff could not prove which defendant had manufactured the drug that actually caused her injuries. While several courts have followed the *Sindell* lead, not all have accepted the "market share" liability theory.

When the defendant's conduct has been grossly negligent, malicious, or utterly reckless with disregard for the consequences of those acts, the courts allow *punitive damages* to be awarded in addition to compensatory damages. The purpose of punitive (or "exemplary") damages is not to compensate the plaintiff, but to punish the defendant and serve a deterrent effect. Unlike compensatory or nominal damages, generally there is no malpractice coverage for punitive damages available to the defendant. Punitive damages, by statute, may be limited by some ratio to actual damages awarded (i.e., 1 : 1 or 3 : 1) and may be made payable in whole or in part to the state. Punitive damages must be reported by the recipient for income tax purposes, whereas compensatory damages are tax free.

As part of the malpractice reform movement during the so-called "malpractice crisis," a number of states modified their damage award procedures. In those situations in which future damages are awarded to cover an extensive period of care and management, the future damages are funded by a paid annuity and divided into monthly payments over the period of the life expectancy of the victim rather than settling with a lump sum. This is to prevent the plaintiff or guardian from wasting the lump award and leaving no funds for care. It also prevents the estate from inheriting a large sum of money as a "windfall" if the patient dies before the anticipated life expectancy period. These are referred to as *structured settlements.*

To avoid a victim obtaining a "double" or excess recovery, statutes in many jurisdictions provide for reduction of damage awards by the amount of compensation received by the plaintiff from "collateral sources" such as insurance or payment for sick leave by the employer.

END NOTES

1. *Tarasoff v. Regents of California.*
2. Prosser & Keaton, *Law of Torts* §§ 30,41 (5th ed. 1984).
3. *Id.*
4. *Pike v. Honsinger,* 49 N.E. 716 (1898).
5. *Nagiv v. News-Sun, Inc.,* 64 Ill. App. 3d 752, 756-757, 381 N.E. 2d 1014, 1017 (1978).
6. *Cooper v. Sisters of Charity of Cincinnati,* 27 Ohio St. 2d 242, N.E.2d 97 (1971).
7. *Gooding v. University Hospital Building, Inc.,* 445 So.2d 1015 (Fla. 1984).
8. *Hizer v. Randolph,* 126 Ariz. 608, 617 P.2d 774 (1980).
9. *Thompson v. Sun City Community Hospital,* 688 P.2d 605 (Ariz. 1984).
10. *Hicks v. United States,* 368 F.2d 626 (4th Cir. 1968).
11. *Hamil v. Bashline,* 481 Pa. 256, 392 A.2d 1280 (1978).
12. *Sindell v. Abbott Laboratories,* 26 Cal. 3d 588, 607 P.2d 924.

GENERAL REFERENCES

Andel, P., *Medical Malpractice: The Right to Recover for the Loss of a Chance to Survival,* 12 Pepperdine L. Rev. 973 (1985).

Brennan, T., and Carter, R., *Legal and Scientific Probability of Causation of Cancer and Other Environmental Disease in Individuals,* 10 J.H.P., Policy and Law, 1, 33-80 (Spring 1985).

Brennwald, S.F., *Comment, Proving Causation in "Loss of a Chance" Cases: A Proportional Approach,* 37 Cath. U. L. Rev. 747-788 (1985).

Delgado, R., *Beyond Sindell: Relaxation of Cause-in-Fact Rules for Indeterminate Plaintiffs,* 70 Cal. L. Rev. 881, 889 (1982).

Glaser, B., *Patients' Rights to Unfettered Treatment, The "Loss of a Chance" Doctrine,* 14 Legal Aspects Med. Prac. 2, 103 (Feb. 1986).

Hirsh, H.L., *Physicians' Potential Liability to Third Parties,* 22 *Med. Trial Tech. Q.* 145-153.

Hirsh, H.L., Shapiro, D., and Lustig, J., *Res Ipsa Loquitur and Medical Malpractice — Does It Really Speak for Patient? Med. Trial Tech. Q.* 410-430.

Hirsh, H.L., Tennery, F.F., and Hanson, V.D., Loss of Consortium, *Med. Trial Tech. Q.* 84-110.

King, J.H., Causation, Valuation and Chance in Personal Injury Torts Involving Pre-existing Conditions and Future Consequence, 90 *Yale L.J.* 1297, 1353-1397 (1981).

Wolfstone, L., and Wolfstone, T., Recovery of Damage for the Loss of a Chance, 28 *Med. Trial Tech. Q.* 21 (1981).

CHAPTER 13 Medical testimony and the expert witness

JOSEPH D. PIORKOWSKI, Jr. D.O., J.D., M.P.H., F.C.L.M.

GENERAL RULES OF ADMISSIBILITY
SPECIAL CONSIDERATIONS
CONCLUSION

The use of medical experts in litigation has increased dramatically in recent years. In medical malpractice and product liability cases, expert testimony usually is necessary to establish one or more of the essential elements of a claim or defense. Similarly, in the criminal context, expert testimony generally is required to support claims of incompetency or insanity, and such testimony may be needed to resolve issues about a defendant's potential for future dangerousness. Even when expert testimony is not required to prove an essential element of a claim or defense, medical experts have been called on increasingly to explain complex scientific concepts to aid the fact-finders' understanding of the evidence.

Much of the popularity of using medical experts undoubtedly stems from the special status the law accords expert witnesses. "Unlike an ordinary witness, . . . an expert is permitted wide latitude to offer opinions, including those that are not based on first-hand knowledge or observation."[1] Because experts today can both offer opinions on ultimate questions of fact and explain fully the bases of their opinions, an expert witness provides a useful vehicle for a skilled trial lawyer to review the evidence on a particular issue and tie it together neatly.

At common law, the presentation of expert testimony was rather cumbersome. Preliminarily, the expert's background, training, and education was reviewed, and the court determined whether the witness was competent to render the proffered opinions. If the witness was found to be competent, the presentation of his or her direct testimony proceeded in a strictly regulated hypothetical question. A Florida court described the common law procedure for presenting an expert witness' direct testimony as follows:

[W]hen an expert is called upon to give an opinion as to past events which he did not witness, all facts related to the event which are essential to the formation of his opinion should be submitted to the expert in the form of a hypothetical question. No other facts related to the event should be taken into consideration by the expert as a foundation for his opinion. The facts submitted to the expert in the hypothetical question propounded on direct examination must be supported by competent substantial evidence in the record at the time the question is asked or by reasonable inferences from such evidence.[2]

The rationale for this procedure was that "[a]dherence to this form for the direct examination of an expert prevents the expert from expressing an opinion based on unstated and perhaps unwarranted factual assumptions concerning the event; facilitates cross examination and rebuttal; and fosters an understanding of the opinion by the trier of fact."[3]

In practice, the use of hypothetical questions was tedious and came under harsh criticism. Wigmore's treatise on *Evidence* contains a sharp critique:

[I]t is a strange irony that the hypothetical question, which is one of the few truly scientific features of the rules of Evidence, should have become that feature which does most to disgust men of science with the law of evidence.

The hypothetical question, misused by the clumsy and abused by the clever, has in practice led to intolerable obstruction of the truth. In the first place, it has artificially clamped the mouth of the expert witness, so that his answer to a complex question may not express his actual opinion on the actual case. This is because the question may be so built up and contrived by counsel as to represent only a partisan conclusion. In the second place, it has tended to mislead the jury as to the purport of actual expert opinion. This is due to the same reason. In the third place, it has tended to confuse the jury, so that its employment becomes a mere waste of time and a futile obstruction.[4]

Rules 702 through 705 of the Federal Rules of Evidence ("the Rules"), which were enacted in 1975, simplified greatly the requirements for the admissibility of expert testimony. The Rules eliminated the requirement that evidence of the facts relied upon by the expert be admitted into evidence; indeed, the Rules expressly permit an expert to rely on facts that are inadmissible. The Rules also obviated the necessity for using hypothetical questions, although hypothetical questions were still permissible. Most states eventually followed the lead of the Rules as applied by the federal courts in eliminating at least some of the common law requirements. Although a great deal of variability still exists among states, the general trend since 1975 has been toward fewer procedural restrictions on the admissibility of expert testimony.

The first section of this chapter reviews the approach courts use in resolving frequently raised questions concerning the admissibility of medical or scientific expert testimony. Although this chapter focuses primarily on medical experts, cases interpreting the law dealing generally with expert testimony are discussed where useful. The major issues include the following: (1) whether the subject matter of the expert's opinion is appropriate to the case; (2) whether the expert is sufficiently qualified to render the proffered opinion; (3) the types of information on which an expert witness can properly base an opinion; (4) the role of general consensus in the scientific community in evaluating the admissibility of expert testimony; and (5) other limitations that pertain to the types of opinions experts can express.

The second section of this chapter reviews some special considerations, including expert testimony in the form of medical literature, the "reasonable degree of medical certainty" standard, discovery of expert witnesses' opinions, and ethical considerations relating to the use of experts.[5]

GENERAL RULES OF ADMISSIBILITY

The law governing the admissibility of expert testimony should be understood in light of two important background considerations.

First, a constant tension exists in the law of evidence generally between the principle that deficient or problematic evidence should be inadmissible and the principle that any problem or deficiency should go to the weight to be given to the evidence rather than to its admissibility. In no other area of the law of evidence is this tension so pronounced as in the area of expert testimony. Many of the rules reflect compromises between these two schools of thought.

Second, it is important to appreciate that the trial judge is accorded broad discretion to determine whether expert testimony should be admitted or excluded in a given case. It is well established that a trial court's decision will be affirmed unless it is "manifestly erroneous."[6]

The subject matter of the expert's opinion

At common law, the courts took a restrictive view of when expert testimony was appropriately introduced into evidence. The standard articulated in *Hagler v. Gilliland*[7] represents the traditional test:

The admissibility of expert opinion evidence is governed by the rule that such evidence should not be admitted unless it is clear that the jurors themselves are not capable, from want of experience or knowledge of the subject, to draw correct conclusions from the facts proved. It is not admissible on matters of common knowledge.[8]

Stated somewhat differently, courts held that "the subject matter must be so distinctly related to some science, profession, business or occupation as to be beyond the ken of the average layperson."[9] If the subject matter was not "beyond the ken of the average layperson," the opinion was deemed unnecessary and, therefore, inadmissible.

The standard articulated in the Federal Rules of Evidence, which has been adopted in form or in substance by most states courts, is much less hostile to expert testimony than the common law standard. Rule 702 provides:

If scientific, technical, or other specialized knowledge will assist the trier of fact to understand the evidence or to determine a fact in issue, a witness qualified as an expert by knowledge, skill, experience, training, or education, may testify thereto in the form of an opinion or otherwise.[10]

As interpreted by the courts, Rule 702 has three distinct requirements for the admissibility of expert testimony. First, the testimony must be comprised of "scientific, technical, or other specialized knowledge."[11] Second, the testimony must help the fact-finder to understand the evidence or to resolve a factual dispute in the case.[12] Third, the witness must be qualified to render the opinion. The first two requirements are considered in greater detail below under the rubric of whether the subject matter of the opinion is appropriate to the case. The courts' approach to qualification is discussed separately in the next section.

In *Daubert v. Merrell Dow Pharmaceuticals,*[13] the U.S. Supreme Court addressed the first of Rule 702's three prongs and noted that "[t]he subject of an expert's testimony must be scientific . . . knowledge." The Court explained:

The adjective "scientific" implies a grounding in the methods and procedures of science. Similarly, the word "knowledge" connotes more than subjective belief or unsupported speculation. The term "applies to any body of known facts or to any body of ideas inferred from such facts or accepted as truths on good grounds." . . . Of course, it would be unreasonable to conclude that the subject of scientific testimony must be "known" to a certainty; arguably, there are no certainties in science. . . . But, in order to qualify as "scientific knowledge," an inference or assertion must be derived by the scientific method. Proposed testimony must be supported by appropriate validation—*i.e.,* "good grounds," based on what is known. In short, the requirement that an expert's testimony pertain to "scientific knowledge" establishes a standard of evidentiary reliability.[14]

The *Daubert* Court emphasized that the approach to "scientific knowledge" is a flexible one.[15] "Its overarching subject is the scientific validity—and thus the evidentiary relevance and reliability—of principles that underlie a proposed submission."[16] The Court also noted that the inquiry must be directed to the principles and methodology used by the expert in reaching his conclusions, not to the conclusions themselves.[17]

To provide guidance to trial judges confronted with the question of whether proposed testimony constitutes "scientific knowledge," *Daubert* identified four factors that bear on the inquiry but do not represent "a definitive checklist or test."[18] First, the Court stated that "a key question to be answered in determining whether a theory or technique is scientific knowledge . . . will be whether it can be (and has been) tested."[19] The second factor is "whether the theory or technique has been subjected to peer review and publication."[20] Third, "the known or potential rate of error" for a particular scientific technique may be an appropriate consideration. Finally, the degree of acceptance of a theory or technique within the relevant scientific community may aid in determining whether expert testimony is admissible under Rule 702.[21]

The second prong of the subject matter inquiry is whether the expert's specialized knowledge will assist the jury in understanding the evidence or determining a fact in issue. That expert testimony may not be *necessary* to prove an element of a claim or defense does not preclude its admissibility if the testimony is otherwise *helpful* to the trier of fact. "*Helpfulness* is the touchstone of Rule 702. . . ."[22]

Courts are divided on the question of whether expert testimony is admissible under Rule 702 when the subject matter of the testimony is within the knowledge or experience of laypersons. In *Ellis v. Miller Oil Purchasing Co.,*[23] the U.S. Court of Appeals for the Eighth Circuit reviewed a ruling in which the trial judge had excluded expert testimony by a qualified accident reconstruction expert. The trial judge had determined "that the expert was in no better position than the jury to determine the

answer."[24] In upholding the ruling, the Eighth Circuit stated that "[w]here the subject matter is within the knowledge or experience of laypersons, expert testimony is superfluous."[25]

Other courts have reached the opposite conclusion. The U.S. Court of Appeals for the Third Circuit has stated that "there is no requirement that expert testimony be 'beyond the jury's sphere of knowledge.' "[26] In *Carroll v. Otis Elevator Co.,*[27] the U.S. Court of Appeals for the Seventh Circuit likewise upheld the admissibility of expert testimony on matters within the jury's ken. The Seventh Circuit considered the admissibility of the testimony of an experimental psychologist with expertise in "human behavior and perception." At trial the expert had testified that "brightly colored, red objects attract small children"; that "[t]his elevator's red stop button was more brightly colored than others" and, thus, "was more attractive to small children than others"; that "a covered stop button is less accessible to children than this uncovered one"; and that "the more difficult a button is to push the less readily it is activated by a small child. . . ." In affirming the trial court's decision to admit this testimony, the Seventh Circuit stated that "[w]hile it is true that one needn't be B.F. Skinner to know that brightly colored objects are attractive to small children and that covered buttons or those with significant resistance are more difficult to activate by little hands, given our liberal federal standard, the trial court was not 'manifestly erroneous' in admitting this testimony. . . ."[28]

The U.S. Supreme Court has stated that the requirement that expert testimony assist the trier of fact to understand the evidence or determine a fact in issue "goes primarily to relevance. 'Expert testimony which does not relate to any issue in the case is not relevant and, ergo, non-helpful.' "[29]

The expert's qualifications

Rule 702 provides that a witness can be qualified by "knowledge, skill, experience, training, or education." It is well established that a witness need not demonstrate all of these bases to qualify as an expert.[30] In some cases, practical experience alone has been held to be a sufficient basis for qualifying as an expert witness.[31] "Whether a witness is qualified as an expert can only be determined by comparing the area in which the witness has superior knowledge, skill, experience, or education with the subject matter of the witness's testimony."[32]

In the context of medical and scientific testimony, the court's approach to an expert's qualification often depends on the nature of the opinion at issue. Courts generally require an expert witness to be a physician before he or she will be permitted to render testimony on the medical standard of care,[33] although courts have been less restrictive in permitting nonphysician witnesses to offer opinions on causation.

[A] distinction must be made between testimony as to cause and testimony relative to the standard of care required of the physician. One need not necessarily be a medical doctor in order to testify as to causation. . . . However, . . . [u]nless the conduct complained of is readily ascertainable by laymen, the standard of care must be established by medical testimony. . . . *Medical* testimony means testimony by physicians.[34]

At common law, an expert testifying about the medical standard of care was required to demonstrate familiarity with the standard in the geographic location in which the defendant physician practiced. That requirement has been relaxed in numerous jurisdictions in cases in which the standard of care is the same throughout the United States.[35] Not all courts, however, follow the more liberal approach.[36]

In most jurisdictions, a physician does not have to be board certified or even a specialist in a particular field of medicine to render an opinion about the standard of care applicable to that field.[37] "The training and specialization of the witness goes to the weight rather than admissibility of the evidence, generally speaking."[38]

An essential prerequisite to offering an opinion about the standard of care, however, is that the expert witness be familiar with the standard of care for the medical problem or procedure at issue.[39] "[M]ore than a casual familiarity with the specialty of the defendant physician is required. The witness must demonstrate a knowledge acquired from experience or study of the standards of the specialty of the defendant physician sufficient to enable him to give an expert opinion as to the conformity of the defendant's conduct to those particular standards. . . ."[40]

In *Hartke v. McKelway*,[41] for example, the plaintiff, over the defendant's objection, was permitted to introduce the testimony of a physician about the standard of care for performing laparoscopic cauterization of the fallopian tubes. Although the expert had performed several hundred tubal ligations, she had never performed a laparoscopic cauterization, she had never assisted in the performance of such surgery, and she had observed such an operation only twice. The court noted that laparoscopic cauterization was a new procedure that was significantly different from the tubal ligation procedure. The court held that "[h]er reading of literature and conferring with other physicians on the eve of trial did not qualify her" and she "should not have been allowed to testify about the standard of care for laparoscopic cauterization."[42] The court concluded that "in order to give an opinion on whether the defendant complied with the applicable standard of care, the witness must be familiar with that standard."[43]

Similarly, in *Northern Trust Co. v. Upjohn Co.*,[44] the court held that a specialist in emergency medicine and internal medicine was not competent to testify on the standard of care to be applied to a defendant, a specialist in obstetrics and gynecology. The court did not make its decision, however, on the basis of the expert witness' field of specialization. Rather, the court examined the expert's knowledge, skill, experience, education, and training to determine whether he was adequately qualified to render an opinion on a pregnancy interruption procedure. The court stated:

He had never worked in an obstetrical or gynecological ward, had attended patients delivering babies "on occasion," but apparently had never been involved in pregnancy interruption procedures. He had never used the drug [that was administered to plaintiff's decedent], never seen it used and never observed the reactions of a patient receiving the drug. In fact, he had never had any experience with the drug in any manner and had not even read the insert and profile for the drug until he was asked to testify in this case.[45]

The court concluded that the expert "was not qualified to give an opinion . . . since he could not know what was customary practice for someone in [the defendant physician's] position."[46]

In *Smith v. Pearce*,[47] the Maryland Court of Special Appeals held that the trial court correctly excluded the testimony of a witness who was admittedly an expert in surgery. The issue in the case involved the standard of care applicable to gastroenterologists. The expert witness was familiar with the standard of care for gastroenterologists at Yale University School of Medicine where he was a professor, but he was not familiar with the national standard of care for gastroenterologists.[48] The court stated that "[w]hile it is well established that a physician may render an opinion on a medical standard of care outside his own specialty, the witness must nevertheless possess the necessary qualifications and sufficient knowledge."[49]

In *Hedgecorth v. United States*,[50] the trial court considered whether two physicians—an ophthalmologist and an emergency medicine specialist—were qualified to give expert testimony regarding the standard of care for performing cardiac stress tests even though they were not cardiologists. The court made a specific finding that both physicians "have demonstrated to this Court that they are familiar with the appropriate standard of care with regard to stress tests. The fact that [these physicians] are not cardiologists does not render their testimony on stress testing inadmissible, but merely goes to the weight given it by . . . the trier of fact."[51]

The principle that emerges from these cases is that a physician's qualification to offer testimony on the standard of care in a particular case does not depend on the witness' title or field of specialization. Rather, it depends on whether the physician has sufficient familiarity with the standard of care applicable to the particular medical problem or procedure at issue to assist the trier of fact in determining what the standard of care is in the case.

As previously mentioned, courts generally have been more receptive to receiving the testimony of nonphysician expert witnesses when the proffered testimony involves the issue of medical causation. In *Owens v. Concrete Pipe & Products Co.,*[52] for example, the court determined that experts in chemistry and pharmacology, both of whom had considerable experience in toxicology, should be permitted to testify "concerning topics such as the risks associated with varying degrees of exposure to certain chemicals."[53] The court stated that "[t]o the extent that their expert testimony is proffered for the purpose of establishing or rebutting causation, and is based on their knowledge of the chemicals rather than on a medical diagnosis of plaintiff's condition, their evidence is admissible."[54] Other courts have reached similar conclusions.[55]

In *Gideon v. Johns-Manville Sales Corp.,*[56] the U.S. Court of Appeals for the Fifth Circuit considered whether the trial court properly admitted in an asbestos case the testimony of the plaintiff's expert, "a biostatistician and epidemiologist specializing in the study of the causes of disease and its effects upon individuals and the public." The defendants had objected that the nonphysician witness had given "medical testimony."[57] The court noted that the witness had not testified about the plaintiff's physical condition or prognosis. In affirming the trial judge's ruling admitting the testimony, the court concluded that the witness was qualified to render opinions about risk of cancer, decreased life expectancy associated with asbestosis, and the date when the toxic effects of inhaling asbestos were first known.[58]

Although courts generally have required witnesses to have medical training to testify about medical diagnoses, courts occasionally have permitted nonphysicians to offer opinions about a diagnosis when the witness' education, training, and experience demonstrate that the witness' opinion will assist the trier of fact. For example, in *Jackson v. Waller,*[59] a will contest case, the court permitted an optometrist to testify about the progressiveness of cataracts he observed while examining the testatrix's eyes for the purpose of fitting her for glasses.

Jenkins v. United States[60] involved an appeal from a criminal conviction in a case in which the defendant had relied solely on the defense of insanity. The defendant had introduced the testimony of three psychologists, two of whom testified that the defendant's mental illness was related to his crime. The trial court instructed the jury that "[a] psychologist is not competent to give a medical opinion as to a mental disease or defect." The U.S. Court of Appeals for the District of Columbia Circuit reversed the defendant's conviction, stating:

> The determination of a psychologist's competence to render an expert opinion based on his findings as to the presence or absence of mental disease or defect must depend on the nature and extent of his knowledge. It does not depend upon his claim to the title "psychologist."[61]

The court acknowledged that "[m]any psychologists may not qualify to testify concerning mental disease or defect. Their training and experience may not provide an adequate basis for their testimony."[62] Nonetheless, the court held that "the lack of a medical degree, and the lesser degree of responsibility for patient care which mental hospitals usually assign to psychologists, are not automatic disqualifications."[63]

One common theme runs through all of these cases: "The trial judge should not rely on labels, but must investigate the competence a particular proffered witness would bring to bear on the issues, and whether it would aid the trier of fact in reaching its decision."[64]

When an expert is proffered to render multiple opinions, the determination of whether the expert is qualified normally should not be made on an "all or nothing" basis. Rather, "expert opinion must be approached on an . . . opinion-by-opinion basis, and the court must . . . carefully examine each opinion offered by the expert to assess its helpfulness to the jury."[65] An expert may be qualified, therefore, to render some opinions but unqualified to render others.

For example, in *Rimer v. Rockwell International Corp.,*[66] a product liability case involving a plane's fuel system, the trial court had permitted a pilot to testify about his experiences as a pilot, the experience of other pilots, and a forced landing that he made as a result of a fuel siphoning problem in a plane similar to that at issue in the case. The trial court had, however, excluded the pilot's opinion that the plane's fuel system had been defectively designed. The U.S. Court of Appeals for the Sixth Circuit concluded that "[t]he district court did not err in excluding the opinion testimony . . . on the design of the [plane's] fuel system."[67]

Similarly, in another product liability case, *Perkins v. Volkswagen of America, Inc.,*[68] the issue was the admissibility of the testimony of a specialist in mechanical engineering who had no experience in designing entire automobiles. The U.S. Court of Appeals for the Fifth Circuit affirmed the trial court's decision to allow the expert to render opinions on general mechanical engineering principles, but not to allow him to testify as an expert in automotive design.[69]

The foundation of the expert's opinion

At common law, ensuring that an expert's opinion had an adequate factual foundation presented little problem. Unless the expert was testifying on the basis of first-hand observation (as in the case of a physician testifying about a patient's diagnosis based on the physician's examination), the facts on which the expert's opinion was based generally had to be admitted into evidence before the expert could state an opinion. Thus, the jury always had before it not only the expert's opinion but also all the testimony, records, and other evidence on which the expert's opinion was based.

The Rules relax the requirement that the underlying facts and data be admissible in evidence. Rule 703 of the Federal Rules of Evidence provides:

The facts or data in the particular case upon which an expert bases an opinion or inference may be those perceived by or made known to the expert at or before the hearing. If of a type reasonably relied upon by experts in the particular field in forming opinions or inferences upon the subject, the facts or data need not be admissible in evidence.

Rule 703 thus continues to permit experts to base their opinions on the traditional foundations, i.e., personal knowledge or facts made known to them at trial. However, Rule 703 expands the common law rule by additionally permitting an expert to base an opinion on facts that have not been admitted into evidence and that are themselves inadmissible. The Advisory Committee explained the rationale behind this modification:

[T]he rule is designed to broaden the basis for expert opinions beyond that current in many jurisdictions and to bring the judicial practice into line with the practice of the experts themselves when not in court. Thus a physician in his own practice bases his diagnosis on information from numerous sources and of considerable variety, including statements by patients and relatives, reports and opinions from nurses, technicians, and other doctors, hospital records, and x-rays. Most of them are admissible in evidence, but only with the expenditure of substantial time in producing and examining various authenticating witnesses. The physician makes life-and-death decisions in reliance upon them. His validation, expertly performed and subject to cross-examination, ought to suffice for judicial purposes.[70]

Rule 703 thus creates the anomalous situation of an expert being permitted to rely on inadmissible facts or data as the foundation for an admissible opinion. The safety net to ensure that the basis of the expert's opinion is reliable is the requirement that the facts or data must be "of a type reasonably relied upon by experts in the field in forming opinions or inferences upon the subject."[71]

Whether the facts or data are "of a type reasonably relied upon" is to be determined by the trial court. "Though courts have afforded experts a wide latitude in picking and choosing the sources on which to base opinions, Rule 703 nonetheless requires courts to examine the reliability of those sources."[72] Until recently, federal courts were divided on the proper level of judicial scrutiny for evaluating whether an expert's opinion is based on facts or data of a type reasonably relied upon by experts in the field. Judge Weinstein's decision in *In re "Agent Orange" Product Liability Litigation*[73] reviews the competing schools of thought:

Courts have adopted two judicial approaches to Rule 703: one restrictive, one liberal. . . . The more restrictive view requires the trial court to determine not only whether the data are of a type reasonably relied upon by experts in the field, but also whether the underlying data are untrustworthy for hearsay, or other reasons. The more liberal view . . . allows the expert to base an opinion on data of the type reasonably relied upon by experts in the field without separately determining the trustworthiness of the particular data involved.[74]

Under either approach,

[t]he trial court's examination of reasonable reliance by experts in the field requires at least that the expert base his opinion on sufficient factual data, not rely on hearsay deemed unreliable by other experts in the field, and assert conclusions with sufficient certainty to be useful given applicable burdens of proof.[75]

At issue in *Agent Orange* was whether expert witnesses proffered by the plaintiffs who were relying on symptomatology checklists completed by the plaintiffs and "prepared in gross for a complex litigation"[76] were basing their opinions on facts or data of a type reasonably relied upon by physicians. The court found that such checklists "are not materials that experts in this field would rely upon and so must be excluded under Rule 703."[77]

Although the result in *Agent Orange* would have been the same regardless of which approach to Rule 703 — restrictive or liberal — the court followed, the court's reasoning reflected the restrictive approach.[78] In particular, the court in *Agent Orange* did not defer to the expert on the question of whether the facts or data he relied on were of a type reasonably relied on by experts in the field. Rather, the discussion focused on the pivotal role of the trial judge in assessing the foundation of the expert's opinion:

[T]he court may not abdicate its independent responsibilities to decide if the bases meet minimum standard of reliability as a condition of admissibility. . . . If the underlying data are so lacking in probative force and reliability that no reasonable expert could base an opinion on them, an opinion which rests entirely upon them must be excluded.[79]

In *DeLuca v. Merrell Dow Pharmaceuticals, Inc.,*[80] the U.S. Court of Appeals for the Third Circuit followed the liberal approach to Rule 703. In marked contrast to the *Agent Orange* court's approach, the *DeLuca* court stated:

Rule 703 has a narrow function; it seeks to delimit the acceptable bases for expert testimony. We have read Rule 703, in conjunction with Rule 104(a), as requiring the district court to "make a factual inquiry . . . as to what data experts in the field find reliable."

In performing this task, the district court must remain mindful that "[t]he proper inquiry is not what the court deems reliable, but what experts in the relevant discipline deem it to be." . . . Further, we have noted that if an expert avers that his testimony is based on data experts in the field rely upon, then Rule 703's requirements are generally satisfied.[81]

The *DeLuca* court found that the plaintiff's expert, who had relied on his own reanalysis of published epidemiological data, was basing his opinions on the same epidemiological data that the defendant's expert used in formulating her opinions.[82] The court held that Rule 703 did not require the plaintiff's expert to accept the conclusions of the authors of the studies on whose data he relied. The court concluded that no basis existed for excluding the plaintiff's expert's opinion under Rule 703.

In *In re Paoli R.R. Yard PCB Litigation,* however, the Third Circuit overruled *Deluca* and its liberal approach to Rule 703.[83] The Court stated: "Judge Weinstein's view is extremely persuasive, and we are free to express our agreement with it because we think that our former view is no longer tenable in light of *Daubert.*"[84] Although the Supreme Court's holding in *Daubert* was based on Rule 702, not Rule 703, the Third Circuit nonetheless held that "[i]t makes sense that the standards are the same, because there will often be times when both Rule 702 and Rule 703 apply."[85] Thus, after *Paoli,* U.S. Courts of Appeals are in agreement that "it is the judge who makes the determination of reasonable reliance. . . ."[86]

Regardless of the type of information on which an expert's opinion is based, courts generally require that an expert's opinion have an adequate factual foundation. At common law, this foundation requirement was easily enforced by the trial judge. If factual assumptions were included in a hypothetical question, but no evidence was contained in the record to support the existence of the assumed facts, then an objection to the hypothetical question would be sustained and the expert's opinion would not be admitted.

Under the Federal Rules of Evidence, expert testimony that lacks an adequate factual foundation has usually been excluded under Rule 703 (for the reasons discussed earlier), Rule 401, Rule 403, or some combination thereof.[87] Rule 403, which is discussed later in the section on additional limitations, permits the trial judge to balance the evidence's probative value against other concerns to determine the admissibility of the evidence. Obviously, an expert's opinion that has no factual basis has little, if any, probative value and thus can properly be excluded. "[E]ven if a witness is eminently qualified, even if there is merit to his views, and even if F.R. Evid. 702, 703, 704, and 705 are most liberally interpreted, there must be and ought to be some reliable factual basis on which the opinions are premised."[88]

Although foundationless expert testimony can properly be excluded by the trial court, it is also generally accepted that "the relative weakness or strength of the factual underpinning of the expert's opinion goes to weight and credibility, rather than admissibility."[89]

The decision of the U.S. Court of Appeals for the District of Columbia Circuit in *Richardson v. Richardson-Merrell Dow*[90] illustrates how courts assess whether an expert's opinion has an adequate factual foundation. In *Richardson* the plaintiffs alleged that the administration of the antinausea drug Bendectin during pregnancy caused their child to be born with birth defects. The trial court had concluded that the plaintiffs' expert's opinion lacked "a genuine basis, 'in or out of the record,'" and "that his 'theoretical speculations' could not sustain the [plaintiffs'] burden of proving causation."[91] The trial court did not, however, exclude the expert's opinion at trial. Rather, after a trial resulting in a jury verdict in favor of the plaintiffs, the trial judge granted judgment notwithstanding the verdict in favor of the defendant.

The court of appeals in *Richardson* agreed with the trial court that the plaintiffs' expert's opinions did not have an adequate foundation. The court stated: "Whether an expert's opinion has an adequate basis, and whether without it an evidentiary burden has been met, are matters of law for the court to decide."[92] The court proceeded to analyze the adequacy of the foundation of the plaintiffs' expert's opinion. The court noted that the expert had "predicated his opinion upon four different factors: (1) chemical structure activity analyses, (2) *in vitro* (test tube) studies, (3) *in vivo* (animal) teratology studies, and (4) epidemiological studies."[93] The court determined that the first three types of studies "cannot furnish a sufficient foundation for a conclusion that Bendectin caused the birth defects at issue in this case."[94] The court then noted that "the drug has been extensively studied and a wealth of published epidemiological data has been amassed, none of which has concluded that the drug is teratogenic."[95] The plaintiffs' expert was able to establish a statistically significant association between Bendectin and the injury at issue only by "recalculating" epidemiological data previously published in peer-reviewed scientific journals.[96] Several other courts have reached conclusions similar to *Richardson.*[97]

Although the issue presented in *Richardson* was decided at the post-trial stage, in light of the court's determination that whether an expert's opinion has an adequate basis is a question of law for the court to decide, there is no reason to believe a different decision would have been reached had the issue been decided pretrial at a Rule 104 *in limine* hearing. Other courts have conducted similar analyses and reached similar results in the pretrial context.[98]

Whether an expert witness' opinion has an adequate factual foundation is an issue that frequently arises in the context of medical causation opinions. The issue can also arise, however, in other contexts such as standard of care opinions.

In *Davis v. Virginia Railway Co.,*[99] for example, the U.S. Supreme Court reversed a judgment in favor of the plaintiff arising from a medical malpractice claim. The Court held that "[n]o foundation was laid as to the recognized medical standard for the treatment [at issue]." The Court held that the opinion of the plaintiff's expert that "he did not 'think that [the treatment] is proper' " did not provide as an adequate foundation for a jury to determine the applicable standard of care.[100]

In *Stokes v. Children's Hospital, Inc.,*[101] the court granted judgment as a matter of law in favor of the defendant because the plaintiff's expert "was required to lay the foundation as to 'the recognized medical standard' " but failed to do so. The court noted that "[i]n a case in which expert testimony is required, it is insufficient for the expert to state his opinion as to what he or she would have done under similar circumstances. . . . Rather, the jury must be informed of 'recognized standards requiring the proper . . . procedures under the circumstances.' "[102]

The role of "general acceptance" of scientific evidence

For the past several decades, many federal and state courts have held that before medical or scientific expert testimony can be admitted into evidence, the principles from which the expert's opinions were derived must have attained general acceptance within the relevant scientific community. This standard was first articulated in *Frye v. United States*[103] and has been referred to as the *Frye* test. The *Frye* test has been applied not only to testimonial evidence but to all forms of scientific evidence.

In *Frye,* the court considered and rejected the admissibility of results of a systolic blood pressure deception test, a precursor of the polygraph test. The court stated:

Just when a scientific principle or discovery crosses the line between the experimental and demonstrable stages is difficult to define. Somewhere in this twilight zone the evidential forces of the principle must be recognized, and while the courts will go a long way in admitting expert testimony deduced from a well-recognized scientific principle or discovery, the thing from which the deduction is made must be sufficiently established to have gained general acceptance in the particular field in which it belongs.[104]

The *Frye* court recognized that jurors can be unduly influenced by evidence that purports to be "scientific." Such evidence, by its very nature, carries with it an aura of accuracy and reliability. The *Frye* test was intended to protect jurors from placing excessive stock in scientific evidence until the principles from which the evidence was derived had gained general acceptance in the appropriate scientific community. "The requirement of general acceptance in the scientific community assures that those most qualified to assess the general validity of a scientific method will have the determinative voice."[105]

The *Frye* test has, however, encountered many difficulties in application.[106] Whether the evidence sought to be admitted has gained general acceptance in the appropriate field can depend on whether the "field" is defined broadly or narrowly. Also, courts have never adequately defined what constitutes "general acceptance." Although courts have recognized that *Frye* "does not require unanimity of view,"[107] no clear standard has emerged for measuring general acceptance among the relevant scientific community.

The Federal Rules of Evidence, which were enacted more than half a century after the *Frye* decision, mention neither the *Frye* test nor any need for scientific evidence to be generally accepted as a precondition to admissibility. Federal Courts of Appeal were sharply divided for years on the issue of whether the *Frye* test survived the enactment of the Federal Rules of Evidence. Some courts reasoned that no common law of evidence survived the enactment of the Federal Rules of Evidence and that the drafters of the Rules intended to abolish *Frye.* Other courts reasoned that the Rules were not intended to be an exhaustive codification of the law of evidence. These courts reasoned that the drafters would not have overruled such a well-accepted, long-standing standard without so much as a comment in the Advisory Committee notes or a statement in the legislative history.

The U.S. Supreme Court finally resolved the question in *Daubert v. Merrell Dow Pharmaceuticals, Inc.*[108] The Court held that the *Frye* test was superseded by the adoption of the Federal Rules of Evidence. The Court made it clear, however, that the *Frye* "general acceptance" test was one of many factors bearing on the reliability of an expert's methodology. The Court stated that " 'general acceptance' can yet have a bearing" on the question of whether evidence is sufficiently reliable to justify its admission.[109] The Court stated:

A "reliability assessment does not require, although it does permit, explicit identification of a relevant scientific community and an express determination of a particular degree of acceptance within that community." . . . Widespread acceptance can be an important factor in ruling particular evidence admissible, and "a known technique that has been able to attract only minimal support within the community," . . . may properly be viewed with skepticism.[110]

The *Frye* test also continues to be important for another reason. State courts, which are not governed by the Federal Rules of Evidence, may still employ the *Frye* test. The Supreme Court of Florida, for example, in a post-*Daubert* decision asserted the continuing vitality of *Frye* as the standard for the admissibility of scientific evidence in Florida.[111]

Additional limitations

Three other limitations on the admissibility of expert testimony warrant brief mention. First, expert witnesses are not permitted to offer legal conclusions. Second, expert witnesses cannot express opinions about the credibility of other witnesses. Third, expert testimony, like all evidence, can be excluded if its probative value is substantially outweighed by other specific considerations.

At common law, expert witnesses were prohibited from giving opinions that embraced an ultimate issue; the rationale was that permitting experts to opine on an ultimate issue would invade the province of the jury. Rule 704 modified the common law rule: "Testimony in the form of an opinion or inference otherwise admissible is not objectionable because it embraces an ultimate issue to be decided by the trier of fact." Thus, under Rule 704, an expert is permitted to offer an opinion on an ultimate issue of fact.[112]

Rule 704 did not, however, open the door to experts opining on legal conclusions. As the U.S. Court of Appeals for the Fifth Circuit explained in *Owen v. Kerr-McGee Corp.*[113]:

> Rule 704, however, does not open the door to all opinions. The Advisory Committee notes make it clear that questions which would merely allow the witness to tell the jury what result to reach are not permitted. Nor is the rule intended to allow a witness to give *legal* conclusions. . . . [A]llowing an expert to give his opinion on the legal conclusions to be drawn from the evidence both invades the court's province and is irrelevant.

Despite the seemingly simplistic distinction between permissible expert testimony on ultimate issues of fact and prohibited expert testimony on conclusions of law, courts have had great difficulty distinguishing between the two in practice. Moreover, courts have not been consistent in applying any set of standards to differentiate opinions of ultimate fact from legal conclusions.

The second limitation is that experts cannot express opinions about the credibility of other witnesses.[114] Evaluating the credibility of witnesses is exclusively the function of the jury. Several courts have excluded expert opinions that effectively tell the jury which witnesses to believe; such opinions are deemed both unhelpful and irrelevant.

In *State v. McCoy,*[115] for example, the Supreme Court of Appeals of West Virginia reversed a defendant's rape conviction based in part on the testimony of a psychiatrist that the alleged rape victim was "still traumatized by this experience."[116] The court stated the psychiatrist's "testimony amounted to a statement that she believed the alleged victim and by virtue of her expert status, she was in a position to help the jury determine the credibility of the most important witness in a rape prosecution."[117] The court determined that the psychiatrist's testimony encroached "too far upon the exclusive province of the jury to weigh the credibility of the witnesses and determine the truthfulness of their testimony. . . ."[118] The court concluded that "admission of her testimony was reversible error."[119]

Courts have held, however, that expert testimony is not inadmissible simply because it may have the indirect effect of bolstering another witness' credibility.[120] "Much expert testimony tends to show that another witness either is or is not telling the truth. That fact, by itself, does not render the testimony inadmissible."[121]

The third limitation is that, in addition to satisfying the standards on the admissibility of expert testimony imposed by Rules 702 through 705 of the Federal Rules of Evidence, expert testimony must not violate any of the other rules governing the admissibility of evidence at trial. A frequent obstacle to the admissibility of expert testimony is Rule 403, which provides:

> Although relevant, evidence may be excluded if its probative value is substantially outweighed by the danger of unfair prejudice, confusion of the issues, or misleading the jury, or by considerations of undue delay, waste of time, or needless presentation of cumulative evidence.[122]

As the U.S. Supreme Court has noted: " 'Expert evidence can be both powerful and quite misleading because of the difficulty in evaluating it. Because of this risk, the judge in weighing possible prejudice against probative force under Rule 403 of the present rules exercises more control over experts than over lay witnesses.' "[123] Thus, even if an expert witness is qualified, the testimony would be helpful, and the basis is proper, the trial court has the discretion to exclude the witness' testimony if it would cause unfair prejudice, confuse the issues, mislead the jury, or waste time.

Preliminary questions of admissibility

An important practical issue with respect to the testimony of medical experts is, "How, procedurally, does a litigant challenge the admissibility of expert testimony?" Court's practices vary greatly; some courts require *in limine* motions concerning such matters to be filed well in advance of trial. Other courts permit challenges to an expert witness' qualifications to be raised for the first time when the witness takes the stand.

Some courts have held that, before excluding expert testimony based on Rule 702, 703, or 403, the trial court must hold an *in limine* hearing to establish a sufficient factual record to support its decision. For example, in *In re Paoli R.R. Yard PCB Litigation,* [124] the U.S. Court of Appeals for the Third Circuit reversed a district court's original order granting summary judgment in favor of defendants because the trial court's rulings excluding evidence pursuant to Rule 702 and 703 were not supported by a sufficiently detailed factual record.[125] The Third Circuit also "reversed the district court's Rule 403 determinations, holding that Rule 403 exclusions should not be granted pretrial absent a record which is a virtual surrogate for a trial record."[126]

On remand in *Paoli,* after a period of discovery, defendants again moved *in limine* to exclude the opinions of plaintiffs' experts and for summary judgment. The district court, pursuant to Rule 104(a) of the Federal Rules of Evidence, held 5 days of *in limine* hearings.[127] At the hearing, 3 of plaintiffs' experts testified and 10 physicians and scientists testified for the defense as to the reliability of plaintiffs' experts' opinions.[128] The district court "filed extensive opinions (totaling 330 pages), setting forth not only findings of fact but also its reasons for again excluding the vast bulk of plaintiffs' expert evidence."[129] In affirming, in part, and reversing, in part, the district court's rulings, the Third Circuit implicitly approved the manner in which the district court conducted the Rule 104 hearing.[130] This decision provides some guidance to trial courts that are attempting to grapple with the appropriate scope of a hearing to decide pretrial motions *in limine* in a complex case.

SPECIAL CONSIDERATIONS
Use of medical and scientific literature as evidence

All state and federal courts in the United States allow medical literature to be used for some purposes at trial. The traditional rule was that learned treatises and articles could be used during cross-examination to impeach or contradict the testimony of a testifying expert; such materials could not, however, be admitted as substantive evidence because of the prohibition against hearsay.

"Virtually all courts have, to some extent, permitted the use of learned materials in the cross examination of an expert witness."[131] Courts vary greatly, however, on what threshold requirement must be met before such materials can be used for impeachment. Courts generally permit a treatise or article to be used for impeachment if the witness relied specifically on that treatise or article in forming his or her opinions.[132] Other courts permit a treatise or article to be used for impeachment in the absence of the witness' reliance if the witness acknowledges that the source is a recognized authority in the field. Still other courts permit such material to be used

for impeachment, even if the witness being impeached does not acknowledge the source as a recognized authority, if the authoritativeness of the source can be established through the testimony of other witnesses or by judicial notice.[133]

The admissibility of medical and scientific literature as substantive evidence has been the focus of heated debate. Opponents of admissibility argue that (1) the field of medicine changes so rapidly that treatises quickly become dated, (2) the trier of fact may be unable to understand complex technical passages that may be presented out of context, (3) the author is not available for cross-examination, and (4) medical literature is unnecessary as substantive evidence when live expert witnesses are available.[134]

However, proponents of the substantive admissibility of medical literature argue that (1) treatises generally are more up-to-date than live experts; (2) attorneys will be able to protect against confusion, the selective presentation of material, or passages being presented out of context; (3) cross-examination of the author is not necessary when a live expert is available to explain the treatise or article; (4) the scrutiny of the peer review process lends a high degree of reliability to opinions or conclusions published in peer-reviewed scientific literature; and (5) the author of a treatise or medical article has no interest in the outcome of the particular case at issue.[135]

The proponents of admissibility succeeded in recent years in having the absolute prohibition against the substantive admissibility of medical literature replaced with a more liberal standard in the Federal Rules and about half of the states. Rule 803(18) of the Federal Rules of Evidence is representative of the prevailing standard.

Although Rule 803(18) creates an exception to the hearsay rule for medical literature, it contains provisions to alleviate some of the concerns of the opponents of admissibility. For example, Rule 803(18) requires that the statements in the medical literature sought to be admitted, either be "relied upon by the expert witness in direct examination" or be "called to the attention of an expert witness upon cross-examination." This requirement ensures that an expert witness is available on the witness stand to explain the passage introduced into evidence, thereby diminishing the concern about the author's unavailability for cross-examination. Rule 803(18) also requires that the proponent of the evidence demonstrate that its source is "established as a reliable authority," either through the testimony of the witness on the stand, another expert witness, or judicial notice. Finally, Rule 803(18) provides that "the statements may be read into evidence but may not be received as exhibits."[136] This provision helps to ensure that the jury does not give undue weight to medical literature vis-à-vis the testimony of live expert witnesses. This requirement also ensures that the jury will not rely on any portion of the treatise or article other than the passages admitted by the court.

The "reasonable degree of medical certainty" standard

Some courts require that an expert hold opinions on causation and prognosis with "a degree of confidence in his conclusions sufficient to satisfy accepted standards of reliability."[137] "A doctor's testimony can only be considered evidence when he states that the conclusion he gives is based on reasonable medical certainty that a fact is true or untrue."[138]

Courts are in general agreement that expert testimony that a conclusion is "possible" does not suffice to meet the standard for admissibility with respect to the party who bears the burden of proof.[139] "A doctor's testimony that a certain thing is *possible* is no evidence at all. His opinion as to what is possible is no more valid than the jury's own speculation as to what is or is not possible."[140]

Courts differ, however, as to how much certainty is enough to constitute a reasonable degree of medical certainty. Some courts have held that the standard requires only that the conclusion is more probably true than not; this formulation renders the phrase synonymous with "more probable than not." Such courts often permit experts to testify in terms of a reasonable probability.[141] Other courts reject that standard. In *McMahon v. Young,*[142] the court stated:

Here, the only evidence offered was that [plaintiff's condition] was "probably" caused [by defendant's conduct], and that is not enough.... Physicians must understand that it is the intent of our law that if the plaintiff's medical expert cannot form an opinion with sufficient certainty so as to make a medical judgment, there is nothing on the record with which a jury can make a decision with sufficient certainty so as to make a legal judgment.[143]

Regardless of which standard is applied, courts generally look to the substance of an expert's testimony, rather than the form, in determining whether the witness has testified with the requisite degree of certainty. In *Matoff v. Ward,*[144] the Court of Appeals of New York stated:

Granted that "a reasonable degree of medical certainty" is one expression of ... a standard [of a witness's degree of confidence in his conclusions] and is therefore commonly employed by sophisticates for that purpose, it is not, however, the only way in which a level of certainty that meets the rule may be stated.... [T]he requirement is not to be satisfied by

a single verbal straightjacket alone, but rather, by any formulation from which it can be said that the witness' "whole opinion" reflects an acceptable degree of certainty.... To be sure, this does not mean that the door is open to guess or surmise....[145]

One important issue is whether a state's requirement that an expert testify "with a reasonable degree of medical certainty" applies in federal court. The applicability of a state standard in federal court depends on whether the state standard is solely procedural or whether it also encompasses a substantive aspect. In *In re Paoli Railroad Yard PCB Litigation,* the U.S. Court of Appeals for the Third Circuit noted that if a state court's standard "were purely a rule of admissibility, [it] would not apply in federal court...."[146] The Third Circuit stated, however, that where a state's requirement for expert testimony held to a reasonable degree of medical certainty sets forth a party's burden of proof, the standard is a substantive rule that is "not in conflict with the Federal Rules of Evidence, and thus governs in federal court."[147] In *Paoli,* the Third Circuit interpreted Pennsylvania's requirement that an expert testify as to causation "with a reasonable degree of medical certainty" as a substantive rule that "constitutes part of the plaintiff's burden of proof"[148] and, therefore, governs in a federal court applying Pennsylvania law.[149]

Discovery of the expert witness' opinions

The Federal Rules' elimination of many of the common law restrictions on the admissibility of expert testimony was premised on the belief that the adversarial system is capable of exposing the deficiencies in an expert's opinions. The drafters of the Federal Rules of Evidence recognized, however, that advance knowledge of the expert's opinions and the bases of the opinions are "essential for effective cross-examination."[150]

In civil cases, Rule 26(b)(4) of the Federal Rules of Civil Procedure "provides for substantial discovery in this area, obviating in large measure obstacles which have been raised in some instances to discovery of findings, underlying data, and even the identity of experts."[151] The vast majority of states also provide for ample discovery of the opinions of testifying experts. However, a few states, such as New York and Oregon, severely restrict pretrial discovery of the identities and opinions of testifying experts.

The law regarding discovery of testifying expert witnesses in civil cases currently is quite varied. The Federal Rules of Civil Procedure were amended effective December 1, 1993. The Rules as amended ("the new Rules") have not been adopted by all U.S. district courts; some federal courts are continuing to follow the rules that were in effect prior to December 1, 1993 ("the old Rules"). Some federal courts permit the attorneys by agreement to opt out of the new Rules and continue to use the old Rules. Most state courts continue to use discovery provisions that closely parallel the old Rules.

Although a detailed review of the law regarding discovery of expert witnesses is beyond the scope of this chapter, a brief review of the applicable provisions of Rule 26 of the old Rules and the new Rules is useful.

Under the old Rules, discovery pertaining to experts who were expected to testify at trial is governed by Rule 26(b)(4)(A). Rule 26(b)(4)(A)(i) allowed a party, through interrogatories, to require any other party to provide four categories of information concerning each expert witness who was expected to testify at trial. These categories were (1) the expert's identity, (2) the subject matter of the expert's expected testimony, (3) the substance of the facts and opinions to which the expert is expected to testify, and (4) a summary of the grounds for each opinion.[152] In practice, at a scheduling conference early in a case, many courts routinely set a date by which each party is required to file a "Rule 26(b)(4) Statement." Typically, the Rule 26(b)(4) Statement is required to set forth the information discoverable under Rule 26(b)(4)(A)(i).

The old Rules also provide that "[u]pon motion, the court may order further discovery by other means, subject to the restrictions as to scope and such provision . . . concerning fees and expenses as the court may deem appropriate."[153] The old Rules do not permit a party to depose another party's testifying expert without first obtaining leave of court. In most jurisdictions, however, it is customary for parties by agreement to take the depositions of each other's experts without obtaining leave of court.

Under the new Rules, discovery of expert testimony is governed by Rule 26(a)(2) and Rule 26(b)(4). Rule 26(a)(2)(A) requires a party to disclose to other parties "the identity of any person who may be used at trial to present evidence under Rules 702, 703, or 705 of the Federal Rules of Evidence."[154] Rule 26(a)(2)(B) then requires a more extensive disclosure than is required under the old Rules:

[T]his disclosure shall, with respect to a witness who is retained or specially employed to provide expert testimony in the case or whose duties as an employee of the party regularly involve giving expert testimony, be accompanied by a written report prepared and signed by the witness. The report shall contain a complete statement of all opinions to be expressed and the basis and reasons therefor; the data or other information considered by the witness in forming the opinions; any exhibits to be used as a summary of or support for the opinions; the qualifications of the witness, including a list of all publications authored by the witness within the preceding ten years; the compensation to be paid for the study and testimony; and a listing of any cases in which the witness has testified as an expert at trial or by deposition within the preceding four years.[155]

Thus, the new Rules place an affirmative disclosure obligation on the party who intends to call the expert as a witness at trial; it is no longer incumbent on other parties to obtain such information through interrogatories.

Rule 26(b)(4)(A) expressly authorizes a party to depose "any person who has been identified as an expert whose opinions may be presented at trial,"[156] thereby harmonizing the rule with the customary practice under the old Rules.

Both the old Rules and the new Rules provide that "the court shall require that the party seeking discovery pay the expert a reasonable fee for time spent in responding to discovery."[157]

The old Rules and the new Rules both also contain a provision governing discovery of nontestifying retained experts. Rule 26(b)(4)(B) provides that "opinions held by an expert who has been retained or specially employed by another party in anticipation of litigation or preparation for trial and who is not expected to be called as a witness at trial" can be discovered only "upon a showing of exceptional circumstances under which it is impractical for the party seeking discovery to obtain facts or opinions on the same subject by other means."[158]

In criminal cases, Rule 16 of the Federal Rules of Criminal Procedure contains the major provisions governing the discovery of an expert witness' opinions. Rule 16(a)(1)(E) provides:

At the defendant's request, the government shall disclose to the defendant a written summary of testimony the government intends to use under Rules 702, 703, or 705 of the Federal Rules of Evidence during its case in chief at trial. This summary must describe the witnesses' opinions, the bases and the reasons therefore, and the witnesses' qualifications.[159]

Rule 16(b)(1)(C) requires the defendant to make a similar disclosure at the government's request "[i]f the defendant requests disclosure under subdivision (a)(1)(E) of this rule."[160] These subdivisions of Rule 16 were added as part of the 1993 amendments; they represent a major expansion of federal criminal discovery. The Advisory Committee explained that "[t]he Amendment is intended to minimize surprise that often results from unexpected expert testimony, reduce the need for continuances, and to provide the opponent with a fair opportunity to test the merit of the expert's testimony through focused cross-examination."[161]

Rule 16 also contains provisions governing discovery of reports of examinations and tests. Rule 16(a)(1)(D) provides:

Upon request of a defendant the government should permit the defendant to inspect and copy or photograph any results or reports of physical or mental examinations, and of scientific tests or experiments, or copies thereof, which are within the possession, custody, or control of the government, the existence of which is known, or by the exercise of due diligence may become known, to the attorney for the government, and which are material to the preparation of the defense or are intended for use by the government as evidence in chief at the trial.[162]

Rule 16(b)(1)(B) imposes a similar, although somewhat different, disclosure requirement on the defendant "[i]f the defendant requests disclosure under subdivision (a)(1)(C) or (D) of this rule, upon compliance with such request by the government. . . ." The defendant's disclosure requirement includes only results of reports of physical or mental examinations and scientific tests *made in connection with the particular case. . . .*"[163] In addition, the defendant is required to produce only materials "which the defendant intends to introduce as evidence in chief at the trial or which were prepared by a witness whom the defendant intends to call at the trial when the results or reports relate to that witness' testimony."[164]

Rule 12.2 imposes a notification requirement on a criminal defendant if the defendant "[i]ntends to rely upon the defense of insanity at the time of the alleged offense,"[165] or "[i]f a defendant intends to introduce expert testimony relating to a mental disease or defect or any other mental condition of the defendant bearing upon the issue of guilt. . . ."[166]

Ethical considerations

Two ethical considerations relating to the use of expert witnesses warrant mention. First, paying a contingent fee to an expert witness is not permitted in most jurisdictions. The American Bar Association (ABA) Model Code of Professional Responsibility includes a disciplinary rule that states that "[a] lawyer shall not pay, offer to pay, or acquiesce in the payment of compensation to a witness contingent upon the content of his testimony or the outcome of the case."[167] The ABA Model Rules of Professional Conduct do not expressly prohibit the payment of a contingent fee to an expert witness, but Model Rule 3.4 prohibits offering "an inducement to a witness that is prohibited by law."[168] The Comment to Rule 3.4 also notes that: "The common law rule in most jurisdictions is that . . . it is improper to pay an expert witness a contingent fee."[169]

The second ethical consideration relates to *ex parte* contacts with expert witnesses in civil proceedings. ABA Formal Opinion 93-378, which was issued in November 1993, concluded:

[A]lthough the Model Rules do not specifically prohibit a lawyer in a civil matter from making ex parte contact with the opposing party's expert witness, such contacts would probably constitute a violation of Rule 3.4(c) if the matter is pending in federal court or in a jurisdiction that has adopted an expert-discovery rule patterned after Federal Rule 26(b)(4)(A). Conversely, if the matter is *not* pending in such a jurisdiction, there would be no violation.[170]

The ABA Standing Committee on Ethics and Profes-

sional Responsibility noted that neither the Model Rules nor the Model Code contains "an automatic bar to lawyers initiating contact with the opposing parties' experts."[171] The committee characterized Rule 26(b)(4)(A) of the Federal Rules of Civil Procedure and similar state provisions as the *"exclusive* procedures for obtaining the opinions, and the bases therefor, of the experts who may testify for the opposing party."[172] Because Rule 26(b)(4) and similar state rules make no provision for informal discovery of expert witness' opinions, the committee concluded that "in those jurisdictions a lawyer who engages in such ex parte contacts would violate Rule 3.4(c)'s prohibition against knowingly disobey[ing] an obligation under the rules of a tribunal."[173]

CONCLUSION

The late 1990s promises to be a dynamic period with respect to the law governing medical testimony and expert witnesses. The U.S. Supreme Court's decision in *Daubert* resolved the long-standing controversy regarding the *Frye* test and provided general guidance about the proper role of the trial court in ensuring the reliability of expert testimony. The full impact of *Daubert* and its practical effect on the practice of litigation involving medical experts, however, remains to be determined.

ACKNOWLEDGMENTS

I would like to express my gratitude to Carolyn Williams and Paul Mogin for providing their insights and editorial suggestions on earlier drafts of this chapter and to Lou Ann Wakeland for her outstanding administrative support.

END NOTES

1. *Daubert v. Merrell Dow Pharmaceuticals,* 113 S.Ct. 2786, 2796 (1993).
2. *Nat Harrison Associates, Inc. v. Byrd,* 256 So.2d 50, 53 (Fla. Dist. Ct. App. 1971).
3. *Id.*
4. 2 Wigmore, *Evidence* § 686, at 962 (Chadbourn rev. 1979).
5. The American Bar Association Section of Litigation published an excellent treatise entitled *Expert Witnesses* written in part and edited by Professor Faust F. Rossi. The treatise includes three parts: first, a careful review of the relevant law of evidence; second, a section that provides general guidance for the litigator on the practical aspects of working with experts; and, third, a section that provides practical guidance on specific types of experts.
6. *Salem v. United States,* 370 U.S. 31, 35, *reh'g denied,* 370 U.S. 965 (1962).
7. *Hagler v. Gilliland,* 292 So.2d 647, 648 (Ala. 1974).
8. *Id.* at 648.
9. *Dyas v. United States,* 376 A.2d 827, 832 (D.C.), *cert. denied,* 434 U.S. 973 (1977).
10. Fed. R. Evid. 702.
11. *Daubert v. Merrell Dow Pharmaceuticals,* 113 S.Ct. 2786 (1993).

12. *Breidor v. Sears Roebuck and Co.,* 722 F.2d 1134, 1139 (3d Cir. 1983).

13. *Daubert v. Merrell Dow Pharmaceuticals,* 113 S.Ct. 2786, 2795 (1993).

14. *Id.* (citation and footnotes omitted).

15. *See id.* at 2797.

16. *Id.*

17. *Id.*

18. *Id.* at 2796.

19. *Id.*

20. *Id.* at 2797.

21. For an excellent review of lower court decisions since *Daubert,* see Hoffman, "Expert Testimony Since Daubert: A Major Shift," Toxics L. Rep. (BNA) 252 (3/3/94).

22. *Breidor v. Sears Roebuck and Co.,* 722 F.2d 1134, 1139 (3d Cir. 1983).

23. *Ellis v. Miller Oil Purchasing Co.,* 738 F.2d 269, 270 (8th Cir. 1984).

24. *Id.* at 270.

25. *Id.*

26. *Linkstrom v. Golden T. Farms,* 883 F.2d 269, 270 (3d Cir. 1989) (*quoting In re Japanese Electronic Products,* 723 F.2d 238, 279 (3d Cir. 1983), *rev'd on other grounds, Matsushita Electrical Industrial Co., Ltd. v. Zenith Radio Corp.,* 475 U.S. 574 (1986).

27. *Carroll v. Otis Elevator Co.,* 896 F.2d 210, 212 (7th Cir. 1990).

28. *Id.* at 212.

29. *Daubert,* at 2795 (*quoting* 3 J. Weinstein & M. Berger, *Weinstein's Evidence* ¶ 702[02], p. 702-18 (1988)).

30. *See American Technology Resources v. United States,* 893 F.2d 651, 656 (3d Cir.), *cert. denied,* 495 U.S. 933 (1990).

31. *Federal Crop Ins. Corp. v. Hester,* 765 F.2d 723, 728 (8th Cir. 1985).

32. *Carroll v. Otis Elevator Co.,* 896 F.2d 210, 212 (7th Cir. 1990).

33. *Shea v. Phillips,* 98 S.E.2d 552 (Ga. 1957).

34. *Rodriguez v. Jackson,* 574 P.2d 481 (Ariz. App. 1977); *but see Harris v. Groth,* 663 P.2d 113 (Wash. 1983).

35. *See McNeill v. United States,* 519 F. Supp. 283, 287 (D.S.C. 1981).

36. In *Falcon v. Cheung,* 848 P.2d 1050, 1054 (Mont. 1993), for example, the court disqualified an expert who had never practiced medicine in Montana and had never practiced at a rural hospital in another state and, therefore, was unfamiliar with the standard of practice in rural Montana.

37. *Frost v. Mayo Clinic,* 304 F. Supp. 285, 288 (D. Minn. 1969).

38. *Baerman v. Reisinger,* 363 F.2d 309, 310 (D.C. Cir. 1966).

39. *Swanson v. Chatterton,* 160 N.W.2d 662 (Minn. 1968); *Hartke v. McKelway,* 526 F. Supp. 97, 101 (D.D.C. 1981), *aff'd,* 707 F.2d 1544, *cert. denied,* 464 U.S. 983 (1983).

40. *Fitzmaurice v. Flynn,* 356 A.2d 887, 892 (Conn. 1975).

41. *Hartke v. McKelway,* 526 F. Supp. 97 (D.D.C. 1981), *aff'd,* 707 F.2d 1544, *cert. denied,* 464 U.S. 983 (1983).

42. *Id.* at 101.

43. *Id.*

44. *Northern Trust Co. v. Upjohn Co.,* 572 N.E.2d 1030, 1041 (Ill. App. 1 Dist.), *appeal denied,* 580 N.E.2d 119 (1991), *cert. denied,* 112 S. Ct. 1172 (1992).

45. *Id.*

46. *Id.*

47. *Smith v. Pearce,* 625 A.2d 349, 359 (Md. App.), *cert. denied,* 632 A.2d 151 (1993).

48. *Id.* at 359.

49. *Id.*

50. *Hedgecorth v. United States,* 618 F. Supp. 627, 631 (E.D. Mo. 1985).

51. *Id.* at 631.

52. *Owens v. Concrete Pipe & Products Co.,* 125 F.R.D. 113, 115 (E.D. Pa. 1989).

53. *Id.* at 115.

54. *Id.*

55. *See Backes v. Valspar Corp.,* 783 F.2d 77, 79 (7th Cir. 1986); *Roberts v. United States,* 316 F.2d 489, 492-93 (3d Cir. 1963).

56. *Gideon v. Johns-Manville Sales Corp.,* 761 F.2d 1129, 1136 (5th Cir. 1985).

57. *Id.*

58. *Id.*

59. *Jackson v. Waller,* 10 A.2d 763, 769 (Conn. 1940).

60. *Jenkins v. United States,* 307 F.2d 632, 643-44 (D.C. Cir. 1962).

61. *Id.* at 645.

62. *Id.* at 644.

63. *Id.* at 646.

64. *Mannino v. International Manufacturing Co.,* 650 F.2d 846, 850 (6th Cir. 1981).

65. *Zenith Radio Corp. v. Matsushita Electric Industrial Co., Ltd.,* 505 F. Supp. 1313, 1333 (E.D. Pa. 1981), *aff'd in part and rev'd in part, In re Japanese Elec. Prods. Litig.,* 723 F.2d 238, *rev'd on other grounds sub nom, Matsushita Elec. Indus. Co. v. Zenith Radio Corp.,* 475 U.S. 574 (1986).

66. *Rimer v. Rockwell International Corp.,* 641 F.2d 450, 456 (6th Cir. 1981), *appeal after remand,* 739 F.2d 1125 (6th Cir. 1984).

67. *Id.*

68. *Perkins v. Volkswagen of America, Inc.,* 596 F.2d 681, 682 (5th Cir. 1979).

69. *Id.*

70. Notes of Advisory Committee on 1972 Proposed Rules.

71. Rule 703, Fed, R. Evid.

72. *Soden v. Freightliner Corp.,* 714 F.2d 498, 505 (5th Cir. 1983).

73. *In re "Agent Orange" Product Liability Litigation,* 611 F. Supp. 1223, 1244 (E.D.N.Y. 1985), *aff'd,* 818 F.2d 187 (2d Cir. 1987), *cert. denied,* 487 U.S. 1234 (1988).

74. *Id.* at 1244 (citations omitted).

75. *Id.*

76. *Id.* at 1247.

77. *Id.* at 1246.

78. *Cf. In re Melton,* 565 A.2d 635, 644 (D.C. App. 1989) (characterizing *Agent Orange* as an "intermediate position"), *vacated,* 581 A.2d 788 (1990), *on reh'g,* 597 A.2d 892 (1991).

79. *In re Agent Orange,* 611 F. Supp. at 1245.

80. *DeLuca v. Merrell Dow Pharmaceuticals, Inc.,* 911 F.2d 941, 952 (3d Cir. 1990), overruled by, *In re Paoli R.R. Yard PCB Litig.,* 35 F.3d 717 (3d Cir. 1994).

81. *Id.* at 952 (*quoting In re Japanese Electronic Products Antitrust Litigation,* 723 F.2d 238, 276-77 (3d Cir. 1983), *rev'd on other grounds,* 475 U.S. 574 (1986)).

82. *See id.* at 953.

83. *In re Paoli R.R. Yard PCB Litig.,* 35 F.3d 717, 747-49 (3d Cir. 1994).

84. *Id.* at 748.

85. *Id.*

86. *Id.*

87. *Lynch v. Merrell-National Laboratories,* 830 F.2d 1190, 1196-97 (1st Cir. 1987).

88. *Johnston v. United States,* 597 F. Supp. 374, 401 (D. Kan. 1984) (quoted in *In re Agent Orange Product Liability Litigation,* 611 F. Supp. 1223, 1250 (D.C.N.Y. 1985).

89. *Taenzler v. Burlington Northern,* 608 F.2d 796, 798 n.3 (8th Cir. 1979).

90. *Richardson v. Richardson-Merrell Dow,* 857 F.2d 823 (D.C. Cir. 1988), *cert. denied,* 493 U.S. 882 (1989).

91. *Id.* at 829.

92. *Id.*

93. *Id.*

94. *Id.* at 830.

95. *Id.* at 832.

96. *See id.* at 831.
97. *See Brock v. Merrell Dow Pharmaceuticals, Inc.,* 874 F.2d 307, 313 (5th Cir. 1989), *modified on reh'g,* 884 F.2d 166 (5th Cir. 1989), *reh'g en banc denied,* 886 F.2d 1314 (5th Cir. 1989), *cert. denied,* 494 U.S. 1046 (1990); *Lynch v. Merrell-National Laboratories,* 830 F.2d 1190, 1194-97 (1st Cir. 1987).
98. *See Lynch v. Merrell-National Laboratories,* 830 F.2d 1190, 1194-97 (1st Cir. 1987).
99. *Davis v. Virginia Railway Co.,* 361 U.S. 354, 357-58 (1960).
100. *Id.*
101. *Stokes v. Children's Hospital, Inc.,* 805 F. Supp. 79, 82-83 (D.D.C. 1992).
102. *Id.* at 82 (*quoting Levy v. Schnabel Found. Co.,* 584 A.2d 1251, 1255 (D.C. App. 1991) (citation omitted)).
103. *Frye v. United States,* 293 F. 1013 (D.C. Cir. 1923).
104. *Id.* at 1014.
105. *United States v. Addison,* 498 F.2d 741, 743-44 (D.C. Cir. 1974).
106. *See* Gianelli, *The Admissibility of Novel Scientific Evidence: Frye v. United States, a Half Century Later,* 80 Colum. L. Rev. 1197, 1208 (1980).
107. *Commonwealth v. Lykus,* 367 Mass. 191, 327 N.E.2d 671 (1975).
108. *Daubert v. Merrell Dow Pharmaceuticals, Inc.,* 113 S.Ct. 2786 (1993).
109. *Daubert,* 113 S.Ct. at 2797.
110. *Id.* at 2797 (citations omitted).
111. *Flanagan v. State,* 1993 WL 347761 (Fla. 1993).
112. Rule 704(b) includes a specific limitation which is applicable only to cases in which an expert witness is testifying with respect to "the mental state or condition of a defendant in a criminal case." This rule precludes an expert witness from stating "an opinion or inference as to whether the defendant did or did not have the mental state or condition constituting an element of the crime charged or of a defense thereto." Rule 704(b), Fed. R. Evid.
113. *Owen v. Kerr-McGee Corp.,* 698 F.2d 236, 240 (5th Cir. 1983).
114. *Henson v. State,* 535 N.E.2d 1189, 1192 (Ind. 1989).
115. *State v. McCoy,* 366 S.E.2d 731 (W. Va. 1988).
116. *Id.* at 737.
117. *Id.*
118. *Id.* (*quoting State v. McQuillen,* 689 P.2d 822 (1984) (Schroeder, J., dissenting)).
119. *Id.*
120. *State v. Myers,* 359 N.W.2d 604 (Minn. 1984).
121. *Id.*
122. Rule 403, Fed. R. Evid.
123. *Daubert,* 113 S. Ct. at 2798 (*quoting* Weinstein, *Rule 702 of the Federal Rules of Evidence is Sound; It Should Not be Amended,* 138 F.R.D. 631, 632 (1991)).
124. *In re Paoli R.R. Yard PCB Litigation,* 916 F.2d 829 (3d Cir. 1990) ("*Paoli I*").
125. *Id.* at 855-59.
126. *In re Paoli R.R. Yard PCB Litigation,* 35 F.3d 17 (3d Cir. 1994) (quoting *Paoli I,* 916 F.2d at 859-60).
127. *Id.* at 736.
128. *Id.*
129. *Id.* at 732.
130. *Id.* at 738-41.
131. McCormick, *Evidence* § 321, at 900 (3d ed. 1984).
132. *Id.*
133. *Id.*
134. *See* 6 J. Wigmore, *Evidence* § 1690 (1979); J. King, *The Law of Medical Malpractice in a Nutshell,* 100-103 (1977); F. Rossi, *Expert Witnesses,* 135-36 (1991).
135. *Id.*
136. Fed. R. Evid. 803(18).
137. *Matoff v. Ward,* 399 N.E.2d 532, 534 (N.Y. 1979).
138. *Palace Bar, Inc. v. Fearnot,* 381 N.E.2d 858, 864 (Ind. 1978).
139. *See Cohen v. Albert Einstein Medical Ctr.,* 592 A.2d 720 724 (Pa. Super. 1991), *appeal denied,* 602 A.2d 855 (Pa. 1992).
140. *Id.* (emphasis in original).
141. *See Parker v. Employees Mutual Liability Insurance Co. of Wisconsin,* 440 S.W.2d 43, 46 (Tx. 1969).
142. *McMahon v. Young,* 276 A.2d 534, 535 (Pa. 1971).
143. *Id.*
144. *Matoff v. Ward,* 399 N.E.2d 532, 534 (N.Y. 1979).
145. *Id.* (citations omitted).
146. *In re Paoli R.R. Yard PCB Litig.,* 35 F.3d 717, 751 (3d Cir. 1994).
147. *Id.* at 752.
148. *Id.* at 751.
149. *Id.* at 750-52.
150. Notes of Advisory Committee on Proposed Rules, F.R.E. 705.
151. *Id.*
152. Fed. R. Civ. P. 26(b) (4) (A) (i).
153. Fed. R. Civ. P. 26(b) (4) (A) (ii).
154. Fed. R. Civ. P. 26(a) (2) (A).
155. Fed. R. Civ. P. 26(a) (2) (B).
156. Fed. R. Civ. P. 26(b) (4) (A).
157. Fed. R. Civ. P. 26(b) (4) (C).
158. Fed. R. Civ. P. 26(b) (4) (B).
159. Fed. R. Crim. P. 16(a) (1) (E).
160. Fed. R. Crim. P. 16(b) (1) (C).
161. Notes of Advisory Committee on Rules, Rule 16, Fed. R. Crim. P.
162. Fed. R. Crim. P. 16(a) (1) (D).
163. Fed. R. Crim. P. 16(b) (1) (B). (emphasis added)
164. Fed. R. Crim. P. 16(b) (1) (B).
165. Fed. R. Crim. P. 12.2(a).
166. Fed. R. Crim. P. 12.2(b).
167. DR 7-109(c), Model Code of Professional Responsibility.
168. Rule 3.4(b), Model Rules of Professional Conduct.
169. Comment 3 to Rule 3.4, Model Rules of Professional Conduct.
170. ABA Formal Opinion 93-378 (November 8, 1993).
171. *Id.*
172. *Id.* (emphasis in original).
173. *Id.*

CHAPTER 14   Liability of health care entities for negligent care

JOHN R. FEEGEL, M.D., J.D., M.P.H., F.C.L.M.

LEGAL BASIS FOR HOSPITAL'S DUTY TO PATIENTS
NONDELEGABLE DUTY
STANDARDS TO MEASURE HOSPITAL CONDUCT
MEDICAL STAFF SELECTION, MONITORING, AND SUPERVISION
EXPANDING HOSPITAL LEGAL DUTIES
MANAGED CARE ORGANIZATIONS
DIRECT LIABILITY OF MCO
CONTRACT AND WARRANTY THEORIES
ERISA
PROFESSIONAL SERVICE CORPORATIONS
CONCLUSION

Corporate liability for the negligent care and treatment by health care providers has historically been limited to responsibility for its employees, acting within the scope of their duties, for the hazardous conditions of its physical plant, and for the equipment it provided. The hospital was considered to be a facility where physicians, contracted privately by patients and usually prior to their arrival, could practice medicine, restricted only by the state regulatory boards. It was the physician and not the hospital who was licensed to practice medicine. The physician, under these circumstances, was considered to be an independent contractor to whom the patient could look for compensation in case of injury due to professional negligence.

When the health care provider was a direct employee of the hospital, however, the hospital could additionally be held liable for injuries to the patient under the doctrine of *respondeat superior*. In this regard, the hospital was treated little differently than other corporate entities who had employees offering services to the public. In general, where the employee acted within the scope of his or her duties, the employer was held responsible for the outcome. In earlier times, some hospitals were run as charitable institutions (eleemosynary) and, as such, were held immune from liability or had damages due to liability greatly reduced on the theory that the charitable contributions were not in-

tended to be used by the donors as compensation for fault. Later, as health care institutions became insured and/or accepted other sources of income, the rationale for these exemptions or restrictions dissolved. Other institutions such as government-run hospitals escaped liability under the sovereign immunity doctrine (the state could do no wrong). No lawsuit could be brought against the state unless the state gave its permission. With a growing recognition of the unfairness of the exemption, local, state, and federal governments enacted legislation allowing claims to be brought for the negligent acts of its employees, albeit with numerous and varied restrictions, conditions, and caps on selected damages.

In our modern era, we are no longer simply concerned with the corporate responsibility of hospitals. We must also deal with the rapidly emerging variants and mutations of organized health care providers. These additional corporate entities now include managed care organizations (MCOs), which include health maintenance organizations (HMOs), preferred provider organizations (PPOs), independent practice associations (IPAs), permutations of all of these based on their internal organizations, and the increasingly popular professional associations (PAs) or professional corporations (PCs) under which one or more physicians can own and be employed by a self-owned third party. Accordingly, this chapter's aim is to recognize the expansion of the concept of corporate liability for negligent health care to include these newer entities, recognizing that health care entities are rapidly changing and adapting to public and private pressures.

Statements and citations that hereinafter mention "the hospital" as the corporate entity should also be considered applicable to the newer varieties of health care organizations—if not perfectly applicable, they should at least be considered as a potential bellweather of things to come.

Under the theory of corporate negligence, the hospital may be held responsible for the acts and omissions of its apparent agents (ostensible agents), under certain circumstances, even when they were thought to be nonemployees or independent contractors. This theory recognizes that the hospital has a *nondelegable duty* to provide reasonable and safe health care to its patients and that *direct* liability can arise for negligent care. Liability for employees may additionally arise out of the doctrine of *vicarious* liability, in which one may be responsible for the actions of others whom he or she controls.

Hence, the responsibility of the health care institution for proper selection, retention, and supervision of professionals on its staff has assumed newer and more hazardous proportions for the corporation. No longer can the hospital simply delegate to a volunteer staff committee the responsibility to examine a staff applicant's credentials and history of prior performance before granting full or restricted staff privileges. Nor can the physician on staff be allowed to practice negligently without some form of reasonable and prudent supervision or review of continued performance. Under the newer doctrine of corporate negligence, the hospital or other health care organization may share responsibility with the negligent physician for the consequences of his or her acts or omissions.

LEGAL BASIS FOR HOSPITAL'S DUTY TO PATIENTS

Case law has expanded the scope of the hospital's independent duty of care to its patients. The law may now impose on the hospital the responsibility for monitoring the activities of its independent medical staff and supervising the quality of medical care provided within it. Where the negligence of its health care personnel is imputed to the hospital under legal theories such as *respondeat superior* and ostensible agency, the hospital may be held liable along with the person whose negligence gave rise to the cause of action.

Under the legal doctrine of corporate liability, a hospital may have a duty to properly select and credential its staff physicians for clinical privileges and a duty to monitor its staff physicians as part of the implied contract between the patient and the hospital. The hospital may even have a duty to intervene actively and affirmatively when a physician is negligent and to prevent the errant staff physician from endangering hospitalized patients. Mere documentation of the problem with the physician may not be enough. Confrontation of the culpable physician is becoming the standard of care for hospitals. Some legal cases have suggested that a hospital has a duty to supervise all persons who provide care to hospital patients and to take reasonable preventive measures or corrective actions for misconduct that would otherwise be considered outside the zone of responsibility of the hospital.

Traditionally, the determination of a hospital's liability for negligent acts of members of its medical staff organization depended on the legal relationship between the hospital and the physician. At one end of the legal continuum was the salaried physician who was a hospital employee. Under the doctrine of *respondeat superior*, the hospital would be jointly liable for the physician's negligence.[1,2] At the other end of the continuum was the independent contractor staff physician who admitted patients under his care to the hospital. In the past, the hospital was seldom liable for an independent contractor staff physician's negligence.[3,4] Hospitals may be sued in medical malpractice actions under either theory of liability. As a general rule, hospitals have not been liable for the actions of staff physicians, even if their negligent actions occurred within the hospital, because those physicians were traditionally considered to be independent contractors. The principle of *respondeat superior*, however, holds hospitals vicariously liable for a physician's negligent care if employed by the hospital. Whether a physician is considered an employee may depend less on the written contract between the institution and the physician, than on the actions and appearances. Thus, if the hospital provides supplies, equipment, uniforms, meals, parking spaces, billing services, and ancillary personnel, a physician who claims to be an independent contractor may be held to be a *de facto* employee, particularly if the physician does not maintain an office elsewhere. The conditions set by the Internal Revenue Service (IRS) may have significance here and should be considered.[5] If a patient seeks treatment directly from the hospital, rather than from the physician who negligently caused the injury, or if the hospital provides no choice to the patient as to which physician provides a particular service as part of treatment, courts may view that physician as an employee and apply the doctrine of *respondeat superior*, even if the treating physician in fact is considered to be an independent contractor for other purposes. If a hospital represents to the patient that a physician is a hospital employee, but the doctor actually is an independent contractor, a court may still hold the hospital vicariously liable for the physician's acts. This legal theory of liability is called *ostensible* or *apparent agency.*

To hold a hospital liable on a corporate liability theory, a plaintiff must show that the hospital knew or should have known that the physician whose negligence caused the plaintiff's injury was providing substandard care to his or her patients. A plaintiff relying on an ostensible agency theory need only show that the plaintiff looked to the hospital for treatment and that the assigned attending physician negligently injured the patient in the provision of the treatment sought.

The hospital's liability for the negligence of a physician whose practice was hospital-based, such as an anesthesiologist or pathologist, was previously determined by the contractual arrangements between the physician and the hospital. These arrangements were referred to in determining whether the physician was more like an employee or an independent contractor, ordinarily a question of fact for the jury to decide.[6–8] Under ostensible agency doctrine, the contract issue is moot.

In *Pederson v. Dumouchel,*[9] the court recognized the need for a hospital to adhere to its own rules and regulations designed to control and regulate a staff physician's conduct. In this case, an injured child was examined by the physician, who diagnosed a fractured jaw. A dentist was called in to perform oral surgery, and the physician who diagnosed the fracture left the hospital. The operation was performed without the diagnosing physician in the operating room. The child suffered intraoperative cerebral anoxia and sustained permanent brain damage. The hospital was found to be negligent because it had not enforced its own rules, which provided that no surgery was to be performed except in the presence of a physician.

The case most often cited, however, as having extended and expanded hospital responsibility to include a direct duty to patients is *Darling v. Charleston Memorial Hospital.*[10] In this Illinois case, a general practitioner who had not treated a leg fracture in several years set and cast a patient's fractured leg. As a result of negligence, the leg had to be amputated. The physician settled with the plaintiff. The hospital was found liable for failing to require the physician to obtain a consultation. *Darling* came to stand for the concept that a patient is entitled to expect that the hospital will provide reasonable care and that the hospital has a duty to monitor and oversee the treatment provided by physicians practicing in the hospital.

Although ambiguities evident in the *Darling* decision have spawned inconsistent judicial pronouncements of a hospital's duty to supervise a physician's rendering of medical care to hospital patients, courts have been more consistent in imposing a duty on hospitals to use reasonable care in the granting of clinical privileges to physicians and in restricting privileges if a physician's misconduct becomes evident.

In *Fiorentino v. Wenger,*[11] the court held that a hospital may be found liable if it allows a physician to provide services to patients in the hospital when those in charge of granting hospital privileges know, or should know through reasonable inquiry, that the physician is likely to commit malpractice. This knowledge may consist of notice that the physician's staff privileges were rescinded at another hospital because the physician had conducted improper and radical surgery.

Mduba v. Benedictine Hospital,[12] held that a nonsalaried physician, despite his contract to the hospital to operate the emergency room, was an employee of the hospital. The reasoning was based on the court's observation that the physician's fees were based on rates guaranteed by the hospital and that he was subject to the rules and regulations of the hospital's governing board.

Subsequent cases have reinforced the proposition that a hospital has a broad duty in granting and rescinding staff privileges. In *Corleto v. Shore Memorial Hospital,*[13] the court held that a hospital could be found liable for permitting a known incompetent physician to perform an operation negligently and for failing to remove him from the case after his incompetence became obvious to the hospital. The court held that the hospital was ultimately responsible for the care of its patients, and therefore, it had a duty to act when it had reason to know that malpractice would probably occur.

Under the corporate negligence theory, a hospital may be liable for negligently failing to establish adequate procedures to ensure the safety and welfare of patients, including when the hospital knew or should have known that the physician who caused injury to the patient was not qualified to practice in the hospital, but nevertheless granted or renewed the physician hospital privileges. Earlier, some courts limited the hospital's duty to supervise staff physicians to situations involving only employee-physicians or to situations of gross negligence by the hospital. Apparently these courts were concerned that the imposition of a broad duty of hospitals to supervise care would impair independent physicians' discretion in purely medical decisions. Other jurisdictions have imposed a duty on hospitals to use reasonable care in the selection of staff physicians if detectable information exists about a physician's incompetence or lack of qualifications. Such notice can be inferred from records related to denying or restricting privileges at other hospitals or the existence of prior malpractice claims against the physician. If there is no notice of a physician's incompetence, and no apparent reason to rescind or deny privileges, a hospital may escape liability. Membership on the medical staff by a physician does not by itself create corporate liability for the hospital or health care organization.

NONDELEGABLE DUTY

One of the landmark decisions in the emergence of hospital liability through the theory of nondelegable duty, for the acts of a nonemployee, independent contractor emergency room physician is *Jackson v. Power*.[14] Jackson fell from a cliff and was airlifted to Fairbanks Memorial Hospital (FMH) where he was examined by Dr. Power, an independent contractor. Severe internal injuries were allegedly missed as a result of Power's negligence. The courts' discussion of ostensible agency centered on whether Jackson or other patients so transported to FMH without their specific request for a designated physician created the requisite appearance of the emergency room (ER) physician as an ostensible agent of the hospital or whether such a patient should have known the treating physician was not an employee of the hospital. The court said that it was a question for the jury. However, in considering the theory of nondelegable duty, the court made an historic decision: that a general acute care hospital has a nondelegable duty to provide non-negligent physician care in its emergency room. Note was taken that FMH was mandated by statute as an acute care facility to provide a physician in the emergency room at all times, and that it was accredited by the Joint Commission on Accreditation of Hospitals (now the Joint Commission on Accreditation of Healthcare Organizations), which imposed standards for operation of the emergency department. In these statutes and standards, along with the hospital's own bylaws, the court found a duty on the part of FMH to provide physician care in its emergency room. Next, the court sought to answer the single question of whether that duty could be delegated. Seeking guidance, the court turned to an air crash case[15] in which Alaska Airlines contended that responsibility had been delegated by subcontract to Chitina Air Service. Looking to the principles governing safety of passengers on common carriers, the Alaska Supreme Court held that the principal carrier would not be allowed to avoid liability by engaging in separate subcontracts to provide food, maintenance, or even supplying crews. In *Jackson,* therefore, the same court saw clear similarities in the responsibility of hospitals in supplying various services to patients and held that the duty to provide physicians and non-negligent care for patients in its emergency room was nondelegable. Such a duty does not extend, however, to situations where a patient is negligently treated in the ER by a physician of the patient's own choice.

In recognizing the doctrine of corporate negligence, the Florida Supreme Court held that a hospital has a duty to select and retain competent physicians who, even though they are independent practitioners, would be providing in-house patient care through their hospital staff privileges. In *Insinga v. LaBella,*[16] the court added that the hospital's responsibility for the acts of the physician do not extend to the physician's acts outside the hospital. This concept is probably not applicable where hospitals enter into direct associations with or purchase the staff physician's private practice, and continue to refer patients to him. Under those limited circumstances, the court may see an inducement of the patient to visit the physician's "private" office due to the referral or the endorsement of the care by the hospital.

STANDARDS TO MEASURE HOSPITAL CONDUCT

Many courts have distinguished the facts involved in determining the standard of care required of a hospital from those of *Darling,* thereby blunting the impact of that case on the hospital's requisite standard of care. Some courts have held that a hospital will not be held liable for an act of malpractice performed by an independently retained physician unless it had reason to anticipate that the act of malpractice would take place. *Lundahl v. Rockford Memorial Hospital,*[17] distinguished the facts of *Darling* on the grounds that the physician in *Lundahl* had been an employee of the hospital and assigned to the emergency room. In *Lundahl,* a boy was taken to a hospital where he was examined by a physician employed by the hospital. The patient was then referred to a staff orthopedist who was not an employee of the hospital. After the orthopedist replaced the moleskin traction with a floating splint, a blood clot formed, eventually requiring an amputation. The boy claimed that the hospital had a duty to review the medical care being given to him by the orthopedist. In *Lundahl,* the appellate court ruled that the decision to treat a patient in a particular manner was a medical question to be made solely by the treating physician, not by the hospital, thus refusing to extend the holding in *Darling.*

Other courts have held that the only way a hospital could be liable for negligent performance of professional services by a member of its staff would be if the plaintiff proved that the hospital had been negligent in its original selection of an unskilled physician.[18] However, in *Pogue v. Hospital Authority of DeKalb County,*[19] a partnership was under contract to staff an emergency room. Although the contract provided that the services performed would be "subject to surveillance by the medical staff of the hospital," and had to be performed in keeping with "good medical practice," the contract also specifically provided that the partners were "independent contractors." In finding that the hospital was not liable for negligence of one of the partnership's members, the court held that the hospital had no right to direct specific medical techniques employed by the physicians. The hospital was not liable when the physician's negligence related to a matter of professional judgment as long as the hospital did not have the right to control his diagnosis and treatment of the patient.

In *Vanaman v. Milford Memorial Hospital,*[20] a case with facts similar to *Darling,* the court came to an opposite conclusion. A mother brought her child to the emergency room with a fractured leg. Her own physician could not be located, so she asked to see the on-call physician, who set the leg, applied the cast, and treated the child in his office after her release from the hospital. The on-call physician, not the hospital, billed for his services. When permanent disability of the leg resulted, the parents sued both the physician and the hospital. In finding that the hospital was not liable, the court said that the medical staff was an organized body with qualifications and privileges approved by the governing board of the hospital for patient care. The court held that the hospital had functioned only as a referral service and had not practiced medicine itself.

However, some courts have recognized and reaffirmed the concept enunciated in *Darling.* In *Ohligschlager v. Proctor Community Hospital,*[21] a patient experienced severe pain and swelling in her arm near the point of insertion of a needle for intravenous infusion. The patient informed a nurse's aide of the pain, but the aide allegedly did nothing. Skin necrosis requiring skin grafting occurred as a result of infiltration of the intravenous medication, which the physician had ordered in an incorrect concentration. The patient brought a malpractice suit charging that the hospital's negligence was the proximate cause of her injuries. The court said that there was sufficient evidence to require submission to the jury of the issues of whether the hospital had failed to heed the patient's complaints and whether it failed to properly supervise the injection ordered by the physician. Citing *Darling,* the court said that the hospital was under the duty to "conform to the legal standard of reasonable conduct in the light of the apparent risk."

In *Tucson Medical Center v. Misevch,*[22] the court restated the duty of the hospital, acting through appropriate committees, to ensure the competence of members of its medical staff. The decision stated that the hospital was responsible to a patient if failure to properly supervise an incompetent physician results in the patient's being injured. In this case, the plaintiff contended that a physician staff member was negligent in administering anesthesia to the plaintiff's wife during disk surgery, and that as a result of this negligence, she suffered cardiac arrest and died. The key contention against the hospital was that the anesthesiologist was under the influence of

alcohol at the time of the operation, and that the hospital was negligent in retaining him on its medical staff.

The court pointed out that among the duties a hospital owes to patients with respect to competence of its medical staff was supervision of the physicians on its staff. The court stated that through the concept of "corporate liability," a hospital and its governing body may be held liable for injuries resulting from negligent supervision of members of its medical staffs. The court reasoned that hospitals assumed certain responsibilities for the care of its patients and thus were required to meet the standards of responsibility commensurate with that trust. If the medical staff was negligent in the exercise of its duty of supervising its members, or in failing to recommend action by the hospital's governing body prior to a patient's injury, then the hospital would be negligent. The court specifically stated that when the hospital's alleged negligence is predicated on an omission to act, the hospital will not be held responsible unless it had reason to know that it should have acted within its duty to the patient. Therefore, knowledge (actual or constructive) is an essential factor in determining whether the hospital exercised reasonable care under the circumstances. The court buttressed this argument by quoting the standards of the Joint Commission on Accreditation of Hospitals, which stated that "In a hospital accredited by the JCAH, the medical staff is responsible to the governing body of the hospital for the quality of hospital patient care. It therefore evaluates the qualifications of applicants and members to hold staff privileges and recommends curtailment and exclusion when necessary."

A hospital's lack of knowledge of a physician's incompetence can also result in liability if the hospital, through the exercise of due diligence, could have acquired such knowledge and acted on it so as to prevent the plaintiff's injury and failed to do so. In the Memorandum of Decision in *Gonzales v. Nork,*[23] the court held that a hospital owed a duty to its patients to protect them from the malpractice of an independently retained surgeon who was a member of the hospital's staff if the hospital knew, had reason to know, or should have known that the negligent acts were likely to occur. In this case, a private physician member of the medical staff had admitted to performing unnecessary and negligent spinal surgery on a hospital patient, a 27-year-old man who had suffered from back pain after being injured in an automobile accident. Three years after this operation, the hospital administrator heard a rumor that the surgeon's malpractice insurance had been cancelled. Because the hospital required staff physicians to have such insurance, it investigated and found that the rumor was true. The hospital promptly placed the surgeon in a monitoring program under which he was forbidden to operate without another qualified surgeon present.

During the trial, the surgeon admitted to performing at least 26 other unnecessary operations over a nine-year period. The court indicated that the liability of the hospital was based on its duty to protect its patients from malpractice by members of its medical staff. Although the hospital had no actual knowledge of the surgeon's propensity to commit malpractice, it was negligent because it had failed to investigate an earlier malpractice case in which the surgeon had been sued. The court concluded that mere compliance with the prevailing standards of the Joint Commission on Accreditation of Hospitals did not discharge the hospital from its duty to its patients because those standards furnished no effective means of detecting a fraudulent physician. The court also concluded that the hospital's system of peer review of the quality of patient care was random, casual, subjective, and uncritical. Therefore, at the time of the surgery on the patient, the hospital had no actual knowledge of the surgeon's fraud and incompetence. The judge, in essence, said that the hospital had a duty to protect its patients from malpractice by members of its medical staff and therefore the hospital governing board was "corporately responsible for the conduct of its medical staff."

The standard of care that the hospital must use to discharge the duty enunciated in *Nork* was detailed and illustrated in *Johnson v. Misericordia Community Hospital,* [24] a case involving the credentialing of a physician member of the medical staff. The court stated that a hospital owes a duty to its patients in selecting medical staff and granting surgical privileges. In this case, a patient contended that the hospital was negligent in appointing the surgeon to the medical staff and in granting him surgical privileges.

Testimony established the surgeon's negligence; this was not challenged on appeal. It was also established that the surgeon misrepresented the truth on his application, and authorized the hospital to verify all information given. The hospital's administrative records were devoid of any procedures utilized in the appointment of the surgeon to the medical staff organization. The court concluded that these procedures would have uncovered, *inter alia,* that at two hospitals the surgeon's privileges were revoked, at another hospital he was denied privileges, he was neither board certified nor board eligible, and 10 malpractice suits had been filed against him.

The appellate court held that a hospital had a duty to exercise reasonable care to permit only competent physicians and surgeons the privilege of using its facilities. It concluded that had the hospital exercised ordinary care in the staff selection process, it would not

have appointed the surgeon to its medical staff, and thus the patient in the instant case would not have been negligently injured. The court enunciated the theory that a hospital owes a duty of care of its patients to refrain from any act that will cause foreseeable harm or an unreasonable risk of danger. The concept of institutional responsibility is interwoven with foreseeability.

Once the duty is established, the standard of care is the degree of care ordinarily exercised by the average hospital in granting staff privileges. The court concluded that the hospital should be charged with constructive knowledge because the hospital could have readily obtained available information if personnel had investigated the surgeon's application. Although a hospital is not the ensurer of competence of its medical staff, it will be charged with gauging and evaluating the knowledge that would have been acquired had it exercised ordinary care in investigating its medical staff applicants. In addition to judicial recognition of the direct duty of a hospital to exercise reasonable care in selecting and retaining staff physicians, some courts have enunciated a duty to supervise the health care provided by physician staff members. The hospital's duty to promulgate regulations to oversee the clinical performance of physicians was enunciated in *Bost v. Riley,* [25] which adopted the concept of corporate negligence for failure to supervise medical treatment. The plaintiff contended that inadequate physician progress notes were evidence of negligent care that resulted in the patient's death. In determining the hospital's liability, the court held that hospitals have a duty to make a reasonable effort to monitor and oversee the treatment prescribed and administered by physicians practicing in the hospital. The court noted that the hospital may have breached its duty to the patient by failing to enforce its own internal rule requiring the keeping of accurate progress notes.

Other legal decisions have tended to limit the hospital's duty to supervise actual medical treatment. In *Cox v. Haworth,* [26] the patient was hospitalized so that his privately retained physician could perform a myelogram. During the course of treatment, the patient sustained permanent injury to the spinal cord. The patient alleged that the hospital was negligent in not obtaining informed consent before the medical procedure was performed. No negligence by the hospital personnel during performance of the myelogram was alleged. The court refused to interpret the doctrine of corporate liability as imposing a duty on a hospital to inform and advise the patient of the nature of the medical procedures to be performed.

The limitations placed on the expansion of the doctrine of corporate liability probably represent judicial recognition that hospitals are not well equipped to actively and concurrently supervise actual patient care.

The personal nature of the physician-patient relationship requires that the physician exercise necessary discretion. Moreover, it is impractical for the hospital to stand over a physician and personally supervise the quality of medical care rendered.

Overseeing the quality of physician performance is a different matter. Review of medical staff clinical performance is a retrospective process because hospitals must ordinarily delegate the review function to a number of medical staff committees (such as quality assurance, risk management, and credentials). The procedure for selection and retention of medical staff members is essentially a retrospective process. To project future performance, the committees use a historical database describing the physician's training, experience, and prior performance. Some courts have conditioned a hospital's duty to supervise the quality of care or competence of its staff on the hospital's knowledge and awareness of a physician's incompetent acts. Thus, for a hospital to be negligent in failing to properly supervise physician performance, it would be necessary to demonstrate that the hospital had either actual or constructive knowledge of the negligent procedures performed or omitted. This approach uses the agency law principle that a corporation is bound by the knowledge acquired by or by the notice given to its agents or officers, who are within the scope of its authority in reference to matters to which its authority extends. In *Fridena v. Evans*,[27] the court held that the negligent physician was an officer of the hospital who held a medical-administrative position as chief of the medical staff. This relationship became the linchpin for imputing knowledge of the physician's incompetence to the hospital. In holding that the hospital had "actual notice" of the physician's incompetence, the court concluded that the hospital had been negligent for failing to supervise the incompetent physician's performance.

Insight into the law's reluctance to create the unusually difficult task of supervising physicians on hospital staffs was provided in *Elam v. College Park Hospital.*[28] The court indicated that the hospital had a duty of "continuing evaluation" of the staff physicians' clinical performance, apparently a less onerous and more achievable modification of the requirement that a hospital supervise the actual medical care. Such a requirement did not necessarily require concurrent supervision and on-line intervention.

Additional modifications of the duty to supervise physicians were expressed in *Pickle v. Curns.*[29] In that case, the court held that a hospital could be charged with negligence for failing to supervise the medical care being given under a physician's care within a hospital. The court rejected, however, the contention that a hospital has a duty to ensure that physicians practicing on its premises never commit negligent acts. Instead, the court formulated the hospital's duty as one to prevent injuries resulting from negligent acts of its staff physicians when it knew, or should have known, that the physician would perform a negligent clinical task.

The trend evinced by these cases is to impose a duty on the hospital to supervise medical treatment only when the hospital has been put on notice by past negligent acts. Thus, the law does not impose on hospitals a duty to concurrently supervise the administration of medical care, but rather to monitor a physician's provision of medical services through patient care assessment committees.

In addition to responsibilities to patients regarding medical staff conduct, hospitals must have adequate policies to protect the welfare of patients receiving care in their institutions and must establish an organizational structure to carry out those policies. A violation of this duty is illustrated in *Polischeck v. United States,*[30] a case in which a hospital was held liable for failing to have the patient examined or her chart reviewed by a licensed physician before her discharge. The hospital permitted emergency room patients to be admitted and discharged by physician assistants, who under the state law were not considered qualified to make such determinations.

In *Ravenis v. Detroit General Hospital,*[31] a court imposed direct liability on the hospital for failing to have appropriate standards of care related to handling tissues to be transplanted from donor cadavers. Several patients were injured as a result of contaminated cornea transplants because the hospital had no policy that required the performance of needed tests on the donor or the donor tissue.

MEDICAL STAFF SELECTION, MONITORING, AND SUPERVISION

Courts have recognized the hospital's duty of selection, monitoring, and supervision of independent contractor members of the medical staff. Although a hospital's overall monitoring system will be closely examined when a hospital is named in a suit, the hospital is not considered to be guarantor of the adequacy of medical care rendered in its facility. Isolated negligent acts of an otherwise competent independent contractor physician are not generally evidence of negligences on the part of the hospital.

In exercising reasonable care in the selection of staff members, the hospital is responsible for obtaining reasonably available information on prospective staff members regarding their credentials and any prior negligent conduct. In *Joiner v. Mitchell County Hospital Authority,*[32] a patient complaining of chest pain was seen at the hospital by an independent contractor member of the medical staff. The physician advised the patient that the condition was not serious and sent the patient home. Shortly after returning home, the patient's condition worsened and he died. The patient's estate sued the hospital directly for its negligence in permitting an allegedly known incompetent physician to continue to serve on its medical staff. The court rejected the hospital's contention that it was relieved of liability by delegating its authority to screen medical staff applicants to the members of the existing staff, reasoning that the medical staff simply acted as an agent for the hospital in screening applicants. The court held that because the hospital knew, or from information in the hospital's possession it was apparent, that the physician was incompetent, the hospital did not act with reasonable care in permitting the physician to remain a member of the staff.

A hospital may also incur liability if it has implemented a data system for evaluating the qualifications of its staff members, but has failed to use this system to restrict the clinical privileges of a physician of demonstrated incompetence. In *Purcell v. Zimbelman,*[33] the court ruled that the hospital had actual "notice" of the surgeon's incompetence, based on evidence that prior similar operations performed by the surgeon had resulted in lawsuits against him and other hospitals. Significantly, the court concluded that the failure of the hospital surgical department, which had reviewed the surgeon's various mishaps in the operating room, to take any corrective action against the surgeon did not relieve the hospital of its duty to protect the patient.

Where a hospital has not implemented review procedures to properly credential and appraise staff physicians' clinical performance, plaintiffs must demonstrate review procedures that would have placed the hospital on notice. *Reynolds v. Mennonite Hospital*[34] involved a negligence lawsuit against several hospitals for damages caused by allegedly unnecessary surgery. The plaintiffs claimed that the hospital failed to comply with certification and review procedures. The court said, however, that such failure, even if the surgeries were unnecessary, was not necessarily sufficient to prove that the hospital was directly negligent. The hospitals had no notice of any flaw in the qualifications or background of the surgeons or of any circumstances existing prior to this plaintiff's surgery that would have caused the hospital to limit or revoke the physicians' privileges to operate. The court pointed out that a hospital is not an insurer of a patient's safety; therefore, because nothing was in the record to indicate that an evaluation of the surgeons' capabilities would have disclosed substandard practices, the hospital was not negligent.

The court declared that the decision to diagnose and treat a patient in a particular manner is a medical question entirely within the treating physician's discretion, and the negligence of a physician in the treatment of a patient cannot be imputed to the hospital where the physician is not an agent or under the direction of the hospital.

In *Braden v. St. Francis Hospital,*[35] the plaintiff alleged that an unnecessary amputation was performed by a staff surgeon, that the hospital had a duty to exercise proper supervision to prevent unnecessary and wrongful surgery, and that it breached this duty. In support of these allegations the plaintiff offered, *inter alia,* statistics showing that the allegedly negligent staff surgeon had performed significantly more amputations than the average number of amputations performed by other surgeons on the hospital staff. The plaintiff also referred to the hospital's bylaws, which documented an elaborate administrative structure of supervision and monitoring to ensure quality care. The court held that a hospital does not generally expose itself to liability for negligence unless it knows or should know of a propensity on the physician's part to commit negligent acts. The court pointed out that statistics do not, in themselves, indicate a proclivity on the part of the staff surgeon to perform unnecessary amputations, because multiple surgeries do not necessarily support a reasonable inference that any one procedure, including the procedure in this case, was unnecessary or negligently performed.

EXPANDING HOSPITAL LEGAL DUTIES

Kirk v. Michael Reese Hospital[36] expanded a hospital's liability beyond its patients to individuals affected by the actions of patients. In that case, the hospital discharged a patient on medication that should not be combined with alcohol, especially if the patient intends to drive. The patient consumed alcohol and subsequently was involved in an auto accident in which an injured third party sued both the patient and the hospital. The court ruled that the hospital had an obligation to that third party, an individual who had not been admitted or treated in the hospital.

In general, hospitals do not have a duty to ensure that its medical staff physicians render medical care competently *outside* the hospital setting. In *Pedroza v. Bryant,*[37] the court held that a hospital is not liable for injuries resulting from malpractice committed in the private office of a nonemployee physician before the patient was admitted to the hospital. The plaintiff charged the hospital with negligence in not ensuring that its staff physician, here the patient's private physician, was competent. Noting that the physician's negligent acts had occurred entirely outside the hospital, the court stated that for the plaintiff to prevail, the court would have to extend the hospital's duty of care under the corporate liability doctrine to patients treated by staff members in their private offices, where the hospital is not involved. The court declined to do so. The court pointed out that acts of malpractice committed by staff physicians outside the hospital are relevant only if the hospital has actual or constructive notice of them and negligently fails to take some action. The court stated that the hospital is not an inspector or ensurer of the private office practices of its staff members. Within the hospital, the delineation of staff privileges may reasonably affect the procedures used by staff members.

The doctrine of corporate liability may encompass a duty for the hospital to inform the patient or the patient's survivors when it is aware of a deviation from the standard of care that has caused an injury. The rationale for the duty is that when a hospital knows that a deviation from the standard of care has caused an injury, the failure to inform the patient or the patient's survivors may constitute fraudulent concealment. In *Kruegar v. St. Joseph's Hospital,*[38] the court held that whether fraudulent concealment was present was a question of fact for the jury to determine. In that case, the plaintiff was advised by her husband's physicians that he had died of heart failure during an operation. Nearly three years later, it was anonymously disclosed to the survivor that malfunction of the respiratory machine used during the operation had contributed to the cause of death. The plaintiff filed suit and alleged that the hospital had a duty to inform her of this fact and was, therefore, precluded from asserting the statute of limitations as a defense. The court noted that fraud can exist without the making of a positive false statement and stated that the suppression of a material fact, which a party is bound in good faith to disclose, is equivalent to a false representation.

A hospital must be sensitive to emerging areas of liability for failure to warn, particularly in areas involving the adverse side effects of radiation and other types of advanced medical treatment and the possibility of contact with communicable diseases. Case law principles governing a hospital's duty to warn in these instances are still developing. *Knier v. Albany Medical Center Hospital*[34] dealt with the hospital's duty to warn the general public that one of its employees has come in contact with a patient with a communicable disease. A nurse's family sued the hospital for failing to warn them that the nurse had been exposed to a contagious disease. The court ruled that it did not have an obligation to warn her family, friends, or the public at large that she had been exposed to scabies.

Far more dangerous than scabies is the threat of AIDS. Duties of the hospital to warn patients of an HIV-positive surgeon were explored in a 1991 New Jersey case, when the hospital restricted the surgeon's privileges until he provided proof of informed consent from his patients. At odds here were the duties of confidentiality to the surgeon as patient and the duties of the hospital to protect other patients from "risk of harm." The superior court held that the restriction and temporary suspension of surgical privileges did not violate the New Jersey law against discrimination.[40] This area of the law is obviously unsettled and further developments in many jurisdictions should be researched before a health care professional or the health care corporation acts. AIDS is considered a handicap in many states, is protected by special laws of confidentiality in others, and is a reportable disease, although not with disclosure of the patient's name, everywhere. How these competing issues will play out remains to be seen. A full discussion may be found in *Dellinger.*[41]

MANAGED CARE ORGANIZATIONS

A managed care organization (MCO) is designed to facilitate the management and financing of health care while delivering services to its enrolled members. The commonest type is the health maintenance organization (HMO), which, in turn, may consist of groups of physicians under contract to an employer or an insurer, independent practice networks, staff model organizations with direct employment of physicians, and open-ended networks that allow enrollees to seek services from within and from outside the organization. Regardless of the variant, the MCOs share a common goal to provide health care services at reduced costs through consumer competition. This concept has been endorsed, at least in theory, by many contemporary "health care reform" measures within and independent of state and federal governments.

Cost containment measures may utilize direct incentive payments to physicians to decrease patient-initiated use of services, reduction of physician involvement where overutilization can be demonstrated, fixed fees for identified procedures, and predetermined annual payments for comprehensive care (the so-called "capitation payment"). These cost containment measures may require the physician to restrict or deny some health care measures requested by the patient. The physician under these conditions becomes the "gatekeeper". Conflicts may arise when the patient feels harm has resulted from the restriction or denial of care. Indeed, the physician may concur that the restrictions are contrary to his or her own medical judgment.

The MCO may face liability for the improper selection and retention of the physicians or other professionals with whom it contracts to provide services to enrollees. This area of liability in similar to that of corporate liability for a hospital's negligence in providing hospital staff privileges, and cases cited elsewhere in this chapter should be reviewed. Because the MCO may function as the provider, the payor, and the quality reviewer, it may be exposed to liability for alleged breaches in each of these areas.

In *Harrell v. Total Health Care, Inc.,*[42] the appellate court found that an HMO had failed in its duty to properly select the physician with whom it contracted to care for the plaintiff, noting a history of malpractice and incompetence. The Missouri Supreme Court found the HMO free of liability on statutory grounds but did not reject the theory of corporate liability.

In *McClellan v. Health Maintenance Organization of Pennsylvania,*[43] the court found the doctrine of nondelegable duty nonapplicable to this HMO, because the HMO did not provide on-site health care services. The court, however, apparently did recognize the theory of corporate liability for negligent staff selection and retention.

Because MCOs are also employers, the theory of *respondeat superior* is applicable to hold the HMO liable for the negligence of its employees and agents acting within the scope of their duties. Staff model HMOs have been held liable for acts of its physicians in *Robbins v. HIP of New Jersey.*[44] In *Sloan v. Metropolitan Health Council, Inc.,*[45] the HMO exercised control over the physician. In *Schleier v. Kaiser Foundation Health Plan of Mid-Atlantic States,*[46] the physician was a consultant rather than an employee, yet the HMO was held liable for his acts, after the appellate court determined that the HMO "controlled" him through its medical director.

Where the physicians were found to be independent contractors and the HMO did not directly treat patients, negligence was not imputed to the organization (*Mitts v. HIP of Greater New York*[47]). A similar conclusion was reached where an HMO contracted with an independent practice association (IPA) and had no direct control over medical decisions. There, the court refused to apply *respondeat superior* (*Chase v. Independent Practice Association*[48]).

Under the theory of apparent or ostensible agency, HMOs have been held liable for negligent acts of affiliated physicians who were not directly employed. Here courts have considered whether the HMO "held out" the physician as an agent, whether the patient looked to the HMO rather than the designated physician for care, whether the physician was provided by lists supplied by the HMO, and whether the HMO restricted the patient's choice of physician,[49] but not when the HMO had exercised no professional control over the physician, such as in *Raglin v. HMO Illinois, Inc.,*[50] or where the state law prohibits the HMO from practicing medicine (*Williams v. Good Health Plus, Inc.*[51]).

Where an HMO physician specifically promised a given result, and the patient relied on that promise, the

HMO could be held liable for breach of contract when the result was not forthcoming from the treatment (*Depenbrok v. Kaiser Foundation Health Plan, Inc.*[52]).

In *Wickline v. State of California,*[53] a patient alleged that her premature discharge from hospital care, based on the utilization review decision to deny additional hospitalization, led to the amputation of her leg. She sued the California Medicaid program (Medi-Cal) for its interference with her physician's judgment to keep her hospitalized longer. The California appellate court held that only the physician could be held responsible for the premature discharge, but allowed that the program could be held liable if there were a defect in its cost containment measures which caused harm. In *Wilson v. Blue Cross of So. California,*[54] the utilization review organization of a private insurer refused extension of the patient's hospitalization for depression. He committed suicide after discharge. The court said the utilization review organization, the insurer, and the utilization review physician could be held liable. Unlike in *Wickline,* there was, *inter alia,* no clear public policy expressed in the statute that required a cost containment utilization review process. The private insurance provisions requiring cost containment review and restriction of services were not public policy.

DIRECT LIABILITY OF MCO

MCOs are also subject to direct liability for organizational or corporate negligence. These cases usually revolve around negligent selection of and retention of incompetent physicians. The theory applied is essentially the same as that of corporate liability of the hospital.[55]

The more recent application of these well-tested decisions to an HMO may be seen in *Harrell v. Total Health Care,*[56] where a Missouri court of appeals upheld a decision against a nonprofit HMO for negligent selection of a physician who was held out to subscribers on its list of specialists.

As courts continue to consider MCOs to be "health care providers," particularly staff model HMOs where care and treatment are actually dispensed, instead of merely financed, one can anticipate that direct liability for negligent supervision and control of its physicians will increase. Establishing a coherent and consistent appropriate standard of care in this area for MCOs may be difficult and as yet remains unclear.[57] It is anticipated that the federal government's efforts to reform health care nationwide may attempt to set practice parameters that some courts may interpret as "standards."

CONTRACT AND WARRANTY THEORIES

Dissatisfied subscribers may seek relief in the courts via legal theories other than negligence. These include breach of contract or warranty or misrepresentation by their MCOs. *Williams v. Health America*[58] and *Boyd v. Albert Einstein Medical Center*[59] provide examples, albeit unsuccessful at the time, of these theories. The more the MCO becomes a "provider" of health care for its subscribers, the more one can expect the court to find contractual or fiduciary relationships between it and the patient. Lawsuits using these business principles and theories will certainly follow.

ERISA

Some claims of malpractice by MCOs may be preempted under the Employee Retirement Income Security Act of 1974 (ERISA).[60] A complete discussion of ERISA is neither possible nor appropriate here. Suffice it to mention that where an MCO, HMO, or PPO plan is offered to an employee as part of a benefit package, it may be qualified as an ERISA program and thus subject to federal regulation. If so qualified, the preempted claims in malpractice are usually those resulting from defective design or implementation of cost-containment or claims handling systems, or those resulting from vicarious or direct liability for negligence by the provider. At present, there does not seem to be any sense of urgency by state or federal courts to preempt medical malpractice claims against MCO providers (see *DeGenova v. Ansel*[61]). However, the issue has not quietly faded away. It may become more popular with further federal involvement in health care and attempts to correct so-called "malpractice crises."[62]

PROFESSIONAL SERVICE CORPORATIONS

Professional service corporations, variously known as a professional corporation (PC) or a professional association (PA), are products of state legislatures. Specific regulations, restrictions, limitations, and liabilities for these corporations and their shareholders, agents, and employees should therefore be researched in the applicable state statutes.

If Florida[63] can be used as an example, then professionals such as physicians, lawyers, accountants, and many others may incorporate for the sole and specific purpose of rendering professional services, provided that its shareholders are duly licensed individually to render the same service. Motivation for incorporation by professionals includes tax benefits, pension plans, group ownership of property or contracts, and to escape the more open liability for the acts of others in a partnership. The corporation cannot legally provide professional medical services, but can be owned by the individual licensed professionals, can contract with others as a provider of health care services, own and convey property, employ persons (who need not be licensed) for managerial purposes, employee licensed professionals who need not be shareholders, sue, and be sued.

Under these professional service corporation arrange-

ments, the individual professionals do not escape liability and responsibility for their own acts. In fact, the professional corporation assumes liability and responsibility for the professional acts of its employees, including the individual licensed professional, ". . . up to the full value of its property."[64]

Professional liability insurance may be purchased by the PA to cover all of its professional employees and others acting within the scope of their duties, and each licensed professional may purchase individual liability coverage. Strict attention should be paid to these variables by all seeking to purchase coverage for the corporation and/or its shareholders and employees, as well as by all those to whom professional employment is offered. The terms may vary significantly from state to state.

Conversely, the liability of individual shareholders for the nonmalpractice liability of the professional corporation has been held in some jurisdictions to be limited to an extent similar to that of shareholders of nonprofessional corporations. For example, for ordinary business debts or nonprofessional contracts entered into solely in the name of the corporation, the assets of the individual shareholders should be exempt. See *We're Associates Co. v. Cohen et al.,*[65] where individual shareholders of a professional corporation of attorneys were not held responsible for the corporation's default on its lease, but compare *South High Dev. Ltd. v. Weiner et al,*[66] where the bar rules made the individual lawyers guarantors for the acts of their professional corporation, when professional duties were concerned.

In the sale or lease of a piece of expensive medical equipment, such as a CAT scan machine, the prudent vendor may require that the individual professionals as shareholders cosign along with the corporation itself.

Notification of the professional corporation at the time of notice to one of its shareholders in an action for malpractice is customary or required in many states, but not necessarily fatal where not done, because the intent of the state legislature in allowing professional corporations was not to provide an escape mechanism for the errant individual.

CONCLUSION

The role of the hospital and other corporations providing patient care has significantly changed in recent years. No longer is the hospital simply a physician's workplace that merely furnishes room, board, operating rooms, sophisticated equipment, nurses, attendants, and other personnel. Today, physicians and the health care corporation both play integral roles in the treatment of the patient. The hospital has assumed the role of a health care center, ultimately responsible for the health care provided within its four walls. The public expectation is that the hospital will act to ensure the overall quality of care rendered. The doctrine of corporate liability is an attempt to pragmatically focus the law on the modern relationships between legal doctrine and social and economic reality. The courts are moving away from an overly strict application of traditional but archaic doctrinal rules and guidelines, in recognition of these changing relationships among the hospital, the health care corporation, patients, subscribers or enrollees, and physicians.

The corporate nature of the modern hospital has demanded recognition of the corporate negligence theory. A common thread running through those legal cases that have applied the corporate negligence theory is the court's role in identifying and analyzing the organizational structure of the hospital. This approach recognizes that hospitals have assumed the dual role of delivering services and reviewing and monitoring the physicians it appoints to its staff. The duty, however, does not automatically render the hospital liable for all malpractice committed by physicians if the hospital has been reasonable in its procedures and has carefully selected and monitored its medical staff.

The movement to assign responsibility for all types of professional malpractice, including acts of independently practicing physicians, to the hospital corporation itself has been slow to develop in the medical care field, although it has become the most common form of legal responsibility in nearly all other aspects of "enterprise liability" in American law during this century.

END NOTES

1. *Bing v. Thunig,* 143 N.E.2d 3 (1957) (N.Y.).
2. *Sepaugh v. Methodist Hospital,* 202 S.W.2d 985 (1946) (Tenn.).
3. *Byrd v. Marion General Hospital,* 162 S.E.738 (1932) (N.C.).
4. *Moon v. Mercy Hospital,* 373 P.2d 944 (1962) (Colo.).
5. 1992-22 I.R.B. 59
6. *Carroll v. Richardson,* 110 S.E.2d 193 (1959) (Va.).
7. *Seneris v. Haas,* 291 P.2d 915 (1957) (Cal.).
8. *Brown v. Moore,* 247 F.2d 711 (1957) (Pa.).
9. *Pederson v. Dumouchel,* 431 P.2d 973 (1967) (Wash.).
10. *Darling v. Charleston Memorial Hospital,* 211 N.E.2d 253 (1965) (Ill.).
11. *Fiorentino v. Wenger,* 227 N.E.2d 296 (1967) (N.Y.).
12. *Mduba v. Benedictine Hospital,* 384 N.Y.S. 2d 527 (1976) (N.Y.).
13. *Corleto v. Shore Memorial Hospital,* 350 A.2d 534 (1975) (N.J.).
14. *Jackson v. Power,* 743 P.2d 1376 (1987) (Ala.).
15. *Alaska Airline v. Sweat,* 568 P.2d 916 (1977) (Ala.).
16. *Insinga v. LaBella,* 543 So.2d 209 (1989) (Fla.).
17. *Lundahl v. Rockford Memorial Hospital,* 235 N.E.2d 671 (1968) (Ill).
18. *Clary v. The Hospital Authority of the City of Marietta,* 126 S.E.2d 470 (1962) (Ga.).
19. *Pogue v. Hospital Authority of DeKalb County,* 170 S.E.2d 53 (1969) (Ga.).
20. *Vanaman v. Milford Memorial Hospital,* 262 A.2d 263 (1970) (Del.).
21. *Ohligschlager v. Proctor Community Hospital,* 303 N.E.2d 392 (1973) (Ill.).
22. *Tucson Medical Center v. Misevch,* 545 P.2d 958 (1976) (Ariz.).
23. *Gonzales v. Nork,* No. 228566 (Cal. Super. Ct. Sacramento Co. (1974) (Cal.).
24. *Johnson v. Misericordia Community Hospital,* 301 N.W.2d 156 (1980) (Wis.).
25. *Bost v. Riley,* 262 S.E.2d 391 (1980) (N.C.).
26. *Cox v. Haworth,* 283 S.E. 392 (1981) (N.C.).
27. *Fridena v. Evans,* 622 P.2d 463 (1981) (Ariz.).
28. *Elam v. College Park Hospital,* 183 Cal. Rptr. 156 (1982) (Cal.).
29. *Pickle v. Curns,* 435 N.E.2d 877 (1982) (Ill.).
30. *Polischeck v. United States,* 535 F. Supp. 1261 (1982) (Pa.).
31. *Ravenis v. Detroit General Hospital,* 234 N.W.2d 411 (1976) (Mich.).
32. *Joiner v. Mitchell County Hospital Authority,* 189 S.E.2d 412 (1972) (Ga.).
33. *Purcell v. Zimbelman,* 500 P.2d. 335 (1972) (Ariz.).
34. *Reynolds v. Mennonite Hospital,* 522 N.E.2d 827 (1988) (Ill.).
35. *Braden v. St. Francis,* 714 P.2d. 505 (1985) (Colo.).
36. *Kirk v. Michael Reese Hospital,* 513 N.E.2d 387 (1987) (Ill.).
37. *Pedroza v. Bryant,* 677 P.2d, 166 (1984) (Wash.).
38. *Kruegar v. St. Joseph's Hospital,* 305 N.W.2d 18 (1981) (N.D.).
39. *Knier v. Albany Medical Center Hospital,* 500 N.Y.S.2d 490 (1986) (N.Y.).
40. *Estate of William Behringer, M.D. v. The Medical Center at Princeton, et al.,* 592 A.2d 1251 (1991) (N.J.).
41. G. A. Reed, and S. W. Malone, *Acquired Immunodeficiency Syndrome, Ch. 13 in Healthcare Facilities Law.* A. M. (Dellinger ed., Little Brown and Company, Boston, 1991).
42. *Harrell v. Total Health Care, Inc.,* 781 S.W. 2d 58 (1989) (Mo.).
43. *McClellan v. Health Maintenance Organization of Pennsylvania,* 604 A.2d 1053 (1992) (Pa).
44. *Robbins v. HIP of New Jersey,* 625 A.2d 45 (1993) (N.J.).
45. *Sloan v. Metropolitan Health Council, Inc.,* 516 N.E. 2d 1104 (1987) (Ind.).
46. *Schleier v. Kaiser Foundation Health Plan of Mid-Atlantic States,* 876 F.2d 174 (1989) (D.C.).
47. *Mitts v. HIP of Greater New York,* 478 N.Y.S. 2d 910 (1984) (N.Y.).
48. *Chase v. Independent Practice Association,* 583 N.E.2d 251 (1991) (Mass.).
49. See *Boyd v. Albert Einstein Medical Center,* 547 A.2d 1229 (1988) (Pa.); *Dunn v. Praiss,* 606 A.2d 862 (1992) (N.J.); Decker v. Saini, 88-361768 NH (1991) (Mich.).
50. *Raglin v. HMO Illinois, Inc.,* 595 N.E.2d 153 (1992) (Ill.).
51. *Williams v. Good Health Plus, Inc.,* 743 S.W. 373 (1987) (Tex.).
52. *Depenbrok v. Kaiser Foundation Health Plan, Inc.,* 144 Cal. Rptr. 724 (1978) (Cal.).
53. *Wickline v. State of California,* 239 Cal. Rptr. 810 (1986) (Cal.).
54. *Wilson v. Blue Cross of So. California,* 271 Cal. Rptr. 876 (1990) (Cal.).
55. See *Darling v. Charleston Community Hospital,* 211 NE 2d 253 (1965) (Ill.); *Purcell v. Zembelman,* 500 P.2d 335 (1992) (Ariz.); *Corleto v. Shore Memorial Hospital,* 350 A.2d 534 (1975) (N.J.); *Elam v. College Park Hospital,* 183 Cal. Rptr. 156 (1982) (Cal.); *Blanton v. Moses Cone Memorial Hospital,* 354 S.E. 2d 455 (1987) (N.C.).
56. *Harrell v. Total Health Care,* 781 S.W. 2d 58 (1989) (Mo.).
57. See D. Kinney, and M. Wilder, *Medical Standard Setting in the Current Malpractice Environment: Problems and Possibilities,* 22 U.C. Davis L. Rev. 421 (1989).
58. *Williams v. Health America,* 535 N.E. 2d 717 (1987) (Ohio).
59. *Boyd v. Albert Einstein Medical Center,* 547 A.2d 1229 (1987) (Pa.).
60. 29 U.S.C.A. § 1001-1461.
61. *DeGenova v. Ansel,* 555 A.2d 147 (1988) (Pa.).
62. W.A. Chittenden III, *Malpractice Liability and Managed Health Care: History and Prognosis,* 26 Tort & Ins. L.J. 451-496 (Sp. 1991).
63. Ch. 621 Florida Stat. (1991).
64. 621.07 Florida Stat. (1991).
65. *We're Associates Co. v. Cohen et al.,* 480 N.E. 2d 357 (1985) (N.Y.).
66. *South High Dev. Ltd. v. Weiner et al.,* 445 N.E. 2d 1106 (1983) (Ohio).

CHAPTER 15

Pharmaceutical product liability

MARTIN J. MACNEILL, D.O., J.D., F.C.L.M.

PHARMACEUTICAL BACKGROUND
GOVERNMENT REGULATION OF THE PHARMACEUTICAL INDUSTRY
STRICT LIABILITY AND PHARMACEUTICALS
CONCLUSION

The concept of strict liability eliminates the need to prove negligence for an injury caused by a defective product.[1] However, policy interests have shaped the unique nature of pharmaceutical case law to provide multiple exceptions to the standard rules of strict liability. Some of the exceptions favor plaintiffs.[2] In such cases, manufacturer liability is easier to prove and is often decided with minimal evidence.[3] Other exceptions favor the defendants in drug-related litigation. The most notable exception is comment k to Section 402A of the Restatement (Second) of Torts.[4] Comment k distinguishes some pharmaceuticals from most other manufactured products by stating that the manufacturer is not held liable for injury from drugs that are seen as unavoidably unsafe.[5] Use of these drugs is seen as justified, even with the apparent medical risks.[6] Certain products are unavoidably dangerous and are incapable of being made safe when manufactured properly. Currently, a majority of courts agree with the Restatement's view and find some drugs dangerous by nature, but it is unclear which drugs are unavoidably unsafe.[7]

Pharmaceuticals are treated differently by the courts than other manufactured products.[8] One reason for this different treatment is the interaction that occurs between the body of the patient and the drug's chemical compound. When a drug is ingested, the response of an individual patient is difficult to predict. Every effect and each adverse reaction is unique. Frequently, the response to the chemical is more dependent on the individual's physiology than on product design. Therefore, a safely designed drug for every situation or every person may be illusory. Some commentators consider the pharmaceutical industry sufficiently unique to be categorized separately from all other forms of product liability.[9] Others believe the drug manufacturer should be held to the same form of strict liability as are other

industries.[10] Still others contend that the pharmaceutical companies should be strictly liable for their products, but define the role of liability differently, usually holding manufacturers to a lesser standard.[11]

PHARMACEUTICAL BACKGROUND
Drug industry

The drug industry in America has changed dramatically since the 1930s and 1940s. Early pharmaceutical companies generally produced a complete line of medication to serve the pharmacist's needs.[12] These companies spent very little money on research, development, or advertising. Customarily, the basic drug ingredients constituted 75% of corporate expenditures.[13]

The impetus for this change was the increasing efficacy of drugs.[14] In the early part of the century, even with hundreds of compounds on the market, few "cures" could be credited to pharmaceuticals.[15] Most drugs sold were for supportive care and did little to affect the course of illness directly. However, by the late 1940s and early 1950s, drugs took the offensive against disease.[16] Penicillin and other broad-spectrum antibiotics heralded a new age, in which medicine could directly attack foreign cells without harming the host. Because most drugs are effective against only one or two conditions, hundreds of drugs are sold. In the United States, the number of physiologically active compounds numbers more than 1000.[17] These compounds in turn are mixed with other compounds which produce hundreds of thousands of products.[18]

Adverse reactions are the unwanted interactions between a drug and a recipient's physiology. Multiple forms of adverse reactions are possible with any allergen.[19] Hypersensitivity[20] or allergic reactions,[21] drug interactions, excessive amounts of the desired effect, unavoidable side effects, and activation of physical illness are a few of the adverse reactions possible with any drug. Wherever possible, a manufacturer should seek to discover and eliminate these unwanted side effects. Adverse reactions to drugs remain one of the major causes of hospitalization, illness, and death in the nation. Some authors believe that more than 140,000 deaths per year are caused by adverse drug reactions in the United States.[22] A product, however, that is highly beneficial to millions of patients may be deadly to a few. Most commentators agree that a prescription drug will not be considered defective if an unusually sensitive user develops an adverse reaction.[23]

1. *Known adverse reactions:* Pharmaceutical manufacturers are required to warn adequately of known dangers in the administration of their product.[24]
2. *Unknown adverse reactions:* Possibly more serious than known side effects are those that remain undiscovered prior to an adverse reaction in the ultimate consumer. Although no national consensus exists on the question, some courts consider an undiscovered side effect to be a defect and impose the same strict liability as with other defects.[25] Others look to comment k of Section 402A and insulate drugs from standard product liability.[26]

GOVERNMENT REGULATION OF THE PHARMACEUTICAL INDUSTRY
History of government regulation

The first attempt at government regulation of the pharmaceutical industry was the passage of the Federal (Pure) Food and Drugs Act of 1906.[27] The act addressed concerns about drug safety and improper advertising practices within the industry.[28] For the first time, the full disclosure of a drug's composition was required.[29]

Congress further strengthened medication regulation by passing the Food, Drug and Cosmetic Act of 1938,[30] which required proof of safety prior to marketing new drugs. Prescriptions were to be used for the majority of drugs and public access to thousands of products was to be restricted. The Food and Drug Administration (FDA) was authorized to police the market and set policy for the sale and distribution of new drugs.

Until the Kefauver-Harris amendments to the Food, Drug and Cosmetic Act were established in 1962,[31] drug manufacturers were not required to prove their drug's efficacy. Due to the widespread concern of drug safety caused by the thalidomide tragedy,[32] the Kefauver-Harris amendments imposed strict guidelines, which led to the removal of 7000 drugs from the market and a stricter labeling of more than 1500 others.[33]

The current regulatory scheme

Since that time, the FDA has experienced great difficulty when trying to identify and communicate the hazards of prescription drugs.[34] The FDA must verify the safety and efficacy of new drugs before approving them for human use. The agency requires a lengthy experimental protocol before a drug may be marketed. Thereafter, the manufacturer must periodically review the drug's safety and efficacy in the population at large.

One of the potentially serious difficulties with the FDA's system is the agency's dependence on manufacturers for the adverse reaction data. It is the manufacturer's responsibility to perform all pre-marketing tests and collect all post-marketing results. In reporting adverse reactions, drug companies have been caught falsifying tests and results.[35] The most recent cases have dealt with fraud within the generic drug industry.[36]

Drug testing. In the United States, bringing a new drug to the point-of-sale to the public is a long and complex process. By the time a new medicine becomes available for general use, it has been tested on both animals and humans under controlled protocols set out by the FDA.[37]

The FDA's protocol for testing drugs only partially shields drug manufacturers from lawsuits. The manufacturers are protected from liability for injuries only if they strictly follow FDA procedures.[38] Within the FDA guidelines a drug manufacturer has significant leeway in deciding how extensively to test a product. Moreover, the manufacturer has almost total discretion to determine what type of experimentation and research is necessary. But in exercising this discretion, the manufacturer takes upon itself additional responsibility and increased liability exposure. For example, the duty to test is a continuing one. The manufacturer is liable if it fails to test adequately all aspects of drug usage. A drug used by consumers on a long-term basis may be deemed insufficiently tested if the only study performed was to evaluate the short-term effect.[39]

Reporting adverse reactions. Continued evaluation of a product after approval by the FDA is a vital part of the regulatory process. Many pathologies become present only after years of drug use in the general population. Indeed, adverse reaction reporting has increased significantly during the past few years.[40] In 1985, the FDA formulated new post-marketing surveillance requirements that will better accumulate data and utilize discovered information on adverse reactions nationwide.[41] Manufacturers are now required to report within 15 days any adverse drug reaction that leads to death, hospitalization, permanent disability, or need for drug therapy. Less virulent reactions must be reported "promptly," but the manufacturer is given a longer period to do so.[42] Manufacturers that do not comply with the reporting requirements are subject to increased liability.[43]

Without government regulation, drug companies

would have neither the incentive nor the ability to police their products in the market. Studies have shown that adverse reactions are grossly underreported by the medical establishment.[44] The reasons for not reporting adverse reactions are numerous. First is the inability to differentiate the adverse reaction from the symptoms of disease. Second is the general reluctance of doctors and patients to report problems.[45] Even after a drug has been proven harmful, the physician may still not wish to report adverse reactions because of fear of malpractice liability. For example, in the mid-1960s, it was estimated that 1700 deaths occurred due to the widespread use of an aerosol asthma medication. However, only six deaths were officially reported as caused by this medication.[46]

STRICT LIABILITY AND PHARMACEUTICALS
Strict liability as applied to pharmaceuticals

Most courts categorize rules of liability that apply to prescription drugs differently than rules for other products. Some courts have held that the rules of strict liability should not apply to some drugs.[47] Other courts apply a limited form of strict liability with less stringent rules applied to drugs. Still other courts do not differentiate between drugs and other manufactured products.[48]

The Restatement (Second) of Torts, Section 402A, comment k, views some drugs as "incapable of being made safe." For example, "the vaccine for the Pasteur treatment of rabies" often "leads to very serious and damaging consequences when it is injected." Such a drug is "properly prepared, and accompanied by proper directions and warning, is not defective, nor is it *unreasonably* dangerous."[49] Comment k does not seek to prevent all suits against drug manufacturers. Although it protects drug manufacturers against liability for design defects, it does not immunize them against suits for manufacturing defects or inadequate warnings.[50]

Multiple policy considerations are behind the adoption of strict liability in torts. Some of these include compensation or spreading of the loss between all consumers of a product, deterrence, encouraging useful conduct by both parties to an action, protecting consumer expectations, and improving the allocation of resources.[51] Multiple approaches have been used by the courts in the development of the concept of defectiveness. One approach is the consumer expectation test,[52] which weighs whether a product is unreasonably dangerous beyond that contemplated by the ordinary consumer. This test has fallen from favor in a majority of courts because it relies on the term "unreasonable" as a requirement of defectiveness. Reasonableness is a negligence concept.[53] If a danger is one generally known to the ordinary consumer, then the product is not per se defective.[54]

Another approach is the risk/utility test.[55] This is a balancing test between the risk of danger associated with a product and the utility of the product to the consumer. It is the most used approach to determine defectiveness.[56] The emphasis is on the safety of the product rather than on the reasonable or unreasonable action of the manufacturer.[57] Some of the factors considered in a risk/utility analysis include the severity of the risk, the likelihood of harm, the benefits of the product, and the feasibility of an alternative design.[58] Once a product is determined to be dangerous, the court then must balance the product's utility against its dangers. Many courts refuse to classify a drug as unreasonably dangerous if the drug's utility to mankind is viewed as greater than the potential for injury to an individual.[59]

Lastly, some jurisdictions offer an alternative test that utilizes a bifurcated standard: either consumer expectation or risk/utility.[60] Use of the disjunctive expands recovery potential for plaintiffs.[61]

Types of defects

We now take a look at types of defects. First, a manufacturing defect might cause one "batch" of the drug to deviate from the norm. Second, a design defect could exist, such as a basic intrinsic flaw in the chemical design.

Manufacturing defects. Manufacturing defects are those that deviate from the manufacturer's design or specifications and thus are different than the usual product that "comes off the assembly line."[62] Manufacturing defects are usually easy to identify because the products are flawed. Even though the cause of the manufacturing defect is usually negligence, difficulty in proof requires a strict liability standard, without regard to the manufacturer's reasonableness in protecting its process from error.[63] The consumer expectation test is utilized because the consumer expects a product to be free of defects.[64]

As an industry, pharmaceutical manufacturers have maintained a good record of keeping manufacturing defects to a minimum. From 1966 to 1971, the FDA ordered 1935 drug recalls for mistaken labeling, contamination, adulteration, or incorrect dosage.[65] Apart from the sulfanilamide disaster,[66] there have been few episodes of death or disability due to manufacturing defects.[67]

Design defects. Whereas a manufacturing defect involves an isolated deviation from the norm, a design defect involves the entire line of products. The product is manufactured according to specifications but remains unreasonably dangerous for its intended use.[68] Difficulty in determining a design defect situation arises when the courts attempt to define "reasonable danger."[69]

If a design is found to be defective, then all of the

products manufactured using that design will be defective. The evaluation of design defect by the jury is based on a four-prong test: (1) feasibility of an alternative design (2) at the time of the manufacture that was (3) commercially available and (4) would not destroy the product's productivity.[70]

Some courts hold that the "FDA's decision of product marketability disposes of the defect issue."[71] These courts conclude that if the FDA disapproves a product, "the product must be considered unavoidably unsafe as a matter of law and thus outside the parameters of strict liability for defective design."[72]

Occasionally, the government accepts responsibility for drug defects. In 1976, the government statutorily accepted liability for any adverse reactions to the swine flu immunization program.[73] The government took the position of the manufacturer for the purpose of liability.[74] This legislation was repealed in 1978.[75] A similar program of "no-fault" compensation was created by the National Childhood Vaccine Injury Act.[76] This legislation has a dual purpose. First, it allows easier access to compensation for those children who have suffered hypersensitivity reactions to vaccines.[77] Second, it provides liability protection for manufacturers of the vaccine to allow them to continue their production.[78]

Warning

Manufacturer's duty to warn. Products that are both properly designed and correctly manufactured may still be dangerous and will be considered defective if not accompanied by a proper warning.[79] The supplier of any product, including the manufacturer of pharmaceuticals, is under a duty to use reasonable care to warn adequately about the risks associated with the use of its product.[80] This duty extends to the risks about which the manufacturer actually knows and to those which, through reasonable care, it should have known.[81]

The duty of a pharmaceutical manufacturer to warn arises when the product is known to cause a particular side effect. The manufacturer is not responsible for unforeseeable or unknown dangers it is unable to discover with reasonable care.[82] Nor is the company a guarantor of the safety of a product that causes an unusual hypersensitivity reaction if that reaction was not known to be a side effect of the product.[83]

The "unavoidably dangerous" protection afforded prescription drugs under the Restatement (Second) of Torts, Section 402A, comment k, is available unless the manufacturer has provided an adequate warning of potential adverse reactions.[84] The protection is not available to those manufacturers who have failed to follow FDA guidelines for testing and marketing of their product.[85]

Drugs are an exception to the rule requiring a warning

of danger to the ultimate consumer.[86] The drug manufacturer's duty to warn includes a warning to physicians of the special risks that accompany normal use.[87] In the majority of cases, there is no duty to warn the patient directly.[88] For the sake of pharmaceutical warnings, the physician is considered the "learned intermediary"[89] and as such the duty to warn, in most instances, ends when an adequate effort is made by the company to instruct physicians of the drug's potential side effects.[90] The pharmaceutical manufacturer has no obligation to warn the ultimate user of danger propensities "where there is an intermediary who is not a mere conduit of the product, but rather administers it on an individual basis."[91] After the manufacturer gives the physician the necessary information, it is then the duty of the doctor to warn the patient.[92]

The manufacturer's duty to warn does not end with the purchase of the drug by the patient. Post-sale warnings are also required. The manufacturer is considered an expert with regard to its product.[93] As an expert, the manufacturer has the duty to stay abreast of the scientific data in the field and the further duty to warn physicians of potential harm caused by the product.[94]

Should an unknown hazard be discovered after the drug has been sold, the manufacturer is required to make reasonable efforts to inform the consumer.[95] This requirement is usually satisfied with warnings to physicians in the form of "Dear Doctor" letters[96] or via detail persons. One court has said that "[a]lthough a product be reasonably safe when manufactured . . . risks thereafter revealed by user operation and brought to the attention of the manufacturer or vendor may impose upon one or both a duty to warn."[97]

The manufacturer is responsible for performing studies of its product when adverse reactions are reported. The results of these studies, if adverse to the product, must be reported to the public (i.e., doctors).[98] This duty to report new adverse findings extends to more than the research of the manufacturer and includes all industry knowledge (i.e., state of the art). Constructive knowledge of potential side effects is presumed with the publication of articles in scientific journals that relate to the product.[99]

Although the duty of drug manufacturers to provide warnings usually extends only to the physician,[100] in cases where the manufacturer knows that the product will reach the public without individualized medical intervention, the drug manufacturer must also warn the public at large.[101] Such an example is immunizations, where everyone is given a standardized dose of the vaccine without individualized dosing by the physician.[102] Likewise, birth control pills are given out without much individual attention. Therefore, no protection exists for the drug producer under the learned intermediary rule in situations where the manufacturer had actual or constructive knowledge of the potential for the public to acquire the product without significant physician intervention.[103]

Adequacy of warning. Adequacy of the warning is a major issue in determining reasonableness. If the warning is adequate, then the defendant drug producer will usually prevail, even if the product is unavoidably unsafe.[104] Adequacy of the warning is achieved when it is obviously displayed, when it gives a fair appraisal of the extent of the danger, and when it properly instructs the user in how to use the product.[105] Likewise, a warning is adequate when it "warns with the degree of intensity demanded by the nature of the risk."[106] A warning, however, may be inadequate if it is "unduly delayed, reluctant in tone or lacking in a sense of urgency."[107]

Even if an adequate warning is given of the risk, it will not insulate the manufacturer from liability when a cure for the defect could have been accomplished with little effort. Moreover, the value of an adequate warning may be diminished by statements that lead the user to minimize the importance of the warning. For example, a warning of one manufacturer concerning birth control pills contained studies showing an increased incidence of thrombosis in British women. The court held that having a study dealing with British women did little to amplify concern of thrombosis in American women and therefore did not adequately warn this group.[108]

In addition, most courts require warnings to be given if an allergic reaction may affect a substantial number of people.[109] Some courts have required a duty to warn of rare adverse reactions if the end result would be exceedingly serious.[110] The Restatement (Second) of Torts states that "[W]here . . . the product contains an ingredient to which a substantial number of the population are allergic . . . the seller is required to give warning . . . and a product bearing such a warning, which is safe for use if it is followed, is not in defective condition, nor is it unreasonably dangerous."[111]

Methods of warning. Warnings may be satisfied in a number of ways. Labeling package inserts, advertising, and interaction with drug company detail persons may all act as adequate warnings to decrease liability.

LABELING. The FDA has numerous requirements for the labeling of pharmaceuticals.[112] These are minimum requirements only and do not relieve the manufacturer of its duty to fully warn of dangers for which it has actual or constructive knowledge.[113] The basic labeling regulation as promulgated by the FDA is that all material facts relating to the drugs are to be presented on the package.[114]

PACKAGE INSERTS. The package insert is the method developed by the FDA for instructing physicians and patients about the makeup, side effects, indications, and dosing of the product.[115] The most important feature of the package insert is the requirement that the information contained therein is completely based on substantial evidence. No "hype" or promotion is permitted to be included. Because physicians have almost unlimited access to drug information through a variety of sources, the package insert is not intended to be the most current repository of information concerning the benefits of a drug. Instead, it has the purpose of informing the physician of any substantial evidence that has been found relating to the drug's benefits or side effects.[116]

The package insert contains information based on data submitted to the FDA by the manufacturer dealing with the safety and efficacy of the drug.[117] A physician is not required to follow the instructions on the package insert. If the doctor chooses not to do so, he or she may be concerned about increased liability.[118] This fear leads many physicians to practice cookbook medicine (i.e., following the product insert instructions implicitly without regard to the patient's individual reactions). However, in general, most physicians are not the dispenser of drugs and so they do not see the product inserts, which can be problematic. Likewise, although pharmacists have access to inserts, they usually rely on computer data for the majority of their product information.

Some courts construe a manufacturer's failure to comply with rules requiring package inserts as constituting negligence per se.[119] Other courts have held that failure to follow statutory regulation concerning inserts is not a controlling issue.[120]

ADVERTISING. Emphasis on product promotion is one of the more controversial actions of the pharmaceutical industry. Manufacturers spend more than one-fourth of their gross income from drug sales on marketing.[121] The majority of this money is spent on advertising and detail persons. The Pharmaceutical Manufacturers Association, realizing the importance of this issue, has promulgated the *Code of Fair Practices in the Promotion of Drug Products.*[122] But, as with many such professional ethical codes, the written word is often overlooked for an improved bottom line.

Drug manufacturers are the dominant, if not the only, source of information about drug risks and benefits for most prescribing physicians. Other independent sources of information, such as medical journals, may be reluctant to publish research criticizing products of drug manufacturers because drug advertising makes up the largest share of the medical journal revenue.[123]

Courts have held drug manufacturers liable for advertisements that dilute proper warnings or reduce reliance of the physician on a package insert.[124] Courts have held that a company incurs liability if it causes a prescribing physician to disregard the warnings that are mandated by the FDA.[125] Some courts have held the manufacturer liable, even when the physician acted in a negligent manner, if the physician's actions were induced through overpromotion.[126]

Drug manufacturers may be held to a warranty standard based on advertising.[127] Drug manufacturers rarely expose themselves to liability by expressly warranting their products.[128] Instead, exposure to breach of warranty liability most often arises through implied warranty and misrepresentation.[129]

DETAIL PERSONS. Detail persons, the sales representatives of ethical drugs, occupy a position different than that of other salespersons. Their potential misrepresentation of the product, rather than being harmless fluff, may lead to death or disfigurement of the ultimate consumer. Detail persons, acting as the liaison between physicians and manufacturer, are the most common transmitters of new information concerning pharmaceuticals. The pharmaceutical industry employs almost 40,000 detail persons.[130]

Detail persons are frequently torn between a desire to increase the substantial profits of the drug manufacturer[131] and a duty to inform the physician of product side effects and possible contraindications. Great potential exists for detail persons to mislead physicians in order to increase sales. Manufacturers are vicariously liable for the actions of the detail persons which are within the scope of their employment.[132] Some courts have held that the liability extends even beyond the scope of employment.[133] An otherwise adequate warning provided by the company can be nullified by an overzealous detail person. High-pressure sales by intense, occasionally knowledgeable, detail persons often determine physician-use patterns. Even though the oral communications of detail persons are difficult to monitor as to completeness or accuracy, drug companies cannot escape liability for improper overpromotion of safety by detail persons.[134]

If the detail person convinces the doctor to disregard warnings provided by the manufacturer, the company may be held liable as to the cause of the injury.[135] At least one court has held that detail persons have a duty to warn of potential adverse reactions.[136] Liability is possible because the doctor might otherwise have been aware of the risks that were involved had the detail persons given adequate warnings.[137]

Causation

As in negligence actions, causation must be proved in strict tort liability. Professor Prosser states that "[s]trict liability eliminates both privity and negligence; but it still does not prove the plaintiff's case."[138] The standard elements of proof, as enumerated in Section 402A of the Restatement (Second) of Torts, are, first, proof that the

product was defective; second, proof that the defect existed at the time it left the control of the defendant; third, proof that the defect created a product that was unreasonably dangerous for the intended or foreseeable use; and, fourth, proof that the defect caused the injury.[139] Within the pharmaceutical industry, the most common ways to prove causation are epidemiological and statistical studies, expert testimony, direct or circumstantial evidence, or a combination of these methods.[140]

In situations where the plaintiff is unable to identify the defective product's specific manufacturer, an industry-wide liability has been devised.[141] Liability may be imposed on every manufacturer of a generic product. It is then the responsibility of the various defendants to prove they did not supply the defective product.[142]

On the other hand, a design defect is easier to prove because all of the same type of drugs are equally defective and available for testing. In a failure to warn case, the plaintiff must prove that lack of proper warning was the proximate cause of the injury. The failure to warn must be the direct link between the product and the injury. The plaintiff must further show that the manufacturer either knew or should have known the danger of harm from the drug.[143] Defendant liability may be severed by the introduction of an intervening cause. In strict liability litigation, courts appear very willing to view intervening causes as being unforeseeable.[144]

Most courts view the terms "user" and "consumer" liberally. Historically, privity was required before permitting recovery. Today, a user may be far removed from the initial privity of contract.[145] If it is foreseeable that a person will be a user, then that person is a potential plaintiff.[146] If, for example, the patient were to ingest multiple drugs, then each drug might be viewed as a cause-in-fact of the subsequent harm. At least one court has held a manufacturer of one defective drug liable for the entire injury sustained by the ingestion of multiple drugs.[147]

The foreseeability of the harm caused by a product is an issue in many courts.[148] Some courts now reject the foreseeability of the harm approach and instead look to the foreseeability of the use.[149]

Physician and/or pharmacist liability

Many physicians and pharmacists are not fully informed of the potential side effects associated with the drugs they prescribe. One study revealed that less than 13% of drug use was evaluated as rational, 21.5% was considered questionable, and, amazingly, more than 65% was judged irrational.[150] Because of the prevalence of drugs in the treatment of patients, many malpractice cases could have pharmaceutical components.

The application of traditional liability rules to pharmaceutical manufacturers is problematic. For example, the defined consumer of prescription drugs is the physician, not the patient. The patient has little input into the drug selected by the physician. The physician holds a position as a "learned intermediary" and as such takes on some of the manufacturer's liability even in the case of product defect.[151]

Physicians and pharmacists who find themselves in a suit resulting from a defective product have some recourse.[152] There is a potential tort action against the manufacturers of the defective products for both the injury to the patient and for damage to reputation and earnings.[153] In many circumstances, this leads to plaintiffs playing one potential defendant against another.[154]

Defenses

Defenses to strict product liability differ from one jurisdiction to the next as discussed on the following subsections.

Assumption of the risk. The Restatement (Second) of Torts describes assumption of the risk as "the form of contributory negligence which consists of voluntary and unreasonable encounter of a known danger."[155] If the consumer knew of the product's defect but disregarded the danger and used the product, he or she is barred from seeking to recover against the defendant. The defendant must prove that the plaintiff knew and understood the danger and that the plaintiff "voluntarily and unreasonably" consented to being exposed to it.[156]

Assumption of the risk is an essential concept for pharmaceutical litigation defense. If adequate warning is given to the doctor and the doctor disregards these dangers, then the physician/patient has assumed some of the risk for potential adverse reactions.

Comparative fault. Comparative fault measures the plaintiff's fault in comparison to the manufacturer's fault and places a percentage value on each. Most states that have comparative negligence systems have applied a comparative fault scheme to strict tort liability litigation.[157] In a pure system, a plaintiff may recover the percent of damage caused by the defendant, regardless of the fault attributable to the plaintiff.[158]

The goal of strict tort liability is not to create in the manufacturer an insurer for product-induced injuries. Comparative fault provides more equity in allocating risks and preventing manufacturers and other consumers from sharing in the costs attributable to those who fail to use products carefully. Most courts that have permitted a comparative fault defense have also permitted defenses of assumption of the risk and misuse.[159] The jury is usually instructed to combine the percentage from each of these defenses and give the percentage of fault as the sum of the three.[160]

Product misuse. The defense of product misuse is permitted when the plaintiff has used a product for a purpose not reasonably foreseeable to the manufacturer.[161] The Restatement (Second) of Torts recognizes the defense of product misuse. Comment h of Section 402A provides that "If the injury results from abnormal handling . . . the seller is not liable."[162] The defense of misuse may be utilized if the plaintiff's misuse of the product was a contributing cause of the injury.[163] To use this defense, the plaintiff's misuse of the product must be unforeseeable.[164] The definition of "unforeseeable" is the important issue. Taking four times the standard dosage of a medication may be foreseeable, but five times may be unforeseeable. There is no standard, fixed, arbitrary cutoff. It is left for the fact-finder to determine foreseeability on a case-by-case basis.

Damages

Similar to negligence litigation, strict liability provides for property and personal damage recovery.[165] With both negligence and strict liability, damage is part of a *prima facia* case.[166]

Commentators have differed in their views of punitive damage awards in strict liability litigation. Some assert that punitive damage awards should be granted as punishment for wanton, willful, reckless, malicious, or "outrageous conduct."[167] Other jurisdictions grant punitive damage awards as a form of deterrence to others who might commit the same outrageous conduct.[168] Most jurisdictions use punitive damages for any combination of the preceding reasons.[169]

Punitive damage awards are common in strict liability litigation involving pharmaceutical products.[170] The plaintiff has the burden of proving the defendant's outrageous conduct by "clear and convincing proof."[171] Punitive damage awards serve to punish inappropriate manufacturing practices and to stop "product suppliers from making economic decisions, not to remedy the defects of the product."[172] The most common type of drug cases in which punitive damages are granted are those in which the manufacturer had knowledge of adverse reactions but failed to properly warn of the danger.[173]

CONCLUSION

The public should be free to purchase goods without fear of defect. Strict tort liability is a valid means to ensure that products function without injury. On the other hand, it is unreasonable for all products to be totally safe and risk free for consumers. A knife with a dull blade might be safer than one with a sharp blade, but part of the sharp knife's efficacy is due to the very cause of its dangerous propensity, namely, its sharpened edge. Ice cream would be safer without the heavy cholesterol content but the joy of eating it comes from its richness, which clogs our arteries. Medication is unique because it is ingested into the body with the knowledge that in a certain number of individuals there will be serious side effects.

It is true that drugs can be made safer, but, even so, certain idiosyncratic reactions will occur that will cause a few to suffer. The answer for those few individuals might be for the government or the manufacturer to set up a trust fund for such reactions, which could be drawn on when a severe reaction occurs. Rather than hamper the medical establishment with increased liability, the courts should take the forefront in the fight to provide a strong defense for drug manufacturers.

END NOTES

1. *Greenman v. Yuba Power Prod.,* 59 Cal 2d 57, 377 P.2d 897, 27 Cal. Rptr. 697 (1963); Restatement (Second) of Torts § 402A (1) (1965) provides: "One who sells any products in a defective condition unreasonably dangerous to the user or consumer or to his property is subject to liability for physical harm thereby caused . . . if (a) the seller is engaged in the business of selling such a product, and (b) it is expected to and does reach the user or consumer without substantial change in the condition in which it is sold."

2. *See Comment, DES and a Proposed Theory of Enterprise Liability,* 46 Fordham L. Rev. 963 (1978).

3. *See Wells v. Ortho Pharmaceutical Corp.,* 788 F.2d 741 (11th Cir. 1986), *cert. denied,* 479 U.S. 950 (1986).

4. Restatement (Second) of Torts § 402A cmt. k (1965). The Restatement defines unavoidably unsafe products as products "which, in the present state of human knowledge, are quite incapable of being made safe for their intended and ordinary use. These are especially common in the field of drugs . . . Such a product, properly prepared, and accompanied by proper directions and warning, is not defective, nor is it *unreasonably* dangerous."

5. *Id.*

6. Restatement (Second) of Torts § 402A, cmt k (1965) further provides: "The same is true of many other drugs, vaccines, and the like, many of which for this very reason cannot legally be sold except to physicians, or under the prescription of a physician. It is also true in particular of many new or experimental drugs as to which, because of lack of time and opportunity for sufficient medical experience, there cannot be assurance of safety, or perhaps even of purity of ingredients, but such experience as there is justifies the marketing and use of the drug notwithstanding a medically recognizable risk. The seller of such products, again with the qualification that they are properly prepared and marketed, and proper warning is given, where the situation calls for it, is not to be held strictly liable for unfortunate consequences attending their use, merely because he has undertaken to supply the public with an apparently useful and desirable product, attended with a known but apparently reasonable risk.

7. *See, e.g., McElhaney v. Eli Lilly & Co.,* 575 F. Supp. 228 (D.S.D. 1983).

8. *See infra* notes 81-82 and accompanying text.

9. *See, e.g.,* Scott, *Medical Product and Drug Causation: How to Prove It and Defend Against It,* 56 Def. Couns. J. 270 (1989); Leighton, *Introduction to the Symposium on Chemical and Food Product Liability,* 41 Food Drug Cosm. L.J. 385 (1986); Schwartz, *Unavoidably Unsafe Products,* 42 Wash. & Lee L. Rev. 1139 (1985).

10. McClellan, *Drug Induced Injury,* 25 Wayne L. Rev. 1 (1978); Maldonado, *Strict Liability and Informed Consent: 'Don't Say I Didn't Tell You So,'* 9 Akron L. Rev. 609 (1976); Merrill, *Compensation for Prescription Drug Injuries,* 59 Va. L. Rev. 1 (1973); Keeton, *Products Liability – Drugs and Cosmetics,* 25 Vand. L. Rev. 131 (1972).

11. Britain, *Product Honesty Is the Best Policy: A Comparison of Doctor's and Manufacturer's Duty to Disclose Drug Risks and the Importance of Consumer Expectations in Determining Product Defect,* 79 NW. U.L. Rev. 342 (1984); Fink, *Education in Pharmacy and Law,* 26 J. Legal Educ. 528, 538 (1974).

12. Many of the pharmaceutical firms are dependent on one to five of their products for the bulk of their profit. A company may produce 50 to 300 drugs but up to 50% of their profit may be produced by the one or two most profitable drugs. *See* Staudt, *Determining and Evaluating the Promotional Mix,* Modern Medicine Topics 8 (July 1957). Few products in this field have any definite assurance of future share in the market. For every 100 products introduced, only 8 will be among the best prescription sellers, another 7 to 10 will pay their own way, and more than 80 will fail. Up to 90% of the total company profit may be from the manufacture of the five top selling drugs.

13. For a competent evaluation of the history of the drug industry, *see* E. Ackerknecht, *Therapeutics from the Primitives to the 20th Century* (1973).

14. *Id.* at 144-45. Another major change that occurred in the pharmaceutical industry was the development of the transnational corporations. Global profit, rather than regional needs, would affect development, research, and marketing strategies. With these and other changes occurring, it became clear that more regulatory efforts would be needed to protect the citizenry.

15. *Id.* at 145. The few exceptions include Salvarsan (a cure for syphilis in Germany) in 1910, sulfonamides (antibiotics in Germany and France) in the late 1930s, and penicillin (an antibiotic in England) in the mid-1940s.

16. *Id.* at 30. Further advances in antibiotics (broad spectrum penicillins, tetracycline, erythromycin, and later the cephalosporins), tranquilizers, steroids, oral contraceptives, cardiac active agents, diabetic medicines, and diuretics all were developed and first utilized in the 1950s and 1960s.

17. U.N. Industrial Development Organization, *The Growth of the Pharmaceutical Industry in Developing Countries: Problems and Prospects,* at 23, U.N. Doc. ID/204, U.N. Sales No. E.78.II.B.4 (1978). The drug market is broken down into over the counter (OTC) and prescription drugs. OTCs are those that are sold directly to the consumer without the need for physician contact. The drugs within this category vary from country to country. Prescription drugs are those that require an order of a physician prior to purchase. This category makes up the largest share of the overall dollar value of drug sales worldwide.

18. Halberstrom, *Too Many Drugs?* F. on Med., Mar. 1979, at 3. While no one knows exactly how many drugs are available on the ethical drug market, it is estimated that between 10,000 and 25,000 different drugs are available for sale.

19. Merck, Sharp & Dohme Research Laboratories, *supra* note 37, at 266. An allergen is any foreign substance capable of eliciting an allergic or hypersensitive response.

20. *Id.* at 270. Hypersensitivity is an exaggerated response to an allergen.

21. *Id.* at 265-287. An allergic reaction is a hypersensitivity to an allergen that builds with repeat exposure.

22. Tally & Laventurier, *Drug-Induced Illness,* 229 JAMA 1043 (1974).

23. *See, e.g.,* Restatement (Second) of Torts § 402A cmt. c (1965).
24. *See id.* at cmt. j (1965).
25. *See, e.g.,* Brochu v. Ortho Pharmaceutical Corp., 642 F.2d 652 (1st Cir. 1981).
26. *See, e.g.,* Johnson v. American Cyanamid Co., 239 Kan. 279, 285, 718 P.2d 1318, 1323 (1986).
27. Ch. 3915, Pub. L. No. 59-384, 34 Stat. 768 (codified as amended in scattered sections of 21 U.S.C. (1982)). This legislation was influenced by the work of the Muckrakers. The Muckrakers were authors who believed government should protect workers from big business. One such author, Upton Sinclair, heavily influenced passage of the Federal Pure Food and Drugs Act. *See generally* A. Craven and W. Johnson, *The United States: Experiment in Democracy* 519-21 (1947).
28. § 1, 34 Stat. 768. ("[I]t shall be unlawful for any person to manufacture . . . any article of food or drug which is adulterated or misbranded. . . ."). *See generally* J. H. Young, *The Toadstool Millionaires: A Social History of Patent Medicines in America Before Federal Regulation* 205-44 (1972).
29. § 8, 34 Stat. 770.
30. Ch. 675, Pub. L. 75-717, 52 Stat. 1040.
31. Drug Amendments of 1962, § 102, Pub. L. 87-781, 76 Stat. 781.
32. Sherman & Strauss, *Thalidomide: A Twenty-Five Year Perspective,* 41 Food Drug Cosm. L.J. 458, 458 (1986). Thalidomide, a medication given to thousands of pregnant women in Europe, caused hundreds of severe birth defects. This drug was in the process of gaining access into the American market when the European findings were brought to the attention of the public.
33. *See* Janssen, *Outline of the History of U.S. Drug Regulation,* 36 Food Drug Cosm. L.J. 420, 439 (1981).
34. *See generally* Safir, *FDA Regulations and Product Liability,* 36 Food Drug Cosm. L.J. 478 (1981); Ryan v. Eli Lilly & Co., 514 F. Supp. 1004 (D.S.C. 1981); Henteleff, *Interrelationships of FDA Laws and Regulations with Products Liability Issues,* 32 Bus. Law 1029 (1977).
35. *See, e.g.,* Blum, *High Stakes: Wonder Drugs Are the Focus of Criminal, Civil Actions; Patients Sue Makers of Psychotropic Drugs,* Nat'l L.J., Oct. 22, 1990, at 1 (LEXIS, Nexis , Omni file).
36. Strickland & Bolar, *A Drug Company Under Siege,* N.Y. Times, Oct. 15, 1989, § 12LI, at 1, col. 3 (LEXIS, Nexis, Omni file). For example, the maker of the generic form of the drug Dyazide was accused of falsifying test data and of paying bribes to FDA inspectors.
37. 21 C.F.R. § 314.1 (1990). This process occurs as follows: (1) Discovery phase: Basic research leads to the synthesis of a new chemical. This phase includes early studies of the compound's chemical properties. (2) Pre-clinical animal testing: A short-term animal toxicity testing for evidence of safety. Tests required at this stage include pharmacodynamics, endocrinology, metabolism, toxicology, and teratology studies. (3) Investigational New Drug (IND) filing: A request is made for authorization to begin human testing. (4) Phase I human testing: Dosage is administered to healthy volunteers for evidence of toxicity in humans. (5) Phase II human testing: Dosage is administered to humans with a particular pathological condition. (6) Phase III human testing: Large-scale tests on humans are performed over a longer period to uncover unanticipated side-effects. (7) Long-term animal studies: To determine the effects of prolonged exposures and the effects on subsequent generations. (8) New drug application: Application for commercial marketing.
38. Ryan v. Eli Lilly & Co., 514 F. Supp. 1004 (D.S.C. 1981). *But see* Stromsodt v. Parke-Davis & Co., 257 F. Supp. 991 (D.N.D. 1966), *aff'd,* 411 F.2d 1390 (8th Cir. 1969).
39. Hoffman v. Sterling Drug, 485 F.2d 132 (3d Cir. 1973).
40. Faich, Knapp, Dreis & Turner, *National Adverse Drug Reaction Surveillance: 1985,* 257 JAMA 2068, 2068 (1987). There were more than 37,000 reports of adverse reactions in 1985.
41. *See* Sills, Faich, Milstein & Turner, *Postmarketing Reporting of ADRs to FDA: An Overview of the 1985 Guideline,* 20 Drug Info. J. 150 (1986).
42. 21 C.F.R. § 314.80 (c)(1) (1990).
43. *Id.* at (k).
44. Faich, *Adverse Drug Experience Reporting and Product Liability,* 41 Food Drug Cosm. L.J. 444 (1986).
45. Merrill, *Compensation for Prescription Drug Injuries,* 59 Va. L. Rev. 1, 50-68 (1973).
46. H. Teff & C. Munro, *Thalidomide: The Legal Aftermath* 109 (1976).
47. *See, e.g.,* Johnson v. American Cyanamid Co., 239 Kan. 279, 285, 718 P.2d 1318, 1323 (1986). (*quoting* Restatement (Second) of Torts § 402A cmt. k (1965)).
48. *See, e.g.,* Brochu v. Ortho Pharmaceutical Corp., 642 F.2d 652 (1st Cir. 1981).
49. Restatement (Second) of Torts § 402A cmt. k (1965) (emphasis in original).
50. *Id.*
51. For an excellent discussion of the policies underlying strict liability, *see* D. Fisher & W. Powers Jr., *Products Liability: Cases and Materials* 50-51 (1988).
52. Restatement (Second) of Torts § 402A cmt. g (1965), which provides: "The rule stated in this Section applies only where the product is, at the time it leaves the seller's hands, in a condition not contemplated by the ultimate consumer, which will be unreasonably dangerous to him. The seller is not liable when he delivers the product in a safe condition, and subsequent mishandling or other causes make it harmful by the time it is consumed. The burden of proof that the product was in a defective condition at the time that it left the hands of the particular seller is upon the injured plaintiff; and unless evidence can be produced which will support the conclusion that it was then defective, the burden is not sustained."
53. Restatement (Second) of Torts § 395 (1965), which provides: "A manufacturer who fails to exercise reasonable care in the manufacturer of a chattel which, unless carefully made, he should recognize as involving an unreasonable risk of causing physical harm to those who use it for a purpose for which the manufacturer should expect it to be used . . . is subject to liability for physical harm caused to them by its lawful use . . ."
54. *Id.* at § 402A cmt. i (1965) (emphasis added). Comment i provides: "The rule stated in this Section applies only where the defective condition of the product makes it unreasonably dangerous to the user or consumer. . . . The article sold must be dangerous *to an extent beyond that which would be contemplated by the ordinary consumer* who purchases it, with the ordinary knowledge common to the community as to its characteristics."
55. *See, e.g.,* Boutland of Houston, Inc. v. Bailey, 609 S.W.2d 743, 746 (Tex. 1980.) (A product must be judged for defectiveness at the time of the harm and based on technology then available).
56. *See, e.g.,* Phillips v. Kimwood Mach. Co., 269 Or. 485, 525 P.2d 1033 (1974); Dosier v. Wilcox-Crittendon, Co., 45 Cal. App. 3d 74, 119 Cal. Rptr. 135 (1975).
57. *See* Britain, *supra* note 25.
58. Wade, *On the Nature of Strict Tort Liability for Products,* 44 Miss. L.J. 825, 829 (1973).
59. *See contra* Brochu v. Ortho Pharmaceutical Corp., 642 F.2d 652 (1st Cir. 1981).
60. Barker v. Lull Engineering Co., 20 Cal. 3d 413, 573, P.2d 443, 143 Cal. Rptr. 225, (1978) (permitting the use of either the consumer expectation test or the risk/utility test).
61. D. Fischer & W. Powers Jr., *supra* note 89, at 91.

62. *Barker v. Lull Engineering Co.,* 20 Cal 3d 413, 429, 573 P.2d 443, 459, 143 Cal. Rptr. 225, 241 (1978) (permitting the use of either the consumer expectation test or the risk/utility test).

63. D. Fischer & W. Powers Jr., *supra* note 89, at 1.

64. *See* Britain, *supra* note 25.

65. M. Silverman & P. Lee, *Pills, Profits and Politics* 333 (1974).

66. A batch of sulfanilamide was improperly mixed with a lethal solvent causing the death of many patients during the 1950s. J. Schnze, *Governmental Control of Therapeutic Drugs: Intent, Impact, and Issues,* in The Pharmaceutical Industry 9-10 (C. Lindsay ed. 1978). For a competent evaluation of the history of the drug industry, *see* G. Porter and H. Livesay, *Merchants and Manufacturer: Studies in the Changing Structure of the Nineteenth Century Marketing* (1971).

67. *Id.*

68. Comment, *Can a Prescription Drug be Defectively Designed?: Brochu v. Ortho Pharmaceutical Corp.,* 31 De Paul L. Rev. 247 (1981).

69. Birnbaum, *Unmasking the Test for Design Defect: From Negligence [to Warranty] to Strict Liability to Negligence,* 33 Vand L. Rev. 593 (1980).

70. Isaacs, *Drug Regulation, Product Liability, and the Contraceptive Crunch: Choices Are Dwindling,* 8 J. of Leg. Med. 533 (1987) (strict liability and duty to warn).

71. *See, e.g., Collins v. Ortho Pharmaceutical Corp.,* 195 Cal. App. 3d 1539, 231 Cal. Rptr. 396 (1986).

72. *Id.* 231 Cal. Rptr., at 404.

73. National Swine Flu Immunization Program of 1976, Pub. L. No. 94-380, 90 Stat. 1113; *see also Ducharme v. Merrill-Nat'l Labs.,* 574 F.2d 1307 (5th Cir.), *cert. denied,* 439 U.S. 1002 (1978).

74. 90 Stat. 1116.

75. Health and Services Amendments of 1978, Pub. L. 95-626, 92 Stat. 3551.

76. Pub. L. 99-660, 100 Stat. 3755 (codified at 42 U.S.C. §§ 300aa-1 to -33 (1986)).

77. 100 Stat. 3758 (codified at 42 U.S.C. § 300aa-10 (1988)).

78. 100 Stat. 3758-59 (codified at 42 U.S.C. § 300aa-11 (1988)).

79. *See, e.g., Basko v. Sterling Drug,* 416 F.2d 417, 426 (2d Cir. 1969). ("[T]here is no strict liability...unless the consumer first establishes a breach of the manufacturer's duty to warn...by showing either (1) that the manufacturer did not warn of a known danger, or (2) that the manufacturer gave inadequate warnings."); *see also Jacobson v. Colorado Fuel & Iron Corp.,* 409 F.2d 1263, 1271 (9th Cir. 1969).

80. Restatement (Second) of Torts § 12 (1965) defines this knowledge requirement as follows: "(1) The words "reason to know" are used throughout the Restatement...to denote the fact that the actor has information from which a person of reasonable intelligence or of the superior intelligence of the actor would infer that the fact in question exists, or that such person would govern his conduct upon the assumption that such fact exists. (2) The words "should know" are used throughout the Restatement...to denote the fact that a person of reasonable prudence and intelligence or of the superior intelligence of the actor would ascertain the fact in question in the performance of his duty to another, or would govern his conduct upon the assumption that such fact exists."

81. *See, e.g., Lindsay v. Ortho Pharmaceutical Corp.,* 637 F.2d 87 (2d Cir. 1980); *Sterling Drug, Inc., v. Cornish,* 370 F.2d 82 (8th Cir. 1966); *Incollingo v. Ewing,* 444 Pa. 263, 282 A.2d 206 (1971), *rev'd on other grounds,* 491 Pa. 561, 421 A.2d 79 (1977).

82. *Griggs v. Combe, Inc.,* 456 So. 2d 790 (Ala. 1984); *Freeman v. United States,* 704 F.2d 154 (5th Cir. 1983).

83. *Gravis v. Parke, Davis & Co.,* 502 S.W. 2d 863 (Tex Civ. App. 1973).

84. *Davila v. Bodelson,* 103 N.M. 243, 704 P.2d 1119 (App. 1985).

85. *Id.*

86. *See, e.g., Buckner v. Allergan Pharmaceuticals,* 400 So. 2d 820 (Fla. Dist. Ct. App. 1981); *Lindsay v. Ortho Pharmaceutical Corp.,* 637 F.2d 87 (2d Cir. 1980). *Id.* at 91. "[T]he manufacturer's duty is to warn the doctor, not the patient. The doctor acts as an 'informed intermediary' between the manufacturer and the patient, evaluating the patient's needs, assessing the risks and benefits of available drugs, prescribing one, and supervising its use."

87. *See, e.g., Fellows v. USV Pharmaceutical Corp.,* 502 F. Supp. 297 (D. Md. 1980) (The manufacturer has a duty to provide warnings to physician but the duty does not extend to the patient); *Ezagui v. Dow Chemical Corp.,* 598 F.2d 727 (2d Cir. 1979).

88. *See, e.g., Fellows,* 502 F. Supp. at 297.

89. In *Reyes v. Wyeth Laboratories,* 498 F.2d 1264 (5th Cir.), *cert. denied,* 419 U.S. 1096 (1974), the court gives an excellent definition of the learned intermediary doctrine. *Id.* at 1276. "[W]here prescription drugs are concerned, the manufacturer's duty to warn is limited to an obligation to advise the prescribing physician of any potential dangers that may result from the drug's use.... As a medical expert, the prescribing physician can take into account the propensities of the drug, as well as the benefits of any medication against its potential dangers.... Pharmaceutical companies...in selling prescription drugs are required to warn only the prescribing physician, who acts as a 'learned intermediary' between manufacturer and consumer."

90. *See Leesley v. West,* 165 Ill. App. 3d 135, 518 N.E.2d 758 (App. Ct.), *appeal denied,* 119 Ill. 2d 558, 522 N.E.2d 1246 (1988); *Stone v. Smith, Kline & French Laboratories,* 447 So.2d 1301 (Ala. 1984); *Mauldin v. Upjohn Co.,* 697 F.2d 644 (5th Cir. 1983).

91. *Bacardi v. Holzman,* 182 N.J. Super. 422, 424, 448 A.2d 617, 618 (1981) (The learned intermediary doctrine protects a prescription drug manufacturer even where the manufacturer knew that the physician might not warn the patient).

92. *See Crain v. Allison,* 443 A.2d 558, 562 (D.C. App. 1982); *Salis v. United States,* 522 F. Supp. 989, 1000 (M.D. Pa. 1981).

93. *Barson v. E.R. Squibb & Sons,* 682 P.2d 832 (Utah 1984).

94. *Id.* at 834 (*citing McEwan v. Ortho Pharmaceutical Corp.,* 270 Or. 375, 528 P.2d 522 (1974)) (actual or constructive knowledge is required).

95. *Schenebeck v. Sterling Drug,* 423 F.2d 919 (8th Cir. 1970).

96. *See* Appendix C for an example of a "Dear Doctor" letter.

97. *Cover v. Cohen,* 61 N.Y.2d 261, 268, 461 N.E.2d 864, 871, 473 N.Y.S.2d 378, 385 (1984) (citations omitted).

98. *See Schenebeck v. Sterling Drug,* 423 F.2d 919 (8th Cir. 1970); *O'Hare v. Merck & Co.,* 381 F.2d 286 (8th Cir. 1967).

99. *Feldman v. Lederle Laboratories,* 97 N.J. 429, 479 A.2d 374 (1984); *see also* Gilhooley, *Learned Intermediaries, Prescription Drugs, and Patient Information,* 30 St. Louis L.J. 633 (1986).

100. *See Brochu v. Ortho Pharmaceutical Corp.,* 642 F.2d 652 (1st Cir. 1981); *Dyer v. Best Pharmacal,* 118 Ariz. 465, 577 P.2d 1084 (Ct. App. 1978).

101. *See Reyes v. Wyeth Laboratories,* 498 F.2d 1264 (5th Cir.), *cert. denied,* 419 U.S. 1096 (1974); *Davis v. Wyeth Laboratories,* 399 F.2d 121 (9th Cir. 1968). This is the standard in vaccines and mass immunizations.

102. *Brazzell v. United States,* 788 F.2d 1352 (8th Cir. 1986).

103. *Williams v. Lederle Laboratories,* 591 F. Supp. 381 (S.D. Ohio 1984).

104. *Formella v. Ciba-Geigy Corp.,* 100 Mich. App. 649, 300 N.W.2d 356 (1980).

105. Madden, *The Duty to Warn in Products Liability: Contours and Criticism,* 89 W. Va. L. Rev. 221, 310-20 (1987); *Richards v. Upjohn Co.,* 95 N.M. 675, 679, 625 P.2d 1192, 1196 (Ct. App. 1980). To be considered adequate:
1. the warning must adequately indicate the scope of the danger;

2. the warning must reasonably communicate the extent or seriousness of the harm that could result from misuse of the drug;

3. the physical aspects of the warning must be adequate to alert a reasonably prudent person to the danger;

4. a simple directive warning may be inadequate when it fails to indicate the consequences that might result from failing to follow it; and . . .

5. the means to convey the warning must be adequate.

106. *Seley v. G.D. Searle & Co.*, 67 Ohio St. 2d 192, 198, 423 N.E.2d 831, 837 (1981).

107. *Id.*

108. *McEwan v. Ortho Pharmaceutical Corp.*, 570 Or. 375, 528 P.2d 522 (1974).

109. *Kaempfe v. Lehn & Fink Prods. Corp.*, 21 A.D.2d 197, 249 N.Y.S.2d 840 (App. Div. 1964), *aff'd*, 20 N.Y.2d 818, 231 N.E.2d 294, 284 N.Y.S.2d 818 (1967).

110. *Tomer v. American Home Prod. Corp.*, 170 Conn. 681, 368 A.2d 35 (1976); *Crocker v. Winthrop Laboratories*, 514 S.W.2d 429 (Tex. 1974) (Drug manufacturers must properly warn of rare adverse reactions if they may be severe).

111. Restatement (Second) of Torts § 402A (1965).

112. 21 C.F.R. § 201 (1990).

113. *Feldman v. Lederle Laboratories*, 97 N.J. 429, 479, A.2d 374 (1984).

114. 21 C.F.R. § 201.5–.10 (1990) ("Labeling of a . . . drug . . . shall be deemed to be misleading if it fails to reveal facts that are . . . material.").

115. *Pharmaceutical Mfr. Ass'n. v. Food & Drug Admin.*, 484 F. Supp. 1179 (D. Del. 1980).

116. *Id.* at 1186. The court in *Pharmaceutical Manufacturers Ass'n* stated that "Congress intended patients using prescription drugs, as well as those using over-the-counter drugs, to receive 'facts material with respect to consequences which may result from the use . . .' When it is determined that the possible side effects of a drug when used as customarily prescribed are sufficiently serious as to be material to the patient's decision on use of the drug, [the FDA] may require disclosure of those side effects on the labeling."

117. 21 C.F.R. § 201.5 (1990).

118. *Ohligschlager v. Proctor Community Hosp.*, 55 Ill. 2d 411, 303 N.E.2d 392 (1973) (The court held that the physician's deviation from the package insert constituted negligence.).

119. *Lukaszewicz v. Ortho Pharmaceutical Corp.*, 510 F. Supp. 961, *amended*, 532 F. Supp. 211 (E.D. Wis. 1981).

120. *See MacDonald v. Ortho Pharmaceutical Corp.*, 394 Mass. 131, 475 N.E.2d 65 (1985), *cert. denied*, 474 U.S. 920 (1985).

121. Harrell, *Pharmaceutical Marketing, in The Pharmaceutical Industry* 80 (C. Lindsay ed. 1978).

122. *See* Appendix D.

123. *See* S. Greenberg, *The Quality of Mercy* 267-83 (1971).

124. *Love v. Wolf*, 226 Cal. App. 2d 378, 38 Cal. Rptr. 183 (1964). *Wolf*, 226 Cal. App. at 399-400, 38 Cal. Rptr. at 196 (citation omitted). The court stated: "[I]f such over-prescription by the doctor was not caused by the over-promotion of Parke-Davis, then, however negligent such over-promotion may have been, Parke-Davis could not be held liable. Its negligence would not have been an inducing, or proximate, cause of the resulting injuries. Dr. Wolf's negligence would have been an intervening, independent, and solely proximate cause. . . . On the other hand, if the over-promotion can reasonably be said to have induced the doctor to disregard the warnings previously given, the warning given is thereby withdrawn or cancelled, and if, furthermore, the jury could have found that the doctor here actually prescribed the drug to cure an infection for which the company's advertising or its detail men could actually have recommended its use, then the pharmaceutical company's negligence remains as an inducing cause coinciding with the negligence of the doctor to produce the result."

125. *See Toole v. Richardson-Merrell, Inc.*, 251 Cal. App. 2d 689, 60 Cal. Rptr. 398 (1967).

126. *See, e.g., Stevens v. Parke, Davis & Co.*, 9 Cal. 3d. 51, 507 P.2d 653, 107 Cal. Rptr. 45 (1973).

127. *Id.*

128. *But see Spiegel v. Saks 34th Street*, 43 Misc. 2d 1065, 252 N.Y.S.2d 852 (Sup. Ct. 1964), *aff'd*, 26 A.D.2d 660, 272 N.Y.S. 972 (1966).

129. *See supra* notes 115-116 and accompanying text. An implied warranty may be breached when a manufacturer fails to warn adequately of known dangers.

130. Pharmaceutical Manufacturers Association, *Prescription Drug Industry Fact Book* 56 (1986).

131. *See generally* J. Lidstone, *Marketing Planning for the Pharmaceutical Industry* (1987); R. Norris, *Pills, Pesticides and Profits* (1982).

132. Restatement (Second) of Agency § 229 (1958).

133. *See, e.g., Schering Corp. v. Cotlow*, 94 Ariz. 365, 385 P.2d 234 (1963).

134. Most physicians tolerate visits and direct sale attempts by detail persons in order to acquire samples of medications. Detail persons frequently use tactics of peer pressure ("all the doctors in this area are using my drug"), bribery ("if you do a study on 200 of your patients using my drug, then the company will award you an honorarium of a trip to Europe to continue your research"), and humiliation ("chiropractors are the only people still suggesting using the other medication") to push their product. Survey of doctors at MacDonald Health Center, Brigham Young University, March 1990 (on file at the BYU *Journal of Public Law* office).

135. *Stevens v. Parke-Davis & Co.*, 9 Cal. 3d. 51, 107 Cal. Rptr. 45, 507 P.2d 653 (1973).

136. *Incollingo v. Ewing*, 444 Pa. 263, 289, 282 A.2d. 206, 220 (1971), *rev'd on other grounds*, 491 Pa. 561, 421, A.2d 1027 (1977): "We think that whether or not the warnings on the cartons, labels and literature of Parke, Davis in use on the relevant years were adequate, and whether or not the printed words of warning were in effect canceled out and rendered meaningless in the light of the sales effort made by the detail men, were questions properly for the jury. Action designed to stimulate the use of a potentially dangerous product must be considered in testing the adequacy of a warning as to when and how the product should not be used; if detail men are an effective means of selling a product and explaining its nature, a jury could find that they also afforded an effective medium of conveying a warning.

137. *See, e.g., Schenebeck v. Sterling Drug*, 423 F.2d 919 (8th Cir. 1970); *Krug v. Sterling Drug, Inc.*, 416 S.W.2d 143 (Mo. 1967).

138. Prosser, *The Fall of the Citadel (Strict Liability to the Consumer)*, 50 Minn L. Rev. 791, 840 (1966).

139. Restatement (Second) of Torts § 402A (1965).

140. Middlekauff, *The Current Law Regarding Toxic Torts: Implications for the Food Industry*, 41 Food Drug Cosm. L.J. 387, 404-05 (1986).

141. Comment, *Industry Wide Liability*, 13 Suffolk U.L. Rev. 980 (1979); *Mulcahy v. Eli Lilly & Co.*, 386 N.W.2d 67 (Iowa 1986) (DES market share liability).

142. Comment, *The Market Share Theory: Sindell's Contribution to Industry Wide Liability*, 19 Hou. L. Rev. 107 (1982).

143. Restatement (Second) of Torts § 402A.

144. *See generally* D. Fischer & W. Powers Jr., *supra* note 89, at 409-11.

145. Restatement (Second) of Torts § 402A cmt. l (1965), which provides: "He may be a member of the family of the final purchaser, or his employee, or a guest at his table, or a mere donee from the purchaser. The liability stated is one in tort, and does not require any contractual relation, or privity of contract, between the plaintiff and defendant."

146. *Winnett v. Winnett*, 57 Ill. 2d 7, 310 N.E.2d 1 (1974).

147. *Basko v. Sterling Drug,* 416 F.2d 417 (2d Cir. 1969).

148. *Helene Curtis Indus. v. Pruitt,* 385 F.2d 841, 859-64 (5th Cir. 1967); *Bigbee v. Pacific Tel. & Tel. Co.,* 34 Cal. 3d 49, 665 P.2d 947, 192 Cal. Rptr. 857 (1983).

149. *See, e.g., Baker v. International Harvester Co.,* 660 S.W.2d 21 (Mo. Ct. App. 1983).

150. M. Silverman & P. Lee, *supra* note 103, at 289-90.

151. Comment, *Strict Tort Liability/Negligence/Prescription Drugs: A Pharmaceutical Company Owes No Duty to a Non-Patient Third Party to Warn Doctors or Hospitals of the Side Effects of a Drug and a Hospital or Doctor Owes No Duty to a Non-Patient Third Party to Warn a Patient of the Effects of a Prescription Drug,* 77 Ill. B.J. 227 (1988); Comment, *Torts—Duty to Warn—Incorrect Prescription of Unavoidably Unsafe Drugs,* 22 Kan. L. Rev. 281 (1984).

152. *See* Merrill, *Compensation for Prescription Drug Injuries,* 59 Va. L. Rev. 1, 50-68 (1973).

153. *See, e.g., Oksenholt v. Lederle Laboratories,* 294 Or. 213, 656 P.2d 293 (1982); Mobilia, *Allergic Reactions to Prescription Drugs: A Proposal for Compensation,* 48 Alb. L. Rev. 343, 364-65 (1984).

154. *See* Willig, *Physicians, Pharmacists, Pharmaceutical Manufacturers: Partners in Patient Care, Partners in Litigation?,* 37 Mercer L. Rev. 755 (1986).

155. Restatement (Second) of Torts § 402A cmt. n (1965).

156. *Smith v. Clayton & Lambert Mfg. Co.,* 488 F.2d 1345, 1349 (10th Cir. 1973).

157. *Daly v. General Motors Corp.,* 20 Cal. 3d 725, 575 P.2d 1162, 144 Cal. Rptr. 380 (1978).

158. *Mulherin v. Ingersoll-Rand Co.,* 628 P.2d 1301, 1303-04 (Utah 1981).

159. *See generally* Fischer, *Products Liability—Applicability of Comparative Negligence to Misuse and Assumption of the Risk,* 43 Mo. L. Rev. 643 (1978).

160. *See, e.g., Duncan v. Cessna Aircraft Co.,* 665 S.W.2d 414 (Tex. 1984).

161. *Perfection Paint & Color Co. v. Konduris,* 147 Ind. App. 106, 107, 258 N.E.2d 681, 682 (1970).

162. Restatement (Second) of Torts § 402A cmt. h (1965), which provides: "A product is not in a defective condition when it is safe for normal handling and consumption. If the injury results from abnormal handling, as where a bottled beverage is knocked against a radiator to remove the cap, or for abnormal preparation for use, as where too much salt is added to food, or from abnormal consumption, as where a child eats too much candy and is made ill, the seller is not liable. Where, however, he has reason to anticipate that danger may result from a particular use, as where a drug is sold which is safe only in limited doses, he may be required to give adequate warning of the danger (see Comment j), and a product sold without such warning is in a defective condition."

163. *Mulherin v. Ingersoll-Rand Co.,* 628 P.2d 1301, 1302 (Utah 1981).

164. *Id.*

165. *See* Restatement (Second) of Torts § 402A (1965).

166. *See generally* W. Prosser, *Law of Torts* § 96 (4th ed. 1971). A prima facie case of negligence requires a duty owed by the defendant to the plaintiff, breach of that duty, causation, and damages.

167. *See* Restatement (Second) of Torts § 908(2) (1965), which provides: "Punitive damages may be awarded for conduct that is outrageous, because of the defendant's evil motive or his reckless indifference to the rights of others. In assessing punitive damages, the trier of fact can properly consider the character of the defendant's act, the nature and extent of the harm to the plaintiff that the defendant caused or intended to cause and the wealth of the defendant."

168. *See, e.g., Malcolm v. Little,* 295 A.2d 711 (Del. 1972).

169. *See, e.g., Miller v. Watkins,* 200 Mont. 455, 653 P.2d 126 (1982); *Newton v. Standard Fire Ins. Co.,* 291 N.C. 105, 229 S.E.2d 297 (1976); *see also* W. Keeton, D. Dobbs, R. Keeton & D. Owen, *Prosser and Keeton on Torts,* § 2, at 9 (5th ed. 1984).

170. *See Hoffman v. Sterling Drug,* 485 F.2d 132, 144-47 (3d Cir. 1973).

171. *Acosta v. Honda Motor Co.,* 717 F.2d 828, 833 (3d Cir. 1983).

172. *Neal v. Carey Canadian Mines,* 548 F. Supp. 357 (E.D. Pa. 1982), *aff'd, Van Buskirk v. Carey Canadian Mines,* 791 F.2d 30 (3rd Cir. 1986).

173. *See G.D. Searle & Co. v. Superior Court,* 49 Cal. App. 3d 22, 122 Cal. Rptr. 218 (1975); *Roginsky v. Richardson-Merrell, Inc.,* 378 F.2d 832 (2d Cir. 1967); *Toole v. Richardson-Merrell, Inc.,* 251 Cal. App. 2d 689, 60 Cal. Rptr. 398 (1967).

CHAPTER 16 Antitrust

DAVID P. CLUCHEY, M.A., J.D.
EDWARD DAVID, M.D., J.D., F.C.L.M.

HISTORY AND INTRODUCTION
CONDUCT VIOLATIONS OF THE ANTITRUST LAWS
DEFENSES
ROBINSON-PATMAN ACT
FEDERAL TRADE COMMISSION
RECENT DEVELOPMENTS IN ANTITRUST AND HEALTH CARE REFORM

HISTORY AND INTRODUCTION

The principal objective of antitrust laws is the prohibition of practices that interfere with free competition in the marketplace. The design of these laws is intended to promote a vigorous competitive economy. Business is expected to compete on the basis of price, quality, and service. The antitrust laws oversee this competition:

The Sherman Act was designed to be a comprehensive charter of economic liberty aimed at preserving free and unfettered competition as the rule of trade. It rests on the premise that the unrestrained interaction of competitive forces will yield the best allocation of our economic resources, the lowest price, the highest quality and the greatest material progress. . . .[1]

The U.S. economy underwent far-reaching and significant change following the Civil War. Technological development and rapid industrialization led to the emergence of a complex economic system. The laissez-faire policy of government during this time led to the amassing of a vast economic power by individuals and certain large firms. Often this power was used to destroy smaller rivals, thus achieving market control.

The public response to this economic system was colored by the changing social conditions of urbanization and immigration. Many felt that business firms should not be permitted to accumulate such wealth and exercise such great control over economic conditions. Discontent was particularly prominent among farmers and workers. The specific targets of their outrage were the giant combinations that came to be called trusts. Chief among these was Standard Oil, apparently the first to use the trust device as a vehicle for merging business into a cohesive entity.[2] Various other trusts followed. The trust device as a legal entity was largely replaced after the turn of the century by the holding company, but the name "trust" remained.[3]

The last two decades of the nineteenth century saw the legal authorities in some states moving to break up some of these business combinations. By 1890, 14 states had constitutional provisions prohibiting monopolies and 13 states had antitrust statutes.[4] These statutes commonly outlawed "any contract, agreement, or combination" to fix "a common price." They also prohibited activity that tended to limit the amount of any product to be sold or manufactured. Although some success was realized, the state constitutional provisions and statutes were for the most part ineffective in controlling or breaking up the large business combinations of the day.[5] This was due in part to the limit of each state's jurisdiction. The corporation would merely reincorporate in another state or otherwise change its practices to avoid specific restrictions. This corporate position of power and control led to public demand that Congress deal with trusts on a national level.[6]

Congressional response to public outrage about monopoly and predatory business practices was the Sherman Antitrust Act of 1890. Despite opposition to the trusts from both political parties, passage of the Sherman Act took several years. Senator Sherman's proposals were strenuously attacked despite the nearly unanimous desire to enact antitrust legislation. The debates focused on the limits of the commerce power as the constitutional basis for such legislation and the meaning of common law restrictions on monopolies and predatory business practices.

The Sherman Act as finally enacted has been described as "as good an antitrust law as the Congress of 1890 could have devised."[7] It was a compromise that essentially restated common law principles prohibiting restraints of trade and monopolization. The Sherman Act went beyond common law in several respects. Unlike common law prohibitions that were entirely civil in nature, the Sherman Act provided for criminal prosecution and penalties of fine and/or imprisonment.[8] The Sherman Act also expressly provided authority to the United States to bring civil actions to enjoin violations of the act and authority to private citizens damaged by violations to seek injunctive relief and treble damages. The nationwide effect of the act and the availability of the federal courts resolved the most serious problems of limited jurisdiction under state law.

Indifference and failure characterized early antitrust policy under the Sherman Act.[9] The drafters of the Sherman Act had intended for it to curb both the power and monopolistic abuses of the great trusts. It had been assumed that the Sherman Act would be self-enforcing because the business community would follow its prohibitions. Assumptions of voluntary compliance proved incorrect. The *Trans-Missouri Freight Association* case was the government's first major antitrust victory.[10] The Supreme Court overturned a determination that the prohibitions of the Sherman Act did not apply to price-fixing agreements between members of a railroad association. This was quickly followed by successful prosecutions in *United States v. Joint Traffic Association*[11] and in *United States v. Addyston Pipe & Steel Co.*[12] Overall, however, results were not impressive and one senator was able to compile a list of 628 trusts formed between 1898 and 1908.[13]

From the beginning of the enactment of the Sherman Act, there was substantial concern about its very general language. In 1911, the Supreme Court decided the *Standard Oil Co. case.*[14] In *Standard Oil,* the Court interpreted Section 1 of the Sherman Act as a prohibition on "unreasonable" restraints of trade and left to the courts the task of applying this "rule of reason."[15] It was the conclusion of some that the ambiguity of the statutory language and the new rule of reason gave excessive discretion to the courts. A movement for elaboration of specific practices inimical to free competition gained momentum and in 1914 the Clayton Act was passed by Congress.[16]

In 1914 the Federal Trade Commission Act was also passed by Congress.[17] The Federal Trade Commission was modeled on the Interstate Commerce Commission and it was anticipated that the commission would provide to businesses notice of conduct that violated the FTC Act through the issuance of cease-and-desist orders without initial penalty. The Federal Trade Commission

Act was another approach to alleviating the uncertainty caused by the general language of the Sherman Act.

The language of these three basic antitrust laws has been little changed since 1914.[18]

CONDUCT VIOLATIONS OF THE ANTITRUST LAWS

Section 1 of the Sherman Act prohibits combinations, contracts, and conspiracies in restraint of trade among the states or with foreign nations.[19] To violate this section, a person must engage in some type of concerted action that restrains trade in interstate commerce or with foreign countries.

Conduct violations should be of particular concern to individuals because of the potential for the award of three times the amount of any antitrust damages found in addition to attorneys' fees and costs of suit. In *Patrick v. Burget,*[20] three Oregon physicians were subject to a jury verdict in excess of $2 million and were reportedly bankrupted by the costs of defending against the allegations of the plaintiff surgeon.

The interstate commerce requirement is a prerequisite to the jurisdiction of the federal courts over alleged antitrust violations. It is necessary that the conduct in question have an appreciable impact on interstate commerce.[21]

In the health care field, the Supreme Court has found that a particular hospital was not "strictly a local, intrastate business" because of the impact that it exerted on the purchases of drugs and supplies from out-of-state sources as well as the revenues derived from out-of-state insurance companies.[22] Denial of staff privileges may satisfy an "effects" test by showing that commerce in the form of medical insurance from out-of-state sources, supplies from out-of-state sources, and interstate patients using a hospital were affected.[23] On the other hand, a number of courts have not found the interstate commerce requirement satisfied in cases involving denial of hospital privileges.[24] Almost all business can be found to have some connection with interstate commerce. This connection, no matter how tenuous, may serve to bring the conduct of a health care provider within the scope of the relevant antitrust statutes. Note, however, that the Clayton Act requires that the prescribed activity be "in commerce." This limits jurisdiction to "persons or activities within the flow of interstate commerce" and incidental effects on interstate transactions are insufficient to confer jurisdiction.[25] This provides little solace to potential defendants because the Sherman Act provisions are broad enough to reach most anticompetitive conduct prohibited by the Clayton Act.

Section 1 of the Sherman Act prohibits restraint of trade, but contains no explicit limiting language. In interpreting this language, the courts initially struggled with the question of whether Congress intended to prohibit all restraints of trade. In 1911, the Supreme Court decided *Standard Oil Co. of New Jersey v. United States,* which held that Section 1 of the Sherman Act was intended to prohibit only unreasonable restraints of trade.[26] What constitutes an unreasonable restraint of trade remains somewhat ambiguous, but since the *Standard Oil* case, the general approach to allegations of illegal restraints of trade has been to evaluate the alleged restraints under the rule of reason. The rule of reason requires a court in applying Section 1 of the Sherman Act to evaluate whether a restraint of trade is in fact an unreasonable restraint on competition. If it is found to be unreasonable, it will be in violation of the statute. The rule of reason was described by Justice Brandeis in *Chicago Board of Trade v. United States:*

Every agreement concerning trade, every regulation of trade, restrains. To bind, to restrain, is of their very essence. The true test of legality is whether the restraint imposed is such as merely regulates and perhaps thereby promotes competition or whether it is such as may suppress or even destroy competition. To determine that question the Court must ordinarily consider the restraint as applied; the nature of the restraint and its effect, actual or probable. The history of the restraint, the evil believed to exist, the reason for adopting the particular remedy, the purpose or end sought to be attained are all relevant facts.[27]

Substantial debate has occurred over what courts may consider in evaluating the reasonableness of a restraint. The current view is that courts are limited to consideration of impacts on competition and may not consider social policy or some worthy purpose allegedly furthered by the restraint. In the application of antitrust principles to the conduct of health care providers, this issue is confronted when a restraint is defended on the grounds that it advances quality of care, or access to care, or some other laudable public purpose.

A good example of the Supreme Court's approach to this issue is found in the discussion of the ban on competitive bidding by professional engineers considered by the Court in *National Society of Professional Engineers v. United States.*[28] The society defended the ban as a means of minimizing the risk that competition would produce inferior engineering work, thereby endangering public safety. Noting that the Sherman Act does not require competitive bidding but prohibits unreasonable restraints on competition, the Court pointed out that:

Petitioners' ban on competitive bidding prevents all customers from making the price comparisons in the initial selection of an engineer, and imposes the Society's view of the costs and benefits of competition on the entire marketplace. It is this restraint that must be justified under the Rule of Reason, and

petitioner's attempt to do so on the basis of the potential threat that competition poses to the public safety and the ethics of its profession is nothing less than a frontal assault on the basic policy of the Sherman Act.[29]

Despite this rather strong statement about the scope of the rule of reason, some lower courts have been willing to consider issues other than impact upon competition in applying the rule of reason to cases involving the health care industry. In *Wilk v. American Medical Association, Inc.*[30] the Court of Appeals for the Seventh Circuit indicated that it would allow a jury to consider issues of patient care in evaluating a prohibition on dealing with chiropractors as a restraint on trade under the rule of reason. The court held that once the plaintiffs had established that the defendant's conduct had restricted competition, the burden shifted to the defendants to show that they had a genuine and objectively reasonable concern for patient care, that this concern had motivated the conduct in question, and that the concern would not have been satisfied with a less restrictive alternative.[31] The court was careful to distinguish this approach from a general consideration of the "public interest" served by the restraint, which would have put its approach in direct conflict with the Supreme Court decisions noted earlier.[32]

In *Hospital Building Co. v. Trustees of Rex Hospital,*[33] the Court of Appeals for the Fourth Circuit used a narrow rule of reason to permit a nonprofit hospital to defend against charges of market allocation and a concerted refusal to deal on the grounds that the planning activities in which the hospital participated were undertaken in good faith and their actual and intended effects were contemplated by federal health planning legislation. This special rule of reason was described by the court as follows:

Because on this view the relevant federal health care legislation is in limited derogation of the normal operation of the antitrust laws, we further think that the burden of proof to show reasonableness of challenged planning and activities under this special rule of reason should be allocated as an affirmative defense to defendants seeking on this ground to avoid antitrust liability. On this basis a claimant, such as plaintiff here, makes out a prima facie case by showing acts that, but for the health care planning legislation, would constitute a per se violation of § 1 under traditional antitrust principles. This establishes liability for appropriate damages unless the defendants then persuade the trier of fact by a preponderance of the evidence that their planning activities had the purpose (and effect if plaintiff proves anticompetitive effects) only of avoiding a "needless" duplication of health care resources under the objective standard of need above defined.[34]

It remains to be seen whether the Supreme Court will be willing to accept considerations of patient care or industry efficiency in rule of reason analysis in the health care industry.[35]

Rule of reason analysis, even limited to issues of competition, can be extremely complex and the burden of proving a rule of reason case in litigation is substantial. This reality was recognized by the courts and a presumption of unreasonableness was established quite early for certain specific categories of anticompetitive conduct.[36] This presumption relieves plaintiffs of the burden of establishing the anticompetitive effect of the conduct at issue and prohibits defendants from introducing evidence on that question. It is widely known as the per se rule.[37]

Per se rule

In contrast to the rule of reason, the courts will apply a per se rule of illegality to practices that have been shown generally to have anticompetitive effects on competition. These practices are presumed to be illegal without substantial inquiry into anticompetitive effect:

There are certain agreements or practices which because of their pernicious effect on competition and lack of any redeeming virtue are conclusively presumed to be unreasonable and therefore illegal without elaborate inquiry as to the precise harm they have caused . . . among the practices which the courts have heretofore deemed to be unlawful in and of themselves are price fixing . . . ; division of markets . . . ; group boycotts . . . ; and tying arrangements. . . .[38]

Although initially the Supreme Court made clear that those found to have taken part in the practices listed by the Court in *Northern Pacific Railway v. United States* would not be given the opportunity to justify their activity, there is now substantial discussion of this point.[39]

In the health care context, the Supreme Court has held that the establishment of a maximum price with the purported goal of holding down health care costs was deemed to be a per se illegal price-fixing agreement in *Arizona v. Maricopa County Medical Society.*[40] The Court in *Maricopa* specifically rejected the argument that it should not apply the per se rule to a price-fixing case involving medical foundations because the judiciary has little antitrust experience with the health care industry. The Court noted that "whatever may be its peculiar problems and characteristics, the Sherman Act, so far as price-fixing agreements are concerned, establishes one uniform rule applicable to all industries alike."[41]

Specific antitrust conduct violations

Price-fixing. Certain conduct has been found by the courts to have "so pernicious an effect on competition" and to be so lacking in any redeeming virtue that it is accorded per se illegal status.[42] One such type of conduct

is price-fixing. As the Supreme Court noted in *United States v. Trenton Potteries Co.,* "The aim and result of every price-fixing agreement, if effective, is the elimination of one form of competition."[43] The economic power to fix a price amounts to control of a market. It does not matter whether the fixing of prices is exercised in a reasonable or unreasonable manner. An agreement that creates such power "may well be held to be . . . unreasonable. . . without the necessity of minute inquiry whether a particular price is reasonable or unreasonable . . . and without placing on the government . . . the burden of ascertaining . . . whether it has become unreasonable through the mere variation of economic conditions."[44]

The agreement to fix prices need not be formal. The agreement itself can be demonstrated by circumstantial evidence.[45] An agreement that "tampered" with price, whether it raised, lowered, or stabilized prices, would be a per se violation.[46] Even agreements that affect price indirectly are often prohibited.[47] Once a practice is characterized as price-fixing it is per se illegal. Making that characterization, however, can be difficult.

In *Chicago Board of Trade v. United States,*[48] the Chicago Board of Trade, a commodities market, had adopted a "call" rule. Members of the board were prohibited from purchasing or offering to purchase during the period between the close of the call session and the opening of the regular trading session on the next business day, any wheat, corn, oats, or rye "to arrive" at a price other than the closing bid at the call session. The United States filed suit under the Sherman Act to enjoin enforcement of the call rule. The Chicago Board of Trade argued that the purpose of the call rule was not to prevent competition or to control prices but to promote the convenience of members by restricting their hours of business and also to break up a monopoly in the grain trade acquired by four or five warehousemen in Chicago. The Supreme Court concluded that this was not price-fixing but was within the right of the board and other trade organizations to impose some restraint on the conduct of business by its members.[49]

In *Broadcast Music, Inc. v. Columbia Broadcasting System, Inc.,*[50] the Supreme Court examined the blanket licensing scheme for copyrighted musical composition utilized by Broadcast Music, Inc. (BMI) and the American Society of Composers, Authors, and Publishers (ASCAP). Although the court of appeals had concluded that the use of a flat licensing fee for blanket permission to play all musical compositions registered with BMI or ASCAP constituted per se illegal price-fixing, the Supreme Court refused to characterize the conduct as price-fixing and instead applied the rule of reason and found the conduct reasonable. The Court noted that the blanket license had a number of unique characteristics, was efficient, and may, in fact, have constituted an entirely separate product.[51]

The leading price-fixing decision in the health care field is *Arizona v. Maricopa County Medical Society.*[52] There the Supreme Court applied the per se rule to an agreement among physicians to set maximum fees pursuant to a foundation program established by the county society. Approximately 70% of the physicians in Maricopa County were involved in the Maricopa plan. These doctors agreed not to charge more than the maximum agreed price for specified services and agreed with insurance companies to provide care to insured patients on that basis. The society defended the foundation plan on the grounds that it fixed only maximum prices, that it was an agreement among members of a profession, that it had procompetitive justifications, and that the courts should further investigate the health care industry before applying a per se rule to conduct by health care providers. The majority in *Maricopoa* rejected each of these arguments and held that the setting of maximum prices constituted per se illegal price-fixing.[53] The majority was unwilling to assign any weight to the unique characteristics of the market for physician services or to the purported cost containment purposes of the plan.[54]

Reimbursement policies of health insurance companies have been challenged as illegal price-fixing agreements.[55] Courts have shown interest in such claims when evidence of provider control over reimbursement rates may exist.[56] When the evidence shows unilateral action with an effect on prices, courts have not been receptive to claims of price-fixing.[57]

Agreements or approaches resulting in the stabilization of prices are considered per se violations. Relative value scales have been challenged as price-fixing mechanisms because they allegedly tend to standardize charges for various types of professional services. The Federal Trade Commission entered into multiple consent orders barring the use of relative value scales in the late 1970s.[58]

The critical issue of rising health care costs has led the purchasers of health care services to take various actions in an effort to stabilize or reduce their costs. Individual action rarely poses antitrust concerns. Collective action including the joint buying of services through preferred provider organizations may, however, trigger antitrust price-fixing concerns. An agreement among buyers not to compete on price in the purchase of goods or services is just as much unlawful price-fixing as is a like agreement among sellers not to compete on price.[59] Joint purchasing programs, although they involve efficiencies, may be unlawful even when their ultimate aim is to reduce the price of the product to consumers. However, the courts have approved joint purchasing arrangements in which the percentage of the market represented by the joint buying group was small. The Supreme Court has implicitly sanctioned wholesale purchasing cooperatives as arrangements seemingly designed to increase economic efficiency and render markets more, rather than less, competitive.[60]

Physicians seeking to avoid price-fixing problems should not agree with competing physicians on any term of price, quantity, or quality. This includes agreement on fee schedules and relative value scales.[61] Although there may be exceptions to this relatively simple statement, the purported exceptions should be carefully examined with the assistance of competent and experienced antitrust counsel.

Tying and exclusive dealing. *Tying* may be defined as the sale or lease of a product or service conditioned upon the buyer taking a second product or service as well. Tying arrangements may be attacked as unreasonable restraints of trade under Section 1 of the Sherman Act.[62] Anticompetitive tying arrangements are specifically prohibited by Section 3 of the Clayton Act[63] and deemed illegal under Section 5 of the Federal Trade Commission Act.[64] The Clayton Act is rarely encountered in suits against physicians and other health care providers because it applies only to the sales of commodities.[65]

The legal standard employed in evaluating tying arrangements may be viewed a modified per se rule. This standard was most recently discussed by the Supreme Court in *Jefferson Parish Hospital District No. 2 v. Hyde.*[66] In *Jefferson Parish,* the East Jefferson Hospital had entered into an exclusive agreement with Roux and Associates for the provision of anesthesiology services at the hospital. Dr. Edwin Hyde, a board-certified anesthesiologist, had applied for admission to the East Jefferson Hospital medical staff and his application had been denied by the hospital's board because of the exclusive contract just mentioned. Dr. Hyde sued the hospital and others, alleging that East Jefferson Hospital had engaged in tying by mandating that any person using services of the hospital requiring anesthesia also use the services of anesthesiologists controlled by Roux and Associates. In *Jefferson Parish,* the Supreme Court described the essential characteristic of an illegal tying agreement:

[T]he essential characteristic of an invalid tying arrangement lies in the seller's exploitation of its control over the tying product to force the buyer into the purchase of a tied product that the buyer either did not want at all, or might have preferred to purchase elsewhere on different terms.[67]

The Court concluded that tying should be subject to per se condemnation when the probability of anticompetitive forcing is high.[68]

In general, to invoke the per se rule against a tying arrangement, it is necessary to establish the existence of two separate products. In addition, it must be shown that the party accused of tying has sufficient market power in the tying product to force acceptance of an unwanted tied product and that it has used that power to tie the products.[69]

In applying this analysis to the facts of *Jefferson Parish,* the Court concluded that East Jefferson Hospital had no significant power in the market for hospital services, the alleged tying product.[70] Without this condition, the Court was unwilling to apply the per se rule against the arrangement. In evaluating the arrangement under the rule of reason, the Court concluded that there was insufficient evidence in the record to support a finding that the arrangement unreasonably restrained competition.[71]

There was substantial debate prior to the Court's decision in *Jefferson Parish* about whether in-patient hospital care could be divided into a number of different products for purposes of a tying analysis. In *Jefferson Parish,* the Court had no difficulty in determining that the evidence amply supported the treatment of anesthesiology services as a separate product for purposes of the tying analysis.[72] The mere fact that services are functionally linked—such as anesthesia to surgery—does not foreclose treating the services as separate products.[73] This determination depends on a realistic appraisal of whether the products are distinct in the view of the purchasers of the products, and whether there is a distinct demand for each of the products.[74]

The utility of *Jefferson Parish* in evaluating the antitrust risks in other factual contexts is limited. The decision in the case turned entirely on an analysis of the market power of East Jefferson Hospital in in-patient services. The Court has, however, once again made clear that there will be no special consideration given to the fact that an alleged antitrust violation occurs in a health care context.[75]

An exclusive dealing arrangement involves an agreement by one party to buy particular products exclusively from another party. This arrangement has the effect of foreclosing to competitors of the seller the opportunity to compete for the purchases of buyers who are parties to exclusive dealing agreements. Exclusive dealing arrangements have been challenged under Section 1 of the Sherman Act,[76] Section 3 of the Clayton Act,[77] and Section 5 of the Federal Trade Commission Act.[78] Generally, exclusive dealing is regarded as a vertical restraint, which is evaluated under the rule of reason.[79] In evaluating exclusive dealing arrangements under Section 3 of the Clayton Act, the Supreme Court has found a violation where the arrangement foreclosed competition in a substantial share of the line of commerce affected.[80] In a more recent case, the Court used the same test but conducted a rigorous structural

analysis and considered a number of unique characteristics of the market in concluding that a substantial share of the market was not foreclosed by the arraignment.[81]

Exclusive dealing agreements are common in the health care industry. A typical example is a contract between a physician or group of physicians and a hospital to provide exclusive services to that hospital in a particular medical specialty, such as pathology, radiology, anesthesiology, and emergency medicine. The arrangement in *Jefferson Parish* between Roux and Associates and East Jefferson Hospital is properly characterized as an exclusive dealing arrangement. In that case the Court did not find sufficient evidence of anticompetitive impact on competition among anesthesiologists from the arrangement to find it unreasonable and noted that Dr. Hyde did not undertake to prove unreasonable foreclosure of the market for anesthesiological services.[82] Nevertheless, Justice O'Connor representing the view of four justices, noted:

> Exclusive dealing is an unreasonable restraint on trade only when a significant fraction of buyers or sellers are frozen out of a market by the exclusive deal.... When the sellers of services are numerous and mobile, and the number of buyers is large, exclusive dealing arrangements of narrow scope pose no threat of adverse economic consequences. To the contrary, they may be substantially pro-competitive by ensuring stable markets and encouraging long term, mutually advantageous business relationships.[83]

In evaluating the facts of *Jefferson Parish* as exclusive dealing, Justice O'Connor readily concluded that there was no potential for an unreasonable impact on competition from the arrangement between Roux and Associates and the hospital.[84]

Prior to the decision in *Jefferson Parish,* a number of lower courts had upheld exclusive dealing arrangements between physicians and hospitals. *Harron v. United Hospital Center, Inc.*[85] dealt with a radiologist's suit following his loss of an exclusive contract because of a hospital merger. The merged entity had contracted with a second physician to operate its Radiology Department. The Fourth Circuit Court of Appeals upheld the right of the new hospital to contract on an exclusive basis with another physician stating that it was "frivolous to urge that the employment of a single doctor to operate the Radiology Department of a hospital invokes the Sherman Act...."[86] The exclusion of an anesthesiologist from a hospital because that hospital had awarded an exclusive contract to the physician group with which the plaintiff had formerly been associated was the focus of concern in *Dos Santos v. Columbus-Cuneo-Cabrini Medical Center.*[87] Plaintiff anesthesiologist sued the hospital and the anesthesiology group under Sections 1 and 2 of the Sherman Act as well as under the Illinois Antitrust

Act. The Seventh Circuit Court of Appeals vacated a preliminary injunction against the exclusive arrangement and remanded the case back to the district court noting that the district court had, in its opinion, improperly limited the relevant geographic market solely to the hospital from which the plaintiff was excluded. The court of appeals suggested "should the instant case proceed to trial, the district court should reconsider on the basis of more complete evidence its preliminary finding regarding the relevant market."[88] The court also suggested that the district court "re-examine the basis of its conclusion that there is no effective competition among hospitals."[89] Although the court of appeals disposed of the case on a finding that the plaintiff had not satisfied other necessary prerequisites for the issuance of a preliminary injunction, it also expressed doubt that the plaintiff would succeed on the merits.[90]

One may anticipate that an exclusive dealing allegation is unlikely to prevail absent a convincing showing that a substantial portion of a rigorously defined relevant market is foreclosed by the arrangement. One may also anticipate that a court will consider seriously and weigh in the balance of a rule of reason analysis any legitimate procompetitive aspects of the arrangement.[91]

Concerted refusals to deal (boycotts). A concerted refusal to deal occurs when a group of competitors or a competitor and others through collective action exclude or otherwise interfere with the legitimate business activities of one or more other competitors. Courts have used the terms "boycott" and "concerted refusal to deal" interchangeably when referring to the exclusion of a competitor by collective action. Boycotts involve concerted action and are generally challenged under Section 1 of the Sherman Act.[92] In general, boycotts have been held to be per se violations of the antitrust laws.[93] In a recent case, however, the Supreme Court has taken a more flexible approach, insisting that the potential for anticompetitive impact be established before the per se rule will be applied.[94]

In *Northwest Wholesale Stationers, Inc. v. Pacific Stationery and Printing Co.*, the Supreme Court concluded that the exclusion of a retail office supply store from a nonprofit cooperative buying association was not a per se violation of the antitrust laws. The Court noted that the per se rule has generally been applied in those cases where "the boycott . . . cut off access to a supply, facility, or market necessary to enable the boycotted firm to compete, . . . and frequently the boycotting firms possessed a dominant position in the relevant market."[95] The Court held that:

A plaintiff seeking application of the per se rule must present a threshold case that the challenged activity falls into a category likely to have predominantly anticompetitive

effects. . . . When the plaintiff challenges expulsion from a joint buying cooperative, some showing must be made that the cooperative possesses market power or unique access to a business element necessary for effective competition.[96]

Since such showing had not been made in *Northwest Stationers,* the Court remanded the case for a review of the rule of reason analysis undertaken by the district court.

Although myriad opportunities exist within the health care arena for boycott activity, the issue has arisen most commonly in cases involving refusals of medical staff privileges at hospitals. Existing members of a medical staff, who would be in direct competition with an applicant for staff privileges, often have significant influence, if not actual control, over the determination whether to grant privileges. In some circumstances a denial of privileges may constitute an effective bar to competition, for example, denial of privileges to a new physician at the only hospital in a community. The privileges issue is complicated by the fact that the training, professional competence, and need for a new physician may be relevant and legitimate issues for the hospital considering an application for privileges and physicians currently active in the applicant's specialty will have substantial expertise and information to contribute on these questions.

The lower courts that have examined boycott allegations in the context of disputes over privileges have adopted a variety of approaches. In *Weiss v. York Hospital,*[97] the Court of Appeals for the Third Circuit concluded that the conduct of members of a hospital medical staff in opposing the granting of hospital privileges to a class of osteopathic physicians was the equivalent of a concerted refusal to deal. Ultimately, the court determined that the per se rule should be applied to this conduct.[98] It suggested, however, that rule of reason analysis would be appropriate if questions of professional competence or unprofessional conduct were at issue or the exclusion was otherwise based on public service or ethical norms.[99]

In *Wilk v. American Medical Ass'n., Inc.,*[100] plaintiff chiropractor sued a number of medical organizations under the Sherman Act for an alleged conspiracy to induce individual medical doctor and hospitals to refuse to deal with plaintiffs and other chiropractors. Although the trial court instructed the jury on the per se rule, the Court of Appeals for the Seventh Circuit concluded that in the context of these facts, "the nature and extent of [the] anticompetitive effect are too uncertain to be amenable to per se treatment. . . ."[101] Moreover, the court determined, the existence of substantial evidence of a patient care motive for the conduct of the organizations made application of the per se rule inappropriate.[102] Other courts have adopted a similar approach.[103] In

Patrick v. Burget,[104] the U.S. Supreme Court reinstated a treble damages verdict in excess of $2 million against three Oregon physicians because of their participation in a peer review process that recommended that the plaintiff surgeon's hospital privileges be revoked. Although the reason given for revocation was substandard care, the evidence strongly supported the conclusion that the true motivation was anticompetitive bias. Although there is some protection for peer review activities under the state action exemption[105] and under the Health Care Quality Improvement Act of 1986,[106] peer review activity stemming from anticompetitive motivation that results in the denial or revocation of hospital privileges may be held to be illegal group boycott activity.

As already noted, boycott activity must involve conduct by two or more participants to constitute a violation of Section 1 of the Sherman Act.[107] In *Copperweld Corp. v. Independence Tube Corp.*,[108] the Supreme Court ruled that for the purposes of the antitrust laws, a parent corporation and its wholly owned subsidiary may not conspire with each other. This reasoning has been applied in concluding that a hospital and its medical staff, a creature of the hospital, do not engage in concerted action for purposes of the antitrust laws.[109] It is, of course, clear that a medical staff is composed of individual physicians, and conduct of physicians either within a medical staff or as individual competitors in the market for physician services will not be protected by the *Copperweld* doctrine.[110]

In evaluating group boycott claims involving the denial or termination of hospital privileges, a number of courts have considered whether the impact on interstate commerce requirement of the Sherman Act has been satisfied. As noted earlier, the Supreme Court in *Summit Health* and *McLain v. Real Estate Board of New Orleans, Inc.*[111] suggested a liberal approach in determining whether this jurisdictional requirement has been met. Factors such as the purchase of supplies, drugs, and equipment from out-of-state sources, the attraction of patients from other states, and the receipt of revenues from sources outside the state appear to satisfy the Sherman Act interstate commerce requirement.[112]

The courts have addressed the interstate commerce issue with some care in hospital privileges cases.[113] They have concluded that it is unnecessary that a plaintiff prove more than that the alleged conduct had a not insubstantial effect on interstate commerce.[114]

Market allocation. Another type of conduct that raises serious questions of restraint of trade is market allocation. Competitors, by agreeing to divide geographic markets or customers, can achieve the benefits of monopoly as to their exclusive market share. In general, the Supreme Court has regarded market allocation agreements among competitors as per se illegal under Section 1 of the Sherman Act.[115] There are, however,

substantial questions of characterization that qualify that statement. It is, for example, clear that territorial or customer restraints that are insisted on by a party operating at a different level of production, such as restraints imposed by a manufacturer on wholesalers, will be evaluated under the rule of reason.[116] There may be a substantial question whether the market allocation scheme is the primary objective of an agreement among competitors or merely ancillary to an otherwise legitimate joint venture. If the latter is the case, the court may well evaluate the entire venture under the rule of reason.[117]

Market allocation agreements among hospitals or physicians could take the form of agreements on geographic placement of institutions or offices. This could be characterized as a geographic market division. Agreements allocating the provision of certain services exclusively to particular hospitals or physicians would be another approach to market division. Evaluation of such agreements is likely to raise complex questions of motivation and anticompetitive effect. For example, some such arrangements may be dictated, or at least approved, by a state agency under applicable health planning statutes. The significance of such approval by a state agency will be discussed in the section on defenses. It is worth noting that no joint venture among hospitals has ever been challenged by federal antitrust enforcement agencies.[118]

Monopolization. Section 2 of the Sherman Act prohibits monopolization, attempts to monopolize, and conspiracies to monopolize.[119] Section 2 does not, by its terms, prohibit monopoly. The antitrust laws promote competition. As a result of competition a successful competitor may achieve a monopoly in a particular market. To declare such a result illegal seems unfair and illogical.[120]

The Supreme Court has suggested that a monopolization offense has two elements: "(1) the possession of monopoly power in the relevant market and (2) the willful acquisition or maintenance of that power as distinguished from growth or development as a consequence of a superior product, business acumen, or historic accident."[121]

Determination of the existence of the first element may be complicated. Monopoly power has been defined by the courts as the "power to control prices or exclude competition."[122] Although the Supreme Court has suggested that monopoly power may be inferred from a predominant share of the relevant market,[123] substantial question remains as to what constitutes a "predominant" share and how the "relevant" market should be defined.[124] Over time, the calculation of market share and the definition of the relevant market have become much more sophisticated.[125]

The second element of monopolization, the willful

acquisition or maintenance of monopoly power, may be similarly elusive. In *United States v. Aluminum Co. of America,*[126] the court suggested that by embracing new opportunities and anticipating the need for new capacity Alcoa had monopolized the market for aluminum ingot. More recently the courts appear to require something more than behavior motivated by legitimate business purposes to support a charge of monopolization.[127] The offense of attempt to monopolize generally requires the proof of three elements: (1) specific intent to control prices or to exclude competitors; (2) predatory conduct directed to accomplishing this purpose; and (3) a dangerous probability of success.[128] Precise definition of conduct that satisfies these elements has proven to be controversial.[129]

In the context of health care, the most common instance of alleged monopolization is the situation in which a hospital with monopoly power is acting to maintain that power and to avoid competition.[130] Similarly, an association of all or most physicians of a given specialty in a relevant market could support a finding of monopoly power in support of an allegation of monopolization.[131] In particular contexts, a health maintenance organization (HMO), preferred provider organization, or other provider organization could face monopolization allegations.

Mergers. Mergers between business entities are generally evaluated under Section 7 of the Clayton Act.[132] Section 7 prohibits mergers in which the effect may be "substantially to lessen competition, or to tend to create a monopoly" in an activity "affecting commerce in any section of the country."[133] The purpose of Section 7 is to reach incipient problems of monopoly, hence the rather broad language noted above.

Section 7 applies to the acquisition of stock or the assets of any person by any other person. It is clear that "person" includes corporations and unincorporated business enterprises[134] and that the section applies to partial acquisitions of assets.[135] Section 7 may apply to joint ventures as well as to more complete integration of business resources.[136]

The determination of whether an acquisition or merger substantially lessens competition or tends to create a monopoly has generated enormous controversy. The Supreme Court in applying Section 7 has engaged in increasingly rigorous structural analyses of the effect of the transaction on competition.[137] This has also been true of merger analysis undertaken by the Federal Trade Commission.[138]

The merger guidelines issued by the Department of Justice in 1968 and substantially revised in 1982, 1984, and 1992 have been exceptionally useful and influential in advancing the analysis of the competitive effect of mergers. The merger guidelines provide a structured approach to defining relevant product[139] and geographic markets.[140] The merger guidelines utilize the Herfindahl-Hirschman index to measure market concentration and provide an outline of enforcement policy for different levels of market concentration and increases in market concentration.[141]

Merger cases brought in the health care context have generally involved for-profit hospitals.[142] At present, hospitals represent the largest economic entities engaged in the provision of health care services, and the expansionary activities of for-profit hospital chains have elicited the interest of antitrust enforcement authorities. Whether the developing merger activities of other types of health care providers will elicit the same interest remains to be seen. It is worth noting that of the approximately 229 hospital mergers that occurred between 1987 and 1991, only 27 were investigated by the federal antitrust enforcement authorities and only 5 were challenged.[143]

DEFENSES
State action exemption

There are a number of defenses or exemptions from liability under the antitrust laws. Although some of these exemptions are the result of action by Congress creating a specific statutory exception to the application of the antitrust laws, perhaps the most important, the state action exemption, was created by judicial decision.

The state action exemption is grounded on the principle of federalism. A state may choose to displace competition in the provision of certain goods or services within its borders and to replace market control with state regulation. As long as this action by the state qualifies under the state action exemption, private parties will be protected from liability under the federal antitrust laws for acting in compliance with this state mandate.

The state action exemption was initially articulated by the Supreme Court in *Parker v. Brown.*[144] At issue in *Parker* was whether a raisin marketing program that had the effect of restricting production and maintaining prices, but which was created by state legislation, was in violation of federal antitrust laws. In refusing to rule against the state program, the Supreme Court noted:

We find nothing in the language of the Sherman Act or in its history which suggests that its purpose was to restrain a state or its officers or agents from activities directed by its legislature. In a dual system of government in which under the Constitution, the states are sovereign, save only as Congress may constitutionally subtract from their authority, an unexpressed purpose to nullify a state's control over its officers and agents is not lightly to be attributed to Congress.[145]

In a number of cases decided since *Parker v. Brown,* the Supreme Court has elaborated on the state action exemption.[146] In *California Liquor Dealers v. Midcal Aluminum Inc.,*[147] the Supreme Court suggested a two-pronged test for determining whether a state regulatory scheme is exempted from the federal antitrust laws. First, the restraint must be "clearly articulated and affirmatively expressed as state policy."[148] Second, the anticompetitive conduct must be actively supervised by the state.[149]

Most recently the Supreme Court has reaffirmed the two-prong *Midcal* test as the appropriate analytical approach for evaluating anticompetitive conduct by private parties acting pursuant to state statute.[150] The Court has also made clear that the second prong of the *Midcal* test is not applicable to municipalities.[151]

The state action exemption has been raised as a defense by defendants in a variety of health care-related antitrust suits. A number of state statutes have been suggested as a basis for the state action exemption, including state certificate of need statutes,[152] state statutes mandating physician peer review,[153] and state authorization to municipal and county-owned hospitals to grant or deny physician privileges.[154]

The lower courts have engaged in substantial debate as to whether a state statute constitutes a clearly articulated and affirmatively expressed state policy to displace competition and whether there is adequate state supervision to satisfy the *Midcal* test.

In several cases in which municipalities were sued for allegedly anticompetitive conduct in contracting for ambulance services, the lower courts have applied only the first prong of the *Midcal* test.[155] While requiring an explicit state policy to displace competition, these courts successfully anticipated the Supreme Court's decision in *Town of Hallie v. City of Eau Claire,* holding that the second requirement of *Midcal,* active state supervision, was not required when a municipality was following an expressed state policy.[156] Liability of municipalities and other political subdivisions for damages under the antitrust laws has now been clarified by statute.[157]

The Supreme Court has recently clarified the active supervision prong of the state action exemption. The clarification was made in the 1992 case *Federal Trade Commission v. Ticor Insurance Co.*[158] The *Ticor* decision allowed the court to explain that state action immunity is "disfavored."[159] Active supervision means more than endowing a state agency with the duty to regulate.

The *Ticor* decision involved title insurance companies practicing in four states. The Federal Trade Commission alleged illegal price-fixing in the setting of fees for title searches and examinations. A rating bureau licensed by the state was authorized to fix rates for the services at issue. The Court of Appeals for the Third Circuit[160] had held that an actively supervised state regulatory program

staffed and funded, granting to state officials ample power and duty to regulate, is sufficient. The Supreme Court disagreed. The Court stated that it was dealing with a "negative option" scheme in which private parties established the rates, which were then filed with the state agencies and became effective unless rejected within a given time period. The Court stated that "the mere potential for state supervision is not adequate substitute for a decision by the state"[161] and that the state must play a more substantial role in determining how the prices are established so that the agreed-on price comes about through deliberate state intervention and not through the agreement of private parties.

Although some initially felt the *Ticor* decision might be limited to price fixing, it has subsequently been extended into other areas.[162] It would appear, therefore, that the tightening of the active supervision prong announced in *Ticor* will be applied in a wide variety of contexts including monopolization, unlawful restraint of trade, and tying.

Explicit and implied exemption

The antitrust statutes are, of course, subject to any limits and exemptions that Congress chooses to place on them. Over the years Congress has enacted a number of specific exemptions for labor organizations,[163] the business of insurance to the extent regulated by state law,[164] agricultural cooperatives,[165] fishery associations,[166] joint newspaper operating agreements,[167] intrabrand territorial restrictions on franchisees of soft drink companies,[168] joint small business programs for research and development,[169] agreements between businesses necessary for the national defense,[170] and joint exporting companies.[171]

In part in response to the decision in *Patrick v. Burget,*[172] Congress enacted the Health Care Quality Improvement Act of 1986.[173] This statute provides a general immunity from damages under the antitrust laws for physicians engaging in professional peer review.[174] In addition, any person providing information to a professional review body[175] regarding the competence or professional conduct of a physician is given immunity from damages under state or federal law.[176] In the event that a suit is brought against a person engaging in professional peer review and is unsuccessful, the statute imposes liability on the person bringing the suit for the costs of suit, including a reasonable attorney's fee, if the claim of the person bringing suit was frivolous, unreasonable, without foundation, or in bad faith.[177]

In addition to the specific exemptions noted, there are express exemptions to aspects of the antitrust laws in the statutes establishing federal regulatory schemes for particular industries. These exemptions are generally specific and limited in scope.[178]

A more difficult question is generated when Congress has not enacted a specific statutory exemption to the antitrust laws, but has entrusted authority over certain matters in an industry to a regulatory agency. The question becomes whether Congress has "by implication" created an exemption from the antitrust laws. In general, implied exemptions from the antitrust laws are disfavored by the courts and are found only when there is a clear conflict between the antitrust laws and other federal statutes.[179]

In the context of health care, the Supreme Court has refused to find an implied exemption from the antitrust laws in federal health planning legislation.[180] In *National Gerimedical Hospital*, Blue Cross defended against a charge of anticompetitive conspiracy in the denial to a hospital of participating status, by arguing that it was acting pursuant to the local HSA plan and furthering the purposes of the National Health Planning and Resources Development Act of 1974.[181] The Supreme Court concluded that in light of the strict approach taken in evaluating the claims of implied exemption to the antitrust laws, Blue Cross would remain subject to the antitrust laws in this case. The Court was unpersuaded that there was "a 'clear repugnancy' between the NHPRDA and the antitrust laws, at least on the facts of this case."[182] The Court left open the possibility that an implied exemption from the antitrust laws might be found in other factual contexts in the health care industry, specifically for activities necessary to make the federal health planning legislation work.[183]

Noerr-Pennington doctrine

The courts have created an exemption from the antitrust laws for conduct by private parties intended to influence governmental action by the legislative, judicial, or executive branches. This exemption is known as the Noerr-Pennington doctrine, drawing its name from two U.S. Supreme Court cases wherein the Court discussed the defense.[184] The underlying purpose of the Noerr-Pennington doctrine is to protect the right of citizens to petition government and to ensure that government's access to information about the desires of citizens remains unimpaired by the threat of liability under the antitrust laws.[185]

While the Noerr-Pennington doctrine is available to protect persons genuinely undertaking to influence governmental action, it is not available where the conduct is "a mere sham to cover what is actually nothing more than an attempt to interfere directly with the business relationships of a competitor...."[186]

Appeals to certificate of need agencies and to physician licensing boards are types of conduct that may be subject to Noerr-Pennington protection unless subject to the sham exception just noted.[187] Hospital peer review committees have not been recognized as governmental agencies for purpose of the Noerr-Pennington doctrine.[188] Unilateral or joint action that does not take the form of an appeal to a governmental decision-maker will not be accorded protection under Noerr-Pennington.[189]

ROBINSON-PATMAN ACT

In light of the recent practice of physicians dispensing medications and the joint venture movement, the Robinson-Patman Act may be pertinent.[190] By the act, vendors are prohibited from selling and customers from buying supplies at discriminatorily low prices—that is, prices not generally available to other customers. The statute forbids price discrimination by vendors among their purchasers so as to lessen competition. However, an amendment to the Non Profit Institutions Act exempts nonprofit hospitals, but only on supplies purchased for the facility's "own use."[191] The exemption allows not-for-profit purchasers to receive discounts of "supplies for their own use." Customarily, nonprofit hospitals have paid less for drugs than the corner pharmacy, with the buyer and seller protected by the statutory exemption.

In *Abbott Laboratories v. Portland Retail Druggists Ass'n,*[192] "for their own use" was interpreted as applying to hospital purchases of drugs dispensed for in-patients, emergency room clientele, patients about to be discharged, some outpatients, and for personal use of employees, students, and physicians, but not for "walk-in" customers. "Own use" has also been defined as being for treatment of hospital emergency room patients, outpatients being treated on hospital premises, and immediate take-home use by discharged patients. These hospitals may also resell products to the medical staff for personal use by physicians and their dependents. Although one should not take lightly the potential liability in damages for defendants in antitrust actions, in the health care field it appears that these suits are more likely to be pursued as a threat in order to alter the defendants' conduct than with the expectation of recovering a judgment. At least, recoveries have been uncommon among reported cases. However, the question has been raised again. Suppliers charge that many nonprofit hospitals are violating the statute by allowing physicians to buy from their discounted stock for use in their offices. Physicians on the staffs of some nonprofit hospitals may lose the privilege of buying medical supplies discounted up to 50% for use in their own offices.

Vendor groups are challenging the practice of hospital product resale or "diversion" on the grounds that it violates federal antitrust laws. Vendors say the practices being scrutinized are:

- Purchases by medical staff members for use in private practice
- Purchases for resale as prescription refills
- Purchases for resale to former hospital patients or walk-ins not being treated at the hospital

FEDERAL TRADE COMMISSION

The Federal Trade Commission (FTC) operates under its own federal statute and may issue cease-and-desist orders against unfair methods of competition.[193] More often the FTC negotiates a consent agreement whereby the party under investigation agrees not to engage in a questioned practice, although without admitting wrongdoing. This administrative agency has had a significant impact on the practice of medicine.

Since the 1940s it has been known that the medical profession is subject to antitrust laws.[194] In a number of instances, the FTC has moved against conduct by groups of physicians. For example, the FTC completed one inquiry by executing a consent decree with the medical staff of a three-hospital organization.[195] Although the FTC does not have jurisdiction over not-for-profit organizations, the medical staff was an unincorporated for-profit association presumed to be subject to FTC powers. The medical staff was charged by the FTC with denying hospital privileges to physicians associated with HMOs, thereby hampering their practice and the viability of the HMOs and denying HMO enrollees access to the hospitals for care by their HMO physicians. The FTC consent agreement, effective for 10 years, provides that applications for staff privileges will not be denied because the applicant is affiliated with an HMO or does not practice on a fee-for-service basis. Neither are applications to be delayed unreasonably nor will different treatment be accorded HMO physicians once admitted to the staff. Copies of the FTC complaint and consent order are to be provided to all staff members and future applicants. Annual compliance reports are to be filed with the FTC. In 1979, the FTC condemned American Medical Association (AMA) ethics rules that banned advertising by individuals and prohibited certain other forms of medical services advertising. The AMA rules also restricted dissemination of price information. The FTC ordered the AMA to cease and desist from enforcing its ethical rules on advertising and to disaffiliate any state or local medical society that continued to ascribe to such rules. Ultimately the Second Circuit Court of Appeals upheld the FTC ruling that such rules violated federal antitrust laws and the ruling was affirmed by an equally divided Supreme Court.[196] The court order allowed the AMA to adopt ethical guidelines prohibiting unsubstantiated, false, and deceptive representation by its members.

The FTC has intervened and condemned relative value guides and has entered into consent decrees prohibiting their use in setting fees or prices.[197,198] It is possible to seek an advisory opinion from the FTC as to whether a contract would, in the (nonbinding) opinion of the FTC, violate the antitrust law.

RECENT DEVELOPMENTS IN ANTITRUST AND HEALTH CARE REFORM

In recognition of the substantial structural change occurring in the health care industry in recent years, the Department of Justice and the Federal Trade Commission have issued statements of enforcement policy regarding mergers and joint activities in the health care area. The first of these statements was issued on September 15, 1993, and addressed six specific areas:
1. Hospital mergers
2. Hospital joint ventures involving expensive medical equipment
3. Physician collaboration to provide information to purchasers of health care services
4. Hospital exchanges of price and cost information
5. Joint purchasing arrangements among health care providers
6. Physician network joint ventures

On September 27, 1994, the Department of Justice and the Federal Trade Commission issued a second "Statements of Enforcement Policy and Analytical Principles Relating to Health Care and Antitrust." The second set of statements addressed nine areas while retaining the basic structure and thrust of the 1993 statements. Statements were added in these areas:
1. Hospital joint ventures involving specialized clinical or other expensive health care services
2. Providers' collective provision of non-fee-related information to purchasers of health care services
3. Providers' collective provision of fee-related information to purchasers of health care services
4. Analytical principles relating to multiprovider networks

The 1994 statements included five of the six statements issued in 1993, replacing physician collaboration to provide information to health care purchasers with two of the 1994 statements.

The statements issued by the federal antitrust enforcement agencies include "antitrust safety zones." Conduct will not be challenged absent extraordinary circumstances when it falls within one of these zones. Analytical principles and illustrations are included for activity falling outside of the safety zones. The statements also commit the agencies to an expedited review process on antitrust issues in health care. The agencies will respond to requests for an opinion on enforcement intentions within 90 days after all necessary information is received regarding matters addressed in the statements, except nonsafety zone merger requests and requests regarding multiprovider networks. The agencies will respond within 120 days to requests on all other nonmerger health care matters.

This extraordinary and unprecedented effort by antitrust enforcement agencies to provide guidance to participants in the health care industry was motivated, in part, by the Clinton administration's health care reform agenda. The Clinton health care proposal envisioned substantial structural change in the health care industry and the statements of enforcement policy were an effort to provide some guidelines to the industry as it anticipated and responded with self-initiated structural change. With the failure of Congress to enact any of the major competing health care reform proposals in 1994, the future of government-initiated structural change in the health care industry is uncertain. Nevertheless, consolidations, mergers, and restructuring continue in the health care industry, driven primarily by market forces. These changes in the health care industry will generate significant antitrust questions for many years to come.

END NOTES

1. *Northern Pacific Railway v. United States,* 356 U.S. 1, 4-5 (1958).
2. Standard Oil adopted the trust format in 1879 and was followed by the rapid development of trusts in other industries. The trust as a vehicle for combining economic power commonly involved a trust agreement among the shareholders of the corporations involved. This agreement gave control over the stock in the corporations to the trustees, in return for which the shareholders received trust certificates evidencing their interest in the property controlled by the trust.
3. *See generally,* E. Kinter, *Federal Antitrust Law* (1980).
4. *Id.* at 130.
5. *Id.* at 128, 130.
6. *See generally* E. Letwin, *Law and Economic Policy in America,* at 53-99 (1965); Kinter, *supra* at 125-29.
7. Letwin, *supra* at 95.
8. Initially a violation of the act was a misdemeanor punishable by a fine of up to $5000 and by imprisonment of up to 1 year. The maximum fine was increased in 1955. In 1974, a violation of the act was made a felony and penalties were substantially increased. A corporation may now be fined up to $1,000,000 and any other person, $100,000. The maximum term of imprisonment is now three years. *See Antitrust Procedures and Penalties Act of 1974,* Pub. L. No. 93-528, 88 Stat. 1708. The Sherman Act is codified at 15 U.S.C. §1-7.
9. *See generally* Letwin, *supra* at 106-42.
10. *United States v. Trans-Missouri Freight Association,* 166 U.S. 290 (1897).
11. *United States v. Joint Traffic Association,* 171 U.S. 505 (1898).
12. *United States v. Addyston Pipe & Steel Co.,* 175 U.S. 211 (1899).
13. 51 Cong. Rec. 14218 21 (1914).
14. *Standard Oil Co. of New Jersey v. United States,* 221 U.S. 1 (1911).
15. *Id.* at 138.
16. Act of October 15, 1914, ch. 322, 38 Stat. 730, 15 U.S.C. §§12-27. The Clayton Act deals specifically with tying, exclusive dealing, price discrimination, and mergers.
17. Act of September 26, 1914, ch. 11, 38 Stat. 717, 15 U.S.C. §§41-51.

18. The most significant change was the amendment of the law of price discrimination by the Robinson-Patman Act in 1936. Act of June 19, 1936, ch. 592, 49 Stat. 1526.
19. 15 U.S.C. §1.
20. *Patrick v. Burget,* 486 U.S. 94 (1988). See discussion at p. 187.
21. *See Summit Health, Ltd. v. Pinhas,* 111 S.Ct. 1842 (1991); *McLain v. Real Estate Board of New Orleans,* 444 U.S. 232 (1980).
22. *Hospital Building Co. v. Trustees of Rex Hospital,* 425 U.S. 738, 743-44 (1976).
23. *Summit Health,* 111 S. Ct. 1842 (1991); *Everhart v. Jane C. Stormont Hospital and Training School for Nurses,* 1982-1 Trade Cas. (CCH) 164, 703 (D. Kan. 1982).
24. *See, e.g., Cardio-Medical Associates v. Crozer-Chester Medical Center,* 536 F.Supp. 1065, 1073-74 (E.D. Penn. 1982), *rev'd,* 721 F.2d 68 (3d Cir. 1983); *Riggall v. Washington County Medical Society,* 249 F.2d 266, 269 (8th Cir. 1957), *cert. denied,* 55 U.S. 954 (1958); *Nankin Hospital v. Michigan Hospital Service,* 361 F.Supp. 1199, 1210 (E.D. Mich. 1973).
25. *See Gulf Oil Corp. v. Coff Paving Co.,* 419 U.S. 186, 194 (1974).
26. *Standard Oil,* 221 U.S. 1 (1911).
27. *Chicago Board of Trade v. United States,* 246 U.S. 231, 238 (1918).
28. *National Society of Professional Engineers v. United States,* 435 U.S. 679 (1978).
29. *Id.* at 695. *See also Fashion Originator's Guild of America v. Federal Trade Commission,* 312 U.S. 457 (1941).
30. *Wilk v. American Medical Ass'n, Inc.,* 719 F.2d 207, 227 (7th Cir. 1983), *cert. denied,* 467 U.S. 1210 (1984).
31. *Id.* at 227.
32. *Id.* at 226.
33. *Hospital Building Co.,* 691 F.2d 678, 685 (4th Cir. 1982), *cert. denied,* 464 U.S. 890 (1983).
34. *Id.* at 686.
35. *See Arizona v. Maricopa County Medical Society,* 457 U.S. 332 (1982) (Health care industry entitled to no unique treatment).
36. The development of this presumption in the area of price-fixing began with *United States v. Joint Traffic Ass'n,* 171 U.S. 505, 568 (1897), continued in *United States v. Trenton Potteries Co.,* 273 U.S. 392, 397 (1927), and reached its high point in *United States v. Socony-Vacuum Oil Co.,* 310 U.S. 150, 221-23, 224 n. 59 (1940).
37. The term "per se" was first used in *Socony-Vacuum,* 310 U.S. at 223.
38. *Northern Pacific Railway,* 356 U.S. 1 at 5.
39. This issue is discussed in the separate sections on conduct violations.
40. *Maricopa County Medical Society,* 457 U.S. at 332.
41. *Id.* at 349 (quoting *Socony-Vacuum,* 310 U.S. at 222).
42. *Northern Pacific Railway,* 356 U.S. 1 (1958).
43. *Trenton Potteries Co.,* 273 U.S. at 397.
44. *Id.* at 397-98.
45. *Eastern States Lumber Association v. United States,* 234 U.S. 600, 612 (1914).
46. *Socony-Vacuum,* 310 U.S. at 221.
47. *But see Broadcast Music Inc. v. Columbia Broadcasting System, Inc.,* 441 U.S. 1, 23 (1979).
48. *Chicago Board of Trade,* 246 U.S. at 231.
49. *Id.* at 241.
50. *Broadcast Music, Inc. v. Columbia Broadcasting System, Inc.,* 441 U.S. 1 (1979).
51. *Id.* at 21.
52. *Maricopa County Medical Society,* 457 U.S. 332 (1982).
53. *Id.* at 357.
54. *Id.* at 351. *Maricopa* was decided by a vote of four to three, two justices not participating. The dissent criticized the failure of the majority to recognize the uniqueness of medical services. *Id.* at 366 n. 13.

55. *See, e.g., Glen Eden Hospital v. Blue Cross & Blue Shield of Michigan,* 740 F.2d 423 (6th Cir. 1984).

56. *Id.* at 430.

57. *See, e.g., Kartell v. Blue Shield of Massachusetts, Inc.* 749 F.2d 922 (1st Cir. 1984).

58. The American College of Radiology, 3 Trade Reg. Rep. (CCH) I21,236; Minnesota State Medical Association, 3 Trade Reg. Rep. (CCH) I21,293; The American College of Obstetricians and Gynecologists, 3 Trade Reg. Rep. (CCH) I21,171; The American Academy of Orthopedic Surgeons, 3 Trade Reg. Rep. (CCH) I21,171.

59. *Mandeville Island Farms, Inc. v. American Crystal Sugar Co.,* 334 U.S. 219, 235 (1948).

60. *Northwest Wholesale Stationers, Inc. v. Pacific Stationery and Printing Co.,* 472 U.S. 284, 295 (1985) (quoting from *Broadcast Music,* 441 U.S. at 20).

61. *See* "Remarks of Charles F. Rule Before the Interim Meeting of the American Medical Association House of Delegates, Dallas, Texas, December 6, 1988."

62. 15 U.S.C. §1.

63. 15 U.S.C. §14.

64. 15 U.S.C. §45.

65. 15 U.S.C. §14.

66. *Jefferson Parish Hospital District No. 2 v. Hyde,* 466 U.S. 2 (1984).

67. *Id.* at 12.

68. *Id.* at 15-16.

69. *Id.* at 17. Justice O'Connor, in an opinion concurring in the judgment in *Jefferson Parish,* which three other justices joined, suggests three prerequisites to an illegal tie: (1) The seller must have power in the tying product market; (2) there must be a "substantial threat" that the seller will acquire market power in the tied product; (3) there must be a coherent economic basis for treating the tied products as distinct products. *Id.* at 1571. She also rejected per se treatment of tying arrangements even if these conditions are met. *Id.* at 37-40.

70. *Id.* at 26-27.

71. *Id.* at 29.

72. *Id.* at 21.

73. *Id.* at 22-24.

74. *Id.* at 23.

75. *Id.* at 25-26, n. 42 (citing *Maricopa County Medical Society,* 457 U.S. 332 (1982); *National Gerimedical Hospital v. Blue Cross,* 452 U.S. 378 (1981); *American Medical Ass'n v. United States,* 317 U.S. 519 (1943)).

76. 15 U.S.C. §1.

77. 15 U.S.C. §14.

78. 15 U.S.C. §45.

79. *Continental T.V., Inc., v. GTE Sylvania, Inc.,* 433 U.S. 36 (1977). See also *Jefferson Parish Hospital,* 466 U.S. at 45 (O'Connor, J., concurring).

80. *Standard Oil Co. v. United States,* 337 U.S. 293, 314 (1949).

81. *Tampa Electric Co. v. Nashville Coal Co.,* 365 U.S. 320 (1961).

82. *Jefferson Parish Hospital,* 466 U.S. at 30 n. 51 (1984).

83. *Id.* at 45 (O'Connor, J., concurring).

84. *Id.*

85. *Harron v. United Hospital Center, Inc.,* 522 F.2d 1133 (4th Cir. 1975), *cert. denied,* 424 U.S. 916 (1976).

86. *Id.* at 1134.

87. *Dos Santos v. Columbus-Cuneo-Cabrini Medical Center,* 684 F.2d 1346 (7th Cir. 1982).

88. *Id.* at 1354.

89. *Id.* at 1355.

90. *Id.* at 1352.

91. *See, e.g., Jefferson Parish Hospital,* 466 U.S. at 45 (O'Connor, J., concurring); *U.S. Healthcare, Inc. v. Healthsource, Inc.,* 986 F.2d 589 (1st Cir. 1993).

92. 15 U.S.C. §1. Section 1 by its terms requires some contract, combination, or conspiracy for a violation of the section to occur. Unilateral action by a businessman has long been recognized as legitimate conduct unrestrained by the antitrust laws. *United States v. Colgate Co.,* 250 U.S. 300 (1919). One significant exception to this proposition would be unilateral action, which could be characterized as monopolization or as an attempt to monopolize.

93. *See Klor's, Inc. v. Broadway-Hale Stores, Inc.* 359 U.S. 207 (1959); *United States v. General Motors Corp.,* 384 U.S. 127 (1966).

94. *Northwest Wholesale Stationers,* 472 U.S. 284 (1985).

95. *Id.* at 2619 (citations omitted).

96. *Id.* at 2621.

97. *Weiss v. York Hospital,* 745 F.2d 786, 818 (3d Cir. 1984), *cert. denied,* 470 U.S. 1060 (1985).

98. *Id.* at 820.

99. *Id.* at 820. The court drew upon language from *Arizona v. Maricopa County Medical Society,* 457 U.S. 332, 348-49 (1982), recognizing some limited vitality for a "learned professions" exemption from the operation of the antitrust laws.

100. *Wilk,* 719 F.2d 207 (7th Cir. 1983), *cert. denied,* 467 U.S. 1210 (1984).

101. *Id.* at 221.

102. *Id.* at 221. See discussion of the rule of reason approach in *Wilk* at p. 182.

103. *See, e.g., Pontious v. Children's Hospital,* 552 F. Supp. 1352 (W.D. Pa. 1982); *Chiropractic Cooperative Association of Michigan v. American Medical Ass'n.,* 617 F. Supp. 264 (E.D. Mich. 1985).

104. *Patrick,* 486 U.S. 94 (1988).

105. See discussion at pp. 188-189.

106. 42 U.S.C. §§11101-11152. This statute was, in part, in response to the verdict in the trial court in *Patrick v. Burget.*

107. 15 U.S.C. §1.

108. *Copperweld Corp. v. Independence Tube Corp.,* 467 U.S. 2731 (1984). For a case involving wholly owned health care subsidiaries, see *Advanced Health Care Services, Inc. v. Radford Community Hospital,* 910 F. 2d 139 (3d Cir. 1990).

109. *See Weiss,* 745 F.2d at 814-17, *cert. denied,* 470 U.S. 1060 (1985); *Feldman v. Jackson Memorial Hospital,* 571 F. Supp. 1000 (S.D. Fla. 1983), *aff'd,* 752 F.2d 647 (11th Cir. 1985); *Cooper v. Forsyth County Hospital Authority,* 604 F. Supp. 685 (M.D. N.C. 1985). *But see Nurse Midwifery Associates v. Hibbett,* 918 F. 2d 605 (1990), *cert. denied,* 112 S.Ct. 406 (1991).

110. *See* discussion of this point in *Weiss,* 745 F.2d at 815-16; *see also Nurse Midwifery Associates,* 918 F. 2d 605 (1990), *cert. denied,* 112 S.Ct. 406 (1991).

111. See discussion at p. 181.

112. *Robinson v. Magovern,* 521 F. Supp. 842, 876-77 (W.D. Pa. 1981), *aff'd,* 688 F.2d 824 (3d Cir.), *cert. denied,* 459 U.S. 971 (1982).

113. *Summit Health,* 111 S.Ct. 1842 (1991); *Cardio-Medical Associates, Ltd. v. Crozer-Chester Medical Center,* 721 F.2d 68 (3d Cir. 1983).

114. 721 F.2d at 75.

115. *United States v. Topco Associates, Inc.,* 405 U.S. 596 (1972).

116. *Continental T.V. v. G.T.E. Sylvania,* 433 U.S. 36 (1977).

117. *Cf. Broadcast Music,* 441 U.S. 1 (1979).

118. *See* "The Role of Antitrust in Improving and Reforming the Health Care System," Remarks of Kevin J. Arquit, Director, Bureau of Competition, Federal Trade Commission, Delivered to the American Bar Association, October 15, 1992.

119. 15 U.S.C.A. §2.

120. *United States v. Aluminum Co. of America,* 148 F.2d 416, 430 (2d Cir. 1945) ("The successful competitor, having been urged to compete, must not be turned upon when he wins").

121. *United States v. Grinnell Corp.,* 384 U.S. 563, 571 (1966).

122. *United States v. duPont & Co.,* 351 U.S. 377, 391 (1956); *accord Grinnel Corp.,* 384 U.S. at 571.

123. *Grinnell Corp.,* 384 U.S. at 571.

124. In *Aluminum Co. of America,* 148 F.2d at 424, Judge Learned Hand noted that: "The percentage we have already mentioned— over ninety—results only if we both include all 'Alcoa's' production and exclude 'secondary.' That percentage is enough to constitute a monopoly; it is doubtful whether sixty or sixty-four percent would be enough; and certainly thirty-three percent is not."

125. *See* in this regard the revised merger guidelines issued by the United States Department of Justice in 1992; §2.1 Product Market Definition; §2.3 Geographic Market Definition; §2.4 Calculating Market Shares.

126. *Aluminum Co. of America,* 148 F.2d at 431.

127. *Aspen Skiing Co. v. Aspen Highlands Skiing Co.,* 472 U.S. 585, 603-05 (1985); *Berkey Photo Inc. v. Eastman Kodak Co.,* 603 F.2d 263, 274 (2d Cir. 1979), *cert. denied,* 444 U.S. 1093 (1980).

128. *See William Inglis & Sons v. ITT Continental Baking Co.,* 668 F.2d 1014, 1027 (9th Cir. 1981), *cert. denied,* 459 U.S. 825 (1982).

129. *See, e.g.,* Cartensen, *Reflections on Hay, Clark and the Relationship of Economic Analysis to Rules of Antitrust Law,* 83 Wis. L. Rev. 953 (1983); Cooper, *Attempts and Monopolization: A Mildly Expansionary Answer to the Prophylactic Riddle of Section Two,* 72 Mich. L. Rev. 373 (1974).

130. *See, e.g.,* Weiss, 745 F.2d at 825, *cert. denied,* 470 U.S. 1060 (1985) (§2 violation reversed because no showing of willful conduct on part of hospital); *Robinson v. Magovern,* 621 F. Supp. at 887 (30% market share does not constitute monopoly power).

131. Allegations of monopolization, *inter alia,* by the attorney general of the State of Maine against an association of anesthesiologists in Portland, Me., resulted in a consent decree restricting the practices of that association. *State of Maine v. Anesthesia Professional Ass'n,* Maine Superior Court, Consent Decree, June 12, 1984. In *Bhan v. NME Hospitals, Inc.,* 772 F.2d 1467 (9th Cir. 1985), a nurse anesthetist alleged violations of §§1 and 2 of the Sherman Act by anesthesiologists and a hospital acting in combination to deny access to the hospital to nurse anesthetists.

132. 15 U.S.C. §18. The Federal Trade Commission may review a merger pursuant to 15 U.S.C. §45 which incorporates the provisions of Section 7. *Stanley Works v. FTC,* 469 F.2d 498, 499 n. 2 (2d Cir. 1972), *cert. denied,* 412 U.S. 28 (1973).

133. 15 U.S.C. §18.

134. 15 U.S.C. §12. In regard to asset acquisitions, the acquiring party must be "subject to the jurisdiction of the Federal Trade Commission." For discussion of this point, *see* Miles and Philip, *Hospitals Caught in the Antitrust Net: An Overview,* 24 Duquesne L. Rev. 489, 664 (1985) and see *FTC v. University Health Inc.,* 938 F.2d 1206 (11th Cir. 1991) and *U.S. v. Rockford Memorial Hospital,* 898 F.2d 1278 (7th Cir. 1990).

135. 15 U.S.C. §18.

136. *United States v. Penn-Olin Chemical Co.,* 378 U.S. 158 (1964).

137. *Cf. United States v. Von's Grocery Co.,* 384 U.S. 270 (1966), *with United States v. General Dynamics Corp.,* 415 U.S. 486 (1974) *and United States v. Marine Bancorporation,* 418 U.S. 602 (1974).

138. *See, e.g.,* Hospital Corporation of America, 3 Trade Reg. Rep. (CCH) I22,301 (FTC Oct. 25, 1985); American Medical International, 3 Trade Reg. Rep. (CCH) I22,170 (FTC July 2, 1984).

139. 1992 Merger Guidelines, §2.1.

140. *Id.* at §2.3.

141. The Herfindahl-Hirschman index (HHI) is the sum of the squares of the individual market shares of all the firms judged to be appropriately included in the market. An HHI of below 1000 in a postmerger market is generally considered unconcentrated, while an HHI above 1800 is generally considered highly concen-trated. An HHI between 1000 and 1800 will be reviewed with emphasis on the increase in the HHI caused by the merger and other factors. This statement is a very summary explanation of the process followed under the Merger Guidelines and reference to the Merger Guidelines is strongly recommended.

142. *See Hospital Corporation of America v. FTC,* 807 F. 2d 1381 (7th Cir. 1986), *cert. denied,* 481 U. 5. 1038 (1987); American Medical International, 3 Trade Reg. Rep. (CCH) 122,170 (FTC July 2, 1984); *United States v. Hospital Affiliates International, Inc.,* 1980-81 Trade Cases (CCH) 163,721 (E.D. La. 1980); *American Medicorp, Inc. v. Humana, Inc.,* 445 F. Supp. 589 (E.D. Pa. 1977).

143. See Statement of Charles A. James, Acting Assistant Attorney General, Antitrust Division, to the Joint Economic Committee of the House-Senate Subcommittee on Investment, Jobs and Prices, June 24, 1992.

144. *Parker v. Brown,* 317 U.S. 341 (1943).

145. *Id.* at 350.

146. *See, e.g., Goldfarb v. Virginia State Bar,* 421 U.S. 773 (1975); *Cantor v. Detroit Edison Co.,* 428 U.S. 579 (1976); *Bates v. State Bar of Arizona,* 433 U.S. 350 (1977).

147. *California Liquor Dealers v. Midcal Aluminum Inc.,* 445 U.S. 97 (1980).

148. *Id.* at 105.

149. *Id.*

150. See *Patrick v. Burget,* 486 U.S. 94 (1988); *see also Southern Motor Carriers Rate Conference v. United States,* 471 U.S. 48, (1985) for *Southern Motor Carriers* the Court rejected the contention that in order to gain the benefit of the state action exemption, the anticompetitive conduct of the private party must be compelled by the state statute.

151. *Town of Hallie v. City of Eau Claire,* 471 U.S. 34 (1985).

152. *See, e.g., State of North Carolina ex rel. Edmisten v. P.I.A. Asheville, Inc.,* 740 F.2d 274 (4th Cir. 1984), *cert. denied,* 469 U.S. 1070 (1985).

153. *See, e.g., Marrese v. Interequal, Inc.,* 748 F.2d 373 (7th Cir. 1984), *cert. denied,* 472 U.S. 1027 (1985); *Quinn v. Kent General Hospital, Inc.,* 617 F. Supp. 1226 (D.C. Del. 1985).

154. *See, e.g., Coastal Neuro-Psychiatric Associates v. Onslow County Hospital Authority,* 607 F. Supp. 49 (D.C.N.C. 1985).

155. *Springs Ambulance Service v. City of Rancho Mirage,* 745 F.2d 1270 (9th Cir. 1984); *Gold Cross Ambulance and Transfer v. City of Kansas City,* 705 F.2d 1005 (8th Cir. 1983), *cert. denied,* 469 U.S. 538 (1985). Both cases involved exclusive contracts for the provision of ambulance services to the citizens of the municipalities.

156. *Town of Hallie,* 471 U.S. at 47.

157. Local Government Antitrust Act of 1984, Pub. L. 98-544, October 24, 1984, 15 U.S.C. §§34-36.

158. 112 S. Ct. 2169 (1992).

159. *Id.* at 2178.

160. 992 F.2d 1122 (3rd Cir. 1991).

161. 112 S. Ct. at 2179.

162. *See, e.g., DFW Metro Line Servs. v. Southwestern Bell Tel. Corp.* 988 F.2d 601 (5th Cir. 1993); *Tri-State Rubbish v. Waste Mgt. Inc.,* 998 F.2d 1073 (1st Cir. 1993).

163. 15 U.S.C. §17.

164. 15 U.S.C. §§1011-1015 (McCarran-Ferguson Act). *See Union Life Insurance Co. v. Pireno,* 458 U.S. 119 (1982); *Group Life & Health Ins. Co. v. Royal Drug Co.,* 440 U.S. 205 (1979); *St. Paul Fire & Marine Ins. Co. v. Barry,* 438 U.S. 531 (1978).

165. 15 U.S.C. §17; 7 U.S.C. §§291-292 (Capper-Volstead Act).

166. 15 U.S.C. §521 (The Fisheries Cooperative Marketing Act).

167. 15 U.S.C. §§1801-04 (The Newspaper Preservation Act).

168. 15 U.S.C. §§3501-03 (The Soft Drink Interbrand Competition Act of 1980).

169. 15 U.S.C. §638(d)(1), (2).

170. 15 U.S.C. §§640, 2158.

171. 15 U.S.C. §§62, 4001-4021 (Webb-Pomerene Act, Export Trading Company Act of 1982).

172. *Patrick,* 486 U.S. 94 (1988).

173. 42 U.S.C. §§11101-11152.

174. The professional review action must meet the standards set forth in 42 U.S.C. §11112(a). This immunity may be lost if a health care entity fails to report information as required by the statute. 42 U.S.C. §11111(b).

175. Professional review body is defined at 42 U.S.C. §11151 (11). It includes a health care entity conducting professional review and any committee of a health care entity or of a medical staff of such an entity conducting such review when assisting the governing body of the institution.

176. Immunity is not provided if the information is false and the person providing it knew it. 42 U.S.C. §11111(a)(2).

177. 42 U.S.C. §11113.

178. *See, e.g.,* The Reed-Bullwinkle Act, 49 U.S.C. §10706 (joint rate filings with ICC by carriers); the Shipping Act of 1916, 46 U.S.C. §813a, 814 (rate agreements between maritime carriers).

179. *See, e.g., United States v. National Association of Securities Dealers,* 422 U.S. 694 (1975); *United States v. Philadelphia National Bank,* 374 U.S. 321 (1963); *Silver v. New York Stock Exchange,* 373 U.S. 341 (1963).

180. *See National Gerimedical Hospital v. Blue Cross,* 452 U.S. 378 (1981).

181. 42 U.S.C. §3001 (National Health Planning and Development Act of 1974).

182. 452 U.S. at 391.

183. *Id.* at 393 n. 18.

184. *Eastern Railroad Presidents Conference v. Noerr Motor Freight, Inc.,* 365 U.S. 127 (1961); *United Mine Workers v. Pennington,* 381 U.S. 657 (1965).

185. *Noerr Motor Freight,* 365 U.S. at 137.

186. *Id.* at 144; *see also Professional Real Estate Investors Inc. v. Columbia Pictures Industries, Inc.,* 113 S.Ct. 1920 (1993); *City of Columbia v. Omni Outdoor Advertising, Inc.,* 111 S.Ct. 1344 (1991); *California Motor Transport Co. v. Trucking Unlimited,* 404 U.S. 508, 513 (1972).

187. *See, e.g., Hospital Building Co.,* 692 F.2d at 687-88; *Feminist Women's Health Center v. Mohammad,* 586 F.2d 530, 542-478 (5th Cir. 1978).

188. *Feminist Women's Health Center,* 586 F.2d at 454.

189. *Virginia Academy of Clinical Psychologists v. Blue Shield of Virginia,* 624 F.2d 476, 482 (4th Cir. 1980), *cert. denied,* 450 U.S. 916 (1981).

190. Robinson-Patman Antidiscrimination Act, ch. 592, §1-4, 49 Stat 1526, 15 U.S.C. 13, 13a, 13b, 21a, 13c (1936).

191. Non-Profit Institutions Act, ch. 283, 52 Stat. 446, 15 U.S.C. 13c (1938).

192. *Abbott Laboratories v. Portland Retail Druggists Ass'n,* 425 U.S. 1 (1976).

193. Federal Trade Commission Act, ch. 311, 38 Stat 717, 15 U.S.C. §44-51 (1914).

194. *A.M.A. v. United States,* 317 U.S. 519 (1943); *see also U.S. v. Oregon State Medical Society,* 343 U.S. 326, (1952).

195. *In re Forbes Health System Medical Staff,* FTC file No. 781-0009, Consent Order, Nov. 13, 1978.

196. *A.M.A. v. FTC,* 638 F.2d 443 (2d Cir. 1980), aff'd, 455 U.S. 676 (1982).

197. *Illinois Podiatry Society, Inc.,* 1977-2 Trade Cas. §761, 761 (N.D. Ill. 1977).

198. *American College of Radiology,* 3 Trade Reg. Rep. (CCH) §21, 23b (1976).

199. "Statements of Antitrust Enforcement Policy in the Health Care Arena," U.S. Department of Justice and Federal Trade Commission, Sep. 15, 1993.

200. *See, e.g.,* "Antitrust Implications of Health Care Reform," American Bar Association Working Group on Health Care Reform, May 14, 1993.

CHAPTER 17

Crimes against and by health care providers and criminal procedures

STAN TWARDY, J.D., LL.M.
S. SANDY SANBAR, M.D., Ph.D., J.D., F.C.L.M.

CRIMES BY HEALTH CARE PROVIDERS
CRIMES AGAINST THE PERSON
CRIMINAL PROCEDURE

Today more than ever before, medicine encounters many situations that spill into the realm of criminal law. Prosecutors, state and federal, are increasingly peering over the shoulders of health care professionals and medical facilities in an effort to ferret out health care fraud and drug abuse. The ongoing unprecedented scrutiny, aided by a high level of computerization, has brought to light a variety of crimes by physicians, nurses, pharmacists, hospitals, clinics, nursing homes, and other health care facilities. Even though small in number, these pill pushers, health quacks, and welfare cheats can give the medical profession a black eye.

Aside from becoming a criminal defendant, the health care provider may be called as an expert witness, may be a victim of a crime, or an innocent bystander. But whatever the nature of the encounter, a rudimentary understanding of criminal law and criminal procedure is often needed in dealing with the multifaceted problems of use, dispensation, and theft of drugs, writing of false and/or fictitious prescriptions, Medicare and Medicaid fraud, rape, homicide (deaths resulting from surgery, drugs, abandonment, improper care, prescribing or injecting drugs, or operating while the physician was intoxicated or on drugs), death or injuries resulting from refusal or failure to provide medical or surgical treatment, reckless nursing or pharmaceutical errors, abuse of children and the elderly, criminal malpractice, income tax frauds, kickbacks for referrals of Medicare patients and from pharmacies, conspiracies, practicing without a license or with a suspended or revoked license, intimacy with minors and psychiatric patients, allegations of assault and battery when a physician is examining or treating a female patient, abortion and fertility prob-

lems, and most recently the wide-ranging debate about assisted suicides and euthanasia.

The criminal liability of physicians, dentists, nurses, and pharmacists frequently results from a high degree of negligent conduct. What the law calls "criminal negligence" is largely a matter of degree, incapable of a precise definition. Whether or not it exists is a question for the jury. The law requires a showing of "gross lack of competency or gross inattention, or wanton indifference to the patient's safety, which may arise from gross ignorance of the science of medicine and surgery, or through gross negligence, either in the application and selection of remedies, lack of proper skills in the use of instruments, and failure to give proper attention to the patient"[1] (e.g., "Practicing fraudulently with gross incompetence and gross negligence," by failing to take and record vital signs of a patient to whom the physician administered anesthesia, utilizing investigational and non-FDA approved substances, etc.). The fact that the patient consented to the specific treatment or operation is no defense to the criminal action against the physician.

The courts have been very careful not to hold physicians criminally responsible for the death of patients as a result of a "mere mistake of judgement in the selection and application of remedies when the death resulted merely from an error of judgement or an inadvertent death."[2] However, a physician was convicted of criminal negligence in the treatment of a mother and her baby for ignoring respiratory stress syndrome.

Criminal responsibility for physical measures and involuntary administration of medications to mentally disordered patients is very broad, especially if the patient doesn't present an imminent danger to himself or others.

Some overzealous prosecutors are also escalating lesser peccadillos and billing errors into major prosecutions. Often, it is a question of intent, and prosecutors are not always the best mind readers—nor are juries—and the consequences to the affected physician can be absolutely devastating if he or she is not believed.

Conviction of a felony, in any state or foreign country, even if not related to medical practice (e.g., tax evasion,[3] possession of an unlicensed machine gun,[4] intimidation of expert witnesses in malpractice action,[5] conspiracy to murder a wife,[6] sexual misconduct with a minor[7] often carries a mandatory revocation and/or suspension of license and/or hospital privileges.

Physicians who are not U.S. citizens, aside from criminal penalties upon conviction and the possible revocation and/or suspension of license, may face the added penalty of losing their resident alien status and being deported. Deportation can often be forestalled when the wife, husband, or children are American citizens.

CRIMES BY HEALTH CARE PROVIDERS
Medicare, Medicaid, and insurance frauds

The federal government, through the Office of the Health and Human Services Inspector General, the FBI, and state and local law enforcement agencies, is targeting health care fraud on a large scale. These cases center on massive, flagrant, and pervasive garden varieties of fraudulent billing and mail and wire fraud. These frauds are usually perpetrated on numerous patients, insurers, and the government with the clearest intent to rip off the health care system with "creative" billing over an extended period of time. These include primarily services that were never performed; repetitive patterns of unneeded procedures and/or hospitalizations; giving and receiving of kickbacks, bribes, or rebates; or false representations for certification of hospitals, nursing homes, intermediate care facilities for the mentally retarded, home health agencies, etc.

Individual physicians are most frequently charged with fraud when using higher billing codes, or "unbundling" CPT codes. Each code describes with specificity the procedure performed. When a physician uses a higher code (this is called *upcoding*), he or she is misrepresenting what was actually done and is billing and getting paid for services that were not performed. Patient visits under the coding system are categorized as brief, limited, intermediate, comprehensive, and extended. These are based on the amount of time spent and services performed. If a physician charges for half an hour for writing a prescription and designates it as an "extensive consultation" instead of a "minimal consultation," the jury will recognize it as a fraud. Also, the hospital records and/or office notes would show what else the physician did. If he or she did nothing else, but consistently used the highest codes, the criminal modus operandi will be obvious to the jury. Testimony that each case was very complex and required the physician to spend an inordinate amount of time with patients is easily refuted. In one case where billing and procedures in one clinic were added up, the incredible discovery was made that there were 25, 30, or even 50 billable hours in a day!

When a physician is "unbundling" codes, he or she is double billing for services performed. The physician is paid once for the whole job (called a "global" fee, which includes all the services rendered) and the second time for the specific things the physician did. In one Texas case, the FBI described it as analogous to charging a global fee of $100 for selling and mounting a tire, and then billing separately and in addition for jacking up the car, unscrewing the lugs, taking off the old tire, mounting a new tire on the rim, putting the tire back on, tightening the lugs, and putting on the hub cap and then charging an extra $100 or so for each step. The defense of "mistakes" in using the codes is not very credible when it can be shown that the same "mistakes" were made on numerous patients, over and over again, and always in favor of the physician. Billing for treatment given to dead patients is increasingly picked up by computers that record the date and time of death.

Other fraudulent transactions have included double billing for fees as attending physician and as a consultant on the same patient at the same time. This is double billing for the same service by any name. Another fraud involves billing separately for different medications prescribed to the same patient. This is a fraudulent imposition of a "royalty" on drugs because the physician was already paid for his diagnosis and treatment, which includes prescribing.

In virtually all cases of Medicare and Medicaid fraud, the courts have ordered full restitution. In addition, heavy fines were imposed in conjunction with jail terms or probation. Federal sentences are based on mandatory guidelines, which leave little discretion to judges.

Allegations of criminality, even where there are no convictions, are almost invariably followed by separate investigations, and often by drastic disciplinary action by state licensing boards, the DEA and state narcotic control authorities, and the barring of reimbursements from Medicare, Medicaid, other federally funded and supported programs, and insurance plans for federal employees. Many HMO and PPO contracts provide for dismissal of physicians tainted by criminality. Theoretically, all such actions should find their way into the National Practitioner Data Bank resulting in denials of licenses and/or hospital privileges to errant physicians.

Prosecution of nurses is rather infrequent. It involves

primarily use, theft, and distribution of drugs. In a few rare cases, nurses have been charged with murder or manslaughter for pulling the plug on patients, recklessly ignoring patients' symptoms and problems, allowing patients to die by not calling physicians in a timely fashion, abandoning patients, and practicing with revoked and/or suspended licenses. Nurses have also been accused of racial bias, as in one case where a nurse called an unruly patient "you black son of a bitch," and removed him from a dialysis machine, leaving dialysis needles in his arm.[8]

Understanding the criminal law

The purpose of criminal law is to define socially intolerable conduct and to make specific prohibitions punishable by law. Criminal procedure deals with constitutional safeguards and the working mechanism of American courts to assure justice and fairness. A health care provider who runs afoul of the criminal law may be consoled by the array of constitutional safeguards that assure a fair trial. The Anglo-American system of justice provides more safeguards to the criminal defendant than any other in the world. In this system, the criminal accused is deemed innocent until proven guilty. In other judicial systems, the criminal defendant must prove innocence.

In a civil case, the standard of proof is that the facts at issue must be proved by a "preponderance of the evidence"; in a criminal case, the state or the federal government must prove its case "beyond a reasonable doubt." Some legal scholars define "preponderance of the evidence" as being merely more likely than not, something more than a 50% probability; this is the standard for civil litigation, which includes most malpractice cases. It means that it is more likely than not that the facts are as the plaintiff argues. In contrast, when a criminal defendant is tried, the prosecution must prove beyond a reasonable doubt that a crime was committed and that the defendant committed that crime. This means that a rational and fair juror would be convinced of the guilt and would have no reasonable hesitation to vote for the conviction. In criminal cases, this usually means that a jury must be unanimous, or that the conviction must be by at least two-thirds of the jurors.

Unlike the federal government, which has only delegated powers to enact and enforce substantive criminal laws, our Constitution gives every state an inherent authority by virtue of its police powers to regulate internal affairs for the protection or promotion of the health, safety, welfare, and morals of its residents. That is why most states have their own, often dissimilar, criminal codes.

Modern criminal law recognizes two major classes of crimes and a number of miscellaneous offenses and violations. By definition, a *felony* is a crime with a potential punishment of imprisonment for one year or more. It includes such crimes as murder (e.g., withdrawal of life support from a comatose patient by a physician or nurse[9], manslaughter, rape, robbery, larceny, kidnapping, arson, burglary, most narcotics and insurance fraud crimes, sex with minors, etc.). Misdemeanors are crimes with a maximum punishment of imprisonment of less than one year. The term *misdemeanor* is applied to the widest range of criminal activity and includes the broadest gradation of offenses and degrees of unpermitted activity (e.g., failure to report child abuse, refusal to allow patients to examine and copy their medical records, willful disclosure of health care information to unauthorized persons, etc.).

Another category of criminal and quasicriminal offenses—both felonies and misdemeanors—are the so-called "strict liability" offenses. The major significance of such offenses is that certain defenses, such as a mistake, are generally not available. These are usually offenses that are part of regulatory schemes, for example, practicing medicine or nursing without a license, writing prescriptions without a valid Drug Enforcement Agency (DEA) registration or state narcotics license, and so on.

In the health care field, both federal and state agencies, under delegation from Congress or state legislatures, have created a multitude of rules and regulations, the violation of which may also be punishable as a crime. These include the DEA's wide-ranging regulations on licensing and supervision of prescribing, storing, and dispensing of controlled substances; the Internal Revenue Service regulations; various health department regulations, including reporting requirements of certain contagious diseases; and so on. Violations of these regulations may be enforced either criminally or administratively by revocation of licenses and heavy fines.

In most states, there exists a third category of offenses and violations, or *prohibited acts,* as they are sometimes called. These acts, though technically crimes, are so minor in nature that the law refuses to classify them as misdemeanors. These include a host of activities such as violating minor traffic laws, allowing dogs to be unleashed, spitting in public, and littering.

After the accused has been apprehended, he or she may be held pending a *preliminary hearing* to determine whether there are sufficient grounds to hold the accused for trial or for a presentation to a grand jury; or the case can be taken directly before a grand jury. The preliminary hearing magistrate may also release the accused on bond or may hold the accused for the grand jury hearing or a trial. The grand jury as well as the magistrate may reject the allegations and free the suspect. Also, the prosecuting attorney may refuse to proceed, which is known as a case of *nolle prosse.*

To establish that the physician is guilty, each and every element of the crime prescribed by the legislature and the culpability of the suspect must be proven beyond a reasonable doubt to the trier of facts—a jury and/or a judge. In prosecuting a crime, the government provides the forum, courtroom, judge, jury, and other necessary functions and functionaries. If the criminal defendant cannot afford a defense attorney or other necessary defense materials, the state will reasonably provide them. The accused must be afforded their constitutional rights, both federal and state (if appropriate), of due process and "equal protection" under the law. At trial the accused may (1) plead guilty, thus obviating the need for an actual trial, (2) plead not guilty and be tried, or (3) plead *nolo contendere* ("I will not contest the charges," while not a guilty plea, is a tacit confession of guilt). After conviction of plea, the judge determines the penalty, if any. Frequently, pleading guilty or *nolo contendere* is based on plea bargaining between the state's and defendant's attorneys.

If the criminal is convicted, the government exacts the penalty—fine, imprisonment, or probation. The victim may also sue the criminal civilly in tort, or the victim may apply to the government for victim compensation in states where such programs exist.

Elements of a crime

The essential elements of a crime are (1) intent *(mens rea)* and (2) the act *(actus rea).* To constitute a crime, the act must be volitional and the intent must be to accomplish the criminal purpose. In the case of misdemeanor offenses and violations, the law does not always inquire whether the criminal intent was present (e.g., the traffic court judge does not inquire into the intent of a person who went through a red light, failed to stop at a stop sign, or made a left turn without signaling). But pulling the plug on a patient presupposes the intent to kill combined with an act to further that purpose. For misdemeanors and petty offenses the element of intent is not normally a consideration.

Lack of intent is not a defense for the category of crimes committed while a person is intoxicated or under the influence of drugs. The law takes the position that such acts are voluntary and that a misconduct in such a state is predictable; therefore, criminal liability should be attached.

Lesser included offenses

Another concept that underlies criminal law in American jurisprudence is the theory of lesser included offenses. For example, the crime of murder usually includes such lesser offenses as manslaughter and battery; the crime of robbery usually includes larceny with the added element of force or threat of force against a person; a burglary includes an unlawful trespass into a dwelling with the intent to commit a larceny or any other crime. By definition, a person cannot commit a burglary unless trespassing has been committed; a person cannot be guilty of robbery unless that person is also guilty of larceny.

The significance of lesser included offenses comes into play when a jury cannot agree on a major crime or when, because of extenuating circumstances, the jury decides to punish the wrongdoer for a lesser included offense. While pulling the plug may be premeditated murder, if there are extenuating circumstances, the jury may only convict of a lesser included offense of manslaughter.

Vicarious culpability

Modern American jurisprudence also tends to disregard distinctions between principals and accessories to a criminal act. The streamlined approach tends to regard an *accessory before the fact* (one who supplies a weapon but does not participate in the murder) not as some quasi-innocent bystander but as an actual participant in the crime. Under this theory, drivers of getaway cars are responsible for murders committed by bank robbers almost to the same extent as if they had pulled the trigger. The *accessory after the fact* is treated differently and is not liable for acts done prior to his or her involvement. Modern jurisprudence is also abandoning the designation of participants in the crime as accessories; instead it regards them as accomplices who are liable for all the foreseeable consequences of the criminal act they intended to aid or in which they participated.

The physician may be vicariously liable for the acts of his or her employees when allowing them unsupervised access to controlled substances, when allowing them to call in prescriptions without consulting him, or when inducing, encouraging, or ordering them to fill out fraudulent insurance claims or to commit other criminal acts.

Under the theory of accomplices, the test of criminal activity is the foreseeability that the crime will be committed and the weight the law attaches to the acts done in furtherance of the conspiracies or crimes. Of special interest to physicians are acts that cannot be committed alone or acts committed by a perpetrator who is legally considered incapable of committing the crime directly because of his or her special status. Examples of such liability include a psychiatrist who told a patient about the problems a certain person was causing him knowing that the patient would promptly proceed to kill that person. In another case, a physician who "allowed himself to be seduced" by a young woman under the age of consent, was subsequently charged with statutory rape. Both physicians were criminally liable. The psychiatrist was convicted of murder even though his patient was acquitted on the basis of insanity. In the case of statutory rape, the young woman, who was technically an accomplice to the statutory rape because of her active solicitation of the seduction, also escaped accomplice liabilities.

In the case of accomplices, it is not necessary that both accomplices to the crime be convicted. If one escapes, is acquitted, or is not caught, the other may nevertheless be convicted as if he or she alone had committed the crime. Secretaries and bookkeepers have often been prosecuted as accomplices when they helped falsify billing records or as accessories after the fact when they helped cover up Medicare frauds. However, when threatened with criminal prosecution, office helpers almost invariably make deals with prosecutors. They are not prosecuted in exchange for testimony against the physician. They are often the most devastating witnesses against physicians.

Accessory after the fact

An accessory after the fact is anyone who renders assistance to a felon after the offense was committed, even though the accessory had no prior knowledge of the commission of the crime. The assistance may involve harboring a fugitive, providing funds for the escape, or hindering the prosecution by delaying the discovery of the crime or apprehension of the felon. In Medicare and insurance fraud cases, this often involves helping to falsify medical records. In modern American jurisprudence, failure to report a felony generally no longer makes one an accessory after the fact.

Assisted suicides. Some states have enacted separate statutes that make it a crime to knowingly assist or encourage a crime. Such crimes include the aiding or abetting of suicide. Recently, Dr. Jack Kevorkian, a Michigan pathologist, has bounced in and out of courtrooms and headlines, first with his "suicide machine" (a low-tech homemade device,) then with all manner of how-to-do-it advice, "counseling," or merely watching some 20 assisted suicides. He also challenged the constitutionality of the Michigan assisted suicide statute. Prosecutors have asked how such "practice of medicine" differs from handing a loaded gun to a suicidal person. Medical licensing boards have asked whether, as a pathologist, Dr. Kevorkian was qualified to diagnose Alzheimer's or evaluate patients with severe depressions, and have revoked his medical license. The DEA wondered whether this was not an abuse of his narcotics license and improper prescribing of controlled substances, whereas the FDA may have wondered

whether his "death machine" required approval by the federal government.

One may even wonder whether Dr. Kevorkian also needed a state license to act as an "executioner." At the time of this writing, Dr. Kevorkian faces multiple charges and has appeals pending. But the questions of being an accessory or of having committed an anticipatory crime, such as in the facilitation of death, may take a long time to be sorted out by other states. Such cases can be prosecuted under the theories of murder, manslaughter, or being an accessory to the crime of suicide in other states where suicide has not been decriminalized, for improper prescription of controlled substances, and so on.

Conspiracies

Conspiracy is a separate and distinct crime from the substantive criminal acts committed pursuant to the plan. Conspiracy consists merely of an agreement or planning of criminal acts by two or more persons who have the specific intent to either commit a crime or engage in dishonest, fraudulent, or immoral conduct injurious to public health and morals. Previously, it was required that in addition to intent, some overt act in furtherance of the conspiracy must have been committed. This has been virtually abandoned in American jurisprudence. For instance, if a hospital administrator and a physician agree to fill hospital beds with nursing home patients to create revenue for the hospital, when these persons do not require hospitalization, the administrator may be convicted of a conspiracy even though his or her acts in furtherance of the conspiracy consisted only of a telephone call, or no act at all. It may suffice that the administrator and the doctor tacitly agreed to defraud Medicare or an insurance carrier. In most states, the proof of the agreement would have been sufficient even if it had not been made in person and there had been no act such as the telephone call. Manufacturers, sellers, and prescribers of unapproved drugs have been convicted of conspiracies (e.g., the laetrile cases[10]).

A factual impossibility to commit a crime is no defense (e.g., when the conspirators agree to kill somebody who is already dead). However, there can be no conspiracy when the objective of the conspiracy is not illegal. The concept of conspiracy involves the accomplishment of an objective prohibited by law. Conspiracies may be punished both as criminal and as civil acts. Thus, a conspiracy to destroy the practice of a physician by excluding that physician from hospitals, or otherwise defaming or disgracing him or her, may be punishable as a crime, even though the mere denial of privileges would not have been a criminal offense. The physician may concurrently seek civil remedies in a lawsuit for damages. In practice, however, in most such cases, unless the circumstances of the cases involving civil wrongs are particularly outrageous, the district attorney will refrain from prosecution, letting the victim seek his or her remedy in civil law.

An interesting example occurred when a physician conspired with the father of an illegitimate child to falsify a blood test to make it appear as if someone else had fathered the child. The conspiracy was prosecuted criminally as a wrong against the state and civilly as a fraud on the mother, which deprived her of child support payments.

Defenses to crimes

Both the substance of the criminal laws and procedures involving criminal trials and convictions are governed by the strict application of the constitutional standards of due process and equal protection. These concepts are constantly redefined by the courts in a tug of war between liberal, socially oriented standards, and the more conservative approaches that balance the rights of the accused against the more important rights of protection of society and victims of crime.

The defense of entrapment is being raised frequently in prosecutions resulting from the increased crackdown on drug overprescribing to "professional patients" and undercover agents, and prescribing without adequate need or examination or in return for sexual favors.

In addition to office charts, the courts allow virtually unlimited production of records by accountants, attorneys, and others. This virtually eliminates the defense of self-incrimination from records held by a third party (hospital, insurance company, or even the physician's professional corporation). The courts also extend virtually unlimited access to bank records when requested under grand jury subpoenas. The courts hold that such compulsion, even though incriminating, is not within the privilege against self-incrimination. The Fifth Amendment privilege against self-incrimination does not protect against compulsion to furnish specimens of body fluids, pubic, or head hair; to provide a handwriting sample or a voice exemplar; to stand in a line-up, or to wear particular clothing;[11] or to provide a hair exemplar.[12] The courts allow great latitude to physicians to conduct physical examinations and tests. These include involuntary minor surgeries for removal of bullets as evidence; rectal and vaginal examinations; penis scraping to reveal menstrual blood of a rape victim's type;[13] scrapings from fingernails and blood testing, provided these are done in a medically acceptable manner.

Because X-rays are potentially harmful and more invasive, the courts are more hesitant to allow them.[14] A forcible taking of impressions of defendant's teeth for comparison with bite marks on body of a homicide victim

was permitted.[15] Procedures requiring general anesthesia or potentially risky procedures are generally not permitted.[16] Statements by criminal suspects can be used against them if they had been warned about self-incrimination (see Miranda rights, *infra*). Statements made to a psychiatrist may not generally be used because they may constitute self-incrimination.[17] The court decided that it was self-defense when a physician shot and wounded an AIDS patient who threatened to bite him. Similarly, a psychiatric nurse claimed self-defense when using a fatal choke hold on a threatening patient.

The defense of faith healing and the question of freedom to choose or refuse medical treatment continue to be litigated. Parents are usually found criminally liable for failure to provide medical care to a minor child where with medical care, the child would have almost certainly survived. Under the guise of protecting the right of the unborn child, a case went all the way to the U.S. Supreme Court, where the Court held that a woman could not be compelled to have a cesarean delivery against her religious beliefs because a physician feared that a vaginal delivery could be harmful to the infant. Many states expressly protect patients who in good faith rely on spiritual means or prayer for healing, although the question of how far such laws may be extended to parents caring for minor children is unclear.

The U.S. Supreme Court has also held that the state has the responsibility of providing a court-appointed psychiatrist to indigents charged with capital crimes.

Causation

Before a criminal defendant can be convicted, it must be shown that his or her act was indeed the cause in fact of the criminal result, or was a substantial contributing factor in causing the criminal result. While the mind may get lost in the labyrinth of contributory factors to the crime, modern jurisprudence focuses on the *sine qua non*, or the so-called "but for" test. This means that without such an act the crime would not have happened. For example, if the defendant had not fired the shot, the deceased would still be alive. In applying the second criterion of a substantial factor, a crime is recognized even though the "but for" test fails. Such an example occurs when the deceased received two injuries from separate and independent sources—he was kicked to the ground by one person and run over by an oncoming car. Another example occurs when three persons play Russian roulette and one is killed. The conduct of the survivors may be deemed a substantial factor, and the two survivors may be charged with manslaughter based on their reckless endangerment of the life of the deceased.

Criminal law recognizes both *acts of commission* and

acts of omission as causes of crime. The gravity of the crime will vary if the physician or nurse who had the duty to care for a patient negligently or intentionally failed to provide him or her with life-sustaining medications or deliberately provided the patient with an overdose causing that patient's death. For purposes of criminal law, a victim's preexisting conditions do not release the defendant from liability. For instance, victimizing a person who has the unusual and unknown fragility of hemophilia or heart disease is a risk that the wrongdoer takes even though the act might not have caused death or serious injury to a healthy individual.

With regard to causation the law also distinguishes between intervening and superseding causes. Other legally recognized multiple causations include concurrent, independently sufficient causes, foreseeable intervening forces that do not break the causation chain, and foreseeable dependent causes for which more than one culprit may be held liable. An *intervening cause* is a cause that occurs after the act of the defendant but before the occurrence of the result. When the intervening cause is sufficient to absolve the defendant from responsibility, it is a superseding cause. An example involves medical complications in which the foreseeable causes may be dependent. An individual stabbed in the arm is hospitalized and contracts blood poisoning from the use of improperly sterilized instruments. The patient dies. The intervening blood poisoning flowed from the stabbing injury and was foreseeable. Most cases hold that medical complications, medical malpractice, and even the victim's refusal to undergo surgery or other treatment are foreseeable dependent causes.

Whatever the defenses, excuses, or justifications, a fundamental principle of criminal law is that these defenses must be asserted to cast a reasonable doubt on the culpability of the defendant. While the burden of proof in a civil case is the mere preponderance of the evidence, variously expressed as 51% or more, the standard in criminal cases is "beyond a reasonable doubt."

Excuses

Among the most frequently invoked defenses excusing criminal culpability are infancy, mental illness, intoxication, mistake, entrapment, and duress. With regard to infancy, most American jurisdictions hold that children under the age of 7 are conclusively presumed to be incapable of committing a crime. This may be a legal fiction, but it is sustained by the courts as essential to protect children. Children between the ages of 7 and 14 are presumed to be incapable of criminal responsibility, but this presumption may be rebutted by evidence of maturity and understanding of the moral and legal consequences of their behavior. Such adolescents are

frequently used by pushers to transport and deliver narcotics or to steal. When it comes to persons older than 14, criminal responsibility attaches, but there is a large body of juvenile law that tempers punishment and provides for rehabilitation. Some states provide that youths younger than 16 years must be tried in special family courts and that juvenile convictions are expunged upon attainment of legal maturity at age 18. In some cases, the law provides that juveniles may be tried as adults upon determination of mental age as opposed to physical chronological age.

Mental illness. Theoretically, mental illness presumes an incapacity to hold the defendant morally responsible for his or her conduct. It is usually defined in law as "insanity." But insanity is not a medical term, and it is beyond the scope of this chapter to get embroiled in the medical and legal quagmires and controversies surrounding the defense of insanity beyond explaining some definitions. Insanity, as defined by the traditional M'Naghten rule, postulates that a person is not guilty by reason of insanity if the following four conditions are met: (1) At the time of the criminal act, (2) the person was laboring under a mental disease or defect (3) that prevented him or her from knowing (4) either the nature and quality of the act or that the act was wrong.

Whereas the M'Naghten focuses on capacity for blameworthiness, the "irresistible impulse" test focuses on volitional controls. It extends the insanity defense to a myriad of situations in which the accused may have known that his or her conduct was wrong and criminal but was supposedly incapable of controlling the conduct. Nor has the question been answered of what constitutes an "impulse." Some courts hold that even if the accused spent a lot of time brooding and reflecting, the acts may still be the result of an impulse. Although the M'Naghten rule is still widely used, one of the newer variations is the American Law Institute's Model Penal Code formulation of "substantial capacity" test. It is a merger of the older M'Naghten rule and the "irresistible impulse." The result is a test that absolves criminal defendants of criminal responsibility if the following three conditions are met: (1) As a result of the mental disease or defect, (2) the defendant lacks substantial capacity (3) to either appreciate the criminality of his or her conduct or to conform it to the requirements of law.

There are virtually hundreds of variations of what constitutes mental disease or defect including organic brain damage, mental retardation, psychosis, addiction to alcoholism, which produces significant *permanent* mental defects (temporary disorientation or emotional frenzy are not sufficient), and various degrees of psychopathic personality.

In the case of retarded persons or others suffering from mental illness short of insanity, a "diminished responsibility" defense may be asserted to mitigate the culpability and reduce the charge. Although traditionally the accused was presumed to be sane and it was the burden of the defendant to plead and prove the defense of insanity, there is a growing trend to shift this burden to the prosecution to prove beyond a reasonable doubt that the accused was sane after the issue of insanity has been raised by the defendant. About half of the states and the federal criminal code have shifted this burden to the prosecution.

There is a growing trend to determine the issue of insanity separately from the guilt. When a defendant is found to be insane, he or she would not be acquitted by reason of insanity but the issue of insanity would be considered in the determination of punishment. In practice, a successful assertion of the insanity defense usually means that the defendant is committed to a mental hospital and kept there until a psychiatrist or judge is convinced that he or she is no longer dangerous and should be released.

Drunkenness. Intoxication by alcohol or drugs may impair the ability to appreciate the significance of the criminal conduct and under certain circumstances may negate culpability. However, voluntary intoxication is increasingly held not to excuse general intent crimes such as rape, battery, or trespass. Performing surgery while under the influence of alcohol or drugs is almost invariably prosecuted as criminal negligence. Nor is voluntary intoxication a defense to strict liability offenses such as statutory rape, mishandling of drugs, or serving liquor to minors. Intoxication may serve as a defense to such subjective intent crimes as larceny in which an honest mistake, which negates the mental state, may operate as a defense.

Mistakes of law. There are a few exceptions to the rule that ignorance of the law is no excuse: (1) when the government has not made information about the law reasonably available to all those who may be affected — this exception applies usually to situations in which the laws punish inaction or omission, such as failure to get a license or permit or failure to file certain information with appropriate governmental agencies (e.g., if reporting of venereal diseases, AIDS, or certain birth defects were made mandatory); (2) when there is reasonable reliance on an official government pronouncement and the defendant has made reasonable efforts to find out about such a law and reasonably believes that his or her conduct is not criminal; or (3) when the defendant reasonably relies on erroneous official interpretation of the law by a public officer or agency responsible for the interpretation and enforcement of the law, such as an erroneous interpretation of controlled substances laws by ranking officials of the DEA.

Entrapment. The defense of entrapment excuses the commission of a crime if a law enforcement officer — federal or state — actually instigated or induced an otherwise innocent person to commit the crime. The test of entrapment is the subjective disposition of the defendant prior to police involvement. This is often the case when undercover agents prevail on gullible physicians to prescribe pain medication without proper examination or need. The authors are aware of a case involving a physician who, without examination, prescribed 20 Tylenol IV to an undercover agent brought to the physician's home in the middle of the night by a "friend" claiming that the woman suffered from severe menstrual cramps.

The defense of entrapment is not available in the case of acts involving personal violence.

Duress. The defense of duress or compulsion is available when a person commits a criminal act under a threat by another, thus causing the accused to reasonably believe that he or she is in danger of imminent death or great bodily harm unless the criminal act is committed. The threat must be present and imminent and may not involve economic-type circumstances in which the person is unable to resist the threat. However, no coercion or threat excuses an infliction of serious physical violence on another.

Privileged conduct

Justification of criminal conduct involving the killing or injuring of another person arises in cases of self-defense, defense of others, crime prevention, defense of property, and necessity. Use of reasonable force and self-defense is permissible if an individual reasonably believes that he or she is in imminent danger of impermissible aggression. The individual may use such force as is necessary to avoid being injured, but use of excessive force may result in criminal liability. Normally being pushed, shoved, grabbed, or hit with bare hands does not justify shooting the aggressor. The use of deadly force in self-defense is permitted only in response to deadly force or a reasonably perceived threat of deadly force.

Courts are divided as to whether a person must retreat from the aggressor before using deadly force in self-defense. Some jurisdictions require what is called "retreat to the wall" before permitting deadly force in self-defense. Such retreat is required only if it is completely safe and makes it possible to avoid the aggressor. The duty to retreat does not apply if the aggressor enters a home or, in some states, the office of the attacked individual. The rights of self-defense and the privilege of using physical force are permissible only to prevent physical bodily harm. The rights do not apply in the case of insults. Self-defense is more liberally interpreted in the western and southern states, and the use of deadly force in self-defense is most severely circumscribed in such states as New York and New Jersey, which have rigid retreat requirements. The right of defense of others varies with th ~ circumstances, but generally the defender of others is protected only if the person he or she helped was truly acting in self-defense.

Prevention of crimes

Private citizens as well as police officers have the right to use whatever nondeadly force is reasonably required to prevent the commission of a crime or the immediate escape of the perpetrator from the scene of either a misdemeanor or a felony. Deadly force may be used only when such force is reasonably believed to be necessary to prevent the commission or completion of such crimes as homicide, violent assaults, kidnapping, robbery, rape and other forcible sex offenses, burglary, and arson. The private citizen who uses force to prevent a crime may be criminally prosecuted if the person killed or injured did not actually commit or attempt to commit a serious, or as the law calls it, an "atrocious" felony. Police officers may use deadly force when they believe that it is necessary to prevent the commission or consummation of what they reasonably believe to be an atrocious felony.

Defense of property

The law allows only the moderate use of nondeadly force in the defense of property. Whereas deadly force may not be used to protect property, it may be used when the person defending the property acts in self-defense, such as in robbery and arson situations.

Necessity

The destruction of private or public property may be justified in reasonable attempts to put out fires and to prevent fires from spreading if the harm that may have been caused by the fire is greater than the harm caused by attempts to avoid it.

Justified killings

The law accepts as a defense the justified killings by public servants such as police officers, soldiers, or executioners in the performance of their duty.

Inchoate crimes

Mere preparation to commit a crime, without actually committing the crime, falls into the category of anticipatory, preparatory, or unsuccessful criminal acts in which the actual intended harm did not develop but the accused did manifest a willingness to cause such harm.

Attempts

Attempted crimes are criminal offenses if some significant act with the intent to commit the criminal act is established. Mere preparation to commit a crime is not enough. A person can be convicted of attempted murder by "pulling the plug," even when the plug was reinserted and the patient didn't die.

Impossible crimes

Criminal liability may attach to an attempt to commit a crime that is physically impossible if the crime would have been committed had the facts been true as the accused believed them to be. Examples include: an attempt to kill someone with an unloaded gun or a gun that jams; a rape attempt that is precluded by the attacker's impotency; an attempt to steal a wallet from an empty pocket.

In some instances, renunciation of a crime acts as a defense when the attempt to commit the crime was abandoned voluntarily, the withdrawal occurred prior to completing the attempted offense, and the defendant made a substantial effort to prevent the attempted crime by either dissuading accomplices or calling the police.

CRIMES AGAINST THE PERSON
Homicide

Homicide is the killing of a human being by another human being. As far as the law is concerned, a homicide may be criminal or innocent. It may be caused by an act of commission (the actual killing) or omission (when one had a duty to take life-saving action but did not do so). To constitute a criminal act, the act that causes the death of another human being must be committed with criminal intent and without lawful excuse or justification. The law divides criminal homicides into three main categories of crimes: (1) murder, (2) voluntary manslaughter, and (3) involuntary manslaughter. Within these categories, the law recognizes various types of crimes and degrees of culpability.

To constitute the crime of murder, voluntary manslaughter, or involuntary manslaughter, it is not necessary that the victim die immediately. The traditional rule was that only if the victim died within one year of the shooting, stabbing, or poisoning, could the perpetrator be charged with murder. Modern American jurisprudence embraces any unlawful causation of death and extends the period to as long as three years.

Deaths resulting from negligent medical treatment, failure to provide treatment, or providing improper or inadequate treatment are seldom treated as murder despite pressures from distraught family members. Absent outrageous or severely aggravating circumstances, even grossly negligent physicians are usually only charged with involuntary homicides.

Homicide laws are also being increasingly affected by advances in medical sciences resulting from successful resuscitation, the ability to revive a heartbeat and respiration, the availability of highly sophisticated artificial life-support systems, and the use of organ transplants.

To sustain a conviction of criminal homicide, the prosecution must establish that the victim was alive at the time of the death-causing act by another person. These thorny questions of when life begins and when life ends are largely a matter of expert medical testimony and/or state law, and they carry with them a Pandora's box of medical and legal problems that will continue to be hotly debated within both professions for some time.

Infanticide

From a standpoint of medical law, one of the most frequently encountered homicides is infanticide. Most states still adhere to the rule that there is no homicide unless the child has been born alive.

The traditional determination of a live birth for purposes of a homicide conviction requires that the child must be physically separated from the mother and must give clear signs of independent vitality, such as breathing or crying. This definition has been repeatedly challenged by prosecutors with the help of medical testimony that seeks to establish that a living fetus is indeed a human being. This has resulted in a number of convictions when some courts convicted individuals on charges of murdering both the mother and the unborn child when they shot or stabbed a pregnant woman.

Some states, led by California, have even modified the homicide laws to include in the definition the unlawful killing of a human being or a fetus with malice aforethought. However, such laws expressly exclude abortion procured with the consent of the mother. Efforts to change laws to include abortions under homicide definition have so far been unsuccessful. Allegations of criminality for failure to treat spina bifida infants have been dismissed.

A physician may encounter infanticide under a great variety of circumstances. Sometimes, he or she may be deemed to have caused the death of the child, and if it was done through neglect or willfulness, the physician may be found guilty. In other cases, suffocation of infants may be disguised as "crib death." Infants' deaths may also have been caused by parents through acts of drowning, scalding, or starvation. Prenatal injuries to the infant resulting in drug abuse by the mother during pregnancy have also led to criminal prosecution in several states (see Chapter 32). If the physician is aware or suspects such infanticides, he or she is legally obligated to report them. Unfortunately, in the majority of cases, physicians are unwilling to become involved, and most infanticides are allowed to pass as "accidents."

Euthanasia

There are two types of euthanasia. The first, *active euthanasia,* or "mercy killing" is a crime in every state. In such cases, the physician takes an active role in the death of a patient by disconnecting a life-support system or giving a lethal overdose. In *passive euthanasia,* a crime may not have been committed, particularly in those jurisdictions in which the concept of a "living will" has been approved by the state legislature. Passive euthanasia simply means taking no further measures, (e.g., therapy) that the patient does not desire. Instead, one merely keeps the patient as comfortable as possible and allows nature to take its course. In California, two respected practitioners faced a murder conviction, later dismissed on technical grounds, for disconnecting the life-support system of an allegedly terminally ill patient.[18] At the Kaiser Foundation Hospital in Harbor City, California, the patient suffered a postoperative cardiopulmonary arrest in the recovery room and, although successfully resuscitated, remained in a coma. It was alleged that there may have been insufficient staff present in the postoperative area (one nurse for five cases). Without the consent of the family, the attending physicians terminated the patient's comatose state after 11 days. The attending physicians not only disconnected the respirator and ordered the nurses not to use endotracheal mist to assist the patient's breathing, which caused the patient to suffocate, but they also removed the patient's intravenous line as well.

To the attending physicians, the choice presented in this medical situation was to permit the patient to die. From the prosecutor's viewpoint, the removal of the respirator and IV amounted to murder. They argued that any shortening of life is a homicide, and, if it is intentional, it should be construed as murder.[19] The prosecutors alleged the following:

1. That the physicians had allegedly lied to the family about the patient's condition;
2. That the physicians had stated that the patient had reached a state of "brain death," when in fact it was argued that they were not certain at all of the actual state of the patient;
3. That the physicians had withheld information about a problem in the recovery room where there was insufficient nursing supervision and inadequate response;
4. That a doctor's order not to treat cardiac arrhythmias (an alteration in the pacing rhythm of the heart) was out of the ordinary, if not conspiratorial, in nature;
5. And perhaps most important, murder charges were filed because the patient had been taken off the IV, dehydrated, and starved to death. This, the prosecutors stated, prevented the patient from ever having a chance to recover.[20]

Even those sympathetic to the physicians who pulled the plug felt that a physician should never take such an abrupt step as pulling the IV. Expert witnesses on the subject of coma and chances for survival described the incident as a medical embarrassment. One of the defendant physicians was quoted as saying: "I will fight to the death to keep bureaucracy and lawyers out of our medical group." By his actions, it appears that this physician achieved just the opposite.

Forcible feeding

In another case, a California district attorney refused to press criminal charges of battery against physicians and nurses for forcibly feeding a suicidally inclined quadriplegic. As a result, the patient sought a civil injunction to stop the intravenous feedings. The patient claimed a right to starve herself to death in order to achieve a death with dignity while in the confines of the hospital. Although the patient failed in her civil suit, it was still possible that the physicians and nurses involved could have been found criminally liable for battery in the unauthorized forced feeding if the patient was not found to be incompetent.

Death certificates

A physician is also capable of imparting an element of criminality to an otherwise lawful act. This is particularly true in cases in which a physician may attempt to spare a family's feelings, further hardship, and suffering by issuing a death certificate and/or failing to report deaths under suspicious or unusual circumstances to the medical examiner or coroner.

Such cases arise many times in the cases of "overdoses." In most states, it is a misdemeanor not to report death under unnatural circumstances to the coroner or medical examiner. In many states there are also misdemeanor charges for failure to report (1) all manner of violent deaths, including thermal, chemical, electrical, or radiational injuries; (2) deaths due to criminal abortion, whether apparently self-induced or not; (3) deaths occurring when a physician was not in attendance; (4) deaths of persons after unexplained comas; (5) medically unexpected deaths during the course of a therapeutic procedure; (6) deaths of prisoners at penal institutions; and (7) deaths of those whose bodies are to be cremated, buried at sea, transported out of state, or otherwise made unavailable for pathological study. Civil and criminal penalties may also be imposed for failure to report diseases that constitute a threat to public health.

Medical fraud

One of the more vigorously prosecuted areas is submission by health care providers of false and fraudulent claims under the Medicaid and Medicare programs. It is a felony to knowingly make false and material statements in the processing of Medicare claims.[21-24] Furthermore, physicians who defraud the government or private insurance companies and use the U.S. Postal Service to do so will face additional penalties.[25] Note also that a physician who is prosecuted in a criminal case for welfare fraud, in which the defendant has defrauded the federal government, may subsequently face a civil action [e.g., under 31 U.S.C.A., § 231, 323(a)],[26] in which those factual matters litigated in the criminal action will act as a bar to their relitigation in civil action through the action of collateral estoppel.[27]

In most instances, criminal prosecutions for health care fraud usually involve the federal government. Physicians should also be aware that criminal responsibility may arise from any material false statements, not only to the federal or state governments, but also to private insurance companies. Conviction for such fraud generally results in suspension or revocation of a medical license.

Medical fraud may also involve misrepresentations of certain cancer, or other treatments, or untested remedies that allegedly produce miraculous cures for other ailments. Criminal prosecutions are often carried out against physicians who offer these false cures to patients either verbally or through the mail, and severe penalties are often invoked. In *People v. Privitera,* several groups challenged California's prohibition on using laetrile to treat cancer.[28] The constitutional challenge raised the issues that the statute was vague and overly broad and violated the equal protection concepts. The vagueness charge, alleging that that portion of the law prohibiting the "prescribing, selling, or administering of any unapproved drug, medicine, compound, or device to be used in the diagnosis, treatment, or alleviation of cancer" was not supported by the court. Defendants argued that it was unclear whether the statute also applied to foods or vitamins naturally occurring in foods, as opposed to drugs. The court stated that the word "compound," using its ordinary interpretation, would cover these substances not considered to be drugs; hence, all substances were prohibited.[29] In addition, because the regulation of such drugs, new or otherwise, has been found to be within the realm of a state's police power, a statute broad enough to protect all citizenry from having an untested compound thrust on them is not overly broad; rather it is proper public safety enforcement.[30]

The defendant's argument that the statute violated the individual's right to privacy, based on arguments issued in *Roe v. Wade,* was also rejected by the court. The court claimed that the abortion statutes were meant to protect individuals from a procedure that was no more dangerous than the alternative procedure of a normal delivery. The statute in question, however, proscribes remedies that may be more harmful than other approved cancer remedies. The court was afraid that individuals faced with cancer may forego approved treatments and instead employ "miracle" cures that do nothing or that may be harmful. It may be that those physicians who design cures outside the mainstream of medicine will face criminal charges simply because they are nonconformists, not because of a standardized scientific analysis of their alleged cures. The last argument in *Privitera* was based on equal protection grounds. Apparently the court believes that the cancer victim has lost all rationality, and therefore is more deserving, whether they like it or not, of legislative protection. Again, the equal protection argument was held without merit.

Criminal prosecutions for medical fraud may also involve multiple violations, which in turn may lead to violations of the Racketeer Influenced and Corrupt Organizations Act (RICO). Such prosecutions not only involve jail penalties and stiff fines, but also permit the government to trace assets and forfeit other private property allegedly purchased with the illicitly obtained funds.

Abusive therapy

The illegality of beatings as therapy is still not a clear area of legal medicine. If the physician makes outrageous claims about the success of such therapies, then the criminal responsibilities are much clearer, even if the defendant is released on a technicality.[31] However, in *State v. Killory*,[32] a psychologist was convicted for administering "therapy" under the guise of beating his naked 15-year-old niece with paddles. The patient was also whipped with a leather belt.[32] While this therapy appears to be of dubious value at best, one wonders whether the issue is the age of the patient as opposed to the therapy used. Such matters are further complicated by the fact that many patients who allege abuse — physical, sexual, or otherwise — are currently, or were in the past, psychiatric patients whose testimony will be regarded dubiously by any judge or jury. Without corroborating evidence, the statements of mental patients often make it difficult to separate fabrications and exaggeration from the truth.

Intimate therapy

Improper or immoral conduct by physicians or dentists toward female patients may result in criminal prosecution for rape or child molestation. Such crimes may also lead to disciplinary measures, including loss of licensure to practice.[33] The courts have repeatedly stated that offenses relating to moral turpitude are not relegated only to actions in the lines of professional practice.[34]

Again, however, because most alleged rape cases against physicians involve psychiatric patients, they are difficult to prosecute. Psychiatric patients have little credibility with a jury. Another obstacle to criminal prosecution is the embarrassment and unwillingness of the witnesses to testify. Unless the suit involves minors, or other unusual circumstances, the defense to such charges is usually that the acts alleged were between consenting adults.

An example of one of the more bizarre criminal prosecutions in this area involved a Chicago dentist. Apparently the patient emerged from the anesthetic to find the dentist in a rather compromising position on top of her. The patient's screams brought the receptionist running into the room, and she saw enough of the dentist's activities to help convict her employer for rape. The defendant further compounded his problems by attempting to bribe his receptionist into repudiating the statements she had made to police.

In *Roy v. Hartogs*,[35] a New York court described criminal prosecutions in sexual abuse cases as having the function of protecting "patients from deliberate and malicious abuse of power and breach of trust by psychiatrists, where the patient entrusts her body and mind in the hope that the psychiatrist will use his best efforts to effect a cure."[36]

Numerous cases involve psychiatrists and other physicians accused of having sexual intercourse with their patients. Although most of these actions are civil suits, rape and/or elements of fraud may be found in cases in which large sums of money were obtained by physicians from their patients under false pretenses. In such cases criminal charges may ensue.

Obviously, although there are many medically related crimes, unique to health care providers, physicians have also been found quite capable of committing a host of other criminal acts that lie totally outside the realm of medical practice.

CRIMINAL PROCEDURE
Burden of proof

In a criminal case, the state or the federal government must prove its case "beyond a reasonable doubt."

As discussed previously, the prosecution must prove beyond a reasonable doubt that a crime was committed and that the defendant committed that crime. This means that a rational and fair juror would be convinced of the guilt and would have no reasonable hesitation to vote for the conviction. In criminal cases, this usually means that a jury must be unanimous, or that the conviction must be by at least two-thirds of the jurors.

Constitutional safeguards

What makes a criminal case different is that the defendant can invoke a broad array of constitutional safeguards that are not generally applicable in civil litigation. Some of these include the following:

1. The Fourth Amendment, which provides protection against unreasonable arrests, searches, and seizures
2. The Fifth Amendment, which provides for a grand

jury indictment and includes prohibitions against double jeopardy and compelled self-incrimination, also guarantees due process of law, which in practice means the application of much more rigid standards than those used in civil trials

3. The Sixth Amendment, which includes the right to a speedy trial, to a public trial by a jury of peers, the right to confront and cross-examine adverse witnesses, the right to subpoena favorable witnesses, and the right to be represented by a lawyer

4. The Eighth Amendment, which prohibits excessive bail and any form of cruel and unusual punishment.

In interpreting these constitutional safeguards, the U.S. Supreme Court has provided definitions of how these safeguards should be applied. Thus, denial of due process may include almost any allegation that law enforcement authorities have engaged in improper behavior. (For example, one court held that due process was violated when a defendant's stomach was forcibly pumped by police officers to extract two morphine capsules. The court ruled that such evidence was not admissible at trial because "it shocked the conscience of the court.")

Legal technicalities

Prosecutors are often frustrated by the legal technicalities, imposed by courts in the strict interests of constitutional due process, that allow criminals to escape convictions. The foremost of these is the "exclusionary rule," which prohibits the use of illegally obtained evidence no matter how strongly it proves that the defendant is guilty. Such cases include finding of bodies of victims, murder weapons, or large quantities of narcotics in areas that were searched without a properly executed search warrant (e.g., trunks of cars or a shed behind the house).

Incriminating evidence against criminal defendants may also be suppressed when the court finds that the defendant's right to privacy was violated. The exclusionary rule also prohibits the use of any information or investigative leads that prove the culpability of the defendant when such information was obtained as a result of illegal conduct on the part of the investigating officers. This is known as the doctrine of "fruits of the poisonous tree."

The gathering of evidence against an accused is also severely limited by court rulings circumscribing electronic surveillance. Thus, in cases in which wiretapping was not properly authorized or the defendant was not advised subsequently that he or she was bugged or not provided transcripts of the bugged conversation, the intercepted conversation may be excluded from use as evidence against the criminal defendant.

Warrants and searches. The validity of a search, even where the incriminating evidence is discovered, can be challenged on the basis that the issuing judge was not "neutral," that the warrant did not exactly describe the things to be seized and/or the place or person to be searched, or that the warrant was not based on a sworn affidavit of a trustworthy or reliable informant establishing probable cause to justify the search. More recently, some common sense rules liberalizing the requirements for warrants and searches under exigent circumstances have been enacted. These exceptions grant police the right to stop and search moving vehicles where they have probable cause to believe that contraband will be found. Even then, most courts continue to hold that once the vehicle is stopped and passengers arrested, a warrant may still be needed to search the immobilized vehicle or open the trunk or to open bags or suitcases in the stopped vehicle.

Other instances for which search without a warrant is permissible include hot pursuit and searches incident to an arrest in which the arrested individual may be searched for any weapons on his or her person and within the area of his or her immediate control. This does not include the trunk of an automobile or adjoining rooms. When police officers assert that the arrestee assented to the search, they must prove by clear and positive testimony that there was no actual or implied duress or coercion.

Persons entering the United States by land, sea, or air, are subject to border searches without a warrant. Courts have also generally upheld searches of airline passengers prior to boarding by holding that passengers may avoid such searches by agreeing not to board the aircraft. Subjecting luggage and mail suspected of containing narcotics to a "sniff test" by trained narcotic detection dogs does not constitute a "search." Also, the "open fields" doctrine allows searches of land outside the dwelling house and outbuildings, where evidence may be in plain view, as in the case of marijuana plants.

Administrative searches without warrants of medical offices, pharmacies, pharmaceutical plants, and storage facilities are often allowed under narcotics laws on the theory that license to handle controlled substances allows governmental agencies to inspect and verify appropriate storage and dispensation of controlled substances. Such searches are also permitted for the seizure of spoiled or contaminated food and in the storage and selling of highly toxic chemicals and in the sale of guns.

Detentions and arrests. A police officer may arrest a person without a warrant when the officer has reasonable grounds to believe that a felony has been committed and that person committed it. An arrest without a warrant can also be made for misdemeanors committed in the presence of police officers. However, nonemergency arrests cannot be made in a private home without a warrant. Without exigent circumstances, all arrests in homes without warrants are presumed to be unreasonable and illegal. The only exception is the detention of occupants of a house or apartment during the execution of a valid warrant for narcotics or contraband.

A police officer may stop a person without probable cause for arrest if the officer has a reasonable suspicion of criminal activity or that person's involvement in a crime. However, the police officer may frisk such a person only if the officer has a reasonable belief that the person may be armed and dangerous. Police officers must also have full probable cause to bring a suspect to a station for questioning.

Miranda warnings. A major safeguard against self-incrimination is the requirement that the criminal defendant be given the Miranda warnings, which inform the criminal defendant of (1) the right to remain silent and not to answer any questions by the police; (2) the possibility that any statement made may be used as evidence; (3) the right to have an attorney present during the questioning; and (4) the possibility that if the accused cannot afford to have an attorney, one will be appointed. Based on the Miranda doctrine, thousands of confessions by criminals have been declared inadmissible because the arresting officer did not adequately provide this warning before questioning the suspect. The question of whether the confessions were tainted or were coercive or illegal is one of the most common grounds for appeal by convicted criminals.

A suspect may waive his or her Miranda rights provided the waiver is done knowingly, voluntarily, and intelligently. This is done mostly in cases in which a suspect wishes to present exculpatory evidence to the police. However, once the suspect starts talking voluntarily, anything the suspect says may be used against him or her.

Right to counsel

The most pervasive right of a criminal defendant is the right to be assisted by an attorney in all criminal proceedings. The courts have defined such criminal proceedings as events "where substantial rights of a criminal accused may be affected." The test is always whether the lawyer's presence would safeguard against any inherent danger of unfairness. The accused always has the right to be represented by a lawyer at a preliminary hearing in which a judge determines whether probable cause to prosecute exists. No such right exists when the accused appears before a federal grand jury, which determines whether there is probable cause to prosecute. A person subpoenaed before a grand jury does not have the right to receive Miranda warnings and may be convicted of additional charges of perjury if

he or she testifies falsely. Although a grand jury witness does not have the right to an attorney in the grand jury room, he or she may interrupt the testimony to step out and consult with an attorney outside the grand jury room. The grand jury system is also used in a number of states east of the Mississippi.

The accused does not have the right to a lawyer when blood samples or handwriting exemplars are taken, when hair samples are taken, or when photographs are shown to potential witnesses. Criminal defendants frequently allege that even though they were represented by a retained or appointed counsel, their constitutional right to effective assistance to counsel was violated or denied because the lawyer was "incompetent." Such allegations are made even against the most highly experienced and competent lawyers after the criminal defendants are convicted.

Starting criminal prosecution

The Fifth Amendment constitutional requirement that the criminal suspect be indicted by a grand jury does not apply to the states. However, it does require judicial determination of probable cause before anyone is deprived of his or her liberty for any extended period of time. Thus, criminal proceedings are frequently started by arrest warrants, probable cause hearings, or grand jury indictments. In some instances, filing of information by the prosecutor is authorized in lieu of a grand jury hearing. In all instances, the accused must be apprised of the nature of all elements of the offense in order to prepare the defense.

The initiation of a criminal prosecution is strictly a matter of prosecutorial discretion, and prosecutors have extremely broad discretion regarding whom to prosecute and what crimes will be charged. It is also a matter of prosecutorial discretion not to prosecute certain individuals or certain crimes, as long as no individuals are singled out for prosecution or are not selectively prosecuted. In most cases, the courts have no power to interfere with a decision not to prosecute, but if the courts find abuse of discretion in cases of selective prosecution, they will dismiss the case.

The law is very strict in that a prosecutor must disclose to the accused any exculpatory information derived from the investigation of the case. This is known as the Brady doctrine and failure to do so constitutes a denial of due process. This information must be disclosed even if the defendant does not ask for it.

The Sixth Amendment guarantee of a speedy trial has been variously interpreted by the courts as prejudicing the defendant by possible loss of defense witnesses resulting in greater likelihood of conviction. The speedy trial provisions come into play only after the charges have been filed. The time period during which charges may be filed is determined by the applicable statutes of limitations. These vary with the specific charges and are governed by federal and state law.

Plea bargaining

Plea bargaining is an agreement between the prosecutor and the defendant. It takes the gamble out of the trial and allows the defendant to plead guilty to a lesser charge in return for a lesser sentence. The courts require that such pleas must be made knowingly and voluntarily. There is no violation of due process if the prosecutors charge the accused with more serious crimes when plea bargaining negotiations break down. However, the courts are usually liberal in allowing an accused to withdraw a guilty plea in order to stand trial. In virtually all cases, the courts refuse to accept plea bargains unless the defendant is represented by a lawyer and thoroughly understands the nature of the plea bargaining agreement.

Right to jury trial

The Sixth Amendment right to jury trial has been held by the Supreme Court of the United States to apply to the states. Exceptions to the right to jury trial are petty offenses that carry penalties of no more than 6 months of imprisonment and do not involve serious offenses. Criminal contempt proceedings provide for a jury trial only if the punishment is more than 6 months in jail.

The traditional doctrine that the jury must be composed of 12 jurors has been ruled not to be a constitutional requirement. Juries of 6 members are increasingly allowed in criminal cases on the basis that they provide sufficient group deliberation. Many defendants prefer 12-person juries because there are greater possibilities of disagreements resulting in acquittals and hung juries. Although in the cases of 6-person juries, unanimity is required, the Supreme Court has upheld noncapital felony convictions based on 10-to-2 and 9-to-3 jury votes for conviction.

The Fourteenth Amendment prohibits racial discrimination in the selection of petit and grand juries. Whereas systematic discrimination in the selection of juries results in reversal and remand for a new trial, the Supreme Court does not require proportional representation of all the component ethnic groups of the community in every jury. In selecting jurors, either the prosecutor or the defense attorney has the right to dismiss a certain number of prospective jurors on peremptory challenges without giving any reason for so doing. Both the prosecutor and the defense attorney may dismiss any number of jurors challenged for cause. These are jurors who indicate that they would not impose the death sentence, would not follow the law, are friends or relatives of either the plaintiff or the defendant or their lawyers, or otherwise indicate a degree of bias and prejudice that would preclude them from judging the case solely based on the evidence presented in court.

The Sixth and Fourteenth Amendments guarantee the right to a public trial. The press cannot be excluded from trials, and state laws vary regarding whether televising of criminal proceedings is allowed or not, regardless of the defendant's objections.

Witnesses

No witness may testify anonymously; the law requires that each person who testifies in a criminal proceeding must give his or her name, address, and such other information as would enable the defendant to determine any possibility of bias and allow the defense to impeach such a witness. *Impeachment* means discrediting of a witness by showing prior inconsistent statements, previous convictions, or untruthfulness.

Medical expert witnesses play a key role in many criminal trials. Most frequently, they are forensic pathologists who testify to the causes of death, the time of death, or the instrumentalities used to commit the crime. Psychiatrists are frequently called to testify when the issue of insanity is raised. When medical expert witnesses give conflicting opinions, the juries are free to accord whatever weight they choose to whichever expert seems more credible.

Protection against self-incrimination

The Fifth Amendment, which protects against self-incrimination, provides that no person shall be compelled in any criminal case to be a witness against himself or herself. Both defendants and witnesses have the right in a legal proceeding to refuse to answer any incriminating questions. While the defendant's right to remain silent may not be challenged, the court may offer immunity to witnesses, thereby forcing them to testify under penalty of being held in contempt.

The trial

Constitutional safeguards of due process require that the accused be presumed innocent and that the prosecution have the burden of proving all of the elements of the criminal offense beyond a reasonable doubt. Before anyone can be convicted of a crime, the prosecution must prove the corpus delicti (the body of the crime) or simply that a crime has been committed. A defendant's confession to a crime without any corroboration is insufficient to satisfy this requirement. Individuals have been known to confess to crimes that they never committed for a variety of reasons, ranging from insanity to a desire for notoriety. In some states, there can be no conviction for homicide unless the body of the victim is found; while in others, there can be no sentence of death in a case where the body has not been recovered.

Although the Constitution does not expressly say so, the most fundamental ingredient of a fair trial in Anglo-American jurisprudence is that the accused is presumed to be innocent until proven guilty and that the prosecution must prove every element of the crime "beyond reasonable doubt." Although the courts have refused to put a percentage figure on "beyond reasonable doubt," the U.S. Supreme Court has ruled that due process is violated if, viewing all the evidence in the light most favorable to the prosecution, no rational judge or jury would have found the defendant guilty of the crime of which he or she was accused.

A guilty plea is a voluntary renunciation of the Sixth Amendment right to jury trial. It has been estimated that up to 95% of all criminal cases are settled by guilty pleas. To ensure that guilty pleas are voluntary, judges use long questionnaires to assure that there was no coercion or promises of a more lenient sentence offered in return for the guilty plea. Theoretically, an accused may not be punished more severely for pleading innocent and asserting his or her right to a jury trial than by pleading guilty. In practice, however, it is often alleged that persons who plead guilty receive lesser sentences.

Double jeopardy

One of the foremost constitutional safeguards is the right against double jeopardy. The Fifth Amendment provides that "no person shall be subject for the same offense to be twice put in jeopardy of life or limb." This provision is intended to protect individuals from harassment, to achieve certainty and finality in criminal proceedings, and to reduce the chances of convicting an innocent person.

Both the state and the federal government can reprosecute the individual if jeopardy has not yet attached. In a jury case, jeopardy attaches when the jury is impaneled and sworn. In a bench trial, jeopardy attaches only when the prosecution has started the presentation of the evidence. The exceptions to these rules include when mistrials are caused by the misconduct of the defendant or defendant's defense counsel; when the jury is unable to reach the verdict; when the judge dies or becomes ill; or, when it is discovered that a juror should be dismissed for cause after the jury has been impaneled. The courts have broad discretion to declare a mistrial if it is found that a trial cannot be fairly continued.

Although this is sometimes perceived as double jeopardy, the same crime may be prosecuted separately by both the state and the federal government based on the doctrine of separate sovereignties. The Supreme Court has upheld the right of a state to convict a bank robber who was tried and acquitted in federal court for the same crime. He was retried by the state when the FBI found considerable additional evidence after the acquittal and turned it over to the state prosecutor.

Nor does the double jeopardy concept apply to separate offenses based on the same crimes. In an Illinois case, the defendant was charged with the murder of his wife and three children. The prosecution tried him first for the murder of the wife and one child, and after he received 20-year and 45-year sentences, the prosecution tried him for the murder of the second child, for which the courts imposed the death penalty. The prosecution could have tried the defendant a fourth time for the death of the third child to maximize the penalty had the death sentence not been imposed.

Exceptions to double jeopardy. As a general rule, if a defendant appeals his or her conviction, the right against double jeopardy is waived. This is usually the case when an appellate court remands the case for a new trial. An exception occurs when the appellate courts hold that the evidence on which the conviction was based was legally insufficient and that the defendant should have been acquitted. Another exception is that a defendant may not be retried for a greater offense of which he or she was found innocent when the conviction is appealed on a lesser included offense.

Although technically a defendant who won a reversal and new trial may be given a more severe sentence after reconviction, this is viewed with great disfavor by the appellate courts; such sentences are usually reduced to the original sentence. It is the courts' way of saying that the defendant should not be punished for exercising the right to appeal. Time served on the original conviction is also credited against the sentence following a retrial.

END NOTES

1. *State v. Lester*, 149 N.W. 297.
2. *Cole v. New York State Dept. of Education*, 465 N.Y.S.2d 637.
3. *Windham v. Board of Medical Quality Assurance*, 104 Cal. App. 3d 461.
4. *Raymond v. Board of Registration in Medicine*, 443 N.E.2d 391.
5. *McDonnell v. Commission on Medical Discipline*, 483 A.2d 76.
6. *Miller v. National Medical Hosp.*, 24 Cal. App. 3d 81.
7. *Haley v. Medical Disciplinary Board*, 818 P.2s 1062.
8. *Hall v. Biomedical*, 671 F.2d 300.
9. 47 A.L.R. 4th 18.
10. *People v. Privitera*, 591 P.2d 919, *cert. denied*, 444 U.S. 949.
11. *Walters v. Secretary of Defense*, 725 F.2d 107.
12. *United States v. Dougall*, 919 F.2d 932.
13. *Brent v. White*, 398 F.2d 503, *cert. denied*, 393 U.S. 1123.
14. *United States v. Ek*, 676 F.2d 379.
15. *Wade v. State*, 490 N.E.2d 1097.
16. *Winston v. Lee*, 470 U.S. 753.
17. *United States v. Leonard*, 609 F.2d 1163.

18. *American Medical News,* Sep. 16, 1983.
19. *Id.*
20. *Id.*
21. *State of Wisconsin v. Kennedy,* 314 N.W.2d 884 (Wis. Ct. App. 1981).
22. *United States v. Matank,* 482 F.2d 1319 (9th Cir. 1973).
23. *People of the State of New York v. Montesano,* 459 N.Y.S.2d 21, 445 N.E.2d 197 (1982).
24. *People of the State of New York v. Chaitin,* 462 N.Y.S.2d 61 (1983).
25. *United States v. Perkal,* 530 F.2d 604 (4th Cir. 1976).
26. *United States v. Zulli,* 418 F. Supp. 252 (1975).
27. *Id.*
28. *People v. Privitera,* 55 Cal. App. 3d Supp. 39, 128 Cal. Rptr. 151 (1976).
29. *Privitera, supra* note 28, 128 Cal. Rptr., at 155.
30. *Id.* at 157.
31. *Hammer v. Rosen,* 181 N.Y.S.2d 805, *modified on other grounds,* 198 N.Y.S.2d 65, 165 N.E.2d 756.
32. *State v. Killory,* 243 N.W.2d 475.
33. *Cadilla v. Board of Medical Examiners,* 103 Cal. Rptr. 455.
34. *Barski v. Board of Regents,* 111 N.E.2d, *aff'd,* 347 U.S. 442.
35. *Roy v. Hartogs,* 366 N.Y.S.2d 297.
36. *Id.*

CHAPTER 18

Countersuits by health care providers

BRADFORD H. LEE, M.D., J.D., M.B.A., F.A.C.E.P., F.C.L.M.

POLICY CONSIDERATIONS
MALICIOUS PROSECUTION
ABUSE OF PROCESS
DEFAMATION
NEGLIGENCE
INTENTIONAL TORTS
CONSTITUTIONAL MANDATE
PRIMA FACIE TORT
APPEALS RESULTS
CONCLUSION

Recent years have seen a precipitous increase in the incidence of medical malpractice litigation. This increase has taken the form of a dramatic rise not only in the number of suits filed but also in the size of judgments and settlements. Although many of the suits filed have some legitimate basis, physicians and their insurance carriers have noted a growing trend in the number of actions filed that lack substantial merit. To counteract these nonmeritorious claims, physicians have sought recourse through countersuits.

Physician countersuits have been conspicuously, although not uniformly, unsuccessful. Countersuits for abuse of process, malicious prosecution, intentional infliction of emotional distress, defamation, barratry, and negligence have been consistently rejected by the courts for numerous reasons.

POLICY CONSIDERATIONS

State and federal courts have to weigh a number of opposing public policy issues when deciding whether to permit countersuits. On one hand, courts have recognized a policy favoring protection of individuals from unjustified and oppressive litigation. On the other hand, courts have sought to protect the public interest by providing injured parties with free and open access to the courts. Countersuits exert a chilling effect on injured persons who would seek legal redress.

Whenever a person with a meritorious claim is faced with the possibility of a countersuit, it is felt by many legal scholars and members of the judiciary that the potential plaintiff's right of access to the courts is threatened. In this situation, the nation's legal system for redress of wrongs would be threatened with failing to protect the rights of the individual, and many meritorious claims for damages would not be pursued. The end result could well be to leave the injured party without adequate remedy. On the whole, courts have given far greater weight to preserving the peace by favoring free access to the courts. That policy choice renders it extremely difficult for wrongfully sued physicians and others to seek an effective remedy via countersuits.

Most physician countersuits are brought against the physician's former patient (plaintiff in the original medical malpractice action) and the patient's attorney. As the countersuit litigation progresses, the focus of attention usually shifts from the former patient to the attorney. This shift occurs because the patient frequently raises the defense that he or she relied on legal advice from the attorney regarding the merits of the case. As a practical matter, because most unsuccessful medical malpractice plaintiffs have limited resources, a judgment against a former patient is often uncollectible. The patient's attorney, however, is frequently covered by a legal malpractice liability policy, so that a judgment against a defendant attorney, if covered in the policy, is usually paid. The lawyer's insurance carrier may be more willing and able to settle than would be its insured. The attorney's defense is weaker than that of the former client. The attorney can usually only claim that, prior to initiating the medical malpractice action, he or she relied on information from the client. The attorney will then claim that such information was inaccurate and led to an unjustified medical malpractice action. Another defense is that the attorney acted reasonably, obtained the advice of medical experts, and relied on their advice before filing suit.

MALICIOUS PROSECUTION

The tort of malicious prosecution has its origin in English common law. It developed as a remedy against persons who unjustifiably initiated a criminal proceeding. Modern English law has not extended this tort to allow redress against persons wrongfully instituting a civil action. A minority of jurisdictions in the United States follow that conservative approach. However, the majority of jurisdictions in the United States currently permit suit based on malicious prosecution should someone have wrongfully initiated a civil lawsuit.

The moving party in a malicious prosecution suit must prove facts that satisfy the four elements of the cause of action: (1) Initial suit was terminated in favor of the plaintiff; (2) it was brought without reasonable or probable cause; (3) it was actuated by malice; and (4) the counterclaimant suffered a "special grievance."

A physician countersuit based on malicious prosecution can be instituted only after the medical malpractice action has been terminated, not while the medical malpractice action is still pending. A formal, favorable determination of the malpractice suit for the physician-defendant must come first. That favorable determination generally need not be a jury verdict for the physician but may be a voluntary dismissal by the patient or an involuntary dismissal by the court.[1] To serve as a basis for a malicious prosecution action, the malpractice action must not have been terminated solely on procedural grounds. "The mere fact that the party complained against has prevailed in underlying action (sic) does not itself constitute favorable termination, though such fact is ingredient (sic) of favorable termination, but such termination must further reflect on his innocence of alleged wrongful conduct; if termination does not relate to merits, reflecting on neither innocence of nor responsibility for alleged misconduct, termination is not favorable in the sense it would support a subsequent action for malicious prosecution."[2]

The most difficult element for a physician to establish in prosecuting a malicious prosecution action is lack of probable cause. Mere failure of a patient to prevail in a medical malpractice action does not by itself indicate lack of probable cause. Courts realize that the complex legal issues and fact patterns surrounding medical malpractice litigation contain substantial uncertainties. In many such cases, questions of liability and damages are not resolved until time of trial. Therefore, a physician must show that the former patient's attorney had no reasonable basis for an ordinarily prudent person to believe that there was merit to the case. It is usually difficult to prove this element, because courts give attorneys a great degree of latitude in pursuing malpractice actions. Courts are even more understanding concerning the early stages of litigation before discovery has progressed. Some courts have liberalized this element by holding that an attorney's failure to investigate and conduct reasonable discovery will support a finding of lack of probable cause.

Malice traditionally implies a motive of ill will. As with the element of lack of probable cause, a showing of malice on the part of the patient or attorney may prove to be an insurmountable barrier. Because of this extreme difficulty, some courts have liberalized the malice requirement. They will find that malice is present if there is a lack of a reasonable belief in the likelihood of success of the malpractice action. Where that suit was begun primarily for a purpose other than adjudication of a reasonably valid claim, malice may be inferred.

The states are divided concerning the damage element. In the majority of jurisdictions that recognize the tort of malicious prosecution, the damage element can only be satisfied by proving "special injury." This requirement is based on the historical origin of malicious prosecution suits. They arose as a redress for the initiation and prosecution of an unwarranted criminal action. Those jurisdictions recognizing the special injury rule require a showing of (1) arrest or imprisonment of the physician, (2) seizure of property, or (3) injury different from that ordinarily sustained by malpractice defendants. Special damages do *not* include the cost of the physician's defense, nor do they include increased liability insurance premiums or injury to the physician's standing in the community. Rather, special damages are those in the nature of business losses. If the physician cannot prove that he or she has lost patients, for example, as a direct result of the groundless malpractice suit, the special damages requirement is not met. The occurrence of one or more of the three types of special injuries is quite rare. To date, no special damages have ever been found in a malicious prosecution suit based on a prior medical malpractice suit in such jurisdictions. As a result, there has been a complete lack of success in prosecuting the tort of malicious prosecution in those states requiring a showing of "special damages."

A number of states that recognize the tort of malicious prosecution, however, require only that the physician demonstrate some injury in order to establish the damage element. This element may include the incurring of attorney's fees to defend the prior medical malpractice action. Other possible damages include the physician's mental anguish, loss of reputation in the community, a decrease in patient flow, and loss of income. Even an increase in liability insurance premiums caused by the prior medical malpractice claim could be sufficient to meet the damage requirement.

A total of three malicious prosecution judgments for physicians have been upheld on appeal. In 1980, an intermediate appellate court in Tennessee allowed a malicious prosecution judgment.[3] The underlying facts surrounding the earlier medical malpractice claim involved an allegation that the defendant doctor negligently and incorrectly diagnosed gonorrhea in the former patient-plaintiff. In the course of prosecution of the medical malpractice action, it was determined that the attorney continued to press the case without his client's consent.

The patient's attorney also made allegations in his original complaint that were not predicated by information from the client; they were fabricated by the attorney. Finally, the plaintiff lost the case, and plaintiff's attorney filed a groundless appeal—again without his client's consent. The key finding was that continued prosecution of a medical malpractice suit, without plaintiff's authorization, constituted clear-cut evidence of lack of probable cause.

A second malicious prosecution action was decided in favor of a physician by the Kentucky Supreme Court in 1981.[4] In that case, the patient-plaintiff had sustained an orthopedic injury before being diagnosed and treated by the defendant doctors. In spite of these facts, the attorney filed a complaint against the two doctors, charging them with negligently causing this patient's injury. The element of lack of probable cause was established by the attorney's filing of a malpractice suit against defendants with full knowledge that plaintiff had suffered the injury before defendants assumed plaintiff's care.

A California intermediate appellate court upheld a malicious prosecution judgment in 1981.[5] The physician-defendant was an orthopedic surgeon who inserted a metal (intramedullary) rod to repair a thigh (femoral) fracture sustained in an automobile accident. The rod broke and had to be removed and replaced by a new one. Plaintiff's law firm filed a product liability lawsuit against the manufacturer of the intramedullary rod. Plaintiff specifically requested that his orthopedic surgeon not be sued, but the patient's lawyer named the surgeon, anyway. The orthopedic surgeon was ultimately dismissed. The court found that suing the surgeon contrary to plaintiff's wishes established lack of probable cause.

In summary, these three cases indicate that the difficult burden of establishing lack of probable cause can be met. These courts upheld judgments for physicians in situations where an attorney prosecuted a suit without the client's consent and where an attorney

recklessly or knowingly maintained suit against a wholly blameless physician.

Since 1981 continuing inroads have been made by appellate courts in furthering the liability of the tort of malicious prosecution. In 1982, the Kentucky Supreme Court[6] reversed a directed verdict for the defendant and returned the case to the trial court level for a rehearing. In 1983, the Kansas Supreme Court[7] reversed a summary judgment for the defendant and returned the case to the state court level for retrial. In 1985, a California intermediate appellate court partially sustained a physician's victory on appeal, but remanded the case to the trial court for a new trial.[8] Finally, in 1986, a California intermediate appellate court[9] reversed a summary judgment for the defendant and returned the case to the state court level for retrial on its merits.

Although none of these recent state appellate court decisions represents a complete victory on the merits by the physician-plaintiff, they certainly indicate a recognition on the part of the appellate courts that malicious prosecution is a viable tort and should be afforded respect at both the trial and the appellate court levels.

A recent opinion in a California Supreme Court case rendered in 1989 dramatically increased the burden of proving a malicious prosecution action.[10] Prior to this ruling, the attorney who filed the prior medical malpractice action had to fulfill a two-part test in order to establish that the prior action was brought with probable cause. First, he or she had to have a subjective belief that the claim merited litigation; second, that belief had to be satisfied by an objective standard of legal tenability.

The California Supreme Court, in a unanimous decision, ruled that the two-part test was invalid. The court stated that what the attorney who previously had prosecuted the medical malpractice action thought (subjectively) was entirely irrelevant to the establishment of the element of probable cause in the subsequent malicious prosecution action. The only standard to be applied was that of objectivity, and if the prior attorney could show that objective tenable evidence supported the prior malpractice claim, then whatever his or her subjective beliefs were at that time was unimportant in establishing a basis for proper probable cause.

Also in that case, the court indicated that the party bringing the action for malicious prosecution could not introduce into evidence opinion testimony of expert witnesses as to whether a reasonable attorney could conclude that the claims advanced in the prior action were tenable. It was the feeling of the Supreme Court that the objective tenability of the prior action was a matter to be determined solely by the present trial judge.

In essence, this important California case has greatly increased the burden of a physician wishing to prove lack of probable cause in a prior medical malpractice action.

It also greatly reduced the defensive burden of the prior attorney in establishing that he or she brought the prior action with necessary probable cause.

Since 1985, a rather interesting development has occurred at the trial court level involving a variation of the tort of malicious prosecution. As previously discussed, the typical defendants in a physician countersuit based on this theory of liability are the original patient-plaintiff in the prior medical malpractice action and his or her attorney. Several recent trial court cases that have not reached the appellate level have involved the naming of the prior plaintiff's expert medical witness as a codefendant in the physician's subsequent suit for malicious prosecution, based on a conspiracy theory of liability.

Conspiracy is a legal theory of liability usually applicable in criminal actions. A conspiracy occurs whenever two or more persons agree to carry out an illegal act. Many jurisdictions permit a conspiracy theory of liability to be pleaded in a civil action. The theory of liability for including the expert medical witness in the malicious prosecution lawsuit is that he or she participated in the prior medical malpractice action by providing expert medical witness advice while knowing that the medical malpractice suit had no merit. In many jurisdictions, a coconspirator such as a participating expert medical witness would be jointly and severally liable for all damages along with the other coconspirators (the former patient and his or her attorney).

It is likely that this new basis of liability for nonmeritorious expert medical witness participation in medical malpractice suits will produce a great deal more caution on the part of physicians to avoid participating in obviously nonmeritorious litigation. Cases of this type should deter many medical expert "hired guns" from participating in those cases in which there is no reasonable basis for believing that medical errors were committed by the treating defendant physician.

ABUSE OF PROCESS

Abuse of process is a cause of action frequently employed by physicians following what is perceived as an unjustified medical malpractice action. The elements of this cause of action include unauthorized use of an otherwise legal process, existence of an ulterior purpose in bringing the original malpractice suit, and resulting damages to the physician-defendant as a result of the abuse of process.

Unlike the tort of malicious prosecution, abuse of process does not require proof of prior favorable determination or lack of probable cause. The principal difficulty faced when successfully prosecuting this cause of action is proof of an ulterior purpose. To establish this element, the physician must demonstrate that the original use of legal process in bringing the medical malpractice action, although justified initially, was later perverted, and the process itself was employed for a purpose not contemplated by the law.

Note that institution of a meritless lawsuit is not sufficient by itself to state a cause of action for abuse of process. Physicians sometimes allege that the original, groundless medical malpractice suit was brought merely to coerce a nuisance settlement. However, a majority of courts have rejected this argument as insufficient to fulfill the requirement of an improper ulterior purpose.

In 1980, the Nevada Supreme Court upheld a countersuit based on an abuse of process.[11] In that case, the defendant doctor was alleged to have been negligent in treatment of bed sores that the patient developed while under the physician's care. A thorough review of the facts indicated that there was absolutely no basis for initiating and/or prosecuting that medical malpractice action. Shortly before trial, the patient's attorney attempted to settle for the nominal sum of $750. The physician refused to settle. The case was tried without the plaintiff's attorney having retained an expert witness, and the plaintiff lost the malpractice case.

The Nevada Supreme Court found that plaintiff's attorney had utilized an alleged claim of malpractice solely for the ulterior purpose of coercing a nuisance settlement. His offer to settle for $750, his failure to investigate the facts properly before filing suit, and the absence of essential expert testimony at trial supported a case for abuse of process. Although this court recognized the threat of litigation to coerce a settlement as satisfying the ulterior purpose element, it is unlikely that other jurisdictions will expand on this holding because of the great weight that courts place on the public policy of providing injured parties free and open access to the courts.

DEFAMATION

The tort of defamation can be found in an oral or written false statement made to a third party about another person that is damaging to that person's reputation and good name. Countersuits based on the tort of defamation rely on the principle that an unfounded suit attacks the professional reputation of the defendant doctor.

Defamation has not proven effective as a cause of action on which to base a countersuit, because of an underlying privilege covering oral and written statements made in the course of judicial proceedings. That privilege immunizes patients and their attorneys from liability for any reasonable communication made in the course of a lawsuit. The purpose of this privilege is to permit the free expression of facts and opinions necessary to decide the merits of a lawsuit. The threat of defamation lawsuits would have a chilling effect on access to the courts and on honest testimony, and would be contrary to the public interest in the free and independent operation of the courts.

A California intermediate appellate court in 1963 did find for a physician in a countersuit based on defamation.[12] However, it should be noted that the fact pattern in this case was very unusual. In the original medical malpractice action, the defendant doctor was charged with negligent diagnosis and treatment of a child, which resulted in the child's death. A local reporter contacted the office of the plaintiff's attorney for information. That attorney reiterated his formal allegations and added additional, unsubstantiated charges. Those charges were incorporated into a subsequent newspaper article. The defendant doctor read that article and contacted the newspaper, demanding that the false allegations be formally retracted in a subsequent article. A newspaper official contacted the attorney who had made the original allegations and asked if the facts set forth in the article were true. The attorney assured the newspaper official that they were true and later supported his claims with formal, written correspondence with the newspaper.

The physician sued for defamation and prevailed at trial. The judgment was upheld on appeal because the attorney's statements to the newspaper were not made in pursuit of the underlying malpractice litigation. The wrongfulness of the attorney's false statements was compounded by his failure to retract them when the newspaper contacted him to substantiate his allegations. Defamation may be a viable form of action in countersuits in which erroneous statements are made outside of usual judicial proceedings. In that circumstance, the privilege covering judicial proceedings will not protect an attorney or patient who makes false statements injurious to a physician.

NEGLIGENCE

The law of negligence requires that individuals not subject other persons to unreasonable risks of harm. A countersuit based on negligence alleges that the patient's attorney was negligent in unreasonably bringing an unfounded lawsuit against the physician. However, under negligence law, the plaintiff must prove that the defendant owed him a duty. No physician has succeeded with a countersuit based on negligence and prevailed to the appellate level.

Courts have consistently held that an attorney owes no duty to a party, other than his or her client, unless that party was intended to benefit from the attorney's actions. In the usual medical malpractice action, an attorney owes a duty to the client (the patient) to zealously represent him or her and to prosecute the claim.

Requiring a concurrent duty to a physician not to file an unjustified suit would create a conflict of interest between attorney and client, denying the latter a right to effective counsel and free access to the courts.

INTENTIONAL TORTS

Intentional torts alleged by physicians in their countersuits against the plaintiffs and their attorneys from the original medical malpractice action include invasion of privacy, intentional infliction of emotional distress, and barratry (persistent incitement of lawsuits). Although the courts have, *in dictum,* lauded the application of these causes of actions as being novel and/or innovative, they have consistently rejected them.

CONSTITUTIONAL MANDATE

Some jurisdictions do not recognize the common law countersuits. Innovative attorneys in those states have attempted to create new theories of liability to permit physicians to bring successful countersuits. In other states that also present major stumbling blocks to countersuits, attorneys have also sought to establish such novel theories.

For example, Illinois courts require proof of a "special injury" in order to prove malicious prosecution. This requirement effectively prevents physicians from winning a countersuit of this nature. However, the Illinois constitution specifically provides that "every person shall find a certain remedy in the laws for all injuries and wrongs which he receives to his person, privacy, property, or reputation. He shall obtain justice by law, freely, completely and promptly."

An attorney representing a radiologist who was sued unsuccessfully seized on this wording to attempt to fashion a new cause of action, based on constitutional mandate. He argued that, because Illinois case law required a showing of special injury, physicians were precluded from successfully bringing a malicious prosecution action. Therefore, any wrongs suffered from unjustified malpractice suits had no remedy. This attorney urged that the Illinois constitution gives a broad remedial right to such plaintiffs who are unable to obtain remedies by more conventional common law causes of action.

An intermediate appellate court in Illinois found that the pertinent section of the Illinois constitution was merely a philosophical expression and not a mandate for a legal remedy.[13] The court ruled that, as long as some remedy for the alleged wrong exists, this constitutional section does not mandate recognition of any new remedy. It so held, even though a physician wrongfully sued is effectively precluded from countersuing. Since the common law remedy of malicious prosecution is technically available to him or her, the courts will not create a new cause of action based on constitutional mandate.

PRIMA FACIE TORT

A form of countersuit recently relied on by creative attorneys attempting to carve out a new countersuit cause of action is the *"prima facie* tort." The elements of this tort are intentional infliction of harm, without excuse or justification, by an otherwise lawful act, causing special damages to the physician.

Innovative attorneys had to resort to this cause of action because of the clear lack of success of the more conventional causes of action. Charges that the patient's attorney was negligent in failing to ascertain the merits of the case prior to filing suit have been summarily dismissed because the patient's attorney is not considered to have a duty of care to an adverse party—the physician. As for claims based on the attorney's breach of the lawyer's oath not to bring frivolous suits, courts generally consider that private citizens are not proper parties to enforce such oaths and that any disciplinary action must come from the organized bar. Charges of barratry—that is, the practice by an attorney of habitually pursuing groundless judicial proceedings—have been dismissed on the ground that barratry is a criminal offense with only a public remedy, not a private one.[14] Casting about for some means of avoiding the strictures of these closely defined causes of action, attorneys in three recent malpractice countersuits have laid before the courts a more novel form of action, the *prima facie* tort. Although in all three instances the physicians ultimately lost, the cases do point the way for possible future physician countersuits.

Prima facie tort is a remedy of fairly recent origin; it grew out of an opinion delivered in 1904 by Supreme Court Justice Oliver Wendell Holmes in a case involving a conspiracy among several Wisconsin newspapers to draw away the advertising customers of a rival paper. In appealing their conviction, the defendants pointed out that their stratagems had been, strictly speaking, perfectly legal, and that they were really being tried for their motives. They argued that motive alone is not a proper line of inquiry for the court. Justice Holmes disagreed, holding that even lawful conduct can become unlawful when done maliciously and that such conduct becomes actionable even when it does not fit into the mold of an existing cause of action.[15]

Out of these general principles there eventually grew the specific cause of action known as *prima facie* tort. Unlike malicious prosecution, abuse of process, or the other torts described earlier, *prima facie* tort has not been accepted or even introduced in all jurisdictions. Ohio, New York, Georgia, Missouri, and Minnesota have recognized the tort by name, whereas Massachu-

setts recognizes the principle without the label. Oregon, on the other hand, once enforced the action but has since discarded it.

No appellate court has thus far upheld a countersuit judgment based on a *prima facie* tort theory. The reason generally stated is that *prima facie* tort should not be utilized to circumvent the requirements of a traditional tort remedy, such as malicious prosecution. The courts stress the need for open access to the judicial system, and state that the *prima facie* tort should not become a catch-all alternative for every countersuit that cannot stand on its own. Appellate courts have refused to accept *prima facie* tort when relief is technically available under traditional theories of liability.

APPEALS RESULTS

Approximately 30 physician countersuits have been decided by appellate courts during the last 10 years. In nearly all these suits, the appellate courts have ruled against countersuing physicians and in favor of medical malpractice plaintiffs and their attorneys. Five appellate decisions have favored physicians who brought countersuits. Specifically, there have been three successful appeals of malicious prosecution actions, one successful appeal of an abuse of process action, and one successful appeal of a defamation action.

CONCLUSION

Although the absolute number of medical malpractice claims has increased dramatically in recent years, there has not been a concommitant increase in the number of successful physician countersuits. Because the courts recognize the strong public policy interest in ensuring that injured parties have free and open access to the judicial system, they are extremely reluctant to allow countersuits because it is felt that countersuits would have a chilling effect on a party's ability to seek legal redress. Despite the application of many innovative and novel causes of action, physician countersuits have been, and will probably continue to be, conspicuously, although not uniformly, unsuccessful.

END NOTES

1. *Raine v. Drasin,* 621 S.W.2d 895 (Ky. 1981).
2. *Lackner v. La Croix,* 25 Cal. 3d 747, 159 Cal. Rptr. 693, 602 P.2d 393 (1979).
3. *Peerman v. Sidicaine,* 605 S.W.2d 242 (Tenn. App. 1980).
4. *Raine,* supra note 1.
5. *Huene v. Carnes,* 175 Cal. Rptr. 374 (1981).
6. *Mahaffey v. McMahon,* 630 S.W.2d 68 (Ky. 1982).
7. *Nelson v. Miller,* 233 Kan. 122, 660 P.2d 1361 (1983).
8. *Etheredge v. Emmons,* no. A014929 (Cal. App. 1985).
9. *Williams v. Coombs,* 86 Daily Journal D.A.P. 1143 (1986).
10. *Sheldon Apel Co. v. Albert & Oliker,* 47 Cal. 3d 836 (1989).
11. *Bull v. McCuskey,* 615 P.2d 957 (Nev. 1980).
12. *Hanley v. Lund,* 32 Cal. Rptr. 733 (1963).

13. *Berlin v. Nathan,* 381 N.E.2d 1367 (1978).
14. *Moiel v. Sandlin,* 571 S.W.2d 567 (Tex. Civ. App. 1978).
15. *Aikins v. Wisconsin,* 195 U.S. 194 (1904).

GENERAL REFERENCES

Logan, *Physician Countersuits,* 32 Med. Trial Tech. Q. 153 (1985-86).
McCafferty, M.D., and Meyer, S.M., *Medical Malpractice Bases of Liability* (Shepard's/McGraw-Hill, Colorado Springs, 1985).

Reuter, S.R., *Physician Countersuits: A Catch-22,* 14 *U. of San Francisco L. Rev.* 203 (1980).
Shipley, W.E., *Medical Malpractice Countersuits,* 84 A.L.R.3d 555.
Yardley, M.J., *Malicious Prosecution: A Physician's Need for Reassessment,* 60 Chi. Kent L. Rev. 317 (1984).

CHAPTER 19

Medical liability insurance

RICHARD F. GIBBS, M.D., J.D., LL.D., F.C.L.M.
RICHARD W. MOORE, Jr., J.D., C.P.C.U.

INSURANCE CONTRACTS AND INTERPRETATION
INSURANCE RATES AND REGULATION
ACCOUNTING REPORTS
POLICY PROVISIONS AND CLAIMS
RISK RETENTION GROUPS

Insurance is a system of protection against the risk of individual loss by distributing, according to the law of averages, the burden of losses over a large number of individuals. In medical malpractice the insured are physicians and other health care providers. They, in turn, add their insurance costs into their fees. For all intents and purposes, patients are self-insured.

In medical practice, insurance is a contract in which, in consideration of a certain payment or premium paid by the insured physician, the insurance company or carrier agrees (in the case of an injury or harm due to negligence) to pay to the aggrieved party a sum of money agreed on or determined by a trier of fact—judge, jury, or arbitration panel—to compensate for the losses resulting from the injury.

INSURANCE CONTRACTS AND INTERPRETATION

In modern society, no written contract is entered into more frequently and read less often than the insurance contract. Even when the contract is read by the purchaser, it is typically not read at the time of purchase, but after a loss has already occurred. The reading is not done to determine what the contract says so much as to determine whether a particular prior incident is covered.

The primary purpose of any insurance contract is to indemnify the policyholder against certain losses that may occur. This absence of any potential gain generally distinguishes insurance contracts from wagering and is the core theme behind many of the limitations within the contract.

The essential concept of the insurance contract is the attempt to define those losses that are covered by the insuring agreement and those that are not. As a result,

certain conditions, limitations, and exceptions are used to limit the general promise to cover losses. Because of the virtually limitless number of factual situations to which an insurance contract may conceivably apply, definitional problems and the attempt to make comprehensible contracts have represented considerable challenges to the legal and insurance communities. Attempts to provide answers to all foreseeable factual situations have resulted in the complexity of insurance language and its interpretation by the courts. In a study by the Pennsylvania Insurance Department based on the FLESCH readability scale (a method of testing the readability of documents by assigning point values for length and complexity), the Bible received a readability score of 66.97 out of a perfect readability score of 100, Einstein's theory of relativity scored 17.72, and the standard automobile insurance policy 10.31.[1]

Aspects of insurance contracts

Although most contracts involve the exchange of goods for money, the insurance contract is an agreement to provide protection or indemnity upon the occurrence of some future event. Since its performance depends on the happening of an event that may or may not occur, it is referred to as an *aleatory contract*. The essential purpose of insurance is to distribute the individual uncertain losses to the group, and, by spreading the risk of loss, increase the certainty of the cost of the loss in the form of the insurance premium.[2] Another aspect of the insurance contract that is important for modern court interpretations is that it is a contract of adhesion. With the exception of very large commercial ventures, the contract is typically drawn up by the insurer. The purchaser has the option of purchasing the contract or not. In recent years, a rule of strict construction has evolved in interpreting insurance contracts. Under this judicial concept, any doubt or ambiguity in the contract is construed against the insurer, because the insurer prepared the contract.[3] As a practical matter, many court decisions, based on seemingly clear language, have determined that the contract is ambiguous when applied to specific facts, because not all contingencies can be anticipated by the drafter of the document. This is one particular area in which the courts have vastly expanded the extent of contractual liability in recent years.[4] Another aspect of the concept of the aleatory contract is that, in some jurisdictions, courts have been willing to recognize the reasonable expectations of the policyholder, even if he or she failed to read the policy. This theory has allowed courts to go beyond the clear and unambiguous language of the policy and to determine in equitable situations that the policyholder is entitled to recovery despite the specific wording of the contract purchased.

Because insurance is an essential element of most commercial and financial transactions of everyday life, courts and legislatures have a much different attitude toward insurance transactions than toward ordinary commercial transactions. Courts have recognized that a contract of insurance requires the highest degree of good faith between the parties; therefore, the failure to disclose vital information, dishonesty, or fraud on the part of either party results in the declaration of the contract as voidable at the option of the innocent party.

As an *executory contract,* an insurance contract will not be performed by the insurer until some future point in time. This has formed the historical basis of the strict regulation of insurance contracts and the insurance industry. Starting in the 1920s, states took an active role in regulating the insolvency of insurance companies to ensure that they had the financial stability to meet their future obligations. This basic goal of insurance regulation has been expanded significantly in the last 10 or 15 years to include many aspects of consumer protection such as limitations on the company's right to cancel agents and insurance policies and establishing regulations on unfair claims settlement practices. Many states also strictly regulate insurance rates.

Formation of insurance contracts

As with any contract, the insurance contract must have a lawful object, must be entered into by competent parties evidencing genuine assent, and must be supported by sufficient consideration. However, in many cases of insurance contracts, these elements are present as a matter of routine commercial transactions. Typically, the first contract made when purchasing insurance

is with an insurance agent. As a general rule, the efforts of an agent are viewed as merely soliciting offers for insurance. However, in dealing with insurance agents, it is important to note that a person described as an "agent" may not be an agent on behalf of the insurance company at all. A clear distinction is made in insurance law between an agent for an insurance company and a broker, who is an agent for the insured.[5] An agent for the company typically has authority under the American Agency System to bind the company to policies, accept payments on behalf of the company, and in other authorized ways represent the interests of the company in dealing with the insured. A broker represents the insured in the procuring of insurance. Because a broker does not represent the insurance company, he does not have the authority to bind the company or accept premiums on its behalf, but is operating as the agent of the applicant for purposes of seeking coverage. This is of particular importance in cases involving the defalcation of an agent and whether coverage is in effect.

In property-casualty contracts, the company typically does not accept the risk until it has received the application in its office and reviewed it. It is of critical importance to determine the exact date and time that coverage became effective, because it is essential for coverage that loss be shown to have occurred within the coverage period. In many situations involving typical business transactions, the time required for this procedure is too long, and the agent is given authority by the company to bind coverage on the occurrence of certain events. The issuance of such immediate binder represents a binding contract to purchase the policy, and provides immediate short-term coverage pending the execution of the completed policy. Although a binder is a brief document, it must contain the basic information needed to reach an agreement and indicate the type of coverage purchased. As a practical point when entering into insurance contracts, it is important to recognize the distinction between a true company agent and a broker, and to determine the extent of the agent's authority to bind the company.[6]

Many courts continue to adhere to the general rule that no acceptance of the application by the insurance company may be inferred from mere silence or delay. However, the majority of courts now hold that the insurer will be liable under the contract when it was negligent in acting on the application in a reasonable time.

In many lines of personal insurance coverage, the policy language is limited by various statutory requirements. In most states, the language of the New York State fire policy of 1943 with its "165 lines" of standard policy provisions is required to be included in all fire and homeowners' policies. In some states, such as Massachusetts, the state has promulgated a uniform automobile insurance policy that all companies must provide.

Fraud

If one party to a contract has been guilty of fraud, the contract is voidable at the election of the innocent party.[7] In this sense, the law distinguishes between fraud and mere folly or carelessness. In most cases, courts require the first four of the following five elements in order for a contract to be rescinded on the basis of fraud. The fifth element is necessary to show damage[8]:

1. False representation—the falsity is of a past or existing fact.
2. Material fact—the materiality is determined by whether the fact influenced or induced the party to enter the contract.
3. Intent to deceive—the party must have intended to deceive, or at least have been recklessly indifferent to the truth or falsity of the statement.
4. Reasonable reliance—the innocent party must have been justified in relying on the statement.
5. Injury or loss must be shown in order to recover damages.

False statements of opinions do not generally constitute fraud. If a person knows that the other is merely stating an opinion, he or she relies on that opinion at his or her own peril.[9] An exception to this involves statements of an opinion by a person who claims to be an expert with particular knowledge of the subject matter. In such cases, false opinions by an expert constitute misrepresentation when dealing with a layperson. By the same token, a statement by a layperson concerning the law is considered a statement of opinion. A statement made by an attorney who is presumed to be an expert can be reasonably relied on by a layperson.

In order for fraud to be found, the party must establish either an intent to deceive or reckless indifference to the truth. Since it is frequently difficult to establish the subjective intent, the surrounding circumstances are typically shown in each case in order to establish the intent.[10]

The requirement of a material fact and reasonable reliance are actually very closely related. Typically, a material fact is one that would influence or cause a party to enter into a contract. It is difficult to see how a person could reasonably rely on a fact that was not material to the contract, but it is typical in these cases that if the fact is actually relied on by the party claiming the fraud, the chances are that materiality will be found.[11] The key question to be asked is whether the fact would have influenced the insurer's decision to accept the application. This question relates to whether or not the concealed facts indicate an increased risk to the insurer, such as the failure to reveal prior losses.

A number of particular types of fraud are found in insurance contracts. A common type of fraud is a situation in which a person impersonates the applicant when taking a medical examination in connection with life or health insurance. In some fraudulent situations, there is collusion between the agent and the third party to defraud the insurance company in ways such as the withholding of adverse information on the application.[12] Closely related to this type of fraud is that of concealment, in which a material fact of importance to the contract is withheld. Although courts generally have not imposed the duty to reveal prior losses or claims, the presence of a specific question regarding loss history may result in a claim of concealment.[13] Most courts agree that an applicant for insurance must be reasonably diligent in notifying the insurer of material facts that come to his or her knowledge even after making the application. However, the person owes no allegiance to disclose facts learned after the insurance contract has been entered into, even though delivery occurs at a later time.

Incontestability clause

Common to life and health insurance contracts is a clause wherein the parties agree that the validity of the contract cannot be contested after the policy has been in effect for a certain period of time. This clause is obviously contrary to the basic aspect of contract law that fraud negates consent. The presence of this clause in life insurance contracts is a result of their long-term nature. It is believed unfair for the company to receive premiums over an extended period of time only to declare the contract invalid at the time of death because of some earlier misrepresentation. The incontestable clause does not extend coverage nor does it preclude a showing that the person had no insurable interest.[14] However, it generally applies to fraud in the application except where it is part of a scheme for profit, such as an attempt to murder the insured or substitute a person to take the insured's medical examination.[15]

Waiver, estoppel, and election

An insurer may deny liability based on one of the reasons previously discussed. However, the insurer may be unable to assert one of its defenses because the insurer has waived the defense, has been estopped from asserting the defense, or has elected not to take advantage of the defense.[16] Although these three concepts are closely related, they have clearly distinctive characteristics. A waiver is an intentional relinquishment of a known right. As such, it is a contractual right, typically contained in the policy, that requires no proof of materiality. An example of a contractual waiver is life insurance policies in which the company agrees to pay premiums during a period of the insured's total disability. An example of a waiver outside the policy is where the company declares a life insurance policy void upon entering the military service. The insured is killed as a result of military service, and a representative of the company writes to the beneficiary stating that the company will waive the defense because the insured died in the service of his or her country. Even a subsequent letter stating that the company has changed its position will not invalidate the express waiver. One primary difference in insurance law is that some waivers are binding even in the absence of consideration.[17]

On the other hand, estoppel in insurance law is a representation of fact relied on by the other party that makes it unfair to allow a party to refuse later to be bound by the representation.[18] A typical example occurs when an agent of the company assures the person that he or she is covered for a certain event, which in fact is not covered by the language of the policy. Of course, in these situations it is necessary that the reliance on the representation was reasonable, the insured was prejudiced as a result, and the fact was material. As distinguished from waiver, estoppel is tortuous in nature and relies on a false representation. By comparison, election is simply the choosing between two available rights that relinquishes the right not chosen. A typical example of an election is when an insurer must decide whether to accept a premium and afford coverage or reject a tender of premium. If the insurer elects to accept the premium, it should be bound by that choice and not permitted to reserve its position.

Reservation of rights

One area of insurance law where the concepts of waiver, estoppel, and election come into play is when a claim is made against the insured for which the insurer may not be liable because of a valid contractual defense. If the insurer elects to defend the insured, as obligated under the contract, there is no problem. However, many instances in which the insurer needs to take action could be interpreted as defending the insured, even before its obligation to defend is determined. A typical example is when the company needs to undertake further investigation to determine whether the facts of the incident fall within the coverage provided in the contract.[19] Since this could be interpreted as a waiver of the right to decline coverage, a company typically notifies the insured by using a reservation-of-rights notice.

The reservation-of-rights notice states that although the company is proceeding with a certain action, it is for the purpose of determining whether there is coverage under the policy, and does not represent a waiver of any future rights of the company to decline coverage. Although this notification clearly should prevent the

insured from being able to rely on the activities of the insurance company to create estoppel since it is a unilateral action, it may not always be effective. To be fully protected, the insurer may seek a nonwaiver agreement. This is a contractual agreement between the insured and the insurance company indicating that neither party will waive any of its rights under the policy as a result of the investigation or initial defense of the action. Typically, both of these procedures are limited in time and scope to information necessary in determining whether there is in fact coverage under the policy.[20]

Bad faith

Regardless of how courts interpreted the provisions of the policy, despite construing the contractual ambiguities against the drafter, or using the reasonable expectations of the insured, it was at least certain that a recovery was limited to the coverage limits of the policy. Recently, however, a number of jurisdictions, led by California, have accepted the rationale that in addition to a contractual remedy for breach of a contract, some types of breach can also result in a tort remedy.[21] These courts have determined that in every contract there is an implied convenant of good faith and fair dealing. This essentially means that neither party can do anything that will injure the right of the other to receive the benefits under the agreement.[22]

These so-called "bad faith" actions have developed during the last 25 years from the landmark California case of *Communale v. Traders and General Insurance Company.*[23] This case held that the insurance company that defends an insured against liability to a third person must compensate the insured for the full judgment if the insured is held liable beyond the policy limits because of the insurer's bad faith in refusing a settlement offer. The result of these cases has been that companies need to be very careful in dealing with claims that could potentially go above the limits of the particular insurance policy involved.[24] Typically, the insured is notified of this possibility, and it is suggested that he or she may wish to retain an independent counsel. As a result, pressure is brought to bear on the insurance company not only by the plaintiff, but by its own insured, to settle the case, when possible, within the policy limits.

In addition, the implication of good faith extends to all dealings between the insurer and the insured. Typical examples include the application of contractual defenses to the insured and the obligation to make first-party payments directly to the insured such as with life and health contracts. The adverse consequences from these types of cases come not only from the fact that damages may be awarded in excess of the policy limits, but also that, in some states such as California, punitive damages are allowed to be based on a bad faith case. In the case of *Frazier v. Metropolitan Life Insurance Company*, the company failed to pay $12,000 in death benefits under a life insurance policy on the grounds that the insured had committed suicide.[25] The jury found that the refusal was improper, and awarded not only the $12,000 under the contract, but also $150,000 for emotional distress and $8 million in punitive damages. Although this award was subsequently reduced and reversed in part on statute of limitation grounds, it shows the potential impact on actuarially determined rates that do not anticipate judgments over the policy limits.

INSURANCE RATES AND REGULATION

Historically, the insurance business can be described as being highly competitive. A large number of sellers, in many cases, provide policies of insurance that are fairly uniform, encouraging price competition.[26] This aspect of the industry helps distinguish it from the public utility area in which a monopoly or semimonopoly has been granted by the state with the addition of rate regulation, which as a practical matter frequently guarantees a rate of return. In contrast, over the years a number of insurance companies have become insolvent and therefore unable to meet their obligations.

Despite the advantages of allowing open market competition to regulate business conduct under the rubric of the antitrust laws, two specific distinctions have created the need for some regulation by governmental agencies. Because insurance is essentially an exchange of the premium for a future promise to perform, the executory nature of these contracts makes the insolvency of an insurance company particularly damaging to the purchasers of insurance. At the same time, the pricing of insurance is based on the gathering of statistical evidence and the use of actuarial science to determine, based on past experience, what the levels of future losses and expenses are likely to be.

Companies have historically combined data because of the limitations on an individual company in gathering statistical information in any one geographical area and for any one class of risks. By applying the law of large numbers, these combined data will more accurately predict future losses than the data from any individual company. Therefore, both the need to regulate companies' solvency to ensure their ability to pay claims and the need to share loss data between companies have placed them outside the conceptual framework of the antitrust laws and required more direct government regulation.

Role of rating bureaus

Particularly prior to World War II, rating bureaus were used by the property-casualty insurance industry to gather actuarial data. These bureaus were composed of insurance company members and had the clear purpose of securing uniformity in premium rates, coverage design, and other matters related to the business of insurance. Many state laws authorized rating bureaus to act in concert with insurance companies in setting rates. Although some of these organizations were limited to the function of collecting and disseminating statistical data and other information (the statistical agent function), other types were allowed specifically to recommend rates or make ratefilings.[27] Prior to World War II these organizations were exempt from the antitrust laws by court interpretation because they were not deemed to be in commerce.[28]

The decision of the U.S. Supreme Court in *Southeastern Underwriters Association v. U.S.*[29] held that bureau activity was subject to the federal antitrust laws, based on an expanded definition of what constituted commerce.

However, in response to the *Southeastern Underwriters* case and the fear that without the ability to share loss data it would simply be impossible to set accurate rates, the U.S. Congress passed Public Law 15, the McCarran-Ferguson Act.[30] This act reaffirmed the desirability of state insurance regulation and the principle that federal statutes should have no application to the "business of insurance" where specifically regulated by the state, except for those federal statutes that dealt specifically with insurance. The McCarran-Ferguson Act also had an exception for boycotts, coercion, or intimidation subject to federal law.

Subsequent to this congressional action, all states specifically authorized rating bureau activity in most lines of property-casualty insurance. Prior to that decision, the practical activities of the states in regulating rates were somewhat limited and focused primarily on ensuring that all rates were sufficiently high to guarantee the continued solvency of companies. In an effort to preempt federal regulation by specifically showing that the states were affirmatively engaged in regulating insurance, a number of states passed fairly specific laws establishing statutory standards for the determination of insurance rates. These laws were fairly uniform because language recommended by the National Association of Insurance Commissioners was adopted by many states,[31] and the laws centered on three statutory criteria that rates not be "excessive, inadequate, or unfairly discriminatory." Many of these laws required the "prior approval" of rates before they could be used. Despite the continued existence of the prior approval laws today, a number of important states, including Illinois and California, continue to allow competition rather than direct state regulation as the method of ensuring fair rates. Even in these states, however, significant regulation of insurance company activities occurs.

Direct regulation

The degree of regulation of rates in the insurance business outside of property-casualty lines has been more limited. Typically no portion of the insurance code provides for direct state regulation of rates for life insurance and most types of health insurance. Part of the reason for this differentiation results from the fact that these lines of insurance have remained independent and there is no equivalent to the types of rating bureaus that once dominated rate-making in property-casualty lines. Some specific lines such as credit life insurance and credit accident and health insurance have been regulated indirectly by the states through the use of their Unfair Trade Practice Acts and the requirement that policy forms be approved.[32]

Because, in part, of the advantages given to Blue Cross and Blue Shield over commercial insurance by virtue of their tax-exempt status, some states have taken a strong position regarding the regulation of their risk classifications. In *Blue Cross v. Insurance Department,* the court allowed a rate to be disapproved that did not include a community rating factor that would reduce the rate differential between those policies issued to elderly individuals and those issued to others, primarily employer groups.[33]

Today, most property-casualty rate regulatory laws place the rate-making initiative with the individual insurance company or rating bureau, with approval or disapproval power resting with the state. In addition to having the authority to determine overall rate levels, most of these laws have been interpreted to include authority over risk classification systems.[34] In most areas of insurance, the risk potentials of individuals fall within certain broad classifications. In automobile insurance, for instance, it has been documented that young male drivers have increased losses as compared with either young female drivers or all adult drivers. It is also clear that drivers operating in congested urban areas have higher loss exposure than operators in rural areas. Therefore, insurance companies have sought to divide the risks they insure into broad classifications that allow the rates for these classifications to more closely match the risk potential of the members of the group.[35] This has resulted, for instance, in the rating of groups and individuals differently for purposes of accident and health insurance and in charging different premiums for medical malpractice coverage based on the type of practice and in some cases geographical considerations.

Particularly in recent years, these rate regulatory laws have been used in some jurisdictions not only to form a basis for the regulation of the solvency of insurance companies, but also to address issues of affordability.

The actuarial method for determining rates is not overly complicated from a mathematics standpoint; it generally involves arithmetic and simple algebra. However, because this method requires predicting future events based on past experience, it is subject to many of the same shortcomings as any economic projection. In the short run the degree of estimation necessary in this process means that it is unlikely for premiums to be exactly right for any given policyholder during that time because of errors in both over- and underestimating. In the long run, this process results in a fairly accurate approximation of the future losses over a number of years.

However, this degree of uncertainty allows some states to exercise their judgment concerning socially and politically acceptable rates for various classes of insureds. Particularly in times of increasing costs, it is tempting for a regulator to determine that physicians cannot pay for the increased cost of medical malpractice,[36] or that the elderly cannot afford the cost of Medicare supplemental insurance. Without a statutory requirement that insurance companies provide this coverage, they will not continue to write coverages for which the approved premium does not cover the cost.

This has resulted in companies withdrawing from offering coverage in some states for such lines as medical malpractice and automobile insurance. In response to these situations during the last 10 years, a number of states have mandated participation of property-casualty companies in various residual market mechanisms. These are basically pooling arrangements that provide coverage the free market economy cannot provide under these circumstances. Some type of pooling or assigning of risks has been established for so-called uninsurable automobile risks in every state of the country.[37] In addition, a number of states have established joint underwriting associations to deal with such unavailable coverages as medical malpractice and liquor liability. Although frequently intended merely to cover high-risk applicants who cannot otherwise be insured in the voluntary market, a number of these have grown to become a major, if not only, source of coverage within a state.[38] Currently in Massachusetts, more than half the drivers, as well as virtually all the doctors and hospitals, are insured through such industry-sponsored joint underwriting associations.

State regulation

In addition to regulating the rates that insurance companies charge, the states have also taken action to regulate insurance companies in other aspects of their operations. Because of some past abuses, many states have regulations involving the handling of claims. These typically set standards for dealing with policyholders who have claims, create administrative procedures to ensure fair treatment, and establish periodic audits by the insurance departments to ensure compliance.

Despite the best efforts of insurance departments to ensure that companies are solvent, insolvencies continue to occur. Therefore, states have established guarantee funds to ensure that claims will be paid, even after an insolvency. All states currently have property-casualty guarantee funds and many states have life and health funds. These guarantee funds require that, when a company becomes insolvent, the rest of the industry step in to ensure that claims will be paid.[39]

A number of states have passed regulations that limit a company's right to cancel or not renew existing policies. While in many cases these regulations establish notice requirements for cancellation so that a person can purchase substitute coverage, they also limit the right to cancel a policyholder, so that that person will not need to be treated as a high risk and insured through a residual market mechanism.[40]

State versus federal regulation

As discussed previously, insurance is one of the highly regulated aspects of our economy that has been left to the states to regulate. Under earlier interpretations of the Constitution, antitrust laws were not applicable to insurance, since insurance was not held to be commerce. As this changed in 1944 with the *Southeastern Under-writers* case, the Congress stepped in quickly to ensure state regulation of insurance by passing the McCarran-Ferguson Act.[41] At the same time, states stepped in to regulate insurance with renewed vigor to establish that they were in fact utilizing the McCarran-Ferguson exception to prevent federal preemption.

More recently, a line of cases has construed the McCarran-Ferguson exception narrowly and has opened the door for increased antitrust scrutiny of insurance practices. Even under McCarran-Ferguson the federal government was always free to regulate insurance by any statute that they passed specifically dealing with insurance. In 1979, the landmark case of *Group Life and Health Insurance Company v. Royal Drug Company*[42] interpreted what constitutes the "business of insurance." This case determined that the business of insurance is "the contract between the insurer and the insured" or to "underwrite and spreading of the risk." Therefore, the exemption did not extend to contracts between insurance companies and drug stores to provide low-cost prescriptions to group insureds. While it may constitute the business of insurance companies, it did not constitute the business of insurance. In another leading case, *Barry v. St. Paul Fire and Marine,* the court expanded the definition of what constituted a boycott within the boycott exception to McCarran-Ferguson.[43] Thus, under present law, unless the activity is core to the concept of insuring a risk, it is subject to antitrust action.

In addition to this indirect regulation through the antitrust laws, the federal government has taken a direct hand in some aspects of insurance that are of national concern. Within the federal government, the Federal Insurance Administration has been involved with a number of federal insurance programs. As a result of the unavailability of crime coverage in the inner city areas following the riots of the 1960s, the federal government established a crime reinsurance program that allowed insurance companies to reinsure those losses with the federal government in certain geographical areas. Currently, almost all of the insurance is written in the New York area and the program has been renewed for only short periods.

Another area of unique concern has been flood insurance. Because the federal government establishes regulations involving the designation of flood plains and limits construction in those areas, it was a logical extension for them also to provide insurance to homes within these flood-prone areas. Originally, this was established as a direct federal program providing flood insurance to eligible policyholders. But recently, the insurance industry has taken a part in marketing and providing the administrative aspects of this program. Although there has been considerable discussion about the appropriateness of these programs as well as future proposals, such as earthquake coverage, these direct federal programs do not currently alter the fundamental concept that insurance is regulated at the state level.

ACCOUNTING REPORTS

The purpose of insurance accounting is to provide information on the financial status of the ongoing business operation to interested parties. It is of critical importance that information be provided to the management of the insurance company in making both day-to-day and long-term decisions. This information needs to be both reasonably accurate and contemporary.[44]

In addition, a number of individuals outside the corporation require current information. For a stock insurance company, the Securities and Exchange Commission imposes requirements concerning the annual statements to aid those contemplating investment in the company. In addition, state insurance departments, which are charged with the responsibility for overseeing insurance company operations within their boundaries, need to have accounting information for the protection of consumers. In this latter role they are assisted by the National Association of Insurance Commissioners (NAIC). The NAIC has established uniform accounting standards to be used by all insurance companies in filing their statements in the various states in which the company is doing business.

In addition to this financial information there is a

parallel system that gathers ratemaking information to be used by the company and insurance departments in setting rates. Although these systems collect similar information, the purpose for which the information is to be used requires different forms of data. Therefore, the accounting data that appear in the annual statement cannot serve as a basis for establishing rates, because the primary purpose of such data is company solvency.

Whereas the ultimate goals of insurance accounting are similar to those of any other business entity, the usual aspects of the insurance industry result in substantial differences in the accounting rules and practices employed.

Insurance problems

Other types of companies, including those involved in manufacturing, use generally accepted accounting principles (GAAP) in producing their financial statements. These rules, with which most readers are familiar, are designed to match revenues with expenses. The revenue received from sales on the one hand is matched against the cost of those same goods sold. This produces, at the end of the accounting period, a bottom line profit or loss, which can either be distributed to shareholders or included in retained earnings. Although some accounting entries, such as depreciation on capital goods, may not accurately reflect current expense, the bottom line is generally an accurate reflection of the firm's profit or loss. Accountants are thus able to measure the per unit cost of goods sold over that period and provide accurate measures to management and shareholders with which their future course may be charted.

In all lines of insurance, particularly in long-tail lines such as medical malpractice, product liability, and hazardous waste, this matching of revenues and expenses is much more difficult. In medical malpractice, for instance, the insurance policy is typically sold for a one-year term based on a fixed premium. Because claims arising out of incidents occurring during the policy period are often not reported until 5 or even 10 years after the term has ended, only a small fraction of the claims to be paid out of that premium will have been reported by the end of the accounting period. Once reported, another 3 to 5 years may transpire before the disposition of the claim. In some states such as New York, it is possible for an individual claim to remain unsettled for as long as 25 years after the policy period has closed.[45] Under these circumstances, it is readily apparent that although the revenue is known at the end of the accounting period, the great bulk of the cost in terms of the payment of losses and accompanying attorneys' fees will remain substantially unknown for a number of years. These facts, however, are of little consolation to the executive planning the company's future or to the shareholder determining whether stock should be held or sold.

Loss reserves

Because claims may not be reported, investigated, and settled for a number of years, the actual paid loss and associated loss adjustment expenses cannot be determined in a timely manner. Therefore, estimates are made of the ultimate value of the claims which are, or will be, filed. By making these estimates it is possible to get an indication of the size of future claims to be paid from present premiums and future investment income. Although this method suffers from problems inherent in making any economic prediction, steps are taken to ensure its accuracy.

A number of ways are used to determine the ultimate value of the claims that have been filed; however, the method typically used in medical malpractice insurance and other "large claim" lines is the individual estimate method. When a loss is reported to the insurer, a reserve is established by the field or home office claims staff. The reserve equals the estimated amount necessary to ultimately settle the claim. The individual estimates on all of the claim files are then aggregated in statistical records by the company. This method works best when claims are definite and the number of claims is too small for the application of reliable averages, particularly because the claims vary greatly in their severity.

For lines involving smaller claims that arise frequently, it is possible to base the reserves on the average value of claims of various types. A third method sometimes used is the loss ratio method in which the ultimate losses in a particular line of insurance are estimated by applying an assumed loss ratio to the premiums earned during the period. This method merely establishes a theoretical reserve and is required in some lines of insurance to establish the minimum statutory loss reserves. This formula approach is not widely used because of its arbitrary nature, yet adjustment of this reserve for actual results in subsequent periods improves the accuracy with time.

Naturally, when a case is first reported to an insurance company, there is very little in the file concerning the facts of the case, statements by witnesses, or other information on which the degree of liability or amount of damage can be estimated. However, over a period of time, the claims staff develops information on the amount of damages involved, such as lost wages, health costs, or the repair of specific damage. Staff members also take statements, talk to expert witnesses, and receive reports from defense counsel. When a claim is initially reported, a reserve is established based on currently available information. As the investigation of the file develops, this reserve is changed to reflect the best estimate of ultimate liability at that time. Thus, on an individual case basis, the reserves that are established for losses change from the time that the file is first opened until the ultimate disposition is made. When these files are aggregated, they produce a statistical loss development pattern that can be used by the actuary to produce a historical record of how reserves tend to change with the age of a case.

It is obvious that the establishment of reserves on individual cases is subjective and requires a great deal of practical experience in handling of similar cases. To improve uniformity, reserves on larger cases are typically set by more senior levels of staff at the company and on a committee basis. An individual adjuster handling a claim will have a relatively low level of reserve authority and must go to a supervisor or manager in order to establish higher levels of reserves. Even the local office does not have authority to establish reserves at the highest claim levels, and usually a committee of senior claim staff at the home office has the ultimate responsibility on very large cases. Despite the very active and high level of consultation that goes into establishing these reserves, some offices and companies may have a bias toward setting reserves higher or lower than necessary in the aggregate.

Aggregate case reserves are not used directly in a financial statement; rather, the information is turned over to an actuary for certain critical adjustments. One of the important functions of the actuary is to analyze in an historical perspective the accuracy with which loss reserves have been established. The actuary compares the record of loss reserves established over time on cases in which the ultimate payments have actually been made. This method enables the actuary to establish statistically the tendency of claims personnel to either overestimate or underestimate the amount it will take to ultimately settle the case. Therefore, from an actuarial perspective, the critical element is not whether reserves are estimated too high or too low, but to ensure that the methods used to establish these reserves result in a uniform approach. This analysis by the actuary produces factors that, when multiplied by the case reserves, produce an adjusted aggregate reserve that eliminates any historical bias.

Incurred but not reported (IBNR)

The methods discussed previously establish reserves on known cases. However, at any time there will be potential claims from incidents that occurred during the policy period but are as yet unreported. A good example is in medical malpractice where fewer than 10% of the claims are reported during the policy year, and almost none of those will result in a final payment. Therefore, at any given time, an insurance company is responsible for incurred losses on incidents that have occurred but have yet to be reported. Although case reserves cannot

be established for claims not filed, to ignore them simply because the company has not received a report would be to significantly understate liabilities and thus substantially overstate income. To accurately view a company's financial position, these future claims must be taken into account. Again, the actuary can make an historical analysis based on past reporting patterns in determining what percentage of claims will be reported at a given point in time after the close of a particular policy year. This produces a statistical estimate of the dollar value of those incurred claims that will be reported in the future.

Thus, a company's loss costs during a particular year are made up of the adjusted reserves on reported cases and the reserves for incurred but unreported claims.

Insurance statutory accounting

The NAIC blank. Annual statements must be filed with the insurance department or other agency within a state where a company is doing business. These forms are required by statute in all states, and are both open for public inspection and used by financial data services such as Bests Insurance Reports: Property-Liability.

The National Association of Insurance Commissioners was established in 1871 to establish, among other things, uniform financial blanks for insurance companies. The association also established rules governing the preparation of the annual statement to ensure uniformity among the states. In effect, these instructions, along with the examiner's manual, provide the source for statutory insurance accounting principles. Currently, the annual statement blank is an oversized booklet containing more than 60 pages of financial statements and exhibits. It bears noting, however, that these statements are filed with the regulators for solvency purposes and do not form the basis for rate-setting activities.

During the 1920s and 1930s, general accounting changed. It became oriented less toward informing management and more toward providing information for potential investors. Statutory insurance accounting did not follow this trend but continued to emphasize solvency considerations. Rather than focusing on accurate measurement of current income, statutory accounting assesses the company's ability to pay all its liability if it went out of business. For this regulatory purpose, the rules concerning statutory accounting are conservative.

Major differences between statutory and GAAP accounting

ADMITTED AND NONADMITTED ASSETS. For federal income tax and GAAP accounting purposes, no distinction is made between assets and nonadmitted assets. Nonadmitted assets in statutory accounting represent types of assets that, though generally considered to have value for noninsurance purposes, are not admitted to an insurance company's statutory balance sheet. Such items as investments not specifically authorized by statute, premiums due over 90 days, prepaid expenses, and office furniture are not included in statutory accounting assets because they are either not legally authorized or not sufficiently liquid. The focus is on whether these assets are liquid enough to be used to satisfy the company's obligations.

Bonds are generally the largest single category of admitted assets of an insurance company and frequently represent more than half the total admitted assets. Typically, many states have statutory rules that limit stock to a prescribed percentage of the insurance company's admitted assets. In addition, property-liability insurance companies normally do not make substantial investments in mortgages because they may be difficult to convert to cash. Reinsurance placed with a company not authorized to transact business in the state is also not recognized under statutory rules. Because bond values are sensitive to interest rate changes as the maturity of the bond increases, bonds in the annual statement are shown at an amortized cost that does not usually represent the true market value of the bonds. This avoids fluctuation in the price of bonds and shields policyholders' surplus from unnecessary fluctuations as long as the company has cash flow sufficient to cover operating expenses without liquidating its investments. Stocks are usually valued at the closing price quotation on the final day of the year.

PREPAID EXPENSES. The expenses attributed to the acquisition of new business, such as agents' commissions, are treated as expenses during the accounting period in which they were incurred. However, the corresponding premium revenue is treated as income over the entire contractual period. In GAAP accounting, acquisition expenses are capitalized and spread over the same period during which the revenues are earned. The insurance approach is conservative because it recognizes the fact that a policy may be cancelled at any time and thus may require a premium refund. However, this conservative approach creates an anomalous situation in insurance accounting. An expanding firm that is rapidly writing new business may find itself in solvency difficulties on its annual statement, not because of an inability to make economic income, but because the acquisition expenses appear on the income statement immediately, whereas the income is reported only over time as it is earned.

TIME VALUE OF MONEY. As we have already discussed, the insurance company's liability for claims that have been incurred but not yet paid is accounted for by the various elements of reserves. Reserves are, in essence, the best estimate as to the ultimate settlement value of these incurred losses. As such, however, these liabilities will actually be satisfied in future years out of the assets represented by the premiums that have been earned, as well as the investment income on those assets between premium payment and claim settlement. Thus, the assets include only the investment income earned to date, whereas the liabilities include the final settlement amount of cases. Because the future expenditure for claims is therefore not matched with the future flow of investment income, the liabilities, particularly in long-tail lines such as medical malpractice, are overstated in relationship to the assets. This difficulty could, of course, be theoretically rectified by simply taking the future claims and discounting them using some assumed interest rate and the time periods indicated by historic loss payment patterns. However, a number of subjective judgments must be made in order to do these calculations. Because companies could overstate their profitability by simply overdiscounting their liabilities, insurance departments have resisted attempts to include discounted liabilities in financial statements for most lines of insurance. Ironically, however, companies are frequently criticized by those outside the industry for overstating their losses as a result of statutory accounting.

Accounting reports furnished by property-casualty companies

Property-casualty companies file a variety of reports with different agencies. The various reports are based on somewhat different rules.

Balance sheet

ASSETS. The major division on the annual statement shows various kinds of invested assets. These primarily include bonds, common stock, cash, and other invested assets. Another important category consists of noninvested assets, primarily agents' balances. These are insurance premiums due on insurance policies written within 90 days prior to the statement date. As discussed earlier, nonadmitted assets either may be excluded entirely from the balance sheet or may have a portion of their values eliminated as being nonadmitted. For instance, agents' balances are considered overdue and nonadmissible after 90 days.

LIABILITIES. Obligations resulting from past or current transactions are liabilities. Historically, property-casualty insurance accounting has used the word "reserves" to describe those liabilities involving money for settling claims. This should be compared with the use of "reserve" in life insurance terminology in which it represents a segregation of retained earnings for specific purposes. This distinction is unfortunate because it causes considerable confusion when discussing an insurer's financial condition. An insolvent company has large reserves, but insufficient assets to pay for them.

Reserves take into account losses, loss-related adjustment expenses, and unearned premiums. They typically equal approximately two-thirds of a company's net admitted assets. As we have already mentioned, the reserves for unpaid losses, established in the claim department as the best estimate of the ultimate cost of disposing of cases, include the actuarial adjustment to correct for overestimates and underestimates.

In addition to loss reserves on known cases currently being adjusted, there are also the reserves for IBNR claims. These represent losses that have already been incurred in the sense that the incident leading to liability has already taken place. However, they are as yet unknown because the report of claim has not been made. Particularly in lines of insurance in which there is a large time lag between incident and claim report, such as with medical malpractice, product liability, or hazardous waste, a substantial portion of the total reserves may in fact be included in this category. The fact that these claims have not yet been reported makes them no less real, although they are actuarial estimates as to the total value of these claims. To ignore them would be to substantially overstate the financial soundness of the company.

In addition to these reserves for unpaid losses, there is also a reserve for loss-adjustment expense. This is made up of two categories: allocated loss-adjustment expense and unallocated loss-adjustment expense. The unallocated loss-adjustment expenses are the general overhead and costs of running a claims operation, which cannot be easily assigned to an individual claim file. On the other hand, the allocated loss-adjustment expenses are, as the name implies, expenses directly attributable to a particular claim. As a practical matter, although some witness fees and other incidental expenses are included in allocated loss-adjustment expense, the great bulk of this expense represents defense counsel fees.

Because of the conservative nature of statutory accounting, a reserve must also be established for that portion of the paid premium that has not been earned during the accounting period. Since a policyholder can cancel the policy and receive a refund of premium, it is necessary to establish a liability for such contingency. While the loss reserves show the company's liability for losses occurring during the period, the unearned premium reserves show the insurer's liability for providing coverage under continuing policies.

Capital and surplus. The admitted assets minus the liabilities equals the "policyholders'" surplus. Initial capitalization provides the resources needed by the insurer to begin business. During continuing operations the policyholder surplus represents the financial protection that guards against insolvency created by fluctuating investment values or underwriting results.

Income statement. The annual statement also includes a summary of operating results entitled "Underwriting and Investment Exhibit Statement of Income." This statement shows the excess of premiums earned over any underwriting losses and expenses that are incurred during the period. The losses and loss-adjustment expenses paid during the year in addition to the new reserves for unpaid losses and loss-adjustment expense are allocated against the period's revenues. Added to this gain from the insurance operations is the net investment income, including realized capital gains and losses. Finally, additional revenues and expenses from sources other than the insurance operation are added.

Reports to the SEC. As a result of the Securities Act of 1933 and the Securities Exchange Act of 1934, all companies with publicly traded securities must comply with certain disclosure requirements. Financial statements of property-casualty insurers filed with the SEC are required to conform to GAAP. In addition, supplemental material must be filed that reconciles the difference between statutory accounting and GAAP.

Federal income tax reports. Because major revisions in the tax code are being considered, it is difficult to review the rules applicable to federal income tax reports. Needless to say, there are special tax rules for determining an insurer's income obligations that recognize the unusual characteristics of insurance companies. To a large extent, these rules have historically conformed with the accounting practices mandated by state insurance regulators.

POLICY PROVISIONS AND CLAIMS
Occurrence versus claims-made policy

Occurrence policies cover incidents occurring within the policy period without regard to when the claims are reported. The policy in effect at the time a service is performed covers a claim based on that service, whenever it is reported in the future. Claims-made policies cover claims reported during the policy period, regardless of when a service is rendered, with some exceptions that are discussed later. Thus claims reported this year are covered by this year's policy; claims reported next year by next year's policy; and so on.

If a policy is maintained with the same company during a person's entire professional life, there is little difference in actual coverage between the occurrence form and most claims-made policies being offered today. However, they are different products having different problems and advantages in specific situations, such as changing policies, changing type of practice, and retirement. They also can result in different comparative costs over a period of years.

The average medical malpractice claim is made 4 to 5 years after the incident, with an additional 2 to 3 years for investigation and settlement. At the outside a claim could be reported much later, and if a jury trial is necessary it may not be closed for 20 years or more after the incident. In these long-tail lines of insurance, it is equally important under either form of coverage that the insurer clearly have the financial stability and backing to be around for at least the period of time it takes for all claims to be closed. It is obvious that since the occurrence form covers all future claims whenever reported, the company must be around to pay the claim.

A typical claims-made policy covers an act or omission, provided the claim is first made against the insured and reported to the company during the policy period.

Additional requirements or limitations to coverage are as follows:

1. The insured has no prior knowledge of the claim at the time the policy went into effect.
2. A retroactive exclusion limits covered claims to those that occur during the policy period or after a retroactive date (normally the date of the first claims-made policy with that company).
3. Prior coverage of the claim for incidents occurring before the commencement of the policy is required, sometimes with the same company.

Prior knowledge of a claim. A claim does not require that suit actually be brought but only that there be a demand for something as the result of a covered activity. It includes the statement that the claimant intends to hold the insured responsible for the cost incurred in correcting a defect or the demand that the insured correct the problem without charge.[46] The idea behind a clause excluding prior claims that the applicant knows about is to permit the company to avoid assuming a known risk. The question that generally must be answered is whether a reasonable professional in similar circumstances would have known of the claim.

Most policies require that the insured provide notice of the claim to the company within the policy period. However, some courts have allowed the notice to be made in a reasonable time where there is "excusable delay," and others have read the clear language of the policy strictly. Some courts have been accused of converting a claims-made policy into an occurrence policy by failing to strictly enforce the notice requirement.[47] Certainly it is in the best interest of the policyholder to inform the company of any incident that he or she has some reason to believe may give rise to a claim.

Retroactive exclusion clause. Most present claims-made policies exclude coverage for any incident that occurred before the date on which the policyholder first took out a claims-made policy with the company. This provision has no practical impact where the young physician takes out his or her first policy (with no prior

incidents to cover), or where the policyholder is switching from an occurrence policy (prior incidents will all be covered under the first policy). There can be severe consequences, however, for others who are not sufficiently informed on how to avoid a gap in coverage.

An unfortunate example of the potential problems of gaps is presented in the case of *Gereboff v. Home Indemnity Company.*[48] This accounting firm had continuous policies with three companies. Home Indemnity covered the period in 1968 when the alleged malpractice occurred. St. Paul Fire and Marine covered the period in 1971 when the malpractice was first discovered by the insureds, and American Home had the coverage in 1973 when the suit was filed. Home Indemnity did not provide coverage because the claim was not reported during the period of its policy, St. Paul did not cover the claim because there was no claim made during the policy period, and American Home did not provide coverage because it had an exclusion for acts that occurred before the retroactive date when its first policy was written. Therefore, despite the significant premium that was paid, the accounting firm in fact had no coverage for this claim.

As graphically illustrated by this case, gaps in coverage can easily occur in claims-made policies. Although they do not occur when switching from an occurrence policy to a claims-made one, gaps can occur when switching from one claims-made carrier to another or when the insured ceases to purchase claims-made policies. If the claims-made policy terminates, for whatever reason, the insured has no coverage for claims arising from incidents before the termination date but reported after that date. Similarly the subsequent carrier would not provide coverage because of the prior act's exclusion. This problem can be remedied by purchasing a "reporting endorsement" to the policy.

Reporting endorsements. The reporting endorsement is an amendment to the policy that provides that all claims occurring during the term of the prior claims-made policies are covered, regardless of when they are reported (assuming as always that they are otherwise covered under the terms and conditions of those policies). In effect, this puts these claims on the occurrence basis.

Typically the reporting endorsement is purchased from the first company to cover these late-reported claims. However, the purchase of the full reporting endorsement may not be guaranteed from that company.

The claims-made insured must not lose sight of the fact that at some point to be fully covered he or she must purchase the reporting endorsement. The endorsement will be priced as of the year of its purchase, so it will be subject to all the accuracy considerations already discussed. Therefore, during periods of rapid increase in cost, the reporting endorsement cost could be much higher than the amount saved in the first four claims-made years even when interest is earned on the savings.

Because these endorsements are typically rather expensive, some companies build the cost of limited reporting endorsements into the basic policy for insureds who have been with the company for some period of time. Usually the policyholder is entitled to this so-called "free tail" on death or disability. In addition, a physician may earn a portion or all of the "free tail" for retirement at a certain age by continuing with that same company for a period of years before retirement. These provisions, however, do not generally help the physician leaving the coverage area, changing companies, or changing practice.

Because medical malpractice coverage is rated based on whether or not the physician is in a high- or low-risk specialty, the reporting endorsement is also rated on a similar basis. To prevent a physician in a high-risk specialty from changing to a low one just before retirement simply to get the benefit of a lower cost-reporting endorsement that would still cover earlier high-risk claims, the company requires the physician to purchase a reporting endorsement any time there is a change to a lower risk specialty. The cost of that endorsement is simply the difference between the cost of the endorsement in the higher rated class and in the lower rated one. This cost reflects the fact that the company will continue to cover subsequently reported high-risk losses. When the physician retires or otherwise changes, he or she will pay only the reporting endorsement for the lower class.

A frequently asked question is whether, rather than purchase the unlimited reporting endorsement, the policyholder should just keep the claims-made policy in effect for the period of the statute of limitations for the type of exposure involved. This is a dangerous practice because of the many exceptions to the absolute statute of limitations in many jurisdictions. In medical malpractice most jurisdictions recognize some exceptions based on the "discovery rule." Under the variations of this rule the statute of limitations does not begin to run until the patient discovers the malpractice or reasonably should have discovered it.[49] In some cases this "discovery" is not limited to the facts of the injury but also includes whether the injury was caused by malpractice and in some cases whether it resulted in irreparable harm. In addition, many statutes are extended for minors and have exceptions for continued treatment or allegations of concealment. All of these exceptions to the general rule mean that in many cases the claim will not be barred no matter how late it is made.

Pricing. Although over years of continuous coverage there is no essential difference as to the totality of claims covered under either type of coverage, their total cost may be quite different. It is apparent that in the first year of coverage with an occurrence policy you are covering 100% of all the claims that arise from the first year of treatment. By comparison the first year of a new claims-made coverage covers in that example only about 30% of the claims from the first year of treatment. As that policy continues in effect through to year 5, the claims-made policy covers larger and larger numbers of potential losses because the cumulative years of past treatment may produce reported and hence covered claims in any policy year. This gradual increase in the number of potentially covered claims results in a gradual increase in the premium for the claims-made policy-holder until in year 5 the policyholder is paying the maximum, or mature, claims-made rate. This rate may be higher or lower than the occurrence rate but probably will be in the same range. The factors affecting the relative cost between the occurrence policy and the mature claims-made rate is discussed later.

It is frequently said that the fundamental difference between these two policies is that the claims-made policy eliminates the tail because it only covers reported claims. Although this is an important aspect of the policy, it is not technically true. The tail of a claim is the time between the incident giving rise to the claim and its ultimate disposition. As such it is made up of the time lag in the claim being made and its report to the company, and then the time required to investigate, settle, or litigate the claim. It is only the delay in the report of the claim that is eliminated in the claims-made policy.

In medical malpractice the average time between the incident and the report to the company is about 4 years. After the report it typically takes an average of 2½ to 3 years to dispose of the claim. Therefore the average lag on an occurrence policy would be around 6 to 7 years as compared with 2½ to 3 for the claims-made policy. The significance for rating purposes is that a 1980 occurrence policy covering 1980 claims must estimate the number of claims and their cost on average through 1986 and for a few claims as far as the year 2000. On the other hand, that same incident in 1980 would be covered by some later years' claims-made policy, on average around 1984. It is obvious, considering the difficulties in projecting future claims from 1980 incidents, that the estimate made in 1984 (in fact, the estimate would be made in pieces between 1980 and 1990 as the reported claims arising from 1980 incidents are reported to the company) will be considerably more accurate than those made in 1980 covering 20 years' worth of claim settlement activity.

In the theoretical world where we know the exact changes in claim cost into the future, both of these rates would be equally accurate regardless of the rate of change from year to year. It is, however, the volatility of these losses in the real world that causes the problems. If in predicting the ultimate cost of 1980 incidents for occurrence policies we end up underestimating the cost of what really happens, the claims-made policy (since its rates are set later in time and hence are more accurate) will appear higher over the course of time. By the same token, if we overestimate the cost of future reported occurrence claims, the accuracy of a claims-made policy results in a lower cost over time. In the last 20 years in medical malpractice we have had both periods of overestimating and underestimating. However, because of the rapid and generally underestimated increases in the underlying cost of medical malpractice during much of that time, the cost comparison has favored the occurrence policy.

The volatility in claims expense itself has also had its impact on the overall cost of these coverages. An objective insurer should receive a higher premium for allocating its scarce resources to a risky line such as medical malpractice. The absence of the risk premium as a result of strict rate regulation has caused the commercial insurers to abandon this market in many states and leave it to the physician companies and residual markets such as joint underwriting associations (required by statute to provide this coverage). Because the volatility of claims-made rates is less than that of occurrence rates, an insurer could write that claims-made policy for less, all things being equal.

Another factor results from the differences between the claims-made and occurrence policies that has a bearing on their relative cost. All insurers take into account the future investment income that they will earn on their premium receipts when they set their rates. This is done by determining the future loss payment pattern for the policy and then discounting these values back to the policy year using an assumed investment yield. The insurer holds the premiums from occurrence policies for a longer period of time, between the payment of the premium by the insured and the payment of the claim. Thus in periods of high interest rates, and particularly where the tail is long, the relative cost of occurrence would decrease. However, these same factors also tend to make the premium savings to the insured in the first four claims-made years more valuable, because the insured could invest the savings at higher rates of interest. Also the long payment pattern makes the cost of the first four years lower because few claims would be reported in that year.

RISK RETENTION GROUPS

During the 99th Congress, the United States was shaken by a crisis in the availability and affordability of commercial liability insurance. Congress was besieged

with complaints regarding huge rate increases, mass cancellations of coverage, and entire lines of insurance virtually unavailable at any price. Crucial activities and services were hard hit. Such activities included those of municipalities, universities, child day care centers, health care providers, corporate directors and officers, hazardous waste disposal firms, small businesses generally, and many others.

To some extent, the "insurance crisis" may be viewed as a repetition of prior experience. It is universally recognized that the liability insurance business is cyclical, with alternating periods of expansion and contraction. In fact, the Product Liability Risk Retention Act of 1981[50] was in large part the result of concerns arising from the last contraction of insurance markets. However, the current insurance problem is far more severe than those previously experienced.

The high cost and limited availability of insurance have been attributed by different observers to a wide variety of causes. Many observers contend that a multifaceted approach is required to deal with the insurance crisis.

The 1981 act was premised on an 18-month study by the Federal Interagency Task Force on Product Liability. It was believed that the proposed risk retention legislation would help deal with the fact that many rates appeared to be based not on actuarial techniques, but on subjective underwriting judgments.[51] Because a risk retention group is simply a group of businesses or others who join together to set up their own insurance company in order to issue insurance policies to themselves, it was believed that by encouraging such groups, the subjective element in underwriting could be reduced. The risk retention group would know its own loss experience and could adhere closely to it in setting rates. It was also believed that the 1981 act, by providing alternatives to traditional insurance, would promote greater competition among insurers to "encourage private insurers to set rates to reflect experience as accurately as possible."[52]

These considerations remain valid and justify expansion of the scope of the 1981 act to include other lines of liability insurance. Congressional hearings indicated the existence of a multibillion dollar insurance capacity shortage, and the creation of self-insurance groups was thought to provide much-needed new capacity. Additionally, according to the Department of Commerce, "[t]he knowledge that substantial insurance buyers can create their own alternative insurance mechanisms is incentive to commercial insurers to avoid sharp peaks and valleys in their costs."[53]

With respect to purchasing groups, risk retention group regulation seeks to enable insurance markets to translate into lower rates and better terms the efficiencies gained from the better loss and expense experience that might arise from the collective purchase of insurance.

Federal legislation alleviated the problems of certain aspects of state law. Some states have created capital and other requirements that make it difficult for risk retention groups to form or to operate on a multistate basis. Many states prevent insurance purchasing groups from achieving the advantages in rates and terms derived from the economic efficiency of collective purchasing that could contribute to resolving affordability and availability problems, or they prohibit purchasing groups altogether. Risk retention and purchasing groups were exempted from state law in order to achieve their beneficial effects.

The federal Liability Risk Retention Act of 1986[54] changed existing law to permit risk retention groups in virtually every line of commercial insurance except workers' compensation. The act preempts state law regulating insurance wherever the federal law applies. Where the federal act is silent, state law remains effective. Cases interpreting the act upheld a number of state requirements on insurers.[55]

Risk retention group enabling legislation is one of many initiatives to address the serious financial and operational problems in the liability insurance industry. Tort reform measures have proliferated and continue to be tested in the courts, legislatures, and marketplace. Most "tort reform" efforts are aimed more at claims limitation and less at liability factors or insurance regulation. However, as a major player in liability disputes, insurers have been intensely interested in such activities.[56]

END NOTES

1. Pennsylvania State Insurance Department, Press Release (Feb. 23, 1973).
2. R. Keeton, *Insurance Law* §1.2, p. 2 (1971).
3. W. Shernoff, S. Gage, and H. Levine, *Insurance Bad Faith Litigation* §1.03 (1986).
4. G. Couche, *Couche on Insurance* §15.83-86 (rev. ed. 1985).
5. *Pieri v. John Hancock Mutual Life Insurance Co.,* 92 R.I. 303, 168 A.2d 277 (1961); *Furlong v. Donhals, Inc.,* 87 R.I. 46, 137 A.2d 734 (1958).
6. *Belanger v. Silva,* 114 R.I. 266, 331 A.2d 403 (1975); *Hancock v. State Farm Mutual Insurance Co.,* 403 F.2d 375 (6th Cir. 1968).
7. *Eisenberg v. Continental Casualty Co.,* 48 Wis.2d 637, 180 N.W. 2d 726 (1970); *Namco, Inc. v. American Employers Insurance Co.,* 736 F.2d 187 (5th Cir. 1984).
8. Couche, *supra* note 4, §35, at 1093; *Carpenter v. Sun Indemnity Co.,* 138 Neb. 552, 293 N.W. 400 (1940).
9. *Vackiner v. Mutual of Omaha Insurance Co.,* 179 Neb. 300, 137 N.W.2d 859 (1965).
10. *Glickman v. Prudential Insurance Co.,* 151 Pa. Super. 52, 29 A.2d 224 (1942).
11. *Burns v. Prudential Insurance Co.,* 201 Cal. App. 2d 868, 20 Cal. Rptr. 535 (1962).
12. *Fisher v. Prudential Insurance Co.,* 107 N.H. 101, 218 A.2d 62 (1966).
13. *Shelter Insurance Co. v. Cruse,* 446 So.2d 893 (La. App. 1984).
14. Couche, *supra* note 4, §72, at 2.
15. *Ludwinska v. John Hancock Mutual Life Insurance Co.,* 317 Pa. 577, 178 A.28 rev'g. 115 Pa. Super. 228, 175 A. 283 (1935).
16. *Clemmons v. Nationwide Mutual Insurance Co.,* 267 N.C. 495, 148 S.E.2d 640 (1966); 1 A.L.R. 3d 1139.
17. *Therrien v. Maryland Casualty Co.,* 97 N.H. 180, 84 A.2d 179 (1951).
18. *St. Paul Fire and Marine Insurance Co. v. Molloy,* 46 Md. App. 520, 420 A.2d 994 (1980), *rev'd on other grounds,* 291 Md. 139, 433 A.2d 1135 (1981); *Sahlen v. American Casualty Co.,* 103 Ariz. 57, 436 P.2d 606 (1968).
19. J. Moore, *Insurers' Preservation of Rights,* 26 For the Defense 23 (1984).
20. D. Wall, *Litigation and Prevention of Insurer Bad Faith* §3.04 (1985).
21. *Id.* at §1.01.
22. Shernoff, *supra* note 3, at §1.07.
23. *Communale v. Traders and General Insurance Co.,* 328 P.2d 198 (Cal. 1958).
24. *Egan v. Mutual of Omaha Insurance Co.,* 24 Cal.3d 809, 157 Cal. Rptr. 482, 598 P.2d 452 (1979) *cert. denied,* 445 U.S. 912, 100 S.Ct. 1271, 63 L.Ed.2d 597 (1980).
25. *Frazier v. Metropolitan Life Insurance Co.,* 169 Cal. App.3d 90, 214 Cal. Rptr. 883 (1985).
26. Comments on the NAIC Program to Monitor Competition, Patricia Danzon (Munch) (1979).
27. P. Danzon (Munch), *The Role of Rating Bureaus in Property-Liability Insurance Markets* (1980).
28. *Paul v. Virginia,* 75 U.S. (8 Wall.) 168 (1868).
29. *Southeastern Underwriters Ass'n v. U.S.,* 322 U.S. 533, 88 L.Ed. 1440, 64 S.Ct. 1162 (1944).
30. McCarran-Ferguson Act, 15 U.S.C. §1011-(1945).
31. J. Mintel, *Insurance Rate Litigation,* p. 4 (1983).
32. *Id.* at 5.
33. *Blue Cross v. Insurance Dept.,* 34 Pa. Commw. 585, 383. A.2d 1306 (1975).
34. Mintel, *supra* note 31, at 113.
35. R. Holton, *Restraints on Underwriting* (1979).
36. *Medical Malpractice JUA v. Comm'r of Insurance,* 478 N.E. 2d 936 (Mass. 1985).
37. F. Lee, *A Profile of the Automobile Shared Market* (1979).
38. L. Soular, *Subsidization of Insurance: A Study of Residual Markets and their Impact on Property-Casualty Insurers* (1980).
39. R. Marcus, *Directory and Chart of State Laws* (1985).
40. Holton, *supra* note 35.
41. McCarran-Ferguson Act, *supra* note 30, at §1011-1015.
42. *Group Life and Health Insurance Co. v. Royal Drug Co.,* 435 U.S. 903, 98 S.Ct. 1448, 47 L.W. 4203 (1979).
43. *Barry v. St. Paul Fire and Marine,* 438 U.S. 531, 57 L.Ed. 2d 932, 98 S.Ct. 2923 (1978).
44. C. and J. Galloway, *Handbook of Accounting for Insurance Companies* (1986); T. Troxel and C. Breslin, *Property-Liability Insurance Accounting and Finance* (2d ed. 1983); R. Strain, *Property and Liability Insurance Accounting* (3d Ed. 1986).
45. J. MacGinnitie, *Malpractice—Where We've Been and Where We May be Going,* National Medical Malpractice JUA Seminar (1984).
46. *Williamson & Vollmer Eng'g., Inc. v. Sequoia Insurance Co.,* 64 Cal. App. 3d 261, 134 Cal. Rptr. 427 (1976); *Continental Casualty Co. v. Enco Ass'n. Inc.* 238 N.W.2d 198 (Mich. App. 1976).
47. *Stine v. Continental Casualty Co.,* 315 N.W.2d 887 (Mich. App. 1982). Windt, *Insurance Claims & Disputes,* §12.02, at 12(1983).
48. *Gereboff v. Home Indemnity Co.,* 383 A.2d 1024 (R.I. 1978).
49. Long, *The Law of Liability Insurance,* §12.02, at 12(1983).
50. Product Liability Risk Retention Act of 1981.
51. House report 97-190, p. 23.
52. House report 97-190, p. 4.

53. July 17, 1986 Congressional Record, pages S9229-S9230.
54. Liability Risk Retention Act of 1986.
55. *Frontier Insurance v. Hager*, S. Dist. Iowa No. 87-645 (1988); *Pennsylvania Insurance Co. v. Corcoran*, Cir. No. 87-7858 (1988).
56. For discussion of such issues, *see* L. S. Maarema, *PUBLIC Regulation of Insurance Law: Annual Survey*, XXIV Tort and Insurance Law J. 472 (Winter 1989); S. Conley and L. H. Vitlin, *The Duties of Good Faith Owed by a Primary Insured to the Carriers Providing Excess Coverage*. 369 PLI/Lit. 337. Practicing Law Institute. 1 January 1989. PLI Order No. H4. 5062; P. B. Weiss, *Comments Reforming Tort Reform*. 38 Catholic Univ. L. Rev. 737 – 1 April 1989; M. Hager, *Civil Compensation and Its Discontents: A Response to Huber*. 42 Stanford L. Rev. 539 (1 Jan 1990); P. W. Huber, *Liability: The Legal Revolution and its Consequences*, (Basic Books 1988).

APPENDIX 19-1   Insurance glossary

ALE Allocated loss expense. See *expenses*.

amortized value See *investments*.

claim A demand to pay. A claim is a demand against a doctor or hospital. It may or may not be insured under a policy, depending on the coverage afforded and the nature of the offense.

claims frequency The number of claims reported in a period, such as a year, ratioed to the number of doctors insured; perhaps "per 100 doctors."

claims-made See *coverage*.

class Short for *classification*. A class is a subdivision of a "universe." To lump all insureds into the same rate grouping would be to overcharge one subgroup (or class) and to undercharge another. In medical malpractice insurance approximately 100 classes are based mostly on medical specialties. However, an insurer may have only seven rate groups, so each rate group contains several classes.

combined loss ratio The sum of (a) the ratio of losses and loss-adjustment expenses incurred to earning premiums and (b) the ratio of all other underwriting expenses incurred to written premiums.

coverage The insurance afforded by the policy and the endorsements or riders attached to it.
Claims-made coverage – the claims-made policy covers only those claims that are *reported* during the term of the (annual) policy, regardless of when the incident occurred.
Occurrence coverage – this policy insures against all incidents that *occurred* during the term of the (annual) policy, no matter how many years later they are *first reported*.

earned premium See *premium*.

expenses I. Loss expense
   A. ALE – Allocated loss expense. That claim expense that can be allocated to a specific claim. This is almost 100% *loss legal*, that is, outside defense attorneys and expert witnesses.
   B. ULE – Unallocated loss expense. The *inside cost* of running a claim department: supervisors, claim examiners, share of executive, heat, light, rent, and so forth.
   II. Commissions – Percentage of premiums paid to brokers.
   III. Taxes – The percent of written premium, paid to the state.
   IV. Administration and overhead – Also includes actuarial, legal, accounting, and investment services, and so forth.

expenses incurred The expenses paid in a period, such as a year, plus the change in expense reserves. Paid expenses, less outstanding expense at the beginning of the period plus the outstanding expenses at the end of the year.

experience A matching of premiums, losses, and expenses. May or may not include investment earnings and/or net profit.
   I. Calendar year experience – brings together the premiums *earned* in a year and the losses *incurred* in the year.
   II. Accident year experience – brings together the losses that *occurred* in a year and the premiums *earned* on policies in effect during that year. Changes over time. See separate definitions of *premium* and *expenses incurred*.

frequency See *claims frequency*.

IBNR Losses incurred but not reported. See *losses*.

investments I. Interest – The interest received on bonds in the portfolio.
   II. Maturity – The date on which a bond matures and the bondholder is paid off at *par*.
   III. Portfolio valuations:
      A. Market value – The value at which we could sell our bonds today. Fluctuates widely, inversely with general interest rates, and directly with quality and other factors.
      B. Par value – The face amount (maturing amount) of each and all of the bonds.
      C. Price or purchase amount – The cost of our bonds, what we paid for them when we bought them.
      D. Amortized value – A straight line trending from the date and amount of purchase to maturity at par. If a bond maturing in 10 years is bought at 90, its amortized value is 91 at the end of the first year, 92 at the end of the second year, and so on, *regardless* of the market values of the bonds at those times. Bonds of insurance companies are valued this way. If not, there would be a good many technical insolvencies, as market values become abnormally depressed.
   IV. Realized capital gain (loss) – The difference between the purchase price of a bond and what you sold it for. By selling the bond, or letting it mature at par, you *realized* a gain or a loss, measured in dollars.
   V. Unrealized capital gain (loss) – The difference between the purchase price of a bond and what it's worth now at market. The bond hasn't been sold or matured, so the gain or loss is *unrealized*.
      Maturity – Unlike stocks, bonds are debts that become due and payable at some time in the future, at which time they are said to *mature*.

ISO Insurance Services Office – A large organization in New York City that gathers and processes the statistics of most insurance companies (not life) in the United States. ISO also publishes rate manuals for most lines of insurance (see *line*) in each of the states.

line Line of insurance – A general kind of insurance, such as Fire, Auto, or Workers' Compensation. The Annual Statement blank provides for 29 lines of insurance and leaves a line blank for some specialty lines. It separates malpractice liability from other liability.

losses The most important statistic:
   I. Losses paid – The losses actually paid on a body of

policies. Calendar year losses paid (see *experience—Calendar year*) are the losses paid out in a given period, say, during 1982, on claims whenever occurred or reported. Does not include loss adjustment expenses which are separate.

After a claim is paid, it is usually *closed,* but not always. There are partial payments on claims that remain open. *Indemnity payments* are those to claimants, and do not include payments to defense attorneys (ALE). Losses paid are indemnity payments only.

II. Losses outstanding—Losses unpaid, and are represented by *loss reserves.* There are two kinds:

A. Case reserves—"Case" is a Claim Department term for "claim" or "file." Technically, it is accompanied by a claim number. When a claim is reported and set up, it gets a claim number and, also, a "case estimate." That is, the Claim Department estimates the final liability of the claim, and that amount goes into reserve, and liability is set up for its ultimate cost. The total of such estimates, minus any amount paid thereon, becomes the losses outstanding reserve for known cases.

B. IBNR—Losses incurred but not reported. Some claims are not reported promptly; others are reported late because the injury takes a long time to become manifest. In any event, provision must be made for such claims, often reported 10 or more years after the event or injury. IBNR reserves, particularly for medical malpractice liability, are substantial, and often exceed the reserves for known cases. They are calculated by the actuary and are based on past patterns of claims emergence, trended to the future.

C. Loss adjustment expenses—see *expenses.*

III. Losses incurred—the sum of losses paid and losses outstanding, with reserves for both case estimates and losses IBNR. The estimated ultimate cost of a body of claims.

market value See *investments.*

maturity See *investments.*

no-pay claims Claims closed without indemnity payment. Also known as CWOP, or closed without payment. There may be some loss adjustment expense paid.

occurrence See *coverage.*

par value See *investments.*

premium The money a policyholder pays for the policy.

I. Written premiums—The sum total of all the premiums for all the policies written for a period, e.g., during 1980.

II. Earned premium—That part of the premium for a policy that represents the expired part of the policy. If a policy has already run for four months, then one-third of its premium is earned and belongs to the company, two-thirds is unearned and refundable to the policyholder if he or she cancels. A proper matching of premiums, losses, and expenses to determine profit includes earned premiums, losses incurred, and expenses incurred.

III. Unearned premium—Premium representing the unexpired part of a policy. Equals written premium minus earned premium. Can become a substantial item on the balance sheet of an insurance company, and is carried as a liability, since it is theoretically refundable.

realized capital gains See *investments.*

reserve A liability on the balance sheet for future payments. See *losses.* There are reserves for unearned premiums, for losses and loss expense unpaid, and for other expenses unpaid. The solvency of a company can be determined only after all reserves and other liabilities have been taken into account.

statutory accounting The system under which insurance companies must report to the state. Many businesses use GAAP, generally accepted accounting principles. Two major differences for joint underwriting associations are (a) under statutory accounting, the JUA may not "discount" its reserves to take into account the investment income they will earn before they are paid out; (b) the JUA may not be given credit for its "equity in the unearned premium reserve." This is the prepaid acquisition expense, or commission paid to brokers. The unearned premium reserve, which is a liability, may not be reduced to reflect this prepaid expense.

ULE Unallocated loss expense. See *expenses.*

underwriting profit (loss) What's left over after subtracting from earned premiums in a period the sum of losses and loss expense incurred in the same period. Investment income is not taken into account; when it is, the result is called *operating* profit or loss.

unearned premiums See *premium.*

unrealized capital gains See *investments.*

CHAPTER 20

Risk management

RICHARD R. BALSAMO, M.D., J.D., F.C.L.M.
MAX DOUGLAS BROWN, J.D.

ORIGIN AND SCOPE OF RISK MANAGEMENT
RISK IDENTIFICATION
RISK PRIORITIZATION
RISK CONTROL
RISK PREVENTION
RISK FINANCING
EXTERNAL RISK MANAGEMENT REQUIREMENTS
CONCLUSION

ORIGIN AND SCOPE OF RISK MANAGEMENT

Risk management programs began in the 1970s as a response to accelerating medical malpractice claims of hospitals, and they have since been adopted by other types of health care organizations. Risk management is the process of protecting an organization's financial assets against losses from legal liability. It is defined by the Joint Commission on Accreditation of Healthcare Organizations (JCAHO) as "clinical and administrative activities that [health care organizations] undertake to identify, evaluate, and reduce the risk of injury and loss to patients, personnel, visitors, and the [organization] itself."[1]

Risk management may be both reactive in its response to events that have already occurred as well as proactive in its prevention of further occurrences. The primary responsibilities of a comprehensive risk management program are identification of legal risk, prioritization of identified risk and determination of proper organizational response, management of recognized risk cases with the goal of minimizing loss (risk control), establishment of effective risk prevention, and maintenance of adequate risk financing. Risk management in a health care organization requires knowledge of the law and of the legal process, an understanding of clinical medicine, and familiarity with the organization's administrative structure and operational realities.

The full scope of risk management encompasses all organizational activity—operational as well as clinical—because liability may originate in either area. This purview includes proper building maintenance and food preparation as well as adverse outcomes of medical care and accurate medical record keeping. This chapter, however, focuses on risk management as it relates to the medical care provided by a health care organization—"clinical" risk management. Clinical risk management requires close cooperation between the legal department and the clinical administrators responsible for quality assessment and improvement and for clinical functional units (e.g., a hospital patient care unit, a medical office, the physical therapy department).

Risk management is usually the prime responsibility of a risk management department or of the legal department, which, in carrying out this function, typically establishes a close working relationship with the clinical administrative staff. Nevertheless, important risk management functions such as risk identification, clinical case review, and clinical risk prevention are the direct responsibility of the clinical staff. Many organizations employ risk managers, who often have training and experience in a clinical field such as nursing, to work with the legal staff and take day-to-day responsibility for some specified risk management functions such as the management of recognized risk cases (risk control) and the coordination of overall risk management activity. In this chapter, the term *risk administrators* refers to those individuals in an organization with formal, organization-wide risk management responsibility, most notably the legal staff and risk managers; in the context of clinical duties, the term's meaning incorporates clinical administrators such as the director of quality assessment and improvement (quality management) and the chief medical staff officer.

Role of risk management

Escalating litigation and the decreasing affordability of liability insurance have generated the demand for increased sophistication in the identification, control, prevention, and financing of medical risk. Today, the trust fund of a self-insured hospital represents a sizable and important asset of that hospital. A highly synergistic commonality of purpose exists between financial management and risk management. A risk administrator seeks to manage what is substantially a financial risk—the loss of financial assets. This loss occurs through the payment of claims for damages and expenses arising from untoward events that become potentially compensable through judgments or settlements and that may erode the hospital's assets and increase the cost of providing health care.[2]

Although the basic purpose of a risk management program is to minimize the cost of loss, there is a tendency to evaluate a risk management program solely from a financial standpoint with regard to current cases and claims. Most administrators of successful risk management programs agree that such a "bottom line" view misses the overriding purpose of a risk management program. Risk management in a health care institutional setting should first and foremost be considered a means of improving and maintaining quality patient care—the cornerstone of risk prevention.[3]

In pursuing this goal, risk administrators must have a close, trusting relationship with the clinical administrators who have direct responsibility for many risk management functions. Effective risk management depends on their active participation. Moreover, formal organizational quality assessment and improvement functions should be operationally linked to the risk management program. This linkage should include the exchange of all relevant information and the sharing of formal risk management responsibilities in order to maximize the understanding of all risk management issues, specific cases, and organizational data. Nonmedical risk administrators must have quick, thorough, and reliable access to medical consultation about clinical issues, specific cases, and organization performance data. The proper relationship should avoid duplication of effort, the potential for misunderstanding between the clinical and legal staffs, and the potential to work at cross purposes in carrying out specific risk management functions.

Risk administrators and quality managers must, in turn, be operationally linked to and influential in the overall management of the organization. For example, tragic consequences can befall a health maintenance organization (HMO) whose risk and quality administrators' efforts to reverse growing risk exposure from poor after-hours access to care are ignored and defeated by a financially driven, organization-wide effort to reduce emergency room utilization.

Despite the necessity of a close working relationship, risk management and quality management are not ideally combined in one department. Risk management is an extension of the legal responsibilities of an organization, so risk management activity should ultimately be directed by an attorney. Fulfillment of quality management responsibilities requires detailed medical knowledge and the trust, respect, and attention of the medical staff. Thus, quality management activity is best led and directed by a physician.

An effective risk management program begins with its system for identifying the specific events likely to result in loss and the general clinical areas of risk exposure. This system should be predicated on a current, thorough understanding of the varied sources of legal risk faced by a health care organization. Risk management then proceeds to risk prioritization, risk control, risk prevention, and risk financing.

Sources of legal risk: new developments and recent trends

Detailed discussion of the varied sources of legal risk that confront health care providers is covered elsewhere in this text and is beyond the scope of this chapter. However, it may be useful here to point out some recent data and trends that indicate the developing legal risks that are especially problematic for health care providers.

The legal risk most commonly associated with a health care organization is medical malpractice. Several recent studies have provided detailed data on the clinical and operational sources of malpractice risk. The Physician Insurers Association of America (PIAA), which consists of 44 professional liability insurers owned or operated by doctors, has been collecting data from member companies since 1985. PIAA conducted an analysis of 78,712 closed claims (malpractice cases that have resulted in a final disposition)[4] (Appendixes 20-1 and 20-2). The most frequently cited medical misadventure was improper performance, which accounted for more than one-third of all misadventure claims. "Errors in diagnosis" was the second most frequent misadventure, most commonly involving cancer of the breast, cancer of the bronchi and lung, appendicitis, acute myocardial infarction, and ectopic pregnancy. When misadventures were ranked according to the size of the indemnity (payout), problems with the proper timing of care (whether too soon or too late) and the proper monitoring of patients appear as major issues. St. Paul Fire and Marine Insurance Company, in its 1993 annual report, offered its policyholders an analysis of claims of their insured hospitals for 1991-1992. These data offer another view of the sources of malpractice risk. Appendixes 20-3 through 20-6 demonstrate, respectively, St Paul's findings as to the top 10 malpractice allegations by average cost, the top 10 malpractice allegations by frequency, all malpractice allegations by location, and major malpractice allegation issues.

The growing use of clinical practice guidelines may develop as a cause of increased medical malpractice risk.[5] Practice guidelines are widely viewed as means to improve the quality and appropriateness of care and, when followed, as shields against liability. Unquestionably, they may provide great benefits to the extent that they improve the quality and efficiency of care. Unfortunately, they also have the potential to stultify and codify the practice of medicine by establishing innumerable sets of micro-standards useful to plaintiffs in proving a departure from the standard of care. In the absence of legal protection accompanying their adoption, fear of deviating from guidelines and the difficulty of remembering their many details may bedevil physicians in years to come.

A developing contributor to medical malpractice risk is the sometimes inordinate deference given to the principle of patient control over treatment choices. Obstetrical care may be the most problematic area. Today, many patients demand home deliveries, impose restrictions on care given to infants, and even refuse cesarean sections, all of which may pose a grave danger to an infant's health and increase the likelihood of an adverse infant outcome. Courts have generally been tolerant of patients' asserting their right to pick and choose how obstetrical care will be provided. At the same time, this attitude causes great unease among risk administrators, who note that the single most costly source of risk to a health care organization is in the area of birth-related infant trauma, which usually can be avoided by cesarean section. In the absence of reasonable limitations on patient choices, it is fully expected that childbirth-related trauma and other adverse outcomes stemming from unlimited patient control over care will grow even more costly to both physicians and their health care organizations.

Failure to obtain informed consent is another important source of risk. It may give rise to an intentional tort or may be a secondary count in a medical malpractice action. States are divided in their approach to determining what information must be provided to patients to enable them to decide whether to accept the risks of proposed treatment. Some states require the disclosure of information that a reasonable physician would disclose to that patient, whereas others require the disclosure of information that a reasonable patient would feel was material to his or her decision of whether or not to accept the risks of treatment. As more clinical outcomes performance data become available, that data may play an increasingly important role in determining the content of disclosure. Risk administrators must be aware of and educate their physicians about the need to meet the legal standard of disclosure, particularly if their organizations are located in states with the "reasonable patient" standard. For example, a patient preparing to undergo heart bypass surgery at a hospital that is a high mortality outlier for this surgery might expect such information to be disclosed when the risks of surgery are discussed. In a recent essay, physicians Topol and Califf argue for more extensive disclosure to patients of institution- and physician-specific outcomes data. Using coronary artery bypass surgery as an example, they suggest the following:

In the future, an ideal approach would be to shift "full disclosure" to inform patients. On the consent forms that patients sign before the procedure, the cardiologist and cardiac surgeon could include their actual risk and success rates, when appropriate, for the past several years, the cumulative number of procedures the physician has done, and the site's overall rate of complications for the procedure. This up-front disclosure to patients would be revolutionary because it is rarely practiced today. . . . Without furnishing such data up front, we are not truly providing informed consent.[6]

Within the context of a patient's right to consent to or refuse treatment, an important question is whether care or treatment may be withheld or withdrawn from certain patients. The law in this area remains in a rather formative stage and varies from jurisdiction to jurisdiction. Generally speaking, care may be withheld if such care or treatment would only be futile or would only delay the certainty of death. Withdrawal of care that has already been initiated is more problematic. In the absence of death, reliance may be given to living wills and durable powers of attorney for health care that, under certain circumstances, allow for care to be withdrawn. One or the other of these two types of advance directives is recognized by most states. In addition, some states have enacted health care surrogacy acts, which permit individuals other than the patient (usually next-of-kin) in the absence of an advance directive to consent to or refuse medical care on behalf of a patient who lacks decisional capacity and who may be terminally ill, in a persistent vegetative state, or suffering from an incurable or irreversible condition that will ultimately cause death. These acts generally provide immunity from suit for health care providers who withdraw care from patients, but on the condition that they follow, in detail, the requirements set forth in the statutes. In the absence of the death of a patient and in the absence of an executed advance directive, withdrawal of care may still be permissible upon the order of a court of competent jurisdiction. Although resorting to courts may be costly, time-consuming, and may generate media exposure, recourse to a court of law in an area that has not been previously clarified in a particular jurisdiction will provide the greatest amount of protection to the hospital as well as to the patient, family members, and other health care providers.

Another developing area of medical-care-associated risk is maintenance of confidentiality. Examination of state law reveals an array of privacy protections, frequently with gaps and areas of uncertainty. Often paper records are presumed, so the status of electronic data is unclear. Consequently, a developing area of risk is the release of electronic patient-level data to government regulators, business coalitions, insurers, and quality monitoring projects. A health care organization's staff in marketing, information systems, and quality management may be insufficiently aware of confidentiality issues and therefore could release data with patient identifiers such as name, address, and social security number linked with personal information such as diagnoses and procedures. All staff should be educated about the importance of maintaining patient confidentiality and should ensure that any electronic patient information released from their organization without specific patient consent be stripped of externally recognizable unique patient identifiers and be allowable under state law. Concern about the inadequacy of many state laws in protecting against the improper release of patient-level electronic data has led to growing support in Congress for a federal law protecting patients' privacy.[7]

Health care institutions will be increasingly held accountable for the actions of providers on their staffs through the expansion of the corporate negligence theory, in which institutions have been held to have duties to properly maintain their facilities, to have available the necessary equipment, to hire, supervise, and retain competent and adequate provider staff, and to develop and implement policies and procedures that will promote quality care. More recently, many courts have enhanced the corporate responsibility of health care institutions through the use of agency theory and a more expansive concept of corporate negligence, incorporating the duty to protect patients from medical staff negligence through the assumption of more control over the quality of care rendered within its facility and the duty to properly credential medical staff members.[8] The federal Health Care Quality Improvement Act of 1986 extended the corporate responsibility of health care organizations by requiring them to make reports to and check with the National Practitioner Data Bank maintained by the Department of Health and Human Services. Failure to check the data bank may subject an organization to the burden of being constructively informed of (i.e., deemed to have knowledge of) the information it would have received had it done so, with this information being admissible in medical malpractice actions.

Finally, an important, developing source of medical liability risk lies in the area of utilization review and benefit determination by insurers. The line between insuring care and directing care is rapidly evaporating. Insurers have exerted leverage through a variety of maneuvers, from obtaining second opinions to outright denial of claims and even to threats of cancelling provider agreements. In the unseemly trade-off of discount prices for patient referrals, the best interests of patients are not always given sufficient consideration. It is likely that this will be an area of increasing controversy between patients and health care organizations. Although a recently decided case[9] in which a verdict was rendered against a managed care organization for $90 million may serve as a wake-up call to all insurers, hospitals and physicians have no immunity from being equally culpable if medical decisions are made on financial grounds. Risk administrators of managed care organizations should be vigilant for the presence of inappropriate financial incentives to limit benefit coverage and utilization of services.

RISK IDENTIFICATION
Importance of early risk identification

Risk of financial loss through legal liability presents itself to an organization in one of two ways. It can appear in the form of an individual patient event that, on inspection, carries with it a significant risk of liability. The actions that may result in liability in a specific case could be unique to that case or could be part of a general pattern of problem care or activity that can be referred to as risk exposure. Risk exposure can be identified in the absence of a specific risk case related to it, because a pattern of activity may be "risky" in terms of liability even though no specific patient injury related to that activity has yet occurred. The earliest recognition of both types of risk are crucial to a health care organization, and as such is a fundamental risk management activity.[10]

The benefit of early risk detection is that it enables risk administrators to conduct the earliest possible investigation of any identified risk cases and to intervene against risk exposure with prevention strategies before any, or at least further, risk cases develop. Successful risk management departments do not wait to be sued before undertaking an investigation of a case and establishing a defense or settlement posture. Within a two-year time period (the period for most statutes of limitations pertaining to medical malpractice), valuable testimony and evidence about a risk case may be lost. All health care organizations should have a set of methods in place to obtain the earliest possible notice or warning of a specific risk case or risk exposure. Quick recognition of a risk case can enable attorneys and risk managers to record the facts of the case when the events are fresh in the minds of the participants and to counsel members of the organization on how to respond to the event. A particular opportunity exists to ensure that the organization delivers subsequent care and administrative services in an expedited and satisfactory way to minimize any patient and family anger over the incident. With proper methods in place, a risk management program should have knowledge of most risk cases long before service of process is made. More sophisticated risk management programs should have notice of 75% or more of the incidents that eventually result in lawsuits filed against the organization.

Methods of risk identification

Most health care organizations employ a variety of means to identify risk cases and risk exposure. In reactive case identification, an organization assesses for risk in cases identified external to the organization as problematic. In proactive case identification, an organization initiates the identification of cases more likely than others to contain risk. Finally, in data-based performance monitoring, an organization moves beyond the individual case as the basis of risk identification and focuses on performance monitoring as the means to uncover risk exposure. Risk administrators should employ each of these three general approaches in their identification of risk cases and risk exposure. These approaches are complementary—risk detected by one may be entirely missed by the others. Risk management programs that rely on only one or two of the approaches run the great danger of failing to recognize all identifiable risk cases and areas of risk exposure. However, some methods within each approach are more likely than others to detect risk, so risk administrators with limited resources should select those methods that are most cost effective in their organizations. Once a case has been identified as a risk case, it is managed according to the principles discussed in the following sections on risk prioritization and risk control.

External case identification

Legal actions. The easiest and most instinctive approach to the identification of risk is the assessment of clinical events that come to an organization's attention in the ordinary conduct of its business. The clearest example of this is a lawsuit. Every organization is com-

pelled to assess and respond to legal actions against it. Such an assessment usually entails a careful examination of the specific circumstances of the clinical case, including a peer review of the medical record. By definition, a lawsuit establishes a case as a risk case because even if an organization feels that the likelihood of loss from liability is small, the cost of preparing for litigation and the cost of the litigation itself is a significant financial loss even without the finding of liability.

Medical record requests. The review of medical records requested by attorneys is another method through which risk can be identified. The fact that an attorney is requesting the records indicates that the case is involved in some legal activity, and some organizations routinely review all such cases. However, reviewing all attorney-requested records, however natural it may seem as a response, can be problematic. First, medical records may be requested for reasons other than suspicion of wrongdoing on the part of the providers or institution (e.g., disputes involving payment of claims or workers' compensation). In the absence of knowledge about the reason for the record request, detailed review of every requested record can be an unfocused activity that may produce a low yield of findings and, hence, may not be cost effective. At the same time, a cursory review of requested records may produce reliable identification of those cases deserving of more detailed review.

Patient complaints. Review of patient complaints is a good way to detect cases with risk and poor quality. Many organizations have a formalized mechanism for handling patient complaints. Often patient complaint descriptive statistics are routinely generated, such as a monthly compilation of all complaints by type, clinical/administrative area, and involved providers. A focused review of complaints that on their face suggest risk or poor quality can be a reasonably productive undertaking when attempting to discover problematic cases.

Billing disputes. Often the reason patients refuse to pay a bill is their belief that the care received was substandard and therefore not deserving of payment. As a result, like patient complaints, review of billing disputes is an excellent method of identifying risk and quality deficiencies. However, the cost effectiveness of reviewing billing disputes is compromised by the fact that some patients make accusations of poor quality simply to justify their refusal to pay for care. Even reviewing the records only from those billing disputes where there is an accusation of poor quality would result in the review of many cases where the accusation was knowingly unfounded. Detailed clinical review of all cases resulting in a billing dispute should probably be reserved for cases involving either large sums of money or significant accusations of substandard quality.

Internal case identification

Occurrence (incident) reporting. Rather than wait for a legal action, a record request, a patient complaint, or a billing dispute to initiate the process of risk identification, most organizations ask their staff to notify the risk management or legal department whenever an untoward or unusual incident occurs. This process is often referred to as *occurrence reporting.* Often a special form, commonly referred to as an *incident report form,* is provided for this purpose. This form indicates specific information that must be provided about the incident (see Appendix 20-7 for an example). Although the information contained in incident reports is commonly protected from legal discovery by state law, some institutions request that reports of patient harm from medical misdiagnoses, therapies, and procedures be reported verbally rather than in writing.

Incident reporting can be useful in identifying areas of risk exposure. Its usefulness as a method of identifying specific risk cases is limited, though, by a number of factors. The reliability of incident reporting can be compromised by the clinical staff's failure to appreciate a risk case or an area of risk exposure, uncertainty about what events to report, fear of getting involved, ignorance of how to file a report, and apathy. Risk administrators must recognize these barriers to reliable incident reporting and take active steps to eliminate them. Risk administrators should work hard to establish a trusting relationship with all physicians, who often see incident reporting as a nursing function and who are wary of admitting the occurrence of adverse clinical outcomes. Physicians should be continually reassured that their communications will be held in the strictest confidence, and that their statements will be protected from legal discovery. Physicians should be allowed to report incidents verbally, which should make it easier to report and somewhat alleviate their fear of reporting.

Progressive organizations actively cultivate a network of risk-sensitive and risk-educated clinical and administrative staff to facilitate incident reporting—a matrix of what can be called risk management "champions." This effort is especially directed at having risk management champions in important areas of patient care and patient interaction. The theory underlying this matrix approach to information gathering is that within an organizational infrastructure (departments, units, sections, and ancillary services), there are certain essential intersections through which potential plaintiffs are likely to pass. Important intersections include a hospital's surgical recovery room, emergency room, intensive care unit, and patient relations department. In addition, the utilization management department, given its expanding role both in hospitals and in managed care organizations and the detailed databases they use, can be one of the best and most reliable sources of information about potential risk cases. Furthermore, the clinical departments of radiology and, perhaps even more importantly, pathology often are recipients of crucial information that medical malfeasance has occurred. Progressive risk administrators aggressively solicit and maintain a network of risk management champions located in important areas of patient contact.

A refinement of incident reporting is *specified occurrence reporting.* With this method, risk administrators specify a set of events that must be reported by staff. This approach takes incident reporting a step further to educate the staff about what specific events should be reported. Staff are nonetheless still encouraged to report any unspecified event or possible area of risk exposure. Specified occurrences can be significant adverse outcomes of medical care (such as significant postoperative complications), accidents or mishaps in the provision of ancillary medical services (such as needlestick injuries), and non–medical care related accidents that occur in the institution (such as slip and fall injuries). Many of the specified occurrences are organization-specific based on the particular risk exposure history.

Random medical record review. Random medical record review was one of the first proactive approaches taken to uncover problem cases. It consisted of unfocused peer review of randomly selected medical records, and for a time was a widespread "quality assurance" activity. However, because of its low yield of positive findings, it has now fallen into complete disfavor as a method of case identification in quality management. It never found use in risk management because the less frequent occurrence of risk, compared to quality deficiency, made this method extremely cost ineffective for risk identification. Nevertheless, a program of random medical record review by providers can be beneficial in educating them to the wide variety of practice styles and approaches present among the staff, and over time may lead to a group consensus on the identification of relatively weak performers.

Occurrence screening. In an effort to avoid the potential unreliability of occurrence reporting, many risk administrators identify groups of cases for screening review without depending on reporting from the staff. This method is to identify groups of cases where the yield of detailed review is likely to be higher than with routine review of cases identified through incident reporting (or its variant of specified occurrence reporting). The criteria used to identify cases for review are event based (e.g., all emergency room deaths) and can be specified as the result of a known institutional area of concern about clinical quality or risk (e.g., all coronary care unit deaths from cardiac arrhythmias). The event that flags a case for review can on its face represent a quality problem (e.g., all medication errors), which may or may not create risk depending on the specific facts of the case, or can be nonspecific ("generic"). The latter events are generic in the sense that they are not particular to a certain type of case or a certain field of medical practice. Commonly used generic screening events, often called *generic indicators,* include unexpected in-hospital death, unplanned postoperative return to the operating room during the same admission, and unplanned postdischarge readmission to the hospital within a specified time period (such as 14 days). The occurrence of a "generic" event does not imply a quality deficiency or the presence of risk in that case. That is, the fact that a patient recently discharged from the hospital needed to be readmitted within 14 days of discharge does not imply a quality or risk problem. Each case identified by a generic occurrence indicator must be carefully reviewed to determine if any quality deficiency or risk is present.

Occurrence screening has found wider use in quality management than in risk management, where the approach to case evaluation is still based primarily on external case identification and occurrence reporting. Even in quality management, though, occurrence screening has met with mixed results as a method for uncovering quality deficiencies. The reason is that most cases that meet a criterion are not found by detailed peer review to have a quality deficiency, leading many to conclude that the expense involved in identifying the cases and then having them all reviewed by busy professionals is not justified by the relatively low yield of findings. The growing consensus is that most cases with quality problems and risk are not detected by the widely used generic screening criteria and that, of the cases that do meet screening criteria, most do not — after careful and time-consuming review — contain risk or a quality deficiency.

Case evaluation

Once a case has been identified as a possible risk case through one of the methods just discussed, the medical record is reviewed clinically. The case should first be reviewed by a physician who is an experienced reviewer of cases and who has an understanding of the potential sources of liability. This physician should recognize the need to be completely objective in assessing for quality of care deficiencies, a risk event, and risk exposure. This physician may have a formal administrative role in the organization, such as the medical director overseeing the quality management activity. If the care is squarely within the field of the experienced physician reviewer, that review may be the only one necessary, especially if the physician finds no arguable evidence of quality deficiency or risk. In any cases of doubt, the physician reviewer should refer the case to another physician for a second review. Risk administrators should realize that

complex cases often involve care in more than one clinical field. Therefore, it is imperative that all aspects of the patient's care be carefully reviewed. This may require a review by an internist or pediatrician (whether general or subspecialized) of surgical cases, because all surgical cases involve at least some "medical" care (but not vice versa).

Evaluation of clinical care by peer review usually includes determination of any culpability of the involved providers and institution. The results of case review can not only help to assess the risk in that specific case, but can also lead to the identification of organizational risk exposure or of substandard providers. Unfortunately, peer case review as a method of identification of risk and quality deficiency is compromised by the understandable reluctance of clinicians conducting the review to criticize the care of colleagues with whom they may practice and socialize. This reluctance is magnified by the frequent defensive posture of clinicians about clinical care in general, and the widespread fear that an adverse assessment will create interpersonal conflicts and be returned in kind when the roles of reviewer and reviewee are reversed in a future case. Moreover, clinicians often vary in the issues which they think are of paramount importance in a specific type of clinical case, which not infrequently results in multiple reviewers of the same case focusing on different events and different aspects of care.[11] These factors create a bias against the recognition of poor quality and risk. This bias may be less problematic in a provider's assessment of system deficiencies, as opposed to provider-related deficiencies, but still could be considerable. Risk administrators must recognize the potential for this bias in provider assessments of individual cases and take decided action to minimize it. Initial review by a trained reviewer and the use of multiple reviewers (especially if the case is surgical) can reduce the effects of this bias. Another way is the use of structured, explicit case review.

Most experienced risk administrators and clinical managers have had the experience of seeing two physicians come to dramatically opposite conclusions in their review of the same case record. Sometimes this discordance stems from a genuine disagreement over the proper clinical care for a specific problem. Not infrequently, however, in complex cases, two physicians (or other clinical providers) focus on entirely different sequences of care and come to different conclusions about the care in question. Informed only that a suit has been filed by the family of a patient who died unexpectedly in the hospital with postoperative sepsis, one reviewer may concentrate on postoperative wound care whereas another may direct most attention to the question of whether the proper prophylactic antibiotics were given.

A second problem with provider peer case review is that, even when providers agree on the specific care to examine, they may not agree on the appropriate standard of care against which to judge the actual care provided. Indeed, some reviewers have difficulty articulating a standard of care at all and may appear to regard all but the most egregious care as acceptable.

A third problem with peer review is that it is often not thorough. Most providers, especially physicians, feel overwhelmed by the time demands of clinical practice and are unwilling to devote much energy to ancillary responsibilities such as peer review. Moreover, physicians in particular are often hostile to the legal process and may have a tendency to diminish the legitimacy of clinical issues identified through it. At times, physicians charged with conducting a case review only cursorily review the record, skimming physician notes and ignoring nonphysician notes all together. (Nonphysician notes are often of crucial importance in understanding the care in a case.) Laboratory data, radiology reports, and pathology data may receive only brief attention.

Risk administrators can do a number of things to increase the usefulness and reliability of peer review. One is to cultivate a network of willing, fair, and thorough case reviewers on which to rely. Risk administrators should continually reinforce the need for thoroughness and fairness in the evaluation of care by peers. Risk administrators should foster the development of this group with informal training and should demonstrate appreciation for the reviewers' efforts.

Another approach is to adopt a structured, explicit method of case review. Structured, explicit case review is designed to reduce the unreliability of case review through explicit identification of questionably problematic sequences of related care and the corresponding standards of care. Case review begins with a "foundation" review by an experienced case reviewer, preferably with a background in quality and risk management, who identifies the major processes of care and any issues associated with them. For each issue identified, a written form is prepared that asks subsequent reviewers to, in writing, explicitly state the standard of care of each sequence of related care in which an issue has been spotted and to assess the care against that standard. Reviewers can be asked to reference applicable published or organizational practice guidelines. Reviewers are given space to identify and comment on issues not identified during the foundation review.

A final technique is to ask more than one reviewer to perform a structured, explicit review. As stated earlier, it is often useful to have reviewers of different specialties assess a case, particularly if it is surgical.

Routine structured, explicit peer review of all cases identified as possible risk cases is too costly and is unnecessary. Although they are an important and indispensable source of information, most cases identified either internally or externally, with the exception of lawsuits, ultimately are not found to contain either risk or a quality deficiency. Therefore, all identified cases should be screened first by an experienced reviewer who can create a structured, explicit case review form if necessary. Structured, explicit case review should be reserved for those cases that appear on initial screening review to have resulted in a serious adverse outcome and a measurable risk of liability.

Strengths and limitations of case identification methods

Although all case identification methods can reveal cases with a risk of loss, some are more useful than others in identifying cases with probable losses. For example, informal studies by hospitals indicate that incident reports are generally poor predictors of lawsuits, perhaps not surprising given the large number that are filed in organizations with aggressive risk management programs. Incident reports remain, however, useful sources of information that can reveal potential risk cases and areas of risk exposure. On the other hand, requests by attorneys for medical records, patient complaints, and billing disputes are factors associated with a higher probability that a lawsuit will follow.

However, keep in mind that case-by-case evaluation does not provide the entire picture of organization-wide clinical risk exposure and quality of care. It paints a picture only of those cases that were identified—not a complete sample of all cases with risk, risk exposure, and quality problems. In particular, cases that result in a patient complaint are a biased sample of patients from which to make inferences about overall organizational clinical risk, because not all patients are equally likely to register a complaint given the same care. Inferences about the general state of clinical risk exposure and quality of care should not be made from a review of cases flagged through external identification methods and by occurrence reporting.

Despite their various strengths and limitations, all of the mentioned methods for case identification should be utilized by a health care organization. Since none is perfect, a case missed by one method may be detected by another. The use of a wide variety of case-specific risk identification methods can be enhanced, but not replaced, as a method of identifying risk exposure by data-based performance monitoring.

Data-based performance monitoring

Data-based performance monitoring is a method of assessing organizational quality of care and risk exposure that is relatively recent and is growing rapidly in importance. It is a method for identifying areas of quality deficiency and risk exposure, as opposed to specific risk cases. Its premise is that an indispensable way to assess organization-wide clinical risk exposure and quality of care is to monitor everyday activity, which has the benefit of avoiding the reporting bias encountered with many of the already discussed methods of risk identification. Data derived from continuous monitoring is used either to identify quality deficiencies and risk exposure or to monitor an organization's response to corrective action taken to remedy previously identified quality and risk problems.

The initial purpose of data-based performance monitoring was the assessment of quality of care. Interinstitutional publicly released data-based assessment of clinical performance began in earnest with the Health Care Financing Administration's report on hospital mortality in the care of selected Medicare patients. Subsequently, many projects have begun ongoing public reporting of comparative hospital performance. Some are done by state agencies (e.g., the Pennsylvania and New York reporting on hospital coronary artery bypass surgery outcomes, and the California reporting on hospital outcomes of acute myocardial infarction and diskectomy) and some are done by voluntary coalitions (e.g., the periodic public reporting of a wide variety of medical, surgical, and obstetrical outcomes for more than 30 hospitals in the Cleveland area by the Cleveland Health Quality Choice Program). Private comparative data are also available (e.g., through the Maryland Hospital Association's Quality Indicator Project). A primary goal of these programs is to stimulate internal quality improvement through comparative performance assessments. Many organizations also gather clinical outcomes data internally and compare their results to published benchmarks or to information obtained from outside databases.

Risk administrators should be aware of all comparative performance data available on their organizations. Proper interpretation of comparative performance data requires a working familiarity with the strengths and limitations of clinical outcomes monitoring.[12] Heretofore, analysis of clinical outcomes data has been the province of clinical quality management staff, in no small part because of its substantial clinical and statistical content. However, comparative clinical outcomes data should be of great interest to risk administrators because they may point out areas of substandard hospital performance and, consequently, of risk exposure. Hospitals with high adverse outcome rates (e.g., mortality) in specific areas of care should aggressively analyze their processes of care in an effort to reduce the rate of adverse outcomes to the lowest achievable levels. The presence of high adverse outcomes in specific clinical areas may flag the presence of unusually high risk exposure in those areas. Although performance data aggregated over hundreds and thousands of cases do not give information about a specific case, a pattern of persistently high risk-adjusted adverse outcomes in a specific clinical area may signal a deficiency in the quality of care, which may have already and could in the future lead to liability in specific cases. For example, a hospital with a high surgical mortality rate, after adjustment for the severity of illness of its patients before surgery, may have clinical problems that result in greater risk exposure than hospitals with low rates. Comparative performance data afford risk administrators an excellent means of risk identification.

Performance data have a second important use. They are indispensable as a tool used inside an organization to continually assess its success in eliminating areas of known risk exposure. This process entails the design and continual measurement of risk indicators and is discussed later in the section on risk prevention.

RISK PRIORITIZATION

Risk administrators must prioritize identified risks in order to expend organizational resources in the most cost-effective way. Organizations usually have limited resources of personnel time and attention. Most risk administrators concentrate risk prevention efforts on events that are infrequent but of great consequence, on the one hand, and to events that are of lesser import but of frequent occurrence.

A rare event of relatively minor consequence can often be handled directly without assembling a quality improvement team. Sometimes the source of risk exposure is suggested by a pattern of events or by data, and the challenge is first to discover the source of the problem. At times the cause of risk exposure is obvious, such as an HMO's failure to have all routine screening mammogram reports reviewed by a physician or nurse, and so preventive efforts can be focused immediately on faulty clinical or operational processes. The intensity of administrative risk prevention efforts should be tailored to the complexity of each individual risk. Clinical problems will usually require a multidisciplinary team, including physicians, with familiarity in all involved clinical and operational areas.

Risk prioritization is important in both assessing the proper response to a recognized risk case (risk control) and in allocating resources for risk prevention. For example, medication errors frequently occur in hospitals. These errors generally include delays in providing patients with prescribed doses of medicine. Identification of such delays are most frequently accomplished through incident reports, but may also be identified through occurrence screening, random medical record review, or patient complaints. The total number of medication delays may then be divided between those delays that actually injured patients and those that had the potential to injure patients. Obviously, risk management personnel must give immediate attention to an error that has resulted in an injury to a patient. In determining the proper response to a medication delay, risk administrators would seek to answer the following questions: Did the error result in an injury to the patient? How significant was the injury? Was the injury of a temporary nature or of a more permanent nature? Has it compromised the care of the patient? Will the adverse effect on the patient extend beyond the current hospitalization? What was the reason for the delay? Was the delay the result of an individual error or a larger institutional problem? Is this an error that has occurred before? On a particular unit? During a specific shift? Caused by a specific health care provider?

The differences between iatrogenic and custodial injuries serve as an illustration of the kind of considerations important in risk prioritization. The distinction between iatrogenic and custodial injuries is relevant when one assesses these two types of injuries in terms of frequency and severity, the two major considerations in prioritizing the organization's response to specific risks. Frequency refers to how often the type of injury occurs and severity refers to how likely that type of injury will result in financial loss. Custodial injuries are estimated to comprise as much as 75% to 85% of all patient injuries in hospitals and ambulatory care areas. However, measured in terms of financial loss, custodial injuries account for less than 25% of aggregate losses. Iatrogenic injuries, on the other hand, while less frequent than custodial injuries, account for approximately 75% to 85% of hospital losses.[13] The lesson to be learned from the distribution of risk between iatrogenic and custodial injuries is not that a concentrated effort should be directed only toward the prevention or management of iatrogenic claims; hospital risk management programs must obviously address both types of injuries. The lesson, rather, is that their relative risks must be carefully evaluated to achieve a balanced approach in preventing and managing both types of injuries.

Identification of major risks

What risks should be considered major risks? For most organizations, a list of major risks can be found in their reporting requirements under excess liability policies. For hospitals, such mandatory reporting is typically required in the event of the following injuries to a patient: unexpected death; brain damage; neurological deficit, nerve damage, or paralysis; loss of limbs; or failure to diagnose a condition that results in a continuous course of treatment. In addition to the aforementioned, a catch-all provision is often included that requires reporting of any claim or medical incident the value of which is equivalent to a certain percentage (e.g., 50%) of the self-insured retention limits. This list is not exhaustive, but if a hospital risk management program is constrained because of financial or staffing limitations, it can serve as a priority list that fulfills most needs.

Key specific risks

Risk management programs of large health care organizations may find it necessary to utilize a more detailed list of key specific risks. Such a list may be compiled based on the individual experience of that organization. Using a hospital as an example, a typical list includes the following major headings: medication errors, patient falls, equipment related, security related, blood related, surgery related, anesthesia related, food related, patient induced, policy related, radiology related, medical record related, laboratory related, intravenous line related, newborn related, maternal related, and physician related. Box 20–1 contains a representative sample of subcategories for each of the aforementioned key specific risks. The categorization of risks associated with a specific hospital will, of course, vary depending on the risk experience of that hospital.

RISK CONTROL

Risk control is the process of managing a recognized risk case to minimize the potential for loss. Most risk administrators find their time primarily directed toward risk control, rather than risk prevention, for an obvious reason. A lawsuit represents an actual loss. Even if successfully defended, a lawsuit will result in expenditures for its defense, primarily in terms of fees for legal counsel and expert witnesses. Tangentially, there may also be an increase in insurance premiums or an increase in the organization's deductible. Consequently, risk administrators find a greater part of their time allocated to risk control than to risk prevention.

Completing the initial investigation

Upon identification of a risk case, an initial investigation is undertaken. This investigation has two purposes: the early assessment of probability and value of loss and the identification of relevant sources of information. The essential steps necessary to complete these objectives are (1) review of the medical record; (2) interview of the potential defendants for whom the organization provides insurance coverage; (3) identification, cataloging, and collection of physical evidence that may be relevant and could otherwise be lost or misplaced (e.g., monitor tracings, temporary logs, and policy and procedures); (4) identification of witnesses who may have information concerning the incident and

BOX 20–1
OPERATIONAL SUBCATEGORIES OF KEY HOSPITAL RISKS

Medication Errors
- Adverse reaction
- Wrong route
- Wrong patient
- Pharmacy error
- Medication not given
- Wrong medication given
- Medication duplicated
- Medication not ordered
- Medication not given at correct time
- Transcription error
- Medication given despite hold order
- Wrong dosage

Patient Falls
- Caused by a liquid or substance on floor
- Fall from bed (siderails up? siderails down? position of siderails unknown?)
- Fall in bathroom
- Fall in room
- Fall outside of room
- Fall off table or equipment
- Fall in elevator
- Fall from crutches or walker
- Fall outside of building
- Fall from chair or wheelchair
- Near fall with assistance

Equipment Related
- Failure of life support or monitor
- Equipment missing or unavailable
- Injury related to medical device

Security Related
- Personal property damage
- Personal property disappeared
- Injury resulting from conduct of another patient

Blood Related
- Wrong blood
- Transfusion reaction
- Delay in transfusion

Surgery Related
- Incorrect needle count
- Incorrect sponge count
- Incorrect surgical instrument count
- Surgical instrument broken
- Loss of pathology specimen
- Unplanned return to surgery
- Removal of retained foreign body
- Unplanned return after readmission

Anesthesia Related
- Respiratory distress reaction
- Related to intubation or related to extubation

Food Related
- Poisoning
- Foreign body
- Improper diet
- NPO order violated
- Burns from foods or liquids

Patient Induced
- Attempted suicide
- Self-mutilation
- Refusal to consent to treatment
- Returned late from approved pass
- Discharge against medical advice
- In possession of drugs, alcohol, or weapon

Policy Related
- Procedural error
- Violation of physician order
- Performance of wrong procedure
- Autopsy signed with no autopsy

Laboratory Related
- Transport delay
- Identification problem
- Loss or damage to laboratory specimen
- Incorrect reading

Intravenous Line Related
- Infiltration
- Wrong solution
- Contaminated or expired solution
- Line disconnected
- Incorrect timing
- Pump malfunction
- Incorrect rate
- Central line complication

Newborn Related
- Apgar scores of less than 3 at 1 minute
- Apgar scores of less than 7 at 7 minutes
- Skull fracture
- Resuscitation
- Transfer from in-house nursery to special care nursery
- Meconium aspiration

Maternal Related
- Maternal injury from obstetrical treatment
- Blood loss

Physician Related
- Failure to diagnose
- Unexpected death
- Brain damage resulting from treatment
- Neurological deficit or nerve injury resulting from treatment
- Injury relating to resident supervision
- Adverse reaction
- Delay in response

Radiology Related
- Reaction to contrast dye
- Unmonitored cardiac or respiratory arrest
- Disappearance of films

Medical Records
- Orders not charted
- Consent not signed
- Disappearance of record

who, because of time constraints, might have to be interviewed at a later time; and (5) collection of medical bills. This five-step initial investigation is not intended to serve as an extensive investigation or to replace the more thorough investigation conducted upon service of process. It is only a preliminary action to determine the essential facts of the case and to identify which personnel have personal information about the incident.

With this information in hand, risk managers and attorneys select and prioritize those incidents that warrant further investigation. This process fulfills the essential risk control functions of gathering and assessing information about potential losses and prioritizing time and efforts toward investigation of probable losses.

Predicting the potential plaintiff

An important part of identifying those risk cases likely to result in loss is to predict which patients will bring a lawsuit. As varied as plaintiffs may be, many of them share certain common characteristics. The following are traits of patients who, in the authors' experience, are most likely to sue a health care organization.

Poor or unexpected results. The most reliable identifying characteristic of the potential plaintiff is that he or she has suffered an unsatisfactory outcome as a result of or despite medical care. The outcome may be direct harm (e.g., a postsurgical complication) or a result that, although not harmful per se, is less than that expected after the care (e.g., unsatisfactory outcome of plastic surgery). A poor or unexpected result from medical care does not mean, of course, that any medical malfeasance has occurred.

Seriousness of injury. Another characteristic of the potential plaintiff is that the injury sustained is permanent and serious, involving death, disability, or disfigurement. Disability may be manifested in various ways; at a minimum, it usually must be sufficient to have resulted in lost wages. The economics of pursuing a legal claim and the impact of medical malpractice reforms have served to impose a modicum of self-regulation and limitation on medical malpractice claims, reducing claims for minor injury and claims that might be called "frivolous."

Weak doctor-patient relationship. A third trait of the potential plaintiff is the absence of a strong relationship with his or her physician. The single greatest deterrent to litigation remains a strong physician-patient relationship rich with positive interactions and communication. A recent study analyzing the demographics and risk of malpractice concludes that the risk of a suit is affected by a physician's gender, specialty, and age. Of note, male physicians were three times as likely to be in a high claims group as female physicians. The investigators surmised that female physicians may in-teract more effectively with patients than their male colleagues.[14]

Uncertain financial future. Many plaintiffs are individuals who face an uncertain financial future. They are often unable to withstand the financial burden of medical expenses attendant with a poor or unexpected result. Therefore, potential plaintiffs are frequently found to be unemployed, underemployed, recently retired, single or recently divorced, or students.

Strong support group. The last trait frequently found among potential plaintiffs is the presence of a strong support group, especially if there are family members who are directly or indirectly associated with medicine or law. As socially acceptable as litigation may be in the United States, persevering through the process of selecting an attorney and initiating legal action still requires a certain degree of motivation and strength, which can be buttressed by supportive family and friends.

In preparing themselves to initiate a lawsuit, potential plaintiffs commonly use similar phrases, with which most risk managers quickly become familiar. Many potential plaintiffs, instead of making a direct threat to sue, often use expressions such as "I want to make sure that this never happens to another patient," "I want to teach you a lesson," and "I am not interested in the money, it's the principle."

Conducting investigations

In conducting investigations, risk administrators need to be aware of legally imposed limits and restrictions. For example, some courts have ruled that risk administrators may not interview subsequent treaters of an injured patient. This theory has been extended by some courts to even prohibit discussions with members of a hospital's house staff and nursing staff. The rationale given is that such *ex parte* discussions violate the sanctity of the physician-patient relationship and are prohibited under physician-patient privilege statutes.[15] A second rationale offered is that a physician has a fiduciary duty to refrain from assisting his or her patient's adversary.

While the aforementioned rationales may be persuasive regarding subsequent providers who care for the patient and who are not employed by the health care organization, application of such a rule that bars an organization from interviewing employees creates a number of practical problems. Such restriction would prevent the organization from being able to respond to a complaint, to develop litigation strategy, to provide accurate or complete responses to discovery requests, to prepare employees adequately for depositions or trial, to depose experts adequately, and to prepare the best presentation at trial.

Of equal concern to an attorney is the protection of investigative reports and interviews from disclosure.

There are two avenues by which such protection may be assured. A recognized principle is that such information constitutes "work product." The work product principle protects a lawyer's representation of his or her client's interest and requires that good cause be shown before a court will allow discovery of a lawyer's preparation of the client's case. Generally, work product includes information prepared by an attorney or his or her representative (e.g., a risk manager) in anticipation of litigation. Such information includes personal knowledge and legal theories along with statements of witnesses. This principle, though, does not necessarily protect information about the location of such information and the names and addresses of witnesses. In applying this principle in the protection of reports and interviews made by attorneys and risk managers, care should be taken to follow the general rules of the work product principle. Disclosure of such information to a third party may result in loss of ability to assert the principle to defeat discovery requests by the other party. If information is gathered by nonattorney risk administrators, the information needs to be forwarded to the attorney, sometimes with the inclusion of a statement that it is being sent to assist the attorney in contemplated litigation.

A second means of protecting such information from discovery by the other party may be available under state statutes that prohibit disclosure of information used internally to improve patient care or to reduce morbidity and mortality. Precise adherence to the rules set forth in a statute usually is critical to protect the information from disclosure. Some statutes may only address hospitals, not having been updated to incorporate HMOs. Generally, information is protected when utilized and discussed within recognized health care organization committees for quality improvement purposes.

Notifying insurance carriers

Risk administrators have the responsibility to properly notify an insurance carrier of a claim or possible claim that exposes its coverage. Reference to the exact wording of the insurance policy will, of course, be critical as to the necessary timing and scope of notification. Generally, the phrasing of the notice requirement is in one of two ways: a policy may require that the insured give the carrier "immediate notice of a lawsuit" or may require notice "when it appears that an occurrence is likely to involve indemnity" under the policy. The second type of notice language can be particularly problematic for a health care organization because it is vulnerable to a subjective interpretation as to when an occurrence is "likely" to involve indemnity. The phrase may be interpreted from both an objective and subjective standard. The controlling rule in insurance law is that if the language of an insurance policy is ambiguous or

otherwise susceptible to more than one reasonable interpretation, it is to be construed in favor of the insured. Notwithstanding this rule, insureds may wish to be cautious and provide notification at the earliest possible moment that it appears a carrier's insurance policy may be exposed.

Selecting defense counsel

The skills expected of a litigator are likely to be different from those of a corporate attorney. Of course, one looks for competency, truthfulness, honesty, and responsiveness in both, as well as the ability to communicate effectively with the client. On the other hand, one might expect a certain aggressiveness in a litigator that might be inappropriate in a corporate attorney. Undoubtedly, one of the greatest assets of a litigator is that he or she possesses the capabilities to take a case to trial, advocate the position of the defendant(s), and, of course, obtain a favorable verdict.

As with the selection of any other consultants, in selecting defense counsel a health care organization would do well to keep in mind the following:
1. Selection should not be made solely on the basis of price.
2. Expectations should be made clear to the defense counsel from the outset.
3. A new defense counsel, regardless of his or her reputation, should always be started on a small project or a single case to make sure a positive working relationship results.
4. The defense counsel should be allowed reasonable professional latitude to do his or her best job, although giving defense counsel freedom of action does not eliminate the organization's responsibility to monitor defense counsel's progress.
5. The results achieved by defense counsel should be fairly evaluated, as both the organization and defense counsel deserve honest feedback from each other.

Assisting defense counsel

A medical malpractice action may be costly to an organization, but it can be extraordinarily disturbing to a health care provider named as a defendant. Generally speaking, physicians and nurses are unaccustomed to the confrontation and adversity that characterize the litigation process. They may be frightened and intimidated by the procedures that, to them, may appear to be geared more toward proving them culpable than to determining what actually happened.

In the discovery or fact-finding stage of the litigation proceeding, risk administrators have a dual role. Both roles serve to reduce the cost of use of outside litigation counsel and the possibility of loss to an adverse verdict or disadvantageous settlement. Risk administrators should assist outside defense counsel in discovery. This task will be made easier depending on the thoroughness with which the initial investigation was conducted. Equally important, risk administrators should help guide the defendant through the litigation process.

Clarification of expectations. The first step in assisting legal counsel is to express the expectations of the organization's risk administrators about how defense counsel will handle the claim. Expectations are best clarified in advance and with a single attorney charged with managing the case. It is important that direction be given to defense counsel in the following five areas: assignment of file, initial review, conduct of discovery, conduct of trial, and arrangement for billing.

If the relationship involves multiple claims, the defense firm and risk administrator should mutually designate an attorney who will have overall responsibility for supervising the various cases referred to that firm. If, because of a conflict or other reason, the defense firm to which a case has been sent is unable to represent the organization, this fact should be communicated immediately to the organization by telephone and the file should be returned promptly. Some organizations defer to the supervising attorney at the defense firm as to the assignment to a particular lawyer. Conversely, some risk administrators prefer matching particular cases to the skills, styles, or personalities of particular lawyers and will retain the right to make the selection. An assignment letter should include the name of the risk administrator covering the file. If a defense attorney other than the one selected to handle the case works on the case, the fact should be communicated to the organization.

As soon as possible after a claim is assigned to a defense firm, an acknowledgment from the primary defense attorney should be received with his or her assessment of the case. This review should include a summary of the pertinent facts revealed to date, a review of medical records, a recitation of the issues presented in the complaint, areas that will require additional research and investigation, and, if there is sufficient information available, a statement of opinion as to liability, verdict potential, and settlement value.

Any motions filed on behalf of the organization should be limited to meaningful issues and receive prior approval from the risk administrator. Any requests by the defense attorney to interview employees of the organization or to retain outside experts should also receive prior approval from the risk administrator. The risk administrator should obtain a status report from the defense attorney no less frequently than twice a year.

Defense attorney requests for approval of travel expenditures should be made in writing and should include the purpose of the trip, the travel destination, the time period required to complete the work, the exact means of travel and the cost, the specific identification, location, and cost of lodgings, and the cost of car rental, if required. In any event, reimbursement should always be supported by receipts. The billing cycle should also be clearly understood and the hourly fees of all defense attorneys working on the case should be provided in writing. Changes in those fees should not be made without the approval of the risk administrator. To enable evaluation of the charge, the bill should provide details of the legal services rendered, including (1) the date of service, (2) a clear description of the service rendered, (3) the actual time expended, and (4) the identity of the lawyer who rendered the service. Charges for review of files should be kept at a minimum and interoffice conferences between attorneys of the defense firm should be discouraged or prohibited. Finally, the defense firm should be informed of which legal expenses will not be reimbursed. Such items might include interoffice conferences, time spent filing papers with the court, secretarial time, copying charges, and unsupported charges for travel.

Distribution of responsibilities. The manner in which the risk administrator and the primary defense attorney share responsibilities during discovery should be clear to both. The risk administrator should help compile answers to interrogatories, if not be entirely responsible for their completion. It is cost effective for risk administrators to undertake as much of this task as possible. Similarly, risk administrators should be responsible for the production of documents such as medical records, billing statements, policy and procedure manuals, incident reports, photographs, laboratory reports, logs, scheduling reports, and other physical evidence.

In most risk management programs, risk administrators automatically assume primary responsibility for drafting answers and production of documents. However, they are probably not as involved as they should be in preparing witnesses for depositions. This task is too often left to defense counsel. As with drafting answers to interrogatories and production of documents, witness preparation should also be a shared responsibility between defense counsel and the risk administrator.

A common complaint of deponents is that they have not been adequately prepared. Unfortunately, at times defense counsel may not have or may not take the time to prepare each witness adequately. To avoid this situation, risk administrators should be trained and ready to prepare witnesses. The two important aspects of this preparation are to provide the general rules of demeanor and conduct of a witness in a deposition, and to review, in detail, the care and treatment rendered by

---

BOX 20–2
TEN RULES FOR THE DOCTOR'S DEPOSITION

From Leaman and Saxton[16]

1. *Know the records intimately*—office records, hospital charts, any statements by other health care professionals, medical literature, and alternative treatments.
2. *The doctor must listen to the question carefully* and respond only when he or she understands it completely. If the doctor does not understand it, then the attorney must be asked to rephrase it. Never help to rephrase it or suggest a more appropriate question.
3. *The doctor should respond thoroughly, but directly and to the point,* and not tell stories, ramble, digress, or volunteer information. On certain topics one may need to be more comprehensive if appropriate to the theme of the defense.
4. *The doctor should use the medical record.* If the record is in order, it can be the best defense tool. For example, the plaintiff's attorney may describe the client's level of pain and suffering. If the doctor's records do not confirm this, the chart can be used to demonstrate it.
5. *The theatrics of the plaintiff's attorney should be disregarded.* Sometimes the attorney will act surprised and shocked by a response, use body language, or repeat certain phrases in an attempt to irritate the defendant. Such theatrics are intended to make the doctor uncomfortable and unsure of the response.
   At times the plaintiff and defense attorneys may resort to arguing with each other. It is important for the doctor not to misinterpret the defense attorney's anger to mean that something has gone wrong or that there is a problem with the responses. Such battles may be a technique for the defense attorney to maintain control of the deposition. If such tactics are to be used, they should be discussed with the doctor prior to the deposition. Their use should also be minimal; professional courtesy is an important part of legal ethics.
6. *The doctor should be consistent.* If the doctor does not give the desired response to a question from the plaintiff's attorney, the attorney may ask the question over and over, each time phrasing it a bit differently, looking for an inconsistent response. The doctor should remember that the plaintiff's attorney has been working on these questions for weeks before the deposition. The doctor's failure to give the anticipated response can be devastating; the attorney will work hard to get the needed response or at least neutralize the damage from an unfavorable, unanticipated response.
7. *The doctor should wait for the next question* after finishing a response. Often the plaintiff's attorney will pause, using body language to urge the doctor to say more. The doctor should not try to fill the void, but should simply wait patiently for the next question.
8. *The doctor should be extremely cautious in responding to leading questions,* such as "Is it a fair statement. . ."; "Let me summarize your testimony as follows. . ."; "Doctor, just so I understand what you are saying . . ." Statements like these mean the plaintiff's attorney is about to reinterpret the doctor's testimony. Usually there is a slight twist to that interpretation, which the attorney is hoping to have affirmed. The doctor should remember that fairness has nothing to do with this process; the interpretation may not correctly reflect what was said. The doctor should agree *only* with those statements with which he or she is comfortable. If the doctor disagrees, then he or she must simply say so, and repeat the previous response.
9. *The doctor should be careful of conversation during breaks.* Although inappropriate, the plaintiff's attorney may try to engage the doctor in conversation. This could have an impact on the case. A deposition is not the time for social niceties. Breaks should be used to relax and regain composure. One must be on guard from arrival at the deposition until departure.
10. *The doctor should be courteous, professional, firm, and credible.* Demeanor should be professional and serious, for a doctor's professional ability has been challenged. As such, a deposition is neither the time nor the place for chitchat and humor. However, under no circumstances should a doctor be offensive, insulting, or argumentative.

---

the deponent, relying in particular on office or hospital records.

Some organizations have shown prospective deponents video tapes of staged depositions. Such tapes are commercially available. In addition, various articles and monographs have been written on the subject. In their excellent book, *Preventing Malpractice: The Co-Active Solution,*[16] Dr. Thomas Leaman and attorney James Saxton provide 10 rules for deposition preparation (see Box 20–2). Although the rules are directed to physicians, they are equally applicable to other health care providers or, for that matter, to any person who is required to give a deposition.

RISK PREVENTION

Effective risk prevention depends on the reliable recognition of risk exposure, the determination of its causes, the implementation of corrective action, and the continual monitoring of risk indicators to determine if risk exposure resolves. This process requires the close and active cooperation of risk administrators and clinical managers.

The following hypothetical scenario illustrates the process of assessment, correction, and prevention of risk exposure identified through the analysis of comparative performance data. Community Memorial Hospital (CMH) is in a state that issues annual public reports on comparative hospital clinical outcomes of care for a variety of conditions. The latest report demonstrated that CMH's comparative risk-adjusted mortality rate for patients admitted with acute cardiac conditions, primarily acute myocardial infarction (AMI) and congestive heart failure (CHF), was statistically significantly higher than expected compared to average care in all state hospitals. A review by CMH of its mortality data from recent years for acute cardiac patients revealed a gradual upward trend of risk-adjusted mortality rates that were higher than expected, but that the CMH rate had never before been a statistically significant high mortality outlier. CMH had not reacted to this upward trend; in fact, it was hardly known among the risk administrators and clinical managers.

A group of CMH clinical managers, quality management staff, and risk administrators formed a multidisciplinary "quality improvement" team to review the report and investigate CMH acute cardiac care. Quality management staff reviewed the report and the CMH data on which it was based, but failed to reveal any basis for challenging the results. Risk administrators then reviewed their records and found that in the past three years the hospital had two lawsuits filed against it involving relatively young patients who experienced sudden death due to cardiac arrhythmias after admission to the coronary care unit (CCU) with what appeared to be stable, mild acute myocardial infarctions. Three cardiologists, aware of the new mortality data, reviewed the care in those cases and concluded that in both cases the care was exemplary and conformed to all clinical standards. These three cardiologists were all members of the CCU quality assurance committee, which routinely reviewed the records from a randomly selected number of CCU deaths each month. A check of CCU quality assurance records during the past 2 years revealed that CCU arrhythmia care was never identified as a problem area. The risk administrators then reported that their informal communication with risk administrators of other hospitals in the city about their experiences with cardiac patients revealed that all other hospitals had at most one similar type of suit. The risk administrators had not noticed any relationship between the two suits, which were filed 18 months apart.

The team then reviewed the pattern of deaths in acute cardiac care patients. It noted that sudden fatal arrhythmias were a relatively frequent cause of death in cardiac patients. After careful deliberation, physicians on the team offered that the percentage might be a bit higher than expected given the clinical condition of the patients in the cases that were reviewed, but stated that they certainly had not noticed such a pattern in their daily practice and that they felt the care of acute cardiac patients to be excellent. Nevertheless, the team embarked on a review of the care of all acute cardiac patients in the last year, concentrating on care that preceded the appearance of potentially life threatening arrhythmias.

After a careful study, the team identified, a bit to its surprise, three potential deficiencies in the care of sudden life-threatening arrhythmias that appeared in acute cardiac patients. One possible problem was an occasional minute or so delay in the recognition of potentially life-threatening arrhythmias by CCU nurses. After review, this problem was determined to be mostly due to inadequate staffing. At times of relatively low staffing, the demands of direct patient care occasionally pulled all nurses away from the monitoring station where each patient's cardiac rhythm was continuously displayed. A second area of concern was discovered with the physicians' care of patients with escalating mild nonlife-threatening arrhythmias. Some physicians were found to be relatively slow in ordering antiarrhythmics in these patients, and a few were still using a drug that, although still accepted as appropriate therapy in these patients, had been abandoned by most physicians in the last 2 years for a newer one that was felt to be slightly more effective. A third possible problem was found with the monitoring equipment. A disproportionately greater number of patients who experienced delayed recognition of acute cardiac arrhythmias were in the few beds that still had an older model of cardiac monitor, whose automatic arrhythmia recognition alarm system was not as advanced as the one in a newer type of monitor used in all of the other CCU beds. The new monitors were purchased one by one in the past three years as the older models wore out. The CCU staff had not thought that the difference in the monitors was significant, and so did not push for the immediate replacement of all of the older models with newer ones.

The risk administrator noted that one of the lawsuits involved a patient treated with the older drug, and the other involved a patient who died during the typically busiest time of the day (during the afternoon change of shift) while on one of the older monitors. Neither of these deaths was thought by the clinical staff at the time to represent a risk case and so neither was reported to the risk administrators. There was no specified occurrence reporting or screening in place for CCU arrhythmia deaths.

The team decided that antiarrhythmic drug use, nurse

staffing levels, nurse attention to monitored rhythms, and type of monitor were process of care issues that needed to be examined. Upon identification of these process elements, but before designing a corrective action plan, the team then developed four indicators to monitor the process of care in acute cardiac patients, and they also decided to review indicator data monthly. The first indicator was the percentage of acute cardiac patients in the CCU who died from a cardiac arrhythmia. This outcome indicator would indicate whether any improvement in the overall results of CCU arrhythmia care occurred after corrective action and, if it did, whether it was sustained over time. The nurse administrator of the CCU recorded the number of CCU patients and whether any died from an acute cardiac arrhythmia, and submitted the data to the quality management department every week. The second indicator was the percent of CCU patients begun on antiarrhythmic therapy who were treated with the older drug. The pharmacy department collected the data and submitted it to the quality management department every month. The third indicator was the ratio of CCU nurses to patients for each shift. Data for this indicator were collected by the CCU nurse administrator and submitted to the quality management department every week. The fourth indicator was the percentage of time that a nurse was physically sitting at the CCU cardiac rhythm monitoring station actively observing patients' cardiac rhythms. Data for this indicator were acquired through unannounced random inspections of the CCU by senior nursing administration staff unconnected to the running of the CCU. These inspections occurred at least once per 24 hours. Data were collected by the nursing administration and submitted to the quality management department each week.

The quality improvement team established expectations for each indicator. The CCU death rate from acute cardiac arrhythmias in acute cardiac patients was anticipated to be at the level expected for the severity of illness for their patients based on the state-wide comparative outcomes monitoring. The use of the older antiarrhythmic drug was expected to fall by 20% per month until its use was eliminated. An expected nurse-to-patient ratio was established, and the expectation was set that a nurse would always be present at the CCU cardiac rhythm monitoring station and be dedicated to observation of cardiac rhythms. The quality management department was charged with collecting the data for each indicator, reviewing each indicator every month to determine whether the performance expectation for the indicator was met, and to reconvene the quality improvement team for repeat investigation and additional corrective action for any indicator that fell below the expected level. The quality management department displayed the data on each indicator graphically, updated each graph with the latest monthly data, and distributed the graphs to all members of the quality improvement team, CCU nursing staff, pharmacy staff, nursing administration, and medical staff members who had CCU privileges.

The quality improvement team then designed a corrective action plan to remedy the particular deficiencies revealed by their investigation. Physicians were counseled to promote the use of the newer antiarrhythmic drug. Staffing levels were adjusted to provide for adequate staff at all times of the day. A program of continual reinforcement to the nursing staff of the need for close monitoring of cardiac rhythms was instituted. And all older model cardiac monitors were replaced. The team decided that it would reconvene for further work if its interventions were ineffectively implemented or, even if well implemented, if they were ineffective in reducing arrhythmia deaths. This information would come through the indicators they had designed.

The quality improvement team never reconvened. Every month, every indicator expectation was met. After 5 months, the use of the older antiarrhythmic drug ceased, and after 9 months the quality management department stopped data collection for and reporting on that indicator. After 4 months, the CCU death rate in acute cardiac patients fell below that rate expected for their patients from the state-wide comparative outcomes monitoring program. The quality management department then discontinued the internal data collection and reporting of the CCU arrhythmia death rate, relying on the annual state report for periodic assessment. The department decided to continue indefinitely with the data collection and reporting on the two indicators related to nursing care.

This scenario illustrates the process of risk prevention based on a continuous quality improvement approach to process improvement and performance monitoring. It demonstrates the importance of a multidisciplinary approach to problem recognition and problem solving. Potential problems were identified, solutions were crafted, and performance was monitored to assess organizational change over time. This approach to risk identification and prevention will be of increasing importance given the growing availability of comparative outcomes data through cooperative projects, state agencies, and the Medicare Peer Review Organizations' new "Fourth Scope of Work" to implement the Health Care Quality Improvement Initiative,[17] as discussed in a later section.

Assessing risk exposure

Risk exposure is identified either by examination of the facts of an individual case, which could reveal a continuing source of liability risk, or from examination of data, which can be trend data of a particular risk indicator or clinical performance data. Once risk exposure is identified, quantitative measures, or indicators, reflective of that exposure should be developed to enable risk administrators to determine the presence of similar risk in other areas of the organization and as a measuring stick to gauge the success of interventional efforts. Literally hundreds of indicators can be measured, so risk administrators must identify a manageable number that will yield the required information.

Indicators are usually rates of selected events, such as hospital falls, medication errors, and adverse clinical outcomes. They may be measured in targeted areas or throughout the entire organization. Data for indicators can be obtained from a wide variety of sources in an organization. Unique databases are often found in claims and billing (whose database typically contains patient encounter data consisting of at least ICD-9-CM codes, visit status, care delivered, and patient disposition), utilization management (often a rich source of data), pharmacy, medical staff office (including the credentialing database), patient relations department (which might have a detailed database of patient complaints and corrective actions), and quality management (which should have all available clinical performance data). The risk administrator should have in his or her own department data on lawsuits, risk cases, incident reports, and specified occurrence reports and screening.

As an example, if a hospital risk administrator identifies falls by patients, staff, and visitors as a source of risk exposure, he or she might determine that much of the problem relates to travel on floors wet from cleaning. Further analysis may lead to the identification of a number of interventions that would serve to minimize or eliminate travel on wet floors. Interventions might include the use of large yellow plastic warning signs placed 6 feet apart around the wet area, confining routine floor cleaning to evenings after visiting hours, and the cleaning of no more than 50% of the width of a walkway at one time. Appropriate indicators for monitoring risk exposure would be the monthly rates of a series of measurements based on routine, random walk-around inspections, such as the percentage of just-mopped floors without proper warning signs, the percentage of floors actually cleaned during visiting hours, and the percentage of floor cleanings where more than one-half of the hallway was mopped. These three represent "process" indicators that reflect the success in executing the interventions. Of course, if the hypothesis that these three interventions will be effective in reducing the rate of falls is wrong, then successful implementation of the interventions will have no effect on the rate of falls. Therefore, it is crucial to include

measurement of an "outcome" indicator that will provide information about whether the problem was ameliorated by the interventions. A useful outcome indicator would be the monthly number of falls by patients, staff, and visitors. Outcome indicators, as opposed to process indicators, should be reflective of the level of risk exposure, and so should be the measure of success of any risk prevention effort.

Clinical quality indicators are often, but not always, risk indicators. Clinical risk indicators are limited to those aspects of medical care that present risk. Quality management, however, encompasses the improvement of medical care that is not felt to present any legal risk. For example, a hospital with the lowest rate of surgical complications in town may seek to lower it even further through an aggressive quality improvement project. If no risk exposure in that area had been identified, the indicators developed to monitor surgical complications would be clinical quality indicators, but not clinical risk indicators. Similarly, not all risk indicators are quality indicators. An institution may identify risk exposure because of the failure of its medical staff to consistently obtain proper *written* informed consent before certain procedures, as required by the staff bylaws. The indicator of percentage of procedures with *written* informed consent forms completed beforehand would be useful to assess risk in this situation. However, failure of the physician to obtain *written* informed consent to a procedure is a legal, not a medical, issue; so an indicator of this failure would be a risk, but not quality, indicator.

Risk indicators should be valid reflections of the clinical or operational activity they are intended to measure. They should be free from measurement bias, and each measured event should be reliably observed. Poorly crafted risk indicators will prevent the accurate recognition of risk exposure and the understanding of its causes, and will doom to failure many risk avoidance efforts.

Defining performance expectations

The next step in risk reduction is to establish for each indicator a target level that will be used as the measure of success in risk reduction. For example, a project to reduce medication errors could establish a target of a 50% reduction in errors over 3 months, and a rate in subsequent months of no higher than 10 incidences per month throughout the organization. These targets are the standards against which the success of the project should be measured, and if the indicator target rate is not met, further corrective action is warranted. Many risk reduction and quality improvement projects ultimately fail despite initial promise because of inadequate long-term monitoring of the risk exposure and the lack of a predetermined commitment to action if expected results are not achieved.

Monitoring the results of action is so important that the necessary indicators and their expected values over time should be established before any action is taken. The measuring sticks (the indicators) and the criteria for success (the expected values) should be established before taking action, so that the determination of whether an intervention is successful will not be biased by the personal stakes acquired by staff in the development and implementation of the corrective action plan.

In particularly troublesome areas, performance expectations can be formalized and reinforced through operational protocols and clinical practice guidelines. These are written formal expressions of courses of action expected in defined circumstances. Classic examples are nursing protocols for initiating blood transfusions and physician practice guidelines for pacemaker insertion. Care must be taken, however, to avoid the possibility of interpreting clinical practice guidelines as strictly defined standards of care. Nevertheless, protocols and guidelines, properly designed, can be an effective way of standardizing selected features of operations and clinical care that can serve to reduce risk exposure. Adherence to them can be measured through indicators.

Taking specific action to reduce risk

Risk prevention depends on the accurate identification of those clinical and operational processes in need of corrective efforts. In their efforts to diagnose the causes of risk exposure, risk administrators should adopt a structured problem-solving technique, predicated on an organized approach to identifying all of the clinical and operational processes that affect the clinical area with risk exposure. This approach may include the construction of process flow diagrams and cause-and-effect diagrams. Input should be obtained from staff with daily working knowledge of each relevant clinical and operational process.

Once an operational or clinical process has been identified as a problem, corrective interventions should be crafted, and each step necessary for their successful implementation should be detailed in a written "corrective action" plan. The plan's formulation should be made with multidisciplinary input, and specific responsibilities and times for completion of each task should be specified. Successful implementation of a corrective action plan will often depend on widespread, continual staff education and committed involvement of managers of all relevant clinical and operational departments.

Adopting general risk avoidance strategies

Risk administrators should develop a general risk avoidance plan, which should include organization-specific strategies. Two universally important components deserve specific mention. The first is to provide *regular general risk management education* to all staff. This program need not go into detail about legal principles, but should keep all staff, clinical and nonclinical, aware of the constant need to avoid risk and report it whenever discovered. This education is particularly important for physicians, given the greater risk exposure encountered in their work. Periodic (e.g., annually) seminars should review the essentials of risk prevention in clinical practice, stressing the crucial elements of good communication and good medical record keeping. The presentation of recent organizational and comparative trend data on risk indicators can be an effective tool to stimulate physician interest and maintain their attention.

A second important component of a risk avoidance plan is to strengthen the medical staff credentialing criteria and procedures. Criteria for good standing should be far beyond mere possession of current licensure and malpractice insurance. Data on quality of care, risk cases, and patient complaints should play a role, particularly data on the clinical outcomes of the physician's care (e.g., surgical mortality and complication rates). It is becoming increasingly perilous for health care organizations to ignore such data in their credentialing process. In their recent review of the impact of performance data on medical practice, physicians Topol and Califf comment that:

> The problem of too many physicians [doing procedures, many of whom perform too few each year to achieve competency,] is compounded by the lack of adequate training for many, who too frequently derive their "training" by attendance at a demonstration course. . . . [C]areful consideration should be given to the criteria for privileges of individual physicians. Low-volume physicians whose patients have poor outcomes should be prohibited from doing procedures. The minimum number of cases per year should be strictly enforced. . . . [For example,] the Joint American College of Cardiology and American Heart Association Task Force recommends that cardiac surgeons do at least 100 bypass operations per year, but in a review of the data now available in New York and Pennsylvania, more than one third of cardiac surgeons did not meet this criterion. . . . Volume is not the only issue; guidelines are necessary for the [corrective] actions that should be triggered when indicators of poor-quality medicine are evident. . . . Indeed, availability of [clinical] outcome data would likely alter the behavior of low-volume or poor-outcome practitioners. However, if these measures are unsuccessful, strategies ranging from admonitory communication to frank termination of procedural privileges could be used.[18]

Continually reassessing risk exposure: the cycle of continuous risk reduction

Risk reduction is a continuous cyclic process, summarized in the schematic in Figure 20-1. The first step of the cycle is the assessment of risk, which includes the identification of risk exposure and its measurement through risk indicators. In doing this, an organization is

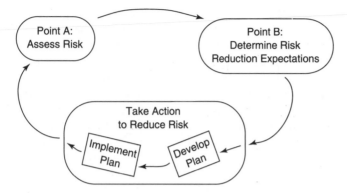

Fig. 20-1. Cycle of continuous risk reduction.

determining its degree of exposure to a certain risk, which is referred to as point A in the diagram. The second step is the creation of expectations of where the level of risk exposure should fall to over time; in this step, the organization determines its risk reduction goal (point B). The third and final step is the taking of action to reduce the risk exposure; that is, to reduce risk exposure from point A to point B. This step requires the development of a corrective action plan and its successful implementation. Once action is taken, the steps of the cycle are repeated as necessary. Risk exposure is reassessed to gauge the success of the intervention and the need for further action. If risk reduction expectations are not met, they are revised as appropriate and further action is taken. Failure to monitor known risk exposure, especially once improvement begins, can allow attention and resources to be diverted to other projects and lead to the ultimate failure of an initially successful intervention.

RISK FINANCING

A health care organization finances the risk of loss from liability in one of two ways. It may retain the risk or it may seek to shift or transfer the risk.[19]

Retaining risk

The use of internal funds to pay losses is referred to as *loss retention* or *retaining risk*. Under this arrangement, a health care organization may either fund or not fund the cumulative value of the risks retained. Of course, the more fiscally responsible approach is to fund the losses in a self-insurance program by which a trust fund is established and the organization makes annual contributions according to actuarial studies as to the estimated value of losses retained. A self-insurance program is most appropriate when a hospital (1) wishes to achieve an advantageous cash flow, (2) has the capacity to satisfy actuarial funding requirements, (3) possesses the sophistication to set appropriate reserves, (4) is able to maintain a reasonably low level of self-retention or

deductible, and (5) finds it otherwise impossible or impractical to transfer the risk.

On occasion, an organization that has a fully funded self-insurance program may, nevertheless, elect to assume a risk for a type of loss not covered under the self-insurance program if insurance for such a risk is either not available or the price is prohibitive. The organization, despite accepting responsibility for it, may neglect to fund it. In the event a loss does materialize, the organization would have to fund it from general operating funds. An alternative is to fund a loss reserve or consider alternative approaches to self-insurance.

Self-insurance programs do pose some inherent problems for the institution. Pressures to achieve short-term financial objectives can place in jeopardy long-term financial viability of the self-insurance program. For example, some institutions limit the funding of a self-insurance fund to actual lawsuits as opposed to probable claims. This approach could eventually result in an inadequate surplus in the trust fund. A similar tendency is for organizations to accept coverage of losses in which the losses are less clear or more unpredictable. Such losses would more prudently be either transferred or covered under a commercial insurance policy. Yet another disadvantage of a self-insurance program is the inability to counteract pressures by excess carriers to increase the self-insured retention limits.[20]

Other insurance arrangements exist that might serve as alternatives to developing a self-insured retention program. These include insurance purchasing groups, risk retention groups, and offshore captive insurance companies.[21] However, these alternative structures may be more expensive and time-consuming to implement and operate than a self-insured trust and may be more applicable to a multihospital system or a physician hospital organization as opposed to a single hospital entity.

Transferring risk

The transfer of risk in whole or in part for most organizations takes place in one of three ways. The most common is to transfer risk to a commercial insurance company under a primary or excess policy. A second approach is to share risk by requiring that physicians who are members of the medical staff or network maintain minimum levels of insurance. These two approaches are commonplace and do not require further elaboration.

The third approach is also fairly common, but has been the subject of misunderstanding and misuse. It attempts to shift liability by use of an indemnification or hold harmless agreement in a contract. Such a provision allows one party to transfer the legal liability to another contracting party, and is a contract clause that is frequently insisted on by vendors, insurers, and managed care programs. Health care organizations should not unwittingly accept such provisions. First of all, many malpractice insurance policies expressly exclude such transfers of liability so that the acceptance of the liability of another may be an uninsured loss. In addition, such provisions are typically worded in an overly broad fashion. An even worse alternative is a mutual indemnification. Neither should be accepted by an organization. A one-way agreement unfairly shifts liability to the hospital, whereas mutual indemnification assures that both parties will become entangled in the question of liability.

When faced with an indemnification provision, an organization's legal counsel should endeavor to have the indemnification provision deleted, should not accept a mutual indemnification, and may suggest the following alternative wording:

It is understood and agreed that neither of the parties to this agreement shall be liable for any negligent or wrongful act chargeable to the other and that this agreement shall not be construed as seeking to either enlarge or diminish any obligation or duty owed by one party against the other or against third parties. In the event of a claim for any wrongful or negligent act, each party shall bear the cost of its own defense.

EXTERNAL RISK MANAGEMENT REQUIREMENTS
Federal requirements

The regulatory environment within which a hospital risk management program operates is an assortment of loosely connected federal laws and programs. The quality of medical care provided in American hospitals is extensively reviewed under the Medicare program's quality review process. Reviews are conducted by peer review organizations (PROs) established in 1982 under the Tax Equity and Fiscal Responsibility Act. The primary role of PROs has been to review medical records to determine whether Medicare beneficiaries are receiving care that is appropriate and of high quality. Great changes, however, are now under way in this program. Under the PROs' new "Fourth Scope of Work," they will implement a program referred to as the Health Care Quality Improvement Initiative (HCQII).[22] The HCQII directs PROs to abandon the old, widely criticized method of generic screens and individual case review based on subjective criteria. Instead, it requires them to use a new approach to the evaluation of hospital care. The core of the new system is the identification of unsatisfactory medical care and clinical outcomes through a computerized review of data from selected medical records (at least in part, data elements identified in Medicare's Uniform Clinical Data Set). PROs will provide physicians and hospitals with data-based comparative performance reports. Where appropriate, a PRO will require physicians and hospitals with unsatisfactory performance to develop and implement correc-

tive action plans. The new method of Medicare PRO review, then, will be founded on data collection, data analysis, comparative performance assessment, and the design and implementation of physician and hospital corrective action plans where necessary.

Although most Medicare review activity is directed at hospitals, health maintenance organizations (HMOs) with Medicare enrollees receive some scrutiny from Medicare reviewers. HMOs with Medicare contracts face periodic detailed reviews of their policies and procedures related to quality assessment and improvement programs, provider credentialing, utilization management, patient complaint evaluation and resolution, and patient grievance procedures.

In enacting the Health Care Quality Improvement Act in 1986, Congress took another step toward improvement of quality of care. The act identified two impediments to the promotion of quality health care: Incompetent physicians often went undetected and many physicians were reluctant to engage in effective peer review out of fear of liability. To address these problems, the act created the National Practitioner Data Bank (NPDB) to retrieve and disseminate information concerning malpractice or disciplinary actions, and provided immunity to physicians who participate in approved peer review activities. Insurers, licensing boards, hospitals, some managed care organizations, and professional societies are mandated to provide reports to the NPDB about payments resulting from medical malpractice actions and disciplinary actions based on reasons related to professional competence. In addition, health care organizations have the responsibility of obtaining information from the NPDB whenever considering applicants for medical staff appointments and every 2 years for practitioners who are already on the medical staff or who have been granted clinical privileges.

Risk management remains a cornerstone of health care reform proposals. Tort reform is expected to include use of alternative dispute resolution systems, requirement that a certificate of merit by a qualified medical specialist accompany a medical malpractice liability action, limitation on amount of contingency fees for attorneys, reduction of awards for recovery from collateral sources, and periodic payments of awards. In addition, a broad-based national effort is expected to develop national measures of quality performance. Such measures would provide information on the accessibility, appropriateness, effectiveness, efficiency, and satisfactoriness of care.

State requirements

Ten states have enacted statutes pertaining to risk management programs: Kansas, Maryland, Rhode Island, Florida, Alaska, Colorado, North Carolina, Massachusetts, Washington, and New York. Two of these states, Washington and New York, refer to a "quality assurance" program in the place of a risk management program. Otherwise, most of the statutes share one or more common characteristics. (Colorado represents an exception because its statute exclusively focuses on the protection of records or reports as part of a risk management program and is used to reduce patient injury or improve quality of patient care.) The remaining statutes all require the establishment of a risk management program in hospitals licensed by the states. In addition, Kansas, Florida, and Washington require that reports be made to a state agency. Maryland, Rhode Island, Alaska, Washington, and New York require the establishment of both a system for reporting and resolving incidents and a system for addressing patient grievances or complaints. Although the American Society for Health Care Risk Management (ASHRM) has not endorsed a state legislative scheme for health care risk management, the Maryland statute most closely resembles the model risk management statute drafted by that organization.[23]

National Committee on Quality Assurance (NCQA)

The NCQA is a not-for-profit organization that offers a voluntary accreditation program for HMOs. Its purview now includes the Health Plan Employer Data and Information Set (HEDIS).[24] HEDIS is a set of specified information about an HMO that employers may find useful in their selection of HMOs with which to contract. In 1991, the NCQA assumed responsibility for coordinating further refinements of the initial version of the HEDIS document, and in November 1993 released the final draft of HEDIS version 2.0. HEDIS includes a set of indicators covering various aspects of clinical care including quality, patient satisfaction, utilization management, and accessibility, as well as nonclinical aspects pertaining to areas such as membership and finance. NCQA review evaluates, among other things, an HMO's explicit quality assessment and improvement program, which should contain clinical risk management functions. NCQA accreditation is growing in importance—it is now required by some national employers of all HMOs that desire to participate in their networks.

The Joint Commission Accreditation of Healthcare Organizations (JCAHO)

The JCAHO is a private organization established by a number of medical societies and the American Hospital Association to develop hospital quality standards and to accredit hospitals according to those standards. Although its gaze is primarily on hospitals, the JCAHO is in the process of extending its scope to integrated delivery systems. In 1989, JCAHO hospital clinical risk management standards were established, and compliance is mandatory for accreditation.[25]

The JCAHO assigns to the hospital medical staff the responsibility for the JCAHO four key clinical risk management standards. Because clinical risk management is a continual activity, the JCAHO will look for documentation of continual medical staff activity in fulfillment of its risk management responsibilities. The JCAHO is focused on content, so medical staff activity that explicitly fulfills clinical risk management responsibilities can be under its "quality assurance" program and not be specifically labeled as "risk management" activity.

The four key clinical risk management duties are:

1. *The identification of general clinical areas that represent actual or potential sources of patient injury.* The "general clinical areas" selected for review should be hospital-specific, based on individual hospital experience and not based on general experience of all similar institutions. JCAHO reviewers will "look for evidence of the medical staff's active participation and the review of national, regional, state, local, hospital-specific, departmental, discipline-specific, and/or professional-liability-underwriter-generated information suggesting actual or potential causes of patient injury." Scoring guidelines stipulate that hospitals must identify at least three general areas of risk.[26]

2. *The development of criteria to identify cases of potential risk and evaluation of these cases.* JCAHO reviewers will "determine whether evidence shows that the medical staff has developed (or participated in developing) measurable criteria/indicators/screens designed to identify undesirable or adverse patient care occurrences. The evidence should also show that criteria/indicators/screens are used to collect data within the [hospital-specific] identified general areas of clinical care that represent significant sources of actual or potential patient injury."[27]

3. *The correction of identified problems.* JCAHO reviewers will look for documentation of medical staff "conclusions, recommendations, actions, and follow-up" as the response to identified clinical risk problems.[28]

4. *The design of programs to reduce risk.* JCAHO reviewers will look for documentation of the medical staff's risk management plans and continuing education activities.[29]

Hospitals have two options on how to structurally assign responsibility for clinical risk management duties. In the first, the medical staff can assume full responsibility for all administrative and operational risk management functions. Alternatively, primary administrative responsibility may be assumed by the hospital administration, but with the close cooperation and support of the medical staff, which retains responsibility for the four key clinical risk management duties. This second option allows a hospital to place administrative responsibility for clinical risk management functions in a legal or risk management department, which also typically has responsibility for all other institutional risk management activity.

The JCAHO's standards focus on whether a hospital achieves the clinical risk management standards—a formalized hospital "risk management" program is not required. No single method of organizational structure, linking clinical risk management to other clinical functions such as quality management, is required by the JCAHO risk management standards.

CONCLUSION

Health care organizations are dynamic entities in which programs, personnel, and priorities are in a constant state of flux. As a result, legal risks can often assume a fluid state. A successful approach to the prevention of injuries caused by a certain set of circumstances may ultimately fail when those circumstances change. The benefits of a fall prevention program successfully instituted in a geriatric unit might disappear with a reduction in nurse staffing, expansion of the unit, change in patient mix, or physical reconfiguration of the unit. When that happens, new solutions and alternative approaches will be required. Risk management programs must be able to modify their efforts in adapting to changing patterns and trends. Risk administrators must realize that problems once solved may reappear and require new solutions, sometimes repeatedly. Constant vigilance through monitoring is essential. Effective risk management requires continual attention to the ever-changing organizational realities and legal milieu.

END NOTES

1. Joint Commission on Accreditation of Healthcare Organizations, *Accreditation Manual for Hospitals* 262 (1992).
2. G. Troyer, and S. Salman, *Handbook of Healthcare Risk Management* 81 (Aspen Systems Corp. 1986).
3. B. Brown, *Risk Management for Hospitals: A Practical Approach* 2 (Aspen Systems Corporation 1979).
4. M. Holoweiko, *What Are Your Greatest Malpractice Risks?*, Medical Economics 144 (Aug. 3, 1992).
5. E. Hirshfeld, *Should Practice Parameters Be the Standard of Care in Malpractice Litigation?*, 266 JAMA, 2886-2891 (1991).
6. E. Topol, and R. Califf, *Scorecard Cardiovascular Medicine: Its Impact and Future Directions*, 120 Ann Intern Med. 68 (1994).
7. *Privacy Fears Place Another Hurdle in Path of Reform*, Modern Healthcare 24 (Nov. 22, 1993).
8. *See* A. Southwick, *The Law of Hospital and Health Care Administration* 554-578 (2nd ed., Health Administration Press, Ann Arbor 1988) for a more detailed discussion of corporate negligence.
9. *Fox v. Health Net of California*, Calif. Super. Ct. (Riverside), No. 219692 (1993).
10. L. Harpster, and M. Veach, eds., *Risk Management Handbook for Health Care Facility* 255 (American Hospital Publishing, Inc., 1990).
11. H. Rubin, et al., *Watching the Doctor-Watchers: How Well Do Peer Review Organization Methods Detect Hospital Care Quality Problems?*, 267 JAMA 2349-2354 (1992).
12. R. Balsamo, and M. Pine, *Twelve Questions to Ask about Your Outcomes Monitoring System*, 20 Physician Executive 13-16, 22-25 (1994).
13. J. Orlikoff, *Preventing Malpractice: The Board's Role in Risk Management*, Trustee 9 (Sept. 1991).
14. M. Tragin et al., *Physician Demographics and Risk of Medical Malpractice*, 93 Am. J. Med. 541 (Nov. 1992).
15. *Petrillo v. Syntex Laboratories, Inc.*, 148 Ill. App. 3d 581, 499 N.E.2d 952 (1st Dist. 1986).
16. T. Leaman, and J. Saxton, *Preventing Malpractice: The Co-Active Solution* 68-70 (Plenum Publishing 1993).
17. S. Jencks, and G. Wilensky, *The Health Care Quality Improvement Initiative: A New Approach to Quality Assurance in Medicare*, 268 JAMA 900-903 (1992).
18. Topol and Califf, *supra* note 6, at 68.
19. A. Sielicki, *Current Philosophy of Risk Management, Topics in Health Care Financing* 6 (Spring 1983).
20. J. Hamman, J. Ziegenfuss, and J. Williamson, eds., *Risk Management Trends and Applications* 73 (American Board of Quality Assurance and Utilization Review Physicians 1988).
21. B. Youngberg, *Essentials of Hospital Risk Management* 145-147 (Aspen Publishers, Inc. 1990).
22. Jencks and Wilensky, *supra* note 17.
23. Harpster and Veach, *supra* note 10, at 19.
24. J. Corrigan, and D. Nielsen, *Toward the Development of Uniform Reporting Standards for Managed Care Organizations: The Health Plan Employer Data and Information Set (Version 2.0)*, 19 J. Quality Improvement 566-575 (1993).
25. The Joint Commission on Accreditation of Healthcare Organizations, *Risk Management Strategies* (1991).
26. Id. at 28.
27. *Id.* at 48.
28. *Id.* at 51.
29. Id. at 14.

APPENDIX 20-1   **Top malpractice allegations by frequency and cost, PIAA data**

	Claims citing misadventure	Percent of all misadventure claims	Paid claims	Average indemnity
1. Improper performance	21,737	35.7%	6,989	$104,260
2. Errors in diagnosis	14,587	23.9	4,800	123,160
3. Failure to monitor case	14,697	7.7	1,649	148,250
4. Procedure not indicated	3,846	6.3	1,287	105,620
5. Medication errors	2,610	4.3	996	81,750
6. Procedure not performed	2,123	3.5	937	160,710
7. Delay in performance	2,049	3.4	781	127,080
8. Failure to recognize complication	2,045	3.4	718	127,080
9. Failure to communicate with patient	1,235	2.0	365	71,240
10. Foreign object left in patient after surgery	1,154	1.9	574	33,650
11. All other misadventures	4,866	7.9	2,129	117,220

Source: Medical Economics 144 (Aug. 3, 1992).

APPENDIX 20-2   **Malpractice allegations with the highest indemnity, PIAA data**

	Average indemnity	Paid claims	Total claims
1. Failure to postpone case when indicated	$303,410	18	63
2. Problems monitoring patient during recovery	299,950	42	106
3. Failure to properly respond	275,480	25	70
4. Not, or improperly, performing resuscitation	263,010	40	151
5. Problems monitoring patient in surgery	244,970	131	291
6. Delay in performance	227,750	781	2049
7. Improper supervision of others	224,100	40	95
8. Errors in anesthetic use or selection	172,090	100	272
9. Intubation problems	166,500	203	450
10. Procedure not performed	160,710	937	2123

Source: Medical Economics 141 (Aug. 3, 1992).

APPENDIX 20-3   **Top ten malpractice allegations by average cost**

Allegation	Number of claims	Average cost
1. Patient monitoring related	324	$105,768
2. Medication: wrong amount/rate/unordered	106	87,003
3. Delayed history, physical, or test (HPT)	55	78,899
4. Delayed/omitted treatment	360	70,769
5. Diagnostic, bad results	97	69,338
6. Amount/rate treatment, incorrect or unordered	92	65,563
7. Treatment complications/bad results	831	61,227
8. Medication: wrong type	87	52,948
9. Wrong diagnosis	343	50,691
10. Misinterpreted results of HPT	162	50,216

Source: St. Paul Fire and Marine Insurance Company, *Update (1993 Annual Report to Policyholders)* 5 (1993).

APPENDIX 20-4   Top ten malpractice allegations by frequency

Allegation	Number of claims	Average cost
1. Treatment complication/bad results	831	$ 61,227
2. Delayed/omitted treatment	360	70,769
3. Injury adjacent to treatment site	348	28,079
4. Wrong diagnosis	343	50,691
5. Patient monitoring related	324	105,768
6. Fall, bed related	225	24,566
7. Type of treatment incorrect	212	40,374
8. Fall, walking related	201	19,475
9. Other diagnostic issue	186	34,909
10. Infection/contamination/exposure	174	29,343

Source: St. Paul Fire and Marine Insurance Company, *Update (1993 Annual Report to Policyholders)* 5 (1993).

APPENDIX 20-5   All malpractice allegations by location

Location/allegation	Number of claims	Percent of total claims	Average cost
Patient care area	1080	29.2	$47,809
Emergency department	1215	19.0	40,741
Inpatient surgery	1115	17.2	39,360
Obstetrical care	775	12.0	96,940
Outpatient services	278	4.3	22,911
Outpatient surgery	231	3.5	49,088
Psychiatric care	228	3.5	26,810
Radiological services	205	3.2	31,309
Therapy services	20	0.3	27,281
Other areas	501	7.8	23,899

Source: St. Paul Fire and Marine Insurance Company, *Update (1993 Annual Report to Policyholders)* 5 (1993).

APPENDIX 20-6   Major malpractice allegation issues

Issues	Number of claims	Percent of total claims	Percent of total cost
Treatment	2793	43.2	51.7
Diagnostic	959	14.8	17.7
Patient fall	912	14.1	6.7
Medication	605	9.4	8.7
Facility/equipment	280	4.3	3.2

Source: St. Paul Fire and Marine Insurance Company, *Update (1993 Annual Report to Policyholders)* 5 (1993).

APPENDIX 20-7   **Unusual incident report**

THIS IS AN INTERNAL QUALITY CONTROL DOCUMENT
DO NOT PLACE IN PATIENT RECORD

NAMEPLATE

I. _____ **PATIENT** _____ **VISITOR** _____ **OTHER** (Check one)

Date of Incident: _____ Time of Incident: _____ A.M. _____
P.M. _____

Location of Incident: _____
(Unit/Area)

Attending Physician: _____

If **NO** addressograph, print
Name, DOB, Unit, Patient, Number;
If visitor: give address.

Witness: _____ Phone No.: _____
Witness: _____ Phone No.: _____

II. **Type of Incident:**   (Check at least one)

_____ Reaction to contrast/dye
Type: _____
_____ Wrong blood given
_____ Unexpected return to the operating room
_____ Brain damage which could be the result
of treatment or medical intervention
_____ Neurological deficit, nerve injury or
paralysis which could be the result of
treatment or medical intervention
_____ Unexpected patient death
_____ Inaccurate needle or sponge count
_____ Unplanned hospital admission subsequent
to outpatient surgery procedure

_____ Informed consent form not signed or inaccurate
_____ Total or partial loss of limb, or the use of limb
_____ Needle stick to patient or visitor
_____ Burns from food, liquid or mechanical equipment
_____ Central line complication/problem resulting in patient injury
_____ Intubation/extubation injury
_____ Damage to or disappearance of personal property
_____ I.V. infiltration (Provide detail in Section III.)
_____ Fall (Provide detail in Section III.)
_____ Medication error (Provide detail in Section III.)
_____ OTHER (Provide detail in Section III.)
_____ Serious illness or injury (including death) to patient which
might have been caused by medical device* (See Section IV)

III. **INCIDENT FACTS/DATA:**   (Should Be Consistent With What Is Written In The Medical Record)

_____
_____
_____
_____
_____
_____
_____

IV. ***PRODUCT IDENTIFICATION:** (this information is required by FDA through The Safe Medical Devices Act of 1990
if the Medical Device has caused serious illness or injury (including death) to patient)

Please list all products/devices connected to the patient at the time of the incident:

Product/Device Name	Lot #/Expiration Date	Serial #	Manufacturer's Name
1) _____	_____	_____	_____
2) _____	_____	_____	_____
3) _____	_____	_____	_____
4) _____	_____	_____	_____
5) _____	_____	_____	_____
6) _____	_____	_____	_____

Disposable items should <u>not</u> be discarded until cleared by Risk Management.

Location of Medical Device/Product: _____

V. **Preparer's Signature:** _____ Date: _____ Time: _____ A.M. _____
P.M. _____

Title: _____
Unit Leader's Signature: _____ Date: _____ Unit: _____

Routing Instructions: 1. Submit original to Office of Risk Management (ORM).
2. Original must be received by the ORM within 24 hrs. of incident.
3. For Patient Care Units — carbon to be maintained by Quality Improvement Coordinating Committee Chairperson.
4. For Ancillary Units — carbon to be maintained by Ancillary Care Evaluation Committee Chairperson.

SERIOUS INCIDENTS — CALL DIRECTLY TO OFFICE OF RISK MANAGEMENT: 2-7828.

THIS FORM MAY NOT BE DUPLICATED

FORM 0325 Rev. 2/92

_____

FOR OFFICE USE ONLY

PART THREE

Medical legal and ethical encounters

CHAPTER 21   # Physician-patient relationship

MATTHEW L. HOWARD, M.D., J.D., F.C.L.M.
LOUIS B. VOGT, M.D., J.D., F.C.L.M.

NATURE AND CREATION OF THE PHYSICIAN-PATIENT RELATIONSHIP
LIMITING THE DUTIES IMPOSED BY THE PHYSICIAN-PATIENT RELATIONSHIP
BREACH OF CONTRACT
THE PHYSICIAN-PATIENT RELATIONSHIP IN SPECIAL SITUATIONS
LIABILITY FOR INJURY TO THIRD PARTIES
RELATIONSHIPS FORMED BY CONTRACT WITH OTHERS
TERMINATION OF THE PHYSICIAN-PATIENT RELATIONSHIP
SPECIAL PROBLEMS IN THE PHYSICIAN-PATIENT RELATIONSHIP
CONCLUSION

Physician-patient relationships presumably have been a source of concern since some unremembered ancestor first claimed special talents or skills in healing. The Hippocratic oath[1] can be thought of as a codification of rules governing the physician-patient relationship, the existence of which suggests that some physicians at least needed to be reminded of proper behavior and bound by oath to enforce their adherence to the social norm. The sanctions[2] of the Code of Hammurabi may be the earliest[3] expression of the idea that physicians should be liable for harm to patients.

Modern professional negligence law, of which medical malpractice is a part, has arisen by application of elements of English common law[4] of contracts and of torts to the same concerns expressed by Hippocrates and Hammurabi. As the twentieth century draws to a close, legislative mandates are increasingly modifying the traditional approaches.

The physician-patient relationship has traditionally been considered a contractual one, although the contract is usually implied by the actions of the parties in seeking and providing advice and care. Written contracts are the exception. The physician is deemed to have promised that professionally acceptable care will be provided, with no guarantee. Unless a specific warranty has been made, courts will not infer that a physician guarantees the success of his or her treatment.[5] That a patient does not pay for services does not affect the existence of the contract or lessen the physician's duties, obligations, responsibilities, or liabilities.[6]

For a physician to be professionally liable to another, four conditions must be met. A person claiming com-

pensation for medical malpractice must show that the professional had a responsibility to that person (duty owed), the duty was not met (an accepted professional standard of care was breached), and the failure to conform to accepted professional standards resulted (causation) in otherwise avoidable damages (injury) to the person making the claim. Each one of these elements (duty, breach of the duty, causation, and injury) must be proven for the plaintiff to prevail. This is true whatever the profession.

The law applied to physicians or other health care professionals is fundamentally the same as that applied to architects, engineers, and attorneys. Before a professional duty can be established, the traditional and general rule has been that a professional relationship must exist. Demonstrating the existence of a relationship between the physician and the person claiming to have been harmed is the keystone of every medical malpractice action.[7]

Under statutes such as COBRA, to be discussed, duties may arise from "hospital-patient" relationships, which, once established in accordance with the terms of the law, impose duties on the physician. When a physician becomes involved in a legal problem that stems from a "hospital-patient" relationship, it is usually because of a special relationship between the hospital and physician.

NATURE AND CREATION OF THE PHYSICIAN-PATIENT RELATIONSHIP

In the absence of a physician-patient relationship, or some other special relationship, physicians are not legally compelled to treat strangers, even during an emergency,[8] in almost all states.*

When a person seeks the services of a physician for the purposes of medical or surgical treatment, that person becomes a patient, and the traditional physician-patient relationship is established.[9] A contract is implied by the mutuality of the relationship.[10] The physician is not an employee of the patient.[11] This traditional relationship is consensual. In other words, a patient has consciously sought out a physician who has affirmatively agreed to provide care. The mutuality of the relationship is independent of who solicits the relationship or who pays for the services provided.[12] As we shall see, many problems arise in situations where the physician is held to a duty to a person for whom he or she has not consciously agreed to provide care.

The creation of the physician-patient relationship usually requires some form of physical contact with the patient. It may be created by a single telephone conversation. Pathologists[13] and radiologists,[14] however, have a duty to the patient to exercise reasonable and ordinary skill and care while rendering their services even though they generally have no personal contact with the patient.

Whether a physician-patient relationship legally exists is a factual determination. For public policy reasons, courts give persons alleging injury from medical malpractice considerable latitude as to the evidence required to establish the existence of the relationship.[15] Courts will determine whether the patient entrusted care to the physician, and whether the physician indicated acceptance of the duty to render care. If the circumstances of the contact caused the patient to have a reasonable expectation of treatment, or if the physician undertook to render treatment, the courts will imply the existence of a relationship.[16]

One legal definition of treatment is "the broad term covering all steps taken to effect a cure of an injury or disease. The word includes examination and diagnosis as well as application of remedies."[17] This broad interpretation, and the willingness of most courts to interpret almost any action as an undertaking-to-treat, may result in a physician-patient relationship that the physician did not intend to create.

LIMITING THE DUTIES IMPOSED BY THE PHYSICIAN-PATIENT RELATIONSHIP

Once established, unless limited or conditioned by agreement, the relationship continues until the services are no longer needed or are properly terminated. Once terminated, the physician is generally not obligated to follow the patient's progress.[18]

Although courts seem quick to establish a physician-patient relationship, they generally recognize the physician's ability to qualify and limit the relationship.[19] The agreement to treat a patient may be limited to one particular treatment or one particular procedure.[20] Physician availability may be restricted to certain times and places.[21] Such limitations must be clearly understood and accepted by the patient.

Physicians are generally free to choose their patients and are not obligated[22] to treat anyone with whom they have no special relationship.[†23] Absent statutorily imposed requirements, physicians are not compelled to practice, to practice under terms other than those the physician may choose to accept, nor does the licensee warrant that he or she will provide care to any or all prospective patients. This principle is recognized by the Principles of Medical Ethics of the American Medical Association and supported by case law.[24]

Once a relationship is legally established however, the physician is liable for any damages legally caused by any breach of the duty. The fundamental duty is to exercise the same degree of knowledge, skill, diligence, and care that an ordinary competent physician would exercise under the same or similar circumstances. There is a concomitant duty to suggest a referral if the physician knows, or should know, that he or she does not possess the requisite knowledge or skill to properly treat the patient.[25] Failure to make a referral is negligence.[26]

The patient is obligated to participate and cooperate in the treatment and to follow reasonable instructions for further evaluation and treatment.[27] If the patient fails to do so, he or she may be prevented from holding the physician solely liable for any resulting injuries.[28] The physician, however, must provide the patient with information necessary to explain why physician recommendations ought to be followed.[29] The physician's relative liability will be determined from the facts and circumstances by the trier of fact. A patient's failure to follow physician instructions does not by itself terminate the relationship or relieve the physician of obligations, nor does the patient's failure to pay the physician's fees relieve the physician from further responsibility.[30]

---

*This chapter is intended to provide an overview of the issues, generally stating the majority view. Case law in particular states may vary, and both case law and statutes in each state should be examined for variance before taking any action with potential legal consequences.

†We must distinguish between duty for professional liability purposes, discussed here, and duties imposed as a condition of licensure. In various states, duties as a condition of continued licensure which restrict a physician's right to choose freely those for whom he will provide care have been imposed. These include abstention from balance-billing of Medicare patients, acceptance of Medicaid patients, and acceptance of HIV-positive patients. Additional restrictions are created by Federal Civil Rights law restricting against discrimination on the basis of race, disability, etc.

BREACH OF CONTRACT

Because the relationship is contractual in nature,[31] an injured party may allege a breach of contract.[32] Where the presumptive patient declines the contract, no physician duty exists.[33] In the medical setting, this claim arises where the physician is alleged to have guaranteed a particular result or has promised to perform in a certain manner.[34] If the physician does not reasonably live up to the guarantee, a valid action for breach of contract may exist, even if the physician's performance was not negligent or deficient under the measure of meeting usual professional standards.[35]

Claims arising in breach of contract are rare because the law allows only compensation for actual damages caused by the breach of contract. Tort damages are far more lucrative for the patient. In addition, most physicians understand the risks of offering guarantees and do not make statements that could be interpreted in such a fashion, although guarantees of physician availability, especially in the obstetrical context, have been a source of suits and are discussed later.

THE PHYSICIAN-PATIENT RELATIONSHIP IN SPECIAL SITUATIONS

"Curbstone" and "sidewalk" consultation. Physicians are not obligated to give gratuitous advice.[36] Once given however, physicians owe a duty of due care to anyone who might reasonably rely on such advice. If the gratuitous advice causes injury, the physician may be liable for the injury.[37] The degree of contact may be determining.[38,39]

"Second opinion" programs. Where a physician receives a referral from a third party for the purposes of a "second opinion," a claim against that physician grounded in medical malpractice can succeed if the patient can demonstrate that the physician either affirmatively treated, or affirmatively advised how treatment should proceed, and harm resulted.[40]

Substitute and covering physicians. As a general rule, physicians may use substitute physicians if they themselves are unavailable. The substitute physician must be competent and qualified,[41] and the patient must be aware, especially where services are particularly personal,[42] that a substitution may take place.[43] Without this understanding, a cause of action for breach of contract and for abandonment may exist. The fact that physicians share after-hours call duty is so widely known that the courts will, in most instances, impose constructive knowledge and consent on the patient, even in the absence of express consent. To be certain that the patient understands and agrees, written consent to "on-call" coverage and substitution should be obtained.

When called on to treat another physician's patient, the substitute physician establishes a separate and independent physician-patient relationship, which in- cludes a duty to diagnose, treat, and manage any identifiable and detrimental condition that may have been negligently caused by the primary physician. Failure to do so may lead to an independent malpractice action against the substitute.[44]

Merely signing a prescription form for another physician has been held insufficient to establish such an independent relationship.[45]

House staff. Generally, interns, residents, and employed staff physicians are treated as employees of their hospital, and as such their liability is vicariously imputed to the hospital. Employees are essentially indemnified by the hospital for acts performed within the usual course of their duties.[46] Physicians working as fellows may not enjoy the hospital's indemnification; their status depends on their contractual agreement with the hospital. They nevertheless have duties to all hospital patients with whom they establish a relationship.

Part-time, volunteer, and clinical faculty. Clinical faculty not employed by the hospital, functioning in an educational capacity for students and house staff, may be liable to patients who serve as teaching examples. In determining whether a physician-patient relationship was created during contact with a patient seen during a teaching session or on rounds, courts will look at the nature of the physician's contact with the patient, and whether the patient had a reasonable expectation that the teaching physician's role included treatment.[47]

As a general rule, the court will determine whether the physician had actual contact with the patient and whether any examination or treatment of the patient was done for the patient's benefit.[48] If an examination causes the patient to reasonably believe that the examination was made for treatment purposes, the court may infer a relationship.[49] In contrast, if a physician conducting a lecture merely discusses a patient's case and recommends a course of treatment that, when followed, results in injury, courts have found no physician-patient relationship and insufficient contact.[50] A teaching physician who supervises the training of a physician-in-training may be held responsible for any negligent care that the instructor ordered and may also be held liable for negligent supervision of the trainee.

Emergency room physicians and other emergency situations. Generally, physicians are not under a duty to treat anyone with whom no relationship exists,[51] even in an emergency situation in which the person will die without aid. The public policy implications of this rule have led to institution of Good Samaritan laws in many states, providing for immunity from professional liability for physicians who intervene in such instances. These laws provide less protection than would be desired by physicians because they are predicated on physician abstention from seeking payment for care rendered, and provide protection from liability for "ordinary" negligence, but not against "gross" negligence. Physicians may be understandably reluctant to risk a court determination as to whether an error committed in the heat of an emergency was "ordinary" or "gross" negligence.

That freedom to refuse treatment does not extend to hospitals, which have a duty to render reasonable emergency medical aid to the extent that hospital facilities will allow.[52] The law in this area has been substantially modified by the Emergency Medical Treatment and Active Labor Act (EMTALA), otherwise known by the name of the law to which it was attached as a rider, COBRA. The law was enacted out of congressional concern that hospitals were refusing to provide care for uninsured patients, sending them instead to public or charity facilities that might be miles away, and thus it was characterized as an "antidumping" law.

As enacted, COBRA provides for fines and suits against hospitals, but only for fines against physicians. Because the law characterizes the fines as civil penalties, trial by jury is not required. Proof of negligence is not required. Each violation may cost a physician $50,000, and this may not be covered by medical malpractice insurance policies.

As COBRA cases have begun to appear in the courts, its scope is being broadened beyond the problems of inappropriate transfers out of emergency rooms of indigents or women in labor. Other emergency room contacts involving persons not transferred because of pay status issues, persons admitted under nonemergency conditions, and persons for whom medical care may ultimately be deemed futile have all led to recent trial court decisions extending hospital liability. It is reasonable to assume that fines against the treating physicians involved will follow. COBRA has been superimposed on the preexisting rule that the private physician who has agreed to be on-call[53] for the emergency room is presumed to have a relationship with the patient based on the public's reasonable expectation of emergency care.[54]

Telephone contacts. Although physical contact is usually required, a relationship may be established even from a telephone call if the court interprets the physician's comments as treatment. Where a covering physician's contact with the patient was limited to informing the patient that his admission could only be arranged by his family physician, and a comment that the family physician's earlier diagnosis seemed reasonable, the court ruled that no relationship had been established.[55] In another case, where a physician questioned his caller, and advised admission to the hospital, a relationship was considered established.[56] Similarly, where a patient, who after talking to a physician about her vaginal infection made an appointment, but was then refused care when she arrived for her appointment, the making of an appointment for the specific purpose of treating the condition which had been discussed over the telephone was deemed sufficient to establish a physician-patient relationship.[57]

Sexual contacts. A sexual component to the physician-patient relationship is universally condemned.[58] Numerous states have passed laws providing for disciplinary action against physicians who engage in such relationships.[59] Although the AMA standard states flatly that all sexual contact between physicians and patients is misconduct, some courts have declined to adopt this view, holding that the sexual relationship must arise out of the physician-patient relationship to fall within the purview of the statute.[60] In other instances, suits grounded in medical malpractice because of sexual conduct have been brought by patients with conflicting results.[61] The increasing social pressure to end such contacts should suggest to the prudent physician that further legislation against such activity is likely and that social relationships should be strictly confined to nonpractice situations.

LIABILITY FOR INJURY TO THIRD PARTIES
Nonpatient relationships with physicians

Not every patient contact results in the creation of a physician-patient relationship. When a physician performs an examination at the request of a third party for sole use of the third party, for example, where an examination is performed for the purposes of determining eligibility for employment or for the issuance of life insurance, courts differ in their interpretation of the physician's duty to the patient. If a physician is employed to perform preemployment examinations, then the physician's duty is owed to his or her employer; no patient-physician relationship is implied. Absence of therapeutic intent is often stated to be the key issue.[62] One court has said that the employed doctor owes no duty to the examinee other than to avoid causing an injury,[63] and is under a duty to use reasonable care to avoid same.[64] Failure to do so may lead to a claim based on ordinary negligence rather than medical malpractice. Another court assumes no duty unless advice is offered.[65] No liability exists for a negligently performed examination, but the employer may be liable to the examinee for the negligent acts of a physician-employee under the doctrine of *respondeat superior*.[66] The physician may in turn be liable to the company under a contract theory for any resulting damages.

As a general rule, a third-party employed doctor is not bound to disclose abnormal findings to an examinee. Possible exceptions to this rule occur if the physician conducts an examination on a person with whom he or she has a prior existing physician-patient relationship,[67] or if the physician completes an attending physician's statement for an insurance company, for which the physician is paid a fee (contrast with physician as salaried employee). Under such circumstances, the physician might have a duty to disclose significant findings to the examinee.

If a physician gratuitously elects to discuss findings with the examinee, he or she must not misrepresent the examinee's medical condition. If the physician recommends treatment, liability may result if substandard advice causes injury to the examinee.[68] Third parties, other than employers, may employ physicians to examine or treat a patient. The courts distinguish between liability to the third party, for the examination itself, and liability to the patient, for the treatment once it has begun.[69]

Indirect relationships with physicians

As previously stated, it is a fundamental legal principle that all persons are required to use ordinary care not to injure others. The duty to take ordinary care is violated when an injury occurs that is reasonably avoidable and is a foreseeable consequence of a person's actions. All physicians have a duty to warn patients about aspects of their medical condition or treatment that could injure others.[70] The physician of a seizure patient, for example, may be liable for injury to a nonpatient if the injury is indirectly caused by negligent treatment, negligent failure to diagnose the condition, or failure to advise the patient of the risks of engaging in dangerous activities.[71] Although the courts reject imposing a physician-patient relationship with the third-party victim, they freely apply ordinary negligence principles and hold that the injury to the nonpatient was a foreseeable consequence of the patient's condition, which imposed on the physician a duty to avoid injury to foreseeable victims.[72] Lack of foreseeability was at issue where a physician treated a police officer for a pituitary gland tumor. A citizen later shot by the officer was not permitted to maintain an action either under malpractice or negligence theories against the treating physician.[73] Liability has resulted when physicians have failed to advise patients of the danger of performing certain acts while taking medications, such as driving while using sedatives[74] or decongestants,[75] or have failed to properly caution patients with communicable diseases to avoid transmitting the disease to third parties.[76] The Michigan Court of Appeals considered a suit against a physician brought by the family of a motorist killed in a motor vehicle accident with the physician's patient. The patient had received a sedating medication by injection and no warning against driving. The Michigan court permitted the suit to proceed, not in negligence as described above, but as a medical malpractice action, ruling that dismissing the suit because of the absence of a physician-patient

relationship between the physician and the deceased would "exalt form over substance."[77] To date, no other court has followed this example.

Where a patient's relative was permitted to remain in an emergency room treatment area, fainted at the sight of blood, and sustained significant permanent sequelae from the resulting head injury, the physician was held to have no liability to the injured relative.[78]

Courts have imposed liability on physicians who bear a special relationship to a dangerous person and a subsequent victim.[79] Such a relationship may support affirmative physician duties for the benefit of a nonpatient third party.[80] The duty to the nonpatient stems from the physician's special relationship with the patient, and the potential for harm to the third party as a result of the patient's behavior. The leading case is *Tarasoff*,[81] which imposed liability on a psychotherapist whose patient had repeatedly expressed hostile intent toward a specific person who was subsequently murdered. Most subsequent cases have limited that liability to the facts of the Tarasoff case; though the victim need not be a patient, where hostile intent has *not* been limited to a specific, readily identifiable person, no liability has been found when harm subsequently resulted.[82]

The duty to protect endangered third persons has been extended to the protection of endangered property.[83]

RELATIONSHIPS FORMED BY CONTRACT WITH OTHERS

If a physician contracts with a third party to treat a patient, the physician-patient relationship is not established with the patient until some overt undertaking occurs. If the physician does not treat the proposed patient, no duty to the expectant patient is created. Physician liability to the third party who relies on the physician's assurance to treat may exist.[84] When a third party contracts with a physician to treat a particular patient and the treatment is undertaken, the physician-patient relationship is established, and the physician's duty is now to the patient,[85] not to the third party. If the physician's agreement to provide care to a patient leads the third party to believe that the patient was being competently cared for, and being reasonably restrained by this belief does not seek care elsewhere, the physician could then be liable to both patient and third party. Liability to the patient would be based on medical malpractice, to the third party on breach of contract. Such a situation could arise in the case of a minor student at college being treated at the request of a parent living elsewhere.

A physician employed by a third party for the sole purpose of obtaining evidence to support the third party's challenge to a claim of injury is under no duty to the examinee.[86] The physician is generally under no duty to inform the examinee of the results of the examination, and is not liable to the examinee if a negligent examination, or negligently prepared report of the examination, later causes injury to the examinee, provided the report was not, as postulated, prepared for the use or benefit of the examinee.[87]

TERMINATION OF THE PHYSICIAN-PATIENT RELATIONSHIP

The duties imposed on the physician by the creation of a physician-patient relationship continue until the relationship is terminated. This may occur through completion of the treatment by virtue of patient recovery,[88] by dismissal of the physician by the patient, by mutual consent, and by formal physician withdrawal.[89] Like any other contract, the parties may terminate the agreement by mutual consent. The patient may unilaterally terminate the relationship for any reason and at any time. This termination may be express or implied by the patient's actions.[90] Even though dismissed, the physician is under a duty to warn the patient of any risk of discontinuing treatment. A prudent physician will carefully document the basis and circumstances of dismissal as protection against a later claim of abandonment by the patient. The relationship may be considered terminated once a patient's care has been properly and completely transferred to another physician so that the services of the transferring physician are no longer needed and the duty of continuing care ends.[91] Once services are terminated, the traditional rule has been that the physician is under no duty either to provide future care or to reestablish the relationship.[92] However, some courts have mandated such liability on the grounds that the physician is in a better position than the patient to keep abreast of changing knowledge.[93]

If, during the course of treatment, a physician concludes that he or she lacks the requisite skill or knowledge to treat the patient competently or, for other acceptable reasons, determines that the patient would be more properly treated by another physician or at another facility, the patient should be so informed. As a practical matter, patients readily accede to their physician's judgment in these circumstances, and termination of the relationship by a mutually agreed on transfer usually results. If transfer is declined, the treating physician is required to inform the patient of the consequences of the refusal, to carefully document the refusal and appropriate counselling, and then to continue care until a proper unilateral termination of the relationship has been accomplished.

Unilateral termination by the physician is permitted.

The patient must be provided sufficient time to arrange care from another physician. Written notice should be provided,[94] preferably by certified mail.[95] The notice should provide an explanation of the patient's condition, and the further services needed, as well as a description of the likely consequences of failure to obtain continuing care. The physician should continue to provide care for such time as it will reasonably take for the patient to secure further care,[96] and this length of time should be specified in the notice letter. Improper withdrawal by physicians has resulted in suits for breach of contract,[97] professional negligence,[98] and abandonment.[99]

Abandonment

Abandonment has been defined as the unilateral severance of the physician-patient relationship by the physician without reasonable notice to the patient at a time when continued medical care is still necessary.[100] Where physician illness or disability is the cause of the withdrawal, abandonment has not occurred. Liability for abandonment may be found where the physician intends to terminate the relationship without the patient's consent, but also where the court finds physician failure to attend the patient as frequently as due care-in-treatment would demand. Such failure denies that patient the benefit of the physician-patient relationship and is referred to as "constructive abandonment."

Abandonment may give rise to an action for either negligence or breach of contract.[101] If a patient is injured because the physician failed to see the patient often enough, or if the physician improperly concluded that the patient's condition required no further treatment, the patient has a cause of action in negligence alone.[102] In an action for negligence, the patient must present expert testimony; such testimony is not required in an action for breach of contract. The remedies vary, however, and negligence is the action generally preferred.

Because abandonment can occur only if there is a valid physician-patient relationship, it does not result if a physician permissively refuses to enter into such a relationship with a particular person.[103]

SPECIAL PROBLEMS IN THE PHYSICIAN-PATIENT RELATIONSHIP

How society perceives the physician-patient relationship is generally reflected in the law. During the past several years, both legislation and case law have tended to perceive the physician as being so able to bear the costs of compensation to injured patients that expansion of physician liability to provide for compensation to more patients is a justifiable public policy. Recent court decisions both support a conclusion that such expansion of physician liability is continuing and equally support a conclusion that the pendulum is beginning to swing in the opposite direction.

Supporting the idea that liability expansion is continuing is the series of cases discussed earlier with regard to COBRA and its extension beyond the situations that presumably led to its adoption, and recent cases in which physicians have been prosecuted under criminal statutes in circumstances that would once have been treated solely as civil professional negligence issues.[104] A case that appears initially to reduce a physician's right to exercise judgment in accepting patients for care, by permitting criminal prosecution for negligently exercising the option to refuse to accept a patient for care, is at the trial stage. The trial court refused to dismiss the indictment.[105]

Supporting the opposite point of view is a recent case in which a deceased patient's family brought suit against treating physicians on the theory that the physician's failure to inform the patient of his prognosis led him to engage optimistically in financial dealings that, due to his subsequent and early death, harmed his heirs.[106] The court declined to hold the physicians liable.

Additional complications have been introduced by the increased role of third-party payors in determining the care provided. In a situation where a third-party payor did not approve a physician's plan of treatment, and declined to pay for continued hospitalization, the court held that the third-party payor could be held liable when medically incorrect decisions resulted from institutional obstacles resulting from attempts to reduce costs. However the third-party payor escaped liability in the particular case[107] because the physician failed to press the patient's case with the payor; the physician was ultimately responsible. In a similar situation,[108] a patient committed suicide following discharge after the insurer declined to pay for further hospitalization. The appellate court reversed a summary judgment for the hospital and remanded for trial on the issue of whether the actions of the insurer led to the death.

An increased duty to treat is being imposed by some states as a condition of licensure. Such statutes modify the physician-patient relationship profoundly, but are outside the scope of this chapter.

CONCLUSION

Physician liability depends on the existence of a physician-patient relationship. Such a relationship may be explicit, implicit, or statutorily imposed. Numerous situations arise in our complex society, in which physician, patient, government, and third-party payor often interact in ill-defined ways, such that physician-patient relationships can arise by implication and without conscious physician intent. Physicians should be cautious in their statements and in their behavior to avoid

creating, contrary to their intentions, a relationship that imposes legal obligations. The legal obligation imposed is the requirement to exercise ordinary professional care in the discharge of professional duties. The plaintiff patient alleging malpractice must establish the existence of the physician-patient relationship, a breach of the duty created by that relationship, and the existence of an injury caused by the breach. Mere reasonable doubt as to these elements may subject the physician to all the financial, emotional, and psychic stress of a suit and its aftermath.

Proof of the elements stated, which requires a mere preponderance* of the evidence, will subject the physician to all of the above, and in addition will trigger National Practitioner Data Bank reports, and may precipitate disciplinary action. Caution is clearly indicated.

END NOTES

1. Attributed to Hippocrates, Greek physician, 4th century B.C.
2. A physician whose patient loses an eye under treatment has his own eye put out.
3. Hammurabi, Babylonian king, lived in the 27th century B.C., or roughly 4700 years before the publication of this work.
4. *Thomas v. Corso,* 265 Md. 84, 288 A.2d 379 (1972) (abandonment, no expert required).
5. *Pike v. Honsinger,* 155 N.Y. 201, 49 N.E. 760 (1898); *Greenstein v. Fornell,* 257 N.Y.S. 673 (1932) (physician not insurer).
6. *Viita v. Dolan,* 155 N.W. 1077 (Minn. 1916) (patient need not pay, physician duty remains).
7. *Kennedy v. Parrot,* 243 N.C. 355, 90 S.E.2d 754 (1956) (preference for tort law over contracts in "due care" situations).
8. *Childs v. Weis,* 440 S.W.2d 104 (Tex. 1969) (physician may arbitrarily refuse to render care to a nonpatient).
9. *Traveler's Ins. Co. v. Bergeron,* 25 F.2d 680, 49 S.Ct. 33 (1928) (relationship established when professional services accepted by another person for purposes of medical or surgical treatment).
10. *Findby v. Board of Supervisors,* 230 P.2d 526 (Ariz. 1951) (consensual relationship); *Brumbalow v. Fritz,* 183 Ga. App. 231, 358 S.E.2d 872 (1987) (patient refused advised admission, then was injured while leaving the emergency room. Suit against physician dismissed.).
11. *In re Estate of Bridges,* 41 Wash.2d 916, 253 P.2d 394 (1953) (physician not employee).
12. *Hoover v. Williamson,* 236 Md. 258, 203 A.2d 861 (1964) (services paid for by employer but duty to employee).
13. *Walters v. Rinker,* 520 N.E.2d 468 (Ind. Ct. App. 1988) (examination of tumor removed from patient establishes physician-patient relationship).
14. *Rule v. Cheeseman,* 181 Kan. 957, 317 P.2d 472 (1957) (radiologist's duty of care).
15. *Viita v. Dolan,* 155 N.W. 1077 (Minn. 1916) (not necessary for patient to know physician, engage his services, or pay for them in ordinary way).
16. *Betesh v. United States,* 400 F. Supp. 238 (D.C. 1974) (preinduction physical physician's recall of rejected examinee to check on progression of disease was sufficient act to indicate treatment).
17. *Kirschner v. Equitable Life Assurance Soc.,* 284 N.Y.S. 506 (1935) (defines "treatment").

---

*Meaning that the jury finds it more likely than not that the physician's action caused the patient's injury.

18. *Fleishman v. Richardson-Merrell, Inc.,* 266 A.2d 843 (N.J. 1969) (no duty to follow patient's progress once relationship terminated).

19. *Osborne v. Frazor,* 425 S.W.2d 768 (Tenn. 1968) (relationship by its terms may be general or limited).

20. *Markley v. Albany Medical Center,* 163 A.D.2d 639, 558 N.Y.S.2d 688 (1990) (duty may be limited to those medical functions undertaken by physician and relied on by patient).

21. *Sendjar v. Gonzalez,* 520 S.W.2d 476 (Texas 1975) (physician had right to refuse hospital calls).

22. *Hoover, supra* note 12 (no duty to nonpatient unless physician affirmatively acts).

23. *Hiser v. Randolph,* 617 P.2d 774 (Ariz. 1980), *overruled on other grounds,* 688 P.2d 605 (1988) (may refuse to treat patient).

24. *Childs, supra* note 8, (right of physician to refuse intoxicated patient); *Childers v. Frye,* 158 S.E. 744 (N.C. 1931) (may refuse to treat nonpatient); *Coss v. Spaulding,* 126 P. 468 (Utah 1912) (employed by third party to examine but also gratuitously advised thereby establishing a relationship).

25. 35 A.L.R. 3d 349 (failure to get consultation).

26. *Shoemaker v. Crawford,* 78 Ohio App. 3d 53, 603 N.E.2d 1114 (1991), *appeal denied,* 64 Ohio St. 3d 1434, 595 N.E.2d 943 (1992) (physician's admitted lack of experience in managing postoperative patient establishes negligence where that lack of experience was proximate cause of patient's injury).

27. 17 A.L.R. 4th 132 (physician-patient relationship for malpractice purposes).

28. 100 A.L.R. 3d 723 (patient contributorily negligent for failure to return).

29. *Truman v. Thomas,* 27 Cal. 3d 285, 611 P.2d 902, 165 Cal. Rptr. 308 (1980) (physician liable for failure to warn of consequences of refusing Pap smear).

30. *Rule v. Cheeseman,* 317 P.2d 472 (Kan. 1957) (neither relationship nor duty dependent on payment for physician services).

31. *Osborne, supra* note 19 (contractual relationship between physician and patient).

32. *Alexandridis v. Jewett,* 388 F.2d 829 (1968) (obstetrician breached contract when he did not deliver baby).

33. *Thor v. Superior Court,* 5 Cal. 4th 725, 855 P.2d 375, 21 Cal. Rptr. 357 (1993) (physician has no duty toward quadriplegic who refuses medically necessary feeding tube).

34. *Guilmet v. Campbell,* 385 Mich. 57, 188 N.W.2d 601 (1971) (physician's representations interpreted as guarantees); *Stewart v. Rudner,* 349 Mich. 459, 84 N.W.2d 816 (1957) (family practitioner breached contract by promising cesarean section that was not performed).

35. *Greenwald v. Grayson,* 189 So.2d 204 (Fla. 1966) (ability to recover in contract even though no negligence shown).

36. *Oliver v. Brock,* 342 So.2d 1 (Ala. 1976) (no obligation to practice or to accept professional employment).

37. *Osborne, supra* note 19.

38. *Ingber v. Kandler,* 128 A.D.2d 591, 513 N.Y.S.2d 11 (1987) (informal opinion offered without review of records or even knowledge of patient's name does not establish relationship).

39. *Grassis v. Retik,* 25 Mass. App. Ct. 595, 521 N.E.2d 411 (1988) (admitting resident not responsible for later negligence of treating physicians where resident had no further contact with patient).

40. *Hickey v. Travelers Ins Co.,* 158 A.D.2d 112, 558 N.Y.S.2d 554 (1990) (cause remanded for trial to determine whether physician was guilty of "negligent omission" for which apparently no liability would be imposed, or "negligent commission" for which liability would be imposed).

41. *Reed v. Gershweir,* 160 Ariz. 203, 772 P.2d 26 (Ct. App. 1989)

(physician not liable for malpractice of covering physician where reasonable care in selecting coverage was exercised).

42. *Alexandridis, supra* note 32 (obstetrician breached contract when resident delivered baby).

43. *Perna v. Pirozzi,* 457 A.2d 431 (N.J. 1983) (patient should be informed of substitution in advance).

44. *Baird v. National Health Foundation,* 144 S.W.2d 850 (Mo. 1940) (substitute physician cannot use other physician's negligence as an excuse for own actions).

45. *Bass v. Barksdale,* 671 S.W.2d 476 (Tenn. Ct. App. 1984) (covering physician signed prescription at request of primary physician).

46. *McKenna v. Cedars of Lebanon Hosp.,* 93 Cal. App. 282, 155 Cal. Rptr. 631 (1979) (malpractice action against resident physician for emergency care rendered to in-patient with whom resident had no prior contact—allowed protection of Good Samaritan statute); *Lethers v. Serrell,* 376 F. Supp. 983 (1979) (intern loses hospital's immunity because he did not function within strict interpretation of statute when he treated nonpatient).

47. *Smart v. Kansas City,* 105 S.W. 709 (1907) (clinical professor examined patient on ward; done with patient's knowledge, consent, and belief the purpose was for treatment—implied relationship).

48. *Rogers v. Horvath,* 65 Mich. App. 644, 237 N.W.2d 595 (1975) (no relationship—exam not conducted for patient's benefit).

49. *Perna, supra* note 43.

50. *Rainer v. Grossmen,* 31 Cal. App. 3d 539 (1973) (lecturing physician gave advice in response to question; no attempt to treat; no relationship).

51. *Pearson v. Norman,* 106 P.2d 361 (Colo. 1940) (license to practice does not require physician to accept all comers).

52. *Clough v. Lively,* 186 Ga. App. 415, 367 S.E.2d 295 (1988) (emergency room nurse checked patient's vital signs and drew blood alcohol at police request; patient died after transfer to jail; physician-patient relationship established by consent to draw blood).

53. *Hiser v. Randolph,* 617 P.2d 774 (Ariz. 1980) (assenting to hospital bylaws, which require participation in emergency room call, altered physician's right to refuse to treat a patient).

54. *Wilmington General Hosp. v. Manlove,* 54 Del. 15, 174 A.2d 135 (1961) (public reliance on hospitals to provide care).

55. *Fabran v. Matzko,* 236 Pa. Super. 267, 344 A.2d 569 (1975) (telephone contact insufficient to establish relationship).

56. *Hamil v. Bashline,* 224 Pa. Super. 407, 305 A.2d 57 (1973) (telephone contact constituted advice and treatment).

57. *Lyons v. Grether,* 218 Va. 630, 239 S.E.2d 103 (1977) (blind patient, staff refuses to permit entry with seeing eye dog, appointment to treat creates duty).

58. Council on Ethical and Judicial Affairs, American Medical Association. *Sexual misconduct in the practice of medicine.* 266 *JAMA* 2741-2745 (1991).

59. For example, Colo. Rev. Stat. Ann. 12-36-117(1)(r), Fla. Stat. Ann. 458.331(1)(j), Ariz. Rev. Stat. Ann. 32-1401(21)(z), Doering's Calif. Bus & Prof Code §756.

60. *Gromis v. Medical Board of California,* 8 Cal. App. 4th 589, 10 Cal. Rptr. 2d 452 (1992) (sexual interaction must breach professional duty in a way "substantially related to the qualifications, functions, or duties of the occupation for which a license was issued").

61. *New Mexico Physicians Mut. Liability Co. v. LaMure,* 116 N.M. 92, 860 P.2d 734 (1993) (insurance company not required to indemnify physician found liable in medical malpractice by jury for sexual misconduct with patient); *Patricia C. v. Mark D.,* 12 Ca. App. 4th 1211, 16 Cal. Rptr. 2d 71 (1993) (psychotherapist not liable in malpractice for sexual misconduct with patient).

62. *Lopspeich v. Chance Vought Aircraft,* 369 S.W.2d 705 (Tex. App. 1963) (employer has liability in *respondeat superior* to employee for physician's negligence; no physician-patient relationship); *Mrachek v. Sunshine Biscuit,* 308 N.Y. 116, 123 N.E.2d 801 (1954) (employer liability for acts of negligent physician; no physician-patient relationship).

63. *Lopspeich, supra* note 62 (no duty to employee except not to injure).

64. *Beadling v. Sirotta,* 41 N.J. 555, 197 A.2d 857 (1964) (preemployment exam, duty of reasonable care; not entitled to results of exam; is entitled to not be injured during exam).

65. *Fleishman, supra* note 18.

66. *Wilmington General Hosp., supra* note 54.

67. *Dowling v. Mutual Life Ins. Co. of N.Y.,* 168 So. 2d 107 (La. 1964) (prior relationship may impose duty).

68. *Keene v. Wiggins,* 69 Cal. App. 3d 308, 138 Cal. Rptr. 3 (1977) (voluntary care or attempt to treat or benefit worker creates a duty).

69. *Maltempo v. Cuthbert,* 504 F.2d 325 (5th Cir. 1974) (promise to parents to treat imprisoned son).

70. *Myers v. Quisenberry,* 144 Cal. App.3d 888, 193 Cal. Rptr. 733 (1983) (failure to warn diabetic of driving risk with missed abortion).

71. *Lemmon v. Freese,* 210 N.W.2d 576 (Ia. 1973) (liable for foreseeable injury to third party resulting from failure to warn patient of dangers of seizures).

72. *New Mexico Physicians, supra* note 61.

73. *Joseph v. Shafey,* 580 So. 2d 160 (Fla. 1991) (no duty or privity of contract between citizen shot by officer, and officer's physician).

74. *Wilschinsky v. Medina,* 108 N.M. 511, 775 P.2d 713 (1989) (physician's duty extends to members of the public who may be injured by sedated driver; the duty is met by warning the patient not to drive).

75. *Kaiser v. Suburban Transportation System,* 398 P.2d 14 (Wash. 1965) (failure to warn bus driver of sedating effect of decongestant).

76. *DiMarco v. Lynch Homes Chester County, Inc.,* 559 A.2d 530 (Pa. 1989) (injured third party relied on incorrect advice provided by physician to patient regarding communicability of hepatitis).

77. *Welke v. Copper,* 144 Mich. App. 245, 375 N.W.2d 403 (1985) (malpractice action allowed despite absence of physician-patient relationship).

78. *McElwain v. Van Beek,* 447 N.W.2d 442 (Minn. Ct. App. 1989) (the duty to warn third parties applies only to dangers arising from the patient).

79. *Duvall v. Goldin,* 363 N.W.2d 275 (Mich. 1984) (special relationship imposes duty on physician that benefits third party).

80. *Id.* (special relationship with dangerous person imposes a duty to warn public).

81. *Tarasoff v. Regents of the University of Calif.,* 17 Cal. 3d 425, 551 P.2d 344, 131 Cal. Rptr. 14, (1976) (failure to warn third party of known threat presented by patient).

82. *Thompson v. County of Alameda,* 27 Cal.3d 741, 614 P.2d 728, 167 Cal. Rptr. 70 (1980) (endangered third party not readily identifiable; no duty to warn); *Sellers v. United States,* 870 F.2d 1098 (6th Cir. 1989) (no duty to injured third party where in-patient psychiatric service had no knowledge of patient's harmful intent to a particular person).

83. *Peck v. Counseling Service of Addison County, Inc.,* 499 A.2d 422 (Vt. 1985) (duty to warn nonpatient third party of possible property damage).

84. *Supra* note 59.

85. *Hoover, supra* note 12, at 250 (relationship between physician and patient no matter who pays).

86. *Davis v. Tirrell,* 443 N.Y.S. 2d 136 (1981) (psychiatrist employed by school district to examine student and advise school district about handicap; no physician-patient relationship).

87. Council on Ethical and Judicial Affairs, *supra* note 58.

88. *Thiele v. Ortiz,* 165 Ill. App. 3d 983, 520 N.E.2d 881 (1988) (duty to evaluate possible complication of surgery 2 weeks postoperatively exists despite presence of other treating physicians).

89. *Peterson v. Phelps,* 123 Minn. 319, 143 N.W. 793 (1913) (termination of duties).

90. *Millbaugh v. Gilmore,* 30 Ohio St.2d 319, 285 N.E.2d 19 (1972) (patient's conduct terminated relationship).

91. *Brandt v. Grubin,* 131 N.J. Super. 182, 329 A.2d 82 (1972) (referral of psychiatric patient terminates duty).

92. *Hoemke v. New York Blood Center,* 720 F. Supp. 45 (SDNY 1989) (physician had no duty to contact past recipients of blood transfusions to warn them that they could be HIV infected and that they could spread the virus to others); *Boyer v. Smith,* 345 Pa. Super. 66, 497 A.2d 646 (1985) (no duty to contact past recipient of medications when new risks discovered).

93. *Tresemar v. Barke,* 86 Cal. App. 3d 656, 150 Cal. Rptr. 384 (1978) (physician required to notify patient of risks of Dalkon shield once such risks became known).

94. *Burnett v. Laymon,* 181 S.W. 157 (Tenn. 1915) (definition of reasonable notice dictated by circumstances of case).

95. *Groce v. Myers,* 224 N.C. 165, 29 S.E.2d 553 (1944) (reasonableness of notice).

96. *Miller v. Dore,* 154 Me. 363, 148 A.2d 692 (1959) (must notify with sufficient time for patient to find substitute).

97. *See* 99 A.L.R. 3d 303 (breach of contract).

98. *Collins v. Meeker,* 198 Kan. 390, 424 P.2d 488 (1967) (improper withdrawal from case).

99. *See Liability of Physician Who Abandons Case,* 57 A.L.R. 2d 432.

100. *Stohlman v. Davis,* 220 N.W. 247 (Neb. 1928); *Mucci v. Houghton,* 57 N.W. 305 (Iowa 1894); *Grace v. Myers,* 29 S.E.2d 553 (N.C. 1944) (abandonment defined).

101. *Chase v. Clinton County,* 217 N.W. 565 (Mich. 1928); *Alexandridis, supra* note 32 (causes of action in abandonment).

102. *Thomas v. Corso,* 265 Md. 84, 288 A.2d 379 (1972) (negligent care distinguished from abandonment).

103. *Easter v. Lexington Memorial Hosp.,* 303 N.C. 303, 278 S.E.2d 253 (1984) (physician-patient relationship required).

104. *State v. Warden,* 784 P.2d 1204 (Utah 1990) (state may prosecute physician for criminal negligence in death of infant, but evidence against physician insufficient for conviction); *People v. Holvey,* 205 Cal. App.3d 51, 252 Cal. Rptr. 335 (1988) (statute providing for criminal prosecution for "contributing to death of elderly dependent adult" is constitutional and applies to physicians; case remanded for trial).

105. *People v. Anyakora,* (N.Y. Cnty Sup Ct., Crim. Term, Part 58), N.Y.L.J. Dec 29, 1993, p. 22, col 1 (chief OB resident indicted both for failure to admit and for falsifying records used to justify refusal).

106. *Arato v. Avedon,* 5 Cal. 4th 1172, 858 P.2d 598, 23 Cal. Rptr. 2d 131 (1993) (physician duty does not extend to liability for inaccurate prognosis as to life expectancy).

107. *Wickline v. State,* 192 Cal. App. 3d 1630, 239 Cal. Rptr. 810 (1986) (physician has duty to advocate for his patient and to challenge inappropriate payor decisions).

108. *Wilson v. Blue Cross,* 222 Cal. App. 3d 660, 271 Cal. Rptr. 876 (1990) (insurer may be liable if refusal to pay for continued hospitalization was clearly contrary to informed medical opinion).

CHAPTER 22

Consent to and refusal of medical treatment

EMIDIO A. BIANCO, M.D., J.D., F.A.C.P., F.C.L.M.
HAROLD L. HIRSH, M.D., J.D., F.C.L.M.

TRADITIONAL CONSENT LAW
SCOPE OF CONSENT
CONSENT BY MINORS
CONSENT BY SPOUSE
CONSENT BY FAMILY MEMBERS
LEGAL DIMENSIONS
INFORMED CONSENT
SCOPE OF DISCLOSURE
PROGNOSIS
CONSENT FORMS
EMERGENCY CARE AND INFORMED CONSENT
CAUSES OF ACTION
EVIDENTIARY PROOF OF ADEQUATE DISCLOSURE
STATUTORY REQUIREMENTS AND DISCLOSURE
DEFENSES TO AN ACTION FOR A LACK OF INFORMED CONSENT
COUNSELING TIPS ON OBTAINING INFORMED CONSENT
A COMPETENT PATIENT'S RIGHT TO REFUSE TREATMENT
RIGHT TO REFUSE LIFESAVING TREATMENT IS NOT ABSOLUTE
REFUSAL OF CONSENT
INFORMED REFUSAL
PHANTOM PHYSICIAN
TESTS REQUESTED BY POLICE
SPECIAL SITUATIONS
CONCLUSION

It is a well-established rule that—absent a serious emergency—a physician must have the patient's consent to proposed treatment before that treatment can be initiated. Two theories of patient consent have evolved: the traditional consent to treatment theory grounded in the law of battery, and the more recent theory of informed consent grounded in the law of negligence. In some jurisdictions, lack of informed consent has been considered a tort in its own right even in the absence of negligence.[1,2] The law protects a person's right to make the decision to accept or reject treatment, whether that decision is wise or unwise.

It is a fundamental principle of our legal system that all persons have the right to make major decisions involving their bodies. The doctrine that a patient who is subject to medical treatment without consent has a cause of action against the physician or surgeon comes from two principles basic to our belief in the inalienable rights of man. The relationship between patient and physician is one known to the law as a "fiduciary relationship" (good faith and trusting). The other principle involved in the doctrine of the right to consent to medical treatment is that a person of sound mind has the right to make the decision about what becomes of his or her body. Neither the state nor another individual has the right to compel someone to accept treatment that he or she does not want.

TRADITIONAL CONSENT LAW

Traditional consent is an inherent aspect of the physician-patient relationship that physicians should clearly understand, not only as a matter of law but as a matter of medical ethics. Consent is either specifically expressed or implied by the surrounding circumstances.

The foundation of the traditional theory of consent to treatment lies in the law of battery and is found in court decisions as early as 1905.[3] Justice Cardozo articulated what has become perhaps the best-known statement of the principle in the 1914 New York case of *Schloendorff v. New York Hosp.*[4]: "Every human being of adult years and sound mind has a right to determine what shall be done with his own body: and a surgeon who performs an operation without his patient's consent commits an assault, for which he is liable in damages . . . ."*Schloendorff* represents the application, in a medical care setting, of the traditional battery law axiom that a person should be free from the physical interference of others. Justice Cardozo's statement is the hallmark of most appellate cases about consent, informed consent, or the right to refuse treatment.

Under the common law, a battery is deemed as an intentional touching of, or use of force upon, another person without the person's consent.[5] Any intentional and unauthorized touching, no matter how slight, may constitute a battery. Unauthorized medical care that may prove beneficial is just as much a battery as a sharp blow to the face. A successful plaintiff in a battery action may obtain punitive damages in addition to compensatory damages.

The expressed or implied consent of the person being touched vitiates the cause of action of battery. Valid consent of the person touched, therefore, is a complete defense to an action of battery.[6] However, an authorization of consent induced by misrepresentation, fraud, or duress is void and of no legal effect. Similarly, a consent may be invalid if the act consented to is unlawful[7] or the consent was given by one who had no legal authority to give it.[8]

Noteworthy is the fact that a battery can occur in the absence of hands-on contact; for example, the administration of medication, the application of X rays and sound waves, or any procedure under the physician's control that does not involve actual body contact. Where the aforementioned conduct occurs in the absence of consent, the courts will probably find a constructive touching that is sufficient for a battery.

To be liable for battery, a person must commit some positive and affirmative act that results in an unpermitted contact.[9] The element of personal indignity is given considerable weight; thus a person is liable not only for contacts that do actual physical harm, but also for those relatively trivial ones that are merely offensive and insulting, such as spitting in another's face, forcibly removing another's hat, or any contact brought about in a rude and insolent manner.[10] Expert medical testimony

is not required in a battery action. Because recovery may be based on the invasion of one's dignitary interest, one may recover from battery even in the absence of physical harm.[11]

Expressed consent

Expressed consent occurs when a patient specifically grants the physician permission to undertake the diagnosis and treatment of a specific problem. Expressed consent may be either in writing or by voice. Written permission creates less of a proof problem in court; vocal permission is legal, but may create a credibility problem in the legal arena.

Implied consent

Consent may be implied from the conduct of the patient in a particular case, or by the application of existing law in certain fact situations. A patient who voluntarily submits to treatment under circumstances that would indicate awareness of the planned treatment authorizes by implication the treatment, even without express consent. A patient who presents himself or herself at the doctor's office for a routine procedure implies his or her consent to treatment.

With the advent of informed consent, the courts have established two prerequisites for a finding of consent implied by a voluntary submission. First, the patient must have some comprehension of the nature of the proposed treatment and must be made aware of the common risks associated with it. Second, the patient must have an opportunity to withdraw from the proposed treatment. *A fortiori,* the same rules would apply to a surrogate with legal authority to consent for the patient.

Implied consent, particularly in the light of informed consent, is risky for physicians and should be relied on only for simple, routine procedures. To avoid the legal risks of implied consent, the physician should carefully document the circumstances of treatment in the patient's record, or document the explanation given the patient concerning the proposed treatment. Note, however, that there are many medical circumstances in which courts will readily find that consent was implied.

Under certain circumstances the law, either by court opinion or by statute, creates an implication of consent.[12] For example, the courts generally find implied consent in a medical emergency. Implied consent is frequently apparent; for example, by some manifestation, by an overt sign, or when the patient fails to object to being touched. In a classic case,[13] Ms. O'Brien brought suit against the steamship line because allegedly she was vaccinated against her will. She held up her arm to be vaccinated. The Massachusetts court found that O'Brien's behavior was such as to indicate consent on her part; thus, in determining whether she consented, the ship's doctor could be guided by her overt acts and manifestations of her feelings.

Some medical situations where implied consent is readily apparent include emergencies, the minor child who requires emergency care, comatose patients requiring immediate treatment, the mentally incompetent, the unavailability of a legal guardian, the intoxicated patient who temporarily lacks the capacity to reason (consent), or a patient who did not sign the consent form but nevertheless allowed treatment to proceed without objection.

SCOPE OF CONSENT

As a general rule, a physician commits a battery if he or she exceeds the scope of consent given by a patient. The problem usually occurs when a surgeon extends a surgical procedure beyond the limits previously discussed with the patient. If the surgeon performs the wrong procedure, clearly he or she is outside the scope of the patient's consent. If he or she performs the wrong procedure in addition to the one authorized by the patient, he or she may be liable for battery. Thus, a physician who performed a nonemergent hysterectomy when he found infected fallopian tubes during surgery on a patient who had consented only to a repair of a lacerated uterus was held liable.[14]

A prominent ear, nose, and throat (ENT) surgeon from St. Paul, Minnesota, advised his patient that she should have a polyp and diseased ossicles removed from her right ear, to which she consented.[15] While the patient was under anesthesia, the surgeon examined her left ear and found a more serious condition than that on the right. He concluded that the left, instead of the right, should have an ossiculectomy, which he performed. The patient filed an action for assault and battery, claiming that her ENT physician had exceeded the scope of her consent. The court observed that if, during the course of an operation, a physician should discover conditions not anticipated, and which, if not removed, would endanger the life or health of the patient, without expressed consent he would be justified in extending the operation in order to remove or palliate morbid disease. The Minnesota court stated that such was not the case at bar; permission to operate on the right ear was not permission to operate on the left ear.

Most jurisdictions have ruled that a physician may extend a procedure beyond the scope of consent to treat an emergency.[16] In many states, a surgeon may extend the surgery if he or she discovers an unexpected abnormal condition during the operation and if prompt treatment of it is reasonably advisable for the welfare of the patient.[17] If the patient authorizes a physician to remedy a condition rather than to perform a specific

procedure, the courts will generally allow the physician to render treatments reasonably necessary to correct the condition.[18] The patient's consent to one procedure does not imply consent to a prohibited extension of such procedure.[19]

CONSENT BY MINORS

The general rule of law is that a minor (age defined by the particular jurisdiction in which one resides) must obtain the consent of a parent or guardian before a physician may proceed with nonemergency treatment. Most jurisdictions have enacted exceptions, however, that allow a minor to consent to selected or limited medical care without the advice or consent of parents:

Minor consent exceptions
Married
Parent but unmarried
Statutory therapeutic exceptions
    chemical abuse
    VD
    contraception
    physical examination for rape
    abortion
    psychotherapy
Emergency

Most of the statutory exceptions are self-evident; however, the emergency medical situation deserves further consideration. Most physicians understand that where there is imminent danger of death without emergency treatment, consent will be implied. On the other hand, what reasonable action can a physician undertake when the medical circumstances require that the physician should anticipate the need to intervene in order to prevent an impending medical disaster? For example, a 14-year-old boy is brought to the emergency department for the evaluation and treatment of a displaced, compound comminuted fracture of the femur. The orthopedist quickly straightens the lower extremity to reduce the potential of permanent neurovascular damage. The patient requires treatment as soon as possible, but the clinical circumstances are not a matter of life or death. The first step is to comfort the patient. The second step is to use all reasonable means, with administrative assistance, to contact the parents. The third step is for the physician to make a reasonable medical judgment, in the best interest of the patient, as to how long one can reasonably wait before encountering a high risk of bone infection and/or neurovascular damage.

CONSENT BY SPOUSE

Consent to treatment by one spouse for the other spouse is not generally recognized by American law, even when the other spouse is incompetent, unless the spouse has been appointed legal guardian by a court of proper jurisdiction.

In a famous 1889 Maryland case,[20] Dr. Housekeeper was consulted by Mrs. Janney about a lump in her breast. Dr. Housekeeper advised a surgical operation, which was scheduled to be performed at her home. Accompanied by two other physicians, Dr. Housekeeper removed Mrs. Janney's right breast. Mr. Janney objected to the surgery stating that he did not consent to the excision of a cancer.

The Janney court simply ruled that the consent of the wife, not that of the husband, was necessary. The Janney decision was momentous because the Maryland Court of Appeals recognized the natural right of a woman to consent for medical treatment irrespective of her husband's wishes in the matter. Noteworthy is the fact that in 1889 a number of jurisdictions had restrictions on the ability of women to own property, to be administrators of their husbands' estates, or to vote.

In 1974, the Oklahoma Supreme Court reviewed a case[21] in which J. C. Murray, husband of Artie V. Murray, sued Dr. D. C. Vandevander, alleging that Dr. Vandevander performed a panhysterectomy on his wife without his consent. The question on appeal was whether a husband can recover from a physician and hospital for damage to a marital relationship resulting from an operation on his wife, consented to by her. The court stated that a married woman, even though living with her husband, has a statutory right to separate earnings and a natural right to her health, strength, skill, and capacity to earn, and that the natural right of a married woman to her health is not qualified by requiring that she have the consent of her husband in order to receive surgical care from a physician. The Oklahoma court cited *Janney v. Housekeeper* and ruled that a married woman in full possession of her faculties has power, without consent of her husband, to submit to a surgical operation upon herself. The husband has no inherent power to consent for his wife, nor does he have a right of refusal that can override his wife's consent to treatment.

In 1976, the U.S. Supreme Court reviewed the constitutionality of a Missouri statute on abortion, which among other things stated:

1. Before submitting to an abortion during the first 12 weeks of pregnancy, a woman must consent in writing to the procedure and certify that her consent is informed and freely given and is not the result of coercion.
2. A woman seeking an abortion must have the co-consent in writing of the spouse unless a licensed physician certifies that the abortion is necessary to preserve the mother's life.
3. An unmarried woman under age 18 must have the

written consent of a parent or person *in loco parentis*.

The court had no problem with the requirement that a woman receive informed consent prior to undergoing an abortion. Mr. Justice Blackmun delivered the opinion of the Court.[22] In *Roe v. Wade*,[23] the Supreme Court held that prior to approximately the end of the first trimester, the abortion decision and its effectuation must be left to the medical judgment of the pregnant woman's attending physician, and that subsequent to approximately the end of the first trimester, the state may regulate abortion procedure in ways reasonably related to maternal health, and at the stage subsequent to viability, the state may regulate and even proscribe abortion except where an abortion is deemed medically necessary for the preservation of the life or health of the mother.

Applying this reasoning to *Danforth*, Justice Blackmun, speaking for the Court, stated:

> The spousal consent provision . . . which does not comport with this standard enunciated in *Roe v. Wade* is unconstitutional, since the State cannot delegate to a spouse a veto power which the state itself is absolutely and totally prohibited from exercising during the first trimester of pregnancy. The state may not constitutionally impose a blanket parental consent requirement . . . as a condition for an unmarried minor's abortion during the first 12 weeks of her pregnancy for substantially the same reasons as in the case of the spousal consent provision.

In the absence of constitutionally acceptable legislation regulating spousal consent, *Janney* and *Murray* clearly state that the common law recognizes a person's natural right to consent for treatment, and that this natural right is not conditioned by marriage. In *Danforth*, the Supreme Court ruled that during the first 12 weeks of gestation, the requirement for a co-consent by the spouse or a parental consent for a minor was unconstitutional on the basis that a state cannot grant to a person veto power that the state itself does not possess.

Although a physician acting in the best interest of a patient may rely on the consent of the spouse of an unadjudicated incompetent patient, the consent of a competent patient's spouse is not a valid substitute for the consent of the patient. Nor is spousal consent a prerequisite for treatment of a competent patient, even if the treatment involves procedures that may affect the patient's marital relationship.[24] However, it is advisable to discuss thoroughly with patient and spouse any procedure that may compromise the patient's ability to reproduce or to perform sexually. Although the husband's consent is not required for artificial insemination of his wife, a husband who is not consulted and does not consent may not be liable for support of the resulting child, and a divorce may be based on adultery.[25] Because the welfare of the child resulting from artificial insemination may be at stake, the physician should not perform such a procedure without the consent of both husband and wife.

CONSENT BY FAMILY MEMBERS

For reasons similar to those cited in the three preceding cases, a family member's right to consent for another family member is not recognized by American law unless the family member is a legal guardian appointed by a court of proper jurisdiction or is the natural guardian of a minor child.[26] Karen Quinlan, approximately age 21 years, overdosed with phenobarbital and Librium. After it became apparent that she would not regain consciousness, her father, Joseph Quinlan, was appointed Karen's legal guardian and ordered the withdrawal of treatment, which her physicians refused to do. Eventually, the New Jersey Supreme Court ruled that Joe Quinlan, acting as Karen's legal guardian, could order the withdrawal of treatment and that such withdrawal of treatment would not be considered homicide, but rather the exercise of a legitimate consent right to refuse treatment in Karen's best interest.

LEGAL DIMENSIONS

At least three legal dimensions surround a person's right to self-determination. The first dimension involves the law of battery, which implies that any unpermitted contact or offensive touching is a personal indignity. The second dimension of modern consent law—informed consent—is concerned with whether a physician imparts that amount of information that a patient has a right to expect prior to making an intelligent, informed choice about whether to accept or reject medical recommendations. The third dimension of modern consent law is based on the right of privacy (right against the invasion of one's privacy). From a medical perspective, the right against the invasion of one's privacy is a doctrine that usually deals with the right of a patient to refuse lifesaving treatment. The Supreme Court found that the right of privacy was evident from the penumbras (shadows cast) formed by emanations from the Bill of Rights, specifically the First, Third, Fourth, Fifth, and Ninth Amendments.[27]

INFORMED CONSENT

The purpose of the doctrine of informed consent, implicit in its name, is to give the patient sufficient information so that he or she has the opportunity to make a knowledgeable and informed decision about the use of a drug or device in the course of treatment. It is part of the duty to warn the patient. The development of the doctrine of informed consent during the past two

decades is evidence of the recent enforcement of this duty to warn.

Informed consent implies joint decision making. The patient's right of self-decision can be effectively exercised only when the patient possesses enough information to enable an intelligent choice. Informed consent is a basic social policy for which exceptions are permitted where risk disclosure poses such a serious psychological threat or detriment to the patient as to be medically contraindicated.[28]

Physicians should be mindful of the fact that the legal doctrine of informed consent has very strong moral and ethical overtones. The AMA's first, second, and fifth Principles of Medical Ethics[29] imply the ethics of informed consent. According to the *American College of Physicians' Ethics Manual,* the patient should be informed and educated about his condition, should understand and approve of his treatment, and should participate responsibly in his own care.[30]

Whereas traditional consent emanates from the law of battery, the prevailing view is that treatment administered in the absence of informed consent is actionable under a negligence rather than a battery theory.[31] Because the doctrine of informed consent is grounded in the law of negligence, a physician's duty to disclose is more than a call to speak merely at the patient's request, or merely to answer the patient's question; it is a duty to volunteer, if necessary, that information needed by the patient to make intelligent decisions.[32]

Whether to disclose

Once the physician-patient relationship is established, the physician has a duty to inform the patient of his or her condition and of the presumptive diagnosis, differential diagnoses, purpose of tests, treatment, risks, alternatives, prognosis, and expectations.[33]

The physician should rarely, if ever, withhold material information, or pressure the patient into making a decision irrespective of the patient's personality makeup, or of any scientific or medical facts. The test for the sufficiency of disclosure is not the length of a catalogue of all information—it is the relevance of the information to the decision being made.

Materiality is the touchstone for determining the adequacy of the disclosure. There are numerous definitions and tests as to what constitutes materiality. In any such test, the crux of the issue is the effect of the nondisclosure on the patient's ability to make an intelligent choice, and as such each case presents the issue as a question of fact.

Elements of informed consent

Based on a number of appellate decisions about informed consent,[34,35] the following elements of informed consent should be understood by practicing physicians:

1. A physician should explain to the patient the nature of the procedure, treatment, or disease.
2. The patient should be informed about the expectations of the recommended treatment and the likelihood of success.
3. The patient should know what reasonable alternatives are available and what the probable outcome would be in the absence of any treatment.
4. The patient should be informed about the particular *known inherent risks* that are *material* to the informed decision about whether to accept or reject medical recommendations.

An inherent risk is one of a number of *known* adverse effects (or injuries) that may occur by the mere use of an indicated drug, or by the mere proper performance of a diagnostic procedure or a surgical operation. A material risk is a particular *inherent* risk a physician knows or ought to know would be significant to a reasonable person in the patient's position in deciding whether to reject or accept treatment.[36]

SCOPE OF DISCLOSURE

The scope and propriety of the disclosure depends on the state of medical knowledge at the time of the disclosure. When appropriate, the patient should also be informed of the identity and responsibility of other persons who will participate in the patient's care and management.

In Florida, pursuant to a civil rights statute, the legislature has determined that every competent adult has the fundamental right to control decisions relating to his or her own medical care, including decisions regarding the provision, withholding, or withdrawal of medical or surgical means or procedures calculated to prolong life.[37] Moreover, there is a recognized fiduciary, confidential physician-patient relationship in Florida that imposes on the physician the duty to disclose known facts.[38]

The limited number of jurisdictions that have specifically addressed this issue, absent extraordinary circumstances, have imposed a duty to inform a patient of an unfavorable diagnosis.[39] Some courts recognize the existence of a therapeutic privilege to withhold the diagnosis in certain situations.[40] In determining whether disclosure of an unfavorable diagnosis is required, the courts have considered such factors as the emotional status of the patient, particularly whether disclosure would seriously jeopardize the chances of recovery— even if slim.[41,42] However, in an ordinary case there would appear to be no justification for suppressing facts, and the physician should make a substantial disclosure to the patient or risk tort liability.[43] Although the *Current*

Opinions of the Judicial Council of the American Medical Association does not specifically mention the issue of unfavorable diagnosis, Opinion 8.11 provides[44]:

The physician must properly inform the patient of the diagnosis and of the nature and purpose of the treatment undertaken or prescribed. The physician may not refuse to inform the patient.

Moreover, a patient's right to know is not necessarily confined to a situation in which "disease is present and has been conclusively diagnosed."[45] In one recent case, a 37-year-old man had seen his doctor with symptoms of exertional chest pain of several weeks' duration, and his physician prescribed nitroglycerine therapy. The court found that the physician had a duty to inform the patient that he suspected coronary artery disease, despite inconclusive tests.[46]

Test results

The right to know also extends to test results. If an abnormal test has clinical significance, as in a Pap smear that may suggest malignancy, the physician is obligated to notify the patient of such a result. Mere failure to notify, in itself, is not actionable. If a physician has made reasonable notification attempts and the patient has related incomplete or misleading identifying information, the patient's negligence might relieve the doctor from liability for the failure to disclose significant test results.[47]

Risks

The disclosure must be viewed in the context of anticipated risks that fall within the expertise of the physician. Discretion consistent with this expertise is greater where the risk of adverse result is relatively slight. Similarly, a full disclosure is not required where the disclosure of all risks would be impractical for therapeutic reasons.

A certain minute incidence of idiosyncratic allergic reactions and unexpected deaths have occurred in nearly all treatments and surgeries, and full disclosure of these unexpected risks has not been required. A minority view holds that all risks potentially affecting the patient's decision should be disclosed.

Complicated medical problems and treatments usually carry more risks and require a more complete explanation.

When a physician wishes to treat a patient's complaint by a method that entails certain definite risks, and knows that a safer alternative treatment exists, the physician is obliged to advise the patient to that effect. As the probability or severity of risk to the patient increases, the physician's duty to inform increases.

When a physician does not wish to perform a procedure that interests the patient because he or she is not entirely convinced that it is the best or safest approach, as long as respectable medical opinion would consider it acceptable, the physician should at least tell the patient that the treatment is available elsewhere, and help the patient contact those who do perform it.

Alternatives

The physician's duty of disclosure has been held to encompass alternative modes of diagnosis and treatment. In other words, there is a duty to apprise the patient of those procedures that represent feasible alternatives to the method initially selected. He or she has a duty to explain available alternatives, and to brief the patient as to the significant pros, cons, disadvantages, and dangers. Physicians should attempt to "walk in the patient's shoes" and consider the patient's hobbies, occupation, and the actual incidence of risks.

An archetypal case involving informed consent would be the treatment of hyperthyroidism. Three modes of treatment are still in vogue — drug therapy, radioactive iodine, and subtotal thyroidectomy. The material risks of drug therapy are a recurrence of hyperthyroidism (up to 72% of patients) and agranulocytosis (less than 1% of patients). The once-feared adverse affect of developing thyroid tumors in later years has not proved to be more likely to develop in radioactive-treated patients than in patients from a randomly selected population; however, the incidence of postradioactive hypothyroidism at 10 years ranges from 40% to 70%.[48] Laryngeal nerve injuries are a well-known risk of thyroidectomy that cause hoarseness. Consequences of superior laryngeal nerve injury are more subtle than recurrent laryngeal injury because vocal cord failure usually does not occur until after protracted use of the voice for approximately 60 minutes, such as opera singing.[49] The most famous case illustrating this point is that of Amelita Galli-Curci, one of the world's great lyrics sopranos of the 1920s whose voice would inevitably fail during the last act of an opera.[50] Vocal cord failure is an inherent material risk of subtotal thyroidectomy that should be disclosed, not only to persons such as Placido Domingo and Luciano Pavarotti, but to anyone, because the "loss of voice" is a devastating injury.

Referrals/consultations

The duty to refer a patient to a specialist is most often imposed on general medicine practitioners. Under some circumstances, however, courts may impose a duty on a specialist to refer the patient to a subspecialist if a higher degree of skill and training is necessary in the management of the patient.[51] An illustrative case is *Logan v. Greenwich Hosp. Ass'n.*[52] In this case an internist suggested that a patient suffering from systemic lupus erythematosus undergo a kidney biopsy to determine the extent of the disease of her kidneys. Following referral to a urologist, the biopsy was performed, but the procedure was complicated by a punctured gall bladder, requiring cholecystectomy.

The court agreed with the plaintiff's contention that the urologist, as the specialist who would perform the procedure, had a duty to disclose all viable alternatives to the method selected, regardless of whether such alternatives might prove more hazardous.[53] The referring internist was found to have reasonably relied on his colleague, a specialist in such matters, to present all viable alternatives.

Similarly, if a physician is not qualified to render necessary treatment, he or she bears a duty to advise the patient to consult an appropriate specialist who can provide the therapy.[54] The physician's duty to consult arises when he or she knows, or reasonably should know, that he or she does not possess the required knowledge and skill to treat the condition.[55] Some courts have held that this duty arises when a physician realizes that a method of therapy is ineffective and alternative modes of treatment are available.[56]

PROGNOSIS

Patients are entitled to know the full prognosis, knowledge of all the complications, sequelae, discomforts, cost, inconveniences, and risks of each option, including no treatment or no action. Patients have a right to know what to expect and what might happen to them. All of this is predicated on the reasonable foreseeability of the events by the physician. Rare or exotic events are not part of informed consent.

Disclosure standards developed by courts

Two approaches have been adopted by the courts in delineating the scope of the physician's disclosure obligation — the professional disclosure standard and the general disclosure standard, or reasonable patient standard.

Under the professional disclosure standard, a physician's duty to disclose is governed by the standard of the reasonable medical practitioner, practicing under the same or similar circumstances. This disclosure standard that is set forth either by statute or common law in a majority of U.S. jurisdictions requires that the physician shall disclose information according to the prevailing standard of care, as established through expert medical testimony. Many courts have established the standard of the reasonably careful medical practitioner in the same or similar community, under the same or similar circumstances. Whether the physician has the duty to disclose facts and, if so, what facts he or she is obliged to reveal largely depends on the usual and customary practice in the local community.

The general or reasonable patient disclosure standard, which is set forth by stature or common law in a significant minority of jurisdictions, imposes a duty on the part of the physician to disclose any information that would reasonably bear on the patient's decision-making process. It should be tailored to the ability of the patient to comprehend. Even in the face of supportive expert medical testimony, a physician may be found to have breached the proper disclosure standard in these jurisdictions if a jury were to conclude that specific information that was not disclosed would have influenced significantly the reasonable patient's decision whether to undergo a particular form of therapy or treatment. The general standard permits the jury to decide whether the physician disclosed enough information for a reasonable patient to make an informed choice about treatment, whereas the professional standard permits physicians to testify whether the physician-defendant disclosed sufficient information, according to community standards of medical practice. The modern trend is for courts to adopt the general standard.

Once it has been established, either by professional or general standard, that a patient did not receive the information that is usually needed to make an informed intelligent choice about whether to refuse or consent to treatment, the court will be interested in the materiality of the lacking information; that is, would a reasonable person have refused or consented under the same or similar circumstances? In other words, did lack of informed consent cause the alleged injury, or would the patient have consented in any event? Depending on the jurisdiction involved, courts have applied one of two standards; that is, the objective standard (the jury decides whether a reasonable patient in the patient's shoes would have refused treatment) or the subjective standard (the jury decides whether the actual patient would have refused treatment). (See the sections about the "but for" rule and burden of proof.)

Most jurisdictions follow an objective standard for the determination of materiality of the risk that requires a determination as to whether a reasonably prudent person in the patient's condition would have given consent had the nondisclosed risk been known.

Who discloses?

Who is responsible for obtaining the patient's informed consent?[57] The courts generally have placed the duty on the patient's attending physician at the time in question.[58,59] The courts generally recognize that the physician, not a nurse or other health care provider, is best qualified to discuss care and management. The nurse or other provider may only supplement or comple-

ment the physician's specific information with general information regarding the patient's situation. A substitute physician covering for the patient's original physician has an independent obligation to inform the patient of risks, benefits, and alternatives to the part of the treatment that he or she is to administer.

Courts are eminently clear in their written opinions that the responsibility to obtain informed consent from a patient clearly remains with the physician, and this responsibility cannot be delegated. The physician *may delegate authority* to obtain informed consent to another physician, but *cannot delegate his or her responsibility* for obtaining a proper informed consent.

Hospital role

A question that frequently arises, particularly for those practicing in a hospital setting, is "Does the hospital have a responsibility to assure that the patient received adequate disclosure even though the courts have placed the primary duty into the physician's hands?"[60]

Under the theory of *respondeat superior,* an employer hospital could be held jointly liable with an employee physician whose failure to obtain informed consent can be shown to have caused injury and damage to a patient. A hospital policy must exist that governs the procedure under which consents are obtained, deviation from which is admissible evidence.[61] Hospital liability can arise when the hospital knew or should have known that the physician did not obtain the patient's informed consent, or for failure to prevent surgery or other treatment from proceeding without the informed consent of the patient. Nurses or other hospital personnel need to delay planned physician treatment if consent previously given is withdrawn by the patient, so that the physician can clarify the patient's decision. Courts tend to impose stricter obligations on hospitals to ensure that physicians obtain consent before performing a procedure. With a nurse acting as its agent, a hospital should monitor that consent has been obtained.

CONSENT FORMS

Hospitals have the duty to assure that informed consent is properly obtained.[62] One court called a hospital's failure to assure that informed consent was properly obtained a "fraudulent concealment."[63]

A patient who consents to surgery by a specific surgeon and is operated on by another surgeon can successfully sue the surgeon who did not operate for malpractice, based on lack of informed consent, and can sue the operating surgeon for battery.[64] One court has allowed recovery on a claim of unnecessary surgery, based on lack of informed consent.[65]

A consent form is not essential, but may be helpful in

establishing at trial that consent was obtained; however, it is not determinative of the issue. The mere signing of a written consent form constitutes only some evidence of a valid consent; the consent must be based on all the elements of true informed consent: knowledge, voluntariness, and competency.

General-purpose consent forms that allow for specific information to be inserted can also be used for numerous procedures and treatments. Most states prohibit by statute or by common law any provisions under which the patient releases in writing the physician and/or hospital from prospective liability that arises from actions or inactions involving the patient's medical care.

Some hospitals and many physicians have developed consent forms that summarize such information and also constitute a permanent record, usually in the patient's medical chart, of the communication between physician and patient. Formats vary considerably according to the treatment setting and particular procedures involved. The American Medical Association (AMA) and other organizations have published consent form manuals that provide sample forms.[66] Witnesses and signed permits are not required; however, a witnessed form is an attestation that an informed consent session took place (however, it is not an attestation that the patient necessarily received adequate disclosure). Even well-drawn consent forms may not prevent allegations of failure to obtain consent in cases involving complex or high-risk treatment.[67] Adequate informed consent is best established by an accurate narrative documentation by the attending physician.[68]

Authority to give consent

Adults are presumed competent and therefore must consent to proposed treatment. An incompetent adult patient who is incapacitated by physical or mental illness and is unable to understand the nature and consequences of his or her actions cannot give a valid informed consent to proposed treatment. As a result, consent must be obtained from someone who is authorized to consent on behalf of the patient. The same is true for minors who, in most instances, lack the legal capacity to consent. Where a court has adjudicated the patient to be incompetent, the patient's court-appointed guardian or conservator must authorize the treatment proposed for the patient. If the physician has determined that the patient is incapable of comprehending the nature and consequences of his or her conduct, but the patient has not been judged incompetent, most courts may decide to accept the consent of the patient's next-of-kin—the closest known relative. In such cases, the guardian or relative is viewed by the courts as standing in the shoes of the patient.

Substituted consent gives rise to a number of problems. The authority of one to consent to treatment for an incompetent patient necessarily implies the right to refuse such treatment. However, the courts have restricted this right of refusal in cases in which consent was unreasonably withheld.[69] In such cases, the physician or hospital may treat the case as an emergency and seek a court order authorizing the necessary treatment. Two issues must be considered: (1) Is there a demonstrable need to proceed before the patient will be able to consider the matter, assuming he or she will become lucid? (2) Is the proposed treatment appropriate for the patient's condition? If there is not time to seek a court order, it is wise for the physician to consult with one or more colleagues and document their concurrence with the proposed therapeutic measures and the need to proceed with the treatment.[70]

If the patient's next-of-kin disagrees with the proposed treatment, or if the patient, although incompetent, takes a position contrary to the family's wishes, the physician must be extremely cautious. There is some indication that the courts will consider the wishes of the patient, even though he or she may be unable to give valid consent.[71] In most cases, it is best to proceed quickly with treatment (1) if a near relative has consented, (2) if it is medically necessary to proceed quickly with treatment, and (3) if there is no applicable prohibitive statute.[72]

The best way to avoid the legal risks of substituted consent for an incompetent adult patient is to place the matter before a court. In most states, any adult citizen of the state, including a near relative of the patient, may petition the court to establish a conservator or guardian of the patient.[73]

Ability to consent

Consent must be given by a patient who is mentally and physically capable of comprehending the information provided by the physician during the dialogue and capable of making a decision concerning the course of treatment. The physical effects of pain or medication must not be so great as to diminish the patient's mental abilities to comprehend the consent process. The fact that the patient is suffering from mental illness or transitory episodes of nonlucidity does not necessarily vitiate the mental capacity to consent to treatment. The mere fact that the patient refuses diagnosis or treatment does not reflect lack of mental capacity to consent to treatment. Coercion must not be used to induce consent. Those patients lacking mental capacity to give informed consent need the consent of a surrogate, usually a close family member or guardian to provide substituted consent.

In the absence of a court-appointed guardian, a third party may be empowered to act on behalf of a principal under the terms of a written power of attorney. Such a document confers authority on a third party to handle specific personal or financial matters on behalf of the principal. In recent years, these documents have been used to permit a third party to make health care decisions on behalf of a principal who has become functionally incompetent. Under numerous state statutes, these powers of attorney are legally effective until there has been a judicial declaration of incompetence or disability. Case law and statutory law do not generally mandate appointment of guardians to provide consent, where interested family members of the patient are available to provide consent for routine day-to-day procedures. No decisions have been reported wherein physicians or hospitals have been found liable for not resorting to court processes to obtain consent to treatment. However, certain types of patients and types of procedures will usually require the appointment and consent of a guardian under the statutes of certain jurisdictions, such as sterilization of a mentally incompetent patient. These statutes must be consulted before unusual procedures such as sterilization, electroconvulsive therapy, psychosurgery, or investigational treatment are undertaken.

The physician whose patient has already received the appointment of a guardian needs to obtain the informed consent of the guardian through the same process of dialogue that the physician would have had with the patient, if competent. Where no guardian for the incompetent patient has been previously appointed by the court, the physician's decision whether to obtain informed consent for nonemergency diagnosis or treatment from family or from a court-appointed guardian will depend on the policy of the hospital.

In most states where the patient is incompetent, the spouse may give consent for the patient in emergency and certain nonemergency situations (custodial medical care). Children, grandchildren, parents, grandparents, siblings, nieces or nephews, or cousins, however, may or may not legally give consent for incompetent patients in medical matters, and court proceedings to designate a guardian may be necessary. In some situations where there is a difference of opinion among family members regarding a patient's care or family members are distant emotionally or geographically, formal legal proceedings may be advisable to determine who can give consent for the incompetent patient.

An exception to the requirement of informed consent is recognized when the patient is incompetent and the procedure contemplated is more of a routine, remedial measure. For example, daily custodial care of incompetent institutionalized psychiatric patients is excepted. However, if informed consent would be required for a specific treatment, for example, the administration of electroconvulsive therapy, the consent of a guardian or appointed substitute decision-maker is required. If the physician has determined that a patient is incapable of comprehending the nature and consequences of his or her conduct, but the patient has not been judged legally incompetent, most courts will accept the consent of the patient's next-of-kin.

Exceptions to material disclosure

There are four generally recognized exceptions to the physician's duty to make prior disclosure of material risks, although all four might not necessarily be available in a particular state.

First, a physician may, in his or her professional judgment, conclude that disclosure of a risk poses such a threat of detriment to the patient that it is contraindicated from a medical point of view. This is known as the "therapeutic privilege" or "professional discretion."[74] The physician may choose to use therapeutic professional discretion to keep medical facts from the patient or surrogate when the physician believes disclosure would be harmful, dangerous, or injurious to the patient. Depending on the circumstances, the physician may,[75] but need not, make the revelations to the next-of-kin.[76]

Second, a competent patient may specifically ask not to be informed.[77] A patient may waive his or her right to make an informed consent.

Third, a physician is privileged not to advise the patient of matters that are common knowledge or of which the patient has actual knowledge, particularly on the basis of past experience.[78]

Fourth, no duty to inform arises in an emergency in which the patient is unconscious or otherwise incapable of giving valid consent, and harm from failure to treat is imminent and outweighs any harm threatened by the proposed treatment.[79]

Opinion 8.07 of the AMA *Current Opinions of the Judicial Counsel*,[80] regarding informed consent, could justify, by analogy, exercising therapeutic privilege by withholding grave prognostic information on the same basis as withholding information regarding risks of treatment.

EMERGENCY CARE AND INFORMED CONSENT

Generally, the law implies patient consent during emergency situations.[81] The courts generally hold that conditions requiring immediate treatment for the protection of the patient's life or health justify the implication of consent if it is impossible to obtain express consent either from the patient or from one who is authorized to consent on his or her behalf.[82] The courts simply assume that a competent, lucid adult would consent to lifesaving treatment. It is essential to document the circumstances that created the emergency.[83] In such cases, the physician must document the following facts: (1) The treatment was for the patient's benefit,[84] (2) an actual emergency existed,[85] and (3) there was an inability to obtain the express consent of the patient or someone authorized to consent on his or her behalf.[86] An emergency is defined as a condition in which there is an immediate threat to the life, person, or health of the patient, and the hazard to the patient will increase without immediate treatment.[87]

The fact that the proposed treatment may be medically advisable, or may become essential at some future time, is not sufficient to allow nonconsensual treatment.[88] If the physician is uncertain whether the patient's condition warrants immediate action without consent, he or she should seek confirmation of the emergency from a colleague. In one case, the court, deciding in favor of the treating physician, relied heavily on the fact that the treating physician had obtained concurring consultations from four surgeons before amputating the patient's crushed foot after a train accident.[89] Generally, the courts have decided in favor of the physician in cases in which immediate treatment was necessary to eliminate an imminent threat of death or harm to the patient.

The general rule concerning consent for emergency treatment applies to the treatment of minors as well as adults.[90] The courts have consistently held in favor of physicians who have treated "mature" minors (usually over the age of 15) who have consented to their own emergency treatment.[91] The courts tend to favor any medical or surgical treatment that is necessary to prevent serious injury to or impairment of the health of a child. However, in any case involving emergency treatment of a minor, it is prudent to make and document an effort to contact the minor patient's parents or legally responsible person.

CAUSES OF ACTION

Conceptually, informed consent merges into and derives from the following:

- Assault and battery
- Negligence involving the duty to disclose
- Simply the tort of lack of informed consent
- The ethical and legal respect for dignity, autonomy, and life.

The early and even some later cases involving patient consent spoke almost exclusively of battery and were concerned with a physician's intentional, unauthorized touching of the patient.[92] A few of the early cases, however, raised the question of whether the action for failure to obtain patient consent ought properly to lie in negligence, rather than battery.[93] In 1957, the California Supreme Court held that an action arising from a physician's failure to give a patient sufficient information

to make an informed decision should sound in negligence, not battery.[94] The court held that a physician violates his duty to his patient and subjects himself to liability if he withholds any facts necessary to form the basis of an intelligent consent. Courts now appear to agree that negligence is the proper cause of action for failure to inform a patient properly about a procedure for which consent is sought.[95] Actions grounded in battery are still found, but usually involve cases in which (1) the patient consented to one procedure, and another was actually performed,[96] (2) the physician failed to disclose a disability that was certain to result from a proposed nonemergency procedure,[97] (3) the physician performed an experimental procedure without advising the patient of its experimental nature.[98]

An increasing number of courts allow the jury to determine whether the physician withheld information necessary to form a reasonable and intelligent decision about proposed treatment. Some courts require no expert testimony,[99] but others allow expert testimony on the question of the materiality of the information withheld and whether the alleged injury is related to the therapeutic or diagnostic process.[100] Depending on the jurisdiction, one of two tests is used by the jury when determining whether the plaintiff/patient would have refused treatment: (1) The subjective test, which requires the jury to ascertain whether the actual patient would have refused, and (2) the objective test, which requires the jury to ascertain whether a reasonable person standing in the patient's shoes would have refused treatment. The fact that the injury has occurred often will color the jury's finding. Courts have recognized this problem.[101]

The ever-present and difficult question for physicians is how much information is legally sufficient? The courts have attempted to give the medical profession some guidance. In *Cobbs v. Grant*,[102] the California Supreme Court stated further that a "lengthy polysyllabic discourse on all possible complications" or a "mini-course of medical science" is not required.

Another view is found in *Canterbury v. Spence,* in which the court stated[103].

The scope of the physician's communication to the patient must be measured by the patient's need, and that need is the information material to the decision. Thus the test for determining whether a particular peril must be divulged is its materiality to the patient's decision: all risks potentially affecting the decision must be unmasked. And to safeguard the patient's interest in achieving his own determination on treatment, the law must itself set the standard for adequate disclosure.

In *Canterbury,* the physician was held liable for failure to divulge a 1% risk of paralysis associated with a laminectomy. The court stressed the serious nature of the undisclosed risk rather than the mathematical possibility of its occurrence.

Numerous courts,[104,105] following the *Canterbury* decision, have followed the reasonable patient standard, but in general the states are pretty much split between the two standards, with a few jurisdictions adopting hybrids of one or the other test.

EVIDENTIARY PROOF OF ADEQUATE DISCLOSURE

Written documentation of the informed consent is of key importance for both parties should litigation later arise. The weight to be accorded to such documentary evidence versus a mere oral consent is a question for the trier of fact. However, a written consent form signed by the patient often provides strong documentary evidence, which, in at least one state, forms a rebuttable presumption that valid consent was obtained. It may be necessary to establish the time, location, and persons present; the content of the dialogue; and the treatment authorized. Much of this information may be contained within the actual consent form, if it is signed by the patient. The evidentiary value of a written consent form that is signed by the patient depends on the specificity of the information in the form viewed in conjunction with the discussions between the physician and the patient. Therefore, standing alone, the form may be insufficient to prove consent. However, any such question of the effect of the form is a factual issue to be determined by the fact-finder.[106] Where the form only speaks in general terms and fails to comply with the relevant statutory provisions requiring specificity, additional evidence is necessary to establish the validity of the consent.

Consent forms and physicians' progress notes should include a statement by the physician which explains that the patient was capable of understanding the nature of his or her physical condition and the proposed diagnostic or therapeutic procedures, and was also capable of understanding the risks of proceeding with the proposal, not proceeding with the proposal, or proceeding with alternative diagnostic or therapeutic procedures. Such statements often contain the acknowledgment that the physician answered all of the patient's questions. The signing of a blank consent form will not support a finding of informed consent. Informed consent will also not be found where the signor is functionally illiterate and there is no indicia that a proper disclosure has been made. It should be noted that an informed consent statute codifies that there is a presumption of validity where there is a written signed consent form.

In handling issues relating to instructions or informed consent in the medical record, any language limitations should be noted as should attempts to work with translators. Notations should be made concerning literature provided to the patient or his or her representative. Notations are necessary to confirm that copies of instructions were relayed to the patient and any failure to comply with the instructions as well as confirmation that the patient was informed of risks of noncompliance should be noted.

Burden of proof

In a medical malpractice case, injury is alleged to have occurred as the result of a treatment error or omission.[107] In the informed consent context, however, litigation may be initiated even where there has been no treatment error or omission, e.g., where treatment that entails foreseeable material risks causes injury. The patient is thus heard to complain not that the treatment was negligently provided, but that had there been full disclosure of the material risks or available alternatives, the patient would not have undergone the treatment and thus would not have been injured (the "but for" rule). As in other medical malpractice cases, it is essential for the plaintiff in an informed consent action to establish that the harm or injury suffered is the proximate result of a breach of duty or violation of the standard of care. When a patient does not receive enough material information to make an informed decision, and is subsequently injured, the patient could successfully sue the physician, even when traditional consent was obtained and the physician's performance was flawless. Noteworthy is the fact that the patient must show that the lack of informed consent (failure to receive sufficient information) was the *cause* of the injury.

"But for" rule

As to proximate cause using a lack of consent tort analysis, the patient must show that an undisclosed risk caused the injury, in the sense that the injury would not have occurred but for the consent that would have been withheld had the patient known of the risk, because if he or she had known, there would have been no consent given[108] (see Chapter 12 on medical malpractice and physician as defendant).

Depending on the jurisdiction involved, courts have taken at least two different approaches in determining whether a lack of informed consent caused an injury: The subjective standard; that is, would the actual patient have refused to consent had the alleged lack of information been disclosed, or the objective standard; that is, would a reasonably prudent person in the same or similar community and circumstances have refused to consent. From a practical point of view, irrespective of which standard is applied, the jury decides whether the patient would have refused treatment if the physician had imparted the alleged missing information.

Knowledge about the varied medical risks that are inherent to the practice of medicine is ordinarily outside the knowledge of layman, and therefore requires the introduction of expert testimony. The expert witness must set forth in testimony that the claimed injury was a result of the diagnosis and treatment, and that the injury is a *known* inherent risk of the treatment that had been rendered. Obviously, if the risk was not a known inherent risk, or there is no medically scientific relationship of the risk to the alleged injury, a lack of informed consent could not have caused the claimed injury.[109] With either standard, the patient has to proffer testimony that would convince a jury that the treatment would have been refused if the withheld information had been received. In those jurisdictions in which a subjective standard is applicable the law requires that the materiality of the nondisclosure to an informed decision be viewed solely from the point of view of the particular patient; in other words, the materiality of a risk to a reasonably prudent person in the patient's shoes cannot be considered.[110]

STATUTORY REQUIREMENTS AND DISCLOSURE

The analysis of any disclosure issue necessarily includes an examination of any statutes of the jurisdiction in which the patient was treated regarding statutory requirements (or exceptions) of adequate disclosure.[111] In some states the duty of obtaining informed consent is codified, giving rise to an additional negligence action for violation of statute.[112] These statutes frequently provide that the health care provider is obligated to inform the patient of the common risks and reasonable alternatives to the proposed treatment or procedure, and that but for failure the claimant would not have consented to the proposed treatment or procedure.

Particular attention must be paid to any statute wherein the risks required to be disclosed are defined by an administrative agency of the executive branch. Disclosure by the physician of such defined risks provides a rebuttable presumption that an adequate disclosure was made by the physician. In at least one state (Hawaii) a physician is not required to explain the realm of potential risks and complications associated with the proposed treatment because by statute the physician is only required to explain the intended result of the treatment.

DEFENSES TO AN ACTION FOR A LACK OF INFORMED CONSENT

One of the best and most cogent defenses against a lack of informed consent is a documented counseling session. The collective experience of the medical profession indicates that many patients forget or misinterpret what physicians say during an informed consent session. There is no question that documentation enhances physician credibility. The note need not be in great detail, but should be a convincing statement that the patient received informed consent.

A second defense may involve the lack of immediate capacity for the person to consent, for example, coma, transitory intoxication, psychosis, or being a minor (who may be competent but lacks the legal capacity to consent). One would not expect informed consent to be an issue during a medical emergency. A third defense involves the "So what!" defense. When asserting the "So what!" defense, the court will give the physician an opportunity to contend that even if his or her patient had been informed of the risk at issue, the patient would have consented to treatment. For example, an intravenous pyelogram (IVP) is of special importance in examining the integrity of the kidney and ureter after blunt or penetrating abdominal trauma.[113,114] A patient who has just sustained severe abdominal trauma undergoes an IVP and subsequently dies from an anaphylactic reaction despite appropriate treatment. The spouse files a lawsuit for a lack of informed consent, alleging that if the decedent had been informed about the approximately 1:50,000 chance of dying from an IVP, more likely than not he or she would have refused the procedure. Applying the "So what!" defense, the physician would argue that even if the decedent had been told about the risk of an IVP, he or she would have consented nevertheless, because the immediate risk of dying from renal trauma far outweighed any very rare risk of death from the IVP.

The *unduly alarming defense* provides the defendant physician with an opportunity to contend that material information was withheld because he or she was acting in the patient's best interest. Acceptance of the unduly alarming defense by a jury would depend on a physician's ability to establish a credible knowledge of the patient's emotional character. The unduly alarming defense has become somewhat sophisticated in terminology by placing it under the rubric of "therapeutic privilege." The physician must prove that he or she exercised the "therapeutic privilege" in the best interest of the patient; otherwise, the patient would have refused necessary and effective treatment and/or would have deleterious effects on the patient's well-being.

Assumption of risk

The doctrine of "assumption of risk" means that the patient understands the possibility of all risks of untoward unpreventable results of either treatment or no treatment, and knowingly consents to the course selected.[115] Where it applies, this is usually a good defense to an action for negligence. Note that this doctrine is related to the doctrine of informed consent and refusal.

A signed consent form or a note in the chart made contemporaneously with the event is presumptive evidence that a valid consent has been obtained. That presumption may be rebutted by the patient if the patient can demonstrate that the quality of the consent was faulted. For example:

- The language was too technical.
- The physician's manner was hostile, antagonistic, pontifical, or condescending.
- The patient was emotionally distressed.
- The patient was sedated.
- There was no time for contemplation and consultation.

There are several statutory defenses to informed consent:

- The patient does not want to be informed or would have undergone the procedure anyway, in at least 12 states.
- The known risks are so commonly appreciated or the risk is too remote a possibility to be substantiated, in 8 states.
- Therapeutic privilege is present in at least 10 states. It prevails when the physician wishes to avoid a substantial adverse impact on, or detriment to, the patient's health.
- An emergency or other compelling circumstances, in at least 15 states.

COUNSELING TIPS ON OBTAINING INFORMED CONSENT

The following list provides some tips when trying to obtain informed consent:

1. *Document the counseling session:* The physician should have documented evidence that informed consent was given to the patient.
2. *Accept the doctrine:* Many physicians resist acceptance of the doctrine of informed consent on practical grounds. On the other hand, there is little or no chance that the doctrine will ever be abolished because informed consent emanates from the right of self-determination and the right to guard against the invasion of one's privacy. Further, informed consent has strong moral and ethical overtones.
3. *Have a third person (health care provider) present at the counseling session:* Patients may be reluctant to question their physicians, but will likely question the witness who, in turn, can inform the physician about the patient's lack of understanding.

A COMPETENT PATIENT'S RIGHT TO REFUSE TREATMENT

The sources of the right to refuse treatment, even when lifesaving, are the following:

1. The law of battery that prevents unpermitted touching of the patient.
2. Informed consent that is grounded in negligence and emanates from the right of self-determination.

3. The spirit of American democracy: Americans have an almost unfettered right to act, provided the act does not interfere with another person's right and does not violate a specific statute or some applicable common law.
4. The U.S. Constitution: According to the U.S. Supreme Court, the right to privacy (right against invasion of privacy) is evident from the Bill of Rights, specifically, the First, Third, Fourth, Fifth, and Ninth Amendments.[116] The Supreme Court has found the right against the invasion of one's privacy to include the right to marry irrespective of race, color, or creed,[117] and the right to possess pornographic literature in the privacy of one's home, even though virtually every process that leads to such possession could be declared illegal.[118]

RIGHT TO REFUSE LIFESAVING TREATMENT IS NOT ABSOLUTE

The right to refuse treatment is not absolute. Occasional exceptions to this principle occur where certain refusals conflict with compelling state interests such as the preservation of life, the prevention of suicide, the protection of third parties, and the protection of the ethical integrity of the medical profession. Increasingly, however, there is a recognized right to die.

A person's right to refuse lifesaving treatment is balanced by the state's interest in human life. When a court is petitioned to override a patient's right to refuse treatment, the process of reviewing the case is not arbitrary. At least four compelling state interests are used by most courts in order to determine whether a state should override a patient's right to refuse treatment. The existence of just one interest is enough to override a patient's right to refuse:

1. Preservation of human life is a paramount state interest.
2. The state has a compelling interest to override a person's right to refuse lifesaving treatment in order to protect innocent third parties (minor children, adult incompetents, and spouses) from not having the opportunity to benefit from having a live healthy parent, guardian, or spouse.
3. The state has a duty to prevent suicide. From a legal perspective, suicide is a direct act or violent measure against one's self, which is specifically designed to end life.
4. The state has an interest in maintaining the ethical integrity of the medical profession. The courts will protect physicians from being forced to treat or not treat without a hearing or the opportunity to withdraw from the case.

Abe Perlmutter[119] was a 73-year-old man with quadriplegia from progressive amyotrophic lateral sclerosis who was unable to breathe without a mechanical respirator. Mr. Perlmutter requested withdrawal of the respirator. His physicians refused to do so because of potential liability for homicide (unlawful killing of another human being). The court stated that a mentally and legally competent patient, having full knowledge of the consequences, may request removal of artificial life support where there is no compelling state interest. When a *Perlmutter* situation arises, however, there is no need to act precipitously and wisdom would recommend consulting the hospital attorney.

Ernestine Jackson was admitted to Mercy Hospital in Baltimore on an emergency basis in February 1984.[120] She was 25 to 26 weeks pregnant and was undergoing premature labor; the fetus was lying in an oblique to transverse position. Cesarean section was recommended. Mrs. Jackson was counseled that there was a 40% to 50% chance she would need a blood transfusion; nevertheless, she steadfastly refused to compromise her religious beliefs and was wholeheartedly supported by her husband. The Maryland Court of Appeals concluded that a competent, pregnant adult has a right to refuse a blood transfusion in accordance with her religious beliefs, where such decision is made knowingly and voluntarily and will not endanger the delivery, survival, or support of the fetus. The court pointed out that its conclusion was consistent with a patient's right of informed consent to medical treatment, and that whether an individual has a right to refuse blood transfusion necessarily turns on facts existing at the moment.

Hubert Hamilton, a 35-year-old Jehovah's Witness, was shot through the chest in 1973. Surgery without transfusion involved a serious risk of death. The judge authorized transfusion after ascertaining that Hamilton fully understood the ramifications of his decision not to consent to blood transfusion, that he was separated from his wife, and that he had a two-year-old child for whom he was the sole support. This case is an example of the state overriding a person's right to refuse treatment based on religious grounds in order to protect an innocent third party (loss of sole support).[121]

REFUSAL OF CONSENT

The corollary of the patient's right to consent to treatment is the right to refuse recommended treatment, after due disclosure by the physician, and the right to withdraw consent previously granted prior to the inception of treatment. The courts generally agree that, in the absence of an emergency, a competent adult patient may refuse medical or surgical treatment.[122] In the Kansas case of *Nathanson v. Kline,* the court summarized the rule.[123]

A man or woman is the master of his or her own body and may expressly prohibit the performance of lifesaving surgery or other medical treatment. A doctor may well believe that an operation or other form of treatment is desirable or necessary, but the law does not permit the physician to substitute his or her own judgment for that of the patient by any form of artifice or deception.

In the vast majority of states, the law upholds a competent adult's right to refuse even lifesaving treatment. The courts generally apply the traditional battery law principle of freedom from unauthorized touchings,[124] or hold that the First Amendment right to free practice of religion precedes a physician's duty to render care.[125] Members of the Jehovah's Witness religious sect, for example, refuse blood transfusions on the basis of their literal interpretation of the Bible's prohibition against drinking blood. However, some courts try to find grounds on which to order the necessary treatment. These courts will usually authorize treatment to protect the life or health of a child or fetus on the grounds that the child will be "neglected" under applicable state statutes if treatment is refused or that the state owes a paramount duty to protect its children.[126] A number of courts have ordered necessary treatment over the objections of competent adult patients.[127] Several courts have held that terminally ill, elderly patients could refuse treatment that would have prolonged their lives, particularly if the treatment were extremely painful, and that the hospital and physician involved would incur no criminal or civil liability for acknowledging refusal.[128]

Refusals of treatment are generally left undisturbed by the courts. The patient's fundamental right of inviolability of the person is controlling in the absence of a compelling state interest. Just as consent to treatment should be properly documented in the patient's medical record, the refusal to consent should be documented.

INFORMED REFUSAL

The corollary of the doctrine of informed consent is often referred to as the requirement of "informed refusal." Courts are expanding the concept of informed consent to include informed refusal. When a patient or his surrogate rejects diagnosis or treatment, he should be advised in a discreet, professional manner of the consequences of the refusal.[129]

If a patient indicates that he or she is going to decline the risk-free test or treatment, then the physician has the additional duty of disclosing all material risks of which a reasonable person would want to be informed before deciding not to undergo the care or procedure. Failure of the physician to disclose to the patient all relevant information, including the risks to the patient if the care and/or test is refused renders the physician liable for any injury legally resulting from the patient's uninformed refusal to take the treatment and/or test where a reasonably prudent person in the patient's position would not have refused if he or she had been adequately informed. This rationale has been applied in at least 11 states and is typified by the thinking of a California court that ruled a patient has the right to be informed of reasonably foreseeable risks that may arise if he or she refuses treatment. In that California case, a woman who refused to have a Pap test done subsequently developed metastases and died of cervical cancer. Her survivors sued, based on the argument that her physician had failed to inform her of the attendant risks in refusing to have the test done. The physician was found liable for failure to disclose the amount of information that was needed for an adequate informed refusal.

"No code" order for competent patient

In the case of a patient who is capable of authorizing or rejecting a do-not-resuscitate order, a "no code" designation should not be issued without the patient's consent. A physician may be liable in damages for failing to determine whether a patient is competent and terminally ill before he or she authorizes the entry of a "no code" on the patient's chart.[130]

PHANTOM PHYSICIAN

A patient who consents to medical care by a specific physician and is treated by another physician may successfully sue the physician who did not operate based on lack of informed consent, and can sue the operating surgeon for battery or negligence predicated on risk of informed consent.[131] Courts have allowed recovery on a claim of unnecessary surgery or medical care based on lack of informed consent. The physician responsible for negotiating informed consent with a patient should be the one who actually will perform the procedure for which consent is being obtained, i.e, not a phantom surgeon/physician. In some jurisdictions, she may, if she sees fit, delegate this duty, but it is still her legal responsibility to make sure that the patient has been properly informed and understands.

TESTS REQUESTED BY POLICE

Two issues of concern to medical personnel arise in connection with tests and physical examinations that police request for criminal suspects: (1) whether such tests constitute a battery for which an examining physician may be held liable and (2) whether such tests constitute a violation of the suspect's constitutional rights.

The extent to which a physician may be liable in battery for performing an examination or test at the request of police but without the patient's consent is unclear. In such cases, a technical battery surely oc-

curs.[132] But the statutes of some states provide that one who operates a motor vehicle on the state's public ways has consented by implication to tests to determine alcohol content in blood.[133] Some of these statutes declare specifically that a person may refuse to take such tests. At least one state, however, provides that an unconscious person is presumed to have consented to such tests.[134] Some states grant immunity to practitioners from any liability arising from obtaining blood samples at the request of a police officer pursuant to applicable state statutes.[135] In the absence of statutes that create such immunity or give rise to implied consent, a physician may be liable for technical battery if he or she performs a test without the patient's consent. However, liability would probably be limited to nominal (extremely small) damages, unless unreasonable force was used or the patient was negligently injured.

The U.S. Constitution places certain restraints on the power of government to interfere with the liberty and property of its citizens. In cases involving the examination of criminal suspects, several of these restrictions arise, including the prohibition against unreasonable search and seizure established by the Fourth Amendment, the privilege against self-incrimination contained in the Fifth Amendment, the right to due process set forth in the Fifth and Fourteenth Amendments, and the right to counsel guaranteed by the Sixth Amendment.

The federal courts have held that a simple physical examination of a suspect does not violate constitutionally based protections against self-incrimination.[136] The admission into evidence of test results from a blood sample taken at the request of a police officer from an unconscious criminal suspect does not violate the Fourth Amendment prohibition against unreasonable searches and seizures or the due process clause of the Fourteenth Amendment.[137] Nor does evidence based on a blood test violate the constitutional prohibition against self-incrimination where a person suspected of violating a motor vehicle code expressly refuses to consent to such a test on advice of counsel.[138] However, the blood sample must be obtained in a simple, medically acceptable manner under the supervision of a physician in a hospital setting; the suspect's request for blood alcohol testing by another acceptable method must be allowed and the physician and police must refrain from using unreasonable force in administering the test.

Scientific analysis of the accused's blood samples, hair, or other similar body materials does not require the presence of the accused's counsel.[139] A search of body cavities for illegally possessed substances is constitutionally permissible as long as there is a clear probable cause and the physician performs the examination under hygienic conditions and in a reasonable manner.[140] Generally, physicians and police officers are given latitude in conducting body examinations during a customs search at a U.S. border.[141]

A blood sample obtained by misrepresentation will make the results inadmissible in evidence and may subject the treating physician to liability in battery. In a case in which a suspect was told by the police that a blood sample was needed to determine intoxication, consent was held invalid because the police actually wanted the sample to determine the suspect's blood type in connection with a rape investigation.[142]

A physician who performs medical examinations or tests at the request of police should remember that the tort liability and constitutional issues involved are usually independent. A test that does not violate the suspect's constitutional rights may nonetheless constitute a technical battery and may subject the physician to tort liability. Although the courts have provided exquisite guidance concerning the constitutional rights of suspects who undergo medical examination, the question of tort liability for those conducting the examination still remains unclear.

The *Mohr v. Williams* case[143] cited earlier established that a physician who exceeds the scope of consent commits a battery. It is common practice for physicians to obtain a group of tests when confronted with a patient in the emergency department. If a physician obtains a blood alcohol that is not medically necessary to evaluate the patient, such an act would constitute a technical battery. In fact, a technical battery is apparent anytime a physician exceeds the scope of consent by obtaining blood tests that are not medically necessary for diagnosis and treatment. Physicians have an overriding concern about whether they should honor police requests, or whether they can be ordered by the police to obtain body fluids that might be used as incriminating evidence where the extraction of such body fluid is not medically necessary. Put another way, under what circumstances can the police direct the suspect to allow the extraction of such body fluid is not medically necessary. Put another way, under what circumstances can the police direct the suspect to allow the extraction of body fluids (pumping the stomach, examining the rectum for glassine bags containing drugs, or obtaining blood specimens) in order to uncover incriminating evidence?

As mentioned earlier, the U.S. Constitution places certain restraints on the power of government to interfere with the liberty and property of its citizens. In cases involving the examination of criminal suspects, several of these restrictions arise, including the prohibition against unreasonable search and seizure established by the Fourth Amendment, a privilege against self-incrimination contained in the Fifth Amendment, the right to due process set forth in the Fifth and Fourteenth Amendments, and the right to counsel guaranteed by the Sixth Amendment.[144]

Three U.S. Supreme Court cases help set the stage to show the boundaries that surround state authority when obtaining body fluids for the purpose of garnering incriminating evidence.

Rochin v. California, 342 U.S. 165 (1952)

Mr. Rochin was a narcotics dealer. Three deputy sheriffs of Los Angeles County forced opened the door to Rochin's room on the second floor of his dwelling. On a nightstand beside the bed, the deputies spied two capsules. The deputies asked Rochin, "Whose stuff is this?" Rochin seized the capsules and put them in his mouth. A struggle ensued, during which the three officers jumped on him and unsuccessfully attempted to extract the capsules. Rochin was handcuffed, taken to a nearby hospital, and at the direction of one of the officers, a doctor forced an emetic solution through a tube into Rochin's stomach against his will. His vomitus contained two capsules, which proved to be morphine. Rochin was convicted of illegally possessing morphine and was sentenced to 60 days in prison. Justice Frankfurter, speaking for the court, said:

> The proceedings by which this conviction was obtained do more than offend some fastidious squeamishness . . . about combating crime too energetically. This is conduct that shocks the conscience. Illegally breaking into the privacy of the petitioner, the struggle to open his mouth and remove what was there, the forcible extraction of his stomach contents—this course of proceedings by agents of government to obtain evidence is bound to offend even hardened sensibilities. They are methods too close to the rack and screw to permit . . . constitutional differentiation. . . . Coerced confessions offend the community's sense of fair play and decency. So here, to sanction the brutal conduct which naturally enough was condemned by the court whose judgment is before us, would be to afford brutality the cloak of law.

In the Rochin case, the U.S. Supreme Court clearly rejected conduct that shocks the conscience, methods close to the rack and screw, and excluded coerced confessions as "constitutionally obnoxious."

Breithaupt v. Abram, 352 U.S. 432 (1957)

A defendant, while driving a pickup truck, was involved in a collision with a passenger car. Three occupants of the car were killed, and the defendant was seriously injured. An almost empty, one-pint whiskey bottle was found in the pickup truck's glove compartment. The defendant was taken to a hospital and while he was lying unconscious in the emergency department, the smell of liquor was detected on his breath. A state police officer requested a blood sample for alcohol. An attending physician, while the defendant was unconscious, obtained a blood sample that displayed an alcohol level of 0.17%. The defendant was convicted and sentenced for involuntary manslaughter. The defendant contended that his conviction, based on the result of the unpermitted blood test, deprived him of his liberty without that due process of law guaranteed by the Fourteenth Amendment, and that the police officer's conduct in the emergency department offended that sense of justice that the U.S. Supreme Court spoke of in *Rochin v. California*. Speaking for the Court, Mr. Justice Clark said:

> We set aside a conviction [in Rochin] because such conduct shocked the conscience and was so brutal and offensive, that it did not comport with traditional ideas of fair play and decency. We, therefore, found that the conduct was offensive to due process. But we see nothing comparable here to the facts in Rochin.
>
> Basically, the distinction rests on the fact that there is nothing brutal or offensive in taking of a blood sample when done, as in this case, under the protective eye of the physician. To be sure the driver here was unconscious when the blood was taken, but the absence of conscious consent, without more, does not necessarily render the taking a violation of a constitutional right.

Schmerber v. California, 384 U.S. 757 (1966)

The defendant was convicted in the Los Angeles Municipal Court of the criminal offense of driving an automobile while under the influence of intoxicating liquor. While receiving treatment for injuries sustained in the automobile accident, he was arrested and, at the direction of a police officer, a blood sample was obtained from the defendant by a physician in the emergency department. Prior to the blood being drawn from his vein, the defendant received his *Miranda* warnings; nevertheless, he objected, *but he did not physically resist*. The blood alcohol level indicated intoxication, which was admitted as evidence at trial. The defendant objected to the admissibility of the blood alcohol test as evidence on the ground that the blood had been withdrawn despite his clear refusal to consent to the performance of the test. He contended that he was denied due process of law under the Fourteenth Amendment, that he was denied his privilege against self-incrimination under the Fifth Amendment, and that he was denied his right not to be subjected to unreasonable searches and seizures in violation of the Fourth Amendment. Justice Brennan delivered the opinion of the Court:

> We thus conclude that the present record shows no violation of petitioner's right under the 4th and 14th amendments to be free of unreasonable searches and seizures. It bears repeating, however, that we reached the judgment only on the facts of the present record. The integrity of an individual person is a cherished value of our society. That we today hold that the constitution does not forbid the state's minor intrusions into an individual's body under stringently limited conditions in no way indicates that it permits more substantial intrusions or intrusions under other condition.

These three cases demarcate the power of government to invade a person's body in order to obtain body fluid for use as incriminating evidence. Conduct that "shocks the conscience" and is "close to the rack and screw" will not be tolerated by the Court because coerced confessions are "constitutionally obnoxious." On the other hand, bodily extractions "taken under the protective eye of a physician" and performed in a medically acceptable manner may fall within constitutional limits, even when the suspect refuses to consent, providing the manner in which the blood was obtained does not shock the conscience. None of these cases discusses the extent of the physician's liability for battery where the suspect refuses to consent.

SPECIAL SITUATIONS
Research involving human subjects

The National Research Act (P.L. 93-348), enacted July 12, 1974, gave the U.S. Department of Health, Education and Welfare (now the Department of Health and Human Services, and the Department of Education) the responsibility for regulating the use of human subjects in biomedical and behavioral research. On March 13, 1975, the Department issued its final regulations entitled "Protection of Human Subjects,"[11,145] which establish in detail the manner in which federally funded research involving human subjects shall be approved and the methods used for protection of subjects. The regulations require that the subject's informed consent be obtained prior to commencing the research. Informed consent is defined as follows:

> (c) "Informed consent" means the knowing consent of an individual or his legally authorized representative, so situated as to be able to exercise free power of choice without undue inducement or any element of force, fraud, deceit, duress, or other form of constraint or coercion. The basic elements of information necessary to such consent include:
>
> 1. A fair explanation of the procedure to be followed and their purposes, including identification of any procedures which are experimental;
> 2. a description of any attendant discomforts and risks reasonably to be expected;
> 3. a description of any benefits reasonably to be expected;
> 4. a disclosure of any appropriate alternative procedures that might be advantageous for the subject;
> 5. an offer to answer any inquiries concerning the procedures; and
> 6. an instruction that the person is free to withdraw his consent and to discontinue participation in the project or activity at any time without prejudice to the subject.[146]

The regulations require documentation of the subject's consent in either a "long" or "short" form.[147] The documentation of consent will employ one of the following three forms:

(a) Provision of a written consent document embodying all of the basic elements of informed consent. This may be read to the subject or to his legally authorized representatives, but in any event he or his legally authorized representatives must be given adequate opportunity to read it. This document is to be signed by the subject or his legally authorized representative. Sample copies of the consent form as approved by the Board are to be retained in its records.

(b) Provision of a "short form" written consent document indicating that the basic elements of informed consent have been presented orally to the subject or his legally authorized representative. Written summaries of what is to be said to the patient are to be approved by the Board. The short form is to be signed by the subject or his legally authorized representative and by an auditor witness to the oral presentation and to the subject's signature. A copy of the approved summary, annotated to show any additions, is to be signed by the persons officially obtaining the consent and by the auditor witness. Sample copies of the consent form and of the summaries as approved by the Board are to be retained in its records.

Either of these forms may be modified, provided that (1) the risk to the subject is minimal, (2) the use of the forms described would invalidate objectives of considerable immediate importance, and (3) any reasonable alternative means for attaining such objectives would be less advantageous to the subject than modifying the consent procedure.[148]

If a physician wishes to treat a patient using medical procedures that depart from established and accepted methods, he or she must be familiar with the federal regulations just discussed and with any applicable laws or regulations of the state.

Consent to experimental procedures

All experimental research involving diagnosis and treatment and the use of investigational drugs or devices must be carefully conducted in conformance with research protocols approved by a hospital's investigations review board and/or research committee. Experimental treatment and procedures are those whose reliability and acceptance have not yet been established in medical practice. Investigational drugs or devices are those the FDA has not yet approved for commercial distribution. The conduct of such investigational diagnosis and treatment, as well as the procurement of informed consent to such treatment, is closely regulated by federal authority. Treatment should not exceed the scope of the patient's consent, unless emergency treatment or a closely related extension of the treatment becomes therapeutically necessary during the performance of the authorized experimental treatment.

Drug research

The Food, Drug and Cosmetic Act[149] authorizes the Department of Health and Human Services to regulate the use of investigational drugs. The regulations issued by the department require the investigator to certify that:

[H]e will inform any patients or their representatives, that drugs are being used for investigational purposes, and will obtain the consent of the subject, or their representatives, except where this is not feasible or, in the investigator's professional judgment, is contrary to the best interest of the subjects.[150]

The regulations define "consent" to mean:

[t]hat the person involved has legal capacity to give consent, is so situated as to be able to exercise free power of choice, and is provided with a fair explanation of pertinent information concerning the investigational drug, and/or possible use of a control, as to enable him to make a decision on his willingness to receive said investigational drug. This latter element means that before the acceptance of an affirmative decision by such person the investigator should carefully consider and make known to him (taking into consideration such person's well-being and his ability to understand) the nature, expected duration, and purpose of the administration of said investigational drug; the method and means by which it is to be administered; the hazards involved; the existence of alternative forms of therapy, if any; and the beneficial effects upon his health or person that may possibly come from the administration of the investigational drug.[151]

Consent is required in all cases in which an investigational drug is administered "primarily for the accumulation of scientific knowledge" or is administered to patients who are otherwise receiving medical treatment.

Any time a patient is enrolled as part of a clinical trial, the duty of the research physician to disclose all possible risks, benefits, and potential consequences must be taken seriously. Where a court finds that the decision to continue a patient in a control group was negligent, serious questions may arise about the validity of exposing control groups to a potentially noxious agent or environment, which in turn may cast doubt on the validity of the concept controlled, and/or the double-blind study.[152]

Elective sterilization using federal funds

To perform a nonemergency sterilization on a male or female patient in a program supported by federal funds administered by the U.S. Public Health Service, a physician must obtain the patient's informed consent. The applicable regulations define "informed consent" as:

[t]he voluntary, knowing assent from the individual on whom any sterilization is to be performed after he has been given (as evidenced by a document executed by such individual):

1. A fair explanation of the procedures to be followed;
2. A description of the attendant discomforts and risks;
3. A description of the benefits to be expected;
4. An explanation concerning appropriate alternative meth-

ods of family planning and the effect and impact of the proposed sterilization including the fact that it must be considered to be an irreversible procedure;

5. An offer to answer any inquiries concerning the procedures; and

6. An instruction that the individual is free to withhold or withdraw his or her consent to the procedure at any time prior to the sterilization without prejudicing his or her future care and without loss of other project or programs benefits to which the patient might otherwise be entitled.[153]

Such consent must be documented in one of two ways: (1) a written consent form describing in detail the information listed in subsections (1) through (6) of the regulations, or (2) a "short form" written consent form that indicates that the six basic elements of consent have been presented orally to the patient, supplemented by a written summary of the oral presentation. The written summary must be signed by the person obtaining the consent and by a witness. Each consent document must prominently display the following language[154]:

NOTICE: Your decision at any time not to be sterilized *will not* result in the withdrawal or withholding of any benefits provided by programs or projects.

Physicians who perform sterilization procedures should be thoroughly familiar with current federal regulations applicable to sterilization. Regulations change so frequently that the previous discussion and extracts are provided as examples only.

Uniform Anatomical Gift Act

The Uniform Anatomical Gift Act, adopted in all states, generally provides that persons aged 18 or older may donate all or part of their bodies after death for research, transplantation, or placement in a tissue bank. Survivors may give authorization for donation, where the decedent had not done so. Consents for donations may be superseded by decisions of state officials to conduct autopsies, in accordance with local statutes or ordinances.

CONCLUSION

The scope and propriety of disclosure to patients is dependent on the state of medical knowledge at the time of the disclosure. When appropriate, the patient also should be informed of the identity and responsibility of other persons who will participate in the patient's care and management. A physician who specializes in psychiatry has the same legal duty as any other physician to exercise reasonable care in selecting, administering, and obtaining informed consent for treatment. A valid consent may be exercised only if the patient giving it is competent enough to engage in the consent process. This can be a particularly critical element for psychiatrists, because they commonly treat patients whose cognitive capacity may be at issue. Once the physician-patient relationship is established, a physician has a duty to inform the patient of his or her condition and of the presumptive and differential diagnoses.[155]

The law in all states requires a physician to obtain the consent of a patient or surrogate before treating that patient. In the absence of that consent, the physician may be held liable in a civil lawsuit for battery, assault, and professional negligence or medical malpractice.

- At least 13 states have professionally articulated disclosure standards, i.e., by physician custom or standard.
- At least 4 states have a reasonable patient standard. This requires no expert witness testimony.
- At least 10 states have no specified standards.
- At least 10 states have a patient comprehension standard, i.e., the reasonable person, or all questions answered.
- Two states, Georgia and Arizona, have abolished or modified the informed consent requirement, the latter possibly by implication.

The process of obtaining a patient's informed consent to a medical procedure requires balancing the need to disclose complete and reliable up-to-date medical information with the practical concern of avoiding undue alarm to patients. The physician may exercise his or her professional judgment with respect to the scope of the disclosure where such is in the best interest of the patient. This exception should be closely limited because it can be contrary to the very basis of the informed consent requirement; that is, the right of self-determination.

Physicians have a moral, ethical, and legal duty to disclose sufficient information to patients in order to obtain a valid informed consent to perform a recommended procedure or treatment.

The moral duty arises from the human person's natural desire to be free to make personal choices about what shall become of his or her body—the right to refuse or accept treatment—thus, the assumption of a definite risk is a highly private and personal matter, rather than a scientific matter. The ethical duty arises from the collective wisdom of the medical profession; mainly, that patients are necessary partners in the diagnostic and therapeutic processes, that physicians have an inherent professional duty to respect a patient's wishes to know about his or her disease, and that patients have a right to know what they need to know prior to making a choice about whether to follow medical recommendations. The legal duty arises from the common law, statutes, and the U.S. Constitution, which recognize that patients have a dignitary interest that does not allow them to be touched in the absence of consent and that Americans have a right to privacy, a right to refuse treatment, and a right to be informed about the benefits and adverse effects inherent in proposed medical care.

The transcending American principle that controls the nature of consent to treatment is the right of self-determination.

END NOTES

1. *Pagan v. State of New York,* 476 N.Y.S. 2d 468 (N.Y. Ct. Cl. 1984).
2. *Salis v. United States,* 522 F. Supp. 989 (Dist. Ct. Pa. 1981); *Taylor v. Wilmington Medical Center, Inc.,* 577 F. Supp. 309 (Dist. Ct. Del. 1983).
3. *Pratt v. Davis,* 118 Ill. App. 161 (1905), *aff'd,* 224 Ill. 300. 79 N.E. 562 (1906).
4. *Schloendorff v. New York Hosp.,* 211 N.Y. 125. 105 N.E. 92 (1914).
5. *Black's Law Dictionary* 193 (rev. 4th ed. 1968).
6. W. Prosser, *Handbook of the Law of Torts* 102 (3d ed. 1964).
7. *Hancock v. Hullett,* 203 Ala. 272. 82 So. 522 (1919).
8. *Moss v. Rishworth,* 222 S.W. 225 (1920).
9. W. P. Keeton et al., *Prosser and Keeton on Law of Torts* 41 (5th ed. 1984).
10. *Id.*
11. J. H. King, Jr., *The Law of Medical Malpractice in a Nutshell* 130 (2d ed. 1986).
12. *See, e.g.,* Ill. Ann. Stat. ch. 95½, para. 11-501.1 (Smith-Hurd Supp. 1976).
13. *O'Brien v. Cunard SS Co.,* 28 N.E. 266 (1891).
14. *King v. Carney,* 204 P. 270 (1922).
15. *Mohr v. Williams,* 104 N.W. 12 (1905).
16. *Wheeler v. Barker,* 92 Cal. App. 2d 776, 208 P. 2d 68 (1949); *Jackovach v. Yocom,* 212 Iowa 914, 237 N.W. 444 (1931).
17. *Barnett v. Bachrach,* 34 A. 2d 626 (N.J. 1943).
18. *McGuire v. Rix,* 118 Neb. 434, 22 N.W. 120 (1929).
19. *Chambers v. Nottebaum,* 96 So. 2d 716 (1957).
20. *Janney v. Housekeeper,* 16 A. 382 (1889).
21. *Murray v. Vandevander,* 522 P. 2d 302 (1974).
22. *Danforth v. Planned Parenthood of Central Missouri,* 428 U.S. 52 (1976).
23. *Roe v. Wade,* 410 U.S. 113 (1973).
24. *Id.*
25. *Gursky v. Gursky,* 39 Misc. 2d 1083, 242 N.Y.S. 2d 406 (1963).
26. *In re Quinlan,* 335 A.2d 647 (1976).
27. *Griswold v. Connecticut,* 381 U.S. 479 (1965); *also see Loving v. Virginia,* 388, U.S. 1 (1967) (the right to marry irrespective of race, color, or creed) and *Stanley v. Georgia,* 394 U.S. 557 (1969) (right to possess pornographic literature in the privacy of one's home).
28. 49 A.L.R. 3rd 501, 505. (1970).
29. American Medical Association's Judicial Council, *Principles of Medical Ethics* ix (1984).
30. Ad Hoc Committee on Medical Ethics, *American College of Physicians' Ethics Manual.* Ann Int Med 101:121-137 (1984).
31. *King, supra* note 11, at 154-55.
32. *Canterbury v. Spence,* 464 F.2d 772 (D.C. Cir. 1972).
33. *King, supra* note 11, at 131.
34. *Cobbs v. Grant,* 502 P. 2d 1 (Calif. 1972).
35. *Sard v. Hardy,* 379 A.2d 1014 (M.D. 1977).
36. *Id.*
37. Civil Rights § 765.02.
38. *Tetstone v. Adams,* 373 So. 2d 362; *Brooks v. Cerrato,* 355 So. 2d 119 (1978).
39. *Dowlings v. Mutual Life Insurance Co.,* 373 So. 2d 362; *Brooks, supra* note 38.
40. *Nathanson v. Kline,* 350 P.2d 1093 (1960).
41. *Nathanson v. Kline,* 354 P. 2d 670 (1969).
42. *Sinkev v. Surgical Assoc.,* 186 N.W. 2d 658 (1971).
43. *Nathanson, supra* note 40.
44. *AMA Current Opinions of the Judicial Counsel* 8.11 (1984).
45. *Gates v. Jensen,* 92 Wash. 2d 246, 250, 595 P. 2d 919, 922 (1979).
46. *Keogan v. Holy Family Hosp.,* 95 Wash. 2d 306, 622 P.2d 1246 (1980).
47. *Ray v. Wagner,* 286 Minn. 354, 176 N.W.2d 101 (1970) (physician not liable when patient's contributory negligence resulted in her failure to learn of suspicious Pap smear result).
48. T. S. Harrison, *Hyperthyroidism, in Textbook of Surgery* 585-93 (D.C. Sabiston ed., 1986).
49. *Id.*
50. *Id.*
51. *Phillips v. United States,* 566 F. Supp. 1 (D.S.C. 1981) (an infant's manifestation of signs of congestive heart failure obligated referral to a pediatric cardiologist under the applicable standard of family practice or pediatric care); *Larsen v. Yelle,* 246 N.W.2d 841 (Minn. 1976); *Id.* at 845. If a physician has every reasonable indication that he or she is fully capable of treating the patient, however, there is no duty to consult another physician. *See Collins v. Itoh,* 503 P.2d 36 (Mont. 1972).
52. *Logan v. Greenwich Hosp. Ass'n,* 191 Conn. 282, 465 A.2d 294 (1983).
53. *Id.* The case was remanded for a new trial on the issue of whether an open kidney biopsy represented a viable alternative.
54. *Osborne v. Frazor,* 58 Tenn. App. 15, 425 S.W.2d 768 (1968). *See Annotation, Malpractice: Physician's failure to advise patient to consult specialist or one qualified in a method of treatment which physician is not qualified to give,* 35 A.L.R. 3d 349 (1971).
55. *Kelly v. Carrol,* 36 Wash. 2d 482, 219 P.2d 79 (1950) (a duty to refer exists when a practitioner knows not only that a therapy will be of no benefit to the patient, but also that an alternative mode of treatment is available elsewhere that is more likely to be successful).
56. *Rahn v. United States,* 222 F. Supp. 775 (S.D. Ga. 1963) (if current therapy is unsuccessful, and if specialty assistance is available, a duty to consult exists).
57. President's Commission for the Study of Ethical Problems in Medicine and Biomedical and Behavioral Research, *Making health care decisions: The ethical and legal implications of informed consent in the patient-practioner relationship. The communication process.* Vols. 1-3 (Government Printing Office 1982).
58. *Price v. Neyland,* 320 F.2d 674 (D.C. Cir. 1963).
59. *Harris v. Robert C. Groth, M.D., Inc., P.S.,* 99 Wash.2d 438, 663 P.2d 113 (1983).
60. *See Cobbs v. Grant,* 104 Cal. Rptr. 505, 502 P.2d 1 (1972); *Green v. Hussey,* 127 Ill. App. 2d 174, 262 N.E. 2d 156 (1970).
61. *Cowman v. Hornaday,* 329 N.W. 2d 422 (Iowa 1983).
62. *Roberson v. Menorah Medical Center,* 588 S.W. 2d 134 (Mo. Appl. 1979).
63. *Garcia v. Presbyterian Hosp. Center,* 593 P.2d 487 (N.M. Ct. App. 1979).
64. *Estrada v. Jacques,* S.E. 2d (N.C. Ct. App. 1984).
65. *Lipsus v. White,* 458 N.Y.S. 2d 928 (N.Y. App. Div. 1983).
66. American Medical Ass'n., *Medicolegal Forms* (1976); Hospital Ass'n of N.Y. State, *Manual of Consent Forms* (1974).
67. *Cross v. Trapp,* 294 S.E.2d 446 (W. Va. 1982).
68. *Archer v. Galbraith,* 567 P.21 115 S (Wash. Ct. App. 1980).
69. *Collins v. Davis,* 44 Misc. 2d 622. 254 N.Y.S. 2d 666 (1964).
70. *Consent to Medical or Surgical Procedures* I Health Law Manual 14-11 (1975).
71. *Petition of Nemser,* 51 Misc. 2d 616, 273 N.Y.S. 2d (1966).

72. For example, the Illinois statute concerning autopsy provides that if one close relative prohibits autopsy, the autopsy may not be performed, even though another close relative had given consent. *See* Ill. Ann. Stat. ch. 91, para. 18-12 (Smith-Hurd 1976).

73. *See, e.g.,* Ill. Ann. Stat. ch. 3. para 112 et seq. (Smith-Hurd 1961).

74. *E.g., Schultz v. Rice,* 809 F.2d 643 (10th Cir. 1986); *Pardy v. United States,* 783 F.2d 710 (7th Cir. 1986).

75. *See Lester v. Aetna Casualty & Surety Co.,* 240 F. 2d 676 (5th Cir. 1957).

76. *Nishi v. Hartwell,* 52 Haw. 188 and 296, 473 P. 2d 116 (1970).

77. *Putenson v. Clay Adams, Inc.,* 12 Cal. App. 3d 1062, 91 Cal. Rptr. 319 (1st Dist. 1970).

78. *E.g., Wachter v. United States,* 877 F. 2d 257 (4th Cir. 1989).

79. *Crouch v. Most,* 78 N.M. 406, 432 P.2d 250 (1967).

80. *AMA Current Opinions of the Judicial Counsel* 8.07 (1984).

81. *Dunham v. Wright,* 423 F. 2d 940 (1970); *Berlinger v. Lackner,* 331 Ill. App. 591. 73 N.E. 2d 620 (1947); *Pratt v. Davis,* 224 Ill. 300, 79 N.E. 562 (1906).

82. 61 Am. Jur. 2D *Physicians and Surgeons* § 159 (1972); 56 A.L.R. 2d 695 § 3.

83. *Restatement of Torts* § 62 (1934).

84. *Luka v. Lowrie,* 171 Mich. 122. 136 N.W. 1106 (1912).

85. *Tabor v. Scobee,* 254 S.W. 2d 474 (Ky. Ct. App. 1952).

86. *Jackovach, supra* note 16.

87. *Luka, supra* note 84.

88. *Tabor, supra* note 85; *Mohr v. Williams,* 95 Minn. 261, 104 N.W. 12 (1905).

89. *Luka, supra* note 84.

90. *Wells v. McGehee,* 39 So. 2d 196 (1949); *Sullivan v. Montgomery,* 279 N.Y.S. 575, 17 N.E. 2d 446 (1935).

91. *Lacey v. Laird,* 166 Ohio St. 12, 139 N.E. 2d 25 (1956); *Gulf and Ship Island R.R. v. Sullivan,* 155 Miss. 1, 119 So. 501 (1928); *Bishop v. Shurly,* 237 Mich. 76. 211 N.W. 75 (2926). *But see contra. Bonner v. Moran,* 126 F.2d 121 (D.C. Cir. 1941), which held that a 15-year-old could not alone consent to donation of blood for benefit of another.

92. *Pizzlotto v. Wilson,* 444 So. 2d 143 (La. 1983); *Mercer v. Chi,* 282 N.W. 2d 697 (Iowa 1979).

93. *See, e.g., Mohr v. Williams,* 95 Minn. 261, 104 N.W. 12 (1905).

94. *Salgo v. Leland Stanford, Jr., Univ. Board of Trustees,* 154 Cal. app. 2d 560, 317 P. 2d 170 (1957).

95. Waltz and Scheuneman, *Informed Consent to Therapy,* 64 Nw. U.L. Rev. 628 (1970).

96. *Bang v. Charles T. Miller Hosp.,* 251 Minn. 427, 88 N.W. 2d 188 (1958); Plante, *An Analysis of "Informed Consent,"* 36 Fordham L. Rev. 639 (1968); McCoid, *A Reappraisal of Liability for Unauthorized Medical Treatment,* 41 Minn. L. Rev. 381 (1957); Leg. Med. Ann. 203.

97. *Bang, supra* note 96.

98. *Fiorentino v. Wenger,* 19 N.Y. 2d 407, 227 N.E. 2d 296 (1967).

99. *Green v. Hussey,* 127 Ill. App. 2d 173, 262 N.W. 2d 156 (1970); *Aiken v. Clarey,* 396 S.W. 2d 668 (Mo. 1965); Bucklin, *Informed Consent: Past, Present, and Future,* Leg. Med. Ann. 203 (1975).

100. *Green, supra* note 99, at 174.

101. *Cobbs v. Grant,* 104 Cal. Rptr. 505, 502 P. 2d 1 (1972).

102. *Id.*

103. *Canterbury, supra* note 32.

104. *Flannery v. Georgetown Univ. Hosp.,* 79 F. 2d 960 (D.C. App. 1980).

105. *Jeffries v. McCague,* 363 A.2d 1167 (Pa. 1970).

106. *Haynes v. Hoffman,* 164 Ga. App. 236, 296 S.E. 2d 216 (1982).

107. *See e.g.,* Alfidi, *Informed Consent, A Study of Patient Reaction,* 216 JAMA 8 (1971); Johnrude, *Informed Consent: An Objective Evaluation of or a Possible Solution,* Radiology (1971).

108. *Small v. Gifford Memorial Hosp.,* 133 Vt. 552. 349 A.2d 703 (1975);

Hunter v. Brown, 4 Wash. App. 899, 484 P. 2d 1162 (1971); *Getchell v. Mansfield,* 260 Or. 174. 489 P. 2d 953 (1971).

109. R. D. Miller, *Treatment Authorization and Refusal, Problems in Hospital Law* 224-25, (Aspen Publications, Rockville, Md., 1990).

110. C. L. Spring and B. J. Winick, *Informed Consent, in Legal Aspects of Medicine,* 61-63 (J. R. Vevaina, R. C. Bone, and E. Kossoff eds., Springer-Verlag, (1989).

111. Alaska Statute § 09.55.556; § 09.55.556 (b).(5). Cal. Health & Safety Code § 1704.5 (1980); Connecticut General Statute § 52-582; Delaware Annotated Code Title 18 § 6852; 18 § 6852(b); Florida Statutes Annotated § 768.46(3)(a); Georgia Annotated Code § 88-2906; Georgia Code Ann. § 31-9-6(d)(1985); Georgia Code Ann. § 31-9-6.1 (1988 Supp.); Hawaii Revised Statutes § 671-3(b); Idaho Revised Statutes § 939-4304; § 939-4304; § 939-4305; Iowa Code Annotated 9 147.137. Iowa Code Ann. § 147.137; Kentucky Revised Statutes § 304 40-320; Louisiana Revised Statutes § 1299 40. A(a); Maine Revised Statutes Annotated Title 24 § 2905; Title 24 § 2905.2; Missouri Statutes 516.280 Revised Statutes Missouri (1978); Nebraska Revised Statutes § 44-2816; Nevada Revised Statutes. § 41 A. 110; New Hampshire Revised Statutes Annotated § 507-c.211. § 507-c:2(b) (4); New York Public Health Law § 2805-d.1 Civ. Procedure Law § 4401-a; North Carolina General Statutes § 90-21.13; § 90-21.13(b); North Dakota Central Code § 26-401-025; Ohio Revised Code § 2317 54A, § 231754; Oregon Revised Statutes § 671.097; Pennsylvania Statutes Annotated Title 40, § 1301.103; Tennessee Annotated Code § 23-3417; Texas Revised Civil Statutes Article 4590; § 6.02 § 98-14-5(2)(d); Utah Code Annotated § 78-14-5(d)(e); Vermont Statutes Annotated Title 12, § 1909(a)(1); 12, § 1909(e) 12 § 1909(d); Washington Code Annotated § 7.70.050.

112. Florida Statutes, § 381.3712(4) (M), (485,324,459.0125) (1984); Georgia Code Section 43-34-21 (G) (1984); Hawaii Revised Statutes, § 671-3 (C) (1983); Kansas Statutes Annotated, § 65-2836(O) (1984); Kentucky House Bill 609 (1984); Louisiana H. Con. Resolution 125 (1983); Massachusetts General Laws Annotated ch. III, § 70E (1979); Minnesota Statutes, § 144.651, Subdivision 9 (1984); New Jersey Revised Statutes, Title 45, ch. 9 (1984); Pennsylvania H.B. 1972 (1984); Virginia Code, Section 54-325.2:2 (1985).

113. A. J. Diethelm. *The acute abdomen, in* Sabiston above, at 796.

114. *Abdominal trauma, in Advanced Trauma Life-Support Instructors Manual.* Published by the American College of Surgeons. Prepared by the Subcommittee on Advanced Trauma Life-Support of the American College of Surgeons, 120 (1989).

115. *Rochester v. Katalan,* 320 A.2d 704 (Del. 1974). *See Annotation, Patient's failure to reveal medical history to physician as contributory negligence or assumption of risk in defense of malpractice action,* 33 A.L.R. 4th 790 (1984).

116. *Griswold v. Connecticut,* 381 U.S. 439 (1965).

117. *Loving v. Virginia,* 388 U.S. 1 (1967).

118. *Stanley v. Georgia,* 394 U.S. 557 (1969).

119. *Satz v. Perlmutter,* 362 SO.2d 160 (Fla. 1978).

120. *Mercy Hosp. v. Jackson,* 489 A.2d 1130 (M.D. 1985).

121. *Hamilton v. McAuliffe,* 353 A.2d 634 (M.D. 1976).

122. *Schloendorff, supra* note 4.

123. *Nathanson v. Kline,* 186 Kan. 393.350 P.2d 1093 (1960).

124. *Schloendorff, supra* note 4.

125. *In re Estate of Brooks,* 32 Ill. 2d 361, 205 N.E. 2d 435 (1965).

126. *Raleigh Fitkin-Paul Morgan Memorial Hosp. v. Anderson,* 42 N.J. 421. 201 A.2d 537 (1964); *State v. Perricone,* 37 N.J. 462, 181 A.2d 751 (1962); *People ex rel Wallace v. Labrenz,* 411 Ill. 618, 104 N.E. 2d 769 (1952); *In re Vasco,* 263 N.Y.S. 552 (1933).

127. *Kennedy Hosp. v. Heston,* 58 N.J. 569, 279 A. 2d 670 (1971); *Application of President of Georgetown College, Inc.,* 331 F. 2d 1000

(D.C. Cir.), *cert. denied*, 377 U.S. 978 (1964); *Collins v. Davis*, 254 N.Y.S. 2d 666 (1964).

128. *Palm Springs General Hosp. v. Martinez*, No. 71-12687 (Dade County Ct. Fla. 1971).

129. *Truman v. Thomas*, 165 Cal. Rptr. 308, 611 P.2d 902 (1980).

130. *Payne v. Marion General Hosp.*, 549 N.E. 2d 2043.

131. *Perna v. Pirozzi*, 92 N.J. 446, 457, A-2d 431 (1983).

132. *See, e.g., Bednarik v. Bednarik*, 18 Misc. 633, 16 A. 2d 80 (1940).

133. *See, e.g.*, Ill. Ann. Stat. ch. 95, ½, para. 11-501.1 (Smith-Hurd Supp. 1976).

134. Fla. Stat. Ann. § 322.261 (c) (West 1975).

135. *See, e.g.*, N.Y. Veh. & Traf. Law § 1194.7.b (McKinney Supp. 1976).

136. *McFarland v. United States*, 150 F.2d 593, *cert. denied*, 325 U.S. 788, *reh'g denied*, 327 U.S. 814 (1945); *Leeper v. Texas*, 139 U.S. 462 (1891); *Battle v. Cameron*, 260 F. Supp. 804 (1966).

137. *Breithaupt v. Abram*, 352 U.S. 432 (1957).

138. *Schmerber v. California*, 384 U.S. 757 (1966).

139. *United States v. Wade*, 388 U.S. 218 (1967).

140. *Rochin v. California*, 342 U.S. 165 (1952); *Rivas v. United States*, 368 F.2d 703, *cert. denied*, 386 U.S. 945 (1966); *Hugues v. United States*, 406 F. 2d 366 (9th Cir. 1968).

141. *See* 22 L.Ed 2d 909 (1970); 16 L.Ed. 2d 1332 (1967).

142. *Graves v. Beto*, 424 F.2d 524 (5th Cir. 1970).

143. *Mohr, supra* note 15.

144. King, *supra* note 31, at 131.

145. 45 C.F.R. § 46.1 *et seq.* (1976).

146. 45 C.F.R. § 46.3 (1976).

147. 45 C.F.R. § 46.10 (1976).

148. 45 C.F.R. § 46.10(c) (1976),

149. 21. U.S.C.A. § 321 *et seq.* (West 1972).

150. 21 C.F.R § 312.1 (A) (13) (1976).

151. 21 C.F.R. § 310.102(b)-(c) (1976).

152. *Burton v. Brooklyn Doctors Hosp. et al.*, 452 N.Y.S. 2d 875 (1982).

153. 42 C.F.R. § 50.202(d) (1976).

154. 42 C.F.R. § 50.202(d) (7) (iii) (1976).

155. *Dowling v. Mutual Life Insurance Co. of New York*, 168 So.2d 107 (La. App. 1964) (physician's failure to inform patient that chest radiograph revealed tuberculous infiltration was actionable in tort).

GENERAL REFERENCES

Flannery F. T., *et al., Consent to treatment*, in *Legal Medicine* 196-207 (1988).

Hirsh, H. L., 5 *Informed Consent: The Journal of Legal Medicine Fact or Fiction?*, 25-27, (Jan. 1977).

CHAPTER 23

Medical records

HAROLD L. HIRSH, M.D., J.D., F.C.L.M.*

PURPOSE AND FUNCTION OF MEDICAL RECORDS
STANDARDS OF RECORD KEEPING
INCIDENT REPORTS
OWNERSHIP AND ACCESS
RETENTION REQUIREMENTS
DESTRUCTION OF RECORDS
COMPUTERIZED MEDICAL RECORDS
PROBLEM-ORIENTED RECORDS AND CONDITION DIAGNOSIS
AUTOAUTHENTICATION OF MEDICAL RECORDS

Medical records are an integral part of patient care — medically, legally, and administratively. They must be up to standard in every way. The medical record of a hospital, clinic, or private physician's patient is often essential to the resolution of issues in nearly every branch of the law — malpractice, personal injury, workers' compensation, and others. Medical evidence is estimated to play a part in about three-quarters of all civil cases and in about one-quarter of criminal cases brought to trial.[1]

A properly kept medical record can serve as the physician's best friend and witness. If improperly maintained, the record may prove to be his or her worst enemy.[2-22]

PURPOSE AND FUNCTION OF MEDICAL RECORDS

The *Accreditation Manual for Hospitals* of the Joint Commission on Accreditation of Healthcare Organizations (JCAHO) has outlined the purposes of medical record as follows:

- To serve as the basis for the patient's care for continuity in the evaluation of the patient's treatment.
- To furnish documentary evidence of the course of the patient's medical evaluation, treatment, and change in condition during the hospital stay, during an ambulatory care or emergency visit to the hospital, or while being followed in a hospital-administered home care program.

- To document communication between the practitioner responsible for the patient and any other health care professional who contributes to the patient's care.
- To assist in protecting the legal interests of the patient, the hospital, and the practitioner responsible for the patient.
- To provide data for the use in continuing education and research.

There are two types of medical records: (1) hospital medical records and (2) physician private office records.

Hospital medical records

The hospital medical record is a complete, current, written record of a patient's history, condition treatment, and the results of hospitalization.[23] The record is used to document chronologically the care rendered to the patient. It is also used in planning for the evaluation of the patient's treatment and in communicating between the patient's physician and other health care professionals in the hospital. Medical and nursing audits and peer review programs measure the quality of care given hospitalized patients by evaluating treatment documented in hospital medical records against established standards or norms.[24]

Hospital medical charts are important legal documents that are utilized in sundry litigation. A good chart enables the hospital and physician to reconstruct the course of treatment and show that the care provided was acceptable under the circumstances.[25]

The contents of the hospital record are usually admissible as evidence for or against the hospital and

*The author gratefully acknowledges work from previous contributors: Claude T. Moorman II, M.D., J.D., F.C.L.M.; David T. Armitage, M.D., J.D., F.C.L.M.; and E. Allen Griggs, M.D., J.D., F.C.L.M.

physician.[26] Therefore, entries to the chart must be made carefully and must have some relevance to the patient's care.[27] All record changes are best made in chronological sequence with an adequate explanation of the change and without altering the original entry.[28] Once the record is complete, no material should be tampered with, removed, or inserted. No attempt should be made to improve the legibility of an original entry by superimposing material on it. Such attempts are often viewed as efforts to alter a record for self-serving purposes.

The Joint Commission on Accreditation of Hospitals (JCAH) requires that the medical records of accredited hospitals contain "sufficient information to identify the diagnosis and treatment and to document the results accurately."[29] Some municipal governments direct hospitals to place certain information on their records.[30]

Medical records vary widely in form and style among hospitals and other health care institutions. Generally, however, all hospital medical charts have two parts: a general information section, dealing with personal matters, and a clinical information section. The minimum information to be included in hospital charts is established by state hospital-licensing regulations, accreditation standards, and hospital and medical staff rules.

To participate in the Medicare reimbursement program, a hospital must have a medical records department that meets the specifications set forth in applicable federal regulations and must maintain medical records which "contain sufficient information to justify the diagnosis and warrant the treatment and end results."[31]

To meet federal requirements for participation, a hospital must include the following information, if applicable to the patient, on its charts: identification data, chief complaint, present illness, past history, family history, physical examination, provisional diagnosis, clinical laboratory reports, X-ray reports, consultation reports, treatment procedures—medical and surgical, tissue reports, progress notes, final diagnosis, discharge summary, and autopsy findings.

A patient's record should contain a contemporaneous recapitulation of what information was obtained and what was actually observed, diagnosed, concluded, and administered. It should also cover details of the treatment plan and of informed consent. Courts tend to accept what is documented as "having occurred" and what is omitted as not having occurred.

Physician's private office records

The purpose and function of medical records created for patients seen in the physician's own private office are the same as the purpose and function of hospital patient records.

Generally, there are no statutory requirements for specific content in private office records. However, as a rule the record should contain a thorough and detailed record of treatment rendered the patient in the office and anywhere else outside of a hospital, which maintains its own records. Instructions given patients by telephone would also be documented in their records. Records should include telephone logs and message and appointment books. The physician should make a note of every call received. Physicians should keep general correspondence and billing records separate from patient medical records.

A physician is the owner of his or her private office records subject to the obligation to furnish them to another physician who assumes responsibility for the patient's care. The estate of a deceased physician is obligated to transfer patient records to successor physicians.[32] However, a physician is not required to transfer a patient's records to an unqualified practitioner, a faith healer, or a chiropractor, who may be treating the patient.[33]

STANDARDS OF RECORD KEEPING

There are recognized standards for record-keeping that are accepted by professional organizations as well as by the courts.[23,24,29,31] The physician must check that, on each sheet of the chart, the name and identification material of the patient are properly filled in for exact identification purposes. These details are important and may be critical.

Entries must be legible and not be vague or ambiguous. The records must be accurate, adequate, and appropriate. They need to be factual, relevant, pertinent, and material. To conform to the standard of care, the physician should record as much as possible, promptly and as often as need be.

The physician and the nurse are now mandated to have separate and complementary admission plans and orders documented in the record concurrent with the admission of the patient. The more urgent the patient's problems, the sooner these documents must be written.

All discharges must include documentation showing that the discharge is medically appropriate with plans for follow-up care and teaching of caregivers of the medical regimen after discharge. Transfers must be documented in a similar manner.

Today, in many hospitals, ward secretaries or clerks transcribe orders. Hospitals must require that a transcribed order be countersigned. A verbal order is legal but is a high risk legally. Verbal orders, oral or telephone, must be countersigned by the physician within 24 hours under a notation "read and approved" with date and time.

Recognized standards for record keeping are accepted by professional organizations and by the courts.

The courts will allow medical records to be introduced as evidence to impugn a health care provider's professional activities. Poorly kept or inadequate records may be considered a breach of the accepted standard of medical care. Hospitals are held responsible for permitting or tolerating poor record keeping.

Information

Generally, office and hospital records of patients must contain the following information:

- Chief complaint or complaints
- Significant historical information, particularly vis-a-vis, medications, allergies, and drug sensitivities
- Social history, including alcohol or drug abuse and family or emotional problems
- Past history of illnesses, surgeries, and injuries
- Physical examination statement including all positive and negative findings
- All diagnostic treatment procedures
- Any laboratory or X-ray report, including the dates ordered, received, and reviewed (Tissue reports include a report of findings on microscopic examination required by hospital regulations.)
- Progress notes, which chronologically represent the patient's progress and are sufficient to delineate the course and results of treatment
- The provisional diagnosis, which reflects the examining physician's preliminary evaluation of the patient's condition
- The consultation report, which is a written and signed opinion of the consultant's findings
- Medications prescribed, treatments provided, and specimens collected as well as where they were sent
- Any reaction or response noted following administration of medication, or following procedures
- Notations concerning lack of patient cooperation, failure to follow advice, and failure to keep appointments (Specifically, follow-up telephone calls and letters should be recorded in the medical record.)
- Consent forms, which have been signed and witnessed for treatments, procedures, or surgeries
- Copies of records or instructions of any kind, including diet and directions to any family member
- Dates and identities of physicians asked to consult as well as a record of the consultant's written or oral responses
- Documentation of patient complaints, the response and times and dates of these matters
- A definitive final diagnosis expressed in the terminology of a recognized system of disease nomenclature
- The discharge summary, which is a recapitulation of the significant findings and events of the patient's hospitalization and condition on discharge

- Autopsy findings in a complete protocol, which are filed in the record when an autopsy is performed
- A chronological summary of the patient's record, which is maintained in the front of the chart.

Nursing personnel records should contain:

- Signed and witnessed consent forms concerning the procedure to be performed
- Notations identifying special problems and instructions such as no oral feeding, allergies, physical limitations, results of laboratory, X-ray, and other examinations, and the status of the patient at the time of arrival in the operating room
- Recordations concerning all preoperative and intraoperative IV solutions, blood or blood products, and medications
- Location of electrosurgical grounding pad
- The prep type and condition of the skin
- Notations concerning disposition of surgical specimens, tissue, or implants
- Identification of all packing, catheters, drains and surgical prosthesis, including serial number, amount, and type
- Instrument, needle, and sponge count

The record should not only be a trail of diagnostic and therapeutic activity, but should also be evidence, in terms of a signed consent form for any intervention, of the patient's participation in the decision-making.

Accuracy

It is critical that medical records be accurate. There is no doubt as to the consequences when a patient is harmed because of an inaccurate record.

In *United States v. Green Drugs,*[34] the Court of Appeals for the 3rd Circuit held that pharmacies may be held strictly liable for record-keeping inaccuracies—however innocent—that violate the Comprehensive Drug Abuse Prevention and Control Act, popularly known as the Controlled Substance Act.[35] The *Green Drugs* case is the first appellate court decision to hold that good faith is no defense to a charge of violating the record-keeping provisions of the Controlled Substance Act.

Corrections and alterations

The general rule is to avoid the need for making corrections. But because few humans are perfect, corrections must be made from time to time. Because the medical record must be completely accurate if it is to provide a sound basis for care planning and recording, errors in charting must be corrected promptly in a manner that leaves no doubt as to the facts of the case. Every health institution should have a written policy and protocol, well publicized among all health care providers. An erroneous chart entry should be labeled as such. The incorrect entry should simply be lined through. A single line through an incorrect entry leaves no doubt as to what has been corrected. The correct information is then entered in the next available space. There should be no attempt to affix it to the original provider. The reason for the change should be noted. The correction should be initialed and the time and date it was made entered (if not otherwise shown in the entry). The incorrect entry should never be obliterated. Pages of the record that contain erroneous and corrected entries are never to be destroyed.

If the patient requests that his or her chart be amended, hospital personnel should advise the patient's physician of the requested changes. The physician should then discuss the request with the patient. If the record is changed, an entry should be added to document that the change was made at the request of the patient, who will thereafter bear the burden of explaining the change.[36]

If possible, a physician or supervisory nurse should correct charting errors that are not caught at the time they are made. They should use the same technique, but should enter their signature near the correction, note the time and the date of correction, and, if appropriate, explain in the record why the correction was made. Mistakes in the chart should not be erased, because erasures could create suspicion concerning the original entry.

Tampering with medical records can be costly to a health care provider's reputation and may also result in large malpractice awards, even if there has been no negligence.[37] At trial, evidence of tampering taints the health care provider's credibility; jurors may then distrust the health care provider.

A most damaging aspect of record keeping concerns purging or upgrading the medical record. Generally any enhancement to the medical record may be more detrimental than helpful in defending a physician or health care provider. Records with obvious alterations, particularly any record that can be shown to have been "fudged," are absolutely deadly in court.[38] Nothing should ever be added, deleted, substituted, removed, or rewritten.[39]

A physician or nurse who improperly alters a medical record may be subject to a license revocation action for unprofessional conduct. In Michigan, for example, it is a crime to deliberately falsify a medical record.[40] Attempting to alter the outcome of a case, civil or criminal, by such methods as altering records under subpoena, or which are likely to be subject to subpoena, is a criminal offense.

Document examination is now a sophisticated science.[41] With skill and uncanny accuracy, experts may be able to determine the time that entries were made in medical records and who made them.

Inappropriate entries

Medical records are sometimes used by hospital personnel and medical staff to convey to colleagues remarks or "editorial comments" that are inappropriate for a patient's chart,[42-45] such as: "Dr. A has mistreated this patient again," "Nurse Y is incompetent and should be fired," "This patient is a chronic complainer and a nuisance," "Mrs. B (the patient) isn't sick—she's crazy." The physician should never record his or her personal feelings about the patient. Only necessary facts should be recorded. Criticisms, witticisms, and derogatory or indiscreet remarks have no place in the chart. Once recorded, however, there should be no attempt to tamper with or alter them. They should be left alone, except for an explanation as to the genesis of the error and an appropriate retraction. That is the lesser of two evils.

Legibility and clarity

Medical record entries should be made in clear and concise language that can be understood by all professional staff attending the patient. Handwritten entries must be legible. An illegible record is worse than no record. Entries should be made in ink or typed. Persons making entries should identify themselves clearly by placing their signatures and printed names and positions after each entry. (A rubber stamp is useful for printed name and position, but care must be taken to ensure that a clear and distinct impression is made.)

Adequate. The medical record must include an adequate account of the treatment given the patient, and it must be sufficiently detailed to enable it to show that the care given meets the hospital's standard of care. Failure to make a complete record of care may lead to a finding that the hospital was negligent in its treatment of the patient.[46]

Timely. It is generally the responsibility of individual practitioners and the hospital's medical staff organization to ensure that patient records are completed within a reasonable time after the patient has been discharged from the hospital.[47]

Medical record entries should be made when the treatment they describe is given or the observations they document are made. Federal regulations governing participation in Medicare require that hospital records be completed within 15 days following the patient's discharge.[48] Hospital accreditation standards specify no precise time limit for completion, but require records to be complete within a reasonable time after discharge.[49] The bylaws of regulations of the hospital medical staff may require staff members to complete records within a specified time and may authorize suspension of members who persistently fail to complete records in accordance with staff rules.[50]

Complete. Incomplete records can be troublesome.

Entries made in a record weeks after the patient's discharge have far less credibility then those made during or immediately after the patient's hospitalization. A physician may be deprived of hospital privileges if he or she fails to maintain adequate records.[51]

Third-party insurance companies, such as Blue Cross-Blue Shield, Medicare, and Medicaid, have been upheld in denying payment for medical services if they are not properly documented and recorded in the patient's record.

Authorization

Although federal regulations governing Medicare state that only physicians are competent to write medical histories and physical examinations in the chart,[52] many institutions authorize nurse practitioners to make such entries, provided they are countersigned by a licensed physician. Licensed house staff may write in the chart as long as their entries are countersigned by the attending physician[53] or the chart shows clear evidence of the attending physician's supervision of the house staff involved.[54] The entries of undergraduate medical students and unlicensed house staff that show the application of medical judgment, medical diagnosis, the prescription of treatment, or any other act defined by applicable state law to be the practice of medicine, should be countersigned by a licensed physician. Similarly, the entries of undergraduate nursing students should be countersigned by a licensed professional nurse, if such entries document the practice of professional nursing as defined by the state's nursing licensure act. Without evidence of proper supervision, a nursing student could be held in violation of the state's nursing licensure act, unless the act specifically authorizes nursing students to practice nursing in the course of their studies toward an R.N. degree.[55] The nursing licensure acts of some states authorize the practice of professional nurses for a limited time without a license by graduate nurses who have applied for a license.[56] Graduate, unlicensed nurses in these states may enter statements in a medical record without countersignature by a licensed nurse. In many hospitals, social workers participate in the care of patients and may make entries in patients' charts.

A physician's verbal orders and other instructions must be transcribed in the medical record and signed by the physician within 24 hours.[57] The accreditation standards of the JCAH and hospital licensing regulations in some states require all physician orders to be written in the patient's medical record.[58]

Appropriate documentation

Methods are available to ensure appropriate documentation of instructions to alleviate any confusion at some future date. Records concerning instructions should include the following:
- Instructions in writing
- A notation concerning reviewing the instruction with the patient, family, or legal guardian
- Document measures taken to assure understanding by the patient or a representative of the patient.

A physician is often asked to countersign entries in patient medical records for house officers, students, and nurses. If the physician's signature appears on the record in a capacity other than having personal knowledge of the particular events, he should explain his capacity and role clearly, and note with signature or initials that he read and approved the entry, so in the event of litigation his position will not be misconstrued. In addition, there is the requirement that each physician is under a duty to maintain and complete medical records in a timely fashion.

It is good medical practice for the physician to discreetly document if she suspects the patient is not following the regimen, making sure she notes her observations as well as patient and family comments generally. The subject of adherence to medical instructions can be significant in medical litigation.

Privacy and confidentiality

Because of the nature of contemporary medical services and related record-keeping practices, a physician's records often contain a vivid sketch of some of the most intimate aspects of a patient's life. As a consequence, accentuated by the fiduciary responsibility of the physician, the law and the medical profession have imposed on a physician and other health care providers the duty of confidentiality and privacy (see Chapter 24).

In addition to constitutional recognition of a person's right to privacy, the Federal Privacy Act has recognized such a right.[59] This statute requires federal agencies to obtain the consent of individuals prior to the disclosure of any record kept by a government agency, including medical records, unless it is for the census or for civil or criminal prosecution.

INCIDENT REPORTS

An *incident* has been defined by the American Hospital Association (AHA) as "any happening which is not consistent with the routine operation of the hospital or the routine care of a particular patient. It may be an accident or a situation which could result in an accident."[60] Hospitals use incident reports in their accident prevention programs to advise their insurers of potential suits and to prepare defense against suits that might arise from documented incidents.

Incident reports are considered hearsay under rules of evidence. Hearsay evidence is generally excluded from a trial unless it qualifies under an exception to the hearsay exclusion rule.[61] The exception most frequently used is the business records exception that is established by statute in most states and in the federal courts.[62] To bring an incident report within the exception, it usually must be shown that (1) the report was made in the regular course of business; (2) it was made at or near the time of the incident; and (3) the sources of information, method, and time of preparation were such as to justify its admission.[63] The courts are split in their construction of such business records statutes. The majority of courts interpret "business" quite narrowly, thus excluding records, such as incident reports, that are not part of the inherent nature of the medical business.[64] However, there is a trend among the courts toward allowing the admission of incident reports generated under circumstances that indicate a high degree of trustworthiness.[65]

In most instances, hospitals are more interested in protecting incident reports from discovery by plaintiff's counsel than in getting them into evidence. The attorney-client privilege has been used to protect incident reports in some states.[66,67]

The protection will customarily attach to hospital incident reports provided (1) they are segregated from other hospital reports and labeled "confidential"; (2) access to the reports is restricted to as few hospital employees as possible; (3) they are generated on standard forms for the primary purpose of presenting or defending lawsuits; and (4) they are transmitted to the hospital's legal counsel in a systematic fashion.[68] The hospital bears the burden of showing that the incident report was prepared in anticipation of litigation (the work product doctrine)[69] rather than being prepared as part of normal hospital routine.

Whether admissible or not, hospital incident reports should be prepared pursuant to published policies and procedures. An incident report is no place for opinion, accusation, or conjecture; it should contain only the facts concerning the incident reported.

OWNERSHIP AND ACCESS

In recent years, the legal status of medical records has changed, as evidenced by court decisions and legislative enactment of statutes making records available to the patient.[68-85] These changes have not disturbed the right of ownership of the patient's original medical record.[86] What the courts and legislatures have done is to recognize two types of ownership. They have separated the traditional ownership of the physical materials, comprising the actual record, from the ownership of the information therein. The former still resides in the health care provider, while the latter is designated to be property of the patient.[87-89] The rules governing patients' rights to inspect or copy their own records vary from state to state, especially regarding psychiatric records.[90] Some statutes permit complete access to the records; some permit it as to only specified portions; and others allows only a summary or report to be given.[91] For details on disclosure of medical information, see Chapter 24, and end notes 92 through 115.

In the absence of statutory authority or applicable court decision, patients have no absolute right to inspect the medical records maintained by their physicians in their offices. A number of states authorize patients to inspect and obtain a copy of their medical record[116]; other states require physicians to provide access to the patient's authorized representatives.[117] It has been suggested that patients carry their own medical records.[118] The patient has a right to the information in the record and is therefore entitled to a copy of his or her hospital record.[119] This privilege has even been extended to the next of kin or executor in the event of a patient's death or incompetence.[120] The right to examine the record also extends to the patient succeeding physician, attorney, or other representative.[121,122] Furthermore, with the rare exception of therapeutic privilege, the refusal of the physician to make records available to persons who are entitled to access them may constitute fraudulent concealment and suspend the running of the statute of limitations.[123]

The courts have held that the hospital, while owner of the original documents,[124] is only the custodian and not the owner of the information constituting the patient's medical record. The patient has a property right in the information appearing or portrayed in the record. This property right may entitle the patient to a copy of the record.[125]

When a patient wants a copy of his or her record, he or she is entitled to all reproducible items even if an outside source is needed for the reproduction. In most jurisdictions, photocopies of the medical record need to be provided to the patient or the patient's representative on request. The provider may require the patient to pay the cost of reproduction but not the bill, and allow a reasonable time for reproduction. The provider should never surrender the original.

Although a patient's right to see her or his record or secure a copy is essentially absolute, it must be reasonable. When a reasonable request is made, patients may, at a convenient time, review or even get a copy of the record. When a patient is given access to the record, the event should be supervised and monitored. Physicians should make themselves available when the patient wants to review records. Hospitals need only advise the physicians when they give the patient access. It should be remembered that patients can always get a court order.

When the patient is discharged from the hospital, only the attending physician retains the right to review the record in perpetuity, unless the patient's (surrogate's) consent is obtained for others.

A patient may assign his or her right of review to anyone, but it should be in writing with the assigned subject entitled to the same considerations as the patient. The authorization is considered valid if, when signed, it refers to the specific type of information to be disclosed, identifies the health care provider the records are being requested from, indicates who is requesting the information, and length of time that the authorization is valid. The authorization may further disclose the purpose for which the information may be used.

The administration of the institution is entitled to review the patient's record for three purposes only: statistical analysis, staffing, and quality of care reviews.

The courts have not recognized a legal right of control by the attending physician over the release of information from the medical records in the hospital. Therefore, neither written nor an oral consent from the physician in the hospital is required prior to disclosure. However, some health care institution associations recommend that the attending physician be notified of the patient's request for access to the medical record and be allowed to intervene if that is possible.

If the physician refuses to make the records available to persons entitled to them, this may be considered fraudulent concealment as an additional cause of action. In any event, it suspends the running of the claim and cause of action. In any event, a patient can always seek a *subpoena duces tecum.*

In those rare instances where the knowledge of the medical facts may be detrimental to the patient, the courts generally recognize the doctrine of "professional discretion or privilege." Courts will not hold the physician liable for failing to reveal the specific information that he or she believes may be detrimental to the patient, providing the physician records the basis for invoking the doctrine.

When a physician acts as the employee of a hospital or clinic, the records usually become the property of the employer in the absence of an agreement to the contrary.[126] The patient could acquire ownership, possession, and control by a contractual agreement with the health care provider.[127]

The peer review organization (PRO) law grants patients access to their records.[128-130] By statue or court decision, every state prohibits disclosure of "proceedings and records relating to the performance of a medical review function."

Access laws

Access laws are discussed in Chapter 24 on disclosures about patients and also in end notes 131 through 156.

Psychiatric records have a special status of discoverability as evidenced by several recent decisions. A physician's personal psychiatric medical records are not discoverable in a malpractice suit against him or her.[157] Nor can a psychiatrist's patient's medical records be discovered by a state agency during an investigation of the psychiatrist.[158]

Legal actions regarding access

Frequently, the plaintiff tries to discover the names, addresses, and case histories of other patients who have been treated by the physician-defendant. Several courts have held that evidence regarding other patients' care can be introduced with the proper protection of those patients.[159-161]

Control of medical records

Transfer. The AMA's judicial council rules of professional conduct have decreed that a physician is ethically obligated to cooperate with and transfer records to the physician who succeeds him or her in caring for a patient.[162]

On the transfer of a practice, including a sale, the records do not automatically go with the practice. The patient information therein belongs to the patient; the physician is only the custodian. However, a blanket notice of the change is sufficient.

Loss. Loss of all or part of the medical record, unless adequately explained so as to prove there was no dereliction of duty, creates a legal inference that the loss was intentional and wrongly motivated.[163] Failure to locate a record is a sure bet for losing a malpractice lawsuit, not being reimbursed for services, and other serious problems.

Spoilation of evidence (medical records). The tort of spoilation of evidence deals with the destruction of evidence, including medical records, and has existed for some time. It is recognized as being established in this country in the 1984 case of *Smith v. Superior Court.*[164] The spoilation may have been deliberate or intentional or negligent.

There are also criminal laws against destruction of evidence, mainly that of obstruction of justice.

Custody and storage. The physician is liable for the proper maintenance, custody, and storage of the record for the required statutory period or for as long as a proper lawsuit can be brought (statute of limitations).[165]

As stated previously, patient medical records are to be considered confidential and must be controlled/stored including protection from unauthorized disclosure (see Chapter 24).

RETENTION REQUIREMENTS

The increased complexity of health care delivery has heightened the importance of medical record retention.

State medical records laws

In most states, there is no specific retention requirement for medical records. State law may dictate specific medical record retention requirements. For example, Maryland law provides that, unless the patient is notified, a health care professional cannot destroy an adult's medical record or laboratory or X-ray report for five years after the record or report is made.[166] In the case of a minor patient, a medical record or laboratory or X-ray report cannot be destroyed until the patient attains the age of majority plus three years or for five years after the record or report is made, whichever is later, unless the parent or guardian of the child is notified, or the minor patient is notified if the care provided was care for which the minor is permitted to consent.[167]

In most states, there is no specific retention requirement for medical charts. Retention periods prescribed by law vary from state to state. Each state's law has unique retention requirements for medical records. Some states provide that such records be maintained permanently, whereas others require retention for a specific period, such as the length of the state's statute of limitation for contract or tort actions. In California, for example, documents that constitute "medical records" generally must be preserved for at least seven years and for minors until after the minor has reached the age of 18, and in any case, not less than seven years.[168,169]

State statutes of limitations

The state's statute of limitations for general civil claims for adults and for minors, should be considered in developing a retention policy. Some states have separate statutes of limitation for adults and for minors for medical malpractice. Statutes of limitations for assault, libel, and slander may also be relevant.[170-172]

Because statutes of limitations establish the time period with which a lawsuit may be brought, providers must be aware of such time limits. Medical records should not be destroyed before the expiration of these periods.

The presence of a latent injury may extend the statute of limitations until the injury is discovered.

Joint Commission on Accreditation of Healthcare Organizations (JCAHO) requirements

JCAHO provides that the length of time for which medical records are to be retained is dependent on the need for their use in continuing patient care and for legal research, or educational purposes, and on law and regulation.[173]

JCAHO requires hospitals to maintain patient care records as a standard of accreditation. In the absence of a specific retention period, it is likely that retention for the period required by state law would be deemed to comply with JCAHO requirements.

AHA and AMRA recommendations

A provider may wish to consider the recommendations of professional associations regarding record retention times. For example, two such associations, the AHA and the AMRA, have recommended that the complete patient medical record, in original or reproduced form, be retained for a period of 10 years. This period would commence with the last encounter with a patient. These associations further suggest that, after 10 years, such records may be destroyed unless destruction is specifically prohibited by statute, ordinance, regulation, or law, and provided that the institution retains certain information for specified purposes.[174]

Alcohol and drug abuse treatment records

The federal regulations protecting confidentiality of alcohol and drug abuse treatment records do not have specific general retention periods. However, the regulations require that the records be maintained in a secure room, locked file cabinet, safe, or other similar container when not in use.[175] In addition, if a program discontinues operations or is acquired by another program, it must purge patient identifying records or destroy the records unless the patient gives written consent to transfer the records or there is a legal requirement that the records be kept for a specific amount of time. The records should be labeled with the name of the program and citation to the court order or law requiring retention and must be destroyed as soon as practical after the end of the required retention period.[176]

Methadone treatment programs must maintain records traceable to specific patients showing dates, quantity, and batch or code marks of the drug dispensed for a period of three years from the date of dispensing.[177] Likewise, when narcotic drugs are administered for treatment of narcotic dependence for hospitalized patients, the hospital must maintain accurate records showing dates, quantity, and batch or code marks for the drug used for at least three years.[178]

Age Discrimination in Employment Act

Under the Age Discrimination in Employment Act, among other records, the results of any physical examination of an employee, where the examination is considered by the employer in connection with a personnel action, must be retained for one year.[179]

Employee medical records

Employee health records should be retained according to specific state and federal retention and statute of limitations requirements.[180] Some state laws guarantee employees and unions the right to review and copy their medical records.

Wrongful death

Since wrongful death is a statutory cause or action, each state has its own statute of limitations. Therefore, the state statute of limitations must be considered in the retention of the patient's medical record.

Malpractice vulnerability/statutes of limitations

It is imperative, apart from any statutory mandates, that a physician maintain comprehensive patient records as long as the threat of a medical malpractice suit exists. The statute of limitations in each state determines what length of time a physician is vulnerable to a malpractice suit. During this period of vulnerability, a physician needs complete and accurate medical records to successfully defend him- or herself in a malpractice action.

All records that have been the subject of an incident that could lead to litigation and all records that have been requested by an attorney or an administrative agency should be excepted from the general retention policy. These records should not be destroyed until the matter is fully resolved. In addition to these considerations, the provider would consult its insurance carriers to determine whether a carrier has specific record retention requirements.

Hospital records

Hospitals generally keep medical records for the period prescribed by law or regulations or for a tie considered appropriate by the individual institution. A hospital must, however, retain radiographic films as part of their regularly maintained records for a period of 5 years; films involved in litigation that commenced before the expiration of the 5-year period must be kept until the litigation has concluded or for 12 years from the date the film was produced, whichever comes first.[181]

Federal regulations governing the Medicare program require participating hospitals to keep patient records for a period of not less then that determined by the appropriate state statute of limitations for tort actions.[182] The AMA recommends retention of records for at least 10 years.[183]

In the absence of statutory or regulatory retention requirements, hospitals should maintain their records at least for the statute of limitations period for tort actions, and preferably for contrast actions, in their respective states.

Public health records

Occupational Safety and Health Administration requirements. The federal Occupational Safety and Health Administration (OSHA) requires that a provider main-

tain documentation of employee's occupational injuries and illnesses, consisting of a log and descriptive summary, a supplementary record detailing such injuries and illnesses, and an annual summary, which is to be posted.[184] All of the foregoing documentation must be retained for at least 5 years following the end of the year to which it relates.[185] However, records pertaining to employee exposure to toxic substances or harmful physical agents must be retained for 30 years.[186]

State requirements. Each state has its own requirements for the maintenance of employee health and health examination records. Such records should be maintained for at least as long as the statute of limitations for workers' compensation or occupational safety claims, even if state and/or federal record retention periods are shorter.

Department of Health and Human Services grants. All financial, programmatic, statistical, and other records of grant recipients that are expressly required to be maintained by the terms of any grant from the Department of Health and Human Services (DHHS) or are reasonably considered pertinent to a DHHS grant must be retained for 3 years from the starting date of the grant. Furthermore, if any litigation claim, federal audit, negotiation, or other action involving such records has been initiated before the expiration of this 3-year period, the records must be retained until completion of the action and resolution of all issues arising from it, or until the end of the minimum 3-year retention period, whichever is later.[187]

Many states have public records laws that apply to public hospitals. Some state statutes explicitly exempt hospital and medical records from disclosure.[188]

Medicare records. All of the following categories of Medicare records are required to be maintained for at least 5 years after a Medicare cost report is filed with the fiscal intermediary.

BILLING MATERIAL. Retain all billings for Medicare services, including form UB-82 (HCFA-1450), and any supporting documents and forms, charge slips, daily hospital or extended care facility (ECF) patients census records, and any other business and accounting records that refer to specific Medicare claims.[189]

COST REPORT MATERIAL. Retain all data necessary to support the accuracy of the entries on the annual cost reports, including original invoices, canceled checks, and all other work papers used in preparing annual cost reports. This would include forms and other similar cost reports, schedules, and related worksheets.[190] Contracts or records of dealings with outside sources of medical supplies and services or with related organizations for which Medicare reimbursement is sought should also be retained.

REVIEWS, REPORTS, AND OTHER RECORDS. Retain hospital and ECF utilization review committee reports, physicians' certifications and recertifications, hospital and ECF discharge summaries, and clinical and other medical records relating to health insurance claims.[191]

The Medicare conditions of participation also place varied requirements on hospitals regarding the length of time records for specific services must be maintained.[192] For instance, a hospital must maintain records of radiologic services including copies of printouts and reports, films, scans, and other image records for at least 5 years. As for laboratory services, the regulations require that records of services performed in a facility certified in accordance with 42 C.F.R. Part 493 be retained for at least 5 years. Part 493 requires that laboratory requisitions or authorizations and records of patient testing including an original report or an exact duplicate of each test report (preliminary and final) must be retained for a minimum of 2 years after date of reporting. Immunohematology records, including reports, must be retained for no less than 5 years.[193] Pathology test reports must be retained for a period of at least 10 years after the date of reporting.

Medicare also has specific retention requirements for (1) long-term care facilities, which is a period required by state law or, if there are no state requirements, for 5 years from the date of discharge for adults and for a minor for 3 years after the resident reaches a legal age under state law; (2) home health agencies, which is 5 years after the month the relevant cost report is filed; (3) comprehensive outpatient rehabilitation facilities, which is 5 years after patient discharge; (4) clinical and rehabilitation agencies (which provide outpatient physical therapy and/or speech pathology services), which is a period determined by the state or, if there is no state requirement, for 5 years after the date of discharge for adults and, for minors, 3 years after the patient becomes of age under state law or 5 years after discharge, whichever is longer, (5) end-state renal disease services, which is as required by state law, or if there is no state requirement, for 5 years from the date of discharge or, in the case of a minor, for 3 years after the patient becomes of age.

Several state regulations provide that records be kept permanently, but some require retention for the period in which suits may be filed. Some states provide that records cannot be destroyed without state agency approval.

Medicare contractors. Medicare regulations also require those who contract with Medicare providers to retain their books, documents, and records for 4 years after the services are furnished under that contract and to require their subcontractors to retain their records for the same period to verify services for which Medicare reimbursement is claimed.[194] This includes physicians who have agreements under Parts A and B.

Notwithstanding the time periods specified here, all records pertaining to any reimbursement issue that is on appeal with the Medicare program should be retained until the conclusion of the appeal.[195]

DESTRUCTION OF RECORDS

Appropriate destruction of medical records should be handled in a manner that optimizes the confidentiality of their contents. Shredding or burning the documents will probably offer the greatest protection. A record should be kept of the patient's name, records destroyed, date of destruction, and person destroying the medical records. It may be advisable to contact the patient in advance of destruction.

Specific state requirements have been noted previously.

COMPUTERIZED MEDICAL RECORDS

The advent of computerized medical records has created some potential legal problems.[196,197] A study of the potential for implementing an automated record system must start with an analysis of state hospital licensing regulations governing the creation, maintenance, and authentication of medical records.[198] The JCAHO recognizes computerization of medical records.[199]

When a hospital contracts with a computer company to automate its medical record system, three primary issues must be considered: confidentiality, privacy, and security. In the opinion of the AMA, there is a breach of medical ethics in making record entries into a computer system whose database is available to more than one user, unless proper security measures are taken.[200] To protect a hospital against potential liability and to protect its staff against charges of legal and ethical violations, it is necessary to design a security system that will prevent unauthorized disclosure of identifiable medical information.

The computer system must have a verification system whereby a physician can authenticate entries and retrieve complete records. This system should be designed so that physicians other than the attending physician can have access only with the consent of the patient or the patient's legal representative. The system should have built-in safeguards to prevent theft or misuse of information.

Two primary legal issues arise when a hospital decides to adopt a computerized medical record system. First, has the health care provider, whose patient records are complied and stored mechanically, produced a "medical record" as defined by state law or regulation? Second, does the system in which the records are stored meet the patient's expectation that the record will remain confidential? Other important legal issues—evidentiary problems, contractual issues, and software patent and copyright issues—must also be analyzed before a hospital computerizes its record system.

Although illegibility can never be a problem, authentication of patient records may prove difficult. Today, there are new processes for user identification, including the development of voice prints and the use of passwords that will alleviate the problem of authentication by ensuring that only authorized individuals have access to patient medical records.

Another legal obstacle in using computerized medical records is the problem of tampering. Safeguards can be built into the process to effectively prevent tampering.

Most statutes mandate that the patient records be written or typed and signed by the physician. Computer systems must therefore be modified to satisfy these statutory requirements.

Computer records generally fall within the definition of discoverable "documents" or "writings" under the laws of most states, and as such are admissible as trial evidence.[201]

Rule 34 of the Federal Rules of Civil Procedure, which is followed by all federal courts throughout the nation, defines the term "document" very broadly, to include data compilations stored on any type of media that can be translated into "reasonably usable form." Court cases across the country have long recognized that, in the absence of evidentiary and procedure objections, computer records are properly admissible as evidence in both civil and criminal cases.[202]

PROBLEM-ORIENTED RECORDS AND CONDITION DIAGNOSIS

The problem-oriented medical record (POMR) is the standard method for recording patient data in many institutions. Its SOAP section, which includes the subjective, objective, assessment, and plan categories, provides a good nucleus of information and has endured the test of time. But it does not provide enough insight into the process of a physician's thinking and his diagnostic efforts. The hospital practice of preparing summaries should be extended to the office and clinic, perhaps on a monthly or annual basis by category. Nontrivial cases should be charted by means of SOAP records.

In an attempt to find a method by which physicians could record more information but take less time to record it, the condition diagram (CD) was developed. It is a shorthand way of recording information and eliminates having to ferret through pages of narrative notes to find essential information. The CD is based on the concept of sentence diagramming: All parts of a sentence have a place on the diagram and would be diagrammed the same way by anyone.

The patient's condition is given in the center of the chart. Arrows point from this box to the patient's description on the left and to two possible outcomes on the right. Above the condition box is pertinent data that led the physician to her diagnosis; directly below that the physician can list the differential diagnoses or the potential conditions. The upper left quadrant lists the induction factors that led to the condition. The upper right quadrant is for listing complications and the lower right for planned treatments.

Experience has shown that the performance of physicians using it improved and that medical students using the CD made fewer errors in diagnosis and had better documentation than those using the POMR.

AUTOAUTHENTICATION OF MEDICAL RECORDS

The term *autoauthentication* refers to a system that allows medical records to be automatically signed on behalf of the health care practitioner, without any assurance that the records have been seen—much less reviewed—by the practitioner after transcription.[203,204] Typically, autoauthentication procedures provide for sending a copy of the transcribed report to the practitioner with an electronic signature affixed; the report will be considered complete if the practitioner does not request corrections within a specified period of time. Although an autoauthentication system may incorporate the use of an electronic signature, the terms are not synonymous, because some health facilities allow use of an electronic signature only after the practitioner has actually reviewed the record.

Regulatory and accrediting issues

Authentication of medical records without verification of their completeness and accuracy by the practitioner is prohibited by the Health Care Financing Administration (HCFA), the Joint Commission on Accreditation of Healthcare Organizations (JCAHO), and many state health departments. HCFA's Medicare conditions of participation[205] and diagnostic related group validation requirements[206] clearly allow electronic signatures, but apparently not autoauthentication, because they appear to require the author of the entry to verify the transcribed report before the signature may be applied. HCFA–Region IX (covering the states of Arizona, California, Hawaii, and Nevada) has verified that it interprets the Medicare conditions of participation to prohibit autoauthentication.[207]

JCAHO standards also allow authentication of medical records using electronic signatures, but likewise appear to require practitioners to affix their signatures after reviewing the reports. JCAHO has confirmed that its standards prohibit auto-authentication of medical records.[208]

A number of states have implemented similar laws and

regulations. For example, in California, the State Department of Health Services (SDHS) has adopted regulations allowing the use of electronic signatures, but these regulations emphasize that only the responsible practitioner can have the ability to apply the signature.[209] In March 1993, SDHS confirmed in an internal memorandum to the district offices in its Licensing and Certification Branch that an electronic authentication system that does not require the practitioner to verify the information in the report after the report is transcribed, i.e., and autoauthentication system, is unacceptable. In other words, authentication may not be done by default (i.e., failure of the practitioner to correct the transcribed report). In accordance with this policy, SDHS has already issued several cease-and-desist orders to California hospitals that had been using autoauthentication systems.

END NOTES

1. Matte, *Legal Implications of the Patient's Medical Record, in Legal Medicine Annual: 1971*, 345-75 (C. H. Wecht ed., 1971).
2. Goldstein, *Hospital Record: Keystone in Malpractice Claims*, 16 Physician's Legal Brief 3 (1974).
3. Holder, *The Importance of Medical Records*, 228 JAMA 118-119 (1974).
4. A. R. Holder, *Medical Malpractice Law*, 394-99 (1975).
5. H. Louisill and D. Williams, *Medical Malpractice* (1960).
6. Harris and Mills, *Medical Records and the Questioned Document Examiner*, 8 J. Forensic Sci. 453-61 (1963).
7. *McGarry v. JA Mercier Co.*, 272 Mich. 501, 262 N.W. 296 (1935).
8. *In re Culbertson's Will*, 292 N.Y.S.2d 806 (1968).
9. *Falum v. Medical Arts Center Hospital*, 160 N.Y. L. J. 2 (1968).
10. Adametz, *Ownership of Physician's Medical Records*, 208 JAMA 1591-92 (1969).
11. Holman, *A Guide to Hospital Records*, 3 Duke L. J. 29-48 (1948).
12. Trostler, *Ownership of Roentgenograms and Medical Records*, 88 American Medical Society 1895-1901 (1927).
13. L. Fleischer, *Ownership of Hospital Records and Roentgenograms*, AMA, Legal Dept., Medicolegal Monographs (1964).
14. U.S. Dep't of Health, Education, & Welfare, Report of the Secretary's Commission on Medical Malpractice, Reports, Studies and Analysis, Access to Medical Records, D.H.E.W. Pub. No. (O.S.) 73-88, at 78-213 (1973).
15. S. W. Donaldson, *The Roentgenologist in Court* (2d ed. 1954).
16. Martin, *Ownership of X-ray Plates*, 46 N.Y. State J. Med, 654 (1946).
17. Wolfstone, *Patient's Right of Access to Inspect and Obtain Copies of Medical Records, in Legal Medicine Annual: 1971*, at 379-86 (C. H. Wecht ed., 1971).
18. *Hurley v. Gage* (Genesse County Circuit Court Mich. 1932).
19. *Emmett v. Eastern Dispensary and Casualty Hosp.*, 396 F.2d 931 (Dist. Ctr. D.C. 1967).
20. Aspen Systems Corp., *Right to Examine Record, in Aspen Hospital Law Manual* 3-17 (1973).
21. *Wallace v. University Hosp. of Cleveland*, 164 N.E.2d 917 (Ohio 1959).
22. *Pyramid Life Insurance Co v. Mason Hosp. Ass'n. of Payne County*, 191 F. Supp. 51 (W. Dist. Ct. Okla. 1961).
23. Aspen Systems Corp., *Medical Records, in Aspen Hospital Law Manual* (1990).
24. Joint Commission on Accreditation of Healthcare Organizations, *Accreditation Manual for Hospitals* 79-92 (1990 ed.).
25. *Foley v. Flushing Hosp. and Medical Center*, 41 A.D.2d 769, 341 N.Y.S.2d 917 (1973).
26. *Medical Records, in Hospital Law Manual* § 3 (1973).
27. *Larrimore v. Homeopathic Hosp. Ass'n.*, 54 Del. 449, 181 A.2d 563 (1962).
28. *Pyramid Life Ins. Co. v. Gleason*, 188 360 P.2d 850 Kan. 95 (1961).
29. S. Chapman, *How Long Should You Keep Your Patients' Medical Records?* Leg. Aspects Med. Practice, 19-33 (Aug. 1979): *Supra* note 24.
30. Chicago Municipal Code § 137.14 (1947).
31. 20 C.F.R. § 405.1026(g) (1976).
32. *In re Culbertson's Will*, *supra* note 8.
33. A. R. Holden, *Physician's Records and the Chiropractor*, 224 JAMA 1071 (1973).
34. *United States v. Green Drugs*, 905 F.2d 694 (3d Cir. 1990).
35. Comprehensive Drug Abuse Prevention and Control Act, Pub. L. No. 91-513, 84 Stat. 1242 (1970); 21 U.S.C. § 801-971.
36. Hirsh, *There's a Right Way and a Wrong Way to Set the (medical) Record Straight*, Modern Medicine, 39, 42. (Apr. 15, 1977).
37. Hirsh, *Tampering With Medical Records*, 24 Med. Trial Tech. Q. 450-55 (Spring 1978); Preiser, *The High Cost of Tampering With Medical Records*, Medical Economics 84-87. (Oct. 4, 1986).
38. S. Gage, *Alteration, Falsification, and Fabrication of Records in Medical Malpractice Actions*, Med. Trial Tech. Q. 476-88. (Spring 1981).
39. Hirsh, *Medical Records: Backbone of Malpractice Prevention*, Physician's Management 159-73 (Oct. 1986); Harris and Mills, *supra* note 6.
40. *See, e.g.*, Mich. Stat. Ann. § 14.624(21) (Callaghan 1976); Tenn. Code Ann. § 63-752(f) (Supp. 1976); Tenn. Code Ann. § 39-1971 (1975) (making it a crime to falsify a hospital medical record for purposes of cheating or defrauding).
41. Hirsh, *supra* note 39.
42. *Hiatt v. Grace*, 523 P.2d 320 (Kan. 1974).
43. *Gotkin v. Miller*, 379 F. Supp. 859 (1974).
44. *Rabens v. Jackson Park Hospital Foundation*, 40 Ill App. 3d 113, 351 N.E.2d 276 (1976); JCAH, *Accreditation Manual for Hospitals* 71 (1986).
45. *Bishop Clarkson Memorial Hospital v. Reserve Life Insurance Co.*, 350 F.2d 1006 (8th Cir. 1965); *Pyramid Life Insurance Co. v. Masonic Hosp. Ass'n. of Payne County*, 191 F. Supp. 51 (West. Dist. Ct. Okla 1961); *Wallace v. Univ. Hosp. of Cleveland*, 171 Ohio St. 487, 172 N.E.2d 459 (1961).
46. *Darling v. Charleston Community Hosp.*, 33 Ill.2d 326, 211 N.E.2d 253 (1964); *Larrimore v. Homeopathic Hosp. Ass'n.*, 54 Del. 449, 181 A.2d 573(1963); *Hansch v. Hackett*, 190 Wash, 97, 66 P.2d 1129 (1937).
47. JCAH, *supra* note 24, at 261; Huffman, *Medical Records Management* 152-54 (6th ed. 1972).
48. 20 C.F.R. § 405.1026(j) (1976).
49. JCAH, *supra* note 24, at 79-92.
50. *Board of Trustees of Memorial Hosp. v. Pratt*, 72 Wyo. 120, 262 P.2d 682 (1953).
51. *Rao v. Auburn General Hosp. et al.*, 573 P.2d 834 (Wash. App. 1977).
52. 20 C.F.R. § 405.1026(h) (1976).
53. 20 C.F.R. § 405.1026(h)-(i) (1976).
54. JCAH, *supra* note 24, at 72-92.
55. Ill. Ann. Stat. Ch. 91 para. 35.33(2) (Smith-Hurd 1966); Tenn. Code Ann. § 63-739(c) (1976).
56. Ill. Ann. Stat. Ch. 91 para. 35.33(5) (Smith-Hurd 1966); Mich Stat. Ann. § 14.694(15) (Callaghan 1976); Tenn. Code Ann. § 63-742(c)(1) (1976).

57. JCAH, *supra* note 24, at 72-92.
58. JCAH, *supra* note 24; Ill. Hospital Licensing Requirements § 3-3.a (1976).
59. Federal Privacy Act, 5 U.S.C., § 552(a) (1974).
60. American Hospital Association and National Safety Council, *Safety Guide for Health Care Institutions* 33 (1972).
61. C. McCormick, *Law of Evidence* § 246.313(a) (2d ed. 1972).
62. Ariz. Rev. Stat. Ann. § 12-2262 (1956); Hawaii Rev. Stat. § 622-5 (Supp. 1974); N.Y. Civ. Prac. b. and R. § 4518 (McKinney 1963); Vt. Stat. Ann. tit. 12, § 1700 (1973); 28 U.S.C.A. § 1732 (1977); 28 U.S.C.S. App. § 803.6 (1975).
63. *See, e.g.,* N.Y. Civ. Prac. L. & R. § 4518 (McKinney 1963).
64. *Hoffman v. Palmer,* 129 F.2d 976 (2d Cir. 1942), *aff'd, Palmer v. Hoffman,* 318 U.S. 109 (1943); Laughlin, *Business Entires and the Like,* 46 Iowa L. Rev. 276 (1961).
65. Comment, *Hospital Accident Reports: Admissibility and Privileges,* 1975 Dick. L. Rev. 493; J. Bromberg, and H. Hirsh, *Medical Records and Hospital Reports,* Med. Law 253-72 (Spring 1982).
66. *See Sierra Vista Hosp. v. Superior Court,* 248 Cal. App.2d 359, 56 Cal. Rptr. 387.
67. 8 J. Wigmore, *Evidence* § 2292 (McNaughton rev. 1961).
68. Bernstein, *Law in Brief: Access to Physician's Hospital Records,* 45 Hospitals 148-52, 170 (1972).
69. Dornette, *Medical Records,* 8 Clinical Anesthesiology 285-91 (1972).
70. *Kabes,* 175 N.Y.S.2d 83 (Sup. Ct. Chemung County 1958).
71. *Wohlgemuth v. Meyer,* 136 Cal. App.2d 326.
72. *Cannell v. The Medical and Surgical Center,* 315 N.E.2d 278.
73. *Musman v. The Methodist Hosp.,* No. C-2051 (1956).
74. Hirsh, *Legal Implications of Patient Records,* 72 Southern Med. J. 726-31 (1979).
75. *In the Matter of Weiss,* 147 N.Y.S.2d 455 (1955).
76. *Jones v. Fakehany,* 67 Cal. Rptr. 810 (1968).
77. J. Hayt, L. Groeschel, and M. McMillan, *Law of Hospital and Nurse,* 317-8 (1st ed. 1958).
78. J. Hayt, E. Hayt, L. Groeschel, *Law of Hospital, Physician and Patient* 652-55 (2d, ed. 1962).
79. *Rabens v. Jackson Hosp. Foundation,* 351 N.E.2d 276, 40 Ill. App. 3d 113 (1976).
80. *Musman, supra* note 73.
81. *Bishop Clarkson Memorial Hosp. supra* note 45.
82. *Gotkin, supra* note 43.
83. University of Pittsburgh Health Law Center, *Hospital Law Manual* §§ 12, 12a (1962).
84. Blanchard, Will You Switch to Problem-oriented Records, 7 *Patient Care* 59-63 (1973).
85. *Medical Records, supra* note 26.
86. In *Hospital Law Manual,* University of Pittsburgh Health Law Center, 1962, §§ 12, 12a.
87. Blanchard, *supra* note 84.
88. Shenkin & Warner, Giving the Patient His Medical Record: A Proposal to Improve the System Sounding Board, 289 New Eng. J. Med. 688-91 (1973).
89. Conn. Gen. Stat. Ann. § 4-104 (West 1974); Colo. Rev. Stat. §§ 25-1-801 to 803 (1975); Fla. Stat. Ann. § 458.16 (West 1974); Haw. Rev. Stat. §§ 622-57 (1977); Ill. Rev. Stat. ch. 51-71-73 & 73(a) (1976); Ind. Code Ann. §§ 34-3-15.54 (Burns 1976); Mass. Ann. Laws ch. 111-70, ch. 123-36, ch. 380 (Law. Co-op. 1977); adds § 144.335 to Minn. Stat. Ann. (West 1977); adding new sections to ch. 629, Nev. Rev. Stat. (1977); N.J. Stat. Ann. §§ 30:4-24.3, 2A:82-42 (West 1978); N.Y. Comp. Codes R & Reg. § 720-20(p) (1971); Rules of the N.Y. St. Bd. of Regents Relating to Definitions of Unprofessional Conduct §§ 29.2(a)(7), 29.1(b)(13) (1977); Okla. Stat. Ann. tit. 76, ch. 18 (West 1978); 1977 Or. Laws

812; Tex. Rev. Civ. Stat. Ann. (Mental Health Code) art. 5547-87 (Vernon 1977); Va. Code Ann. § 8.01-413 (1978).
90. Cal. Op. Att'y Gen. 151 (1976); Cal. Welf. & Inst. Code § 5328 (West 1976); D.C. Code Ann. § 21-562 (1980); Ga. Code Ann. § 88-502.10 (1978); Me. Rev. Stat. Ann. § 34-1-13 (1976); Mich. Comp. Laws Ann. § 14.800(748) (West 1976); N.J. Stat. Ann. § 30.4-24.3 (West 1976); Utah Code Ann. § 78-25-25 (1977); *see also* Ga. Code Ann. § 88-502.10 (1978); Ky. Rev. Stat. Ann. § 210.235 (Baldwin 1978); Me. Rev. Stat. Ann. § 34-1B; Meh Comp. Laws.
91. Wolfstone, *supra* note 17; *Right to Examine Record, supra* note 20.
92. Bernstein, *supra* note 68; Dornette, *supra* note 69.
93. E. Hayt & J. Hayt, *Legal Aspects of Medical Records* 58-62 (1964).
94. Hayt, Groeschel, and McMillan, *supra* note 77; Hayt, Hayt, and Groeschel, *supra* note 78.
95. *Current Opinions of the Judicial Council of the American Medical Association* (1981).
96. Hirsh, *Medical Records — Their Medico-legal Significance,* 2 J. Fam. Pract. 69-75 (1975).
97. *Gaernmer v. State of Michigan,* 187 N.W.2d 429 (Mich 1971), aff'd. 180 N.W.2d 308 (Mich 1970).
98. Bernstein, *supra* note 68.
99. Dornette, *supra* note 69.
100. *Kabes,* 175 N.Y.S.2d 83 (Sup. Ct. Chemung County 1958).
101. *Wohlgemuth,* 136 Cal. App.2d 326, 293 P.2d 816 (1956).
102. *Cannell v. The Medical and Surgical Clinic,* 315 N.E.2d 278 (Ill. 1974).
103. *Musman v. Methodist Hosp.,* No. C-2051 (Ind. 1956) (unreported case).
104. Donaldson, *supra* note 15; Trostler, *supra* note 12; Fleischer, *supra* note 13.
105. Hayt, Groeschel, and McMillan, *supra* note 77.
106. Hayt, Hayt, and Groeschel, *supra* note 78.
107. 42 Pa. Cons. Stat. Ann. § 151 (Purdon Supp. 1987).
108. Turkington, *Legal Protection for the Confidentiality of Healthcare Information in Pennsylvania Patient and Client Access Testimonial Privilege, Damage Recovery for Unauthorized Extra-legal Disclosure,* 32 Vill. F. Rev. 288(1987).
109. *Id.* at 292.
110. 55 Pa. Code s 5100-33 (C) (1986); *see generally* 55 Pa. Code § 5100-33 (b)-(d), (g)-(j) (1986).
111. Miller, *Confidentiality or Communication in the Treatment of the Mentally Ill* 9 Bull Amer. Acad. Psych. Law 54-59 (1981).
112. Miller, *Outpatient Civil Commitment of the Mentally Ill: An Overview and an Update,* 6 Behav. Sci. Law 99, 111 (1988).
113. *Tarasoff v. Regents of the Univ. of California* (1976), 118 Cal. Rptr. 129, 529 P.2d 553 (1974); 17 Cal. 3d 425, 551 P.2d 334 (1976).
114. Melville, *Confidentiality: Widened Disclosure in the Clinical Context,* 45 U. Toronto Fac. L. Rev. 179-186 (1987).
115. *See, e.g.,* Ill. Ann. Stat. ch. 48, para. 138.8(a) (Smith-Hurd Supp. 1977); Wis. Stat. Ann. § 804.09 (West 1977).
116. *See* Ill. Ann. Stat. Ch. 51, para. 73 (Smith-Hurd Supp. 1977); *Rabens, supra* note 44; Blanchard, *supra* note 84.
117. Shenkin & Warner, *Giving the Patient His Medical Record: A Proposal to Improve the System Sounding Board,* 289 New Eng. J. Med. 688-91 (1973).
118. Hirsh, *supra* note 39.
119. Hirsh, *supra* note 74.
120. Hayt, *supra* note 77.
121. Hayt, *supra* note 78.
122. *Rabens, supra* note 79.
123. *Musman, supra* note 73.
124. *Bishop Clarkson Memorial Hosp., supra* note 45.
125. *Hospital Law Manual, supra* note 86.
126. Blanchard, *supra* note 84.

127. 5 U.S.C.A. § 552 (1977 & 1989 Supp.).
128. 5 U.S.C.A. § 552a (1977 & 1989 Supp); 5 U.S.C.A. § 552a (1974) (Federal Privacy Act; Peer Review Improvement Act of 1982, Pub. L. No. 97-248, §§ 141-150, 96 Stat. 382 (1982) (codified at 42 U.S.C.A. §§ 1320c-1320c-12); Pub. L. No. 98-21, § 602, 97 Stat. 167 (1983).
129. 42 U.S.C.A. §§ 1381-1383c (1983 & 1989 Supp.).
130. 42 U.S.C.A. § 1320a-7b (1989 Supp.).
131. Matter of Grand Jury Subpoena Duces Tecum, dated December 14, 1984 c/o *M.D., P.C. v. Kuriansky,* 505 N.E.2d 925 (1987).
132. 42 C.F.R. pt. 2 (1988).
133. *E.g.,* Iowa Code Ann. § 22.7 (West 1989 Supp.); *Head v. Colloton,* 331 N.W.2d 870 1983).
134. *Eugene Cervi & Co. v. Russell,* 184 Colo. 282, 519 P.2d 1189 (1974).
135. *Head v. Colloton,* 33, N.W. 2d870 (Iowa 1983).
136. *Wooster Republican Printing Co. v. City of Wooster,* 56 Ohio St.2d 126, 383 N.E. (1978).
137. *E.g.,* Fla. Stat. § 415.504 (1987); Iowa Code Ann. § 232.75(2) (West 1985); Cal. Penal Code § 11166 (West 1982); Mich. Comp. Laws Ann. § 722.625 (West 1987) *E.g.,* Fla. Stat. § 415.103 (1987).
138. *E.g.,* Iowa Code Ann. § 85.27 (West 1984).
139. *E.g.,* Acosta v. Cary, 365 So.2d 4 (La. Ct. App. 1978).
140. Pub. L. No. 91-596, 84 Stat. 1590 (1970) (codified as amended at 29 U.S.C.A. (1985) and in scattered sections of 5, 15, 29, 42, and 49 U.S.C.).
141. Medicare Program, Acquisition, Protection and Disclosure of Utilization and Quality Control Peer Review Organization (PRO) Information, 49 Fed. Reg. 14977 (1984) (to be codified at 42 C.F.R. § 476). et seq.; *e.g.,* Ore. Rev. Stat. § 677.415 (2); Mich. Comp. Laws 333.21515.
142. *Corleto v. Shore Memorial Hosp.,* 138 N.J. Super. 302, 350 A.2d 534 (1975)
143. *Jordan v. Court of Appeals for the Fourth Supreme Judicial District of Texas, Supreme Court of Texas,* 701 S.W.2d 644 (1988).
144. *Marzen v. U.S. Dept. of Health and Human Services,* 632 F. Supp. 785 (N.D. Ill. 1986), aff'd 825 F.2d 1148 (7th Cir. 1987); *see also* S. Rep. No. 1219, 88th Cong., 2d Sess. (1964) reprinted in 1974 Source Book 86.
145. *Atwell v. Sacred Heart of Pensacola,* 520 So.2d 30 (Fla. Sup. Ct.) 1988.
146. *Leslie v. Barnes,* _____ N.E.2d _____, *(DC Maine, 1988.)*
147. *Peritz v. Kay,* 530 N.Y.S.2d 761 (City Court, City of N.Y., Queens County) 1988.
148. In the Matter of A-85-04-38, _____ N.Y.S.2d _____ (N.Y. Sup. Ct.) 1987.
149. *Kincaid v. Harper-Grace Hospital,* _____ N.W.2d _____ (Mich. App.) 1988.
150. Joseph, *Modern Visual Evidence* (Law Journal Seminars Press, New York, 1987); Fed R Evid. 1006.
151. DeGeorge, *A Physician's Anticipatory Release of Patient Medical Records to a Professional Liability Insurer,* 9 J. Legal Med. 123 (1988).
152. *Rea v. Pardo,* 133 Misc.2d 516, 507 N.Y.S.2d 361 (1986); *rev'd* 522 N.Y.S.2d 393 (1987).
153. DeGeorge, *supra* note 151.
154. *Marion v. N.P.W. Medical Center,* _____ F. Supp. _____ (DCMD Pa.) 1987.
155. *Community Hosp. Assn. v. District Court,* 194 Colo. 98, 570 P2d 243 (1977); *Ziegler v. Superior Court,* 134 Ariz. 390, 656 P2d 1251, 1255 (1982); *Rudnick v. Superior Court,* 11 Cal. 3d 924, 114 Cal. Rptr. 603, 523 P2d 643, n. 13 (1974); *Hyman v. Jewish Chronic Disease Hospital,* 15 NY2d 317, 258 NYS2d 397, 206 NE2d 338 (1965); *Osterman v. Ehrenworth,* 106 N.J. Super. 515, 256 A2d 123 (1969); *Shepherd v. McGinnis,* 257 Iowa 35, 131 NW2d 475, 481 (1964);

contra: Argonaut Ins. Co. v. Peralta, 358 So2d 232 (Fla. App., 1978); *Parkson v. Central Dupage Hosp.,* 105 Ill. App. 3d 850, 61 Ill. Dec. 651, 1135 NE2d 140 (1982); *Gunthorpe v. Daniels,* 150 Ga. App. 113, 257 SE2d 199 (1979); *Hospital Corp. of America v. Superior Court of Pima County,* _____ S.W.2d _____ (Arizona App.) 1988.
156. *Lieb v. Department of Health Services,* 14 Conn. App. 552 (1988).
157. *Allen v. Smith,* S.E.2d 924 (W VA S Ct of App) 1988.
158. *Danielson v. Superior Court of the State of Arizona,* _____ S.W.2d (1987).
159. *Doe v. Stephens,* _____ F. Supp _____ (D.C. App.) 1988.
160. Community Hosp & Zeigler *supra* note 155.
161. Hirsh, *supra* note 74.
162. *Current Opinions of the Judicial Council of the American Medical Association* (1981).
163. Hirsh, *supra* note 74.
164. *Smith v. Superior Court,* 151 Cal. App. 3d 491, 198 Cal. Rptr. 829 (1984).
165. Maryland Health General Article, § 4-403(b), Health General Article, § 4-403(c).)
166. 22 California Code of Regulations ("CCR") § 70751(c).
167. 22 CCR § 70749, *See also, Bondu v. Gurvich,* 473 So.2d 1307 (Fla. 3d DCA 1984); *supra* note 146.
168. *E.g.,* Iowa Code Ann. § 614.8 (1989 Supp.); *contra* Fla. Stat. § 95.11(4)(b) (1987).
169. *E.g., McDonald v. United States,* 843 F.2d 247 (6th Cir. 1988); *Muller v. Thaut,* 230 Neb. 244, 430 N.W.2d 884 (1988)
170. *E.g.,* Carr v. Broward County, 541 So.2d 92 (Fla. 1989); *McDonald v. Haynes Medical Lab. Inc.,* 192 Conn. 327, 471 A.2d 646 (1984); *contra Hardy v. VerMeulen,* 32 Ohio St. 3d 45,512 N.E.2d 626 (1987); *Shessel v. Stroup,* 253 Ga. 56,316 S.E.2d 155 (1984).
171. JCAHO Standard MR 4.2.
172. American Hospital Association and American Medical Record Association, *Statement on Preservation of Medical Records in Health Care Institutions* (1975).
173. 42 C.F.R. § 2.16.
174. 42 C.F.R. § 2.19(a).
175. 21 C.F.R. § 291.505(d)(13)(ii).
176. 21 C.F.R. § 291.505(f)(2)(u).
177. 42 C.F.R. § 1627.3.
178. Illinois Hospital Association, *Record Retention Guide for Illinois Hospitals* 9 (1977).
179. Ill. Ann. Stat. ch. 111 ½, para 157-11 (Smith-Hurd 1977).
180. 20 C.F.R. § 405.1026(b) (1976); For example, Fla Const art 1, § 23 provides that "Every natural person has the right to be free from governmental intrusion into his private life except as provided herein."
181. Hirsh, *Will Your Medical Records Get You Into Trouble? Legal Aspects of Medical Practice,* Sept. 1978, at 51.
182. 29 C.F.R. §§ 1904.2, 1904.4, 1904.5
183. 183 29 C.F.R. § 1904.6.
184. 29 C.F.R. § 1910.20.
185. 45 C.F.R. §§ 74.20, 74.21, 74.22.
186. *Supra* note 184.
187. *See, e.g.,* Medicare Intermediary Manual, HIM-10, §§ 480-80.1.
188. HCFA-2540-86, HCFA-2540S, HCFA-2552-84, and HCFA-2552-85.
189. 42 C.F.R. § 482.24.
190. 42 U.S.C.A. § 1395x(v) (1)(I) (1989 Supp.).
191. *Supra* note 189.
192. *Supra* note 189, at § 480.1.
193. 42 C.F.R. § 420.320.
194. *Supra* note 187.
195. *Supra* note 193.

196. M. Hiller, *Computers, Medical Records, and the Right to Privacy,* J. Health Policy Law, 463-85 (Fall 1981).

197. Godes, *Computer Records and Communications. May Not Be Confidential As You Think,* Health Care Newsletter 7-10 (Dec. 1990).

198. G.S. Giebink & L. L. Hurst, *Consumer Projects in Health Care* (1975); Tenn. Code Ann. §§ 1301, 1320, 1321, 1323 (1974); Hirsh, Rosenfeld, Taffet, and Passerelli, *Physician's Medical Records: Why, Whether, Wherefore, How, and Their Longevity,* 4 Med. Law 145-54 (1984); E.W. Springer, *Automated Medical Records and the Law* (1971); *Computerized Medical Records,* 25 Buffalo L. Rev. 75 (1975); Kuhn, *Hospitals,* JAHA, at 145 (October 1977).

199. JCAH, *supra* note 24.

200. American Medical Association, *AMA Computers & Medicine Special Report: Confidentiality of Computerized Patient Information* (Resolution 38, A-77 of A.M.A.) (1979).

201. *See e.g.,* N.C. Gen - Stat. § 37.1; Iowa Code Ann § 622.28.

202. *See e.g., Monarch Federal Savings & Loan Ass'n v. Genser,* 383 A.2d 475 (N.J. Super. Ct. 1977).

203. State Agency Letter Number 93-8, *supra; Joint Commission Perspectives,* Sep./Oct. 1991.

204. Kodzielski and Reynolds, *Auto-Authentication of Medical Records: The Risks Still Outweigh the Benefits,* 8 Health Care Law Newsl. 3-7, (Sep. 1993).

205. 42 CFR § 482.24 (C) (1).

206. 42 CFR § 412-46 (b).

207. HCFA Division of Health Standards and Quality-Reyes K, State Agency Letter Number 93-8, issues April, 1993.

208. Joint Commission Perspectives, Sept./Oct. 1991. 22 CCR § 70751 (g); *see also Bond v. Gorrich,* 473 So. 2d1307 (Fla. 3d DCA 1984).

209. California Code of Regulations (CCR) § 70751(c).

CHAPTER 24

Disclosure about patients

HAROLD L. HIRSH, M.D., J.D., F.C.L.M.*

RIGHT OF PRIVACY AND CONFIDENTIALITY
EDUCATIONAL USE OF PATIENT INFORMATION
PRIVILEGED COMMUNICATION
TESTIMONIAL DISCLOSURES
APPROVED DISCLOSURES
STATUTORY DUTY TO DISCLOSE/REPORT/RECORD
DUTY TO WARN
LIMITATIONS OF DISCLOSURE
DISCOVERY
REASONABLE AND "LEGITIMATE INTEREST" DISCLOSURES
TORTS
PROFESSIONAL AND HOSPITAL LICENSING LAWS
DEFENSES

RIGHT OF PRIVACY AND CONFIDENTIALITY

A patient's right to privacy and confidentiality has been protected since the time of early civilization. Privacy is a patient's right to have peace of mind regarding the exposure and revelation of his or her body, or depictions thereof, to unauthorized persons; whereas, confidentiality is the identical right to the protection of information or records. The term *privacy* is often used to refer to both situations without clear distinction. A patient's right to privacy and confidentiality has one of the highest priorities in our legal system. Statutes and court decisions proclaim the duty to provide, maintain, and enforce a patient's right to privacy and confidentiality, and also the perils of failing to do so. The Supreme Court has recognized it as a constitutional right. No longer is privacy and confidentiality merely a moral, ethical, professional obligation; it is a legal duty.

The medical profession recognizes the sanctity of the confidential physician-patient relationship, as noted in the Hippocratic Oath, the Principles of Medical Ethics of the American Medical Association,[1] and numerous state medical societies, e.g., New York.[2]

The information disclosed to a physician during the course of the relationship between physician and patient is confidential to the greatest possible degree. The

*The author gratefully acknowledges work from previous contributors: Steven B. Bisbing, Psy.D., J.D.; Marvin Firestone, M.D., J.D., F.C.L.M.; Richard S. Goodman, M.D., J.D., F.C.L.M.; and Joseph T. Smith, M.D., J.D., F.C.L.M.

patient should feel free to make a full disclosure of information to the physician in order that the physician may most effectively provide needed services. The patient should be able to make this disclosure with the knowledge that the physician will respect the confidential nature of the communication. The physician should not reveal confidential communications or information without the express consent of the patient, unless required to do so by the law.

Most states have statutory provisions regulating the conduct of medical professionals and specifically delineating privacy and confidentiality. A health care provider has a fiduciary duty (highest legal degree of obligation or duty) to protect a patient's privacy and confidentiality except when required not to do so by law. In recent years, this has been modified by judicial doctrines that impose a duty to warn their patients when the patient's condition presents a danger to self or others. Because of the nature of the relationship of a physician with a patient, the physician may be civilly, and possibly criminally, liable for disclosure of confidential information to another without permission, particularly socially, or gossip about a patient, even if it is true. In essence, confidentiality refers to the right of a person (e.g., patient) not to have communications given in confidence revealed, without authorization, to outside parties.

Even before the physician-patient relationship was considered a contractual one, it was confidential. No distinction is made between information orally communicated to the physician and observations made by the physician. It does not even expire at the death of the patient.

When the patient consults the physician for diagnosis or treatment, the patient gives information with the expectation that it will be kept confidential. The confidential nature of the communication is inferred from the fact of the physician-patient relationship. However, if the physician is employed by someone other than the patient and the visit is not for the purpose of treatment, the privilege will not attach. For example, when a physician is appointed by the court or employed by opposing counsel, an insurance company, or by plaintiff's own counsel to examine a party in preparation for trial, communications to the physician are not considered confidential. Also, in the absence of a special statute protecting the information, records of a patient's participation in a research project, as opposed to treatment records, are not privileged.

Communication between physician and patient held to be confidential includes *all* data that the physician has found by direct examination of the patient or while performing objective studies of the patient through chemical or physical tests or production of images, or electrical studies. Such information is properly reported to the patient and no one else, unless released by the patient or appropriately by a surrogate or as required by statute or court order.

If a physician fails to reveal to a patient an unfavorable diagnosis, and discloses this information to other individuals, including family members, he or she may be held liable for medical malpractice if such nondisclosure departs from accepted medical standards and practices. Furthermore, he or she may be held liable for breach of the physician-patient relationship for disclosing such information to other individuals, including the patient's family, without the patient's consent.

Health care team responsibility

The courts have delineated and circumscribed access to both the patient's body and records in the furnishing of health care services to members of the "health care team."[3] The examination must be humane, reasonable, decent and discreet, exposing only the body parts under examination.

Access to a patient's body and to confidential medical information is limited to the primary health care team specifically rendering care to the patient, and to others with special permission.[4] Members of the team include the attending physician, assigned house officers (if they represent), and all of the nursing personnel, including nursing associates and affiliates (licensed practical nurses and nurses' aides) involved in the care of the patient. Also included are house officers, technicians, orderlies, ward clerks, therapists, social service workers, patient advocates, and comparable officer personnel.

Consultants, students (medical and nursing), and chaplains are not automatically members of the health care team. The patient must be informed of their involvement and given the opportunity to agree to or reject them. Students should not be identified by the staff as a doctor or nurse, but rather as a student doctor or nurse.

Practices such as examining patients in the presence of unidentified students and others and discussing patients at professional conferences for educational purposes should not be permitted.

Ward rounds and conferences, even for educational purposes, may be attended only by members of the health care team. Visiting experts, regardless of their background or purpose, may attend or participate only with the patient's prior consent.

The administration of the health care institution is entitled to review the patient's records for three purposes only—statistical analysis, staffing, and all quality of care reviews. This does not include "doctor" talk!

Erosion of patients' rights

Although in some ways the issues of confidentiality and privacy are still hallowed concepts, emphasized both medically and legally, they are constantly being eroded.

As the complexity of health care has increased, physician-patient confidentiality has been greatly undermined. Patients' records in hospitals, clinics, and physicians' offices are handled and perused daily by numerous known and unknown parties directly involved in patient care or under the supervision of the hospital, the physician, or the clinic. These include nurses, ward clerks, secretaries, therapists, and technicians. In addition, representatives of "review" agencies, organizations, and committees peruse, review, and critique these records. To all of these, disclosure of the information occurs by the nature of their functions. In addition, reports of consultations, laboratory studies, images, and other findings are transcribed, typed, and filed by numerous secretaries and clerks who have access to this information and to whom disclosure is not avoidable. Similarly, employees of insurers, including those involved in health insurance, disability insurance, liability insurance, workers' compensation, insurance carriers, and others have a right by contract to review in detail these confidential records.

EDUCATIONAL USE OF PATIENT INFORMATION

Publication of information or pictures or discussion of a patient without consent, even with obfuscation of the identity, if he or she is or can be identified by name, description, or appearance, may lead to a successful lawsuit for invasion of privacy, even if the pictures or information are published in a medical journal for legitimate educational or scientific purposes.[5] If the patient is recognized, the medical practitioner is vulnerable to a lawsuit for breach of confidentiality or invasion of privacy. Problems can be avoided by getting the patient's, parental, or guardian's prior approval in the case of a minor.

A patient may very well give consent to the taking of photographs to be used in medical journals.[6] However, if the scope of the use of the films to which the patient has consented is violated, he or she may have a cause of action. Even if the patient consents to the use of photographs or information, the physician is obliged to protect the patient's privacy as much as possible. Unless the patient expressly forbids photographs, physicians may take photographs of the patient for the medical record expressly for professional purposes and restricted educational situations.

The highest court of Massachusetts enjoined public showing of a film of inmates of an institution for insane persons charged with crimes or delinquency, but permitted continued showings to audiences of a specialized or professional character with a serious interest in rehabilitation.[7] The court observed that the public interest in having these people informed outweighs the rights of the inmates to privacy. However, the Maine Supreme Court ruled that when a patient had expressly objected to being photographed, there could be liability for photographing the patient even if the photograph was solely for the medical records.[8] It is prudent to obtain express consent for taking and using photographs, but liability for photographs taken without express consent is not likely if the patient does not object and uses are appropriately restricted. However, a New York court permitted a physician and nurse to be sued for allowing a newspaper photographer to photograph a patient even though the patient was informed of the identity of the photographer and did not object.[9] Of course, public or commercial showing without consent can lead to liability.[10]

A New York appellate court ruled that representatives of an incompetent patient do not have a right to photograph the patient in the hospital.[11] The petitioners failed to show a sufficient need to justify a court order that they be permitted to film an eight-hour videotape of their comatose daughter in an intensive care unit for use in a suit.

Later a New York court ruled that a patient had no right, before filing a malpractice suit, to a videotape of the patient's operation.[12] It was found not to be a part of the medical record because the physician had taken it for his personal use.

PRIVILEGED COMMUNICATION

In common law, a physician who was called as a witness had no right to decline or refuse to disclose any information on the grounds that it had been communicated to him confidentially in the course of his attendance upon or treatment of his patient in a professional capacity. Neither could the patient, in case the physician proved a willing witness, by objection, exclude such information, or as a witness himself, refuse to disclose any communication made by him to the physician.

"Privileged communication," or "testimonial privilege," is a specific and narrow application of the right of confidentiality. In effect, a testimonial privilege is a statutorily created rule of evidence that enables the holder of the privilege to prohibit the person to whom the confidential information was entrusted from testifying in a judicial proceeding without the consent of the person who provided that information. In the physician-patient relationship, the patient holds the privilege and may generally bar the physician from testifying about confidential matters. Testimonial privilege applies only in a judicial proceeding.

Although confidential communications between patient and physician have traditionally been considered secret, they were not accorded the status of legal privilege.[13]

In 1928, the New York legislature enacted the first physician-patient privileged communication statute.[14] California followed closely thereafter with its Code of Civil Procedure. These early statutes laid the groundwork for the legislated privilege.

At present, every state except South Carolina has enacted some form of physician-patient, psychiatrist-patient, or psychotherapist-patient privilege. However, there is considerable variation among the states regarding the circumstances in which the privilege is available and under which providers are covered. It is embodied in the statutes of 43 states and the District of Columbia. In seven of these jurisdictions, statutes provide for a distinct psychiatrist/psychologist-patient privilege. In others, evidentiary privileges may be extended to physicians' assistants, nurses, social workers, dentists, rape counselors, and secretary/receptionists acting as agents of a physician.[15,16] Seven states have not codified this right.

According to an eminent authority, four canons must be present to protect a communication from disclosure[17]:

- The communication ought to originate in a confidence.
- Confidentiality must be essential to the full and satisfactory maintenance of the relationship between the parties.
- The relationship must be one that the community seeks to foster.
- The injury that would inure to the relationship by the disclosure of the communications must be greater than the benefit gained in the litigation.

These criteria are reflected in the privilege status in most states, where the terms of each element of the privilege are specifically defined.

Courts agree when interpreting the privilege that the essential elements that must exist before the privilege applies are (1) a physician-patient relationship, (2) information acquired during the relationship, and (3) the necessity and propriety of the information to enable the physician to treat the patient in his or her professional capacity.

A communication is a disclosure of information that may be given verbally by the patient or may be diagnostic data gathered by the physician through observation and examination of the patient. Identifying data such as a patient's name and address is a communication, although this information may or may not have been revealed with the anticipation that it would be kept confidential. Certain types of medical and diagnostic data, however, are not considered communications. For example, a tissue sample, surgically removed and submitted to a laboratory for examination and testing, was not considered a communication by the patient to the physician. Contents of reports of adverse drug reactions have been held to be confidential communications between patient and physician. Dental records have been held not to be communications between physician and patient.

The type of information barred by the testimonial privilege is, typically, information learned in the course of treatment or an examination leading to treatment. The coverage would include the physician's diagnosis, conclusions, and even the acknowledgment that a particular person is in treatment. But not all information or communications made to the physician receive blanket coverage. Courts require a clear and definite connection between the patient's communication and the implementation of treatment. On one hand, it is likely that any communication made to the psychiatrist within the course of treatment would be considered privileged. However, disclosures made for purposes other than obtaining treatment (e.g., to qualify for insurance or employment) are not likely to be protected.

In a fascinating case[18] in which a physician saw 1170 patients per day using an assembly line technique involving only a brief interview, the court held that this did not create a confidential physician-patient relationship so as to give rise to the privilege.

A rule of privilege is a rule of evidence, not of substantive law, and applies only in the judicial context. There is no physician-patient privilege under the Federal Rules of Evidence and none at federal common law. In the federal courts, the issue of privilege is determined by the law of the state in which the court is located.[19,20] State privileges do not apply in most federal suits concerning federal law.[21] Generally, a physician may not invoke the privilege; it may be done only by the patient

and almost always through the patient's attorney. However, the physician-patient and psychiatrist/psychologist-patient privileges have been asserted by physicians on behalf of their patients.[22]

In *Scull v. Superior Court*,[23] a psychiatrist was charged with four counts of sexually molesting a teenage female patient. The court perceived that the mere disclosure of a patient's identity may serve to dissuade others from seeking psychotherapy because of perceived societal stigmas. The court's holding reaffirms the psychotherapist-patient privilege by endorsing the rationale on which it is based, as well as the societal values that originally caused it to be recognized since it is intended to encourage those in need of treatment for emotional or mental problems to seek the services of psychotherapists.

A mother has been allowed to assert the physician-patient privilege on behalf of her infant in an obstetrical malpractice case,[24] and a parent can assert the privilege on behalf of his or her minor child.[25] Further, a drug company has used the privilege in a products liability case to preclude production of records of third-party patients containing information about adverse effects of the drug.[26] The privilege has been held not to terminate or be waived on the death of the patient. Thus, it also can be asserted by a representative of the decedent's estate.[27]

Courts have also held that a nonparty witness may invoke the privilege during a deposition prior to trial to avoid revealing confidential communications made to her physician, but may not refuse to testify as to relevant medical incident or facts.[28]

It is generally conceded that the physician-patient privilege extends to information contained in medical and hospital records.[29] Thus, courts hold that hospital personnel may assert the privilege on behalf of those patients whose records are being sought. In fact, at least one court upheld that hospitals have a duty or obligation to maintain the confidentiality of patient records.[30]

Other courts hold that a hospital may not use the physician-patient or social worker-client privilege in opposition to the subpoena for hospital records, where the hospital is the subject of a grand jury investigation for possible commission of crimes against its patients.[31]

The privilege will be lost if it is not asserted in a timely manner. If the opposing party attempts a disclosure of a confidential physician-patient communication, an objection must be made at the time or it cannot be asserted later. Therefore, the patient, the patient's attorney, or the attending physician must actively defend the privilege.

If it frequently advantageous and necessary to assert the physician-patient privilege to control the scope of informal discovery by the opposing attorney.[32] Attending physicians are often approached by attorneys adverse to their patients, *ex parte*, without notice to the attorney representing the patient. Such contacts all too often lead to the inadvertent and unauthorized disclosure of information that could not be obtained through normal discovery procedures. The *ex parte* contacts may be upheld by the courts for economic reasons or by balancing the importance of the privilege against other factors.

The lawyer who represents an injured patient must take precautions to protect his or her client's privilege. The lawyer may consider cautioning the treatment physician at the earliest stages of the case. One method is to send a letter accompanying the medical authorization to inform the physician that by filing a lawsuit the patient does not waive all privilege of confidentiality.

A physician is admonished to respond as follows:

- Release only the information authorized to be released.
- Release information only to the persons to whom it is authorized to be released.
- Do not discuss information obtained during the physician-patient relationship with any third party except the patient and the patient's attorney unless specifically authorized to do so.
- Do not discuss such information with any other physician except as necessary for treatment by you or in order to seek consultation with the other physician unless specifically authorized to do so.

The burden of proof is on the party seeking to establish the existence of the privilege. Where the privilege is claimed by the patient who is also a party, it is widely held by statutory and common law that no adverse inference as to the facts suppressed may be drawn from the claim of the privilege.

In most jurisdictions privilege statutes are strictly construed as they are in derogation of common law. A number of states, however, have interpreted privilege statutes liberally and held them to be remedial in nature.

Attorneys for plaintiffs and defendants have attempted to assert the physician-patient privilege to prevent the admission of a physician's medical records and reports, as well as oral testimony from physicians, in almost every type of action imaginable. Where all criteria for its application are met, the privilege is recognized in civil action. In addition to medical malpractice cases, the privilege is also raised in cases involving auto accidents and workers' compensation claims. It may be involved in disputes by beneficiaries over wills or insurance policies, investigations into Medicare or Medicaid fraud, medical licensure and staff privilege contests, child custody disputes, child abuse actions, and all types of individual criminal prosecutions and grand jury investigations.[33] In all of these actions, the privilege may be raised either during the course of pretrial discovery or to contest admissibility of evidence or impeach the witness during trial. The privilege applies to production and admissibility of evidence during judicial proceedings.[34]

When local law enforcement officials conducting a criminal investigation demand names, addresses, or other information about a hospital patient, health care professionals and hospital staff may be inclined to assume that he or she is obligated to cooperate. Disclosing such information without the consent of the professional and/or the patient may, however, violate the right of confidentiality in a professional-patient relationship and lead to legal liability.

In *State v. Jaggers*,[35] a state licensing board was precluded from obtaining a list of patients under the care of a chiropractor. The court found that the chiropractor had a duty to assert the patient-physician privilege and to refuse to release the list to the board.

Similarly, the physician-patient relationship can limit a physician's right to submit affidavits to the court. In *Mississippi State Board of Psychological Examiners v. Hosford*,[36] the doctor's license was suspended following his submission of an affidavit to a court during a divorce proceeding regarding his counseling of the couple.

In New York, however, the privilege did not protect a physician's records from a grand jury subpoena investigating Medicaid fraud.[37]

The scope of the privilege varies. Pennsylvania limits the privilege to communications that tend to blacken the character of the patient,[38] whereas Kansas extends the privilege to all communications and observations.[39] Michigan limits the privilege to physicians,[40] but New York extends the privilege to dentists and nurses.[41] When a nurse is present during a confidential communication between physician and patient, some states extend the privilege to the nurse, while other states rule that the communication is no longer privileged for the physician. Generally, the privilege extends to otherwise privileged information recorded in the hospital record.[42] However, information that is required to be reported to public authorities has generally been held not to be privileged unless the public authorities are also privileged not to disclose it.

The privilege usually does not apply to court-ordered examinations or other examinations solely for the benefit of the third parties, such as insurance companies.

Alaska established a common psychotherapist-patient privilege for criminal cases.[43]

Evidentiary privilege

Many state jurisdictions, as well as the federal courts, recognize an "evidentiary privilege," similar to the well known physician-patient privilege, under which psychotherapists are prohibited from divulging confidential information about their patients obtained in the course of treatment. In recent years, the continued viability of this privilege has been questioned, but a recent California appellate decision indicates that the privilege is still alive and well, at least in that jurisdiction.

TESTIMONIAL DISCLOSURES

Courts generally refuse to impose liability for testimonial disclosures.[44] Physicians and hospitals are not obligated to risk contempt of court to protect confidences (except for substance abuse records), although they may choose to do so.

Practically all communications between the professional liability carrier and the attorney for the health care provider are privileged and not subject to discovery by the opposition.[45]

Many states' statutes specifically impose restrictions on the testimony of physicians as to privileged data when no authorization has been given.[46] The physician should expect that a court may order a physician to reveal certain information even though the physician must comply or face contempt charges.[47]

Patient names

The Michigan Supreme Court ruled that patients' names are protected by the physician-patient privilege.[48] Courts have refused to disclose to patients the names of persons with matching tissues who refuse to be donors or are blood donors with AIDS. Most courts have not permitted the discovery of nonparty patient names. Similarly, the Arizona Supreme Court ruled that the physician-patient privilege does not protect patient names in Arizona, but still refused to order release of other names because it did not consider them relevant.[49]

Committee reports

Many states have enacted statutes protecting quality assurance and peer review activities and committee reports from discovery or admission into evidence. These laws are designed to permit the candor necessary for effective peer review to improve quality and reduce morbidity and mortality. Courts have found these laws constitutional,[50] although they have allowed access when the plaintiff had a need to know.

In many jurisdictions, statutes particularly declare the confidentiality of hospital review boards and specifically protect the records of such committees against discovery through judicial fiat or subpoena, and the courts have been generous in honoring the privilege thus conferred.[51] In still other states and some federal courts, a similar status of confidentiality has been fashioned out of the common law on grounds of public policy (the need

for the patient to come "clean").[52] Together, hospital review committee records and administration incident reports have been made inviolable by the law, and nonparty patient records have been similarly protected.[53]

Some courts have strictly interpreted statutory protections, reducing their effectiveness. For example, a New Jersey court refused to apply the statutory protection for "utilization review committees" to related committees, such as the medical records and audit, tissue, and infection control committees.[54] Some courts have interpreted statutory protections broadly. For example, the Minnesota Supreme Court found that a complications conference report was protected under a statute that protected "the proceedings and records of a review organization."[55]

Some courts have recognized a common law qualified privilege based on the public interest in peer review activities. A District of Columbia court refused to order release of information concerning a peer review committee's activities.[56] However, other courts have refused to recognize a common law privilege for peer review.[57]

Because the status of committee reports is still an open question in many states, these reports should be carefully written so that, if they must be released, they will not inappropriately increase liability exposure.[58]

Of significance is the fact that whatever the scope of the privilege, it extends only to the minutes and records generated during peer review. Thus, anticipatory committee oversight records, such as those generated by tumor boards, have been held to be confidential. On the other hand, if the attending physician deviated from the panel recommendation, this could provide serious evidence of a violation of the standard of care.

Even if a particular record might be privileged and immune from discovery, the raw data and other factual aspects that underlie the committee's final conclusions may well be subject to disclosure. Certainly the testimony of the relevant witnesses and supporting documentation—unless independently subject to a claim of confidentiality—would be available to the adverse party.

For publicly supported hospitals, including those receiving legislatively allocated funds under one of many statutory health care programs, other relevant peer review reports and investigative reports may be obtained pursuant to Freedom of Information acts. Once information is obtained by and filed with a public agency, it might be disclosed at the discretion of the agency even if disclosure is not mandated by Freedom of Information acts.

Most other types of records, even those generally deemed privileged, can be both discovered in advance of trial and then used at trial to prove negligence on a theory of custom, habit, or the selection of an inappropriate standard of care. Thus, a hospital's "incident reports"[59] routinely prepared by the staff for inclusion in the patient's chart (not purely for administrative purpose) after an untoward result, a physician's personal (not patient) office records kept for his or her own edification, the report of a noninvolved hospital's committee assigned to review the propriety of continued staff privileges for a physician charged with malpractice in a different hospital, and statements made by physicians to their attorneys in preparation for malpractice litigation have all been deemed discoverable. The only barrier has been one applicable in other contexts as well, a showing of either materiality, relevancy, or good cause.

More surprising are cases holding that despite the physician-patient privilege, a physician's patient treatment records are discoverable merely by taking the precaution of preserving or obfuscating the identity of the patients.[60] Then treatment failure with these other nonparty patients would be admissible at trial to show that the physician should have anticipated injury from a particular course of treatment or to demonstrate a pattern of professional incompetence. Although the jury would be instructed to use this damaging information only for a limited purpose, such limiting instructions are not regarded as particularly efficacious.

The policy of the law in most jurisdictions is to promote a full and free disclosure of all information by a patient to the treating physician. Consequently, of the courts that have specifically addressed this issue, the majority have imposed liability on a physician for disclosing confidential information without the patient's consent based on the following theories: (1) invasion of privileged relationship between patient and physician, (2) violation of a statutory requirement governing licensing of physicians preventing disclosure of confidential information, and (3) violation of a state testimonial privilege statute regarding confidential information gained through the physician-patient relationship.

Nonetheless, the courts are far from unanimous on this subject. Although espousing weighty considerations of public policy, by using different rationales or finding a basis for a variance from the policy, some courts have reached contrary results and refuse to recognize any right of confidentiality.[61] Those courts that have judicially created a doctrine of "privilege" for these documents carefully note exceptions in cases of "exceptional necessity" or under "extraordinary circumstances."[62] Courts have also made exceptions when the information sought is "at the heart of the litigation," as well as when the material sought is not the specific minutes but rather material used in the committee proceedings.[63]

Exceptions

With the emergence of new case law regarding the scope and limitations of, and exceptions to confidentiality and testimonial privilege, it is obvious that this area of the law is far from settled.

As a rule of thumb, based on sound clinical judgment, a physician should presume that confidential information is privileged and that he or she is barred from disclosing any information unless it is evident that the privilege has been waived or testimony is legally compelled.

The privilege is subject to many exceptions and circumstances of waiver. Even when the privilege does not exist, it may be so narrowly construed as to be of little value to an individual seeking to prevent disclosure of medical records.

The number of situations in which a patient may not invoke the testimonial privilege may constructively neutralize the value of the statute. Some of the more common situations excepted include (1) civil commitment proceedings, (2) child custody disputes, (3) litigation in which a patient places his or her physical and or mental status at issue (known as the "patient-litigation exception"), (4) contest of a will, (5) the law requires the physician to file a report (e.g., cases involving child abuse, communicable disease, or a patient who threatens himself or others), and (6) certain legal actions between the physician and patient (e.g., physician sues to collect unpaid bills for treatment, or the patient sues the physician for malpractice).

Where medical information is sought by a legislative or administrative body, the privilege may provide no protection at all.

The Arizona Court of Appeals has upheld a lower court's order allowing the plaintiff patient, who alleged she unnecessarily had a heart pacemaker implanted, to review the charts of 24 other nonparty patients to determine whether the two defendant physicians did this with regularity.[64] All clues of the identities of the patient were removed. Of the 24 charts, the plaintiff's medical expert found unnecessary implementation in 20. The appellate court also ruled this evidence could be introduced at trial.

A special public policy exception to the privilege may have been carved out by the courts or the legislature. Recently, the New Jersey Superior Court ruled in a medical malpractice action that an *in camera* inspection of the consultation notes of the plaintiff's psychologist was the best way to accommodate the antithetical policy interests favoring liberal pretrial discovery of relevant information and the necessity of protecting the plaintiff from needless exposure.

Several additional situations exist in which courts have held that the release of confidential information may be valid without the patient's authorization. For example, if a patient is involved in some form of legal action, including a civil commitment proceeding, portions or the entire medical record may be held discloseable.[65,66] Similarly, records that have been ordered by the court may require disclosure. However, it is not a subpoena but a judge's ruling that generally controls release. The subpoena merely gets the records to the court.

Current Opinion 5.05 of the Judicial Council of the American Medical Association states:

The obligation to safeguard the patient's confidences is subject to certain exceptions which are ethically and legally justified because of overriding social considerations. Where a patient threatens to employ serious bodily harm to another person, and there is a reasonable probability that the patient may carry out the threat, the physician should take reasonable precautions for the protection of the intended victim, including notification of law enforcement authorities. Also, communicable diseases, gunshot and knife wound should be reported as required by applicable statutes or ordinances.[67]

State law is in total conformity with the Current Opinion of the Judicial Council. Disclosure has been permitted if a patient presents a danger to self or other[68]; if necessary to prevent the spread of a contagious disease[69]; and in other circumstances in which the public interest or private interest of the patient so demands.[70]

Except in those states that recognize the "therapeutic privilege exception," physicians have no right to prevent release of information from the medical records when such release is authorized by the patient or by law. Therefore, neither a written nor an oral consent from the patient is required prior to disclosure.

Waivers

Like the various exceptions enumerated, the right and scope of patient waivers differ from state to state. Generally speaking, if an adult is legally competent, only he or she may execute a valid waiver of the privilege. Persons legally declared incompetent are typically said to have vested their power of waiver in a legal guardian. Similarly, waiver decisions regarding minors are generally made by the parent or legal guardian. Implied waivers are recognized by the courts and usually defined in individual cases rather than by statute. A patient may also release a physician from the obligations of the privilege by explicitly waiving the privilege. Again, state laws may differ considerably. For instance, a patient who testifies about privileged matters may not bar a physician from doing so. Valid waiver in a separate case, or disclosure of privileged information outside the courtroom, may in some states constitute a permanent waiver but may have no impact on the original right of privilege in other states.

Another well-established exception to the privilege applies when an individual files suit, as in *Duflinger v. Artiles,*[71] for damages due to alleged mental and emotional injuries. Under such circumstances, the litigant is assumed to have waived the privilege.

Waiver of the privilege may be expressly stated or implied, such as when a patient institutes a malpractice action. Where plaintiffs place their medical condition at issue by filing a products liability action, plaintiffs waive the privilege as to disclosure of relevant condition evidence. The question then may become whether plaintiffs will allow defendants to implement the waiver by conducting *ex parte* interviews of their physician, instead of depositions. In one decision under District of Columbia code sections pertaining to the medical privilege, plaintiffs were required to execute authorizations permitting their physicians to engage in informal *ex parte* interviews with representatives of the defendant.[72] This may be the result where the court finds the plaintiffs have attempted to limit defense counsel's access to plaintiffs' physicians as a trial tactic. This is not the intent of the privilege statutes and may be construed by the court as an attempt to use the privilege to impede the judicial process.

In a Pennsylvania case,[73] a federal district court held that when a patient signs a consent to treatment form, which promises confidentiality in accord with the state privilege law, and that patient later files a personal injury suit, the patient's abrogation of the privilege by filing a lawsuit overcomes the promise of confidentiality contained in the consent form. In such a case, the plaintiff-patient has placed his or her medical history at issue and, therefore, has waived the right of confidentiality.

In some states, when a patient files a personal injury action, the state privilege statute often will indicate that the plaintiff, by filing a lawsuit bringing his or her health status into question, has waived the right to assert the privilege.

However, the privilege is not automatically waived in most jurisdictions by merely filing a lawsuit; the waiver may be limited to a specific subject matter or area. Where the privilege is not waived, the courts have upheld the patient's right of confidentiality by awarding sanctions against the opposing party or by issuing protective orders.

The patient may, of course, consent to the disclosure or waive the privilege, permitting the physician to testify. The privilege can also be waived by contract. Insurance applications and policies often include waivers. Other actions can constitute implied waiver. Introducing evidence of medical details or failing to object to physician testimony generally waives the privilege.[74]

Authorization of disclosure outside the testimonial

context usually does not waive the privilege.[75] Thus, the patient generally may authorize other persons to have access to medical records outside of court and still successfully object to having them introduced into evidence unless other actions have waived the privilege. In a few states, authorization of any disclosure to opposing parties waives the privilege.[76]

Waiver of the privilege usually permits only formal discovery and testimony, not informal interviews. Express patient consent is generally required before informal interviews are permitted.[77] However, other courts have permitted informal interviews based on waiver of the privilege.[78] Prudent providers limit disclosures to formal channels unless express patient consent is obtained.

APPROVED DISCLOSURES

A patient's valid informed authorization to disclose certain information will legally protect a physician. The physician should keep three important considerations in mind. First, is the authorization truly informed? Second, does the authorization comport with any relevant state requirements? Third, even with a patient's authorization, a physician should provide only the minimum amount of information necessary to answer the questions posed by a third party. Furthermore, unnecessary revelation regarding the patient's condition without authorization could subject the individual revealing the information to a variety of legal actions. A medical practitioner is charged with the responsibility of providing continuity of health care for his or her patients. No patient should suffer by the failure to transfer adequate information to the succeeding health care provider to ensure continuity of care.[79] Exchange of patient information between health care providers does not diminish any of the requirements of the law to protect the patient's confidentiality.[80]

As has been noted, the right to confidentiality is not absolute; it has been abridged by the courts.[81] As to ordinary patients, the physician may respond to telephone or personal inquiries as to the patient's presence and status in vague and ambiguous terms only. As to so-called newsworthy patients, the medical practitioner may respond to telephone or personal inquiries regarding the patient's presence, the diagnosis, and status in vague and ambiguous terms. Hospitalization may be revealed. But the patient (surrogate) may interpose or object to even these disclosures.

STATUTORY DUTY TO DISCLOSE/ REPORT/RECORD

Sometimes information such as a child abuse or contagious disclosure report is required to be disclosed by law. These disclosures are not an invasion of privacy because they are legally authorized.

Even if the patient or representative opposes information release, health care providers are required by law to *permit access* to medical information in many circumstances. Providers are required to report many patient conditions to law enforcement or public health authorities.

Most states have enacted laws that compel or authorize hospitals and physicians to release information from patient records for certain specific purposes. The law compels disclosure of medical information in many contexts other than discovery or testimony.[82] Reporting laws have been enacted that require medical information to be reported to governmental agencies. The most common examples are vital statistics, communicable (contagious) disease, child abuse, wounds, venereal disease, injuries sustained in accidents or violence, occupational diseases, and cancer. The fact that such reports may involve release of confidential information usually will not act as a bar to the statutorily required reports.[83]

Familiarity with these and other reporting laws is important to assure compliance and to avoid reporting to the wrong agency. Reports to the wrong agency may not be legally protected, resulting in potential liability for breach of confidentiality.[84]

Obviously, statutes that require reporting of these cases make it incumbent on the physician to do so[85]; a physician not only has the right to disclose the information to proper authorities, he or she has the *duty* and is immunized against legal liability. Persons who could have avoided injury if information had been disclosed have won civil suits against providers who failed to disclose such information.

The health care provider's failure to conform to the statutory requirement has made the provider liable to administrative and criminal penalties. It has also been held to be negligence per se (not requiring proof of negligence) in civil suits brought by the injured patients and/or third parties.

Some statutes do not mandate reporting, but authorize access to medical records, without the patient's permission, on request of certain individuals or organizations or the general public.

Vital statistics

All states require the reporting of births and deaths.[86] The reporting of a death generally must be accompanied by a medical certificate describing the cause of death. These laws are a valid exercise of the state police power. Some states treat death certificates as public records; other states do not routinely make them public, but do not specifically protect their confidentiality. As a general matter, death certificates report both the immediate cause of death (for example, pneumonia) and the ultimate cause that produced the immediate cause (for example, AIDS). Some states significantly restrict the disclosure of the cause of death, whereas other states freely allow it under their freedom of information laws.

Wounds, accidents, and violence

Many states require the reporting of certain wounds. Some states specify that all wounds of certain types must be reported. For example, New York requires the reporting of wounds inflicted by sharp instruments that may result in death and all gunshot wounds.[87] Other states limit the reporting requirement to wounds caused under certain circumstances. For example, Iowa requires the reporting of wounds that apparently resulted from criminal acts.[88] Thus, wounds that are clearly accidental or self-inflicted do not have to be reported in Iowa. Some states require reports of accidents and radiation incidents.

The Oklahoma Supreme Court has held[89] that a physician could not be sued by a patient who was convicted of rape after the physician informed police that he suspected the patient was the rapist the police were seeking. The disclosure was protected by public policy.

Abuse

Most states require reports of suspected cases of child abuse or neglect.[90] Some professionals, such as physicians and nurses, are required to make reports as mandatory reporters. Anyone who is not a mandatory reporter may be a permissive reporter. In some states any report arising out of diagnosis or treatment in an institution must be made through the institutional administration. Most child abuse reporting laws extend some degree of immunity from liability for reports made through proper channels.[91] A mandatory reporter who fails to report child abuse is subject to both criminal penalties[92] and civil liability for future injuries to the child that could have been advised if a report and been made.[93]

There have been disputes in some states over whether some behavior, such as sexual activity of younger minors, must be reported as child abuse.[94]

Child abuse reports made under mandatory state laws obviously can be made without patient consent or a court order, but release of records to child abuse agencies may require consent or an order.

Some states have enacted adult abuse reporting laws for spouses and the elderly that are similar to the child abuse reporting laws.[95] Adult abuse reporting *generally* requires agreement from the victim.

Substances and devices

National reporting laws apply to hospitals that are involved in manufacturing, testing, or using certain substances and devices. For example, fatalities due to blood transfusions must be reported to the Food and Drug Administration (FDA).[96,97] A sponsor of an investigational medical device must report to the FDA any unanticipated adverse effects from use of the device.[97] Device manufacturers have a duty to report to the FDA when a death or serious injury has occurred in connection with the device.[98]

Workers' compensation

Some state statutes grant all parties to a workers' compensation claim access to all relevant medical information after a claim has been made.[99] In some states, courts have ruled that filing a workers' compensation claim is a waiver of confidentiality of relevant medical information.[100] In states without such statutes or rulings, medical records should not be released until authorized by the patient or the patient's representative or until legally subpoenaed.

Governmental agency access

Some federal and state statutes give governmental agencies access to medical records on request or through administrative subpoena. For example, peer review organizations (PROs) have access to all medical records pertinent to their federal review functions on request. A federal district court has ruled that Medicare surveyors have a right of access to records of non-Medicare patients, as well as to those of Medicare patients.[101] Hospital licensing laws often grant inspectors access without subpoena for audit and inspection purposes.

State public records laws

Many states have public records laws that apply to public hospitals. Some state statutes explicitly exempt hospital and their medical records from disclosure.[102] A court ruled that Colorado's law did not permit a publisher to obtain all birth and death reports routinely.[103] The Iowa Supreme Court has decided that names of unselected potential bone donors could be withheld from disclosure and that although the potential donor had never sought treatment at the hospital, the potential donor was a patient for purposes of the exemption because the medical procedure of tissue typing had been performed.[104] However, in an Ohio case the state law was interpreted to require access to the names and the dates of admission and discharge of all persons admitted to a public hospital.[105] In states that follow the Ohio rule, it is especially important to resist discovery of nonparty records because removal of "identifiers" does not offer complete protection when dates in the records may make it possible to identify the patient from the admission list.

Freedom of information act

The federal Freedom of Information Act (FOIA) applies only to federal agencies.[106] A hospital does not become a federal agency by receiving federal funds, so the FOIA applies to few hospitals outside of the National Institutes of Health, Veterans Administration, and Defense Department hospital systems. When the FOIA applies, medical information is exempted from disclosure only when the disclosure would "constitute a clearly unwarranted invasion of personal privacy." Thus, the act provides only limited protection of confidentiality of medical information in the possession of federal agencies. However, the Federal Privacy Act may provide some additional protection to such information.[107]

Public health

Communicable disease. Most states require reports of venereal disease and other communicable diseases.[108] A California court observed that in addition to criminal penalties and administrative sanctions for not reporting a contagious disease, civil liability is possible in a suit by persons who contract disease that might have been avoided by proper reports and warnings.[109] At least one state requires reports to private individuals.[110] Florida requires hospitals to notify emergency transport personnel and other individuals who bring emergency patients to the hospital if the patient is diagnosed as having a contagious disease.[111]

Cancer and noncontagious diseases. Some states require reports of cancer and other selected noncontagious diseases.

Convulsive disorders. A few states require reports to state driver licensing agencies of conditions with seizures whose presence could lead to loss of license.[112]

Occupational diseases. Some states require occupational diseases such as asbestosis to be reported.[113] Under the federal Occupational Safety and Health Agency (OSHA), two types of record keeping are required—a medical record and a training record.[114] A detailed *medical record* for each employee with occupational exposure must be kept until 30 years after termination of employment. The record should contain the staff member's name and social security number. Training records need to include the dates of sessions, training materials, and name and qualifications of the individual performing the training and of the employee (including job title) who attended. These records must be kept for 3 years following the date of training.

Medical and training records must be available for inspection and copying by any employee as well as by OSHA representatives. Even if a practice is closing its door permanently, OSHA must be provided three months advance notice prior to destroying the records.

Hepatitis B vaccine (HBV) vaccination status and any related medical records including dates of all vaccinations, records related to any exposure incidents including results of examinations and testing, the written post-

exposure evaluations, and copies of the information provided to the evaluating physician must be available to an OSHA representative. These files must be kept confidential and not disclosed to anyone (including other practice employees) without the individual's written consent.

DUTY TO WARN

A physician's duty of care includes the duty to warn patients[115] and others who might be reasonably foreseeable potential third-party victims of the dangers incident to their patient's health problems.[116] It is increasingly recognized that a health care provider has the responsibility to identify any reasonably foreseeable harmful situation and, if possible, to prevent it. Failure to advise the patient or the others of the known or reasonably foreseeable dangerous situation resulting in harm is negligence.

Depending on the circumstances, the warning should be made to the patient and to third parties known to be in proximity to or to have appropriate contact with the patient, such as relatives, associates, an employer or fellow employee, and/or to the proper authorities. This provides an opportunity to prevent the harm, for example, of spread of the communicable disease.

When the health care provider breaches this duty and the patient or third party suffers a causally related injury, the health care provider may not only be liable for negligent care, he or she may be rendered liable for the breach of the duty to warn. The failure of the physician to warn the patient or the interested others is a separate and distinct negligent act. This is true whether the condition is completely diagnosed or still under study.

Threats to others

A number of courts have ruled that there is a duty to warn potential identified victims or to identify someone who can intervene when a patient has made a credible threat. The first decision to impose this duty was *Tarasoff v. Board of Regents.*[117] When the Tarasoffs sued for the death of their daughter, the California Supreme Court found the employer of a psychiatrist liable for the psychiatrist's failure to warn the daughter that his patient had threatened to kill her. The court ruled that he should have either warned the victim or advised others likely to apprise the victim of the danger. Four years later the same court clarified the scope of this duty by ruling that only threats to readily identified individuals create a duty to warn, so there is no duty to warn a threatened group.[118] During the next few years this philosophy was extended.[119] The Arizona Supreme Court ruled that foreseeable victims had to be warned even without specific threats.[120] The Washington Supreme Court ruled that the duty to warn extended to unidentifiable victims.[121] The Vermont Supreme Court extended the duty to warn to include property damage, imposing liability on a counseling service when a patient burned his parent's barn.[122] Some courts have declined to establish a duty to warn even readily identified individuals.[123]

Under the laws of most states, communications made in the course of psychotherapy are confidential and are protected against disclosure by a patient-psychotherapist privilege. However, in many states, if the psychotherapist reasonably believes that disclosure of the patient's otherwise confidential communications is necessary to prevent a threatened danger to an identifiable victim, the psychotherapist will be protected if he or she discloses the communications in order to protect the victim, the privilege not applying to such disclosures.

In such situations, the psychotherapist is not only permitted to disclose the confidential communications but may have an affirmative duty to warn an identifiable victim of the danger. This duty to give a so-called *Tarasoff* warning is widely recognized across the country. Under *Tarasoff*, a psychotherapist must inform the intended victim or appropriate other that the potential victim is in danger, but need not provide any rationale for his or her belief.

Patient-psychotherapist privilege versus duty to warn victims. Two recent criminal cases, *Menendez v. Superior Court*[124] and *People v. Wharton*,[125] illustrate the courts' continuing efforts to balance a patient's expectation of confidentiality and the societal interest in fostering that expectation against the professional's recognized obligation to protect potential victims of a patient's known violent intentions. California has tipped the balance in favor of disclosure.

In *Menendez*, two brothers, Lyle and Erik Menendez, were charged with the August 20, 1989, murder of their parents in their Beverly Hills home. The brothers had been patients of psychotherapist Dr. L. Jerome Oziel for some time prior to the death of the parents. During the first of four psychotherapy sessions between the boys and Dr. Oziel several months after the murders, one of the brothers confessed that both committed the murders, and the other told Dr. Oziel that, because he now knew of their crime, they had to kill him and anyone associated with him.

Dr. Oziel, considering his life and the lives of his family to be in danger, disclosed the confession to his wife and to a business associate who had been present in his office during his sessions with the Menendez brothers. Dr. Oziel also prepared audio tapes of his notes from the first three sessions, and made an actual recording of the last session.

Dr. Oziel's tapes eventually were seized by the district attorney. At a hearing to determine whether the tapes were protected by the patient-psychotherapist privilege, the court found that Dr. Oziel's first two sessions with the Menendez brothers constituted psychotherapy, and that, absent an applicable exception, any communications made in the course of those sessions would be privileged. However, the court concluded that California's "dangerous patient" exception applied and, therefore, the disclosures contained in the tapes of the first two sessions were not privileged.

Had the court stopped there, its holding would have been unremarkable as an application of *Tarasoff*. However, *Menendez* also holds that the psychotherapy relationship ends once a patient clearly expresses a desire to kill the therapist and has the ability to carry out the threat. The court found that Dr. Oziel's last two sessions with the Menendez brothers did not constitute psychotherapy because any therapeutic relationship that might have existed disintegrated once the brothers threatened Oziel's life. Recognizing that the patient-psychotherapist relationship must be based on trust, the court observed that once the brothers had expressed unequivocally a desire to kill Oziel, he could not reasonably be expected to maintain an effective professional relationship with them. Thus, the court concluded that the tapes of the last two sessions also were not protected by the patient-psychotherapist privilege.

Moreover, the court expanded the permissible extent of the *Tarasoff* warning by stating that where, as in the case before it, a "generic" *Tarasoff* warning is insufficient to convince anyone of the seriousness of the threat, specific information about the threatened crime may be revealed without breaching the patient-psychotherapist privilege. In the court's opinion, without including such specifics, Dr. Oziel would have been hard pressed to convince anyone of the seriousness of the threat. The court also found that Dr. Oziel's periodic updates to his wife and business associate about the Menendez brothers' disclosures were within the "dangerous patient" exception to the patient-psychotherapist privilege.

In *People v. Wharton*, defendant Wharton was convicted of the first-degree murder of Linda Smith. Prior to the murder, Wharton had seen two psychotherapists, and had confided to both that he feared he would harm Ms. Smith and/or himself. Both considered Wharton a sufficient threat to Ms. Smith to warn her that she was in danger, and did so, but unfortunately to no avail.

At trial, the court permitted both psychotherapists to testify not only about the substance of the warnings given Ms. Smith, but also about certain of Wharton's statements that had triggered the warnings. The California Supreme Court affirmed the admissibility of the therapists' testimony notwithstanding the patient-psychotherapist privilege, concluding that once a warning is made in a unprivileged communication to a third person — her, the victim — the substance of the warning is no longer confidential. Under the *Wharton* reasoning, once a *Tarasoff* warning is given, a psychotherapist may be compelled to testify not only about the content of the warning, but also about the patient's communications that triggered it. The court agreed with the defendant that application of the "dangerous patient" exception does not completely remove the privilege from a defendant's confidential communications, but only those that give rise to the *Tarasoff* warning. The court, however, provided no guidance as to how to distinguish such communications from others that remain privileged.

The *Wharton* and *Menendez* cases are important for several reasons. First, *Menendez* is a significant restriction on the scope of patient-psychotherapist confidentiality because it permits a psychotherapist to disclose patient communications in as much detail as he reasonably believes necessary to prevent the threatened danger. The case thus gives psychotherapists wide latitude to disclose any communications, including a patient's confession of a crime, that they reasonably believe necessary to convince others of the seriousness of the threatened harm, and also to continue providing updates to potential victims. Presumably, it would be permissible under this standard to disclose some of the patient's history and diagnosis if relevant. Moreover, under *Wharton* these communications will be admissible in any later legal proceedings. Removing the privilege on such a wholesale basis raises serious questions about whether it is possible for psychotherapy to continue once a *Tarasoff* warning has been given. It also leaves unanswered the question of what must be said to the patient, after a *Tarasoff* warning has been given, about the confidentiality of any future communications related to the threat of violence.

Second, *Menendez* raises interesting questions by attempting to define at least one factor that terminates psychotherapy for purposes of the patient-psychotherapist privilege. In effect, *Menendez* says that because psychotherapy is necessarily based on trust, there can be no genuine therapeutic relationship once a patient seriously threatens the therapist's life. *Menendez* permits a court to step in after the fact and decide, at least for limited purposes, whether a therapeutic relationship did or did not exist at a given time. Such second-guessing raises the possibility of even greater incursions into a broad reading of the patient-psychotherapist privilege, and again raises a question as to how psychotherapy can continue once a patient who is capable of carrying out a serious threat against a psychotherapist's life makes such a threat. Indeed, under the reasoning of *Menendez,* a court could find that any sessions conducted after such a threat do not constitute psychotherapy. In such case,

no communications made in the course of the sessions would be privileged.

Menendez and *Wharton* narrowed the scope of the patient-psychotherapist privilege, and *Menendez* attempted to enunciate the limits of the patient-psychotherapist relationship, at least in some situations. The *Menendez* case significantly expands the permissible content of the *Tarasoff* warning to include any of the patient's privileged statements that the psychotherapist reasonably believes are necessary in order to convince the intended victim, law enforcement agency, etc., of the extent and seriousness of the danger.

In Delaware, the court ruled in *Laird v. Naidu*[126] that the treating psychiatrist had a duty to protect the public from a potentially violent patient, noting that the psychiatrist had "first hand knowledge of the patient's long standing and continuing dangerous propensities," and that such a release of information did not violate public policy.

On the other hand, a court ruled in *Kirk v. M. Reese Hosp. and Medical Emergency*[127] that the physicians only need warn identifiable, potential victims, and not the general public. Similarly, in *Purdy v. Public Administration v. County of Westchester,*[128] the court ruled that the physician had no duty to protect the public after an elderly woman patient injured a third party while driving from the health facility.

Certain medical conditions

Similarly, when a health care provider ascertains a medical condition with dangerous propensities, for example, diabetes mellitus or cerbrocardiovascular disease, which may impair the patient's control of his or her activities, the health care provider has a duty to warn.[129] This is true whether the condition is completely diagnosed or still under study. Epilepsy and other convulsive disorders were the medical conditions that health care providers have ignored to their legal detriment.[130,131]

Medications

The courts have imposed the duty to warn on a health care provider when medications with potentially dangerous therapeutic or side effects are administered.[132] If a drug is administered that might affect a patient's functional ability, even one as simple as ambulating, the health care provider is obliged to explain the hazard to the patient and/or to someone who can control the patient's movements such as the family or others who can reasonably be expected to come into contact with the patient. The administration of antihistamines and psychotropic drugs without adequate warning have been the health care provider's downfall in several cases. This duty also applies to patients engaged in any activity that may be hazardous, such as operating a motor vehicle.

Contagious diseases

A particular concern arises out of the decisional law that requires a provider to take reasonable steps to avoid transmission of a contagious disease and to protect third parties exposed to the disease.[133] When a contagious disease is diagnosed, there is a duty to warn persons at risk of exposure unless forbidden by statute, e.g., AIDS.[134,135] Hospital staff, family members, and others caring for or in contact with the patient should be warned.[136] The general rule is that a health care provider is liable for negligence in permitting persons to be exposed to communicable disease to their harm.[137,138] The courts have applied this rule for the protection of health care workers and of other patients of the provider.[139,140] Providers must consider whether disclosure in addition to the express statutory requirements is warranted.[141,142]

As early as 1928 a court ruled that a physician could be liable for the death of a neighbor who contracted smallpox while assisting in the care of the physician's patient with smallpox because the physician failed to warn the neighbor of the contagious nature of the disease.[143] However, in most states there is no duty to warn all members of the public individually. A California court observed that liability to the general public might result from failure to make a required report to public health authorities.[144] In at least one state there may be a duty to warn a broader range of individuals. The South Carolina Supreme Court ruled that a hospital could be sued by the parents of a girl who had died of meningitis.[145] Her friend had been diagnosed and treated at the hospital for meningitis, and the hospital had not notified persons who had had prior contact with its patient during the likely period of contagiousness.

In one case,[146] a physician in attendance on a case of typhoid fever was found to have a duty to notify attendants of the nature of the disease, warn them of the danger of infection, and instruct them about the usual methods approved by the profession for preventing the spread of the disease.

In another decision,[147] the plaintiff alleged that the hospital that employed his wife as a nurse was negligent in failing to follow proper procedures and to warn her about the contagious disease of a patient under her care. The wife, husband, and two children contracted the disease—scabies. The trial court granted the hospital's motion for summary judgment on grounds that the hospital's duty ran to patients and possibly its staff, not to the staff's family and friends. The court reasoned that it would be impractical to require a hospital to warn the general public that one of its personnel had been exposed to a contagious disease; and that limiting the duty to members of the staff's household would unreasonably cause the hospital to invade the private lives of its employees.

Courts have ruled in favor of health care providers in cases where disclosure was intended to prevent the spread of contagious diseases.[148] Under the common law duty to disclose information, there could be liability in some circumstances for failing to disclose a contagious disease.

HIV/AIDS. Many states have statutes that specify when an HIV test result or diagnosis of AIDS may be disclosed.[149] An individual who has an HIV infection still has the reasonable expectation that this condition will not be unreasonably disclosed to third parties without his or her consent. A cause of action for invasion of privacy for the HIV patient may be predicated on that expectation. The statutes are often strictly interpreted. A California physician was sued for writing a patient's HIV status in a medical record without the written consent required by state law even though the patient had given oral consent.

This right to privacy, however, is not unlimited. Statutorily mandated reporting procedures for contagious or infectious diseases such as HIV infections would act to limit the right to privacy of patients with those diseases. It is not unreasonable to disclose this status on a need to know basis to spouses, family members, sexual partners, other health care providers, public health officials, caregivers, potential adoptive/foster parents, or appropriate state health authorities. This does not give rise to an invasion of privacy. Special medical records should and need not be kept for this information.

For those involved in research relating to AIDS, any research records that identify the research subject are strictly confidential. Such records can only be disclosed to third parties with the written consent of the research subject and, in the absence of written consent, to medical personnel if needed to meet a medical emergency of the research subject, and to the health department for purposes of certain special investigations. Prior to participation in any research study, a detailed written consent, including revelation, must be obtained from the research subject.

Applicants for grants to support counseling and testing programs regarding HIV infection must agree to comply with federal, state, and local laws aimed to ensure confidentiality of information and records of those counseled or tested.

As to information required to be transmitted to the federal Centers for Disease Control and Prevention (CDC), the federal Freedom of Information Act prohibits the disclosure of personnel and medical files that would constitute a clearly unwarranted invasion of privacy. The Federal Privacy Act states that no agency shall disclose to any person any individual's record within its systems without prior consent of the individual. However, disclosure may occur if one could show compelling circumstances that affect the health and safety of an individual.

Unjustified breaches of confidentiality attract civil monetary penalties, civil claims for damages, or other remedies and criminal penalties.

There are civil penalties for the negligent or willful disclosure of test results that in any way identify the test subject. Willful or negligent disclosure of their type also exposes the disclosing party to liability for damages, including damages for economic, bodily, or psychological harm to the test subject. The negligent or willful disclosure may also expose the disclosing party to misdemeanor criminal prosecution.

Once the diagnosis of AIDS is absolutely established, in most jurisdictions health care providers must immediately report all confirmed cases to the local health officer. A few states require a healthcare provider to report AIDS-related complex (ARC) and HIV-positive patients. This is a legally accepted exception to the principle of confidentiality based on public health needs.

Although requirements of mandatory reporting are far from uniform, especially those for AIDS, ARC and HIV infection, the health care provider's failure to conform to the statutory requirement makes the provider liable to civil, administrative, and/or criminal penalties. It has also been held to be negligence per se (not requiring proof of negligence) in civil suits brought by the patients injured, including third parties, who suffer as a result of the failure to report.

AIDS cases must be reported to the public health department in all jurisdictions. In some, the duty arises under the requirement to report venereal or sexually transmitted disease; in others, it is under a specific AIDS reporting statute.

The laws of most states, including those for AIDS or ARC, require that names and addresses be supplied. A few states require reporters of HIV infections to identify individuals by a code or initials only.

Blood bank. In most jurisdictions, blood banks and plasma centers are required, upon retesting for confirmation, to provide the health department with the identities of donors who test reactive for HIV antibodies (as well as for those who have markers for hepatitis B or syphilis).

The "Look Back" programs require blood banks to notify all hospitals of donors whose blood has been found to have HIV antibodies. The hospitals determine who the recipients of that donor blood were and notify them.

Disclosure. Special legislation has been enacted in some states concerning disclosure of any information relating to screening for the HIV antibody. The state statutes vary significantly.

A health care provider who erroneously disclosed to a third person that a person has an HIV infection may be subject to a suit for defamation providing the untruth is believed and acted on to the detriment of the reportee.

A health care provider may be the object of a suit for negligent infliction of emotional injury if an individual is erroneously advised that he or she has an HIV infection.

Notification. "Notification" refers to the process of informing an individual of exposure to a communicable disease. "Partner notification" means notifying known individuals who have had sexual contact with a person infected with a venereal disease. "Contact tracing" is used to mean medical investigation, which seeks to identify the individuals who have been exposed to venereal disease. Contact tracing and partner notification are traditional devices for combating venereal diseases.

Some states require health care providers to prepare a written notification to accompany the body of a decedent infected with HIV and to inform funeral directors of the illness. Other states require a more generic notification when the body is infected with any disease that may be transmitted through contract. The CDC now recommends that morticians use universal precautions.

Warning. The duty to warn and notification have a common denominator. A medical provider has a duty to warn a patient of HIV positivity. There is an implied exception to confidentiality that allows a limited power of disclosure when necessary to protect life, safety, well-being, or other important interests based on the duty to warn.

The courts have developed a legal doctrine that a person must disclose knowledge of a sexually transmitted disease including HIV infection to other partners. The legal duty to third parties is a corollary of the duty to warn and an example of the abandonment of the doctrine of privity. It is an enforcement of the public health responsibilities of a health care provider to adequately warn the public of the hazard of the communicability of a contagious disease.

Right to know. As important as the principle of confidentiality is, it must yield when clearly necessary for the public health. People are claiming a right to be informed of a potential exposure to HIV, ranging from sexual and needle-sharing partners to health care and emergency workers. The right to know takes on increasing importance with the brightening prospects for effective early intervention that can slow the progression of disease and potentially provide years of a fuller life.

A Texas court allowed discovery of donor names in an AIDS case, but prohibited contact with the donors.[150] The Colorado Supreme Court ordered disclosure to the court clerk of the name of a donor with AIDS so that the plaintiff could submit written questions to the donor through the clerk.[151] Thus, there is a risk that records obtained without identifiers could be linked later to patient names through another exception.

In a landmark case, the question passed was "Does a patient who contracts AIDS after a blood transfusion have a right to ascertain the identity of the donor?" A Florida appellate court in south Florida said no.[152] The court said the donor's right to confidentiality and privacy was protected by both the federal and state constitutions and was superior to those of the recipient.

In this case, the defendant was hit by a vehicle. To save his life, he was given 51 units of blood during emergency treatment. A year later, he was diagnosed as having AIDS. The possibility that 51 donors might be subject to humiliation, embarrassment, and discrimination compelled the court to protect them from any kind of intrusion into their private lives.

The chief judge dissented; he argued that the plaintiff merely wanted the names and addresses of donors. He said that he could think of no reason why the 51 persons would have any objection whatsoever to the patient's relatives merely having their names. And for the donors who have AIDS, their right to privacy must take second place to revealing and paying the price for the immense harm they have done. The dissent was the forerunner of the recent decisions.

Consider *Howell v. Spokane & Inland Empire Blood Bank.*[153] On October 1, 1984, before blood screening tests for AIDS were available, John Doe X made a voluntary blood donation at Spokane and Inland Empire Blood Bank (SIEBB). At that time, SIEBB was routinely asking donors to self-screen and to refrain from donating blood if they were members of any high-risk group, which groups SIEBB identified to donors.

On October 8, 1984, Howell received two units of blood at Deaconess Medical Center. The blood was provided to Deaconess by SIEBB. One of the units had been provided to SIEBB by John Doe X. Two years later, in August 1986, John Doe X again donated blood. At that time, blood screening tests were available to detect antibodies to the HIV virus, which is known to cause AIDS. John Doe X's donation was tested and found to contain such antibodies, and SIEBB notified John Doe X of the test results. Both John Doe X and Howell currently test seropositive.

On December 4, 1987, Howell sued SIEBB, John Doe X, and others on a number of theories. On August 5, 1988, before John Doe X appeared in the action, the trial judge ruled orally that SIEBB must disclose John Doe X's identity. John Doe X then appeared and moved for reconsideration of the order. The trial judge reversed and ruled that discovery could proceed through interrogatories, requests for production of documents, and depositions upon written questions, but the identity of John Doe X would remain confidential. If the initial round of discovery indicated a need for disclosure of John Doe X's name, a motion for disclosure could be brought at that time. If disclosure of John Doe X's identity was indicated, it would be provided to only one of Howell's counsel and to no one else absent court order. None of John Doe X's relatives or acquaintances could be contacted without court order. Finally, John Doe X's identity would not be placed in the record of the court until after a final judgment was obtained.

Following the entry of this order, Howell was provided 10 years' worth of John Doe X's and his wife's medical records and their dental records. Howell has deposed John Doe X's wife, his treating physician, and a physician who has counseled John Doe X. John Doe X has also answered 19 interrogatories propounded to him by Howell and 80 by SIEBB. Although John Doe X desired to have his deposition taken by written question, Howell was allowed to conduct a videotaped deposition with John Doe X's face obscured so Howell and his counsel could observe John Doe X's body language. This deposition lasted five hours. John Doe X testified that he is not a member of a high-risk group, and that his alleged exposure to the AIDS virus must have happened during a separation from his wife in 1982, during which period he had vaginal sex with one woman three times. John Doe X's physician testified that the likelihood of a casual heterosexual contact resulting in the transmission of AIDS is remote.

John Doe X also testified that before he made the 1984 blood donation, he read a handout given him by SIEBB entitled "An Important Message to All Blood Donors". This handout identified high-risk groups and asked members of those groups to refrain from donating blood. A copy of John Doe X's donor card, which lists, among other things, his weight, blood pressure, and pulse was produced by SIEBB. However, the medical questionnaire that is routinely given to donors was not produced because SIEBB claimed that it was unavailable.

On October 12, 1989, the trial judge granted summary judgment of dismissal of Howell's claims against John Doe X for negligence, res ipsa loquitur, negligent infliction of emotional distress, outrage, assault, and loss of consortium. Howell appealed the entry of this summary judgement, the order preventing John Doe X's face-to-face deposition, and the discovery order preventing disclosure of John Doe X's identity.

The Supreme Court held that (1) recipient did not meet burden of presenting some evidence that donor should not have given blood because he knew he was at risk of carrying virus and (2) trial court did not improperly limit recipient's pretrial discovery by withholding name of donor.

Howell has a legitimate interest in being compensated for his injuries. Howell is an asymptomatic carrier of the virus, who may never develop the disease. However, he must continue to live with the knowledge that he may someday develop AIDS and suffer a terrible death from the disease.

The Court held that trial court did not improperly restrict scope of discovery by recipient of blood donation from donor infected with HIV virus. He was not prejudiced by being limited, in his ability to challenge donor's statement that he was not a member of a high-risk group for becoming infected with HIV virus at the time he made the donation. By court order Howell was precluded from discovering the name of the donor without showing of need, and from contacting relatives or acquaintances of donor; recipient had been furnished with full medical records of donor and his wife, had deposed donor through television with his face obscured but with opportunity to witness donor's "body language," and deposed donor's wife and treating physicians. John Doe X had answered 19 interrogatories propounded by Howell and 80 interrogatories propounded by SIEBB. John Doe X has offered evidence that he did not have reason to believe he should not be donating blood in 1984.

Donor John Doe X has a significant interest in avoiding intrusion into his private life. Because the HIV virus is known to be transmitted through sexual contact, intravenous drug use, and blood transfusion, Howell would undoubtedly wish to ask highly personal questions of John Doe X's relatives, friends, coworkers, and others. In addition, persons associated with AIDS are known to suffer discrimination in employment, education, housing, and even medical treatment.

In *Doe v. Puget Sound Blood Center,*[154] the case involves a discovery order that directed defendant Puget Sound Blood Center to disclose the name of the person (Donor X) who donated blood to the blood center; that blood was later transfused to plaintiff during emergency surgery. Plaintiff alleges that the blood he received was contaminated with the AIDS virus. Plaintiff alleges, as one of several liability theories, that the blood center failed to design and implement reasonable screening and/or testing procedures that would have prevented the dissemination and administration of blood contaminated with the AIDS virus to the plaintiff.

Plaintiff died in June 1988, allegedly as a result of his AIDS condition. The record discloses that the donor died from complications associated with AIDS. The actual names of the plaintiff-blood recipient and his wife were disclosed in the original pleadings. Those names have been changed to John and Jane Doe and John Doe's estate substituted for the deceased blood recipient. The file was sealed pursuant to stipulation. The donor is not a party to this suit, and has not been named as a "John Doe" defendant.

The blood transfusion to plaintiff Doe occurred in August 1984. Almost a year later, Donor X, who had donated before, planned to donate blood to the Blood Center. However, Donor X tested positive to a test (ELISA) which indicated the presence of the human immunodeficiency virus. The blood bank later determined that Donor X was the source of the blood earlier transfused to plaintiff. Two years after Donor X tested positive, the blood center advised the plaintiff that the blood he had received may have been HIV contaminated.

Plaintiff contends the identity of Donor X is necessary to investigate the blood center's contention that thorough screening had occurred, and to pursue his claims against the blood bank, and if the circumstances warrant, an independent negligence action against the donor.

The Supreme Court held that a physician-patient privilege did not apply to blood donations. The donor is not attended by a physician, is not seeking medical treatment, nor was information acquired to enable the blood center to prescribe for the "patient."

The trial court entered the following order. The defendant blood center shall disclose to plaintiff in writing identifying information that it may possess concerning the blood donor including his or her name, address, telephone number, and social security number. Such information shall be kept confidential until such time as the donor is named a defendant herein. The donor shall not be joined as a defendant without prior court approval.

The blood center sought reversal of the discovery order, contending that the order was an abuse of the trial court's discretion. The blood center appealed in its right and also asserted rights and privileges of Donor X. The Court emphasized that Donor X, deceased, was not a party to this suit, no action by plaintiff is pending against Donor X or his estate; indeed, there has been no disclosure of the identity of Donor X. The Court affirmed that the ultimate issue was whether the trial court abused its discretion by ordering disclosure of the identity of Donor X, subject to the conditions and limitations of the order, upon the record before the court. It had not.

LIMITATIONS OF DISCLOSURE

Access to a patient's records is limited to law enforcement authorities on subpoena only, except for the Criminal Division of the Internal Revenue Service, or in the unlikely event that the law enforcement officers are in "hot pursuit."[155] Government agencies charged with providing and receiving reimbursement may have access to a patient's records only when investigating the patient's care (quality of care review), but not when investigating the physician; they need a court order under these circumstances.

Some courts have recognized that disclosures are sometimes against the best interests of the patient's health. The provider may invoke therapeutic professional discretion and deny disclosure. Courts have overruled the physician. When in agreement, they generally insisted that medically contraindicated information be made available to the patient's representative. Some courts have ruled that the provider is permitted to withhold medically contraindicated information from patients only when they had representatives, provided by the state if necessary.

In a New York case, a mental hospital attempted to enforce its policy of releasing records only to physicians.[156] The court ruled that the records could be protected from disclosure only if the hospital proved release would cause detriment (1) to the patient, (2) to involved third parties, or (3) to an important hospital program. Since none of these was proved, the court ordered disclosure to the persons authorized by the patient.

In 1986 a Pennsylvania court found that inappropriate denial of access could be held to be intentional infliction of emotion distress.[157]

Substance abuse

Access to medical information is limited by some federal and state statutes, such as federal substance abuse confidentiality laws and state licensing and confidentiality laws.[158]

Special federal rules deal with confidentiality of information concerning patients treated or referred for treatment for alcoholism or drug abuse.[159] The rules apply to any facility receiving federal funds for any purpose, including Medicare or Medicaid reimbursement. The regulations preempt any state law that purports to authorize disclosures contrary to the regulations, but states are permitted to impose tighter confidentiality requirements. The rules apply to any disclosure, even acknowledgment of the patient's presence in the facility. Information may be released with the patient's consent if the consent is in writing and contains all of the following elements: (1) the name of the person or program to make the disclosure, (2) the name or title of the person or organization to receive the information, (3) the name of the patient, (4) the purpose of the disclosure, (5) how much and what kind of information is to be disclosed, (6) the patient's signature, (7) the date signed, (8) a statement that the consent may be revoked, and (9) the date when the consent will automatically expire. One exception to the general rule permitting disclosure of admission and discharge information concerns information about substance abusers. With few exceptions, federal regulations prohibit disclosure of information concerning patients being treated for substance abuse or related conditions.[160]

DISCOVERY
Discovery rules

Discovery in the law gives the opposing party the right of access to certain information available to the other party or their witnesses.[161] All matters that are not privileged are discoverable by opposing parties if they are relevant or can be reasonably calculated to lead to relevant information.

As with most matters, discovery depends on the jurisdiction involved. Some jurisdictions have placed a limit on the time within which the discovery rule could operate.

In a case where the discovery rule is applicable, when the statutory period of limitations begins to run remains unclear for many jurisdictions. For example, the period may commence (1) upon discovery of the injury alone; (2) when the plaintiff discovers both the injury and how it was caused; (3) after the plaintiff discovers the injury, its cause, and the fact that it was caused by the wrongful conduct of another; or (4) after all of these have occurred and the identity of the wrongdoer becomes known. Because the law is constantly changing in this regard, it should always be rechecked whenever a new suit is initiated.

If a party is required to submit to a physical examination under discovery, the examined party may request and obtain a copy of the examination results, and the party ordering such examination is then entitled to receive medical reports from the examinee's attending physician. The presence of the party's attorney during the physical examination also helps to protect the physician from unwittingly and improperly disclosing medical information about the patient.

Where a party in a malpractice action seeks to discover medical information about the patients of a defendant or other treating physician, courts generally will uphold the privilege and refuse to allow disclosure of the names and addresses of patients not involved in the litigation. However, dates from the medical records on nonlitigant patients of a defendant physician may be discoverable, as long as the names and addresses are kept confidential so that innocent third parties will not be harassed or drawn into the dispute.

Entries made directly into the patient's chart concerning communications with legal representatives or insurance carriers may be discoverable.[162]

Formal discovery

In lawsuits and administrative proceedings the parties are authorized by law to demand relevant *unprivileged* information in the control of others. This is called the "discovery" process. The most frequent discovery demand is by a subpoena.

Subpoenas. A physician may release *confidential* information under proper legal compulsion. This is an exception to disclosure. However, the issue of legal compulsion is often misunderstood by many physicians.

Generally, a subpoena or discovery order in itself is not proper legal compulsion. It is simply a legal order, to appear in court, but not to testify. Typically subpoenas are signed by the clerk of the court at the request of an attorney. Therefore, a physician who receives a subpoena should continue to safeguard the confidential interests of a patient until the relevant legal issues regarding testimonial privilege are properly addressed.

A subpoena accompanied by a patient's authorization will, in theory, release a physician from the prohibition of privilege. However, it is at least an ethical duty of the professional to verify that the consent by the patient was informed and consistent with any statutory requirements.

In most, but not all, circumstances courts will not permit discovery of information concerning health care of persons who are not parties.[163] Some attorneys have sought such information to establish what happened when similar treatment was given to other patients. Providers have resisted these attempts on the basis that they invade patient privacy, violate the physician-patient privilege, and are not relevant because of the uniqueness of the condition and reaction of each patient.[164]

Sometimes challenges to subpoenas are successful. A New Jersey court refused to order a woman or her psychiatrist to answer questions concerning nonfinancial matters in a marriage separation case because the husband had failed to demonstrate relevance or good cause for the order.[165] When judges are not certain whether to order a release, they may order that the information be presented for court review before ruling. An Illinois court ruled that this review should be by a judge, not an administrative hearing officer.[166]

In some situations, the only way to obtain prompt appellate review of an apparently inappropriate discovery order is to risk being found in contempt of court. In one case a physician challenged a grand jury subpoena to the records of 63 patients.[167] The trial court found him to be in contempt for failing to comply. The Illinois Supreme Court held that he must release the records of the one patient who had waived her physician-patient privilege, but reversed the contempt finding on the other 62 records. They were protected by the physician-patient privilege in Illinois until a showing of a criminal action relating to the treatment documented in the records was made.

Valid subpoenas should never be ignored and should never be challenged except on advice of an attorney. An Illinois court affirmed a $1000 fine assessed against an orthopedic surgeon for ignoring a subpoena and refusing to appear at a trial involving his patient.[168] In a Kansas case a treating physician was jailed for refusing to testify until he was paid an expert witness fee.[169] However, the Iowa Supreme Court ruled that an expert witness who is a stranger to the litigation may not be compelled to give opinion testimony without a demonstration of compelling necessity.[170]

A subpoena may require that medical records (or copies) be provided to the court or to the other side in the suit.[171,172] Under the current liberal discovery practices, medical records of parties can nearly always be subpoenaed if the mental or physical condition of the party is relevant. However, sometimes the medical records custodian has a duty to refuse to provide records in response to subpoenas. For example, federal rules require a court order before substance abuse records may be released.

When records can be subpoenaed, those who provided the health care usually can also be ordered to give depositions.[173]

A court order, including a subpoena, does not permit release of information unless the requirements of the regulations have all been met. The regulations require a court hearing and a court finding that the purpose for which the order is sought is more important than the purpose for which Congress mandated confidentiality. The regulations have been interpreted to permit hospitals to tell the court why they cannot comply with the order until after a hearing. After a hearing, courts have ordered disclosures to assess probation, revocation, and child abuse proceedings.[174] A federal district court ordered disclosure to assist an Internal Revenue Service investigation of a surgeon. Courts have declined to order disclosure when the information was sought to challenge the credibility of witnesses.[175]

Under West Virginia law,[176] the release of patient information without patient notification or consent is generally prohibited.[177] However, the state does permit medical records to be released pursuant to an order of any court, based on a finding that the information is sufficiently relevant to a preceding before the court to outweigh the importance of maintaining the required confidentiality.[178]

In California,[179] unlike West Virginia, the general patient confidentiality statute expressly permits the release of patient records without patient consent in response to a *subpoena duces tecum,* provided certain notice and procedural requirements are met. Relying on this statute, a California appellate court recently reached an opposite conclusion from that of the West Virginia court in a case involving virtually the same facts.

In *Inabnit v. Berkson,*[180] the court focused on a notice requirement imposed by California law, which had been complied with by the party issuing the subpoena prior to the release of the records. California Code of Civil Procedure 1985.3 generally provides that persons seeking access to medical records in connection with a civil proceeding must give notice to the patient, allowing reasonable time for the patient to object to the release before the medical records are produced. In the *Inabnit* case, the court indicated that the patient had received the required notice and had had sufficient opportunity to object, but had not done so.

The state's statutory law is critical to the analysis of the factual context, including the types of records being sought, the nature of the patient's illness or treatment, the identity of the party seeking the information, and the type of proceeding in which the information will be used. Similarly, federal law imposes strict disclosure requirements with respect to any patient records involving substance abuse treatment.[181]

The physician should also consider the scope of disclosure of a consent that accompanies a subpoena. A vigilant and sensitive physician should refuse to disclose information clearly irrelevant to the legal issues or outside the scope of the patient's authorization. Absent an order from the court, or a more specific consent from the patient, a physician should remain steadfast in a refusal to disclose information of questionable relevancy, unless ordered to do so.

All unprivileged matters are discoverable by opposing parties if relevant or if reasonably calculated to reveal relevant information.[182] The formal procedures set forth in Rules 26 to 35 of the *Federal Rules of Civil Procedure* have been adopted in the majority of states and in all federal courts. Under these rules, a party is entitled to inquire into the extent of injuries by ordering physical and mental examination, deposing attending physicians, and obtaining medical records and reports. Private conversations between a patient's attending physician and counsel adverse to the patient are not mentioned in these formal discovery rules.[183]

Rules of civil procedure involving discovery are designed to enhance and enforce the methods of discovery. The methods of discovery are set out in Rule 26(a), which provides:[184]

If the physician is expected to be called as an expert witness, certain information may be obtained by the way of interrogatories, pursuant to Rule 26(b)(4)(A). If the party is examined under Rule 35, and the examined party requests a copy of the examination results, the party ordering the examination is then entitled to receive medical reports from the examinee's attending physician.[185]

Informal discovery

In many, if not most cases, facts are discovered informally. The privilege statutes were enacted to protect the privacy of the patient, prevent future embarrassment, and enable the patient to discuss problems candidly with his or her physician.[186]

In light of the preceding cases, and the duties imposed by the AMA's Principles of Medical Ethics and privilege statutes, nonparty physicians who attend to patients are not free to discuss all information and opinions with counsel adverse to the patient. Physicians may assert the physician-patient privilege to protect the confidentiality of the patient's records[187]; they may even have a duty to assert the privilege.[188]

Rulings on ex parte discovery

The District of Columbia federal court, in an unreported order without opinion, held the *ex parte* discussions by adverse counsel with an attending physician were permitted.[189] A malpractice plaintiff in this case objected to defense counsel's informal interview with her treating physician. The court held that such informal discovery was justified because it was less cumbersome and much less expensive than formal discovery.

This court's ruling is remarkable because it conflicts with substantial authority to the contrary. In several cases, courts have held that opposing attorneys cannot informally interview the treating physician, even if the physician-patient privilege has been waived. In *Jaap v. District Court,*[190] the Supreme Court of Montana held that the district court lacked authority to order private interviews of the patient-plaintiff's physicians; the opinion relied on the discovery rules as the exclusive manner for such discovery. The Supreme Court of Minnesota, in the medical malpractice case of *Wenninger v. Muesing,*[191] held similarly that the rule that established procedure for disclosing medical testimony after a compulsory waiver of the medical privilege because a patient is placing his or her health in issue provides exclusive means by which an adverse party may obtain pretrial discovery of medical testimony relating to a patient's physical or mental health or blood condition. Private nonadversary interviews with a patient's attending physician by the inquiring party's counsel are not contemplated under this rule.[192]

The Supreme Court of Colorado articulated a similar

attitude in *Fields v. McNamara*,[193] as it criticized a broad authorization for disclosure of medical information.[194]

The Federal District Court of North Dakota, in *Weaver v. Mann*,[195] considered the formal discovery rules the exclusive means of eliciting information from an attending physician, admonishing opposing attorneys to "refrain from engaging in private conversation with the doctors."[196] The court cited *Garner v. Ford Motor Company*, and earlier an Alaska federal district court case, in which the holding was the same on the identical issue. But in a later case, *Trans-World Investments v. Drobny*,[197] the Alaska Supreme Court, although not overruling the *Garner* case, felt "that informal discovery methods were to be encouraged and were preferable to the more formal method utilized in *Garner*.[198] The Alaska Supreme Court, citing Rule 26(b)(1) of the Federal Rules of Civil Procedure, gave broad interpretation to what information would be considered relevant in medical matters.[199] This Court severely criticized the physician-patient privilege. Quoting Professor Wigmore from *Wigmore on Evidence* (Vol. 8, §2380a at 831), the court stated[200]

[The application of the privilege had] fostered problems collateral to those it sought to cure. . . . [T]he practice employment of the privilege has come to mean little but the suppression of useful truth — truth which ought to be disclosed and would never be suppressed for the sake of any inherent repugnancy in the medical facts involved. . . . There is little to be said in favor of the privilege, and a great deal to be said against it. The adoption of it in any other jurisdiction is earnestly to be deprecated.

Quoting *McCormick on Evidence* (§105 at 228, 2d ed., 1972), the court reasoned that "more than a century of experience with the statutes [creating the privilege] had demonstrated that the privilege in the main operated not as a shield of privacy, but as the protector of fraud." Consequently the abandonment of the privilege seems that best solution.[201]

The holding by the District of Columbia court in *Teital v. Reynolds* is buttressed by the Alaska Supreme Court opinion, which ruled that there was no jurisdiction for treating a physician any differently from any other witness.[202] The District of Columbia court indicated that the physician, like any other third-party witness, may insist on a subpoena or formal deposition if he or she wishes. This court, as does the Alaska Supreme Court, treats the rules of discovery as the exception rather than the rule. Neither the physician's duty of confidentiality nor the extent of waiver is discussed in either of these opinions.

Considering the inconsistency of the cases and the apparent difficulty of trial judges in understanding the issues involved, lawyers who represent an injured patient must take some precautions to protect their clients' privilege. At the earliest stages of the case, the lawyer may send a letter cautioning the treating physician that by filing a lawsuit the patient does not waive all privileges of confidentiality.

Ex parte contacts by adverse counsel may be a basis for legal and ethical action against both attorney and physician involved in the abrogation of the patient's rights.[203] If such information is obtained with advance notice to the patient's attorney as required, a complaint against the opposition's attorney could include allegations of fraud if the disclosure is obtained by misrepresentation of the applicable law related to privilege. This act may also constitute other intentional torts, such as invasion of privacy, infliction of emotional distress, or outrageous conduct.[204]

Medical records

Some states have statutes that establish a general responsibility to maintain the confidentiality of medical records.[205] Some states have statutes that address only records regarding treatment for certain conditions, such as venereal disease.[206] In *Von Goyt v. State of Alabama*,[207] the state brought a petition to terminate the defendant's parental rights, alleging that the defendant could not properly care for her children because of her mental condition. At the hearing, the state introduced into evidence the defendant's medical records from two mental hospitals, although the defendant had never authorized the release of these documents. The defendant's parental rights were terminated, and she appealed on the basis that the information contained in the records about her treatment was protected by the psychologist-client privilege, and that therefore the record should not have been admitted into evidence.

On appeal, the Court of Appeals of Alabama held that a court may disregard the psychologist-client privilege in a custody proceeding. The court based its decision on the fact that since it must determine what is in the best interest of the child, it must similarly be able to inquire into the mental fitness of the parent. In this case, because substantial evidence was introduced that cast doubt on the defendant's stability, the court properly reviewed the records to determine her present mental fitness, as well as the likelihood of her future mental fitness.

The Alabama court balanced the patient's interest in privacy and confidentiality against the state's interest in the well-being of the two children whose custody was at issue, and found that the children's best interest was of paramount concern.

Not all releases of information violate the right of privacy. For example, the Minnesota Supreme Court has ruled[208] that even though the patient had requested that information not be released, it was not an invasion of privacy to disclose orally that the patient had been discharged from the hospital and that she had given birth when the information was disclosed in response to a direct inquiry concerning that patient at the time near her stay in the hospital. The better practice would be to attempt to avoid release of discharge and birth information when the patient requests nondisclosure.

Most states provide some confidentiality for the identities of biological parents of children who are adopted,[209] but this statutory protection does not usually extend to children who were not legally adopted.

Medical records are also hospital business records. Many hospital staff members must have access to them to operate the hospital.[210] Hospitals have authority to permit internal access by professional, technical, and administrative personnel who need access. Examples of uses that require access include auditing, filing, billing, replying to inquiries, and defending potential litigation.

A Missouri court upheld the authority of hospitals to review records for quality assurance purposes.[211] A federal appellate court has ruled[212] that a public hospital could not permit a chaplain to review records without patient consent. A Texas court[213] permitted a hospital to be sued for allowing a person assisting a patient's investigations to review her medical records without her express consent. A federal district court in Oklahoma ruled[214] that insurers have a right to copy hospital records upon proper patient authorization. The court found that the hospital's refusal to provide access to the patient's records constituted unlawful interference with the insurer's business.

Hospitals can refuse to release records until presented with a release form that complies with their reasonable policies. A Missouri court upheld a hospital's refusal to release records to an attorney who presented a form with an altered date.[215] The general practice is to permit staff members to use the medical records for bona fide research. Research by nonstaff members should be subject to a review and approval process. The Department of Health and Human Services recognized this practice in its human studies regulations by conducting some federally funded research that involved only records that otherwise were not eligible for review or expedited review.[216]

REASONABLE AND "LEGITIMATE INTEREST" DISCLOSURES

In true emergencies, reasonable disclosures may be made in the hope of contacting appropriate persons and getting information in turn.

Disclosures must be made on court order and to appropriate persons, such as the insurance carrier and attorney, under the "legitimate interest" doctrine, when the medical practitioner is being sued for malpractice. Other health care providers may access any record of a patient when they are the target of the patient's lawsuit. When patients are allowed to authorize their own access, they may also authorize access by others.

The disclosure of the minimum amount of information necessary is a good rule of thumb when a situation requires disclosure without the patient's consent. Such situations include instances in which a court compels disclosure, or in certain emergency conditions involving danger to the patient or some third party. The latter situation may deleteriously affect the therapeutic relationship, but a physician may be ethically (if not legally) obligated to act in the public's and patient's best interest by breaching confidentiality, e.g., the duty to be warned.

Courts have found limitations on permissible disclosure based on the implied promise of confidentiality in the physician-patient relationship, violation of the right of privacy, and violation of professional licensing standards.[217]

Disclosures to family

People, friends, and relatives often seek to obtain information about patients. Most often, there is particular interest in the condition and treatment of the individual.[218] Family members are interested in their relatives. There is implied consent to keep the immediate family informed of patient progress unless the patient directs that no information be released or a statutory prohibition applies, such as the federal substance abuse confidentiality rules.

A medical practitioner is best advised to secure permission from the patient to discuss a medical condition with spouse, parents, and children, including minors, unless the patient is incompetent. Suits against a physician for disclosure of confidential information to a family member are very limited.

Release of psychiatric information is subject to special restrictions in some states.[219] A New York court has stated that a spouse should not be given psychiatric information, even when there is no estrangement, unless (1) the patient authorizes disclosure or (2) a danger to the patient, spouse, or another person can be reduced by disclosure.[220] Some states authorize disclosure of psychiatric information to spouses and others in additional circumstances.[221]

The New York court, however, reasoned that unless justified, such as if there is a danger to the patient or another person, confidential information should not be disclosed without authorization.[222] In this case, *MacDonald v. Klinger*, the plaintiff underwent two extended courses of treatment with the defendant psychiatrist, during which patient-plaintiff revealed intimate details about himself.[223] The defendant psychiatrist, without justification and without consent, subsequently divulged those intimate details to the plaintiff's wife. As a consequence of the disclosure, the plaintiff lost his marriage, his job, and his financial stability, and suffered severe emotional distress requiring further psychiatric treatment.

In its opinion for the plaintiff, the court noted that a physician-patient relationship is one of trust and confidence, out of which springs a duty not to disclose. Breach of this duty is not merely a broken contractual promise, but a violation of the fiduciary responsibility implicit in the physician-patient relationship. A Louisiana court held that a husband has the right to obtain medical information concerning his wife from his wife's physician during marriage, even if the couple lives apart.[224]

Disclosures to other parties

Requests for medical information by third parties such as insurance companies or employers require, in most states, that full disclosure be made only after an informed authorization has been given by a patient. It is the responsibility, both ethically and legally, of the treating physician to be sure that the patient's consent to disclosure is voluntary, informed, and competent. Similarly, in order to avoid ethical conflicts as well as possible liability for defamation or invasion of privacy, a professional should act with discretion in releasing sensitive information.

Insurance companies compile computerized medical records that are readily available for scrutiny.[225] Insurance applications themselves often contain a section euphemistically entitled "Your Right to Privacy." The section states that the company may collect or verify information pertaining to age, occupation, physical condition, health history, and avocation, and that it may be necessary to share such information with other individuals or organizations without the expressed written authorization of the applicant. Insurance companies assert that, although the information will be treated as confidential, brief reports may be made to the Medicine Information Bureau, a nonprofit membership organization of life insurance companies that operates an information exchange service on behalf of its members.

One of the major problems concerning confidentiality involves completing various insurance forms for reimbursement, health and accident benefits, and even life insurance applications.[226] No forms should be completed without a release signed by the patient or a surrogate, such as the next-of-kin if the patient is medically incapable. Spouses may not sign for one another unless there is medical incompetence or there is an agreement to do so. The signature must be verified by comparison with a known signature to be certain that it is not fraudulent.

If the request is more than one month old, it is suspect and its authenticity should be promptly confirmed with the patient or a surrogate. A new release should be requested. Releases that state "I authorize any and all

information" have been interpreted by courts to mean any and all *pertinent* information. Unless the patient clearly intended a broader release, only that information pertinent to the claim should be furnished.

Information that is not relevant to a third party's request should be carefully deleted so as to avoid unwarranted disclosure and to protect the patient's right of confidentiality.

Disclosure to the patient's employer or insurance company has resulted in lawsuits.[227] The Alabama Supreme Court ruled that disclosures to an employer without authorization violated the implied promise of confidentiality and could result in liability.[228] However, a New York court ruled that when a patient authorized partial disclosure to his employer the physician was not liable for giving a complete disclosure.[229] The prudent practice is to refuse to release any information when only a misleading partial release is authorized.[230]

Some courts have found implied authorization to release information to an insurance company based on patient actions.[231] In a Colorado case, submission to a medical examination at the insurance company's request was considered implied authorization.[232] However, the prudent practice is to obtain the patient's written authorization.

Some individuals can have a significant effect on affairs of business and state, and their conditions are valuable information. The general interest in unusual health conditions and conditions of those involved in public events focuses media attention on health information. The health condition of individuals is an important element of many insurance coverage determinations and legal proceedings.

Some courts have allowed release of nonparty information on an anonymous basis. Information about the nonparty that is not relevant to the third party's request should be carefully deleted so as to avoid unwarranted disclosure and protect the patient's right of confidentiality.[233]

This general rule of maintaining confidentiality is by no means absolute. Many states provide exceptions: Authorized access is given to the executor or administrator of the decendent's estate. The next-of-kin is granted access by some states.

Disclosure by surrogates

Someone other than the patient must authorize access by nonhospital personnel whenever the patient is unable to authorize access because of incapacity, minority, or death.

Minors

The scope of parent and guardian access to the information of minors is less clear.[234] Some state statutes specify that information regarding certain types of treatment, such as treatment for venereal disease and substance abuse, cannot be disclosed without the minor's consent. Some statutes specify that parents must be informed before minors can obtain certain kinds of services.[235]

When minors legally consent to their own care, it is likely that parents do not have a right to information concerning the care.[236] If the minor fails to make other arrangements to pay for the care and relies on the parents to pay, the parents may be entitled to more information. However, providers can release information concerning immature minors to their parents without substantial risk of liability unless state statutes expressly prohibit release. When a mature minor wishes information withheld from parents, the provider must make a professional judgment concerning information release to the parents except in the few circumstances where the law is settled, such as when a constitutional statute requires or forbid notification. Disclosure is generally permitted when there is likelihood of harm, such as contagious disease, to the minor or others and avoidance of the harm requires parental involvement.

Mentally incapacitated patients

Guardians of mentally incompetent patients are entitled to access when circumstances mirror those in which competent patients can obtain access. However, some state courts have suppressed family confidences and information that may upset the patient severely.[237]

When a mentally incapacitated patient does not have a guardian, the hospital generally may rely on authorization by the next-of-kin or other responsible person who is authorizing medical treatment, especially for access by the responsible person or by others for continuity of patient care or payment of charges. When the mental incapacity is temporary and the release of the information can reasonably wait, it is usually prudent to wait for the patient's authorization.

Deceased patients

In a few states the legal responsibility to maintain confidentiality ends with the patient's death. It is still prudent to insist on appropriate authorization. After the patient's death, if there is an executor of the estate, the executor's authorization should usually be sought before releasing information. If there is no executor, authorization should be obtained from the next-of-kin, such as a surviving spouse or a child.[238]

In most states, only the executor or administrator of the decedent's estate has the authorization to request or authorize the release of medical information concerning a deceased patient.[239] Many states, additionally, provide that the spouse of the decedent may have access to the information.

A physician is best advised to check the state's statutes to determine whether or not there are any more specific requirements for the release of this information (such as a court order).

Discharged patients

When a patient is discharged, only the attending physician retains the right to review the records in perpetuity unless the patient's (or surrogate's) consent is obtained for others.[240]

Consent to disclosures

The release of confidential information is based on the authorization or consent of the patient or surrogate, the judicial mandate of the courts, and any statutory mandate. The patient should be told of the need to share information with other health care persons and agencies if sharing is required, and the patient should sign the appropriate consent form.

Questionable disclosures to third parties

Preemployment physicals. What obligations, if any, does a physician have to disclose results of a preemployment or annual physical examination to an employee? In the past, courts have ruled that there is no physician-patient relationship created in the context of these employment physicals; it is only a nonconsensual relationship.

Recent cases indicate that the courts are changing their perception of the physician-patient relationship. A person coming to a physician for employment examination purposes under the auspices of an employer does get involved in an ostensible or apparent physician-patient relationship. This imposes on the physician and/or the institution he or she represents an affirmative duty to reveal health problems or potential hazards to the examinee.[241] This is part of the public health function of a health care practitioner. This is part of the "duty to warn."

Certainly there is no question, that except under certain selected circumstances, a physician has a duty to inform his patient of medical problems. Now the courts are imposing a similar duty on the "pure examining" physician and the sponsor—the prospective or actual employer he or she represents.

Causes of patient action. Under common law, neither physician nor patient has a privilege that precludes communication between them from being disclosed to a third party. However, of the courts that have specifically addressed this issue, the majority has upheld the right of a patient to recover for unauthorized disclosure of confidential information.

This is well articulated in the New York case of *Doe v. Roe*.[242] A physician who violates the duty not to disclose may be liable for damages in tort or contract.

TORTS

Privacy torts, in relation to the practice of medicine, have been recognized for many years.[243] The invasion of privacy or breach of confidentiality may be by means of the taking of an undesired photograph by a physician, thus giving rise to an intrusion claim. If the media is involved, the suit may involve a claim for publication of private facts, a claim that the patient was represented in a false light, or that the patient's name and likeness was misappropriated for commercial use. A physician's liability in a privacy case is predicated on the extent of his or her activities or participation in the tortious invasion.[244] However, in other cases in jurisdictions where communications between patients and physicians are not considered privileged, the courts have refused to recognize any liability for such disclosure.

Breach of privacy

Privacy has been defined as the right to keep information about oneself or access to one's personality inaccessible to others.[245,246] All but a few states have recognized a right to privacy that is actionable at law. The standard applied to determine whether liability exists is that the action or matter made public must be one that would be offensive and objectionable to a reasonable person of ordinary sensibilities.

Breach of confidentiality

Discussing a patient's problem with an unauthorized third party is an unlawful disclosure, and breach of confidence is a well-recognized cause of action against the physician. A patient has the absolute right to assume that information given to a physician will not be transmitted without his or her knowledge and consent.[247] This, in truth, applies to all health care providers—nurses and medical or physicians' assistants.

A minority of courts have upheld claims for breach of confidentiality based on the fiduciary duty of the physician or patient to safeguard against unauthorized disclosures of information gained during treatment.

Breach of loyalty

Breach of loyalty by a physician to a patient by relating confidential material to an uninvolved party is not dissimilar, in the law's eyes, to breach of the fiduciary relation. The obligation in a "trust" relationship between physician and patient (i.e., the fiduciary relation) necessarily involves good faith on the part of the physician in dealing with a patient. Failure to uphold the fiduciary duty may lead to charges of deceit and fraud.

Statutory breaches

Patients have argued that physician licensing statutes and patient privilege statutes provide a remedy for unconsented disclosures of confidential information. In cases based on this theory, damages have typically been restricted to economic losses flowing directly from the breach and excluding compensation based on any residual harm [for example, emotional distress, marital discord (loss of consortium), or loss of employment].

Breach of contract

A physician who has made an unauthorized disclosure of confidential information can be sued not only in tort, but also for breach of contract arising from the existence of the self-imposed ethical principles of the medical profession not to disclosure information received from patients.

The physician's culpability may also be based on violations of other doctrines, such as breach of an implied contract of confidentiality and the jurisdiction's statutory evidentiary privilege against disclosure of information obtained in the course of the physician-patient relationship.

Court cases and decisions

Several courts have enforced the patient's right of confidentiality, finding not only an ethical duty, but also a legal duty, of the physician.

The following states have established that a patient may bring an action against a physician for disclosing confidential medical information without consent: Alabama, Georgia, Illinois, Nebraska, New Jersey, New York, Ohio, Oregon, South Dakota, Utah, and Washington. The law in other jurisdictions remains unclear.

Courts have based their action on the Oath of Hippocrates, the AMA's Principles of Medical Ethics, the applicable state licensing and disciplinary statutes, the fiduciary nature of the relationship, and the implied covenant of confidentiality in the contract between the patient and physician. Other courts have recognized the existence of a fiduciary and confidential relationship between patient and physician.[248] The relationship provides an "aura of trust and the expectation of confidentiality . . . and undivided loyalty," as the court in *Hammonds v. Aetna Casuality & Surety Co.* expressed it.[249]

For example, physicians should not, by verbal or written reports, expose a patient to ridicule or humiliation. An unusual situation arose in the Utah case of *Berry v. Moench*,[250] in which the physician sent a report containing unfavorable character observations to a medical colleague, breaching his duty of confidentiality and loyalty to his patient. The patient succeeded in winning damages for libel and defamation of character.

The case of *Humpers v. First Interstate Bank of Oregon*[251] involves a plaintiff who gave up her daughter for adoption. When the daughter reached the age of 21, she attempted to find her biological mother. Although the daughter was unable to gain access to the confidential court file of her adoption, she did locate the defendant, who had been her mother's attending physician. The defendant agreed to help the daughter locate her biological mother. To this end, he gave the daughter a letter stating that although he could not locate his records, he remembered giving the plaintiff diethylstilbesterol (DES) and that the possible consequences of this medication made it important for the daughter to locate the plaintiff. The information regarding the DES was fabricated to help the daughter gain access to the confidential records concerning her birth and adoption. Hospital personnel, relying on the defendant's letter, allowed the daughter to make copies of the plaintiff's medical records, which enabled her to find the plaintiff.

The mother was extremely upset by the unexpected appearance of her daughter, and brought an action against the defendant to recover for her emotional distress. On review, the Supreme Court of Oregon held that the plaintiff had a valid cause of action against the defendant for breach of a confidential relationship. The court recognized that under certain circumstances a physician would have a valid defense to breach of confidentiality, such as child abuse or a duty to report a disease. However, the court held that the duty of confidentiality could not be disregarded solely to satisfy the curiosity of a person who sought her biological mother.

In *Alexander v. Knight*, the Pennsylvania Supreme Court considered the action of a physician in submitting a report on a patient to a doctor employed by the patient's antagonist in litigation. The court stated:

We are of the opinion that members of a profession, especially the medical profession, stand in a confidential or fiduciary capacity as to their patients. They owe their patients more than just medical care for which payment is exacted: there is a duty of total care that includes and comprehends a duty to aid the patient in litigation, to render reports when necessary and to attend court when needed. That further includes a duty to refuse affirmative assistance to the patient's antagonist in litigation. The doctor, of course, owes a duty to conscience to speak the truth; he needs, however, speak only at the proper time.[252]

In *MacDonald v. Klinger*,[253] a patient brought action for breach of fiduciary duty of confidentiality against a physician for disclosing confidential information to the patient's wife. He alleged that his marriage subsequently deteriorated, that he lost his job, suffered financial difficulty, and was caused such severe emotional distress that he required psychiatric treatment. The court

discussed *Hammonds* and *Doe v. Roe*[254] and *Heller,*[255] and concluded that such disclosure "in the absence of an overriding concern would deter the one in need from obtaining the help required. Disclosure of confidential information . . . to a spouse will be justified whenever there is a danger to the patient, the spouse, or another person; otherwise information should not be disclosed without authorization."[256] In such instances, revelation of confidential information by a physician constitutes a breach of this confidential relationship, and the law may hold the physician liable. The confidential and fiduciary relationship between physician and patient has been found to stem from a physician's ethical obligation or from an implied contract not to disclose confidential information obtained while treating a patient.

In *Simonson v. Swenson,*[257] the physician diagnosed a patient's condition as syphilis, but told the patient that to be certain of the diagnosis he would need to perform a Wasserman test, which he could not do in his own office. Fearing that the disease was in a highly contagious state, the physician told the patient to move out of the small hotel where he (the patient) was staying. When the physician discovered that the patient had not moved out of the hotel, he informed the proprietor of the hotel that the patient had a contagious disease, and the proprietor then forced the patient to move. The Wasserman test eventually proved that the patient did not have syphilis, and the patient sued the physician for wrongful breach of confidence.

The court said that a wrongful breach of confidence would give rise to a civil action for damages but that in this case the physician had a duty to disclose the diagnosis to prevent the spread of the disease.

States that have enacted a physician-patient testimonial statute have generally also allowed a cause of action for unauthorized disclosure.

PROFESSIONAL AND HOSPITAL LICENSING LAWS

In a few jurisdictions, the courts have indicated that liability for a physician's unauthorized disclosures of confidential information about a patient constitutes a violation of statutory provisions governing the licensing or regulating the conduct of physicians and is unprofessional conduct and grounds for discipline by the licensing board.[258,259] Such a violation may cause the physician to lose his license, suspension or revocation for unjustified dissemination or willful disclosure of confidential information. Approximately 23 states have made the willful betrayal of a professional secret or the willful violation of a confidential or privileged communication a ground for the revocation of a physician's license to practice in that state. The example is the Iowa rules pertaining to physicians and nurses.

It is also a criminal offense in at least one state. It may also give rise to a cause of action on behalf of the patient in negligence per se.

Misuse of confidential information without disclosure can also lead to sanctions. A New York psychiatrist was indicated for securities fraud because he traded in stocks allegedly based on inside information received from a patient.[260]

Hospital accreditation requirements

Hospitals are required, as a condition of accreditation, to maintain the confidentiality of their patients' records and to release patient information only to authorized persons. This point is aptly reflected in the ethical codes of the various health institutions and organizations[261] (see earlier sections above for exceptions).

Professional responsibilities

This obligation of confidentiality is a fundamental right of the patient, and therefore is of great concern to all physicians. To that end, all state medical societies have principles of professional conduct, indicating that the doctor of medicine should safeguard the patient's confidences within the constraints of the law.

In some states a hospital, its personnel, and medical staff are bound by professional ethics, staff bylaws, or licensure requirements to keep information in a medical record confidential. Failure to keep such information confidential would be considered unprofessional conduct sufficient to justify revocation of a license to practice medicine.

Hospital staff members have been discharged for unauthorized disclosure of medical information about patients. However, courts and arbitration panels tend to reinstate them unless there has been a consistent pattern of enforcement. Institutional policies concerning confidentiality should be followed; some courts will impose liability for failure to follow institutional rules. Some courts have supported dismissal of employees for confidentiality violations. Disclosing whether the patient is in the institution is also prohibited. Staff who are involved with substance abusers should be familiar with these regulations and know how to comply with them.

A decade ago a Minnesota court addressed a nurse who had been dismissed for a breach of confidentiality. The court found that she was not guilty of misconduct and, thus, should receive unemployment compensation because the hospital's policy had not been adequately enunciated to the staff.[262]

Recently, the Iowa Supreme Court addressed a case in which a medication aide had been fired for disclosing confidential patient information while complaining to a member of the county board of supervisors about patient care.[263] The court ruled that the disclosure was miscon-

duct that disqualified the aide from unemployment compensation.

Actions against physicians for releasing information gained while treating patients are rare in American jurisprudence; this paucity of cases is something of a tribute to the medical profession.[264]

DEFENSES

A number of defenses are available to the physician charged with making an unauthorized disclosure of confidential information about a patient. The physician may not be held liable if he or she can show that the disclosure was made for certain overriding interests to which the law affords greater protection than to the interest of the patient in keeping the information undisclosed, such as when the public interest demands the disclosure of such information for health reasons or when public policy permits disclosure to the patient's spouse. In addition, a physician cannot be held liable if required by law to make such a disclosure. Finally, in a number of jurisdictions, liability against a physician will be denied unless it can be shown that the disclosure was made maliciously.

As a general overview, most litigation stems from cases where the media has published the story or likeness of a patient without consent. A threshold question in these cases is whether the patient can be recognized as a particular individual. The patient may recover damages, but they may be mitigated because the patient is recognizable to only a few people.

Furthermore, although lack of consent alone would seemingly prove the patient's privacy claim, courts have accorded the media a "newsworthiness" privilege if the material reported is deemed to be of legitimate public interest. This privilege is consistent with the underlying value, recognized by both the medical and general community, of being informed of new developments in medical science. However, in some cases courts have recognized that publication may be actionable regardless of its news value because it may be offensive to a person of ordinary sensibilities. It should be noted that although the media may have the availability of a newsworthiness defense it is not at all clear whether a physician can claim its benefit. Physicians who are party to an invasion of privacy or breach of confidentiality may have a more difficult time defending themselves. Recent cases indicate that the newsworthiness defense will enjoy greater vitality, but that decision can only be made with respect to the facts of each individual case.

END NOTES

1. *AMA Current Opinions of the Judicial Council,* Opinion 5.05 (1984).
2. *Principles of Professional Conduct, Medical Society of the State of New York* 277 (reprinted 1985).

3. Hirsh, *Legal Aspects of Nursing Administration* 31-33 (S. Dienemann, ed., Appleton & Lange, Norwalk, Conn. 1990).

4. Hirsh, *Privacy and Confidentiality,* 31 Nursing Homes 30-32 (Mar./Apr. 1982).

5. *Wenninger v. Muesing,* 307 Minn. 405, 240 N.W. 2d 33 (1976).

6. 22 J. Health & Hosp. L. 291 (1989).

7. *Commonwealth v. Wiseman,* 356 Mass. 251, 249 N.E.2d 610 (1969); *see also Adams v. St. Elizabeth Hosp.,* No. 87-CA-180, 1989 Ohio App. LEXIS 913 (Mar. 16, 1989); *as discussed in* 22 J. Health & Hosp. L. 291 (1989).

8. *Estate of Berthiaume v. Pratt,* 365 A.2d 792 (Me. 1976).

9. *Anderson v. Strong Mem. Hosp.,* 531 N.Y.S.2d 735 (Sup. Ct. 1988).

10. *E.g., Feeney v. Young,* 191 A.D. 501, 181 N.Y.S. 481 (1920); *Vassiliades v. Garfinkels,* 492 A.2d 580 (D.C. 1985).

11. *In re Simmons,* 112 A.D.2d 806, 492 N.Y.S.2d 308 (4th Dep't 1985); *but see North Hosp. Dist. v. ABC,* No. 86-026514 (Fla. Cir. Ct. Broward County Oct. 20, 1986).

12. *Hill v. Springer,* 132 Misc. 2d 1012, 506 N.Y.S.2d 255 (1986).

13. *Dutchess of Kingston's Case,* 20 How. St. Trials, 355 (1976).

14. N.Y. Rev. Stat. Part III, ch. VII, art. 8 573 (1828).

15. Iowa Admin. Code §470-135.401(10) (1979); §590-1.2(d)(6) (1980).

16. *E.g.,* Kan. Admin. Regs. §28-34-9(b)(1974).

17. Wigmore, *Evidence* §2292 (M'Naghten rev. 1961).

18. Unreported case.

19. *Alder v. State of Indiana,* 154 N.E.2d 716 (1958).

20. *State of New Jersey v. Amaniera,* 334 A.2d 398, 132 N.J. Super, 597 (1974).

21. Fed. R. Evid. 501; *United States v. Bercier,* 848 F.2d 917 (8th Cir. 1988).

22. *Tihani v. Bronx-Lebanon Hosp. Center,* 69 App. Div. 2d 759, 415 N.Y.S.2d 5 (1979).

23. *Scull v. Superior Court,* 206 Cal. App. 3d 784, 254 Cal. Rptr. 24 (1988).

24. *Grosslight v. Superior Court of Los Angeles County,* 72 Cal. App. 3d 502, 140 Cal Rptr 278 (1977); *in Matter of Handicapped Child,* 118 Misc. 2d 137, 460 N.Y.S.2d 256 (1983).

25. *Rudnick v. Superior Court of Kern County,* 11 Cal. 3d 924, 114 Cal. Rptr. 603, 523 P.2d 643 (1974).

26. *See* 81 Am. Jur. 2d *Witnesses* §235 (1976) and cases cited therein; *Annot,* 10 A.L.R. 4th 552 (1981) and cases cited therein; *see also Tucson Medical Center, Inc. v. Rowles,* 21 Ariz. App. 424, 520 P.2d 518 (1974); *In re June 1979 Allegheny County Investigating Grand Jury,* 490 Pa. 143, 415 A.2d 73 (1980).

27. *Allegheny County Investigating Grand Jury, supra* note 26.

28. *Williams v. Roosevelt Hosp.,* 108 App. Div. 2d 9, 487 N.Y.S.2d 767 (1985).

29. *In Matter of Application to Quash a Subpoena Duces Tecum in Grand Jury Proceedings,* 56 N.Y.2d 348, 452 N.Y.S.2d 361, 437 NE2d 1118 (1982).

30. *Rasmussen v. South Fla. Blood Serv.,* 500 So.2d 533 (Fla. 1987); See also: *Banta v. Superior Ct.,* 112 Ariz. 544, 544 P.2d 653 (1976); *accord Mason v. Regional Medical Center,* 121 F.R.D. 300 (D. Ky. 1988); *Tarrant County Hosp. Dist. v. Hughes,* 734 S.W.2d 675 (Tex. Ct. App. 1987), *cert. denied,* 108 S.Ct. 1027 (1987); *Belle Bonfils Mem. Blood Center v. District Ct.,* 763 P.2d 1003 (Colo. 1988).

31. *E.g., Ex parte Abell,* 613 S.W.2d 255 (Tex. 1981).

32. *E.g., Huzjak v. United States,* 118 F.R.D. 61 (N.D. Ohio 1987); *Transworld Investments v. Drobny,* 554 P.2d 1148 (Alaska 1976).

33. *See, e.g., In re Grand Jury Subpoena Duces Tecum Dated December 14, 1984,* 113 App. Div. 2d 49, 495 N.Y.S.2d 365 (1985), *appeal dismissed,* 67 N.Y.2d 756, 490 NE2d 1233 (1986) *and appeal after remand* 119 App. Div. 1016, 500 N.Y.S.2d 223 (1986); *in Matter of Application to Quash a Subpoena Duces Tecum in Grand Jury Proceedings,* 56 N.Y.2d 348, 452 N.Y.S.2d 361, 437 N.E.2d 1118

(1982); *in Matter of Camperlengo v. Blum,* 56 N.Y.2d 251, 451 N.Y.S.2d 697, 436 N.E.2d 1299 (1982); *Board of Medical Quality Assurance v. Hazel Hawkins Memorial Hosp.,* 135 Cal. App. 3d 561, 185 Cal. Rptr. 405 (1982); *People v. Doe,* 116 Misc. 2d 626, 455 N.Y.S.2d 945 (1982).

34. *State v. Thresher,* 122 N.H. 63, 442 A.2d 578 (1982).

35. *State v. Jaggers,* 514 N.Y.S.2d 407 (1987).

36. *Matter of Grand Jury Subpoena Duces Tecum dated December 14, 1984; M.D., P.C. v. Kuriansky,* 505 N.E.2d 925 (1978).

37. Pa. Stat. Ann. tit. 42. §5929 (Purdon 1982).

38. Kan. Stat. Ann. §60-427 (1988 Supp.).

39. Mich. Comp. Laws §600.2157 (1986).

40. N.Y. Civil Practice L. & R. §4504 (McKinney 1989 Supp.).

41. *E.g., In re New York City Council v. Goldwater,* 284 N.Y. 296, 31 N.E.2d 31 (1940).

42. *Allred v. State,* 554 P.2d 411 (Alaska 1976).

43. Winslade, *Confidentiality of Medical Records: An Overview of Concepts and Legal Policies,* 3 J. Legal Med. 497, 503 (1982).

44. McCormick, *McCormick on Evidence* (3rd ed. 1984).

45. Holder, *Medical Malpractice* (2nd ed. 1978).

46. *Annot,* 10 A.L.R. 4th (1981).

47. *Schechet v. Kesten,* 372 Mich. 346, 126 N.W.2d 718 (1964); *Banta v. Superior Ct.,* 112 Ariz. 544, 544 P.2d 653 (1976); *accord Mason v. Regional Medical Center,* 121 F.R.D. 300 (D. Ky. 1988).

48. *Id.*

49. *E.g., City of Edmund v. Parr,* 587 P.2d 56 (Okla. 1978); *Jenkins v. Wu,* 102 Ill.2d 468, 468; N.E.2d 1162 (1984); *but see Southwest Community Health Servs. v. Smith,* 107 N.M. 196, 755 P.2d 40 (1988); *Young v. King,* 136 N.J. Super. 127, 344 A.2d 792 (Law Div. 1975); *Warrick v. Giron,* 290 N.W.2d 166 (Minn. 1980).

50. *Bredice v. Doctors Hosp., Inc.,* 50 F.R.D. 249 (D.D.C. 1970); *e.g., Davison v. St. Paul Fire & Marine Ins. Co.,* 75 Wis.2d 190, 248 N.W.2d 433 (1977).

51. Gregory, *Immunity for Physicians in Peer-Review Committees: Can Confidentiality Be Ensured?* 11 Legal Aspects Med. Prac. (Sep. 1983).

52. Kadzielski and Dickinson, *Lack of Uniformity of State Approaches to Protecting Peer Review Confidentiality,* Health Care Newsletter 15-20 (Feb. 1994).

53. *Young v. King,* 136 N.J. Super. 127, 344 A.2d 792 (Law Div. 1975).

54. *Warrick v. Giron,* 290 N.W.2d 166 (Minn. 1980).

55. *Bredice, supra* note 51.

56. Davison, *supra* note 51.

57. *Schechet v. Kesten,* 372 Mich. 346, 126 N.W.2d 718 (1964); *e.g., City of Edmund v. Parr,* 587 P.2d 56 (Okla. 1978); *Jenkins v. Wu,* 102 Ill.2d 468, ___ N.E.2d 1162 (1984); *but see Southwest Community Health Servs. v. Smith,* 107 N.M.___ 755 P.2d 40 (1988); *Young v. King,* 136 N.J. Super. 127, 344 A.2d 792 (Law Div. 1975); *Warrick v. Giron,* 290 N.W.2d 166 (Minn. 1980); *Bredice v. Doctors Hosp., Inc.,* 50 F.R.D. 249 (D.D.C. 1970); *Davison v. St. Paul Fire & Marine Ins. Co.,* 75 Wis.2d 190, 248 N.W.2d 433 (1977).

58. Kadzielski and Dickinson, *supra* note 53.

59. *E.g., Head v. Colloton,* 331 N.W.2d 870 (Iowa 1983).

60. Romanowich, *Patients and Their Privacy—Sh! A Balancing Act Between the Public Interest and the Individual,* 12 Legal Aspects Med. Prac. (Aug. 1984).

61. Mills, *Medical Staff Peer Review,* II Legal Aspects of Medical Practice 5-8 (Sep. 1983); *Mayfield v. Gleichert,* 484 S.W. 2d 619 (C.A. Tex. 1972).

62. *See, generally,* Anton and Devries, *Confidentiality of Medical Information,* XII CTLA Forum 172-73 (1982).

63. *Hospital Corporation of America v. Superior Court of Pima County,* ___ S.W.2d ___ (Ariz. App. 1988).

64. Miller, *Outpatient Civil Commitment of the Mentally Ill: An Overview and an Update,* 6 Behavioral Sci. Law 99, 111 (1988).

65. Miller, *Confidentiality or Communication in the Treatment of the Mentally Ill,* 9 Bull. Amer. Acad. of Psych. & Law 54-59 (1981).

66. AMA, *supra* note 1.

67. *Schwartz v. Thiele,* 242 Cal. App.2d 799 (1966).

68. *Simonsen v. Swenson,* 177 N.W. 831 (1920).

69. *Hague v. Williams,* 181 A.2d 345 (1962).

70. *Duflinger v. Artiles,* 234 484, 492-99, 673 P. 2d 86, 93-99 (1983); see also: *Britt v. Superior Court,* 20 Cal. 3d 844, 856, 143 Cal. Rptr. 695 (1978); *Bond v. District Court in and for Denver Cty.,* 682 P.2d 33, 38 (Colo. 1984).

71. *See, e.g., Doe v. Eli Lilly & Co., Inc.,* 99 FRD 126 (D DC, 1983); *but see also Stempler v. Speidell,* 100 NJ 368, 495 A2d 857 (1985) and *State ex rel. Klieger v. Alby,* 125 Wis 2d 468, 373 NW2d 57 (Ct App 1985); *appeal denied,* 127 Wis. 2d 572, 383 N.W.2d 64 (1985).

72. *Dennie v. Univ. of Pittsburgh School of Medicine,* 638 F. Supp. 1005 (W.D. Pa. 1986).

73. *E.g., Inabnit v. Berkson,* 199 Cal. App. 3d 1230, 245 Cal. Rptr. 525 (5th Dist. 1988).

74. *E.g., Cartwright v. Maccabees Mut. Life Ins. Co.,* 65 Mich. App. 670, 238 N.W.2d 368 (1975).

75. *E.g., Willis v. Order of R.R. Telegraphers,* 139 Neb. 46, 296 N.W. 443 (1941).

76. *E.g., Loudon v. Mhyre,* 110 Wash.2d 675, 756 P.2d 138 (1988); *Nelson v. Lewis,* 130 N.H. 106 534 A.2d 720 (1987); *Wenniger v. Muesing,* 307 Minn. 405, 240 N.W.2d 333 (1976); *see also Ritter v. Rush-Presbyterian-St. Luke's Medical Center,* 177 Ill. App. 3d 313, 532 N.E.2d 327, 126 Ill. Dec. 642 (1st Dist. 1988).

77. Hirsh, *supra* note 4.

78. AMA, *supra* note 1.

79. Anton and Devries, *supra* note 63.

80. Romanowich, *supra* note 61.

81. *See, generally,* 33A C.J.S. *Health & Environment* §§19-20; 39 Am. Jur. 2d *Health* §§23, 26, 32-33.

82. Hirsh, *supra* note 4.

83. *E.g., Hope v. Landau,* 398 Mass. 738, 500 N.E.2d 809 (1986).

84. *See, e.g.,* Ariz. Rev. Stat. Ann. §§ 36.621 to 36.623 (1986); Cal. Health & Safety Code §§ 3122.3124-3125 (West 1979); Colo. Rev. Stat. §§ 25-1-647, 25-1-649, 25-4-402 (1982); Ala. Code §§ 22-11-3, 22-11-15, 22-12 (1975); Conn. Gen. Stat. Ann. §§ 19a-207, 19a-221 (West 1986); Del. Code Ann. tit. 16 §§ 505-508 (1983); Fla. Stat. Ann. §§ 741.051 to 741.0593 (West Supp. 1986); Ga. Code Ann. § 19-3-40 (1982); Hawaii Rev. Stat. § 572-7 (1984 Supp.).

85. *E.g.,* Fla. Stat. §§382.16, 382.081 (1987). *E.g., Robinson v. Hamilton,* 60 Iowa 134, 14 N.W. 202 (1882).

86. N.Y. Penal Law §265.25 (McKinney 1980).

87. Iowa Code Ann. §147.111 (West 1989).

88. *Bryson v. Tillinghast,* 749 P.2d 110 (Okla. 1988); *see also State v. Beatty,* 770 S.W.2d 387 (Mo. Ct. App. 1989); *Porter v. Michigan Osteopathic Hosp. Ass'n,* 170 Mich. App. 583, 428 N.W.2d 718 (1988); Ohio Att'y Gen. Op. No. 88-027 (Apr. 21, 1988).

89. *E.g.,* Fla. Stat. §381.231 (1987) §384.25 (1987); D.C. Code 2-1352(a)(b).

90. *E.g., Thomas v. Beth Israel Hosp.,* 710 F. Supp. 935 (S.D. N.Y. 1989); *Krikorian v. Barry,* 196 Cal. App. 3d 1211, 242 Cal. Rptr. 312 (2d Dist. 1987); *Ackerman v. Tri-County Orthopedic Group,* 143 Mich. App. 722, 373 N.W.2d 204 (1985).

91. *E.g., Gladson v. State,* 258 Ga. 885, 376 S.E.2d 362 (1989).

92. *E.g.,* Iowa Code Ann. §232.75(2) (West 1985); *Landeros v. Flood,* 17 Cal. 3d 399, 551 P.2d 389 (1976).

93. *E.g., People v. Stockton Pregnancy Control Medical Clinic,* 203 Cal.App.3d 225, 249 Cal. Rptr. 762 (3d Dist. 1988); *Planned Parenthood v. VandeCamp,* 181 Cal.App.3d 245, 226 Cal. Rptr. 361 (1st Dist. 1986).

94. Fla. Stat. §415.504 (1987).

95. 21 C.F.R. §606.170(b) (1988).

96. 21 C.F.R. §812.150(b) (1988).

97. 49 Fed. Reg. 36,326-51 (1984); 59 Hosps., 76 (Mar. 10, 1985).

98. *E.g.,* Iowa Code Ann. §85.27 (West 1984).

99. *E.g., Acosta v. Cary,* 365 So.2d 4 (La. Ct. App. 1978).

100. *O'Hare v. Harris, Medicare & Medicaid Guide* (CCH) ¶31,054 (D.N.H. Mar. 12, 1981).

101. *E.g.,* Iowa Code Ann. §22.7 (West 1989 Supp.); *Head v. Colloton,* 331 N.W.2d 870 (Iowa 1983).

102. *Eugene Cervi & Co. v. Russell,* 184 Colo. 282, 519 P.2d 1189 (1974).

103. *Head v. Colloton,* 331 N.W.2d 870 (Iowa 1983).

104. *Wooster Republican Printing Co. v. City of Wooster,* 56 Ohio St. 2d 126, 383 N.E.2d 124 1983). (1978).

105. 5 U.S.C.A. §552 (1977 & 1989 Supp.).

106. 5 U.S.C.A. §552a (1977 & 1989 Supp.).

107. *E.g.,* Fla. Stat. §381.231 (1987); §384.25 (1987).

108. *Derrick v. Ontario Community Hosp.,* 47 Cal. App. 3d 154, 120 Cal. Rptr. 566 (4th Dis. 1975).

109. California Health and Safety Code 1701.1 (West 1979).

110. *E.g.,* Fla. Stat. §395.0147 (1987).

111. Cal. Health & Safety Code § 1799.100 (West 1987).

112. Chan, *Status Epilepticus: Timing Is the Standard of Treatment,* 33 Trauma 83-91 (Oct. 1991).

113. Pub. L. No. 91-596, 84 Stat. 1590 (1970) (codified as amended at 29 U.S.C.A. §§651-678 (1985) and in scattered sections of 5, 15, 29, 42, and 49 U.S.C.).

114. DC Code 207.

115. Pub. L. No. 91-596, 84 Stat. 1590 (1970) (codified as amended at 29 U.S.C.A. §§651-678; (1985) and in scattered sections of 5, 15, 29, 42, and 49 U.S.C.); 29 USCS §651-678 (1982); 52 Fed. Reg. 41818 (October 30, 1987, 54 Fed. Reg. 23,042 (May 30, 1989); 29 U.S.C.A. §§201-219 (1978 & 1989 Supp.).

116. H. L. Hirsh, *Physician's Liability to Third Parties: A Kaleidoscopic View,* XI Scalpel and Quill (Feb. 1977).

117. H. L. Hirsh, *Duty to Warn and Duty to Recall Revisited Nursing Homes* (May/June 1983).

118. *Tarasoff v. Regents of Univ. of California,* 7 Cal. 3d 425, 433-44 (1976).

119. *Thompson v. County of Alameda,* 27 Cal. 3d 741, 614 P.2d 728 (1980); *Hamman v. County of Maricopa,* 775 P.2d 1122 (Ariz. 1989).

120. *See, e.g., Eckhardt v. Kirts,* 179 Ill. App. 3d 863, 128 Ill. Dec. 734, 534 N.E.2d 1339; *appeal denied,* 126 Ill. 2d 558, 133 Ill. Dec. 667, 541 N.E.2d 1105 (1989); *Tamsen v. Weber,* 166 Ariz. 364, 802 P.2d 1063 (Ariz. Ct. App. 1990); *Schuster v. Altenberg,* 144 Wis. 2d 223, 424 N.W.2d 159 (1988); *McIntosh v. Milano,* 168 N.J. Super. 466, 403 A.2d 500 (1979).

121. *Peterson v. State,* 100 Wash. 2d 421, 671 P.2d 230 (1983).

122. *Peck v. Counseling Serv.,* 146 Vt. 61, 499 A.2d 422 (1985).

123. *E.g., Shaw v. Glickman,* 45 Md. App. 718, 415 A.2d 625 (1980).

124. *Menendez v. Superior Court,* 228 Cal. App. 3d 1320 (1991).

125. *People v. Wharton,* 53 Cal. 3d 522 (1991)

126. *Laird v. Naidu,* 539 A.2d 1064, 1988.

127. *Kirk v. M. Reese Hosp. and Medical Emergency,* 513 N.E.2d 387, 1987.

128. *Purdy v. Public Administration v. County of Westchester,* 514 N.Y.S.2d 407, 1987.

129. *Whitfield v. Canuld Construction Co.,* 83 S.E. 2d 460 (S.C., 1954); *Kaiser v. Suburban Transportation System,* 398 P.2d 14, 65 Wash. 2d 461; *amended,* 401 P.2d 350 (1965).

130. Barrow, and H. D. Fahey, *Epilepsy and Law,* (rev. 2d ed., Harper and Row, New York 1966).

131. *Freese v. Lemmon,* 210 N.W. 2d 576 (Iowa 1973).

132. A. R. Holder, *Medical Malpractice Law* 121 (John Wiley & Sons, New York 1975).

133. *Jones v. Stanko,* 118 Ohio St. 147, 160 N.E.456 (1928); *see also S.A.V. v. K.G.V.,* 708 S.W.2d 651 (Mo. 1986) (*en banc*).
134. *Gill v. Hartford Accident and Indemnity Co.,* 337 So.2d 420, Fla. Dist. Ct. of App. (Sep. 24, 1976).
135. *Wojick v. Aluminum Co. of America,* 18 Misc.2d 740, 183 N.Y.S.2d 351 (Eric County Sup. Ct. 1959).
136. *Derrick v. Ontario Community Hosp.* 120 Cal. Rptr. 566 (Cal. Ct. of App. Apr. 11, 1975).
137. *Hoffman v. Blackmon,* 241 So.2d 752 (Fla. 1970).
138. *Skillings v. Allen,* 173 N.W. 663, 143 Minn. 323, 5 A.L.R. 922 (1919).
139. *Jones v. Stanko,* 160 N.E. 456, 118 Ohio State 147 (1928).
140. *Fostage v. Corona,* 330 A.2d 355 (N.J. Super. Ct. Dec. 18, 1974).
141. *Simonsen v. Swenson,* 177 S.W. 831 (Sup. Ct. Neb. 1920).
142. *Cochran v. Sears Roebuck and Co.,* 34 S.E. 2d 296, 1945.
143. *Derrick v. Ontario Community Hosp.,* 47 Cal. App. 3d 154, 120 Cal. Rptr. 566 (4th Dist. 1975).
144. *Phillips v. Oconee Mem. Hosp.,* 290 S.C. 192, 348 S.E.2d 836 (1986).
145. H. L. Hirsh, *Human Immunodeficiency Virus Confronts the Law, Ethics and Society,* 22 Annals Acad. Med. 69-85 (Jan. 1993).
146. Unreported case.
147. *Knecht v. Vandalia Medical Center, Inc.,* 14 Ohio App. 3d 129, 470 N.E.2d 230 (1984).
148. *Supra* notes, 81, 83, 84.
149. *See, generally,* H. L. Hirsh, *A Visitation with AIDS, Part II: Major Clinical Manifestations and Syndromes, Med. Trial Tech. Q. 1989; 36:151-68; H. L. Hirsh, A Visitation with AIDS, Part III. Further Major Clinical Manifestations and Syndromes.* Med. Trial Tech. Q. 1990; 36:281-320; H. L. Hirsh, *A Visitation with AIDS, Part IV. Minor Clinical Manifestation and Syndromes.* Med. Trial Tech. Q. 1990; 36:321-58; H. L. Hirsh, *A Visitation with AIDS, Part V. Management.* Med. Trial Tech. Q. 1990; 36:450-64; H. L. Hirsh, *A Visitation with AIDS, Part VI. Medical Dilemma, Legal and Ethical Quagmire,* Med. Trial Tech. Q. 1990; 36:464-95; H. L. Hirsh, *A Visitation with AIDS, Part VII. Medicine Dilemma, Legal and Ethical Quagmire (cont'd), Med. Trial Tech. Q. 1990; 37:1-60; H. L. Hirsh, A Visitation with AIDS, Part VIII. Medical Dilemma, Ethical Quagmire (cont'd), Med. Trial Tech. Q. 1990; 37:146-86; H. L. Hirsh, A Visitation with AIDS, Part IX. Medical Dilemma, Legal and Ethical Quagmire (cont'd), Med. Trial Tech. Q. 1990; 37:27-327; H. L. Hirsh, A Visitation with AIDS, Part X. Medical Dilemma, Legal and Ethical Quagmire (cont'd), Med. Trial Tech. Q. 1991; 37:47-150; H. L. Hirsh, A Visitation with AIDS, Part XI. Medical Dilemma, Legal and Ethical Quagmire (cont'd), Med. Trial Tech. Q. 1991; 38:1-43; H. L. Hirsh, A Visitation with AIDS, Part XII. Medical Dilemma, Legal and Ethical Quagmire (cont'd), Med. Trial Tech. Q. 1991; 38:154-85; H. L. Hirsh, AIDS and the Law. A Summary and Conclusion.* JLM 1988; 10:169-210; H. L. Hirsh, AIDS Updated: a Review – Part 1, Trauma 1989; 31:85-106; H. L. Hirsh, *AIDS Updated: a Review – Part 2,* Trauma 1990; 31:65-102; H. L. Hirsh, Health Practitioners Transmit HIV, Trauma 1991; 33:1-7; H. L. Hirsh, *HIV-infected Emergency Room Patients Pose Risk for Hospital Staff.* Trauma 1991; 33:1-4; H. L. Hirsh, *On Guard and Suspicious, Managing AIDs in the Emergency Room.* Trauma 1988; 30:1-6; H. L. Hirsh, *Professional Ethical Duty to Treat HIV-Infected Patients,* Trauma 1990; 32:1-5.
150. Cohen, *Doctor Is Accused of Inside Trading on Patient's Data,* WALL ST. J., July 28, 1989, at B8, col. 3.
151. *See* note 150.
152. *South Florida Blood Service, Inc. v. Ramussen,* 467 S.2d 798 (1985).
153. *Howell v. Spokane & Inland Empire Blood Bank,* 117 Wash. 2d 619, 818 P.2d 1956 (1991).
154. *Doe v. Puget Sound Blood Center,* 819 P 2d 370, 117 Wash. 2d 772, 60 U.S.L.W. 2351 (1992).
155. *Anton and Devries, supra* note 63.
156. *Cynthia B. v. New Rochelle Hosp. Medical Center,* 60 N.Y.2d 452, 458 N.E.2d 363, 470 N.Y.S.2d 1221 (1983).
157. *Pierce v. Penman,* 357 Pa. Super. 225, 515 A.2d 948 (1986).
158. *AMA Diagnostic and Treatment Guidelines Concerning Child Abuse and Neglect,* 254 J.A.M.A. 796-800 (1985); Cal. Penal Code §11166 (West 1982); Cal. Penal Code §11172 (West 1982); Mich. Comp. Laws Ann. §722.625 (West 1987); *Ackerman v. TriCounty Orthopedic Group,* 373 N.W. 2d 204, (Mich. Ct. of App., 1985); Miss. Code Ann. 93-21-25 (1987).
159. 42 C.F.R. pt. 2 (1988).
160. Supra note 146.
161. Firestone, *Sh! Patient Privacy and Confidentiality in a Lawsuit: Physician Privilege v. Discovery,* 13 Legal Aspects Med. Pract. 1-3 (Feb. 1985).
162. McCaman and Hirsh, *Medical Records – Legal Perspectives,* 6 Primary Care 685-87 (1979).
163. *Franco v. District Court for City & County of Denver,* 641 P. 2d 922 (Colo. 1982).
164. *Id.*
165. *Ritt v. Ritt,* 52 N.J. 177, 244 A.2d 497 (1968).
166. *Laurent v. Reglji,* 74 Ill. App. 3d 214, 392 N.E.2d 929, 30 Ill. Dec. 164 (4th Dist. 1979).
167. *People v. Bickham,* 89 Ill.2d 1, 431 N.E.2d 365 (1982).
168. *Schmoll v. Bray,* 61 Ill. App. 3d 64, 377 N.E.2d 1172, 18 Ill. Dec. 536 (4th Dist. 1978).
169. *Swope v. State,* 145 Kan. 928, 67 P.2d 416 (1937).
170. *Mason v. Robinson,* 340 N.W.2d 236 (Iowa 1983); *see also Bible v. Jane Phillips Episcopal Hosp.,* No. 86-C-461-B (N.D. Okla. Oct. 23, 1987), *as discussed in* 21 J. HEALTH & HOME 61 (1988).
171. Hirsh, *Medical Records – Their Medico-legal Significance,* 2 J. Fam. Pract. 69-75 (1975).
172. Daley, *Medical Reports and Their Admissibility Under Section 52 of the Evidence Act.* Advocates Quar. 207-211 (1980); *see also e.g., Group Hospitalization & Medical Servs., Inc. v. Blankfeld,* No. HM-87-2088 (D.Md. Feb. 10, 1988), *as discussed in* 16 HEALTH L. DIG., Apr. 1988, at 17; *Fagan v. Department of Professional Regulation,* 534 So.2d 802 (Fla. 3d DCA 1988); *Krygier v. Airweld, Inc.,* 137 Misc. 306, 520 N.Y.S.2d 475 (Sup. Ct. 1987); *Community Hosp. Ass'n v. District Ct.,* 194 Colo. 98, 570 P.2d 243 (1977); *State ex rel. Lester E. Cox Medical Center v. Keel,* 678 S.W.2d 813 (Mo. 1984) (*en banc*).
173. *Id.*
174. *In re Baby X,* 97 Mich. App. 111, 293 N.W.2d 736 (1980).
175. *United States v. Providence Hosp.,* 507F Supp. 519 (E.D. Mich. 1981).
176. W. VA. Code §27-3-1.
177. *Allen v. Smith,* 368 S.E.2d 924 (W. Va. 1988).
178. W. VA. Code §27-3-1(b)(3).
179. CAL. CIV. Code §56.10(b)(3).
180. *Inabnit v. Berkson,* 199 Cal. App. 3d 1230, 245 Cal. Rptr. 525 (5th Dist. 1988).
181. 42 U.S.C. §§290dd-3, 290ee-3; 42 C.F.R. §§2.1 *et. seq.*
182. *Fed. R. Civil P. 26(a).*
183. *Id.* at 26-35.
184. *Id.* at 26(a).
185. *Id.* at 26(b)(4)(A) and 35.
186. *Community Hosp. Ass'n. v. District Court,* 570 P.2d 243 (1977).
187. *Osterman v. Ehrenworth,* 106 N.J. Super. 515, 256 A.2d 123, 127 (1969).
188. *Roberts v. Superior Court of Butte County,* 9 Cal. 3d 330, 508 P.2d 309, 107 Cal. Rptr. 309 (1973).
189. *Teital v. Reynolds,* Dist. Ct. D.C., c.m. No. 81-2687 (1975), *not fd.*
190. *Jaap v. District Court,* 623 P.2d 138 (Mont. 1981).
191. *Wenninger v. Muesing,* 307 Minn. 405, 240 N.W. 2d 33 (1976).

192. Hirsh, *supra* note 4, at 410-411, Weininger, 240 N.W.2d at 336-37.
193. *Fields v. McNamara,* 189 Colo. 284, 540 P.2d 327 (1975).
194. *Id.* at 286, 540 P.2d at 328-29.
195. *Weaver v. Mann,* 90 F.R.D. 443 (D.N.D. 1981).
196. *Id.* at 443.
197. *Garner v. Ford Motor Co.,* 554 P.2d 1148 (Alaska 1976); *see also Trans-World Investments v. Drobny.*
198. *Id.* at 1148 and 1152.
199. *Id.* at 1151-1152; *see also Federal Rules of Civil Procedure*
200. *Id.* at 1150; *see also Wigmore on Evidence,* Vol. 8, §2380a at 831.
201. *Id.* at 1151; *see also McCormick on Evidence,* §105 at 228 (2d ed. 1972).
202. *Teital, supra* note 190.
203. *See Horne v. Patton,* 331 P.2d 814; *Simonsen v. Swenson,* 104 Neb. 224, 177 N.W. 831, 9 A.L.R. 1250 (1920); *Smith v. Driscoll,* 94 Wash. 441, 162 P. 472 (1917); *Clark v. Geroci,* 208 N.Y.S.2d 5654; *Berry v. Moench,* 331 P.2d 814; *Hammonds v. Aetna Cas. & Surety Co.,* 237 F. Supp. 96; *Hague v. Williams,* 37 N.J. 238, 181 A.2d 345 (1962); *but see Colins v. Howard,* 156 F. Supp. 322 (S.D. Ga 1957); *Quarles v. Sutherland,* 215 Tenn. 651, 389 S.W.2d 249 (1965).
204. *See, generally,* Anton and Devries, *supra* note 63.
205. Grossman, *Confidentiality in Medical Practice,* Ann. Rev. Med. 43-55 (1977).
206. *E.g.,* Iowa Code Ann. ch. 140 (West 1989); *e.g., In re Arsalone,* 512 A.2d 1383 (R.I. 1986); *Coleman v. Wiener,* 139 Misc.2d 26, N.Y.S.2d 480 (Sup. Ct. 1988).
207. *Von Goyt v. State of Alabama,* 461 So.2d 821 (1984).
208. *Koudski v. Hennepin County Medical Center,* 317 N.W.2d 705 (Minn. 1982).
209. *Supra* note 6.
210. McCaman and Hirsh, *supra* note 163.
211. *Klinge v. Lutheran Medical Center,* 518 S.W.2d 157 (Mo. Ct. App. 1975).
212. *Carter v. Broadlawns Medical Center,* 857 F.2d 448 (8th Cir. 1988).
213. *Cassingham v. Lutheran Sunburst Health Servs.,* 748 S.W.2d 589 (Tex. Ct. App. 1988).
214. *Pyramid Life Ins. Co. v. Masonic Hosp. Ass'n,* 191 F. Supp. 51 (W.D. Okla. 1961).
215. *Thurman v. Crawford,* 652 S.W.2d 240 (Mo. Ct. App. 1983).
216. 45 C.F.R. §46.101(b)(5) (1988); 46 Fed. Reg. 8,392 (1981).
217. *E.g., Crippen v. Charter Southland Hosp.* 534 So.2d 286 (Ala. 1988); *Tower v. Hirshhorn,* 397 Mass 581. 492 N.E.2d 728 (1986).
218. McCaman and Hirsh, *supra* note 163.
219. Miller, *supra* note 65; M. B. DeKraii, and B. D. Sales, *Confidential Communications or Psychotherapists,* 21 Psychotherapy—Theory/Research/Practice/Training (1984); M. Lewis, *Confidentiality in the Community Mental Health Center,* 37 Am. J. Orthopsychiat. 946-955 (1967).
220. *MacDonald v. Klinger,* 84 A.D.2d 482, 446 N.Y.S.2d 801 (4th Dep't 1982).
221. E. A. Plaut, *A Perspective on Confidentiality,* Am. J. Psychiat. 1021-24 (1974).
222. *MacDonald v. Klinger,* 84 A. D. 2d 482, 446 N.Y.S. 2d 801 (4th Dep't 1982).
223. *Hammonds v. Aetna Casualty and Surety Co.,* 237 F. Supp. 96 (1965).
224. *MacDonald, supra* note 223.
225. M. Siegler, *Confidentiality in Medicine: a Decrepit Concept,* 307 N. Engl. J. Med. 1518-21 (1982).
226. Hirsh, *Patient Confidentiality,* Physician's Management (Oct. 1988).
227. McCaman and Hirsh, *supra* note 163.
228. *Horne v. Patton,* 291 Ala. 701, 287 So.2d 824 (1973).

229. *Hyman v. Jewish Chronic Disease Hosp.,* 15 N.Y.2d 317, 258 N.Y.S.2d 397, 399 (1965).
230. *Id.*
231. *E.g., Alberts v. Devine,* 395 Mass. 59, 479 N.E.2d 113 (1985); *Clark v. Geraci,* 29 Misc. 2d 791, 208 N.Y.S.2d 564 (Sup. Ct. 1960).
232. *Conyers v. Massa,* 512 P.2d 283 (Colo. Ct. App. 1973).
233. *Franco, supra* note 164; *see also Community Hospital Assn. v. District Court,* 194 Colo. 98, 570 P2d 243 (1977); *Ziegler v. Superior Court,* 134 Ariz. 390, 656 P2d 1251, 1255 (1982); *Rudnick v. Superior Court,* 11 Cal. 3d 924, 114 Cal. Rptr. 603, 523 P2d 643, n. 13 (1974); *Hyman v. Jewish Chronic Disease Hospital,* 15 NY2d 317, 258 NYS2d 397, 206 NE2d 338 (1965); *Osterman v. Ehrenworth,* 106 N.J. Super. 515, 256 A2d 123 (1969); *Shepherd v. McGinnis,* 257 Iowa 35, 131 NW2d 475, 481 (1964); *contra: Argonaut Ins. Co. v. Peralta,* 358 So2d 232 (Fla. App., 1978); *Parkson v. Central Dupage Hospital,* 105 Ill. App. 3d 850, 61 Ill. Dec. 651, 1135 NE2d 140 (1982); *Gunthorpe v. Daniels,* 150 Ga. App. 113, 257 SE2d 199 (1979).
234. Am. Med. News 28 (Mar. 17, 1989).
235. *E.g., H. L. v. Matheson,* 450 U.S. 398 (1981).
236. Buxbaum and Hirsh, *Minors and Health Care—Who Decides?,* 2 Med Law 335-45 (1983); *e.g., Gaertner v. State,* 385, Mich. 49, 187 N.W.2d 429 (1971).
237. Miller, *supra* note 65.
238. Holder, *Medical Malpractice Law* 270-277 (2nd ed. 1978).
239. *See* Lane Med Lit Guide §§3.51-3.63 (1986).
240. Hirsh, *Medico-Legal Implications of Medical Records,* IX Scalpel and Quill 13-15 (Dec. 1975).
241. McCaman and Hirsh, *supra* note 163.
242. *Doe v. Roe,* 93 Misc. 2d 201, 400 N.Y.S.2d 668 (Sup. Ct. 1977).
243. Louise II & D. Williams, *Medical Malpractice* (1960).
244. *Supra* note 17. McConnell, *supra* note 202.
245. L. D. Hankoff, *Clinical Confidentiality: Dilemmas and Guidelines,* 83 New Jersey Med. 655-59 (1986).
246. E. Zenoff, *Confidential and Privileged Communications,* 182 JAMA 160-166 (1982).
247. Wachsman, *Hear All, See All, But Silence May be Golden: Confidentiality, Privacy, and Privileged Communication,* 13 Legal Aspects Med. Pract. 5-8 (Feb. 1985).
248. Wigmore, *supra* note 17.
249. *Hammonds v. Aetna Casualty and Surety Co.,* 243 F.Supp. 7933 (D.C. Ohio, 1965).
250. *Berry v. Moench,* 8 Utah 2d 191, 331 P.2d 814 (1958).
251. *Humphers v. First Interstate Bank of Oregon,* 696 P.2d 527 (1985).
252. *Alexander v. Knight,* 177 A 2d. 142 (1962).
253. *MacDonald v. Klinger,* 446 N.Y.S.2d 801.
254. *Doe v. Roe,* 400 N.Y.S.2d 668 (1977).
255. Heller, *Some Comments to Lawyers on the Practice of Psychiatry,* 30 Temple L. Rev. 401, 405-06. (1990).
256. McDonald, *supra* note 221, 84 A.D. at 488, 446 N.Y.S. 2d. at 805.
257. *Simonsen v. Swenson,* 177 N.W. 831 (1920).
258. Siegler, *supra* note 226.
259. Feldman, *Privacy, Privacy, Where Art Thou Privacy? The Laundry is Hung Out to Dry,* 12 Legal Aspects Med. Pract. 5-7 (Sept. 1984).
260. Cohen, *supra* note 151.
261. Joint Commission For Accreditation of Health Care Organizations, *Accreditation Manual For Hospitals* 79-92 (1990 ed.).
262. *Group Health Plan, Inc. v. Lopez,* 341 N.W.2d 294 (Minn. Ct. App. 1983).
263. *Hill v. Iowa Dep't of Employment Servs.,* 442 N.W.2d 128 (Iowa).
264. A. R. Holden, *Medical Malpractice Law* 270-277 (2d 668 (Sup. Ct. 1977).

CHAPTER 25 — Telephone contacts and counseling

WILLIAM R. WICK, J.D.
HARVEY KATZ, M.D.

THE IMPACT OF THE TELEPHONE ON MEDICAL PRACTICE
DEVELOPMENT OF STRUCTURED TELEPHONE MANAGEMENT
PRINCIPLES OF TELEPHONE MANAGEMENT
ANATOMY OF A TELEPHONE CALL
MEDICAL AND LEGAL IMPLICATIONS OF TELEPHONE MEDICINE
CONCLUSION

THE IMPACT OF THE TELEPHONE ON MEDICAL PRACTICE

The piece of equipment used most frequently by physicians in the United States is probably the telephone. With technological advances such as the cellular phone, a doctor can engage in just about any activity and still be available for professional consultation. Such availability can be both a blessing and a curse. Patients naturally turn to the telephone to obtain prompt medical advice. Reliance on the telephone in all phases of medical care is increasing dramatically. Telephone contacts regarding medical concerns are so frequent that procedures used for telephone advice must be closely scrutinized to avoid patient dissatisfaction and to avoid giving improper advice.

The impact of the telephone on medical practice cannot be denied. The telephone is relied on for prompt access to medical care. Doctors schedule both professional and nonprofessional activities around telephone accessibility. A patient's most immediate access to his or her doctor is the telephone. Telephone contacts account for between 11% and 50% of all medical encounters.[1] Another study reported that 12% to 28% of all primary medical care is delivered over the phone and up to one-half of physician-patient telephone contacts result in further evaluation.[2] In 1971, 13% of all patient-care contacts in the United States was reported to be by telephone. A decade later, "among primary care specialties, telephone calls account for 19.4 percent of all patient encounters in family/general practice, 24.6 percent in general internal medicine, 28.5 percent in pediatrics, and 19.6 percent in obstetrics/gynecology."[3]

Although the telephone is used extensively in all primary care specialties, most studies regarding physician-patient telephone contacts are related to pediatric care. The average pediatrician receives 1 to 2 hours per day of incoming calls seeking medical advice.[4] In a busy primary practice of six doctors, an average of one new phone call is received every 90 seconds.[5] In a 1987 study of Denver and Baltimore pediatricians, approximately 51% of the respondents considered the telephone the most frustrating part of their practice.[6] After-hour phone calls are generally inconvenient, and the sheer volume of calls can be overwhelming.

DEVELOPMENT OF STRUCTURED TELEPHONE MANAGEMENT

Telephone contacts in primary practice run the gamut from requesting care for medical emergencies to handling routine administrative details. Because the volume of calls is large, telephone management is an essential part of every medical practice. Phone calls must be managed so as not to be obtrusive during office hours. Patient telephone contacts must be handled promptly and efficiently and coverage must be provided at all times when doctors are away from the office.

It is impractical, if not impossible, for a physician to speak to every patient who calls. Delegation of telephone responsibility to nonphysicians occurs whether it is planned or not. Although there is some controversy about whether nurses or other trained personnel should do telephone triage or give advice,[7] it is clear that nonphysician personnel already perform both functions. In many settings, the delegation of telephone responsibility to nonphysicians is unstructured. Telephone advice given without procedural parameters encourages assumption of more responsibility by nonphysicians than the physician assumes. Lack of documentation and inappropriate follow-up may occur even when advice is given by a doctor. In this context, it is clear that a structured approach to telephone advice and counseling is required.

Concerns with telephone management began to appear in the literature in the late 1960s and early 1970s. The early literature involved time motion studies and frequency of physician-patient phone contacts. This progressed to recognition of the need for training, specialization of personnel, and development of protocols and procedures to handle telephone contacts.

Beginning in the early 1970s and with more emphasis recently, attempts were made to formalize telephone counseling procedures. Systems to handle telephone contacts were developed for nonphysician personnel. These systems recognized that a registered nurse or other personnel specifically trained for telephone counseling could provide prompt, accurate advice to meet the patient's needs, allowing more efficient use of the physician's time for direct patient care.[8]

In 1972, the American Academy of Pediatrics in its work *Standards of Child Health Care* included a chapter on telephone techniques.[9] The academy said "the handling of telephone calls concerning minor illness is the most urgently felt pressure of pediatric practice and the patient care-taking tasks most frequently delegated by pediatricians to allied health personnel."[10] Guidelines were developed for handling patient telephone contacts. Physicians were advised to make sure that every pediatric setting formulated its own decision-making rules and standing orders and that a set of written guidelines was available.

A registered nurse, Sally Tripp, was one of the early authors and advocates of guidelines for telephone counseling systems.[11] She found nurses were making health care decisions using the telephone, and the time had come to establish guidelines to determine when patient care could be managed via the phone. A system to evaluate the effectiveness of that management was also needed. Tripp focused on the use of the telephone in pediatric practice. The guidelines she developed were to assist the nurse in decision-making concerning whether a child should be seen immediately by a doctor, needed to be seen by the doctor but not immediately, whether the doctor should talk to the mother, or if the situation was appropriate for home management.

During the 1970s, Dr. Harvey Katz recognized the role of the nurse practitioner in pediatric health care and the need for assessing the quality of telephone care given by nonphysician personnel.[12-14] Comprehensive works in the field of pediatric telephone management by Dr. Jeffrey L. Brown[15] and Dr. Barton Smith[16] appeared in 1980. In 1982, Katz published the *Telephone Manual of Pediatric Care.*[17] Katz recommended that pediatricians develop procedures for dealing with patient problems over the telephone. In this context, guidelines were developed for commonly encountered questions and symptoms. The materials were developed in response to a lack of published material on telephone use. This need was particularly evident in pediatrics where a high volume of patient contact was by telephone. According to Dr. Brown, programs for training physicians and nurses were either ignored or gave cursory attention to the principles of screening and treating patients over the phone.[18]

In a 1986 publication, *Management of Pediatric Practice,* the American Academy of Pediatrics observed that the office telephone system was "an integral part of pediatric practice, yet too often it is neglected or left to chance."[19] Organization of a telephone system that included specialized training, protocols, and supervision was advocated.

In 1990, Scott and Packard authored *Telephone Assessment with Protocols for Nursing Practice*[20] in response to perceived needs in nursing practice. They viewed their work as a tool for nursing management rather than a medical tool used by nurses. The procedures were designed for use by experienced nurses in a formalized telephone consultation setting.

Once protocols and systems were developed to handle telephone management, attention shifted to evaluation of the effectiveness of the system and the performance of personnel. Simulations were used to evaluate telephone decision-making by primary care physicians. The hypothesis was that experienced physicians would make correct management decisions more frequently when performing telephone triage. The study concluded that most physicians obtained information sufficient to determine the severity of the illness but that factors other than the type or amount of information obtained could account for deficiencies in telephone management.[21] A recent study of an after-hours pediatric telephone triage system in Denver was analyzed retrospectively. In 4 years, 107,938 phone calls were managed without adverse clinical outcome.[22] Given the volume of medical care delivered over the telephone, the volume of literature evaluating the success of this form of medical management is surprisingly small.

PRINCIPLES OF TELEPHONE MANAGEMENT

After the medical community acknowledged that patients were managed over the telephone, organized and efficient methods for appropriately handling this aspect of medical practice were needed. Although the physician is the most qualified person to give medical advice, the focus of telephone management has been on procedures for nonphysician personnel. Delegating telephone management allows for more efficient use of the physician's time and provides better access to medical services.

An organized procedure for telephone management separates patient calls related to routine administrative matters from those needing medical assessment. The procedure developed is, in essence, one of timing, prioritizing, or triage. The person performing the telephone function, whether a physician or nonphysician, determines if the call presents a true emergency, if the patient must be seen immediately or later in the day, or in the near future, if home management is appropriate, or if the caller needs to be referred elsewhere.

The telephone system is an extension of the physician and the practice. The effectiveness of a practice is often judged by its telephone encounters. Procedures for telephone management must reflect the overall patient care philosophy of the practice. These procedures should provide efficient access to appropriate care, continuity of that care, and the necessary follow-up.

Telephone management is, in reality, triage. The purpose of a telephone encounter is to assess the need for medical care in terms of immediacy rather than to diagnose and treat. Standard procedures should help decide the immediacy of the need for health care and assist the patient in making health care decisions.

The elements of a telephone management system include the following:

1. Delegation of responsibility to a person specifically designated for the function
2. Standard protocols and guidelines for telephone assessment
3. Specialized training for telephone assessment
4. A system for documentation specifically designed for telephone encounters
5. Proper coverage, supervision, review, and evaluation.

Delegation of responsibility

Most procedural systems for telephone management involve delegating the majority of telephone calls to an individual other than a physician. In many settings, this is a nurse or a nurse practitioner. However, some physicians use specially trained, non-nurse personnel in this capacity. Qualifications for the position generally include intelligence, warmth and compassion, a calm personality, and sound judgment. If a person is to be trained for this function, some experience or interest in the area of practice is helpful.

Telephone management requires that the individual involved be a skilled communicator. This is often a product of personality and requires a "people" orientation. Any telephone encounter has the usual requirements of any interpersonal contact. The person with telephone responsibility must be polite, interested, business-like, and must speak clearly and distinctly.

Standard protocols and guidelines for telephone assessment

Protocols have been developed for use in telephone encounters to provide guidelines for assessing callers and assisting in the management. A number of manuals have been developed for telephone counseling and triage.[23-26] Each practice should formulate its own decision-making guidelines and rules, and the persons responsible for telephone assessment should be familiar with these guidelines. Protocols provide suggestions for patient teaching and self-evaluation when home management is elected. These protocols will aid in providing consistent patient care and appropriate prioritizing. However, protocols cannot teach assessment skills and do not diagnose. They simply provide a means to be used in assessing problems and directing appropriate care.

Although the telephone encounter has been described as a triage or "sorting out," it is more than that. Telephone assessment involves an exercise in independent and informed judgment. Not all patients who are ill need to see a doctor. In many cases, all the patient needs is assurance and directions for personal assessment.

The primary purpose of a telephone encounter is to identify the immediacy of the patient's need. Telephone decision-making either by a physician, nurse, or other trained telephone counselor attempts to determine the appropriate disposition of the problem. Calls requesting health care advice are separated by degree of urgency. Telephone management personnel must be able to differentiate among severe life-threatening emergencies, in which the patient should be seen immediately, and dangerous conditions, in which the person can be transported to an office or emergency room within 20 to 30 minutes, and those in which the situation can be handled either by immediate appointment, appointment on the same day, or a future appointment. Guidelines and protocols are designed to assist the telephone manager in identifying the urgency of each situation.

Specialized training for telephone assessment

Effective telephone systems incorporate training programs to familiarize personnel with the telephone system, techniques for telephone management, and the protocols and guidelines. Such training is required not only prior to the time the person is placed in the position but should be an ongoing part of any telephone management system. Training methods include a review of protocols and manuals, formal lectures, role-playing, monitoring actual patient contacts, and enactment of troublesome situations.

In addition to the professional education required generally of all health care personnel, ongoing training and evaluation specifically directed toward telephone management must be part of any telephone system.

A system for documentation specifically for the telephone encounters

Documentation of the telephone encounter is essential. The method of documenting telephone contacts is no different from the documentation required for any other medical assessment. Entries should be made in ink, errors noted as such, late entries designated, and significant information noted. An adequate medical record requires that a history be obtained and recorded and the disposition specified. Entries should be made immediately after the encounter.

The form of document used for the telephone encounter must be adapted to the needs of the practice. In some cases, entries are made in a telephone logbook. Other practices use a form with self-adhesive backing. A specialized telephone encounter notepad that can be carried in a lab coat pocket allows for easier reporting.

The reasons for documenting the telephone encounter are obvious. Information conveyed during a phone conversation may be essential to future medical care. If additional information needs to be conveyed or if instructions need to be modified, this information is available. Without a record of the encounter, the appropriateness of the care cannot be evaluated and the effectiveness of the system cannot be assessed.

Procedures for coverage, supervision, review, and evaluation

Every telephone management system that delegates calls to nonphysician personnel requires physician availability. Telephone management systems must have someone available to take calls at all times. A physician must also be available or on call continuously. In addition, physician supervision in terms of review and follow-up is essential.

Although protocols provide assistance in proper management, certain calls must invariably be referred to a physician. These include emergency calls, a nonemergency call where the patient feels it is an emergency, and any time the patient asks to speak to a doctor.

Every telephone system should be monitored on a regular basis. It has been recommended that a physician should review the charting related to telephone dispositions at least twice a day and calls should be reviewed with the nurse or nurses handling them before they go off duty.[27] The frequency of review is best determined by the requirements of the individual practice, the personnel involved, and the degree of responsibility that has been delegated, but every telephone system staffed by nonphysician personnel must have a system for physician review.

ANATOMY OF A TELEPHONE CALL

Each telephone encounter has a basic anatomy that can be divided into three parts:
1. Identification
2. History and assessment
3. Disposition.

The first part of the conversation usually begins with a greeting, identification of the caller, and the person receiving the call. The next step is an inquiry about the reason for the call and an offer of help.

Taking a history and obtaining relevant information is obviously more difficult over the telephone than in face-to-face encounters. Visual clues and physical findings are absent. During the telephone encounter, reliance must be placed on tone and expression, how messages are phrased, and the choice of words. Information must be obtained to make an appropriate assessment and recommendation. Protocols are used after sufficient information is obtained about the problem to direct the focus of the inquiry. Major concerns and symptoms should be recorded. The telephone counselor must be alert to situations where the first reason given for the call may not be suggestive of the ultimate problem.

Telephone responsibility for non-nurse medical assistants is to provide access to care rather than treatment. Therefore, diagnosis is not the goal. The patient must join in and assist the decision-making process. The major goal of the nonphysician is to assist the caller in the decision-making. The initial approach is open-ended in an attempt to determine the general reason for the call. When the general reason for the call is ascertained, questions can be asked to focus the inquiry. These questions should lead the caller to elaborate on significant points. Silence may also encourage the caller to elaborate.

Based on the information received, a mutual decision should be reached on how to proceed. A record must be made of the instructions given. If information was given from a reference source, that should be noted. When home care is suggested, instructions should be given and reviewed with the caller to be sure the instructions are understood. The caller must be advised of what to look for, why it is significant, and that any change in circumstances should be reported immediately. It has also been recommended that every phone call have an alternate solution, for example, a directive that there be a call back if the symptoms do not improve within a specified period.[28]

MEDICAL AND LEGAL IMPLICATIONS OF TELEPHONE MEDICINE
Special concerns with telephone encounters

As soon as a medical practice gives advice and counseling over the telephone, a legal duty to the patient arises. Medicolegal aspects of patient care extend to advice given over the telephone and provide yet another avenue of potential liability. Procedures for telephone practice have been developed in an effort to ensure that patients are handled appropriately and in a way that will be scrutinized favorably when challenged in court.

Like any other aspect of medical practice, the telephone encounter may provide the basis for a malpractice claim. To be liable for action taken in a telephone encounter, the health care provider must violate the standard of care. The standard of care is generally considered to be the degree of care, skill, and judgment usually exercised by the average practitioner in the circumstances presented. The same standard, that of average care, applies to advice given in person or over the telephone.

The difficulty of telephone assessment cannot be denied. The telephone encounter has been described as assessing a patient with your eyes closed and hands tied. There are health care providers who advise against telephone assessment. If no advice is given, no duty arises.[29]

The board of directors of the Emergency Nurses Association approved a position statement on telephone advice on April 27, 1991:

ENA believes that, in the best interest of the patient, the nurse should not render opinions regarding diagnosis or treatment by the telephone. The emergency nurse should inform the person calling that conditions cannot be diagnosed by telephone and that the caller should either come to the emergency department for examination and treatment or see a private physician or health care provider. In some cases, it may be necessary for the nurse to assess the urgency of the situation and determine if it is life threatening. In life threatening situations, it may be appropriate for the nurse to teach CPR or other life saving measures by phone. In these situations, emergency medical services should be assessed. The nurse should carefully document each conversation.

ENA recognizes that some institutions have developed sophisticated telephone triage programs. These programs should be predicated on clearly defined protocols, with medical direction by experienced, professional emergency staff members. Staff members should have specialized education in triage, telephone assessment, legal aspects and limits, and capabilities of the service. A quality assurance program is essential to ensure quality control of the telephone triage program.[30]

Although controversy exists as to whether telephone advice should be given, studies evaluating telephone care have generally demonstrated that the systems function well. The Denver study showed that in 4 years 107,938 cases were successfully managed without an adverse clinical outcome.[31] Evaluation of primary care physicians indicated that inadequate telephone triage may be related to factors other than type or amount of information obtained.[32] The inability to obtain adequate information by telephone may correlate with an inability to elicit information with the patient present.

Three basic rules should be followed in telephone contacts:
1. If there is any doubt about the seriousness of the condition, the person should be seen.
2. If more than one phone call is received about one individual on the same day, the patient should be seen.
3. If the patient requests an examination, the patient should be examined.

As long as patients contact physicians by telephone, advice will be given, and whenever assessments are made that require judgment, the potential exists for a claim that the judgment is in error. In telephone encounters, like all other aspects of medical care, judgments will be required. Organized procedures, protocols, training, and an evaluation system can reduce the potential for claims but cannot eliminate them. Exposure to liability for telephone encounters is no different from other aspects of medical practice, and the potential for liability does not justify abandoning this form of access to health care.

Recording phone calls

In some multispecialty clinics, all telephone encounters are tape recorded to document patient contacts. Although this practice may be helpful to the practice, it may not be legally useful or practical. In some jurisdictions, recorded telephone calls are inadmissible unless the caller is specifically aware of the fact that the telephone conversation is being recorded. For example, Wisconsin has a statute that provides that evidence obtained from recording a telephone conversation is "totally inadmissible" in civil actions unless the person is informed that the conversation is being recorded and that it may be used in court.[33] As a practical matter, most medical practitioners do not wish to provide this type of information to their patients. In some jurisdictions, a recorded telephone encounter may not be admissible in the defense of a medical negligence claim.

Inquiry about medication

Questions about medications present a potential for liability. Health care providers may provide advice about medications commensurate with their training. A doctor can give directions concerning the use of prescription medications. Registered nurses cannot prescribe but can engage in teaching about the appropriate use of medications.[34] A consistent policy for handling questions related to medications should be part of any telephone management system.

Cases involving telephone encounters

Few appellate court decisions deal specifically with the issue of whether telephone management has met the standard of care. Reported cases have considered legal issues raised in the context of telephone management. There are decisions that consider whether a telephone contact is sufficient to create the physician-patient relationship necessary for liability and whether telephone calls extend the statute of limitations. A telephone encounter may determine the place of trial. Improper telephone advice may provide the factual basis on which liability is predicated.

A telephone call for the purpose of initiating treatment may be sufficient to create a physician-patient relationship. Most courts dealing with the issue have decided that telephone advice may, depending on the content of the conversation, create such a relationship. A telephone call merely to schedule an appointment with a health care provider does not itself establish a physician-patient relationship where there is no ongoing relationship and no medical advice is sought.[35]

A physician's refusal to see a patient in response to a late-night phone call may not create a physician-patient relationship sufficient to provide the basis for liability. In *Clanton v. Vonhamm*,[36] the patient went to a hospital emergency room complaining of back pain, was examined by a physician, and released. Later, the patient reached the physician at home. After listening to the symptoms, the physician, according to the plaintiff's allegations, refused to see her, told her it was too late, and that she should see him in the morning. The plaintiff's back condition resulted in paraplegia. The issue was whether the telephone conversation created a physician-patient relationship. Plaintiff interpreted her conversation with the doctor as a "total refusal of her efforts to secure (the doctor's) medical services." The plaintiff did not believe the doctor took her case, did not rely on any medical advice, and was not dissuaded from seeking medical attention as a result of anything the doctor said. In denying liability, the court concluded that a physician-patient relationship did not arise from the phone call.

Consultation on a treatment plan over the phone may be sufficient to allow the jury to consider whether a physician-patient relationship exists. A medical malpractice action was initiated to recover damages for severe birth injuries suffered by the infant plaintiff.[37]

The defendant, an obstetrician/gynecologist, rendered prenatal care to the plaintiff but did not attend the delivery. The mother was admitted to the hospital after her membranes ruptured. She remained in the hospital for 2 days. Labor did not progress. She was discharged. Plaintiff later contacted the defendant doctor who advised her to return to the hospital. He then called the attending physician and made recommendations for treatment including induction of labor. Plaintiffs based their allegations of medical negligence on the telephone recommendations. The court concluded there was, at least, a question of fact on the negligence issue in light of the defendant's participation in the treatment through the telephone recommendations.

Factual disputes may relate to medical advice given over the telephone. In *Howat v. Passaretti*,[38] an action was commenced by the deceased's estate seeking damages for improper treatment of a fractured left leg. The defendant orthopedic surgeon made the diagnosis. Unfortunately, the patient died from massive pulmonary emboli. The facts concerning phone calls to the defendant physician's office were disputed. There was evidence that the deceased made two calls and was told each time by the doctor's receptionist to keep his leg elevated, take aspirin, and keep his next appointment. The defendant denied receiving the calls and denied that any of his employees gave such advice.

Plaintiff's expert witness testified that if the calls were made, the patient should have been told to come in for examination. The receptionist had no recollection of any contact with the decedent, and there were no telephone message slips regarding the decedent's calls. The jury found for the health care provider, and the verdict was sustained on appeal.

A claim of medical malpractice for loss of a testicle was allegedly due to improper telephone advice.[39] The patient contacted the physician and complained of testicular and abdominal pain. The patient's pain persisted, and he had a number of telephone contacts with the defendant doctor. The doctor assumed the patient had recurring subacute prostatitis. It was subsequently discovered that the patient had an infarcted testicle due to torsion. Plaintiff's claim presented an issue of fact for the jury on whether it was negligent to provide treatment over the telephone without insisting on a physical examination.

Another factual dispute concerning information given over the phone arose in an emergency room setting.[40] The patient was brought to the emergency room following an automobile accident. The hospital had no residents or interns. Physicians voluntarily made themselves available on a rotating basis to treat patients in the emergency room.

After the emergency room nurse telephoned the

doctor on call, it was his duty to diagnose the patient's condition, prescribe treatment, and determine whether to admit the patient to the hospital. As frequently happens, the nurse and the doctor disputed the frequency of the telephone contacts and the information conveyed. The patient died, and the death was attributed to traumatic shock. The doctor on call did not come to the emergency room to examine the patient stating that he relied on information given by the nurse over the phone. There was no dispute that the physician was told that the patient had been in an accident and had sustained more than a slight or insignificant injury. The conflicting testimony about the phone call may have lead to the jury verdict in favor of the patient.

Telephone calls have also been considered by courts in determining whether actions are time barred by the statute of limitations. Although the plaintiff did not have a firm appointment for future treatment when she left the hospital, the patient's telephone call to arrange a further appointment indicated a continuous relationship necessary to extend the statute of limitations.[41]

A telephone call to a physician requesting a release letter that involved no advice or consultation did not create an issue as to whether or not the statute of limitations was extended.

Factors considered in determining whether treatment ceases include the following:
1. Whether there is a relationship between the patient and physician with regard to the condition
2. Whether the physician is attending and examining the patient
3. Whether there is something more to be done.[42]
Telephone consultations may constitute proof of a continuing physician-patient relationship.[43]

Whether the statute of limitations is extended depends on the statutory language, which can vary from jurisdiction to jurisdiction. In some states the statute of limitations does not begin to run until the end of a continuing course of treatment. A telephone call may be considered part of the continuing treatment or provide evidence of a continuing physician-patient relationship, which extends the statute.

A telephone call may also create an issue regarding the place of trial. Advice given in a telephone call from the patient's home in one county to the health care provider in another county provided the basis for a malpractice claim. The plaintiffs initiated the action in the county where they placed the call and where they received the advice. The court concluded that the proper venue was in the county where the caller received the advice.[44]

The authors are aware of an unreported case that focused directly on the procedural system for telephone advice given by a registered nurse working in a pediatric group practice. The advice was given by a trained pediatric nurse counselor. The counseling system had been in existence for 2 years prior to the incident that gave rise to the medical negligence action. The suit was brought 10 years after the incident. The nurse counseling system included specialized training, a training manual, and protocols and guidelines. The nurses worked closely with the pediatricians who were available for consultation if questions arose and for appointments if examinations were necessary.

The case involved a claim of misdiagnosis of hemophilus influenza type B meningitis. A 27-month-old girl presented to her pediatrician with a fever of 104 degrees. She was diagnosed as having the flu and aspirin was prescribed. The child did not improve, and her parents called the pediatric office 48 hours after her initial evaluation. The testimony differed as to the telephone encounter. The nurse felt it was acceptable for the parents to observe the child and call the next morning if there was no improvement. The log entry did not document the offer of an appointment or the parents' refusal. The clinic was not contacted the following morning but a day later, 4 days after the original visit and 2 days after the telephone call, and the child's condition had worsened. The parents contacted the on-call physician who suspected meningitis and directed the parents to take their daughter to the local hospital where a lumbar puncture confirmed the diagnosis.

The child responded to antibiotic therapy but sustained significant neurological sequelae including profound deafness, mental retardation, right-side hemiparesis, poor speech, and retarded language development. The jury found the clinic negligent and awarded $2.5 million dollars in damages.

From a survey of the jurors, it was learned that the liability finding was based not on the fact that advice was given over the telephone, but the nurse's failure to follow the practice's established guidelines and protocols. The jury felt it was reasonable and appropriate to give medical advice over the telephone. They were not critical of the organization and structure of the nurse counseling system. The jurors responding to the inquiry felt that people seeking advice from a medical clinic did not always need to speak to a doctor, and it is appropriate for a person with a nursing background to perform the telephone counseling role. The criticisms offered by the jurors are those frequently heard in medical negligence litigation: that the assessment was inadequate and the documentation needed improvement.[45]

CONCLUSION

From the standpoint of potential liability, telephone counseling systems do not differ significantly from other aspects of medical practice. An organized procedure must be adopted and implemented by well-trained and skilled personnel. Identification of potential high-risk problems can serve as "red flags" for the phone counselor. Certain circumstances are more likely to lead to serious adverse outcomes. These tend to be life-threatening diseases that are difficult to diagnose at early stages because of nonspecific symptoms. These potential cases must be identified so that phone counselors can be trained to be aware of them and respond appropriately.

A number of measures can be taken to improve the quality of telephone encounters and reduce liability. All medically relevant telephone encounters must be documented. Specific personnel must be designated and trained for the function. Guidelines and procedures must be adopted. High-risk situations must be identified and discussed. The system needs a low threshold for examination and appointment. When nonphysician personnel are performing the telephone counseling function, physicians must be available for supervision, consultation, and examination. The system must provide a procedure for evaluation of quality and service as well as follow-up.

Finally, it has been recognized for more than two decades that medical advice is given over the telephone. In that time, it has been recognized that nonphysician personnel can be specifically trained to deal successfully with telephone evaluation and management. In the same period, litigation involving medical assessment and evaluation has skyrocketed. As long as health care providers are required to make judgments over the telephone, lawsuits are likely to follow. However, no data are available to suggest that telephone management has emerged as an area of greater medicolegal concern than any other area of practice.

END NOTES

1. P. D. Sloane et al., *Physician Decision-Making Over the Telephone,* 20 J. Fam. Prac. 279 (1985).
2. S. Z. Yanovski et al., *Telephone Triage by Primary Care Physicians,* 89 Pediatrics 701 (Apr. 1992).
3. S. E. Radecki et al., *Telephone Management by Primary Care Physicians,* 27 Med. Care 817 (Aug. 1989).
4. A. B. Bergman et al., *Time Motion Study of Practicing Pediatrics,* 38 Pediatrics 254 (1966).
5. H. P. Katz, *Telephone Manual of Pediatric Care* (Slack, Inc. 1982).
6. P. Fosarelli and B. Schmitt, *Telephone Dissatisfaction in Pediatric Practice: Baltimore and Denver,* 80 Pediatrics 28-31 (1987).
7. J. M. Dunn, *Warning: Giving Telephone Advice Is Hazardous to Your Professional Health,* Nursing 40-41 (Aug. 1985).
8. J. Strain and J. Miller, *The Preparation, Utilization, and Evaluation of a Registered Nurse Trained to Give Telephone Advice in Private Pediatric Office,* 47 Pediatrics 1051-56 (1971).
9. Committee on Standards of Child Health Care American Acad-emy of Pediatrics, *Telephone Techniques in Pediatric Practice,* in Standards of Child Health Care (2nd ed. 1972).
10. *Id.*
11. S. Tripp, *Telephone Techniques in Pediatric Practice,* 71 Am. J. Nursing 1722-24 (1971).
12. H. P. Katz, et al., *Quality of Telephone Care: Assessment of a System Utilizing Non-Physician Personnel,* 68 Am. J. Pub. Health 31-37 (1978).
13. H. P. Katz, *Telephone Utilization in a Prepaid Multispecialty Group Practice.* Abstract presented at Eleventh Annual Meeting, Ambulatory Pediatric Association, 42 (1971).
14. H. P. Katz et al., *Night Call—An Extended Role for the Nurse Practitioner.* Abstract presented at Fourteenth Annual Meeting, Ambulatory Pediatric Association 70 (1974).
15. J. L. Brown, *Telephone Medicine, a Practical Guide to Pediatric Telephone Advice* (C. V. Mosby Company 1980).
16. B. D. Schmitt, *Pediatric Telephone Advice: Guidelines for the Health Care Provider on Telephone Triage and Office Management of Common Childhood Symptoms,* (Little, Brown and Company 1980).
17. Katz, *supra* note 5.
18. J. L. Brown, *Pediatric Telephone Medicine: Principles, Triage and Advice* vii (J. B. Lippincott Company 1989).
19. E. J. Saltzman and D. W. Shea, *Management of Pediatric Practice* 28 (American Academy of Pediatrics 1986).
20. M. P. Scott and K. P. Packard, *Telephone Assessment with Protocols for Nursing Practice* (W. B. Saunders Company 1990).
21. S. Z. Yanovski et al., *supra* note 2, at 705.
22. S. R. Poole et al., *After Hours Telephone Coverage: The Application of an Area-Wide Telephone Triage and Advice System for Pediatric Practices,* 92 Pediatrics 670 (Nov. 1993).
23. J. L. Brown, *Pediatric Telephone Medicine: Principles, Triage, and Advice* (J. B. Lippincott Company 1989).
24. Schmitt, *supra* note 16.
25. H.P. Katz, *Telephone Medicine Triage and Training: A Handbook for Primary Health Care Professionals* 4 (Slack, Inc. 1990).
26. Scott and Packard, *supra* note 20.
27. Schmitt, *supra* note 16, at 11.
28. Scott and Packard, *supra* note 20, at 11.
29. Dunn, *supra* note 7, at 40.
30. Emergency Nurses Association, *Position Statement: Telephone Advice,* 17 J. Emergency Nursing 52A (Oct. 1991).
31. S. R. Poole et al., *supra* note 22.
32. Yanovski et al., *supra* note 2.
33. Wis. Stat. § 885.365.
34. Scott and Packard, *supra* note 20, at 9.
35. *Weaver v. Univ. of Michigan Board of Regents,* 506 N.W.2d 264 (Mich. App. 1993).
36. *Clanton v. VonHaam,* 177 Ga. App. 694, 340 S.E.2d 627 (1986).
37. *DeJesus By Negron v. Parkchester General,* 161 A.D.2d 465, 555 N.Y.S.2d 374 (1990).
38. *Howat v. Passaretti,* 11 Conn. App. 518, 528 A.2d 834 (1987).
39. *Craft v. Wilcox,* 180 Ga. App. 372, 348 S.E.2d 894 (1986).
40. *Thomas v. Corso,* 265 Md. 84, 288 A.2d 379 (1972).
41. *Ward v. Kaufman,* 120 A.D.2d 929, 502 N.Y.S.2d 883 (1986).
42. *Giles v. Sanford Memorial Hosp. & Nursing Home,* 371 N.W.2d 635 (Minn. App. 1985).
43. *Grondahl v. Bulluck,* 318 N.W.2d 240 (Minn. App. 1982).
44. *Anthony v. Forgrave,* 337 N.W.2d 546 (Mich. App. 1983).
45. K. P. Katz and W. Wick, *Malpractice, Meningitis, and the Telephone,* 20 Pediatric Annals 85-89 (Feb. 1991).

CHAPTER 26 # Ethics and bioethics

BERNARD J. FICARRA, M.D., SC.D., LL.D., F.C.L.M.*

BASIS FOR ETHICAL CONDUCT
ETHICAL AWARENESS WHEN GIVING ADVICE
ETHICAL NORMS IN SCIENTIFIC WRITING AND SPEAKING
BIOETHICS AND LAW
SCIENTIFIC RESEARCH, CLINICAL INVESTIGATION, AND INNOVATIVE THERAPY
RATIONING OF SCARCE MEDICAL RESOURCES
LIFE, DEATH, AND EUTHANASIA

[T]he consideration that human happiness and moral duty are inseparably connected, will always continue to prompt me to promote the progress of the former, by including the practice of the latter.

GEORGE WASHINGTON (1732-1799)
IN A LETTER TO THE BISHOPS, CLERGY, AND LAITY OF
THE PROTESTANT EPISCOPAL CHURCH IN NEW YORK,
WRITINGS, VOLUME 30, PAGE 383.

Moral behavior and ethical ideas are as complex as human relationships. Bioethics is exhibited basically in two fashions—that of the theorists and the practicalists. The theorists represent the views of speculative thinkers immersed in hypotheses. They reflect on ethical matters and formulate various theories and explanations thereof. The practicalists present practical dicta expressed by those who lived the experiences under question—experiences that often demanded an immediate command decision. Such persons are moored to eternal verities which sanctify sacred essentials that inure character against faulty invectives.

For the Dominican theologian Thomas Aquinas (1225-1274) a primary datum of moral knowledge is that men and women are unique beings. They are different from, although related to, everything else in the visible universe. This uniqueness is manifested in all their actions. Human beings choose, select, and propose conclusions as they adapt various means to attain them. By virtue of intelligence and free will the individual person is the judge and master of every indigenous, personal act performed.

Because an obtained good end adds perfection to nature, only those actions have merit insofar as they are suited to promote perfection. Contemporaneously, every good end lends luster to life. Because an arrived-at end is dependent on intellectual activity, the hierarchy of good must be pursued to preserve the primordial dignity of human intelligence. A worthy moral life is nothing more than the free direction of human actions to obtain good ends.

BASIS FOR ETHICAL CONDUCT

Internal morality and the external performance of duties to others form the structure of human sociability that molds a person into the being that he or she is. Because human beings are self-subsistent as well as self-possessed of virtue, they have intentional control over their actions.

All things produced by humanity are really true and good only if they correspond to and are consistent with the ultimate origin of truth. But not every person is a strong champion for truth and fit to take up the challenge in the cause of preserving truth. Many people—either from ignorance or insufficient zeal for truth—have joined the forces of error to become enemies of truth. Hence they have surrendered to the multiple subtleties of error that incarcerate flexible, upright judgments and thereby inhibit theodicy.[1]

All the great moral systems which have exercised much influence have been fundamentally the same; all the great intellectual systems have been fundamentally different. In

*The author gratefully acknowledges work from previous contributors: Alan L. Dorian, M.D., A.C.L.M., and Cyril H. Wecht, M.D., J.D., F.C.L.M.

reference to our moral conduct. There is not a single principle now known to the most cultivated Europeans which was not likewise known to the ancients. In reference to the conduct of our intellect, the moderns have not only made the most important additions to every department of knowledge that the ancients ever attempted to study, but besides this they have upset and revolutionized the old methods of inquiry.[2]

Despite the potency it possesses, the workings of the intellect can be indecisive and lack the acuteness to make a differentiation between right and wrong. Although the human intellect is essential for the production of an act, it may be used ineffectually in the division of human acts into good and bad.

Differentiation between good and evil is founded on personal morality. Proper morality is derived from ideals of the highest caliber. Morality gives direction to human behavior even when it appears to be fragile and questionable.

The morality of conduct is determined not only by the content of the act as such, but also by its goal and its foreseeable consequences. Every human person by means of his or her singular, distinct nature is the recipient of basic human rights. This gift is derived from the intrinsic nature of humanity. Right reason determines that which is inherent to being human. To have reason is part of the nature of humankind.

In reference to certain bioethical standards that are threatened, a strong, unyielding moral mentality is needed. A kind of thinking that is neo-Manichaean has surfaced.[3] It threatens to treat the human body as a biological shell. As such it has nothing to do with actual humanity. Therefore any moral good is absent. Natural law becomes distorted by teleologism, proportionalism, and consequentialism.[4]

Moral conduct speaks to the educated conscience to behave in accordance with native intelligence that leads away from impropriety that importunes truth. Traditional professionalism engenders an atmosphere that is harmonious with uplifting ethical conduct and honorable moral deportment.

With all its magnetic attractions and seductive pleasures, modernism has mesmerized humanity. Hence, the capacity to know the truth may be diminished. Free will is sometimes obtunded as the power to select truth with submission to it is weakened. Hence, skepticism dominates the thinking process as mental stagnation allows emotionalism to direct actions.

The conscience can be hardened against truth, which fortifies goodness. Expression of conscience is founded on its propaedeutic reality. It is an act of individual intelligence. The function of conscience is to apply the universal knowledge of the good in a specific situation and to arrive at a judgment as to the conduct to be chosen when a decision is required.

The individual conscience has the option to determine the criteria for what is good and what is evil. Unfortunately this creates confusion in social actions, which easily become aimless without constructive purpose. When the elasticity of human conscience favors the self, goodness may be detoured. Such a situation is quite congenial to the establishment of an individualistic code of morality. The ultimate consequences of this individualism can lead to a denial of the concept of human nature and its essential attributes.

Criticizing the misuse of intelligence and the presence of moral imperfections is inherent in the duties of persons enrolled in a learned profession. Whispers intimate that physicians are not as concerned about bioethics as they should be. In a writing of major significance, a university sociologist charges that her contact with doctors of medicine indicates that there is a widespread insensitivity to ethical issues.[5] Blame is placed on the American medical education system, which accentuates clinical instruction over moral principles.

Another caveat arises when consideration is given to the union between universities and the biomedical industry. This linkage is not an ethical example for medical students during the formative years in their chosen profession. The relationship between academia and commercial bioscientific corporations is tinged, at times, with questionable conduct. Businesses have not hidden the fact that many scientists have been seduced by "offering professors consulting fees, stock holdings, and percentages of profits in return for rights to their bioengineering breakthroughs that lead to new drugs or other medical developments."[6]

Recently, medical schools have become aware of deficiencies in teaching medical ethics in their curricula. Deans are encouraging medical students to take sociology classes and courses in communication skills and medical ethics.

Within the unity of the medical community, the promotion and preservation of the highest standards of professional conduct is the task of those who have leadership in the multitiered medical societies. It is their obligation to advocate the ethical catechesis of Hippocrates and the precise rules of ethical conduct published by the American Medical Association.

With these preambles, some ethical disquietudes are to be reviewed under the discerning microscope of nature's way. First we must disallow skepticism to dominate thinking that permits emotionalism to rule the mind. When this occurs, truth is avoided. Human intelligence is suppressed and free will is less effective. Bioscientists must not encode into their own morality that which is a deceptive deviation from known ethical propriety. This threatens idealism to be dethroned by opportunism. It is a denouncement of a cautious con-science and the abandonment of judicious wisdom.

> And if riches be a desirable possession in life,
> what is more rich than Wisdom, who produces all things?
> And if prudence renders service,
> who in the world is a better craftsman than she?[7]

ETHICAL AWARENESS WHEN GIVING ADVICE

Among the privileges derived from the licensed title of "doctor of medicine" is advising patients. Clinical physicians are in the forefront of bioscientists who are consulted for information on many subjects, not all of which are of a strictly medical nature. Some may be medicolegal. Others are oriented to societal stress.

Physicians, psychologists, psychiatrists, medicolegalists, and similar counselors are unable to ignore their ethical responsibility when giving advice. The difficult dilemmas of patients should not be of minimal concern to the professional adviser. Some specific examples include adult children's need to be guided in matters such as placing elderly parents in a nursing facility and writing a living will.

Even at the social and domestic levels, aiding a person to arrive at a moral decision is a grave responsibility. When an experienced professional assists anyone in making a decision, due ethical considerations must be used. An obligation exists to advise wisely with consideration given to the welfare of all those involved. Paucity and gravity of benefits must be of equal importance to each person involved. No personal benefit is to be considered that can revert to the counselor by any advice given. Whenever a moral decision can affect people's lives—their personal character, social relationships, family unity, and daily living—the counsel given is one of major importance. It is not to be taken lightly, casually, and nonsensically. Bioscientists carry the heavy burden of rendering advice that involves life and death.

ETHICAL NORMS IN SCIENTIFIC WRITING AND SPEAKING

Persons of education, learning, and teaching ability are human beings like all others. But their talents require deportment commensurate with the intellectual status achieved. Therefore, what they write, say, and do must be impeccable. They are imitated by youth and emulated by students. Thus, they are instruments in the molding process of many who are seen and unseen by the speaker or writer.

Recognizing the touchstone blessing of academic acclaim some researchers worship the false gods of notoriety, public acclaim, and the news media. Electrified by the propulsion to achieve greatness, they choose

to follow the devious pathways of the illusive rainbow that may lead to failure. In the interim they have embraced dishonesty, chicanery, and deception. Superior intelligence starts with accurate facts and then pursues a research project with fairness, accuracy, and objectivity without any falsehood.

Conscience is the monitor watching over behavior. Unfortunately, it is too easy to favor one's own conscience. When gain is available the authority of conscience can be disobeyed easily. Each person can stifle the ethical governor of conscience by subjective domination. Contemporary immoral forces lend strength to unethical autarky.[8]

Cheating is an evil learned early in schools, colleges, and universities. It commences as cheating on examinations. Starting with little "crib notes," it increases to gigantic proportions. After an academic career of studying is completed and the terminal degree obtained, the chronic cheating infection does not vanish. Another form of cheating in scholarship is in writing. The most common way is to have papers, theses, and dissertations ghostwritten. This serious form of cheating is most difficult to control because such activity has evolved into a business enterprise with many customers. Hence, some persons receive acknowledgment for work they did not do.

Each individual is the master of decision making. Those with pure moral integrity will be noncheaters. The entire responsibility is a personal one in terms of deciding to be a cheater or a noncheater.[9] Cheating is fundamentally deplorable because it leads to the gain of something—in this case, knowledge—without working for it.

Cheating in science comes in four major categories. Arranged alphabetically they are as follows:

- *Cooking* is the elimination of negative results by choosing only data that suit the researcher to arrive at a sought-after conclusion or to prove a predetermined point.
- *Forging* is the act of recording observations that were never made, citing experiments that were never carried out, quoting nonexistent manuscripts, and plagiarism.
- *Fudging* is the act of rearranging data to suit the purpose of the performer, investigator, and author.
- *Trimming* is the manipulation of data to look better by amplification, such as recording the use of 100 animals in an experiment when only 10 were studied, and using a lesser number of controls than the number stated. Trimming is also known as massaging and fudging data.

Incentives for fraud include trying to secure a research position, to prove that public funds and/or grants for a research project were used properly, and to convince grantors of funds that a certain drug, appliance, or procedure is safe and therefore acceptable.

Scientific writing is not exempt from ethical norms. There is no simple answer as to the frequency of deception in the sphere of writing for publication. Four issues seem to be thrust on editors of scientific journals:

1. Submission of the same manuscript to two journals under different titles. This is done to increase the number of publications listed in a *curriculum vitae*. A more serious deviation is outright falsity in a manuscript that reports fabricated data.

2. An excessive number of authors on one manuscript. This allows each name to take credit for a literary contribution, adding another writing to his or her bibliography. Credit as author should go only to those who have contributed to it.

3. The sending of reprints of scientific articles published to newspapers, health magazines, and other nonscientific publications to obtain free publicity, which is not in keeping with traditional professionalism.

4. The lack of appropriate application of statistics, which can be manipulated to serve a preconceived purpose. Falsified statistics give misinformation. They give validity to research when it is unwarranted and misleading. Data obtained unscientifically is intellectual misconduct worthy of censorship.[10]

The publication of false information detours honest scientists from real pathways that may produce end products that are life-saving. Care must be taken not to encourage fraudulent science. When it is discovered, the punishment never fits the crime.[11]

Professional men and women are not permitted to create a device that insulates them from adhering to the normal ethical standards of human conduct expected of those who are learned. Danger lies in faulty bioscientific promulgations that when accepted as truth may destroy someone's life. There is no justification for publishing falsity and half-truths. A scientist's moral task is quite prosaic, basic, and mundane. It is to report research honestly.

A classical example of a scientist out of step is Philippus Aureolus Theophrastus Bombast von Hohenheim (1493-1541). Known more familiarly as Paracelsus, he is marked in medical history as one who separated himself from the accepted medical views and traditions of his generation. Historical rumor suggests that "his proclivity towards verbosity and ostentation has made his middle name Bombast synonymous with pretentiousness in the languages of the West. His contempt for many of his fellow physicians marked him as an unpopular innovator."[12] Paracelsus gained historical fame for his bombastic personality, not for his contributions to science, which by comparison are minimized.

Only human beings can lie. It is not an animal achievement. Chronic liars can become pathological and self-destructive. Many behavioral specialists treat lying as a natural by-product of psychological growth. Such thinking wears out the moral fabric that binds society into a unit of respectable citizens. "Removing the distinction between speaking the truth and telling a lie eliminates the expectation of ethical behavior because no framework of either truth or reason for abiding by it has been established."[13]

BIOETHICS AND LAW

Law as a monitoring ombudsman assists in preserving ethical medical behavior through the judicial vehicle of legal redress. This is accomplished by allegations, lawsuits, and constructive criticism.

Legal medicine warns against ethical distortions that may bring about legal recriminations. Legal medicine has become a potent, positive force in the preservation of moral medical prestige.

Distaste for legal invectives has engendered within bioscientists an adverse emotionalism. Disturbing pressures from socioeconomic restrictions have forced all persons rendering health care to be aware of the rules, regulations, and restrictions imposed on them by the law. The beginning of their career is marked by state scrutiny prior to receiving a license, certificate, and other testimonial authorizing performance in their health field.

Law and medicine as two learned disciplines know the need for a harmonious relationship between them. In some jurisdictions physicians and lawyers have agreed to a joint code of professional behavior. Such codes are prepared by the Joint Medicolegal Committee of the state medical society and the state bar association.

The purpose of these mutually accepted codes is to establish standards of practice and of ethical conduct for physicians and lawyers where there are interrelationships between the medical and legal professions. The standards presented are founded on the principles set forth in the canons of ethics of the state bar association, and the principles of professional conduct of the medical society of the state.

The trend for applying old laws and new ones to controversial moral medical controversy is discernible. "Through an evolutionary process that seems peculiar to broad-based laws that are enacted to combat one set of problems and end up being applied to a host of others, the Federal racketeering act now finds itself the weapon of choice in the struggle against violence at abortion clinics."[14] Established in 1970 to combat crime, the Racketeer Influenced and Corrupt Organization Act, known as RICO, has had many applications beyond the original intention. It is currently used in commercial disputes and routinely in criminal cases that have no connection to organized crime. In December 1993 the Supreme Court heard arguments in a case that requires an answer as to whether advocates of abortion rights can bring the legal force of the RICO statute against antiabortion protesters who have demonstrated outside abortion clinics.

A further example of legal expression on the abortion issue was noted in Germany. "The post–World War II German constitution explicitly guarantees the right to life, and according to the 1975 abortion decision, which applied that guarantee to unborn life, the drafters of the constitution did so in reaction against the Nazi doctrines of destruction of a life unworthy to live and the final solution."[15] On May 28, 1993, the Constitutional Court of Germany upheld the right to life for unborn children.

Postwar investigations disclosed the atrocities committed by infamous experimenters such as Mengele under the surveillance of the SS (Schutzstaffel). Nazi law encouraged inhuman acts, giving immunity to physicians who were politically correct. Thus they were motivated to perform horrendous acts.

Doctors under Hitler gained academic rank by complying with an SS requisite. "To qualify for university teaching the physician conducted human experiments on concentration camp inmates, including orphaned children."[16] When such inhumanity is protected under a nation's law, only disaster will result.

Overreaction to a perceived evil may bring about laws to stamp it out by a counterforce of immoral punishment. Saint Paul, in the Epistle to the Galatians, gave us the ultimate judgment on all evil when he wrote that we ought not to "delude [y]ourselves into thinking God can be cheated: where a man sows, there he reaps."[17]

The law has issued a caveat to bioscientists on another subject. Physicians especially may be accused of conflict of interest when investing in areas dealing with medicine. The Ethics in Patient Referrals Act of 1989 is a legal bill that restricts physician ownership of health care facilities. A spokesperson for the American Medical Association has expressed an opinion that the Ethics in Patient Referrals Act is superfluous. "The restrictions in reimbursements, the expense in providing health care, and the number of physician-owned entities and joint ventures have heightened the visibility of something that always existed. The AMA's own ethical guidelines, which maintain that physicians should disclose any conflict of interest to the patient, are sufficient in restricting activity or egregious abuse. The acid test is utilization review, not prohibition."[18]

The purpose of law is to do good. Natural human impulses, when uninfluenced by evil, are to lead to morally ethical conclusions. Without detractions law and ethics seek the same end, which is satisfactory performance that sustains good and shuns evil. Legal medicine and philosophical ethics "cleave to that which is good."[19]

SCIENTIFIC RESEARCH, CLINICAL INVESTIGATION, AND INNOVATIVE THERAPY

By virtue of their accomplishments in their chosen discipline, bioscientists are deemed to be persons of exceptional intelligence. Under the guidance of the intellect, such individuals are possessors of an educated conscience that differentiates between what is naturally good and that which deviates from goodness. Upon these unbiased, learned disciplinarians of mental integrity the burden is placed to be the champions of proper ethical conduct in their personal behavior and professional deportment.

Medical ethics has become sensitive and responsive to social, economic, and technological changes. Novel legal actions based on new technological accomplishments have collided with bioethicists. In many instances the law has the final word. Legal decisions are sometimes in disagreement with ethical thoughts, allowing technology to overshadow medical tradition and time-honored custom.

After World War II the Nuremberg trials brought into public view the horror of human experimentation and clinical investigation on unfortunate victims of war. Ever since these trials, debate over moral and ethical controversy has continued. Medical researchers and other scientists have been made aware of the legal, ethical, and moral dangers of illegal human experimentation.

Reaction to the Nuremberg revelations and involuntary human guinea pigs caused reactions in the formation of codes for medical conduct. Among these were the Declaration of Helsinki Codes and Guidelines and the World Medical Association International Code of Medical Ethics. Passage of time has brought changes to these codes. However, they served a valuable purpose. In some way these codes forced scientists to take a second look at what they were doing and calmed down some researchers who were on the verge of being carried away by enthusiasm for a specific research project.

In 1973, a statement was made that many human experiments were outside the confines of bioethics and were prompted by the desire to further the interest of science rather than to bring a benefit to a patient.[20] Presently, no scientist has the power to sanction that which is morally wrong.

It is a false premise to believe that whatever works must be good. There must always be an ethical reality for a physical practicality. Three central elements apply to the positive force that leads to good scientific results: moral truth, positive value judgments, and upright performance. All aim for the common good. Any biological discipline worthy to treat human society must be founded on strong moral truths compatible with the fundamental nature of honesty.

Bioscientists engaged actively in their professional endeavors do not need any ethical anagnorisis.[21] Neither should they employ circumlocution nor boasts to defend untenable ethical misconduct. No words can change that which is evil into goodness.

Unless scientific conduct is of the highest caliber, conscience becomes crenated, leading to the evanescence of ethics. Such unsavory umbra breeds diminished discretion. Then human performance becomes self-serving and protective of self-glory that faults opposition to a healthy mindset. A self-proclaimed ethical standard is formulated and becomes an individualized personal guidon under which a new order of rules reigns and altruism vanishes. Judgment based on truth fails to be the ultimate *imprimatur*. It is the beginning of the end of bioethical good conduct because "the least deviation from the truth is multiplied later a thousandfold."[22]

Unprecedented progress in the biomedical sciences has excited researchers into wanting to know what more can be done in the research laboratory and through clinical investigations. Ironically this progressiveness is attacked and questioned as bioethical impediments are discerned. Adequate ethical self-discipline is often lacking as some scientists lose sight of the evil inherent to what they are doing.

A sampling of this type of bizarre behavior was presented as an editorial in a highly respected scientific journal. "Is there no end to the revisionist impulses of the age? Animals/insects found frozen for thousands of years [may be] revitalized by cloning DNA from the insects [by finding] a DNA strand long enough to include a gene. Insert the gene into a fruit fly and resuscitate proteins of long-extinct species. Now, if the resuscitated was to come from the blood cells of the dinosaur that unwittingly had been the source of the mosquito's last meal? What would happen?"[23] *Mirabile dictu.*

In the specialty of obstetrics many bioethical questions arise that elicit different answers that beget confusion. One such question centers about amniocentesis. In itself

amniocentesis is a morally indifferent undertaking . . . . [I]t is of great value in managing the pregnancies of women who have become sensitized to the Rh positive cells. By injecting Rh negative women with Rhogam, highly concentrated Rh antibodies, at any time they are at risk for exposure to Rh positive cells, they can be prevented from becoming sensitized themselves. Amniocentesis has other uses that are of significant benefit to the preborn child. The most frequent indication for this helpful use of the technique occurs during the last three months of pregnancy when the mother is experiencing medical problems which are a threat to herself and the baby. For

example when severe hypertension is present, the obstetrician may elect to deliver the infant several weeks before the due date to be certain the baby can survive outside the womb. To ensure that the baby can survive outside the womb, the doctor will order an amniocentesis and have the fluid analyzed for evidence of lung maturity before accomplishing the delivery. Amniocentesis has been blackened and called by many degrading names. While studies were being performed on amniocentesis, simultaneously efforts were made in chromosome and gene research.[24]

Prenatal testing has value and objections to it are diminishing. With the success of amniocentesis came intrauterine transfusion, early delivery, and other treatments. The end in view is to assist the intrauterine child. Another prenatal test that has ethical implications is chorionic villus sampling [CVS]:

Morally, it has no redeeming features. The scientific advancement offered by CVS is that it is performed in the nine to eleven week window of pregnancy. The accuracy and safety of CVS is less than that of amniocentesis, and while the differences are not huge, they raise concerns. So what is the advance? The results of this test are available in the third month of pregnancy rather than the fifth.[25]

Psychiatric care has been criticized in some places. Ethical disregard for the patient has been aimed at psychiatrists. In regard to the homeless a moral responsibility seems to have been avoided. The homeless mentally ill have been living on streets for the past 20 years. This social disgrace commenced in the late 1960s when the large state mental hospitals were phased out. Better care was to be provided in small community-based facilities. Here the dispossessed patient was to be given shelter, supervision, rehabilitation, and required psychiatric treatment. However good intentioned, the community-based program is a failure. The law is no help in this matter because it forbids involuntary treatment unless the mentally ill are either dangerous or are unable to survive in freedom. Moral duty proposes that the homeless who are mentally ill require paternalistic intervention within the parameters of the law to give them human care.

Fundamental ethics supports the medicolegal overseeing of the domestic violence syndrome child and spousal abuse. Awareness of this epidemic has been made to all those involved in administering health care.[26] Friction has arisen among the three major systems involved: criminal justice, social service, and health care. The ethical responsibility to report such violence is intimidated by the fear of legal involvement and physical reprisal. The protection of confidentiality is needed for all those involved when records are subject to subpoena. Often what is ethically proper is foiled by fear.

Concerning innovative therapy, attention has been directed to the topic of ectopic pregnancies. There are advocates of implanting the fetus in tubal pregnancies into the uterine cavity. Because of the success with *in vitro* fertilization, an impetus has been given to the idea. This approach to save intact ectopic pregnancies when subjected to moral analysis is not ethically deficient. The surgical procedure assists in the physiological mission of allowing a newly generated life to grow in its normal anatomic habitat.

In the continuing saga on obstetrics the new reproduction era climaxes with the process of surrogate motherhood. Converse to artificial insemination, medicolegal and ethical barriers are not alien to it. Surrogate motherhood, frozen human embryos, and fetal tissue transplants were not envisioned in the pretechnology medical past. Human interference in the biologic function of reproduction borders on chaos until the law and bioethics start to agree with each other on what is permissible.

Surgeons specializing in artificial and transplanted organs are not free from legal and ethical hazards. The growing shortage of transplantable human organs has awakened a renewed interest in obtaining organs from non-heartbeating cadavers. This issue focuses on the ethical, psychosocial, public policy, and legal questions engendered by this probability. A method has been proposed to minimize the ischemia time associated with procuring organs from cadavers. Procurement would be anticipated from patients who die after choosing to forego life-sustaining therapy. Another series of complex ethical issues is sure to arise around this controversial method of securing human organs.

These will be added to the existing medicolegal and ethical unsolved issues now present, some of which are stained by scandal. A government effort to outlaw trade in human organs exposed commercialism in kidneys for cash at a private London hospital in 1989. This revelation prompted legislation by Parliament. "The legislation (makes) it a crime to pay or receive payment for a human organ, act as broker in such transactions, or solicit buyers or sellers. It . . . [permits] voluntary donors to be reimbursed for the costs of removing a kidney."[27] The law was prompted by reports that Turkish peasants were paid to donate kidneys at a private hospital. Donors were paid $3200 to $5600.

Therapeutic medicosurgical acts and invasive research procedures are moral acts because they express and determine the goodness or evil of the individual who performs them. Because these acts are deliberate choices, they give moral definition and identification to scientists who perform them. Thus character is formed by the decisions made.

Research initiatives, innovative technology, and progressive learning threaten to penetrate the barriers of space, time, and nature. Biotechnology, molecular engineering, and nuclear physics are so awesome as to their potential that the social impact of their future performance has not been realized.

The affatus[28] of intellectual restlessness at times has ignored the commitment of science to ethical restrictions that in past decades placed universal confidence in research scientists, clinical physicians, and all renderers of health care. It was a time when conscience monitored, influenced, and directed judgment. Accumulated, repeated deviations from morality can destroy the long, distinguished tradition of excellence in the biosciences. The ethical stability of past generations solidified scientists in their professional relationships and was the envy of every other profession. Bioscience is a discipline that gathers talent into an eclectic, ecumenical group of dedicated people whose principal concern is to serve humanity.

Now this group finds itself at a turning point in the history of science. The moment has arrived when an assessment is needed to determine where science is going. It must recapture that scholarly dignity and probity in activity that has been indigenous to noble professions. The contemporary panorama of biomedical research anticipates spectacular future accomplishments that will be startling. The magnitude of predictable discoveries may receive a plethora of praise, but treading carelessly on morality can tarnish easily the expected glamor. That which may bring ephemeral acclaim also may degrade to an everlasting lower rank.

Pervasive acceptance of self-reliance on decision making without common moral standards is not withering away. This trend away from morality and ethical restraints is due in part to the forceful influence of ongoing technological progress. The idea has surfaced "that whatever we can do we should do."[29] The worshippers at the shrine of technology do not accept restraints. "It's hard for the moralist to say this is not permitted. People get the idea that morality is simply an attempt to put restraints on progress. They want as much as they can get as quick as they can get it."[30]

Scientific research that seeks the ultimate truth is unable to deviate from the affirmations of moral truth. Even when a majority prevails in disagreement, pure truth will survive. Consensus of peers and the approbation of the general public can become a minority oppression that destroys an intended good. The Hippocratic oath is the template chrestomathy[31] for all those associated with medicine in particular and the biosciences in general.

Scientists can be easily caught in the web of self-importance. In the sweeping history of biotechnology, these persons may become enshrined but that is not the door into heaven. They may enjoy the captivating excitement of coupling science with technology by applying new knowledge to the sacramental value of birth, reproduction, and death, but all this munificence is deficient if it is not encased in truth and is bereft of all commercialism. No person worthy of the appellation of scientist manufactures himself or herself into a *golem*[32] that glorifies the self. There is more to being a scientist than engaging in experimentation, theorization, clinical observation, and treating patients. The social consequences of bioscientific innovation may be beyond the immediate present. Therefore, ethical monitoring is essential to prevent widespread havoc resulting from the fruits of bioscientific studies and performances. The monitors should be highly talented individuals endowed with a sense of moral responsibility and who possess the courage of unyielding honesty.

Research and clinical scientists serve themselves best if they are wary not to enter areas where even angels fear to tread. If they do, they may suffer the loss of ethical and spiritual graces that can lead to their destruction. Good ethical principles should not bend to the mutability of whims. The code of scientific chivalry does not condone wimpishness. The *lares* and *penates*[33] of a master scientist are relentless integrity and accurate skillful performance. May it never be said of bioscientists anywhere:

Indeed the idols I have loved so long
Have done my credit in this world much wrong:
Have drowned my glory in a shallow cup,
And sold my reputation for a song.[34]

RATIONING OF SCARCE MEDICAL RESOURCES

Currently, no prudent politician wishes to be seen as an advocate of *rationing*. As a society we may have become wary of the economic and emotional costs of medical technology, yet the great majority of us—like the medical profession itself—is committed to its fundamental place in patient care. We have nurtured a variety of quibblers and questioners, but few Luddites.[35] ". . . But our collective efforts still remain disproportionately thin in comparison with the centrality of the issues raised by the past century's growing 'reign of technology.'"[36] Among the great impediments to the attempt to establish cost containment in medical care is the use, and sometimes abuse, of medicosurgical technology.

Two fundamental approaches for restraining health care costs are competition and regulation. The race for patients has prompted many medical specialists to lower their fees to the level prescribed by insurance carriers, Medicaid, and Medicare. Regulations are disguised under peer review, utilization committees, ambulatory surgery, 1-day surgical procedures, etc. The overt regulators are the diagnosis related group (DRG) system promulgated under the Tax Equity and Fiscal Responsibility Act and fixed payments based primarily on diagnosis rather than on services performed.

State control of medical care as represented by the federal government is the aim of many politicians and other social groups of diverse compositions. Their purpose is to lower the high price paid for medical diagnosis, treatment, and in-hospital care. Cost containment has become a priority with cost effectiveness not given the consideration it deserves.

Rationing is an inevitable component of any medical plan that aims at the reduction of health costs. American citizens are not totally prepared psychologically to accept government regulations of health care. Placing limitations on many health benefits will be inevitable. The geriatric age group will be the first victims of rationing.

The director of the Hastings Center in New York makes some predictions regarding the elderly:

The time has come in the case of medicine and the care of the aging to develop a more purposeful agenda, one that asks just what it is we are after. The short-term successes of medicine continue to divert attention from the now-recognized cumulative social burdens of an aging society they are creating . . . . We can no longer afford to avert our eyes from what that signifies. . . . Though they would face a denial of life-extending medical care beyond a certain age, the old would not necessarily fear their aging any more than they do now, nor would the young—even knowing that life-extending equipment would be cut off at a certain age.[37]

This sentiment is not original; Marcus Tullius Cicero (106-43 B.C.), the Roman statesman, law-giver, and orator, intimates this concept in his writing *De Senectute*.

Although the fundamental principles have not changed, the environment in which physicians and surgeons practice outside the hospital ambiance has. Daily changes occur as a result of governmental directives, FDA warnings, new rules from insurance carriers, Medicare/Medicaid notices, etc. "Despite the projected effect of health maintenance organizations and other alternate delivery systems, health care costs will continue to escalate. . . . Finally the philanthropic support for the variety of patient-care, educational, and research programs that typify the unique organization of the American health-care system can be expected to decline."[38] These thoughts sustain the opinions that costs for rendering health care are out-of-hand and practically uncontrollable. Falling is the number of anonymous *pro bono popolo*[39] donors to medical causes. Private persons of wealth no longer give large sums of money to the legions of scientists who request assistance for research, clinical investigation, and establishment of free health clinics.

High patient expectations and advanced medical technology have outstripped the public's ability to pay for what they expect. This is the background of the reason why rationing of medical care is being considered seriously in the United States. The elementary basis for rationing is that there is insufficient money to pay for the demanded and needed medicosurgical services. Every aspect of this nation's medical system has been biased in favor of compassion. With the onset of rationing, compassion will yield to some socioeconomic assumption unknown at present.

Life that can be saved, ought to be saved. This ethical principle is general in nature, but its immediacy and pertinence bears most heavily upon the field of medicine.[40]

LIFE, DEATH, AND EUTHANASIA

Hippocrates, the founder of formalized medicine, believed it to be of the utmost importance that each and every physician preserve the name and honor of medicine by working conscientiously, even reverently, in accordance with the maxim he set down: "Medicine is the science of healing, not of harming."[41]

Life in all stages is a precious gift that should not be treated lightly. This includes the inception of life, which has not received its proper respect. The eminent expositor of English common law, Sir William Blackstone (1723-1780) summarized this thought in his famous *Commentaries:*

An infant *in ventre sa mere,* or in the mother's womb, is supposed in law to be born for many purposes. It is capable of having a legacy, or a surrender of a copyhold estate, made to it. It may have a guardian assigned to it; and it is enabled to have an estate limited to its use, and to take afterwards by such limitation, as if it were then actually born. And in this point the civil law agrees with ours.[42]

So under English common law,[43] according to Blackstone, "life begins in contemplation of law as soon as an infant is able to stir in the mother's womb."[44]

Plato taught that birth to death were the boundaries for mortal life prior to entering the realm of immortality. Interference with this natural existence has been altered by advocates of abortion, right-to-die, and euthanasia. When these protagonists for death propagandize, they fail to express the viewpoint that a person's right to human dignity is never more pertinent than when he or she is dying. Death is an immediate, final, irreversible event. Dying may be a prolonged process with much emotional upheaval that prompts some people to control it.

The law recognizes that a competent person may control his or her dying by hastening it. Shortening the dying time occurs when the person elects to refuse treatment and/or nourishment. Added to these methods is the current tendency to issue a "no code" order on in-hospital patients. It is a frequent request for patients to instruct physicians that no resuscitating measures be used on them.

In keeping with these thoughts, we must consider the intransigency of ordinary versus extraordinary medicosurgical treatment. Many headlines were written in the daily press on this subject, which continues to be divisive. Over the years no better answer has been given than that expressed by an expert in *pastoral medicine* as it was termed in those years. Bioethics is the descendant of that discipline, which received little notice and less publicity by comparative study in the 1950s. An utterance heard almost four decades ago is memorable and applicable today:

But normally one is held to use only ordinary means— according to circumstances of persons, places, times, and culture—that is to say, means that do not involve any grave burden for oneself or another. A more strict obligation would be too burdensome for most men and would render the attainment of the higher, more important good too difficult. Life, health, all temporal activities are in fact subordinated to spiritual ends. On the other hand, one is not forbidden to take more than the strictly necessary steps to preserve life and health, as long as he does not fail in some more serious duty.[45]

This dictum when applied may lessen the number of neomorts[46] and possibly eliminate them entirely in future years.

The sanctity of human life is not to be considered a sentiment of past generations. It is both sad and frightening to see the recognizable trends in society of the diminished appreciation of life. So in a strange way, compassion is extended to criminals facing death. Many persons in high places are opposed to the death penalty. Religious groups have sought a more humane, hopeful, and effective response against violence than the threat of execution. They support and urge the abolition of capital punishment. Serious discussions on the death penalty include the disproportionate infliction of legal death on minority and disadvantaged persons. Other arguments are the unproven effectiveness of the death penalty in deterring criminal behavior, and the absence of exemption legislation for either juveniles and/or those who are mentally retarded. Thus these advocates uphold the belief that "the punishment for murder in the first degree shall be life imprisonment without the possibility of parole or death."[47]

Added to the list of objections is the claim that execution, especially by lethal gas, violated the Eighth Amendment prohibition on cruel and unusual punishment. Opponents of the death penalty insist that executing criminals neither deters illegal behavior nor does it advance morality. Opposing views of persuasive argumentation maintain that certain crimes are so grievous an affront to humanity that the only adequate response is the death penalty.

Another thought advanced in support of the death penalty is that to deny capital punishment in principle negates and denies the fundamental equality of distributive justice for all human beings. Without capital punishment, a person may behave toward all others with impunity, because the perpetrator does not fear having to share the same fate as the deceased victim. Such circumstances accord to the criminal a more superior status than the victim. This untouchable privilege was reserved for ancient royalty. Today it is reserved for capital criminals.

With a prison population close to 1.3 million, including 2500 on death row, overcrowding has become the flint that can spark unrest. Depending on the location, the annual cost for housing one prisoner ranges from $35,000 to $60,000. "Adding to the problems in state prisons, . . . the administration has signaled a slowdown in the massive prison-building program."[48] A tallied opinion on the death penalty indicates that the majority of law-abiding citizens favors capital punishment. A Gallup poll showed that 78% of the American public supports the death penalty.[49]

Western civilization expressing itself through its legal system had considered active euthanasia a crime. The basis for this conviction was the Anglo-American common law that by inherited tradition recognized the indigenous value of human life as a sacred, unique, unalterable gift. Many persons believe that the regard for human life was pulverized with the legalization of abortion in 1973.

A new Dutch law allowing euthanasia under certain circumstances was approved with a narrow margin. Under this legislation euthanasia remains a crime; however, if physicians follow a checklist of 28 requisites they will not be prosecuted for assisting at a suicide.[50] The results of the Netherland's experiment have been associated with abuses. Official findings by government officials unfolded violations of the limits set by Dutch courts. Judicial demands are that all cases of euthanasia be reported to prosecutors, so that they can determine that it was voluntary. "Only about 200 cases are reported to the prosecutors annually. Yet the Dutch government has found that physicians [euthanized] well over 2,000 patients at their own request and helped another 400 commit suicide."[51]

In the Netherlands the definition of euthanasia only extends to acts, although the phrase "the deliberate action to terminate life" could include withdrawal or omission of treatment. This leads to consideration of the much criticized active/passive (act/omission) distinction in relation to euthanasia—the distinction between active euthanasia and passive euthanasia by either not providing or withdrawing treatment. The total incidence of euthanasia and physician-assisted suicide in the Netherlands (both voluntary and involuntary) is more than 6000 per year, or 4.7% of all deaths in that country.[52,53]

A consistent ethical conduct in life does not deal with moral concerns ephemerally. All uplifting ethical behavior operates on a systematized experience guided by conscience-formulated general principles. This should be noted especially when solutions are sought on social issues involving human life. Recognition must be given to a growing social tendency that when life becomes less valuable in one area, a diminishing attitude toward life is manifested in regard to other issues. The irreplaceable value of human life in all its stages must not be downgraded in an era of intellectual progressiveness in scientific technology.

Euthanasia is not a private matter that arises out of the false reason of right-to-privacy. It involves ethical standards fostered on the general public that is sustained by the law.[54] The Dutch legislation is branded as the most permissive euthanasia policy in the industrialized world. Many human beings take lightly the most precious gift they possess. Recognizing "the societal value that the life of every individual has worth in and of itself and is not to be devalued by reason of an individual's incapacity or perceived diminished quality of life," the State of Maryland passed a bill for advance directives on life-saving, and dying decisions.[55]

In 1991 a so-called "aid-in-dying" initiative was on the ballot of the State of Washington.[56] The opposition has stated, "Whether you sugarcoat the word euthanasia or not, it still spells killing at the tomb end of the womb-to-tomb cycle irreverence for life."[57] If passed, it would have made it legal for physicians to give lethal injections to terminally ill patients with less than six months to live.

In centuries past the annals of history disclose that an attempt to commit suicide was a crime. During these twilight years of the twentieth century adversarial debates continue on the morality, professional ethics, and legality of assisted suicide. Today there remains a risk of criminal liability for aiding and abetting a suicide.[58] This peril exists for physicians as well as family members, and household companions of a patient. Now there are enthusiasts who desire to technologize euthanasia. "[I]n the much publicized case of Dr. Jack Kevorkian assisting Mrs. Janet Adkin's death, why did [the pathologist] Dr. Kevorkian and Mrs. Adkin, resort to a suicide machine which was even given a special, trademarked name, the Thanatron?[59] One obvious reason is in order to try to avoid prosecution for murder by eliminating the possibility that Dr. Kevorkian could be held, in law, to have caused Mrs. Adkin's death. Through use of the machine, Mrs. Adkin could be regarded, in law, as causing her own death, in which case the situation was one of suicide—and if anything, assisting in suicide on the part of Dr. Kevorkian, was not at that time a crime in Michigan."[60] Since the Mrs.

Adkin event, legislation has been passed in Michigan making it a crime to assist a person to commit suicide.[61]

In 1993, Zimmerman noted that "Since ancient times, doctors bound by the Hippocratic Oath have pledged to cure patients. Dr. Kevorkian believes that doctors should have the right also to help those who are experiencing great physical or mental suffering to end their lives. So far, Dr. Kevorkian has assisted or been present at the suicides of 20 people since 1990."[62]

A euthanasia experience of historical note refers to King George V of England. It has been written that the British king's physician hastened what was assumed to be the king's imminent expiration so that the story might appear first "in the morning papers rather than the less appropriate evening journals." This quotation is from disclosed notes made by the royal physician. Lord Dawson wrote that he hurried the king's death on the night of January 20, 1936, by administering injections of morphine and cocaine. King George V, grandfather of Queen Elizabeth II, died approximately 40 minutes later, in time for the morning paper. Foremost among the morning tabloids was *The London Times,* which carried the dignified and appropriate headline "Death of the King. A Peaceful Ending at Midnight."[63] This is disturbing to those who see life's exodus as the final act in the physiologic drama of human nature's normalcy; and that it should not be accelerated pathologically.

Postscript

Sir William Osler (1849-1919), a satellite in the galaxy of medicine, said:

I have three personal ideals. One, to do the day's work well and not to bother about to-morrow. . . . The second ideal has been to act the Golden Rule, as far as in me lay, toward my professional brethren and toward the patients committed to my care. And the third has been to cultivate such a measure of equanimity as would enable me to bear success with humility, the affection of my friends without pride, and to be ready when the day of sorrow and grief came to meet it with the courage befitting a man.[65]

Faithfulness to honest values is a mark of distinction that is unreserved. It is an asset discerned in persons of distinct erudition and worn as a badge of courage to preserve what is good, right, and morally correct. Life is constant warfare. To win the many daily battles one must carry the cardinal virtues as pierceless armor against spiritual invectives. These insignia are not simple garnitures to be an ostentatious embellishment for display to attract notice and notoriety. Rather they are the lines of defense against evil in all its disguises.

The four cardinal virtues are the quadruple qualities of justice, prudence, fortitude, and temperance that emanate out of the fountainhead of truth. Hence, virtue is the quality of moral excellence, righteousness, and

responsibility. It is probity at its best, radiating sublime goodness that obliterates evil. Conformity to standard morality, mores, and modes of impeccable personal behavior are its beacon lights. Abstention from vice marks virtue's rectitude. Virtue is a means of controlling one's life and destiny guiding them in the right direction.

Medicine and law should adapt themselves to the highest possible standards of professional ethics that are expected in persons of intelligence. Such moral patterns will bring to both disciplines the respect they deserve. Learned associations, like the American College of Legal Medicine, have the grand opportunity to be in the forefront of leadership toward this ideal — which is easily said and more difficult to perform, but not beyond fulfillment. Morality and ethics will flourish in both professions when the splendor of truth is recognized, pursued, and adopted. Attached to this appreciation is the expression of thanksgiving for past accomplishments, perseverance for present bioscientific efforts, and trust in future scientists. By an ethical resurgence, morality will be rekindled that will substitute need for greed, commitment for compromise, and promise for platitudes.

END NOTES

1. *Theodicy* is a vindication of divine justice in the face of the existence of evil. From the French *Théodicée,* title of a literary work by Leibnitz written in 1710.
2. From *Moral Versus Intellectual Principles In Human Progress* from the *History of Civilization in England* by English writer Henry Thomas Buckle (1821-1862). Found in *A Library of the World's Best Literature,* published in 1897 by International Society, New York, Vol. 6, p. 2677.
3. *Manichean* is a generic word for any dualistic philosophy considered to be heresy by certain religions.
4. *Teleologism* is the dictum of teleology, which is the philosophical study of manifestations of design or purpose in natural processes or occurrences, under the belief that natural processes are not determined by mechanism but rather by their utility in an overall natural design. Proportionalism is defined as the moral theological doctrine which holds that the moral quality of an action is determined by whether the evils brought about by a proposed action are proportionate to the goods the action effects. Consequentialism holds that the action which brings about the best effects is morally preferable, without referring to the goodness or evil of the act itself.
5. Wendy Carlton, *In Our Professional Opinion: The Primacy of Clinical Judgment Over Moral Choice* (University of Notre Dame Press, Indiana 1990). Dr. Carlton is a member of the sociology faculty.
6. David Stipp, *Schools Rein in Faculty Stakes in Biomedicine,* Wall Street J., Mar. 12, 1990, at B1, B6.
7. Book of Wisdom, ch. 8, verses 11 to 16.
8. *Autarky* is a policy of self-sufficiency. In economics it means nonreliance on outside assistance such as imports or economic aid. Applied to human conduct it signifies self-sufficiency in use of conscience whereby it is the ultimate, supreme tribunal for judging right from wrong.
9. 6 *The Surgical Team* 8-11 (Feb. 1977).
10. The four issues are based on an editorial by P. J. Palumbo, M.D.,

Editorial, Transition: A New Editor, in 62 *Mayo Clinic Proceedings* 230 (Mar. 1987).

11. Daniel Greenberg, *Publish or Perish — or Fake It,* U.S. News & World Report, June 8, 1987, at 72, 73.

12. J. P. Dolan, *Paracelsus,* 71 *J. So. Carolina Medical Soc.* 175 (1975); *also* M. G. McGuinn, *The Writings of Paracelsus.* In Reynolds Historical Library, Birmingham, UAB, (1993) and exhibit on Paracelsus in Waring Library, Medical University of South Carolina.

13. Cal Thomas, *Lying in the Rights Vineyard,* Washington Times, June 2, 1988, at F3.

14. Stephen Labaton, *Ideas and Trends. Old Laws Have a Way of Learning New Tricks,* N.Y. Times, December 19, 1993, at 14E.

15. Jake Novak, *The German Abortion Rights Decision: Formally Restrictive, Practically Much Like the U.S.,* 5 Woodrow Wilson Center Report 3, 4 (Sep. 1993). The author quotes German Justice Benda who stated: The constitutional restriction of abortion reflects Prussian common law instituted in the eighteenth century by Frederick the Great.

16. Michael H. Kater, *Doctors under Hitler,* 124 (University of North Carolina Press, Chapel Hill 1989).

17. Galatians, ch. 6, verse 7.

18. James Todd, M.D., senior deputy executive vice president of the American Medical Association.

19. Romans 12:9.

20. H. K. Beecher, *Ethics and Clinical Research,* 52 New Eng. J. Med. at 12 (June 8, 1973). Dr. Beecher achieved acclaim as a professor of anesthesiology at Harvard Medical School. He was a pioneer in bioethics serving the Council on Drugs of the American Medical Association. Professor Beecher published *Experimentation in Man* as a report to the AMA.

21. *Anagnorisis* is a term used by Aristotle (384-322 B.C.) in the *Poetics* to indicate the moment of recognition in which a character moves from ignorance to knowledge.

22. Aristotle in *De Coelo,* 1.5. 271b, 9-10.

23. *The Sciences* (New York Academy of Sciences Mar./Apr. 1993).

24. William F. Colliton, Jr., M.D., Medical Affairs Director for American Life League, Inc., Stafford, Virginia 22554 in *All About Issues* at 3,4, March/April 1992/35.

25. The Doctor Has Advised You, *supra* note 20.

26. The State of New York Dept. of Health as modified the Health Code 10NYCRR405.34. Now it mandates that physicians, social workers, and nurses include this type of teaching in their in-service hospital training programs.

27. Associated Press report from London, Wall Street J., July 10, 1989, at B6A.

28. *Affatus* is defined as creative impulse.

29. Public lecture at Fordham University, New York, by Rev. Avery Dulles, S. J., reported by George W. Cornell, Associated Press, in Washington Post, Oct. 24, 1992, at B7 under title "Theologian Fears for the Future of Democracy."

30. *Id.*

31. From the Greek word "khrēstomatheia" meaning *useful learning.* In English chrestomathy is the selection of literary passages used in studying literature, i.e., samples as outstanding examples.

32. *Golem* in Jewish folklore is an artificially created human being endowed with life by supernatural means.

33. *Lares* and *penates* are esteemed household possessions from two kinds of household Roman gods. Lar was a tutelary deity or spirit of an ancient Roman household. Penates were the Roman gods of the household, the guardians and protectors of the home and the state whose cult was closely connected to and identified with the lares. It is derived from the Latin word *penus* meaning the interior of a house.

34. From the *Rubaiyat,* stanza 93, by Omar Khayyám.

35. Luddites were a group of British workmen who, between 1811 and 1816, rioted and destroyed textile machinery in the belief that it would diminish employment. Probable origin is from Ned Lud[d], a late eighteenth century worker who destroyed stocking frames in England.

36. Charles E. Rosenberg, *From the President. Technology and Modern Medicine,* Newsletter of the American Association for the History of Medicine, July 1993, No. 42, at 1.

37. Daniel Callahan, *Setting Limits* (Simon and Schuster, New York 1987).

38. Address given at the 13th commencement exercise of the Mayo Medical School, Rochester, Minnesota, May 21, 1988, by Virginia V. Weldon, M.D., Deputy Vice-Chancellor for Medical Affairs, Washington University, School of Medicine, St. Louis, Missouri, under the title *An All-Consuming Journey.*

39. Latin translation is *for the good of the people.*

40. Oliver A. Cvitanic, *Inquiry into the Moral Prerogatives of the Potential Human Life,* 49 The Pharos 13, 17 (Spring 1986).

41. Edmund D. Pellegrino and Alice A. Pellegrino, *Humanism and Ethics in Roman Medicine: Translation and Commentary on a Text of Scribonius Largus.* Presented in abbreviated form before the Washington Society for the History of Medicine, April 30, 1983, and the American Osler Society, Minneapolis, May 3, 1983. Published in 7 Literature and Medicine 22-38 (Johns Hopkins University Press, Baltimore 1988).

42. Blackstone, *Commentaries on the Laws of England,* Book I, ch. 1, at 130.

43. Common law is decisional law, i.e., the body of legal precedents constituted by reported cases decided by courts, wherein no statute is involved. American common law is derived in large measure from English common law, as it was prior to the Revolution. Taken from a paper delivered September 1, 1966, at the annual convention of the International Academy of Law and Science, at the University of Madrid, Spain.

44. Blackstone, *supra* note 42, at 129.

45. Spoken to an audience of international physicians (anesthesiologists) by Pope Pius XII (Pontiff from 1939-1958) on November 24, 1957, during meetings in Rome of the International Catholic Physicians Guilds from the Americas and Europe.

46. *Neomorts* is the name given to patients who are brain-dead, referred to in nonscientific writing as "living" dead.

47. Pub. L. 102-382, District of Columbia, approved Oct. 5, 1992, 102nd U.S. Congress.

48. *The Trouble in America's Prisons,* U.S. News and World Report, April 26, 1993, at 14.

49. R. T. Edwards, *A Look at the Death Penalty from Behind the Prison Walls,* 43 The Catholic Standard No. 42, 3 (Oct. 22, 1992).

50. The defense available to Dutch physicians to justify euthanasia is one of necessity *(overmacht)* contained in Article 40 of the Dutch Penal Code.

51. Richard Doerflinger, *Dutch Government Study Shows the Danger of Legalized Euthanasia,* 41 The Catholic Standard 7, 15 (Oct. 24, 1991).

52. A. M. Capron, *Euthanasia in the Netherlands: American Observations,* 22 Hastings Center Report 30, 31 (1992).

53. Margaret A. Somerville, *The Song of Death: The Lyrics of Euthanasia,* 9 J. Contemporary Health Law Policy 1-76 (School of Law, The Catholic University of America, Washington, D.C. 1993).

54. J. Keown, *On Regulating Death,* 22 Hastings Center Report 40 (1992).

55. The Health Care Decision Act took effect in the State of Maryland on October 1, 1993.

56. Washington State Initiative 119, November 1991.

57. Editorial, *Cause for Concern,* 42 The Catholic Standard No. 46, 11 (Nov. 14, 1991).

58. Harold L. Hirsh, *Death and Dying,* Trauma 1:24 (Matthew Bender, Conklin, N.Y. 1993).

59. A. Hister, *Kevorkian Offers Cold Comfort on Euthanasia Debate,* Globe and Mail (Toronto), Sept. 14, 1991, at C8. *Thanatron* is derived from *Thanatos,* which is death as a personification or as a philosophical notion. When used without a capital T it is an alleged instinct to self-destruction, i.e., the death wish. A meditation on death is termed *thanatopsis.* It arises from *thanatos* meaning death in Greek.

60. Somerville, *supra* note 53, under subtitle *Why Do We Technologize Euthanasia?,* at 33, 34.

61. Act 84, Public Acts of 1992, 1992 Michigan ALS84; 1992 Mi. P.A.84; 1992 Mi. HB5501.

62. Mark Zimmermann, *Dr. Death Isn't Fascinating,* The Catholic Standard 11 (Dec. 16, 1993).

63. Editorial, *A Death in Time,* Washington Post, Nov. 30, 1986, at C6. In the same editorial is stated that Lord Dawson's biographer, Francis Watson, who examined the notes after the doctor's death omitted any mention of them from his book published in 1950. The biographer disclosed the information years later in an article written for the British publication called *History Today.* Mr. Watson remarked: "I am certain Lord Dawson was convinced he was acting correctly and I have no doubt he had no qualms about it at all." A different view was taken by Kenneath Rose, biographer of George V, who said Lord Dawson's act was "nothing short of murder in the eyes of the law."

64. Sir William Osler, *Aequanimitas* 445 (P. Blakiston's Son & Co., Philadelphia 1932).

CHAPTER 27

Fetal interests

FREDERICK ADOLF PAOLA, M.D., J.D., F.C.L.M.

ETHICAL CONSIDERATIONS
THE LAW AND FETAL INTERESTS

When does the American legal system grant rights to the unborn human? Whose interest predominates when conflicts arise between the rights of the mother and those of her fetus? Who decides what should be done with the tissue removed during an abortion or miscarriage? Because the unborn are unable to assert their own interests, who should serve as their representative? These issues are among those undergoing critical analysis in light of recent scientific advances, judicial decisions, and legislative enactments.

Although in legal contexts the term *fetus* has been used to refer to the conceptus throughout all stages of development, *fetus* more properly refers to "the product of conception from the end of the eighth week to the moment of birth."[1] Prior to this (that is, from the moment of conception until approximately the end of the eighth week) the developing human is more properly referred to as an *embryo*. In this chapter, we use the terms *fetus* and *conceptus* interchangeably.

ETHICAL CONSIDERATIONS
The moral standing of the unborn

Underlying the legal controversy over fetal interests is an essentially ethical question: "Does the human fetus have moral standing?" "To attribute moral standing to a creature . . . is to say that it deserves or merits or qualifies for the protections of morality."[2]

One approach has been to equate moral standing with "personhood."[3] Under this approach, a fetus has moral standing and thus a right to life and freedom from infliction of bodily harm, if he or she is a person; thus, it becomes morally relevant to ask, "When does the embryo/fetus achieve personhood?" Three responses to this question have been suggested. One submits that the embryo is a person from the moment of conception. A second claims that personhood is not achieved until the moment of birth, when "independent life and human relationships are possible. [A] third . . . adopts the middle ground . . . recogniz[ing] the status of the embryo as linked to certain stages of biological development."[4] Under this third view, the fetus becomes a person somewhere between conception and birth—perhaps when he or she becomes recognizably human, or perhaps when heart or brain activity appear, or perhaps when he or she becomes viable (capable of surviving outside the womb).

A second approach recognizes that deciding on *when* the developing human achieves personhood does not answer the ethical question, because nonpersons may still have moral standing. Stated otherwise, personhood is a *sufficient* but not necessarily a *necessary* condition for having moral rights:

Personhood is important as an inclusion criterion for moral equality: any theory which denies equal moral status to certain persons must be rejected. But personhood seems somewhat less plausible as an exclusion criterion, since it appears to exclude infants and mentally handicapped individuals who may lack the mental and social capacities typical of persons.[5]

Under this approach, the moral standing of the fetus

might be grounded in respect for the intrinsic value or inherent dignity of life in general or human life in particular (since, "while there may be an ongoing discussion as to [the] personhood [of the embryo/fetus], no one denies that the human embryo constitutes human life"[6]); or the moral standing of the fetus might be grounded, beginning in the second trimester, in respect for sentient beings.[7]

Alternatively, it might be argued that, even assuming the fetus is not yet a person, he or she is a *potential* person, and that this potential to become a person endows the fetus with the same basic moral rights enjoyed by persons.

Meta-ethics and fetal interests. Just what are we doing when we make a judgment that the fetus has moral standing; that, for example, abortion is immoral?

Moral skeptics espouse the ethical theories that assert "there are no right answers to moral questions [such as abortion] — only *accepted* answers," and include *moral nihilists* and *irrealists. Nihilists* believe that there are no such things as moral facts and "that without moral facts moral practice is all a sham."[8] *Irrealists* agree that there are no such things as moral facts, but maintain that such facts are not necessary for moral practice. There are several different versions of *irrealism,* including *subjectivism* (which asserts that, in making a moral judgment about abortion, people are doing nothing more than expressing their personal feelings on the subject — i.e., "I don't like abortion") and *relativism* (which asserts that moral truth exists only in relation to one's particular society or culture).

In contrast to moral skepticism is the view epitomized by the idea of *natural law,* "the view that there is an unchanging normative order that is a part of the natural world . . . , that there is a natural foundation to moral beliefs."[9]

Clearly, our understanding of what it means to make a moral judgment will affect the way we answer the question "How ought I act toward those whose judgment on the moral standing of the fetus is different from my own?" Corresponding to the meta-ethical theories just discussed are normative theories addressing this question.

Consider the position of those who believe that abortion is morally wrong because it is the taking of life that has moral status. Within this group some seem undisturbed by the fact that there is deep disagreement over the moral status of the fetus. They wish to prohibit abortion. But others in this group, while holding that abortion is wrong, [maintain] that reasonable persons could disagree with them and that human reason seems unable to resolve the question. For this reason, they oppose legal prohibitions of abortion. The former believe that the latter do not take the value of human life seriously, while the latter believe that the former fail to recognize the depth

and seriousness of the disagreement between reasonable persons.[10]

Thus, *normative relativists* are likely to believe that it is wrong to judge those who hold different values, or to try to make them conform to one's values, because their values are as valid as one's own. At the other end of the spectrum, *universalists* or *absolutists,* taking the position that both sides of the abortion debate cannot be right and that there is only one moral truth with regard to the moral standing of the unborn, are likely to believe that whatever intrinsic value an ethic of nonjudgmental tolerance may have is outweighed by the gravity of the fetal interests at stake.

THE LAW AND FETAL INTERESTS
Constitutional rights of the unborn

In *Roe v. Wade,*[11] the U.S. Supreme Court determined that the unborn were not "persons" as far as the U.S. Constitution was concerned. Consequently, the unborn were denied constitutional protection from deprivation of life, liberty, or property. The *Roe* Court also found a constitutionally fundamental "right of privacy broad enough to encompass a woman's decision whether or not to terminate her pregnancy." Such a right could be abridged only where such abridgement was needed in order to achieve a compelling state interest. Whereas *Roe* recognized the state's interest in the "potential" human life represented by the fetus, *Roe* did not recognize any rights of the unborn themselves; and *Roe* asserted that the state's interest in protecting potential human life becomes compelling only at the point of fetal viability. The effect of *Roe* was to strike down state laws criminalizing abortion.

In the 1992 decision dealing with the abortion issue, *Planned Parenthood v. Casey,*[12] the Supreme Court reaffirmed a woman's constitutional right to abort a fetus before viability without "undue"[13] state interference, as well as the state's right to prohibit abortion after viability except to preserve the life or health of the woman.

[T]he *Casey* Court held that the state had a legitimate interest in protecting fetal life from the onset of pregnancy. Accordingly, it was legitimate for government to act [throughout pregnancy] to undermine abortion, so long as it did not . . . "unduly burden" the woman's ability to choose it. This position contrasted sharply with *Roe v. Wade's* holding that only during the third trimester could government enact regulations designed to preserve the life of the fetus.[14]

Fetal rights under tort law

Although early common law recognized fetal rights under criminal law and property law, it did not recognize fetal rights under tort law.

The first American case to address an individual's

right to bring an action for harm sustained while *in utero* was *Dietrich v. Inhabitants of Northampton.*[15] In this case, a woman who was five months pregnant slipped and fell on the defendant's negligently maintained road. She prematurely delivered a baby that lived only about 15 minutes. The legal issue was whether the child could maintain a cause of action in negligence. The Massachusetts Supreme Judicial Court, in an opinion by Justice Holmes, answered in the negative, reasoning that the "unborn child did not have standing to sue because it was part of its mother, and not a separate being, at the time of the injury."

In *Allaire v. St. Luke's Hospital,*[16] a pregnant patient was severely injured by a negligently operated hospital elevator. The baby was born severely and permanently disabled several days later. The Illinois Supreme Court, citing *Dietrich,* denied a cause of action.

In a vigorous dissent, however, Justice Boggs distinguished *Dietrich* by narrowly interpreting its holding as applicable only to the nonviable fetus. Boggs argued that the fetus in *Allaire,* being viable, had an existence separate from that of its mother; he concluded that the hospital, therefore, owed it a duty of due care.

Finally, in *Bonbrest v. Kotz,*[17] the Federal District Court for the District of Columbia held that a child sustaining an injury while a viable fetus could maintain a cause of action against a third party. The court, as had Justice Boggs, distinguished *Dietrich* on the ground that, in *Bonbrest,* the infant plaintiff was viable at the time of the injury.

The *Bonbrest* decision opened the floodgates to what is now the majority rule favoring recovery for prenatal injuries. Every jurisdiction now permits recovery for prenatal injuries where the child is born alive. Furthermore, even the conditions considered key for recovery in *Bonbrest*—that the fetus be viable at the time of injury and that the plaintiff survive delivery—have been removed in some jurisdictions. Thus, the majority of state courts have now rejected the viability requirement of *Bonbrest* and now allow recovery for prenatal injuries inflicted at any point during gestation.[18]

Preconception tort liability. The rejection of the viability requirement has made it possible for courts to recognize tort liability not only before viability, but even before conception. Preconception tort liability refers to "those situations in which the defendant's tortious actions prior to the plaintiff's conception result in harm to the infant plaintiff."[19]

In *Jorgensen v. Meade Johnson Laboratories,*[20] the U.S. Court of Appeals for the 10th Circuit held that plaintiff children, alleging that their mother's preconception use of defendant Johnson's oral contraceptives had caused their Down's syndrome, could maintain a cause of action for preconception tort liability. Likewise, the Supreme Court of Illinois, which had denied recovery to an infant plaintiff on the basis of no separate legal existence at the time of injury in *Allaire* (overruled in 1953 by *Amann v. Faidy*), has now broadened its range of potential plaintiffs to include those not even conceived yet at the time of the injury. In *Renslow v. Mennonite Hosp.,*[21] the court found "a right to be born free from prenatal injuries foreseeably caused by a breach of duty to the child's mother." Emma Renslow was 13 years old and Rh negative when she negligently received transfusions of Rh positive blood. Her daughter was born nearly eight and one-half years later and required exchange transfusions because of her mother's sensitization. Permanent damages were alleged to have occurred due to blood incompatibility and resulting hemolysis. In extending a tortfeasor's duty to those who have not yet been conceived, the court termed it "illogical to bar relief for an act done prior to conception where the defendant would be liable for this same conduct had the child, unbeknownst to him, been conceived prior to his act."

In contrast, the New York Court of Appeals, in *Albala v. City of New York,*[22] concluded that New York law did not recognize a cause of action for preconception negligence. Likewise, the Appellate Division of the Supreme Court of New York has held that New York does not recognize a preconception strict liability cause of action.[23]

A relatively new subset of preconception tort claims is illustrated by the so-called third-generation DES lawsuits. In *Enright v. Eli Lilly & Co.,*[24] a plaintiff injured as a result of premature birth alleged that her grandmother's ingestion of DES while pregnant with her (plaintiff's) mother damaged her mother's reproductive system and in turn caused plaintiff's prematurity. The New York Court of Appeals, citing *Albala,* held that the plaintiff had no cause of action. Likewise, in *Sorrels v. Eli Lilly & Co.,*[25] a woman and her infant daughter alleged that use of DES by the infant's grandmother had caused the infant's prematurity and consequent severe hearing loss. The U.S. District Court for the District of Columbia, saying that Maryland law did not recognize a preconception duty, dismissed the plaintiff's preconception claims.

Wrongful death of fetuses. Historically under the common law, liability was imposed on tortfeasors whose victims survived, but tortfeasors who killed their victims escaped liability, since the cause of action "died" with the victim. Wrongful death statutes were enacted as a legislative response to this perceived loophole in the common law, and allowed survivors to seek compensation for the death of the victim. Where an injured fetus is born alive and dies subsequently, every state now permits a wrongful death action to be brought on his or her behalf.[26]

When the victim is stillborn, courts have disagreed over whether a fetus is a "person" within the meaning of state wrongful death statutes. *Verkennes v. Corniea*[27] was the first opinion to allow a wrongful death action on behalf of a stillborn child. Recovery was still conditional on fetal viability at the time of the injury. As of 1992, approximately 36 jurisdictions allowed recovery for the wrongful death of a fetus. The majority of these jurisdictions, like *Verkennes,* have held that only a viable fetus is protected under wrongful death statutes; only three (Georgia, Louisiana, and Rhode Island) have indicated that recovery is not conditional on fetal viability. Twelve other jurisdictions still deny recovery to the stillborn infant, concluding that even the viable fetus is not a "person" within the meaning of the applicable wrongful death statute.[28]

Parental tort liability. Although the courts have been willing to compensate the unborn for injuries caused by negligent acts of tortfeasors, especially professionals responsible for the care of the mother and fetus, few have imposed liability on those individuals whose actions most commonly are hazardous to the unborn. Pregnant women who, for example, smoke, use cocaine, or abuse alcohol impair the development of their infants. Most who do so are aware of the potential for harm to their babies.

The reluctance to compensate children injured prenatally by their mother's conduct stems largely from a desire to avoid intruding on the privacy interest of the pregnant woman, but also reflects the parental immunity doctrine. Intrafamily tort immunity was intended to promote the societal goal of family harm and unity.

In 1980 in *Grodin v. Grodin,*[29] the Michigan Court of Appeals overruled the doctrine of parental immunity and expanded fetal rights to allow a cause of action for damages against a child's mother for the mother's negligence during pregnancy. In holding that "the litigating child's mother would bear the same liability for injurious, negligent [prenatal] conduct as would a third person," the court in essence "pitted the legal rights of the pregnant woman and the fetus against each other, rather than conceptualizing them as one legal entity."[30]

Fetal rights and criminal law

Early Anglo-American law recognized fetal rights under criminal law. As early as 1628, Lord Coke proposed that an individual should be criminally liable for injuring a child *in utero* if that child were later born alive. "Thus, if a pregnant woman took a harmful potion or if a man beat a pregnant woman, the wrongdoer would be charged with murder if the woman later delivered a baby who subsequently died of the resulting injury."[31]

The criminal law continues to recognize the fetus as a person with regard to the criminal acts of third parties.

Eighteen states now have "feticide" statutes, and another two states recognize a common law crime of "feticide," thus treating the killing of a pregnant woman as two counts of homicide.[32] In 1984, in *Gloria C. v. William C.,*[33] a New York family court recognized a fetus as a person for the purpose of issuing a protective order. In that case, a pregnant woman sought a protective order to protect her fetus from her allegedly abusive husband.

Criminal prosecution of pregnant women. With regard to recognition of the fetus as a person in terms of the criminal acts of mothers, the Center for Reproductive Law and Policy has reported that, as of 1992, approximately 167 women in 24 different states had been charged with crimes against their fetuses.

Because no state has a statute specifically criminalizing drug abuse by the pregnant woman, prosecutors have unsuccessfully attempted to prosecute maternal substance abuse under the guise of other laws, such as those dealing with child abuse, child support, manslaughter laws, or the delivery of a controlled substance.

Pamela Rae Stewart-Monson, for example, had placenta previa. She was advised by her physician to stay off of her feet, to abstain from sexual intercourse, and to seek medical attention if she bled vaginally. She delivered a brain-damaged baby that died within six weeks. Mrs. Stewart-Monson was arrested and charged under Section 270 of the California Penal Code, an 1872 child support statute that prohibited the intentional omission of "necessary . . . medical attendance [to children]." Since its enactment, the statute had been extended, in 1925, to cover fathers who failed to support "a child conceived but not yet born," and in 1974 to cover mothers.

California alleged that Mrs. Stewart-Monson failed to maintain bedrest, engaged in sexual intercourse, used amphetamines on the day of delivery, and failed to seek medical attention promptly once vaginal bleeding began. The indictment was dismissed on a pretrial motion on the grounds that the child support statute did not encompass the conduct alleged.[34]

Likewise, Elizabeth Levey was eight and one-half months pregnant when she crashed her car, allegedly driving while intoxicated. On the day after the accident, she delivered a stillborn baby. The district attorney charged Mrs. Levey with vehicular homicide, relying on the Massachusetts rule that a fetus is a person under the homicide law.[35] The charges were later dropped.[36]

Diane Pfannenstiel was charged under a Wyoming statute that prohibits intentionally or recklessly injuring a child.[37] Pfannenstiel was 4 months pregnant when arrested. The case, therefore, differed from the cases above in that the mother was charged with child abuse before the child was even born. The court dismissed the charges against Ms. Pfannenstiel because the district attorney could not prove that the fetus, still *in utero* and thus unavailable for examination, had been injured.

In 1989 in Florida, Jennifer Johnson was charged with and convicted of delivering (postnatally through the umbilical cord) a controlled substance (cocaine) to a minor (her newborn infant), notwithstanding defense counsel's argument that the drafters of the applicable Florida delivery law did not intend for that law to apply to the unborn.[38] The conviction was upheld by Florida's 5th District Court of Appeals,[39] but was reversed unanimously by the Florida Supreme Court. The court found that there was insufficient evidence to support the trial court's finding of fact that cocaine had been delivered postnatally to the neonate through the umbilical cord, and that the state legislature had not intended to treat drug-dependent mothers as criminals.

Forced medical intervention on behalf of the unborn

Judicial intervention and the viable fetus. It has been reported that since 1981 health care providers have, on more than 21 occasions, asked courts to order unwilling women to submit to cesarean sections, and that 86% of these requests have been granted.[40] The following cases are illustrative.

In *Raleigh Fitkin-Paul Morgan Memorial Hosp. v. Anderson,*[41] a court ordered a Jehovah's Witness woman, eight months pregnant and hemorrhaging, to submit to a blood transfusion to save her life and the life of her fetus. Likewise, in *Jefferson v. Griffin Spaulding County Hospital,*[42] a court ordered a full-term woman with placenta previa to submit to a cesarean section after her physicians informed her of a 99% chance that her baby would not survive a vaginal delivery.

In contrast, in *In re A.C.,*[43] A.C. was in her twenty-sixth week of gestation and dying of cancer. The District of Columbia District Court ordered a cesarean section against the wishes of A.C. and her husband, and the surgery was performed. The baby girl lived less than three hours and A.C. died within two days.

The District of Columbia Court of Appeals vacated the district court's order, and held that "in virtually all cases [where maternal and fetal health interests conflict] the question of what is to be done is to be decided by . . . the pregnant woman . . . on behalf of herself and the fetus,"[44] regardless of the age of (i.e., viability) the fetus.

Just recently, a 22-year-old Illinois woman was told by a maternal-fetal medicine specialist that her 32-week-old fetus was not receiving enough oxygen. The physician advised the woman to undergo either induction of labor or a cesarean section. The woman, a Pentecostal Christian, refused for religious reasons, insisting that the child be born naturally and asserting that God would protect her unborn child. The hospital informed Cook County officials, who sought to have a court order the

pregnant woman to undergo the cesarean.[45] An Illinois Appellate Court confirmed a lower court ruling that the state could not force the woman to undergo a cesarean. The case was appealed to the Illinois Supreme Court, which on December 16, 1993, refused to enter the dispute. On December 18, 1993, the U.S. Supreme Court declined the request of the fetus's representative (the Cook County public guardian) that they hear the case.[46] On December 29, 1993, a baby boy was delivered to the couple, identified as Mircea and Tabita Bricci. Although the baby appeared to be well physically, obstetricians warned that "it will be more than six months before any signs of any mental abnormalities or retardation would be detectable."[47]

Judicial intervention and the previable fetus. In *Taft v. Taft,*[48] the husband of a woman 16 weeks pregnant sought a court order requiring his wife to submit to a "purse string sutures" process in order to maintain cervical competency and save the fetus's life. Although the appellate court refused to override the mother's (religious) objections, it did so on the narrow grounds that no evidence was offered to support the medical necessity of the medical treatment in question.

In a second case, *In re Jamaica Hosp.,*[49] the court ordered a woman 18 weeks pregnant to submit to a blood transfusion in order to save both her own life and the life of her fetus. The woman had refused for religious reasons. The court determined that while the fetus was not yet viable and the state's interest in protecting his or her potential life therefore not yet compelling, the state's interest was "highly significant" and outweighed the mother's right to refuse treatment for religious reasons.

Fetal protection by third parties

An interesting area of the law of fetal interests concerns its treatment of fetal protection by third parties. As a general rule, "[T]he duty to do no wrong is a legal duty . . . [whereas t]he duty to protect against wrong is, generally speaking and excepting certain intimate relations in the nature of a trust, a moral obligation only, not . . . enforced by law."[50] American law, while traditionally imposing no affirmative duty on individuals to rescue strangers, is "in a steady movement toward requiring acts of Good Samaritanism . . . by whittling away at the concept of 'stranger.' "[51]

As such, while not penalizing the failure to rescue complete strangers, the law recognizes rescue as a normal human reaction. As Judge Cardozo wrote in *Wagner v. International Railway Co.,* "Danger invites rescue. The cry of distress is the summons to relief. The law does not ignore these reactions of the mind in tracing conduct to its consequences. It recognizes them as normal."[52] "The law's tendency is to compel men to act like good neighbors and to leave heroism to individual option."[53]

Against this background, the law's treatment of the fetus's right to be abetted by third parties is somewhat uneven, a phenomenon no doubt attributable to the unique nature of the "maternal-fetal dyad."[54]

Johnson Controls. In *UAW v. Johnson Controls,*[55] a company excluded from employment in its battery factory all women younger than 70 unwilling or unable to produce medical documentation of sterility. The company, concerned that lead used in the battery-making process would result in fetal abnormalities, professed an interest in the health of its employees' fetuses, as well as concern about legal liability. The U.S. Court of Appeals for the 7th Circuit upheld the policy.

Determining that protecting the safety of fetuses (or other noncustomer third parties) is not reasonably related to either the "essence of the [battery-making] business" or the "essence of the job," the U.S. Supreme Court held that Johnson Controls' fetal protection policy was illegal under Title VII of the Civil Rights Act of 1964[56] as amended by the Pregnancy Discrimination Act of 1978.[57] In essence, the effect of the Court's restrictive interpretation of Title VII was the following: whereas before *Johnson Controls* employers were free to act so as to protect fetal safety (though they had no duty to do so), after *Johnson Controls* employers were legally prohibited from doing so.

Rights of conscience. Congress and 44 state legislatures have enacted *conscience clauses*—statutes intended to protect health care providers' rights to refuse to provide or participate in certain procedures [including abortion] to which they have moral or religious objections."[58] While these clauses exist to protect the rights of health care providers with moral objections to abortion, fetuses clearly have an interest in seeing such rights protected. Unfortunately, the existing statutory protection of rights of conscience is inadequate from the point of view of fetal protection.

For example, not all conscience clauses protect all classes of persons. Some state conscience clauses protect "individuals,"[59] but not institutions. Many of the conscience clauses that do extend their protection to institutions protect only private institutions.[60] Only 10 states' conscience clauses prohibit discrimination in admission to residency training programs because of an applicant's refusal to participate in "the controversial service."[61] Furthermore, there is a substantial body of evidence that the existing rights of conscience of health care providers are being ignored[62]; and, to make matters worse, most courts view conscience clauses with disfavor and interpret the involved statutory language narrowly.[63]

Frozen embryos

The development of technology for creating embryos through *in vitro* fertilization (IVF) and freezing those embryos for later disposition has created new ethical and legal issues. Once created, what may ethically be done with these so-called "preembryos"? What does existing law have to say on the subject? What should the law have to say on the subject?

We should point out that American constitutional law, as interpreted by *Roe* and later abortion cases, has nothing to say about what may or may not be done with preembryos.

First, the viability standard cannot be applied to a technology that allows an embryo to be sustained indefinitely outside the mother's body; and second, when an embryo is outside the mother's body and frozen, its existence is no longer in conflict with [the woman's] constitutionally protected privacy interests.[64]

Specifically, *Roe* and progeny do not preclude the state from protecting these preembryos. "*Roe* merely holds that the state cannot force a woman to physically bear a child . . . until the point of viability has been reached."[65]

In assessing the constitutionality of laws regulating the disposition of frozen embryos, the standard to be applied by the courts will depend on whether or not they view the right to avoid genetic parentage as a fundamental right. If that right is determined not to be fundamental, then state action will be upheld if reasonably related to a legitimate state interest. In contrast, if that right is deemed to be fundamental, then state action "unduly burdening" that right will be struck down as unconstitutional unless such action is necessary to achieve a compelling state interest.

In perhaps the most famous IVF case to date, the Tennessee Supreme Court, in *Davis v. Davis,*[66] was forced to decide on the custody of seven cryopreserved embryos in a divorce case.

The trial court had held that the embryos were "children *in vitro*" and, invoking the doctrine of *parens patriae,* granted temporary custody to the mother. The Court of Appeals of Tennessee reversed and, in granting joint legal custody to Mr. and Mrs. Davis, implied that the cryopreserved embryos were property to be distributed equitably rather than persons.[67] The Tennessee Supreme Court, in affirming the decision of the appeals court, held that the embryos were not persons under the law, but that neither were they property. Rather, they were something in between, deserving of special respect. In addition, the court wrote that

the gamete providers should execute prior agreements [dealing with the disposition of the embryos] that may be modified later by agreement. Absent such modification, the agreement is enforceable. If no prior agreement is made, . . . where the gamete providers disagree on disposition . . . the case should be decided in favor of the party objecting to becoming a parent if the opposing party has any other reasonable way to become a parent.[68]

In effect, the court found that the right to avoid

genetic parenthood is a fundamental right, and seemed to echo the American Fertility Society's characterization of preembryos as something in between person and property:

The preembryo deserves respect greater than that accorded to human tissue but not the respect accorded to actual persons. The preembryo is due greater respect than other human tissue because of its potential to become a person and because of its symbolic meaning for many people. Yet, it should not be treated as a person, because it has not yet developed the features of personhood, is not yet established as developmentally individual, and may never realize its biological potential.[69]

Louisiana has a statute that treats cryopreserved embryos as legal persons prior to implantation.[70] Under this statute, transfers of frozen embryos are treated as adoptions.

Protection for preembryos under the criminal law. It has been suggested that preembryos might possibly enjoy protection under the criminal law of certain jurisdictions. Thus, Missouri implicitly affords preembryos the protection of its homicide statute by defining them as legal "persons":

[T]he laws of this state shall be interpreted . . . to acknowledge on behalf of the unborn child at every stage of development, all the rights, privileges, and immunities available to other persons, citizens and residents of this state, subject only to the Constitution of the United States, and decisional interpretations thereof by the United States Supreme Court. . . .[71]

In contrast, under New York State law a "person" is one "who has been born and is alive."[72] A fetus, therefore, could not claim to be a "person" for the purposes of New York's homicide law. Nevertheless the destruction of a fetus beyond 24 weeks of gestation is considered a homicide under New York law. Theoretically, the reach of the homicide law could be extended to include other nonpersons, such as preembryos.

Wisconsin illustrates another approach. Under Wisconsin law, the destruction of an unborn child (a human being from the time of conception until live birth), though not characterized as a homicide, is punishable by a $5000 fine and/or up to 3 years in prison where the offender is not the mother, $200 and/or 6 months in prison where the offender is the mother.[73]

END NOTES

1. *Stedman's Medical Dictionary* (Williams and Wilkins, Baltimore, 23rd ed. 1976).
2. T. Beauchamp, *The Moral Standing of Animals in Medical Research*, 20 *Law, Med. Health Care* 7-16, at 9 (1992).
3. "Persons" generally are capable of reason, self-awareness, social involvement, and moral reciprocity. *See* Beauchamp, *supra* note 2.
4. B. M. Knoppers and S. LeBris, *Recent Advances in Medically Assisted Conception*, 17 *Am. J. L. & Med.* 329-61, at 335 (1991). Thus, the embryonic heart begins to beat by about day 21 of gestation. Brainwaves are detectable by day 40. There is evidence of fetal respiratory movement ("breathing" amniotic fluid) by the end of the third month of gestation, which, it is thought, prepares the lungs for extrauterine life.
5. M. A. Warren, *Abortion, in* Singer P, ed.: *A Companion to Ethics* 311 (P. Singer ed., Blackwell 1993).
6. Knoppers and LeBris, *supra* note 4, at 337.
7. "Many neurophysiologists believe that normal human fetuses begin to have some rudimentary capacity for sentience at some stage in the second trimester of pregnancy." *See* Warren, *supra* note 5, at 309.
8. M. Smith, *Realism, in A Companion to Ethics* 403 (P. Singer ed., Blackwell 1993).
9. S. Buckle, *Natural Law, in A Companion to Ethics* 162, 170 (P. Singer ed., Blackwell 1993).
10. D. Wong, *Relativism, in A Companion to Ethics* 448 (P. Singer ed., Blackwell 1993).
11. *Roe v. Wade,* 410 U.S. 113 (1973).
12. *Planned Parenthood v. Casey,* No. 91-744 and 91-902, U.S. Sup. Ct. (1992).
13. Under the "undue burden" test, state laws are invalid if they have the purpose or effect of placing a substantial obstacle in the path of a woman seeking to abort a nonviable fetus.
14. M. A. Field, *Abortion Law Today* 14 *J. Legal Med.* 13 (1993).
15. *Dietrich v. Inhabitants of Northampton,* 138 Mass. 14 (1884).
16. *Allaire v. St. Luke's Hospital,* 184 Ill. 359. 56 N.E. 638 (1900).
17. *Bonbrest v. Kotz,* 65 F. Supp. 138 (D.D.C. 1946).
18. *See, e.g., Kelly v. Gregory,* 125 N.Y.S.2d 696 (App. Div. 1953).
19. M. L. Mascaro, *Preconception Tort Liability: Recognizing a Strict Liability Cause of Action for DES Grandchildren,* 17 *Am. J. L. & Med.* 435-55, at 437 (1991).
20. *Jorgensen v. Meade Johnson Laboratories,* 483 F.2d 237 (10th Cir. 1973).
21. *Renslow v. Mennonite Hosp.,* 67 Ill. 2d 348, 367 N.E.2d 1250 (1977).
22. *Albala v. City of New York,* 54 N.Y.2d 269, 429 N.E.2d 786, 445 N.Y.S.2d 108 (1981).
23. *Catherwood v. American Sterilizer Company,* 126 A.D.2d 978, 511 N.Y.S.2d 805 (N.Y. App. Div. 1987).
24. *Enright v. Eli Lilly & Co.,* 77 N.Y.2d 377, 570 N.E.2d 198, 568 N.Y.S.2d 550 (1991).
25. *Sorrels v. Eli Lilly & Co.,* 737 F. Supp. 678 (1990).
26. W. Prosser & W. Keeton, *The Law of Torts,* §55, at 368 (5th ed. 1984).
27. *Verkennes v. Corniea,* 38 N.W.2d 838 (Minn. 1949).
28. G. A. Meadows, *Wrongful Death and the Lost Society of the Unborn,* 13 *J. Legal Med.* 99-114, at 103 (1992).
29. *Grodin v. Grodin,* 102 Mich. App. 396, 301 N.W.2d 869 (1980).
30. R. I. Solomon, *Future Fear: Prenatal Duties Imposed by Private Parties,* 17 *Am. J. L. & Med.* 411-34, at 412 (1991).
31. 3 E. Coke, *The Third Part of the Institutes of the Laws of England* 50 (1628 and photo reprint 1979).
32. Solomon, *supra* note 30, at 413.
33. *Gloria C. v. William C.,* 124 Misc. 2d 313, 476 N.Y.S.2d 991 (N.Y. Fam. Ct. 1984).
34. G. J. Annas et al., *American Health Law* 978 (Little, Brown & Co., Boston 1990).
35. *Commonwealth v. Cass,* 392 Mass. 799. 467 N.E.2d 1324 (1984), construing Mass. Gen. Laws Ann. ch. 90, §246(a) (1984 & Supp. 1991) to include a fetus as a person.
36. Washington Post, November 25, 1989, at A4.
37. Casper Star-Tribune, Jan. 25, 1990, at B1, col. 1.
38. *Florida v. Johnson,* No. E89-890-CFA slip op. (Seminole Cty., Cir. Ct. July 13, 1989).
39. *Johnson v. Florida,* No. 89-1765 (Dist. Ct. App., 5th Dist., Apr. 18, 1991).
40. M. A. Field, *Controlling the Woman to Protect the Fetus,* 17 *Law, Med. & Health Care* 114 (1989).

27 Fetal interests **371**

41. *Raleigh Fitkin-Paul Morgan Memorial Hosp. v. Anderson,* 201 A.2d 537, *cert. denied,* 377 U.S. 985 (1964).

42. *Jefferson v. Griffin Spaulding County Hosp.,* 274 Ga. 86, 247 S.E.2d 457 (1981).

43. *In re A.C.,* 573 A.2d 1235 (D.C. 1990).

44. *Id.* at 1237.

45. Patrick T. Murphy, the public guardian in Cook County, Illinois, and the representative of the fetus, maintained that the woman should not be physically compelled to undergo a cesarean; rather, it was his position that if she disobeyed a court order to have the operation, she should be fined.

46. N.Y. Times, December 15, 1993, at A22, col. 5; *see also* N.Y. Times, December 19, 1993, at 35, col. 1.

47. Newsday, December 31, 1993, at 7, col. 1.

48. *Taft v. Taft,* 446 N.E.2d 395 (Mass. 1983).

49. *In re Jamaica Hosp.,* 491 N.Y.S.2d 898 (S.Ct. Queens Co. 1985).

50. *Buch v. Armory Mfg. Co.,* 69 N.H. 257, 44 A. 809 (1897).

51. E. Cahn, *The Moral Decision* 190 (Indiana University Press, Bloomington 1955). These "intimate relations" or exceptions to the no-duty rule, which have been deemed to create or impose an affirmative duty to rescue, include the following situations: (1) cases where a special relationship exists between the plaintiff and defendant; (2) cases where the defendant is bound contractually to rescue plaintiff; (3) cases where the danger or injury to the plaintiff is due to the defendant's own conduct; (4) cases where the defendant has already undertaken to rescue the plaintiff; and (5) cases where the defendant is required statutorily to rescue plaintiff.

52. *Wagner v. International Railway Co.,* 232 NY 176 (1921).

53. Cahn, *supra* note 51, at 191.

54. S. S. Mattingly, *The Maternal-Fetal Dyad,* 22 *Hastings Center Report* 13-18 (Jan.-Feb. 1992).

55. *International Union, UAW v. Johnson Controls,* 886 F.2d 871 (7th Cir. 1989)(en banc), *cert. granted,* 110 S.Ct. 1522 (1990), *rev'd,* 111 S.Ct. 1196 (1991).

56. 42 U.S.C.A. §2000e (West 1981 & Supp. 1991).

57. Pub. L. No. 95-555, §1, 92 Stat. 2076 (codified as amended at 42 U.S.C.A. §2000e(k)).

58. L. D. Wardle, *Protecting the Rights of Conscience of Health Care Providers,* 14 *J. Legal Med.* 177-230 (1993).

59. *See, e.g.,* Iowa Code Ann. §146.1; 42 U.S.C. §300a-7(a).

60. Wardle, *supra* note 58, at 184-85.

61. *Id.* at 193.

62. *Id.* at 219-21.

63. *Id.* at 199.

64. Saltarelli, *Genesis Retold: Legal Issues Raised by the Cryopreservation of Preimplantation Human Embryos,* 36 *Syr. L. Rev.* 1021 (1985-86).

65. C. Perry and L. K. Schneider, *Cryopreserved Embryos: Who Shall Decide Their Fate?,* 13 *J. Legal Med.* 463-500, at 471 (1992).

66. *Davis v. Davis,* No. 34, slip op. (Tenn. Supreme Court, June 1, 1992).

67. *Davis v. Davis,* 1990 Tenn. App. LEXIS 642 (13 Sept. 1990).

68. *Davis v. Davis,* No. 34, slip op. (Tenn. Supreme Court, June 1, 1992).

69. Ethics Committee of the American Fertility Society, *Ethical Considerations of the New Reproductive Technologies,* 53 *Fertility & Sterility* 37S, 58S, Supp. 2 (June 1990).

70. La. Rev. Stat. Ann. §9:123 (West 1991).

71. Mo. Rev. Stat. §1.205(2) (Supp. 1992).

72. N.Y. Penal Law §125.05 (McKinney 1987).

73. Wis. Stat. Ann. §940.04 (West 1982).

GENERAL REFERENCES

Blank, R. H., *Maternal-Fetal Relationship: The Courts and Social Policy,* 14 J. Legal Med. 73-92 (1993).

Capron, A. M., *Fetal Alcohol and Felony,* 22 Hastings Center Report 28-9 (May-June 1992).

Capron, A. M., *Parenthood and Frozen Embryos: More Than Property and Privacy,* 22 Hastings Center Report 32-3 (Sep.-Oct. 1992).

Garcia, S. A., *Drug Addiction and Mother/Child Welfare: Rights, Laws, and Discretionary Decisionmaking,* 13 J. Legal Med. 129-203 (1992).

Merrick, J. C., *Maternal Substance Abuse During Pregnancy,* 14 J. Legal Med. 57-71 (1993).

Robertson, J. A., *Casey and the Resuscitation of Roe v. Wade,* 22 Hastings Center Report 24-28 (1992).

CHAPTER 28 Organ donation and transplantation

VICTOR WALTER WEEDN, M.D., J.D., F.C.L.M.*
EDWIN KELLERMAN, M.D., J.D., F.C.L.M.

STATE ANATOMICAL GIFT ACTS
ROUTINE INQUIRY/REQUIRED REQUEST
PRESUMED/IMPLIED CONSENT
CADAVER ORGANS: DETERMINATION OF DEATH
ORGANS AND TISSUES FROM FETUSES AND ANENCEPHALICS
LIVING RELATED DONORS: DONOR CONSENT
INCOMPETENT DONORS
CONFIDENTIALITY OF POTENTIAL DONORS
ARTIFICIAL AND ANIMAL TRANSPLANTS
DONOR SCREENING
FEDERAL LEGISLATION
SELECTION OF ORGAN RECIPIENTS
COST AND PAYMENT CONSIDERATIONS
MALPRACTICE SUITS
RECENT DEVELOPMENTS

Transplantation is one of the most exciting, rapidly changing, dramatically successful, expensive, and visible areas of medicine. This is why it is also probably the area subject to the most intense scrutiny by public policy-makers. Transplantation has been a serious therapeutic option for kidneys only within the last three decades and within the last decade for other organs, particularly since the advent of the immunosuppressant cyclosporine in the mid-1980s. Nonetheless, transplantation has largely moved beyond the stage of experimentation.

In 1988, there were 9123 kidney transplants, 1647 heart transplants, 74 heart-lung transplants, 1680 liver transplants, and 243 pancreas transplants in the United States. The heart and liver transplants more than doubled from three years before.[1] In addition, 36,900 corneas[2] and countless other tissues such as heart valves, blood, skin, bone, and dural tissue were transplanted.

The one-year patient survival rate for living related kidney transplants is now 96% and for cadaveric kidney transplants it is 90%, up from 50% one decade before. The one-year survival rate is 80% for heart transplants, 65% for liver transplants, and 35% for pancreas transplants.[3]

Transplantation centers have multiplied and no longer are limited to academic institutions. As of the beginning of 1990, 250 medical institutions have been operating an organ transplant program, including more than 200 centers capable of kidney transplants, 150 capable of heart transplants, and 80 capable of liver transplants. Approximately 50 organ procurement organizations operate in 11 designated regions.[4]

In general, the demand for tissue and organs far outstrips the supply. In the United States, over 16,000 patients were on kidney waiting lists at the beginning of 1989, over 1,400 patients were on heart waiting lists, and over 900 were on liver waiting lists.[5] An estimated 4000 were awaiting corneal tissue transplants.[6]

Potential demand, particularly for vital organs, is vastly greater than present demand. As the procedures and reimbursement mechanisms become better established, more potential recipients may avail themselves of the opportunity. The Senate report on the National

*The opinions or assertions contained herein are those of the author and are not to be construed as official or as representing those of the U.S. Army or the Department of Defense.

Transplant Act stated that "It is estimated that with recent improvements in transplantation surgery and medical management as many as ten percent of our population at some time may be candidates for transplantation surgery in the future."[7]

The traditional procurement policy of "voluntarism" has been inadequate. The potential supply of organs is limited to the approximate 20,000 patients declared brain-dead in the United States each year, but organs are actually harvested from only about 15% of these.[8] The increasing need for organs and the inadequacy of initial voluntary efforts have been the driving forces behind much of the legislation concerning transplantation. In 1968 the Uniform Anatomical Gift Act (UAGA) was promulgated to facilitate cadaver donations. Later statutes were amended to allow for donation by a signature on the back of drivers' licenses. Brain death statutes were passed to allow removal of vital organs from artificially maintained bodies. Medicare funding and the Joint Commission for Accreditation on Healthcare Organizations (JCAHO) accreditation standards now mandate that hospitals have protocols for routinely approaching families for organ donations. States have passed required request and routine injury laws. Implied consent for corneas from medical examiner cases has been adopted in many states. As the pressure for organs mounts, policy-makers will increasingly move away from voluntary to compulsory systems of procurement.

The major legal problems that arise pertinent to transplantation are consent or authorization to donate, the determination of death in the case of procurement from a cadaver, and the rationing of organs and medical resources.

STATE ANATOMICAL GIFT ACTS

The foundation for the law on organ procurement in this country is the UAGA, which provides the legal authorization for the system of voluntary donations and specifically defines the legal mechanisms for organ and tissue donations. In an effort to promote organ and tissue procurement, the National Conference of Commissioners on Uniform State Laws (NCCUSL) and the American Bar Association, after three years of deliberation, drafted the model act in 1968.[9] By 1972, all 50 states, the District of Columbia, and Puerto Rico had adopted the UAGA, spurred on by the excitement over heart transplantation. Many of the states modified the UAGA during enactment or by later amendments. A substantially altered 1987 version of the UAGA, embodying new legal developments and other legislation, has been promulgated by the NCCUSL (see Appendix 28-2).[10] As of March 1990, it had been adopted by 10 states (Arkansas, California, Connecticut, Hawaii, Idaho, Montana, Nevada, North Dakota, Rhode Island,

and Utah), and it is anticipated that it will be adopted widely.

The UAGA authorizes persons or their families to make an "anatomical gift" of all or part of his or her body to take effect upon death. The legally binding right to direct the disposition of one's own remains after death is a new right created by the UAGA. Previously, as a carryover from the original common law of England, one had no property rights in his or her body after death. Individuals could not clearly bequeath their bodies, and heirs could nullify or overrule bequests. Even families did not have full property rights in bodies, but rather a limited right to possess the body for burial purposes. Bodies were considered "quasiproperty."[11,12]

According to the 1968 UAGA, any person 18 years of age or older and "of sound mind" can execute an anatomical gift. Many states have substituted different age requirements. The requirement for a "sound mind" has been deleted from the 1987 UAGA. An anatomical part includes organs, tissues, eyes, bones, arteries, blood, other fluids, and other portions of the human body. Any condition can be imposed on the gift, but if the condition is inappropriate or unacceptable, it should be declined.

Gifts by a decedent

The decedent's wishes, if known, are to be carried out despite the wishes of the next-of-kin. Knowledge of religious beliefs may constitute knowledge of the decedent's intentions. In *In re Moyer's Estate,*[13] the Utah Supreme Court found this posthumous control over one's body was "in the public interest" so long as it was not "absurd" or "preposterous." In *Holland v. Metalious,*[14] the deceased in her will donated her eyes to an eye bank and her body to one of two medical schools. The New Hampshire Supreme Court stated that the wishes of the decedent should usually be carried out, but since the medical schools had declined to accept the donation (because of objections of the spouse and children), the court ruled that the surviving spouse could determine the disposition of the body. No survivor has the legal right to veto a valid gift by the decedent; however, as a practical matter, if the family objects to the donation over the expressed desire of the decedent, it may be prudent to decline the decedent's donation.

Gifts by next-of-kin

When a deceased has not indicated his or her intentions, then the UAGA spells out specifically who among those available at the time of death may make an anatomical gift of the body or body parts. The UAGA first designates the spouse, and if the spouse is not available at the time of death, then an adult son or daughter, followed by either parent, then an adult sibling. If none of the above is available, a guardian of the person of the decedent at the time of the death or any other person authorized or under an obligation to dispose of the body (e.g., the medical examiner or anatomical board) may donate the body or body parts.

Consent by one next-of-kin (e.g., one brother) is legally negated by the objection of another of the same class of next of kin (another brother), although inquiry of all of a class is not required to exclude the possibility that someone might object, as confirmed in *Leno v. St Joseph Hospital.*[15] New York allows any family member to veto a gift by any other family member; in Florida a spouse cannot make a donation over the objection of an adult son or daughter.

The statute is silent in regard to the status of divorced or separated spouses, stepparents, stepchildren, other dependents, designated caretakers, those appointed power of attorney, and others. The list of next-of-kin to be approached for organ donation in the UAGA is not necessarily the same as that for inheritance, autopsy consent, or even required request statutes. Consent by next-of-kin must be timely; the specified individuals must make the gift "after or immediately upon death." This provides little guidance as to the time and diligence necessary in attempting to contact these persons before considering them "unavailable." Time limits for the harvest of particular organs and tissues are clearly relevant.

Execution of the gift

The gift may be executed by a will or other document. Such provisions in typical estate wills are discouraged because they are usually not immediately available at the time of death. The use of "living wills" is preferred because they are immediately available as part of the medical record. Two witnesses are necessary to validate a gift during the donor's lifetime, but none is required in the case of a gift by next-of-kin. Some states have relaxed or eliminated (as in the 1987 UAGA) this witness requirement, whereas other states have statutorily specified witness requirements. The next-of-kin can make gifts by a signed document or by telegraphic or recorded message. The 1987 UAGA would also allow other forms of communication reduced to writing and signed by the recipient. Neither delivery nor public filing is necessary to make the gift effective. The gift can be revoked or amended by a signed statement, an oral statement in the presence of two witnesses, or a statement to an attending physician.

Any card, form, or even a sticker may be carried by the donor to evidence the intention of the gift. During the mid-1970s, 44 states incorporated legislation to enable organ and tissue donation by the mere signing of the back of a driver's license. Most organ procurement agencies and transplant surgeons do not accept such a signature by itself (so-called pocket wills) but rather require the contemporaneous consent of the next of kin. They speculate that the decedent may have changed his or her mind since the signing and that they could not afford the negative publicity that might occur in the face of objections by the family. Use of donor cards is mandated in the 1987 UAGA, which requires law enforcement officers and emergency rescue personnel to make a reasonable search for a document of gift and then requires the hospital to cooperate in the implementation of the anatomical gift. Routine inquiry further emphasizes acceptance of documents of a decedent's wishes and provides a mechanism to check the currency of the card.

Persons accepting a gift

Any specified person, physician, hospital, accredited medical school or university, tissue bank, or procurement agency can accept an anatomical gift for education, research, therapy, or transplantation. Several states additionally allow donation to anatomical boards, which generally receive unclaimed bodies for educational purposes. In Connecticut, the State Commissioner of Health must approve recipients. The attending physician is the presumed donee if a donee is not specified. The attending physician who makes a determination of death is excluded from participating in any part of the transplant procedures, although it does not prevent him or her from communicating with the transplant team. "Hospital" is substituted for "attending physician" in the 1987 version of the act.

The intentions of the donor must be respected, including any condition imposed on the gift. A donee can accept or reject a gift. The donee of the entire body can authorize embalming and funeral services. One provision authorizes any postmortem examination necessary to ensure medical acceptability of the donated organ, including an autopsy. The donee of a part must remove the part without unnecessary mutilation and then relinquish custody to the next-of-kin or other person under obligation to dispose of the body. The drafters chose not to deal with the issue of compensation for processing the gift.

The UAGA does not qualify in any way the legal right of a physician, organ procurement organization, or transplant team who receives a donated organ to do with it what they perceive as properly carrying out the intentions of the family. It has been argued that the donee holder of an organ is the "owner" of the organ and thus has the absolute right, limited only by any express covenant of purpose, to choose the ultimate organ recipient. It has also been argued that the intermediary party is an agent of the donor or the donor's family and is liable for failure to comply with their wishes. It has even been espoused that the donee is a public trustee, who is liable for negligence (or perhaps conversion) to a prospective recipient for an inappropriate selection.

Medical examiners

Most vital organs are retrieved from patients who are declared brain-dead because most natural deaths render organs unsuitable for transplants. These brain deaths usually result from motor vehicle accidents or other violence and therefore generally fall under the jurisdiction of the coroner or medical examiner. The UAGA states that it is subject to other state laws governing autopsies; hence medical examiner and coroner laws take precedence. Comments to the original 1968 NCCUSL act state that it "is necessary to preclude the frustration of the important medical examiner's duties in cases of death by suspected crime or violence . . . it may prove desirable in many if not most states to reexamine and amend, the medical examiner statutes to authorize and direct medical examiners to expedite their autopsy procedures in cases in which the public interest will not suffer." The 1986 National Task Force on Transplantation also recommended enactment of laws that would encourage coroner and medical examiners to give permission for organ and tissue procurement from cadavers under their jurisdiction.

Many states have "implied consent" statutes that allow harvest of corneas from medical examiner cases when no known objection to the harvest exists. The 1987 version of the UAGA provides that the medical examiner may authorize removal of an organ or tissue for transplant purposes if it will not interfere with the postmortem investigation and if the medical examiner does not know of an objection to the donation after making a reasonable effort, and taking into account the useful life of the part, to find documentation of the decedent's intention and to contact the next-of-kin.

Immunity

The physician who removes an organ in good faith is protected from civil and criminal liability by the UAGA. Mississippi and Montana grant civil immunity only; South Carolina makes an exception for malpractice. In *Nicoletta v. Rochester Eye and Human Parts Bank*,[16] parties recovering organs were protected when they relied on the good faith belief that a person consenting to donation was a surviving spouse when, in fact, she was not. This provision of immunity withstood constitutional attack in *Williams v. Hofmann.*[17]

The provision applies only to valid gifts. The UAGA takes effect only after death has been declared; hence it does not afford protection to the pronouncement of death itself. Failure to comply with the provisions of the

act (e.g., no unnecessary mutilation of the body) may itself demonstrate bad faith. However, the act's provisions are to be construed liberally in order to achieve its stated goal of promoting organ and tissue donations. In *Ravenis v. Detroit General Hosp.,*[18] the Michigan Court of Appeals ruled that the protection did not preclude liability for the negligent failure of a hospital to adequately screen a donor for disease that was subsequently transmitted to a recipient. Thus courts may interpret this provision of immunity to be inapplicable to malpractice.

Most states also have protective clauses in their blood banking statutes that specifically maintain that blood transfusions, organ procurement procedures, and transplants are to be regarded as services rather than sales of products; accordingly members of the transplant team are exempt from strict product liability.

The 1987 UAGA revision

The 1987 NCCUSL model act, among other things, added provisions for routine inquiry, required requests, presumed consent for medical examiner cases, and prohibition of the sale of organs (see Appendix 28-2).[19] These constitute substantial new provisions that codify in the UAGA legislation that which has to some extent been adopted elsewhere. These issues are discussed in the following sections.

ROUTINE INQUIRY/REQUIRED REQUEST

Possible policy solutions to increase voluntary organ and tissue donations include "routine inquiry," "required request," and "presumed or implied consent" legislation. Only 1 of 25 hospital deaths provide material suitable for organ donation, although 24 out of 25 deaths provide material suitable for tissue donations.[20] It has been estimated that 17,000 to 26,000 potential organ donors die each year in the United States.[21] Only 15 to 20% of potential donors become actual donors; in 1984 this amounted to just over 2600 donors.[22,23] However, approximately 70% to 75% of families were approached for permission to grant donation.[24] The limiting factor appears to be the inadequate request and referral by the health care team.[25-28]

Recognizing the problem, Arthur Caplan called for "required request" legislation, which would force providers to approach families for donation in appropriate cases.[29] This focuses on the consent of surviving family members. "Routine inquiry," on the other hand, refers to the asking of a patient upon hospital admission if he or she is an organ donor. This focus is on the advance decision of the individual and his or her right to self-determinism, which is the proper priority according to the UAGA. Furthermore, it saves valuable time by preempting the need to contact the family before procurement. However, some have argued that queries during admission to the hospital are poorly timed because potential patients may feel apprehensive either that the care they receive might be substandard if they fail to comply with a request for donations or that medical providers might be less vigorous in resuscitative attempts if they do comply.[30]

Required request is now found in the state law of 44 states, federal Medicare/Medicaid conditions of participation,[31] and the JCAHO standards of accreditation.[32] Both the JCAHO and Medicare merely require that a hospital have written protocol. Most current state legislation has been enacted in the form of amendments to state anatomical gift acts and rather closely tracks the federal law. State laws are typically more detailed and sweeping, and apply to non-accredited, nonparticipating hospitals. However, state laws are generally weak; few states even require documentation of the request that might allow for enforcement, and several create institutional exemptions and wide discretionary exceptions for requests. These state laws vary greatly and are summarized in Table 28-1.[33] Approximately half the states have weak versions of required request, in which the sole requirement is a mere written hospital policy of routine requests of family members. In some states the request is to be made by the physician, whereas in others the request is to be made by a designated member of the hospital or of the regional organ procurement agency. Appropriate training of the requestor is sometimes required. Half the states require documentation of the inquiry and its disposition: In many states this documentation is in a log book, a central registry, or a place other than the medical record.

There are numerous exceptions for the requirement of request, based on considerations such as medical criteria, known objection, or religion. In Alabama, the attending physician can decide that inquiry should not be made. In Massachusetts, exception is allowed where discussion would cause the family undue emotional distress. Lobbying efforts have exempted hospitals in several states. Kentucky is the only state that has an explicit penalty for failure to comply with state routine inquiry legislation.

To date, the effect of various early measures requiring request has been to double and triple overall tissue procurement, but vital organ procurement, which was the target of the legislation, has increased only modestly. Legal sanctions may be imposed if these provisions are not followed or are insufficient. Indeed, the Health Care Financing Administration (HCFA) is trying to find ways to assess compliance with its Medicare/Medicaid required request regulations.[34]

The 1987 UAGA has provisions for both routine inquiry (Section 5[a]) and required request (Section 5[b]). Documentation is to be placed in the medical record. The hospital administrator is responsible for implementation, and the Commissioner of Health has responsibility for oversight. Furthermore, the legislation mandates that donor cards are to be sought and respected. Law enforcement and emergency personnel as well as hospital personnel are to make a reasonable search for a donor card or other documentation of gift at the time of death or "near the time of death." When they find evidence of a desire to donate, the hospital is to cooperate in the implementation of the gift. Administrative (but not criminal or civil) sanctions are to be imposed.

PRESUMED/IMPLIED CONSENT

Presumed consent laws, in which consent is presumed in the absence of actual knowledge of objection, are common in Europe. It is a policy of "opting out" instead of "opting in." It has not been a popular notion in the United States, but as demand continues to outstrip the supply for organs and tissues, presumed consent will be increasingly favored by policy-makers. Even in countries with implied consent laws, families are regularly asked permission for donations anyway.[35]

Eighteen states have enacted legislation authorizing medical examiners to have corneas removed based on presumed consent. These laws allow removal of the corneas when the death falls under jurisdiction of the medical examiner, when removal of the corneas will not interfere with the investigation or disturb the appearance of the body, and when there is no known objection from the next-of-kin. Maryland passed the first such law in 1975. These presumed consent laws have been highly effective in increasing the supply of corneas.

Statutes vary remarkably in the degree of diligence required in attempting to locate family members. Some states require no effort, others require "reasonable effort," some require "a good faith effort," some specify attempts for a 4-hour period, and some specify 24 hours unless the organ or tissue would become unfit earlier. Numerous instances of families becoming outraged after corneas have been retrieved from their loved ones have resulted in litigation and, in Texas, in a change in the law.[36]

In *Powell v. Florida*,[37] the implied consent statute for removal of corneas by medical examiners was upheld by the Florida Supreme Court. Two sets of parents sued when the corneas of their sons were removed by medical examiners without their consent or without any attempt to give them notice. The court found that the legislation was reasonable, did not violate due process or equal protection requirements, and served a public purpose. It noted that the state of Florida was spending $138 million per year to support its blind citizenry and that corneal

TABLE 28-1. State required request/routine inquiry legislation as of April 1, 1988

Enactment date	AL 86	AZ 86	AR 87	CA 85	CO 87	CT 86	DE 86	DC 86	FL 86	GA 86	HI 86	IL 86	IN 86	KS 86	KY 86	LA 86	MA 86	ME 85	MD 86	MI 86	MS 87
Type of legislation:																					
Required request	+	+						+	+	+						+		+	+[1]	+	
Routine inquiry, required		+	+	+	+	+	+				+	+	+	+	+		+		+[2]		+
Application of legislation:																					
Hospital qualification	+			+[3]	+[4]	+[5]	+[3]		+[6]			+[3,7]	+	+	+[8]						
Exclusion, medical criteria	+			+	+	+	+	+	+	+		+				+	+	+	+	+	+
Exclusion, known objection	+				+		+	+	+	+		+				+	+		+	+	
Exclusion, judgment of attending	+			+										+				+		+	
Exclusion, religious (required)						+		+				+					+		+		
Other miscellaneous exclusions								+				+									
Requestor:																					
Hospital administrator	+	+						+	+	+	+	+	+		+	+	+	+	+	+	+
Organ procurement agency		+								+					+						
Attending physician																		+		+	+
Training required		+			+		+		+[12]	+[12]						+[12]		+[12]			
Requestees:																					
UAGA classification	+	+		+	+				+	+	+		+	+	+		+	+		+	+
Otherwise specified							+	+				+				+			+		
Request:																					
On admission	+	+	+	+																	
Upon death		+	+	+	+	+	+		+	+	+	+	+	+	+	+	+	+	+	+	+
Notify OPO if no request		+				+	+	+		+				+	+			+	+	+	+
Required by hospital protocol								+											+		
Documentation:																					
Medical record	+			+	+		+		+			+	+		+	+		+	+		
Central registry																+					
Hospital log book						+											+			+	
Other							+			+											
Miscellaneous:																					
Encourage sensitivity	+	+		+	+		+			+		+	+	+		+	+	+	+	+	+
Exculpatory clause					+									+							+
Penalties															+						
State funding									+												

Continued.

TABLE 28-1. State required request/routine inquiry legislation as of April 1, 1988—cont'd

	MO 86	MN 87	MT 87	NE 87	NV 87	NH 86	NJ 85	NM 87	NY 85	NC 87	ND 87	OH 86	OR 85	PA 86	RI 86	TN 86	TX 87	VA 88	WA 86	WV 86
Enactment Date																				
Type of legislation:																				
Required request	+	+				+	+	+	+		+		+							+
Routine inquiry, required			+	+	+					+		+		+	+	+	+	+	+	+
Application of legislation:																				
Hospital qualification		+[8]				+[9]							+[3,10]			+[3]				
Exclusion, medical criteria	+	+	+	+	+	+			+				+	+	+	+	+	+	+	+
Exclusion, known objection	+	+	+	+	+				+		+[11]		+	+		+	+			+
Exclusion, judgment of attending			+		+						+	+	+							
Exclusion, religious (required)	+	+	+	+					+			+				+	+			+
Other miscellaneous exclusions		+	+									+		+						
Requestor:																				
Hospital administrator	+	+	+	+	+				+		+	+				+		+		+
Organ procurement agency	+	+										+								
Attending physician	+	+	+	+	+	+		+	+	+	+	+	+	+	+	+	+		+	+
Training required	+	+	+	+	+	+		+	+[12]		+	+[12]	+[12]	+[12]	+	+				+[12]
Requestees:																				
UAGA classification	+	+	+	+	+	+		+						+	+	+			+	+
Otherwise specified							+		+											
Request:																				
On admission	+	+	+	+	+	+						+	+	+	+	+	+		+	+
Upon death	+	+	+	+	+	+		+		+	+				+	+	+	+	+	
Notify OPO if no request		+							+											
Required by hospital protocol	+	+	+	+	+	+	+	+	+											+
Documentation:																				
Medical record	+	+	+	+								+		+		+				
Central registry		+		+																
Hospital log book			+						+			+			+		+			
Other			+					+												
Miscellaneous:																				
Encourage sensitivity	+	+	+	+				+	+	+	+			+	+	+	+	+	+	+
Exculpatory clause	+	+	+	+	+			+	+			+		+				+	+	
Penalties		+																		
State funding																				

From V.W. Weeden and B. Leveque, *Routine Inquiry for Organ and Tissue Donations.* 84 Tex. Med. 30-37 (1988).

[1]For minors only
[2]For nonemergent admission of adults and minors
[3]General acute care only
[4]Exemption may be requested
[5]Excluding short-term children's general hospital
[6]Verified trauma center or hospital that provides emergency or acute medical care
[7]Hospitals of more than 100 beds
[8]State agency compliance condition of licensure
[9]Hospitals licensed under Revised Statutes Annotated #151
[10]Specified exemptions
[11]Attending must document exception in medical records
[12]Nonstatutory rules established by state agency

transplantation is in great demand and is frequently successful in restoring sight. The court determined that recovery from medical examiner autopsy cases was the most important source of quality tissue and that removal of the corneal tissue was an insignificant bodily intrusion compared with the autopsy itself, which did not affect the decedent's appearance. The court cited California statistics that approximately 80% of the families of decedents could not be located in time for medical examiners to remove usable corneal tissue. The court further held that the next-of-kin has no property right in the remains of the decedent but merely a limited right to possess the body for burial purposes.

Similarly, medical examiner implied consent statutes have withstood constitutional challenge in Georgia[38] and Michigan.[39]

In *Kirker v. Orange County,*[40] a mother was awarded damages for the intentional infliction of emotional distress caused by the "mutilation" of her daughter's body when the medical examiner granted permission to remove the child's eyeglobes despite an expressed refusal for corneal donation in the medical record. The medical examiner should have known of the objection. An attempted coverup was also shown.

As previously mentioned, the 1987 model act includes a provision authorizing any organ or tissue donation by a medical examiner for transplantation based on a presumed consent provided that reasonable effort is made to discover any appropriate objection. Maryland and California have expanded presumed consent beyond medical examiner situations to include patients dying in hospitals.

CADAVER ORGANS: DETERMINATION OF DEATH

Most kidneys (80%) and necessarily all livers and hearts for transplantation are harvested from cadavers; the vast majority of these organs are from patients who have been declared brain-dead, usually while in the neurosurgical intensive care unit. This allows for the timely harvest of cadaver organs that are well perfused and have been little affected by untoward diseases (kidneys can be stored for one to two days; hearts and livers for only a few hours). In such cases a determination of death is necessary. The premature removal of organs may subject the physicians to civil and criminal liability.

The law has always held that a person is dead when a licensed physician pronounces him or her dead, if the determination is based on accepted medical standards. Brain death has become an accepted standard, and every court that has examined the question has held it a legally proper determination, regardless of the presence or absence of a state brain death statute. However, medical standards for determination of brain death have become

rigorous in many jurisdictions, and failure to adhere to methods for determination specified by such standards may result in liability.

The physician who removes an organ in good faith is possibly protected from civil and criminal liability by the Uniform Anatomical Gift Act. This act appears to take effect only after death has been declared. However, it is to be construed liberally in order that its stated goal of promoting organ and tissue donations may be achieved to avoid conflicts of interest (Section 7[b]), and specifically states that the physician who makes the determination of death "shall not participate in the procedures for removing or transplanting a part."

In *Tucker v. Lower,*[41] the brother of an organ donor alleged that the organs had been removed before the donor was legally dead. At the time Virginia had not yet adopted a brain death standard. The jury found for the surgeon, based on a jury instruction that death could be determined if there was complete and irreversible loss of brain function.

However, in *Strachan v. John F. Kennedy Memorial Hosp.,*[42] the court ruled that the hospital was liable for delaying the release of a body while attempting to change the parent's decision not to donate, when an emergency room physician had diagnosed brain death three days before the official pronouncement of death and disconnection of the respirator.

ORGANS AND TISSUES FROM FETUSES AND ANENCEPHALICS

The national organ shortage is much more critical for pediatric organs (especially livers) than for adult organs. Less than 5% of organ donations are from donors under 5 years of age.[43] It has been estimated that the potential demand each year for infant organs is approximately 1000 livers and 500 hearts and kidneys.[44] This is a conservative estimate because approximately 7500 infants with life-threatening congenital heart defects are born each year.[45] In 1989 the United Network for Organ Sharing listed 83 patients under 5 years of age who were waiting for a kidney, 148 patients waiting for a liver, and 10 patients waiting for a heart or heart-lung block. Half the transplant candidates die before an organ becomes available. In comparison with adults, a very low number of infants and children die with transplant-suitable organs.

Anencephalic infants represent an important potential source of fetal organs. Organs from such infants could meet the bulk of the current demand for infant organs. Organs from stillborns and infants dying from other diseases are not generally suitable for procurement and transplantation.

Anencephaly is an abnormality of primary neurulation commencing within the first month of gestation that results in the congenital absence of a major portion of the brain, skull, and scalp. Cranial neural tissue is exposed and often protrudes from the skull defect. Both cerebral hemispheres are absent or unrecognizable. Although some rudimentary cerebral development can occur, there is no functioning cerebral cortex. Anencephalic children cannot reason and presumably cannot suffer. The term *monster* has been applied to this anomaly, which represents the most severe form of neural tube defect (spina bifida). Anencephaly is a universally fatal condition. Two-thirds of anencephalic infants die *in utero*. Very few survive beyond one week after birth. Infants provided maximal support may survive somewhat longer, but it appears that when strict diagnostic criteria are applied, survival still does not exceed two months. Longer survival periods have been reported; however, the diagnostic criteria were not well documented. Cases of amniotic band syndrome, ruptured encephalocele, and iniencephaly (per se) are sometimes confused with the diagnosis of anencephaly, and probably account for the rare cases of prolonged survival reported in the literature.

Between 13% and 33% of infants born with anencephaly have defects of the nonneural organs. These defects may complicate care and render their organs unsuitable for donation.

Estimates of the incidence of anencephaly have varied from 0.3 to 7 per 1000 births.[46] Differences are due, among other things, to different diagnostic criteria, true geographical differences, and prenatal screening programs. Prenatal detection of anencephaly usually results in early termination of pregnancy; thus screening programs can dramatically reduce the incidence of anencephaly at birth. The Centers for Disease Control cites an incidence of 0.3 per 1000 births (live births and stillbirths).[47] Extrapolation of this figure would indicate that more than 1000 infants are born with anencephaly annually in the United States, but this figure would drop to less than 100 if screening and induced abortion were uniformly applied.

The first transplant of the heart of an anencephalic infant occurred in October 1987 at the Loma Linda University Medical Center in California without legal incident. Subsequently, other parents requested that their anencephalic children be used as donors to help other children. This meant that the pregnancy was allowed to be carried to term rather than terminated. With parental permission, the live-born anencephalic children were then placed on respiratory support, and their organs donated if brain-death criteria were fulfilled within one week. Only 1 of 12 anencephalic newborns met brain death criteria and no recipient could be found for his organs; consequently, the program was sus-

pended. One of the infants survived for two months after the respirator was removed.[48]

The Medical Task Force on Anencephaly reported in March 1990 that it was able to identify 80 anencephalic infants who were involved in transplantation protocols.[49] Only 41 infants were used as sources of organs, providing 37 kidneys, 2 livers, and 3 hearts.

A major problem with organ donation from anencephalic infants is that legal criteria for brain death are not easily applied. Brain-death criteria are derived from the Uniform Determination of Death Act, in which a declaration of brain death is based on irreversible cessation of all brain functions, including those of the brain stem (so-called whole-brain death). Although anencephalic infants have no higher cortical function, they may have good brain stem function. Therefore they have intact circulatory and respiratory function and good reflexes; may cry, swallow, and regurgitate; and may respond to pain, vestibular stimuli, and sometimes sound. Frequent malformations of special sense organs and facial muscles may complicate neurological evaluations or render them impossible.[50]

Although technically incorrect, some have argued that anencephalics are "brain absent," and so the brain death concept is simply not applicable. Some have argued that anencephalic infants have no capacity to reason and thus are not "persons" within the meaning of governing statutes. They may be considered nonviable fetuses. Several states have introduced bills to allow a determination of death in anencephalic infants. One approach is for states to amend their brain death acts to declare anencephalic babies brain-dead. Another approach is to change the UAGA so that the term *donor* includes those with either brain death or those who are diagnosed as anencephalic. If an anencephalic child is a person born alive, then the baby Doe handicapped infant regulations may apply, requiring "appropriate nutrition, hydration, and medication," and arguably may prevent organ procurement until natural death.

Many commentators have alluded to a "slippery slope"; that is, by creating a special category of brain death for anencephalic infants, we may be opening Pandora's box. If anencephalic babies are seen to have a marginal existence that can be sacrificed for the good of society, then who else can be sacrificed? Why not extend brain death equivalence to other handicapped infants, particularly to those who are suffering from their handicap? Why limit such rationalization to neonates? What of other brain dead–like patients, such as those in chronic persistent vegetative states? These commentators feel that the law should be consistent, that the less fortunate ought not to be treated with lesser justice. If an anencephalic infant is a person and is alive, then he or she is ethically worthy of respect and has legal rights.

The Medical Task Force on Anencephaly noted that anencephaly differs from persistent vegetative state (PVS) in that (1) anencephaly is an embryological malformation, whereas PVS is an acquired condition with various etiologies; (2) in anencephaly the extent of neurological malformation is readily demonstrable by clinical examination, whereas in PVS the extent of permanent neurological damage is not always observable; (3) anencephaly can be diagnosed with certainty, whereas the diagnosis of PVS may be problematic; (4) the prognosis for anencephaly is measured in days to weeks, but patients with PVS may live for months to years.[51]

The Medical Task Force on Anencephaly recognized four general approaches to organ procurement from infants with anencephaly: (1) The infant is immediately placed on maximal life support systems at birth, and the organs are removed as soon as possible without regard to presence or absence of brain stem function; (2) the infant is immediately placed on maximal life support systems at birth, and the organs are removed after brain stem functions are observed to stop; (3) the infant is given standard (minimal) care until he or she develops hypotension, hypoxia, bradycardia, or cardiac arrest, is placed on maximal life support systems, and the organs are removed after brain stem functions are observed to stop; (4) the infant is given standard (minimal) care until the infant dies, and then the organs are harvested. Of 34 anencephalic infants who were on transplantation protocols and could be thus categorized, the success rate for transplantation was 100% for the first approach but 0% to 11% for the other three approaches.[52]

There is a conflict of interest between the clinician's duty to maintain the health of the donor and the duty to preserve organs for a potential recipient.

Fetal tissue has uses other than for pediatric organ transplants. Fetal tissue is plastic, immunoprivileged, and available. It has been used to treat diabetes and bone marrow disorders and is a possible consideration for the treatment of Parkinson's disease, Alzheimer's disease, and almost any genetic metabolic disease.

The 1973 *Roe v. Wade* decision did not deprive the fetus of all legal protections, and subsequent regulations and judicial case law have furthered fetal rights. In particular, federal regulations regarding the protection of human subjects may apply. The 1975 Department of Health and Human Services section 46.201 states that HHS regulations apply to "research, development, and related activities involving . . . the fetus." The 1985 Health Research Extension Act prohibits federally supported research on nonviable, living fetuses *ex utero* unless (1) that research is for the benefit or health of the

fetus; (2) the research will pose no added risk of suffering, injury, or death to the fetus; and (3) the research cannot be accomplished by other means. Some states limit experimentation on aborted fetal remains, although transplantation research is arguably not research on the remains themselves, within the meaning of the statutes. The 5th Circuit Court of Appeals has declared unconstitutional Louisiana's statute prohibiting experimentation on an unborn child or a child born as a result of abortion.[53]

Potential sources of human fetal tissue include tissue from stillbirths, ectopic pregnancies, spontaneous abortions, and elective abortions. The tissue must be viable; sufficiently differentiated for use; of sufficient quantity for extraction and implantation; free from major genetic abnormalities or diseases; and free from bacterial, fungal, and viral contamination. These requirements generally render all fetal tissue useless, except that derived from elective abortions. In other words, as a practical matter, only tissue from elective abortions is of sufficient availability and quality to serve as a significant source of fetal tissue for transplantation.

On March 22, 1988, then Secretary of Health and Human Services Robert Windom, sparked by an NIH proposal to implant fetal tissue into patients with Parkinson's disease, imposed a moratorium on further NIH funding of experiments using fetal tissue, pending a report from a special NIH advisory panel to examine the medical, ethical, and legal implications of using aborted fetuses for research. After several meetings, 18 of 21 panel members concluded that the use of fetal tissue from induced abortions for transplantation research would be acceptable. The panel recommended that appropriate guidelines be established and that the decision to terminate a pregnancy be kept independent from the decision to use the tissue for research. Nonetheless, on November 2, 1989, Secretary Louis Sullivan disregarded the panel's recommendations and extended the moratorium indefinitely. He indicated that such research might provide justification for women to decide to have an abortion and would likely result in an increased incidence of abortions across the country.[54-56]

The moratorium does not affect use of fetal tissue not involving transplantation into human subjects with NIH funds. The NIH may fund research using fetal tissue from spontaneous abortions or may fund transplants of human fetal tissue (even from induced abortions) into animals. Moreover, the policy letter has no legal bearing on transplantation of any fetal tissue that is not federally funded.

Several instances of women desiring to become pregnant to supply relatives, friends, or themselves with fetal tissue have been reported. The expressed language of the UAGA authorizes a parent of an aborted fetus to donate the remains to a specific individual for transplantation. In these cases, the interests of the mother are manifestly not those of the fetus.

Concern has also been raised over a market in fetal tissue for transplantation, which might result in conceptions and abortions for profit or in manipulation of abortion decisions to the risk of pregnant women. Hana Biologicals of Alameda, California, applied to the Food and Drug Administration for permission to market fetal pancreatic tissue. Jeremy Rifkin petitioned the Department of Health and Human Services to declare such a sale prohibited by the National Organ Transplant Act. As of yet, there has been no response.[57]

The British Medical Association has promulgated guidelines on the use of fetal tissue, including the condition that tissue may be obtained only from dead fetuses resulting from therapeutic or spontaneous abortion. Death of a fetus was defined as an irreversible loss of function of the organism as a whole.[58]

LIVING RELATED DONORS: DONOR CONSENT

Legal requirements for transplantation by a living related donor primarily revolve around issues of consent of the donor for organ procurement. The rights of privacy and self-determination demand that adults of legal age and sound mind must give informed consent for donation of their organs or tissues. Competent adults should give consent voluntarily, knowingly, and intelligently after being fully informed of potential risks.

In the typical case, the HLA-matched sibling is asked to donate a kidney. The sibling may have considerable trepidation concerning the risk, pain, and disfigurement of the surgery as well as the potential future compromise of his or her remaining kidney. Although consent is usually granted, the potential donor may decide to refuse. There is no legal duty to be a Good Samaritan. Family and community pressure may significantly cloud the voluntariness of this consent. On the other hand, noncadaveric donations from people outside the family are often viewed with suspicion, and centers are reluctant to avail themselves of such opportunities.

In the case of *McFall v. Shrimp*,[59] Robert McFall, a victim of aplastic anemia and in need of a bone marrow transplant, sued to compel his cousin, David Shrimp, the only person found on initial testing to be a compatible donor, to complete his compatibility testing and, if compatible, to donate a portion of his marrow. The marrow harvest was described to Shrimp as consisting of inserting a curved needle into his hip at least 200 times. McFall's counsel argued that there is a duty to aid another in peril of his life; the court disagreed. McFall never received a transplant and died shortly thereafter.

In the case of a vital organ transplant, a psychiatric or psychological assessment of the donor and donee may be advisable to negate possible future allegations of duress and also because of the high rates of psychiatric morbidity and suicide in recipients.

Organ donors have failed in their suits against transplant surgeons because of the absence of a physician-patient relationship.

In *Sirianni v. Anna*,[60] a mother, who donated a kidney to her son after his kidneys were negligently removed by a surgeon, was not allowed to recover against the surgeon for her impairment of health, which she sustained as a result of the loss of her kidney. She undertook the operation with full knowledge of the consequences.

INCOMPETENT DONORS

In the case of minors and incompetents (e.g., mentally retarded persons), a court order is usually necessary for the organ transplantation. Although parents and guardians may generally consent to medical treatment of their children and wards, it is not clear that they have the same authority when surgery is not medically indicated. As a practical matter, most surgeons refuse to perform such surgery without a court order. The consent of guardians or parents is often additionally sought, but the court may overcome their refusal.

In most cases involving intrafamilial transplants, judicial approval has been granted. Often judges have conducted these hearings in chambers, and, if so, have almost always allowed the harvest procedure and foregone the need for a written explanation of the court's findings. Even where a record is present, courts have not always articulated well the basis for their decision. Perhaps this is best categorized as simple judicial approval of parental consent.

In a 1972 Connecticut case, *Hart v. Brown*,[61] the court approved a transplant between two identical 7-year-old twins, considered the medical ramifications, and stated that the parents' motivation and reasoning had met with approval of the guardians ad litem, physicians, clergymen, and the court itself.

Courts also invoke the equitable doctrine of *parens patriae* to give consent on behalf of minors and incompetents. The court often appoints a guardian ad litem in such cases to argue on behalf of the incompetent.

If the court focuses on the interests of the potential donor with a protective eye, it may find that there is no objective reason for the donor to submit to the risk and bodily intrusion of an organ harvest. Indeed, it has been argued that the court has no power to authorize the surgery in the absence of specific enabling legislation.

In the 1973 Louisiana case, *In re Richardson*,[62] a husband brought suit against his wife to compel her consent to the removal of a kidney from their mentally retarded child for donation to the boy's older sister. The 4th Circuit Court held that neither the parents nor the courts could authorize surgical intrusion on a mentally retarded minor for the purpose of donating organs, that such would invade the minor's right to freedom from bodily intrusion and that it was not shown to be in the minor's best interest.

In 1975, the Supreme Court of Wisconsin in *In re Guardianship of Pescinski*[63] held that the court had no power to compel a 39-year-old catatonic schizophrenic to donate a kidney to a 38-year-old sister in the absence of any showing of benefit to the incompetent: "[An] incompetent particularly should have his own interests protected. Certainly no advantage should be taken of him." Medical testimony indicated that the risk to the donor at that time was one death in 4000 kidney transplants. The dissent stated that requirement of consent was inappropriate as applied to an incompetent without lucid intervals.

Other courts have authorized donation by applying a "best interest" test and finding psychological benefit (or absence of detriment) and asserting consent.

In a 1979 Texas case, *Little v. Little,*[64] a mother sought judicial consent for the removal of a kidney from her 14-year-old daughter with Down's syndrome for her son. The guardian was opposed. The mother argued that the daughter was the only suitable donor for her brother, that there was no threat to her life, and that the daughter would have wanted this for her ill brother. Medical testimony alleged that the daughter was a "perfect match," despite the fact that brother and sister were not identical twins, and that the chances of finding a suitable cadaver kidney was extremely remote. The judge authorized the transplant on the basis of "substantial psychological benefit" to the donor.

Courts have increasingly utilized the doctrine of "substituted judgment" to decide cases of sticky ethical issues in medical cases involving incompetents. Specifically, the court must substitute itself, as nearly as possible, for the incompetent, to act with the same motives and considerations as would have moved the incompetent.

In 1969, in *Strunk v. Strunk,*[65] the mother of a 27-year-old mentally retarded male with an IQ of 35 petitioned the court for a kidney removal to be used for his 28-year-old brother. The court, based on psychiatric testimony that the death of the donor's brother would have an extremely traumatic effect on the donor, allowed the transplantation to avoid the detriment. The court reached this result despite testimony from the director of the renal division at the local institution that if something happened to the retarded donor's remaining kidney, he would not meet the selection criteria necessary for hemodialysis or transplantation. The dissent stated that "it is common knowledge that the loss of a close relative or a friend to a six-year-old is not of major importance. Opinions concerning psychological trauma are at best most nebulous."

CONFIDENTIALITY OF POTENTIAL DONORS

Potential donors are often HLA-matched to attempt to find an immunocompatible host and thereby achieve a greater chance of graft survival. Modern immunosuppressive therapies generally obviate this need except in the case of bone marrow transplantation. The need for matched organs has given rise to expensive HLA registries. There is great pressure to give out names of those matching phenotypes to potential recipients.

In the case of *Head v. Colloton,*[66] the plaintiff, William Head, was a leukemia victim who sued to demand disclosure of the only potential donor who had a matching HLA type in the institution's bone marrow transplant registry. The potential donor had been HLA-typed as a possible platelet donor for an ill family member. She was telephoned by the registry and asked in general terms if she would be interested in being a bone marrow donor, whereupon she responded that she would be interested only if it was for a family member. The court maintained the anonymity of the potential donor and refused further inquiry, but did so on narrow legal grounds relating to the interpretation of the Iowa Freedom of Information Act. The plaintiff died during the court proceedings without having had a marrow transplant.

Names of potential donors should be placed on registries with the informed consent of the donors who should be able to withdraw their names at any time. Disclosures should be restricted to necessarily involved medical personnel only.

ARTIFICIAL AND ANIMAL TRANSPLANTS

In the immediate future, artificial organs and heterografts (except porcine heart valves) will continue to play only a minor role in transplantation and will remain largely experimental. Baboon hearts and livers have always been rejected and thus have fallen from favor. Artificial hearts also have a poor overall record but may be used for temporary replacement until a human transplant can be performed. Left ventricular assist devices, on the other hand, have become popular.

Failure to obtain adequate informed consent has been a major criticism of most pioneering efforts. Today, this issue is better recognized, and more appropriate consent procedures are being followed. All human experimentation must be reviewed by a medical institutional internal review board (IRB). The first artificial heart transplant precipitated a lawsuit, *Karp v. Cooley,*[67] which remains the leading authority on the issue of informed consent for an experimental therapy.

There are special considerations regarding artificial

organs. The Medical Device Amendment[68] was enacted in 1976 to ensure the safety of medical devices and subjects manufacturers of artificial organs placed into interstate commerce to complex regulations. The DHHS and the FDA have responsibility to promulgate regulations under this act. These regulations were not enforced in cases of early artificial heart transplants but have since been and will continue to be enforced. Another consideration is the possible application of strict product liability to these implants.

DONOR SCREENING

Donors must be screened to determine suitability of donation. Transmission of disease from an organ or tissue donation is relatively rare (except for cytomegalovirus infection, which is likely to be of little consequence). Transplantation personnel must maintain constant vigilance against bacterial and fungal infections from organs and tissue derived from septic patients and from contamination during handling. The implant itself may act as a nidus for infection. Other serious disease that can be transmitted via transplantation include cancer or infections from the human immunodeficiency virus (HIV), hepatitis B, tuberculosis, toxoplasmosis, and Jakob-Creutzfeldt disease. Also, the organ itself may be impaired by nontransmissible disease such as atherosclerosis.

Screening for transmissible disease involves chart review, specific laboratory tests, and examination of the donor. The United Network for Organ Sharing, discussed later in this chapter, requires documentation of certain tests and evaluations as minimal acceptable standards for an independent organ procurement agency.

Inadequate screening can give rise to litigation. Ordinary negligence liability results if the disease or defect is discoverable by standard medical practices. Failure to test for HIV antibody would be a breach of standard medical practice in cases of heart transplantation, but it would result in liability only if the donee subsequently developed an HIV infection. If there were no results available by the time a transplantation would need to proceed, liability might not attach because a court might find that a surgeon acted reasonably. However, a court may find that the brain-dead cadaver should have been maintained until a result could have been obtained or that if a risk factor were present in the donor's record the donation ought to have been declined. Liability should not attach if, as is known to happen, HIV is transmitted despite a negative HIV antibody test; donor screening is imperfect. Faulty testing or specimen mixups may result in incompatible organs being transplanted, in which case liability is likely. The immunity statutes previously mentioned may pro-

tect an organ procurement agency or a transplantation team.

In *Ravenis v. Detroit General Hosp.,*[69] the hospital was found negligent in two cases in which patients lost the sight remaining in an eye following transplantation of an infected cornea transplant. No hospital official was responsible for selection, slit-lamp examinations were not performed despite availability of equipment, and the appropriate information for the surgeon to determine the unsuitability of the tissue for transplantation was missing from the patient's chart.

FEDERAL LEGISLATION

Health matters are generally the province of state law. Because of ongoing developments in the field, the need for centralized national allocation of organs, and funding issues, the federal government has become increasingly involved in transplantation. The federal government has attempted to enhance and coordinate private and local government initiatives, such as sponsoring the establishment in 1983 of the American Council on Transplantation, a group of private-sector organizations and individuals to promote organ donation (recently dissolved).

The National Organ and Transplantation Act was enacted in 1984.[70] It called for the creation of a national Organ Procurement and Transplantation Network (OPTN) to match prospective donors to prospective recipients, the creation of a special advisory task force, and the prohibition of the sale of organs.

The network, the heart of the law, was to create a fair and equitable system of organ allocation that could optimize matches between organs and patients anywhere in the country. The original intent was to accomplish this by facilitating regional independent organ procurement agencies (IOPAs). Grants for the establishment of new procurement agencies and the improvement of existing procurement agencies were authorized to form an adequate base of a truly national network. This network was then to "assist organ procurement organizations in the distribution of organs which cannot be placed" locally, to develop organ procurement standards, and to help coordinate transport.

The United Network for Organ Sharing (UNOS), a private nonprofit entity solely devoted to organ procurement and transplantation, was awarded the federal contract to run the OPTN in September 1986. Federal oversight of UNOS is provided by the Division of Organ Transplantation under the Health Resources and Services Administration, within the Public Health Service and the DHHS.

The Task Force on Organ Transplantation was created by Secretary Heckler in January 1985. It rendered its final report in April 1986 and was dissolved.

The 78 recommendations largely define federal policy.

The Omnibus Budget and Reconciliation Act (OBRA) of 1986[71] built on the 1984 legislation and the Task Force recommendations by amending the Social Security Act. First, it mandated as Medicare and Medicaid conditions of participation that hospitals institutionalize a "required request" policy (as previously explained) to increase the voluntary supply of organs. Second, also as Medicare and Medicaid funding requirements, it stated that hospitals performing transplantations must be members and must abide by the rules and policies of the OPTN (i.e., UNOS).

The statutory requirement that transplantation centers must be members and abide by the OPTN gives UNOS great regulatory power. In fact, UNOS is considered by many to be a unique experiment in self-regulation within the health care field. UNOS requirements are more stringent than DHHS regulations. The policies of UNOS, equivalent to conditions of participation, are subject to review and approval by the DHHS and are subjected to public "notice and comment" in the *Federal Register.* Despite lip service to the contrary, the system appears to operate in a very centralized manner, rather than the flexible, pluralistic decentralized system originally envisioned in the 1984 Transplant Act.[72]

Membership in UNOS as a qualified IOPA was a great organizational challenge. The task force recommended that competition between organ procurement organizations be discouraged. IOPAs were required to have defined and exclusive service areas. The response was for all IOPAs in given areas to merge into single entities. As of 1990 it appears that this has been accomplished; a true regional system of IOPAs is in place across the nation. Anticipated litigation never materialized.

Membership in UNOS as a transplantation center qualified by procedure will continue to be problematic. To become members new programs must already have performed a particular procedure many times, which is almost impossible without federal funding. Thus the UNOS membership guidelines tend to entrench existing members who helped establish the guidelines. The governmental umbrella that UNOS enjoys might to some extent shield its members from antitrust considerations.

Sale of organs

The National Organ Transplant Act of 1984 prohibited the transfer of "any human organ for valuable consideration if the transfer affects interstate commerce."[73] The term *human organ* is defined as the human kidney, liver, heart, lung, pancreas, bone marrow, cornea, eye, bone, skin, and any other organ included by the Secretary of the DHHS for regulation. It is not intended to include replenishable tissues such as blood

or semen. The term *valuable consideration* does not include the "reasonable" payment associated with removal, transportation, implantation, processing, preservation, quality control, and storage, or the expenses of travel, housing, or lost wages in connection with donation of the organ.

The commerce clause reflects an attempt to fit the regulation into the federal constitutional commerce powers. This language, in other situations, has been interpreted so broadly as to include almost any interstate or intrastate transaction. Nonetheless, several states have also passed such prohibitions.

A 38-year-old leukemia victim needed a bone marrow transplant, but could not find a suitable donor. His older brother was homeless and earned money by serving as a subject in medical experiments. He initially refused to be tested for compatibility. An anonymous donor offered him $1000 to undergo testing and $2000 to donate. He was tested and was found not to be an HLA match. If he had matched, the prohibition against "the transfer of any human organ for valuable consideration" arguably would have been applicable and would have barred his marrow donation to his brother.[74]

Food and Drug Administration

The FDA has jurisdiction over tissue banking and has maintained a task force on transplantation since 1983. The regulation of the safety and efficacy of human tissue is analogous to regulation of manufactured materials for use in therapy. The agency is developing proposals for regulating cryopreserved semen, dura mater, and heart valves. The FDA is not concerned with solid organs except possibly for disease transmission by improper screening of donors. The FDA is also concerned with organ perfusion solutions.[75]

On October 5, 1993, the U.S. House of Representatives passed H.R. 2659, the Organ and Bone Marrow Transplantation Amendments of 1993, to revise and extend programs relating to the transplantation of organs and bone marrow. The proposals would amend 42 U.S.C., Sections 273 and 274. The amendments would extend for three fiscal years the authorization of appropriations for the National Organ Transplant Act (NOTA), authorizing the expenditure of 20 million dollars in fiscal year 1994 and "such funds as may be necessary" in fiscal years 1995 and 1996. This legislation, which is administered by the Health Resources and Services Administration of the DHHS, made the following changes to strengthen the organ transplantation system and to assure more effectively the equity and effectiveness of organ procurement and allocation procedures.

The Secretary of Health and Human Services is required to issue regulations establishing enforceable procedures for the procurement, allocation, and transplantation of solid organs and bone marrow. Such regulations also would establish that criteria that must be satisfied for membership in OPTN. In issuing such regulations, the secretary is directed to take into consideration existing policies and guidelines issued by UNOS and the National Bone Marrow Registry.

The secretary is required to review and approve any changes in the amount of patient registration fees imposed by the private contractor administering the system of solid organ procurement.

Organ allocation policies of the OPTN and the member organ procurement organizations (OPOs) are required to maintain for each solid organ a single list of patients referred for transplants, and give preference to patients who are U.S. citizens or permanent resident aliens. Other foreign nationals may receive an organ from an unrelated donor only if no U.S. citizen or permanent resident alien is found to be a medically appropriate recipient of such organ.

Expansion of the system of patient advocacy for bone marrow transplant patients is provided with an inclusion for case management services. The General Accounting Office is required to perform studies of the National Marrow Donor Program.

Last, the Secretary of Health and Human Services is required to study the feasibility, fairness, and enforceability of allocating solid organs to patients based solely on the clinical need of the patient involved and the viability of organs involved.

Legislation and administrative rule-making in the areas of organ donation and transplantation are undergoing continual revisions. The reader is recommended to consult the appropriate federal and state reference source materials, in addition to current medical-legal periodicals to keep apprised of these revisions and updates.

SELECTION OF ORGAN RECIPIENTS

The scarce supply of organs and tissues relative to demand, as well as the economic considerations of transplantation, thrust grave ethical decisions concerning rationing on the medical community. The allocation of organs must be perceived by the public to be fair and equitable or else the national organ and tissue supply (which depends on voluntary contributions) will be jeopardized.

Regulation of recipient selection for organs is now imposed nationally through funding requirements. The National Organ Transplant Act of 1984 created the OPTN for the equitable distribution of all available organs in the United States.[76] The Omnibus Budget Reconciliation Act (OBRA) of 1986 now requires all hospitals to abide by the policies of the OPTN as

conditions of Medicare/Medicaid payment.[77] The federal OPTN contract was awarded to UNOS.

The basis of the UNOS system is a computerized point system for allocation. The point system is an objective method of patient selection determined primarily by probability of success, time on the waiting list, logistic factors, and medical need, modified from the proposal by Starzl.[78] Variances can be granted for "fair patient selection criteria" to accommodate local concerns.

Kidneys require more stringent testing than other solid organs because potential donees can be maintained on dialysis while awaiting an optimal kidney. "Tragic choices" must be made for nonpaired vital organs. Kidneys will be offered first to the recipient located anywhere in the country who has a perfect antigenic match. Only 15% to 25% of kidneys will have such a match. Otherwise, cadaveric kidneys will be allocated on a point system based on time of waiting, quality of antigen match, and panel-reactive antibody screen. Medical urgency is not considered for kidney allocation.

Extrarenal organs will be allocated based on organ size, ABO typing, time of waiting, degree of medical urgency, and logistic factors. Pancreata will be offered solely on the basis of distance to a potential recipient and time on a waiting list.

Pediatric organs and patients are given special consideration. Dual transplants (e.g., kidney-pancreas simultaneous transplants) are also handled outside the usual schema.

Patients on local waiting lists are offered organs in descending sequence with the highest number of points receiving the highest priority. Only if an organ is not accepted locally will it be offered regionally, and then nationally. Organ sharing arrangements between interregional and intraregional OPOs may be entered into on approval of UNOs. The OPTN (UNOS) patient waiting list is open only to direct UNOS-member OPOs, and such members cannot offer organs to non-UNOS–member transplantation centers. A potential recipient may be placed on multiple listings, even though it is known to confer some advantage.

The final decision to accept an offered organ remains the prerogative of the transplantation surgeon and/or physician responsible for the care of the patient. A transplantation center has one hour to accept an offered organ, or the offering procurement agency will be free to offer the organ to another recipient.

The issue of whether the patient with the greatest chance of survival or the one with the greatest urgency should receive an organ has been a source of continuing debate. The very fact that a potential heart recipient deteriorates and becomes suddenly much more ill means that he or she is at once more critically in need of a new heart and less likely to survive the transplantation. This question is largely moot with respect to kidneys, because patients can be placed on dialysis (except in the rare case of exhaustion of vascular access sites). However, the issue of deterioration is paramount with respect to hearts and livers. Limited points are given to heart and liver patients for urgency in the UNOS system.

Highly sensitized patients or "responders" are patients who have antibodies against most histocompatibility antigens. A negative crossmatch may give a responder his or her only chance to receive a surviving transplantation. However, the chance of organ acceptance is lower than for similarly matched nonresponders. The transplantation community generally feels an obligation to offer to this patient his or her last small chance at a tolerable organ.

Matching is a significant criterion, based on sound immunological principles. HLA compatibility is unavoidably discriminatory to blacks and Hispanics (who have a several times higher rate of end-stage renal disease) because most available kidneys have been donated by whites. On the basis of histocompatibility alone, most kidneys from large urban centers would go elsewhere to white suburban areas. HLA compatibility is of debatable significance to other organs.

Other criteria, such as age and lifestyle, although not a part of the UNOS point system, may be locally operative. Valid medical justifications for these gray areas exist; for instance, is a young patient a better surgical risk than an alcoholic who continues to drink and is likely to damage the new liver and not likely to take medications regularly? However, discrimination based on age or social position raises issues of fairness. Such subjective criteria are also prone to capriciousness. These do not seem to be primary selection criteria.

After a patient receives a transplant, he or she is usually given greater consideration for a subsequent organ, but the chances for long-term success fall as a patient receives more transplants.

As mentioned in the last section, persons from other countries may not simply come to the United States and pay for a transplant and deplete our national organ resources. Payment for organs per se is now prohibited. Currently aliens are held to about 5% of current waiting lists, but those on the lists are to be treated like American citizens and not to be discriminated against based on political influence, national origin, race, sex, religion, or financial status. UNOS members are not to enter into contractual arrangements with foreign agencies or governments or perform transplants on nonresident aliens for financial advantage. Exportation and importation of organs are to be strictly arranged and coordinated through UNOS. Although thousands are maintained on the United States waiting lists, several hundred kidneys are shipped abroad because they are unacceptably old by rigorous U.S. standards.

Lawsuits can be filed against hospitals, transplant surgeons, and committees on behalf of patients who fail to obtain vital organs because others have received the organs first. This is increasingly likely because criteria might be attacked as arbitrary, capricious, or otherwise unreasonable. The implication that one recipient is chosen over another for financial reasons might be argued as an illegal sale of an organ and thus a basis of liability. Another problem area involves cases in which a sudden decline in health precipitates a recipient's "jumping the queue," being ranked higher priority, and receiving an organ that would have gone to another, whereas the sudden deterioration may suggest a poorer prognosis (meanwhile others in the queue are at increasing risk for sudden death). The potential liability for choosing between who shall live and die is enormous, and the absence of suits to date is surprising.

COST AND PAYMENT CONSIDERATIONS

The expense of vital organ transplantation is enormous. The approximate range for a typical kidney transplant is $25,000 to $30,000; for a heart transplant procedure, $57,000 to $110,000; for a heart-lung transplant, $130,000 to $200,000; for a liver transplant, $135,000 to $238,000; and for a pancreas transplant, $30,000 to $100,000.[79] Perhaps the most expensive single item is the cost for time spent in the intensive care unit.

Transplantation failures and ancillary costs (such as transportation and lodging for the patient and family when the patient does not live near the transplantation center) markedly elevate these figures. Almost all vital organ transplant patients require lifetime maintenance on immunosuppressant therapy, although this may be changing. The cost of conventional immunosuppression maintenance (steroids and azathioprine) averages $1000 to $2000 per year and for cyclosporine, $5000 to $7000 per year. (However, because cyclosporine decreases overall complications, it does not raise overall costs. The Omnibus Budget and Reconciliation Act of 1986 enabled Medicare and Medicaid to cover outpatient immunosuppressive therapy, particularly cyclosporine, for one year after transplant.[80] Before it was repealed, catastrophic health insurance legislation also provided coverage of immunosuppressive agents.)

The cost of transplantation is, of course, generally prohibitive for individuals, and they must rely on third-party reimbursement. Furthermore, many, if not most of those in need of a solid organ transplant, are incapable of employment. Thus transplants can be viewed as treatment for a catastrophic life-threatening illness.

It is instructive to look at the Medicare End-Stage Renal Disease Program (ESRDP) established in 1972 to provide treatment to kidney-failure victims regardless of their ability to pay.[81] This was the first disease specifically singled out for funding through its own special program by the federal government. The cost of the ESRDP, primarily for long-term dialysis, continues to escalate as the number of beneficiaries accumulates; it is presently 70,000 people.[82] Current expenditures are estimated to be over $2 billion per year. This is far greater than anticipated, and the ESRDP is often pointed to as an expensive program run amok.[83,84]

Kidney transplants are easily shown to be cost-effective, with the initial large investment generally being paid back in four years, when compared with the alternative, hemodialysis. The long-term costs of maintaining patients with functioning grafts are only one-third of those for dialysis patients.[85,86] Furthermore, the quality of life is improved and allows more people to become productive citizens again. There is no alternative for heart or liver transplants.

It has been estimated that a national heart transplant program would cost $5 billion annually for an anticipated 17,000 to 35,000 patients.[87] A national liver transplant program would cost an additional $1 billion annually for an estimated 5000 patients.

In this era of cost containment, many find it hard to justify the expense of transplantation for the few, while sacrificing more widespread financing of health care. The juggernaut is difficult to stop because our society finds it difficult to deny individual pleas for a specific and lifesaving treatment. Increasingly, the federal government is looked to for subsidization of transplants, but federal fiscal restraints will make this difficult.

At present the costs of transplantation are high, but not higher than the costs of taking care of the typical AIDS patient or cancer patient, and the results are much better. As a result of the organ shortage, the total costs to the government are now relatively low and predictable. However, the government's ability to pay for organ transplants may not continue, particularly because of a growth in the supply of organs, increase in demand, and technological innovations, such as usable artificial organs. Over time, pressures will undoubtedly grow to relax the standards for patient reimbursement. The history of the ESRDP demonstrates this process of ever more lenient selection standards tending toward universal access.

Medicare pays for kidney transplants and heart transplants (as of 1987) if the patient has been unable to work for at least two years because of the heart condition, and liver transplants in children under seven years of age with biliary atresia. Kidney transplants constitute approximately 80% of all organ transplants, and so the federal government funds the bulk of transplantation efforts. Medicare does not pay for

procedures it considers to be experimental. Based on a report by the Office of Health Technology Assessment that liver transplants are no longer experimental, the HCFA reported in the March 8, 1990, *Federal Register* that it will begin to pay for some adult liver transplants, including those needed because of alcoholic cirrhosis, but excluding any end-stage liver disease produced by a chemical or toxic agent or hepatitis B antigen-positive cirrhotic disease.[88]

States pay for transplantation procedures for low-income persons through Medicaid (subsidized by the federal government). The states vary greatly in their coverage and payment policies: 48 states pay for residual kidney costs, 40 for liver transplants, 32 for heart transplants, 15 for heart-lung transplants, and 8 for pancreas transplants.[89] Furthermore, 47 states pay for outpatient immunosuppressive drugs, and 35 pay for organ procurement services.[90]

Under Medicare and Medicaid (and most private health insurance plans) the funding eligibility trigger is "medical necessity" for the treatment. Thus the government will pay for a transplantation if, like other medical therapy, it can be shown that the procedure is reasonable and necessary for the illness and that such treatment is not experimental.

Patients have successfully sued for reimbursement from state agencies when policies or administrative regulations have unfairly denied coverage. In *Brillo v. Arizona*,[91] Mrs. Brillo successfully sued the state to provide coverage for her liver transplantation. The service director's policy determination was that the state would not pay for adult liver transplants because they were experimental, although they would pay for pediatric liver transplants. The court found the policy to be arbitrary and capricious, and a denial of equal protection of the law.

In *Allen v. Mansour*,[92] the Michigan court ordered Medicaid funding for an alcoholic with cirrhosis, holding that the recipient selection criterion of a two-year abstinence from alcohol in cases of cirrhosis owing to alcoholism was arbitrary and unreasonable as formulated and applied. The court noted that this criterion was developed on meager experience and that "medical necessity of the procedure is the touchstone for evaluating the reasonableness of standards in state Medicaid plans."

In *Lee v. Page,* the Florida Medicaid program refused to fund a liver transplant to be performed at the University of Nebraska for a medically qualified 26-year-old woman with a "fatal liver disease." The state's position was that the high cost of the liver transplant procedure, which would divert substantial funds from other needy persons, and the minimal benefit to the population of all eligible recipients made the refusal to pay reasonable. The court indicated that states have considerable leeway to implement federally backed Medicaid programs. States must adopt "reasonable standards," but they cannot exclude coverage for "medically necessary" treatments. A state can legitimately argue in support of its refusal to fund a treatment as unnecessary either because the treatment is experimental or because it is inappropriate. The court held that liver transplantation is no longer experimental. Then the court held that an unfavorable cost/benefit determination is not a medical appropriateness criterion and thus is not a reasonable standard from which to refuse funding:

> This is not a question of the limits on the amount Medicaid will pay for a procedure, but rather a case where Medicaid refuses to pay the entire amount based on the cost of the procedure. . . . [States] cannot eliminate one health-related service while leaving others intact. . . . It does not appear that federal law permits Florida to refuse to fund all liver transplants. . . . Florida voluntarily entered the federal Medicaid cooperative program and must comply with the standards.[93]

In *Todd v. Sorrell*,[94] a Virginia child was determined to be a suitable candidate for a liver transplantation by the Children's Hospital of Pittsburgh. Eighty-five percent of the child's liver had been removed because of cancer, and secondary biliary cirrhosis had developed. The hospital required an advance payment ($162,000). The Virginia Medicaid program refused to pay because its policy was to pay for pediatric liver transplants in cases of biliary atresia but for no other diseases. The U.S. Court of Appeals for the 4th Circuit overturned the district court's holding and granted an injunction ordering the state to pay for the transplantation pending a final three-judge panel review. Nonetheless, citing the high costs of liver transplants ($250,000), other priorities, and the poor outcomes of liver transplants, Virginia decided to stop Medicaid funding of all liver transplants (May 1988).

Oregon decided to not spend any Medicaid monies on transplantations except for kidneys and corneas. It reversed its controversial stand after an enormous storm of public protest was raised.[95,96]

MALPRACTICE SUITS

For a number of reasons malpractice suits involving transplantation of vital organs have been almost nonexistent. First, in the past transplantations were considered largely experimental, and as such customary standards were not well established. Second, failure was a well-recognized risk. Third, the careful attention by physicians in these cases resulted in generally good relationships and good communication with patients and their families. Fourth, the surgeons and institutions involved were of high stature and esteem. Fifth, the physicians practicing this art were few and closely knit, making opposition testimony difficult to find. Sixth, damages were difficult to prove, given the ill health of the patients. However, a marked increase in suits may be anticipated in the future because these conditions will no longer hold true as vital organ transplants become commonplace.

In *McDermott v. Manhattan Eye, Ear & Throat Hosp.*,[97] the appellate court reversed a lower court's finding of negligent corneal transplant, holding that there was insufficient evidence to support a malpractice claim that the surgeon lacked the skill or experience to perform the operation, that the operation was of extreme delicacy with a high incidence of failure, and that the situation was one of desperation.

The degree to which courts are reluctant to find liability in favor of transplant efforts can be found in *State of Missouri ex rel. Wichita Falls General Hosp. v. Adolph*.[98,99] A Missouri transplant team flew to Wichita Falls, Texas, to harvest a heart from a donor and then returned to Missouri to transplant the heart into a recipient. During the transplant they discovered that the Texas hospital had incorrectly typed the donor as type A rather than type B. The patient died shortly thereafter, despite a second transplant. A Missouri appeals court refused to let a Missouri trial court assert jurisdiction over a Texas hospital for fear of a chilling effect on future transplants.

Several problem areas are particularly likely to be litigated in the future, especially the issues of informed consent and suitability of the organ for transplant.

Theoretically, strict liability (in which the court may award damages without a finding of fault by the defendant) might apply to injuries sustained from implants of diseased or defective organs as an unreasonably dangerous defective product or from an implied warranty. Plaintiffs in early cases of hepatitis and adverse reactions to transfusions of blood and blood products successfully argued theories of strict liability. Later decisions rejected the notion, holding that provision of blood is a service and not the sale of a product.

Most states now have statutes that specifically protect hospitals and blood banks from strict liability. Such laws hold that transfusions of blood and blood products are not sales and hence no warranties attach and that liability may be imposed only for negligence or willful misconduct. Many statutes further include transplantations of other tissues and organs in these provisions. The states that specifically mention blood but fail to mention other tissues and organs might risk the interpretation that their legislatures intended to exclude organ transplantations from such protection. Otherwise, strict liability is unlikely to be applied to organ transplantation, because transplantation will be construed to be a hospital and physician service instead of the sale of a product, in light of the blood banking court decisions and the federal and state proscriptions against sales of organs. Statutory immunity conferred by the UAGA might also apply to negligent procedures, as was discussed above.

RECENT DEVELOPMENTS

The House of Delegates of the American Medical Association (AMA) on December 7, 1993, adopted a report from the Council on Ethical and Judicial Affairs that was subsequently revised in response to comments received from peer reviewers.[100] This report recommended that mandated choice, in which individuals would be required to state their preferences regarding organ donation when they renew their drivers' licenses, file income tax returns, or perform some other task mandated by the state, should be pursued by the AMA in working with state medical societies to draft model legislation for adoption by state legislatures. The Report raised ethical objections to the alternative of presumed consent in which it is assumed that an individual would consent to be an organ donor at death unless an objection from the individual prior to death, or from their next-of-kin after death, is known to the health care provider. A federal circuit court has adopted this approach.[101] In this case the circuit court of appeals, in reversing the district court, determined that a widow could maintain a civil rights action filed against the coroner based on his removal of the decedent husband's corneas for their use for transplantation without the widow's consent, in that consent was presumed to be present when the coroner claimed a lack of knowledge as to any objection to such removal of organs for transplantation prior to performing the procedure.

Recent dialogue between medical examiners and transplant coordinators in cooperating to maximize the lawful retrieval of organs and tissues for transplantation is occurring.[102,103] Representatives from the Association of Organ Procurement Organizations, the North American Transplant Coordinators Organization, the American Society of Transplant Surgeons, and the National Association of Medical Examiners have met for the purpose of agreeing on guidelines for their respective members. This need for cooperative efforts is underscored by estimates that currently approximately one suitable transplant candidate in this country is dying every four hours for lack of a suitable organ for recommended transplantation. These guidelines are needed to protect concerns that forensic evidence will not be lost or affected by the subsequent transplantation surgery. The results of a retrospective study during the years 1990 through 1992 of information received from responding organ procurement organizations in this country indicated that as many as 2979 individuals may have been denied transplants due to medical examiner denials.[104] Such denials were generally the result of a perceived need by the medical examiner to preserve forensic evidence that could later be necessary in documenting the cause of death of an individual.

In today's managed care medical practice environment with intensified scrutiny of health care costs, questions have been raised as to the possible current surplus of transplantation centers in this country. At the first joint annual meeting of UNOS and the DHSS Division of Organ Transplantation such questions were discussed.[105] Statistics presented indicated that 40% of kidney transplant centers were performing fewer than 25 transplants a year, and that 40% of liver transplant centers were performing fewer than 15 transplants per year, accounting for only 8% of livers transplanted in the nation. In contrast, statistics were presented indicating that the 20 largest liver transplant centers were performing 76% of the liver transplants in the nation. Some evidence presented indicated that a better outcome occurred from centers that had a higher volume of cases. Therefore, performance criteria were suggested as a basis for determining whether a new transplant program should be approved, or whether an existing program should be allowed to continue with government support. It was also pointed out at this joint meeting that the cost of a transplant generally goes down as the volume of cases increases at a center. The future of the availability of nearby transplant centers for many citizens will of necessity be determined by these considerations.

END NOTES

1. *Transplant Statistics* [fact sheet from information packet], UNOS. Richmond, Va., undated (1990).
2. *Eye Banking Activity: 1988* (Eye Bank Association of America, Washington, D.C. 1990).
3. National Task Force on Organ Transplantation, *Organ Transplantation: Issues and Recommendations* (U.S. Dept. of Health and Human Services, Washington, D.C., GPO# 1986 O-160-709, 1986).
4. *Supra* note 1.
5. *Supra* note 1.
6. *Supra* note 2.
7. *Supra* note 3.
8. *Supra* note 3.
9. Uniform Anatomical Gift Act (1968), National Conference of Commissioners on Uniform State Laws, Chicago, Ill. (1968).
10. Uniform Anatomical Gift Act (1987), National Conference of Commissioners on Uniform State Laws, Chicago, Ill. (1987); 8A ULA 16, 1989 (Suppl.).
11. *New Developments in Biotechnology: Ownership of Human Tissues and Cells — Special Report* (Office of Technology Assessment, U.S. Government Printing Office, Washington, D.C. 1987).
12. P. Matthews, *Whose Property?: People as Property.* Current Legal Problems 193-239 (1983).
13. *In re Moyer's Estate,* 577 P.2d 108 (1978).

14. *Holland v. Metalious,* 198 A.2d 654 (1964).
15. *Leno v. St Joseph Hosp.* 302 N.E.2d 58 (1973).
16. *Nicoletta v. Rochester Eye and Human Parts Bank,* 519 N.Y.S. 2d 928 (1987).
17. *Williams v. Hofmann,* 223 N.W.2d 844 (1974).
18. *Ravenis v. Detroit General Hosp.,* 234 N.W.2d 411 (1976).
19. *Supra* note 10.
20. Maximus, Inc., *Assessment of the Potential Organ Donor Pool: Report to Health Resources and Services Agency* (Washington, D.C., Department of Health and Human Services 1985).
21. *Organ Transplantation Q & A* (U.S. Dept. of Health and Human Services, Division of Organ Transplantation, Washington D.C., DHHS Pub. No. (HRS-M-SP) 89-1, 1988).
22. K. J. Bart, et al., *Increasing the Supply of Cadaveric Kidneys for Transplantation,* 31 Transplantation 383-87 (1981).
23. S. W. Tolle, et al., *Responsibilities of Primary Physicians in Organ Donation,* 106 Ann. Int. Med. 740-44 (1987).
24. J. Prottas, *The Structure and Effectiveness of the U.S. Organ Procurement System,* 22 Inquiry 365-76 (1985).
25. J. M. Prottas, *The Organization of Organ Procurement,* 14 J. Health Politics, Pol. & L. 41-55 (1989).
26. A. L. Caplan, *Professional Arrogance and Public Misunderstanding,* 18 Hasting Center Report 34-37 (1988).
27. S. J. Youngner et al., *Brain Death and Organ Retrieval,* 261 JAMA 2205-10.
28. J. Prottas and H. L. Batten, *Health Professionals and Hospital Administrators in Organ Procurement: Attitudes, Reservations, and Their Resolution,* 78 Am J Pub Health 642-45 (1988).
29. A. Caplan, *Ethical and Policy Issues in the Procurement of Cadaver Organs for Transplantation,* 314 N. Engl. J. Med. 981-83 (1984).
30. J. F. Childress, *Ethical Criteria for Procuring and Distributing Organs for Transplantation,* 14 J. Health Politics, Pol. & L. 87-113 (1989).
31. Omnibus Budget Reconciliation Act (OBRA) of 1986, Pub. L. 99-509, §9318 amending Title XI of the Social Security Act adding §1138, Hospital protocols for organ procurement and standards for organ procurement agencies [H.R. 5300]; further clarification in 53(40) *Federal Register* 6526-51 (Mar. 1, 1988).
32. Joint Commission on Accreditation of Healthcare Organizations Standards, MA.1.4.13 & MA.1.4.14 (1988).
33. V. W. Weedn and B. Leveque, *Routine Inquiry for Organ and Tissue Donations,* 84 Tex. Med. 30-37 (1988).
34. *Transplant Action* (American Council on Transplantation, Alexandria, Va. July-August 1989).
35. A. Caplan, *Organ Procurement: It's Not in the Cards,* 14 Hastings Center Report 9-12 (1984).
36. *Supra* note 33.
37. *Powell v. Florida,* 497 So.2d 1188, 1986, *cert. denied,* 107 SC 2202 (1986).
38. *Georgia Lions Eye Bank v. Lavant,* 335 S.E.2d 127, 1985, *cert. denied,* 475 US 1084 (1986).
39. *Tillman v. Detroit Receiving Hosp.,* 360 N.W.2d 275 (1984).
40. *Kirker v. Orange County,* 519 So.2d 682, 1988.
41. *Tucker v. Lower,* No. 2831, Law & Eq. Ct., Richmond, Va. (May 23, 1972).
42. *Strachan v. John F. Kennedy Memorial Hosp.,* 538 A.2d 346 (1988).
43. *Transplant Action* 4 (American Council on Transplantation, Alexandria, Va. Sept./Oct./Nov. 1989).
44. J. R. Botkin, *Anencephalic Infants as Organ Donors,* 82 Pediatrics 250-56 (1988).
45. J. W. Walters, *Anencephalic Organ Procurement: Should the Law Be Changed?* 2 BioLaw S83-S89 (1987).
46. D. A. Stumpf et al. (The Medical Task Force on Anencephaly), *The Infant with Anencephaly,* 322 New Engl. J. Med. 669-74 (1990).

47. Centers for Disease Control, *Congenital Malformations Surveillance,* January 1982–December 1985 (Dept. of Health and Human Services, Washington, D.C. 1988).
48. *Loma Linda Stops Program to Retrieve Transplantable Organs from Anencephalic Newborns,* BioLaw §13-1, U:1127 (1988).
49. *Supra* note 46.
50. *Pediatric Brain Death and Organ/Tissue Retrieval* (Plenum Publishing Corp.).
51. *Supra* note 46.
52. *Supra* note 46.
53. P. King and J. Areen, *Legal Regulation of Fetal Tissue Transplantation,* 36 Clin. Res. 187-222 (1988).
54. J. Palca, *Fetal Tissue Transplants Remain Off Limits,* 246 Science 752 (1989).
55. M. W. Danis, *Fetal Tissue Transplants: Restricting Recipient Designation,* 39 Hastings L. J. 1079-1152 (1988).
56. C. Marwick, *Committee to Be Named to Advise Government about Fetal Tissue Transplantation Experiments,* JAMA 259:3099, 1988.
57. *Committee on Fetal Tissue Transplantation Established,* BioLaw §13-1, U:965 (1988).
58. *BMA Guidelines on the Use of Fetal Tissue,* The Lancet 1119 (May 14, 1988).
59. *McFall v. Shrimp,* Allegheny Cnty Ct. Common Pleas, 10 Pa.D.&C.3d 90 (1980).
60. *Sirianni v. Anna,* 285 N.Y.S. 2d 709 (1967).
61. *Hart v. Brown,* 289 A.2d 386 (1972).
62. *In re Richardson,* 284 So.2d 185 (1975).
63. *In re Guardianship of Pescinski,* 226 N.W.2d 180 (1975).
64. *Little v. Little,* 576 S.W.2d 493 (1979).
65. *Strunk v. Strunk,* 445 S.W.2d 145 (1969).
66. *Head v. Colloton,* 331 N.W.2d 870 (1983).
67. *Karp v. Cooley,* 349 F Supp 827 (1972), *aff'd,* 493 F.2d 408 (1974).
68. Medical Device Amendment, Pub. L. 94-295 (1980).
69. *Ravenis, supra* note 18.
70. National Organ Transplant Act, Pub. L. 98-507, 98 Stat 2339, 42 U.S.C. 201 (Oct. 1984).
71. *Supra* note 31.
72. J. F. Blumstein, *Government's Role in Organ Transplantation Policy,* 14 J. Health Politics, Pol. & L. 5-39 (1989).
73. *Supra* note 70.
74. *Payment to Homeless Man to Donate Bone Marrow to Brother,* BioLaw §13-3, U:881 (1988).
75. *Transplant Action,* supra note 43, at 2.
76. *Supra* note 70.
77. *Supra* note 32.
78. T. E. Starzl, et al., *A Multifactorial System for Equitable Selection of Cadaver Kidney Recipients,* 257 JAMA 3073-75 (1987).
79. *From Here to Transplant . . . Introductory Information for Patients and Families* 19 (American Council on Transplantation, Alexandria, Va., rev'd Oct. 1989).
80. *Supra* note 32.
81. End-Stage Renal Disease Program (ESRDP), Pub. L. No. 603, §86 Stat. 1329 (1972).
82. *Supra* note 64.
83. Angell, *Cost Containment and the Physician,* 254 JAMA 1203-07 (1985).
84. J. Aroesty and R. Rettis, *The Cost Effects of Improved Kidney Transplantation,* Rand Rep. No. R-3099-NIH/RC (1984).
85. *Id.*
86. P. E. Eggers, *Effect of Transplantation on the Medicare End-Stage Renal Disease Program,* 318 New Engl. J. Med. 223-29 (1988).
87. *Supra* note 84.
88. *HCFA Notice,* 55 Fed. Reg. 8547 (Mar. 8, 1990).
89. P. H. Schuck, *Government Funding for Organ Transplants,* 14 J. Health Politics, Pol. & L. 169-90 (1989).

90. *Id.*
91. *Brillo v. Arizona,* cited in *ACT Transplant Action* (July/Aug., 1986).
92. *Allen v. Mansour,* 681 F. Supp. 1232 (D Ct. E. D. Mich. 1986).
93. *Lee v. Page,* No. 86-1081-Civ-J-14, U.S. Dist. Ct., Middle Dist. of Florida, Jacksonville Division (Dec. 19, 1986).
94. *Todd v. Sorrell,* No. 87-3806, U.S. Ct. of App., Fourth Circuit (Mar. 4, 1988).
95. H. G. Welch and E. B. Larson, *Dealing with Limited Resources: The Oregon Decision to Curtail Funding for Organ Transplantation,* 319 New Engl. J. Med. 171-73 (1988).
96. R. Crawshaw et al., *Organ Transplants: A Search for Health Policy at the State Level,* 150 West. J. Med. 361-63 (1989).
97. *McDermott v. Manhattan Eye, Ear & Throat Hosp.,* 270 N.Y.S. 2d 955, *aff'd without opinion* 224 N.E.2d 717 (1966).
98. *Missouri ex rel. Wichita Falls General Hosp. v. Adolph,* 728 S.W.2d 604 (1987).
99. R. M. Baron, *Asserting Jurisdiction over the Providers of Human Donor Organs: State of Missouri ex rel. Wichita Falls General Hospital v. Adolph,* 92 Dick. L. Rev. 393 (Winter 1988).
100. Council on Ethical & Judicial Affairs (AMA), *Strategies for Cadaveric Organ Procurement Mandated Choice and Presumed Consent,* 272 JAMA 809-12 (1994).
101. *Brotherton v. Cleveland,* 923 Fed.2d. 477 (6th Cir. 1991).
102. D. Jason, *The Role of the Medical Examiner/Coroner in Organ and Tissue Procurement for Transplantation,* 15 Am. J. Forensic Med. & Path. 192-202 (1994).
103. R. Voelker, *Can Forensic Medical and Organ Donation Co-exist for Public Good?* 271 JAMA 891-92 (1994).
104. T. Shafer et al., *Impact of Medical Examiner/Coroner Practices on Organ Recovery in the United States,* 272 JAMA 1607-13 (1994).
105. A. Skolnick, *Are There Too Many US Transplantation Centers: Some Experts Suggest Fewer, Cheaper, Better,* 271 JAMA 1062-64 (1994).

APPENDIX 28-1 **Organs used in transplantation***

CORNEAS

The clear "window" in front of eye allowing light to enter

The first cornea transplant was performed in 1905

More than 250,000 people have received cornea transplants in the last 30 years

Some 40,000 people receive cornea transplants annually in the United States

At any given time 3,000 to 5,000 people await corneas

The body does not reject a transplanted cornea

Cornea donors range in age from newborn to age 70 or older

KIDNEYS

The kidney is the most frequently transplanted organ

More than 60,000 kidney transplants have been performed in the United States since 1981

Approximately 75% of kidneys are from non-related, deceased donors; approximately 25% come from living-related donors

More than 20,000 people in the U.S. are on waiting lists for kidney transplants

Kidneys have functioned normally after transplantation for more than 30 years with living-related donors

Kidneys have functioned normally after transplantation for more than 20 years with non-related cadaver donors

HEART

Since 1967 more than 10,000 heart transplants have been performed in the United States

Several thousand people are currently awaiting heart transplants in the United States

The one-year survival for heart transplants currently averages 80%

Survival rates of up to 17 years have been documented for heart recipients

Currently several thousand heart transplants are being performed annually in the United States

LIVER

An estimated 5,000 people die each year in the United States from end-stage liver disease who would have been acceptable candidates for liver transplantation

More than 10,000 liver transplants have been performed since 1986

The one year success rate for liver transplants is about 75%

Patient survival of over 15 years is documented

Living-related partial liver transplants, usually involving a parent donating a portion of his or her liver to a child have been done

---

*From U.N.O.S. Annual Reports on the U.S. Scientific Registry for Organ Transplantation and the Organ Procurement and Transplantation Network.

LUNGS

The lung is the most complicated type of transplant performed, and may be transplanted along with the heart depending on the nature of the illness

Almost 1,000 lung transplants are currently being performed annually in the United States

The success rates of single and double lung transplants are improving dramatically

PANCREAS

A pancreas transplant can cure diabetes

If a patient undergoing a kidney transplant has diabetes, the pancreas may be transplanted along with the kidney

More than 800 pancreas transplants have been performed in the United States since 1982

BONES

About 300,000 bone graft procedures are performed annually in the United States

An estimated 500,000 people await some form of bone transplant procedure in the United States

Most bone transplants last the life of the individual

Bone can be preserved and stored indefinitely by a "bone bank"

SKIN

Skin can be used as a temporary covering for severe burns

Donor skin is generally from the back or thigh

Skin can be cryo-preserved for up to 4 weeks for use with burn victims. It can be preserved via a freeze-drying process for up to 5 years for use in periodontal work

BONE MARROW

Transplanted bone marrow is used to treat patients with leukemia or other forms of cancer, certain types of anemia, and certain genetic diseases

Close relatives are the best potential donors

When a match can not be found from a relative, the odds of an unrelated person being a close match are 20,000 to 1

APPENDIX 28-2   Amended Uniform Anatomical Gift Act (1987)*

NOTE: Words or phrases enclosed in square brackets [   ] indicate instances in which each state is to supply its own appropriate terms.

SECTION 1. **Definitions.** As used in this [Act]:

(1) "Anatomical gift" means a donation of all or part of a human body to take effect upon or after death.

(2) "Decedent" means a deceased individual and includes a stillborn infant or fetus.

(3) "Document of gift" means a card, a statement attached to or imprinted on a motor vehicle operator's or chauffeur's license, a will, or other writing used to make an anatomical gift.

(4) "Donor" means an individual who makes an anatomical gift of all or part of the individual's body.

(5) "Enucleator" means an individual who is [licensed] [certified] by the [State Board of Medical Examiners] to remove or process eyes or parts of eyes.

(6) "Hospital" means a facility licensed, accredited, or approved as a hospital under the law of any state or a facility operated as a hospital by the United States government, a state, or a subdivision of a state.

(7) "Part" means an organ, tissue, eye, bone, artery, blood, fluid, or other portion of a human body.

(8) "Person" means an individual, corporation, business trust, estate, trust, partnership, joint venture, association, government, governmental subdivision or agency, or any other legal or commercial entity.

(9) "Physician" or "surgeon" means an individual licensed or otherwise authorized to practice medicine and surgery or osteopathy and surgery under the laws of any state.

(10) "Procurement organization" means a person licensed, accredited, or approved under the laws of any state for procurement, distribution, or storage of human bodies or parts.

(11) "State" means a state, territory, or possession of the United States, the District of Columbia, or the Commonwealth of Puerto Rico.

---

*From National Conference of Commissioners on Uniform State Laws (July 1986).

(12) "Technician" means an individual who is [licensed] [certified] by the [State Board of Medical Examiners] to remove or process a part.

SECTION 2. **Making, Amending, Revoking, and Refusing to Make Anatomical Gifts by Individual.**

(a) An individual who is at least [18] years of age may (i) make an anatomical gift for any of the purposes stated in Section 6(a), (ii) limit an anatomical gift to one or more of those purposes, or (iii) refuse to make an anatomical gift.

(b) An anatomical gift may be made only by a document of gift signed by the donor. If the donor cannot sign, the document of gift must be signed by another individual and by two witnesses, all of whom have signed at the direction and in the presence of the donor and of each other, and state that it has been so signed.

(c) If a document of gift is attached to or imprinted on a donor's motor vehicle operator's or chauffeur's license, the document of gift must comply with subsection (b). Revocation, suspension, expiration, or cancellation of the license does not invalidate the anatomical gift.

(d) A document of gift may designate a particular physician or surgeon to carry out the appropriate procedures. In the absence of a designation or if the designee is not available, the donee or other person authorized to accept the anatomical gift may employ or authorize any physician, surgeon, technician, or enucleator to carry out the appropriate procedures.

(e) An anatomical gift by will takes effect upon death of the testator, whether or not the will is probated. If, after death, the will is declared invalid for testamentary purposes, the validity of the anatomical gift is unaffected.

(f) A donor may amend or revoke an anatomical gift, not made by will, only by:
(1) a signed statement;
(2) an oral statement made in the presence of two individuals;
(3) any form of communication during a terminal illness or injury addressed to a physician or surgeon; or
(4) the delivery of a signed statement to a specified donee to whom a document of gift had been delivered.

(g) The donor of an anatomical gift made by will may amend or revoke the gift in the manner provided for amendment or revocation of wills, or as provided in subsection (f).

(h) An anatomical gift that is not revoked by the donor before death is irrevocable and does not require the consent or concurrence of any person after the donor's death.

(i) An individual may refuse to make an anatomical gift of the individual's body or part by (i) a writing signed in the same manner as a document of gift, (ii) a statement attached to or imprinted on a donor's motor vehicle operator's or chauffeur's license, or (iii) any other writing used to identify the individual as refusing to make an anatomical gift. During a terminal illness or injury, the refusal may be an oral statement or other form of communication.

(j) In the absence of contrary indications by the donor, an anatomical gift of a part is neither a refusal to give other parts nor a limitation on an anatomical gift under Section 3 or on a removal or release of other parts under Section 4.

(k) In the absence of contrary indications by the donor, a revocation or amendment of an anatomical gift is not a refusal to make another anatomical gift. If the donor intends a revocation to be a refusal to make an anatomical gift, the donor shall make the refusal pursuant to subsection (i).

SECTION 3. **Making, Revoking, and Objecting to Anatomical Gifts, by Others.**

(a) Any member of the following classes of persons, in the order of priority listed, may make an anatomical gift of all or a part of the decedent's body for an authorized purpose, unless the decedent, at the time of death, has made an unrevoked refusal to make that anatomical gift:
(1) the spouse of the decedent;
(2) an adult son or daughter of the decedent;
(3) either parent of the decedent;
(4) an adult brother or sister of the decedent;
(5) a grandparent of the decedent; and
(6) a guardian of the person of the decedent at the time of death.

(b) An anatomical gift may not be made by a person listed in subsection (a) if:
(1) a person in a prior class is available at the time of death to make an anatomical gift;
(2) the person proposing to make an anatomical gift knows of a refusal or contrary indications by the decedent; or
(3) the person proposing to make an anatomical gift knows of an objection to making an anatomical gift by a member of the person's class or a prior class.

(c) An anatomical gift by a person authorized under subsection (a) must be made by (i) a document of gift signed by the person or (ii) the person's telegraphic, recorded telephonic, or other recorded message, or other form of communication from the person that is contemporaneously reduced to writing and signed by the recipient.

(d) An anatomical gift by a person authorized under subsection (a) may be revoked by any member of the same or a prior class if, before procedures have begun for the removal of a part from the body of the decedent, the physician, surgeon, technician, or enucleator removing the part knows of the revocation.

(e) A failure to make an anatomical gift under subsection (a) is not an objection to the making of an anatomical gift.

SECTION 4. **Authorization by [Coroner] [Medical Examiner] or [Local Public Health Official].**

(a) The [coroner] [medical examiner] may release and permit the removal of a part from a body within that official's custody, for transplantation or therapy, if:

(1) the official has received a request for the part from a hospital, physician, surgeon, or procurement organization;

(2) the official has made a reasonable effort, taking into account the useful life of the part, to locate and examine the decedent's medical records and inform persons listed in Section 3(a) of their option to make, or object to making, an anatomical gift;

(3) the official does not know of a refusal or contrary indication by the decedent or objection by a person having priority to act as listed in Section 3(a);

(4) the removal will be by a physician, surgeon, or technician; but in the case of eyes, by one of them or by an enucleator;

(5) the removal will not interfere with any autopsy or investigation;

(6) the removal will be in accordance with accepted medical standards; and

(7) cosmetic restoration will be done, if appropriate.

(b) If the body is not within the custody of the [coroner] [medical examiner], the [local public health officer] may release and permit the removal of any part from a body in the [local health officer's] custody for transplantation or therapy if the requirements of subsection (a) are met.

(c) An official releasing and permitting the removal of a part shall maintain a permanent record of the name of the decedent, the person making the request, the date and purpose of the request, the part requested, and the person to whom it was released.

SECTION 5. **Routine Inquiry and Required Request; Search and Notification.**

(a) On or before admission to a hospital, or as soon as possible thereafter, a person designated by the hospital shall ask each patient who is at least [18] years of age: "Are you an organ or tissue donor?" If the answer is affirmative the person shall request a copy of the document of gift. If the answer is negative or there is no answer and the attending physician consents, the person designated shall discuss with the patient the option to make or refuse to make an anatomical gift. The answer to the question, an available copy of any document of gift or refusal to make an anatomical gift, and any other relevant information, must be placed in the patient's medical record.

(b) If, at or near the time of death of a patient, there is no medical record that the patient has made or refused to make an anatomical gift, the hospital [administrator] or a representative designated by the [administrator] shall discuss the option to make or refuse to make an anatomical gift and request the making of an anatomical gift pursuant to Section 3(a). The request must be made with reasonable discretion and sensitivity to the circumstances of the family. A request is not required if the gift is not suitable, based upon accepted medical standards, for a purpose specified in Section 6. An entry must be made in the medical record of the patient, stating the name and affiliation of the individual making the request, and of the name, response, and relationship to the patient of the person to whom the request was made. The [Commissioner of Health] shall [establish guidelines] [adopt regulations] to implement this subsection.

(c) The following persons shall make a reasonable search for a document of gift or other information identifying the bearer as a donor or as an individual who has refused to make an anatomical gift:

(1) a law enforcement officer, fireman, paramedic, or other emergency rescuer finding an individual who the searcher believes is dead or near death; and

(2) a hospital, upon the admission of an individual at or near the time of death, if there is not immediately available any other source of that information.

(d) If a document of gift or evidence of refusal to make an anatomical gift is located by the search required by subsection (c)(1), and the individual or body to whom it relates is taken to a hospital, the hospital must be notified of the contents and the document or other evidence must be sent to the hospital.

(e) If, at or near the time of death of a patient, a hospital knows that an anatomical gift has been made pursuant to Section 3(a) or a release and removal of a part has been permitted pursuant to Section 4, or that a patient or an individual identified as in transit to the hospital is a donor, the hospital shall notify the donee if one is named and known to the hospital; if not, it shall notify an appropriate procurement organization. The hospital shall cooperate in the implementation of the anatomical gift or release and removal of a part.

(f) A person who fails to discharge the duties imposed by this section is not subject to criminal or civil liability but is subject to appropriate administrative sanctions.

SECTION 6. Persons Who May Become Donees; Purposes for Which Anatomical Gifts May be Made.

(a) The following persons may become donees of anatomical gifts for the purposes stated:

 (1) a hospital, physician, surgeon, or procurement organization, for transplantation, therapy, medical or dental education, research, or advancement of medical or dental science;

 (2) an accredited medical or dental school, college, or university for education, research, advancement of medical or dental science; or

 (3) a designated individual for transplantation or therapy needed by that individual.

(b) An anatomical gift may be made to a designated donee or without designating a donee. If a donee is not designated or if the donee is not available or rejects the anatomical gift, the anatomical gift may be accepted by any hospital.

(c) If the donee knows of the decedent's refusal or contrary indications to make an anatomical gift or that an anatomical gift by a member of a class having priority to act is opposed by a member of the same class or a prior class under Section 3(a), the donee may not accept the anatomical gift.

SECTION 7. Delivery of Document of Gift.

(a) Delivery of a document of gift during the donor's lifetime is not required for the validity of an anatomical gift.

(b) If an anatomical gift is made to a designated donee, the document of gift, or a copy, may be delivered to the donee to expedite the appropriate procedures after death. The document of gift, or a copy, may be deposited in any hospital, procurement organization, or registry office that accepts it for safekeeping or for facilitation of procedures after death. On request of an interested person, upon or after the donor's death, the person in possession shall allow the interested party to examine or copy the document of gift.

SECTION 8. Rights and Duties at Death.

(a) Rights of a donee created by an anatomical gift are superior to rights of others except with respect to autopsies under Section 11(b). A donee may accept or reject an anatomical gift. If a donee accepts an anatomical gift of an entire body, the donee, subject to the terms of the gift, may allow embalming and use of the body in funeral services. If the gift is of a part of a body, the donee, upon the death of the donor and before embalming, shall cause the part to be removed without unnecessary mutilation. After removal of the part, custody of the remainder of the body vests in the person under obligation to dispose of the body.

(b) The time of death must be determined by a physician or surgeon who attends the donor at death or, if none, the physician or surgeon who certifies the death. Neither the physician or surgeon who attends the donor at death nor the physician or surgeon who determines the time of death may participate in the procedures for removing or transplanting a part unless the document of gift designates a particular physician or surgeon pursuant to Section 2(d).

(c) If there has been an anatomical gift, a technician may remove any donated parts and an enucleator may remove any donated eyes or parts of eyes, after determination of death by a physician or surgeon.

SECTION 9. Coordination of Procurement and Use.

Each hospital in this State, after consultation with other hospitals and procurement organizations, shall establish agreements or affiliations for coordination of procurement and use of human bodies and parts.

SECTION 10. Sale or Purchase of Parts Prohibited.

(a) A person may not knowingly, for valuable consideration, purchase or sell a part for transplantation or therapy, if removal of the part is intended to occur after the death of the decedent.

(b) Valuable consideration does not include reasonable payment for the removal, processing, disposal, preservation, quality control, storage, transportation, or implementation of a part.

(c) A person who violates this section is guilty of a [felony] and upon conviction is subject to a fine not exceeding [$50,000] or imprisonment not exceeding [five] years, or both.

SECTION 11. Examination, Autopsy, Liability.

(a) An anatomical gift authorizes any reasonable examination necessary to assure medical acceptability of the gift for the purposes intended.

(b) The provisions of this [Act] are subject to the laws of this State governing autopsies.

(c) A hospital, physician, surgeon, [coroner], [medical examiner], [local public health officer], enucleator, technician, or other person, who acts in accordance with this [Act] or with the applicable anatomical gift law of another state [or a foreign country] or attempts in good faith to do so is not liable for that act in a civil action or criminal proceeding.

(d) An individual who makes an anatomical gift pursuant to Section 2 or 3 and the individual's estate are not liable for any injury or damage that may result from the making or the use of the anatomical gift.

SECTION 12. **Transitional Provisions.** This [Act] applies to a document of gift, revocation, or refusal to make an anatomical gift signed by the donor or a person authorized to make or object to making an anatomical gift before, on, or after the effective date of this [Act].

SECTION 13. **Uniformity of Application and Construction.** This [Act] shall be applied and construed to effectuate its general purpose to make uniform the law with respect to the subject of this [Act] among states enacting it.

SECTION 14. **Severability.** If any provision of this [Act] or its application thereof to any person or circumstance is held invalid, the invalidity does not affect other provisions or applications of this [Act] which can be given effect without the invalid provision or application, and to this end the provisions of this [Act] are severable.

SECTION 15. **Short Title.** This [Act] may be cited as the "Uniform Anatomical Gift Act (1987)."

SECTION 16. **Repeals.** The following acts and parts of acts are repealed:

(1)

(2)

(3)

SECTION 17. **Effective Date.** This [Act] takes effect _____.

APPENDIX 28-3   National Organ Transplant Act*

AN ACT

To provide for the establishment of the Task Force on Organ Transplantation and the Organ Procurement and Transplantation Network, to authorize financial assistance for organ procurement organizations, and for other purposes.

Be it enacted by the Senate and House of Representatives of the United States of America in Congress assembled, That this Act may be cited as the "National Organ Transplant Act."

TITLE I—TASK FORCE ON ORGAN PROCUREMENT AND TRANSPLANTATION

ESTABLISHMENT AND DUTIES OF TASK FORCE

Sec. 101. (a) Not later than ninety days after the date of the enactment of this Act, the Secretary of Health and Human Services (hereinafter in this title referred to as the "Secretary") shall establish a Task Force on Organ Transplantation (hereinafter in this title referred to as the "Task Force"). (b)(1) The Task Force shall—

(A) conduct comprehensive examinations of the medical, legal, ethical, economic, and social issues presented by human organ procurement and transplantation.

(B) prepare the assessment described in paragraph (2) and the report described in paragraph (3), and

(C) advise the Secretary with respect to the development of regulations for grants under section 371 of the Public Health Service Act.

(2) The Task Force shall make an assessment of immunosuppressive medications used to prevent organ rejection in transplant patients, including—

(A) an analysis of the safety, effectiveness, and costs (including cost-savings from improved success rates of transplantation) of different modalities of treatment;

(B) an analysis of the extent of insurance reimbursement for long-term immunosuppressive drug therapy for organ transplant patients by private insurers and the public sector;

(C) an identification of problems that patients encounter in obtaining immunosuppressive medications; and

(D) an analysis of the comparative advantages of grants, coverage under existing Federal programs, or other means to assure that individuals who need such medications can obtain them.

(3) The Task Force shall prepare a report which shall include—

(A) an assessment of public and private efforts to procure human organs for transplantation and an identification of factors that diminish the number of organs available for transplantation;

*From Pub. L. 98-507, 98th Congress.

(B) an assessment of problems in coordinating the procurement of viable human organs including skin and bones.

(C) recommendations for the education and training of health professionals, including physicians, nurses, and hospital and emergency care personnel, with respect to organ procurement;

(D) recommendations for the education of the general public, the clergy, law enforcement officers, members of local fire departments, and other agencies and individuals that may be instrumental in affecting organ procurement;

(E) recommendations for assuring equitable access by patients to organ transplantation and for assuring the equitable allocation of donated organs among transplant centers and among patients medically qualified for an organ transplant;

(F) an identification of barriers to the donation of organs to patients with special emphasis upon pediatric patients, including an assessment of—

(i) barriers to the improved identification of organ donors and their families and organ recipients;

(ii) the number of potential organ donors and their geographical distribution;

(iii) current health care services provided for patients who need organ transplantation and organ procurement procedures, systems, and programs which affect such patients;

(iv) cultural factors affecting the facility with respect to the donation of the organs; and

(v) ethical and economic issues relating to organ transplantation needed by chronically ill patients;

(G) recommendations for the conduct and coordination of continuing research concerning all aspects of the transplantation of organs;

(H) an analysis of the factors involved in insurance reimbursement for transplant procedures by private insurers and the public sector;

(I) an analysis of the manner in which organ transplantation technology is diffused among and adopted by qualified medical centers, including a specification of the number and geographical distribution of qualified medical centers using such technology and an assessment of whether the number of centers using such technology is sufficient or excessive and of whether the public has sufficient access to medical procedures using such technology; and

(J) an assessment of the feasibility of establishing, and of the likely effectiveness of, a national registry of human organ donors.

MEMBERSHIP

Sec. 102. (a) The Task Force shall be composed of twenty-five members as follows:

(1) Twenty-one members shall be appointed by the Secretary which:

(A) nine members shall be physicians or scientists who are eminent in the various medical and scientific specialties related to human organ transplantations;

(B) three members shall be individuals who are not physicians and who represent the field of human organ procurement;

(C) four members shall be individuals who are not physicians and who as a group have expertise in the fields of law, theology, ethics, health care financing, and the social and behavioral sciences;

(D) three members shall be individuals who are not physicians or scientists and who are members of the general public; and

(E) two members shall be individuals who represent private health insurers or self-insurers.

(2) The Surgeon General of the United States, the Director of the National Institutes of Health, the Commissioner of the Food and Drug Administration, and the Administrator of the Health Care Financing Administration shall be ex officio members.

(b) No individual who is a full-time officer or employee of the United States may be appointed under subsection (a)(1) to the Task Force. A vacancy in the Task Force shall be filled in the manner in which the original appointment was made. A vacancy in the Task Force shall not affect its powers.

(c) Members shall be appointed for the life of the Task Force.

(d) The Task Force shall select a Chairman from among its members who are appointed under subsection (a)(1).

(e) Thirteen members of the Task Force shall constitute a quorum, but a lesser number may hold hearings.

(f) The Task Force shall hold its first meeting on a date specified by the Secretary which is not later than thirty days after the date on which the Secretary establishes the Task Force under section 101. Thereafter, the Task Force shall meet at the call of the Chairman or a majority of its members, but shall meet at least three times during the life of the Task Force.

(g)(1) Each member of the Task Force who is not an officer or employee of the United States shall be compensated at a rate equal to the daily equivalent of the annual rate of basic pay in effect for grade GS-18 of the General Schedule under section 5332 of title 5, United States Code, for each day (including travel time) during which such member is engaged in the actual performance of duties as a member of the Task Force. Each member of the Task Force who is an officer or employee of the United States shall receive no additional compensation.

(2) While away from their homes or regular places of business in the performance of duties for the Task Force, all members of the Task Force shall be allowed travel expenses, including per diem in lieu of subsistence, at rates authorized for employees of agencies under sections 5702 and 5703 of title 5, United States Code.

SUPPORT FOR THE TASK FORCE

Sec. 103. (a) Upon request of the Task Force, the head of any Federal agency is authorized to detail, on a reimbursable basis, any of the personnel of such agency to the Task Force to assist the Task Force in carrying out its duties under this Act.

(b) The Secretary shall provide the Task Force with such administrative and support services as the Task Force may require to carry out its duties.

REPORT CENTER

Sec. 104. (a) The Task Force may transmit to the Secretary, the Committee on Labor and Human Resources of the Senate, and the Committee on Energy and Commerce of the House of Representatives such interim reports as the Task Force considers appropriate.

(b) Not later than seven months after the date on which the Task Force is established by the Secretary under section 101, the Task Force shall transmit a report to the Secretary, the Committee on Labor and Human Resources of the Senate, and the Committee on Energy and Commerce of the House of Representatives on its assessment under section 101(b)(2) of immunosuppressive medications used to prevent organ rejection.

(c) Not later than twelve months after the date on which the Task Force is established by the Secretary under section 101, the Task Force shall transmit a final report to the secretary, the Committee on Labor and Human Resources of the Senate, and the Committee on Energy and Commerce of the House of Representatives. The final report of the Task Force shall include —

(1) a description of any findings and conclusions of the Task Force made pursuant to any examination conducted under section 101(b)(1)(A),

(2) the matters specified in section 101(b)(3), and

(3) such recommendations as the Task Force considers appropriate.

TERMINATION

Sec. 105. The Task Force shall terminate three months after the date on which the Task Force transmits the report required by section 104(c).

TITLE II — ORGAN PROCUREMENT ACTIVITIES

Sec. 201. Part H of title III of the Public Health Service Act is amended to read as follows:

PART H — ORGAN TRANSPLANTS

ASSISTANCE FOR ORGAN PROCUREMENT ORGANIZATIONS

"Sec. 317. (a)(1) The Secretary may make grants for the planning of qualified organ procurement organizations described in subsection (b).

"(2) The Secretary may make grants for the establishment, initial operation, and expansion of qualified organ procurement organizations described in subsection (b).

"(3) In making grants under paragraphs (1) and (2), the Secretary shall —

"(A) take into consideration any recommendations made by the Task Force on Organ Transplantation established under section 101 of the National Organ Transplant Act, and

"(B) give special consideration to applications which cover geographical areas which are not adequately served by organ procurement organizations.

"(b)(1) A qualified organ procurement organization for which grants may be made under subsection (a) is an organization which, as determined by the Secretary, will carry out the functions described in paragraph (2) and —

"(A) is a nonprofit entity.

"(B) has accounting and other fiscal procedures (as specified by the Secretary) necessary to assure the fiscal stability of the organization,

"(C) has an agreement with the Secretary to be reimbursed under title XVIII of the Social Security Act for the procurement of kidneys.

"(D) has procedures to obtain payment for non-renal organs provided to transplant centers,

"(E) has a defined services area which is a geographical area of sufficient size which (unless the service area comprises an entire State) will include at least fifty potential organ donors each year and which either includes an entire standard metropolitan statistical area (as specified by the Office of Management and Budget) or does not include any part of such an area,

"(F) has a director and such other staff, including the organ donation coordinators and organ procurement specialists necessary to effectively obtain organs from donors in its service area, and

"(G) has a board of directors or an advisory board which— "(i) is composed of—

"(I) members who represent hospital administrators, intensive care or emergency room personnel, tissue banks, and voluntary health associations in its service area,

"(II) members who represent the public residing in such area,

"(III) a physician with knowledge, experience, or skill in the field of histocompatibility,

"(IV) a physician with knowledge or skill in the field of neurology, and

"(V) from each transplant center in its service area which has arrangements described in paragraph (2)(G) with the organization, a member who is a surgeon who has practicing privileges in such center and who performs organ transplant surgery,

(ii) has the authority to recommend policies for the procurement of organs and the other functions described in paragraph (2), and

(iii) has no authority over any other activity of the organization.

"(2) An organ procurement organization shall—

"(A) have effective agreements, to identify potential organ donors, with a substantial majority of the hospitals and other health area entities in its service area which have facilities for organ donations,

"(B) conduct and participate in systematic efforts, including professional education, to acquire all usable organs from potential donors

"(C) arrange for the acquisition and preservation of donated organs and provide quality standards for the acquisition of organs which are consistent with the standards adopted by the Organ Procurement and Transplantation Network under section 372(b)(2)(D),

"(D) arrange for the appropriate tissue typing of donated organs,

"(E) have a system to allocate donated organs among transplant centers and patients according to established medical criteria,

"(F) provide or arrange for the transportation of donated organs to transplant centers,

"(G) have arrangements to coordinate its activities with transplant centers in its service area.

"(H) participate in the Organ Procurement Transplantation Network established under section 372,

"(I) have arrangements to cooperate with tissue banks for the retrieval, processing, preservation, storage, and distribution of tissues as may be appropriate to assure that all usable tissues are obtained from potential donors, and

"(J) evaluate annually the effectiveness of the organization in acquiring potentially available organs.

"(c) for grants under subsection (a) there are authorized to be appropriated $5,000,000 for fiscal year 1985, $8,000,000 for fiscal year 1986, and $12,000,000 for fiscal year 1987.

ORGAN PROCUREMENT AND TRANSPLANTATION NETWORK

"Sec. 372. (a) The Secretary shall by contract provide for the establishment and operation of an Organ Procurement and Transplantation Network which meets the requirements of subsection (b). The amount provided under such contract in any fiscal year may not exceed $2,000,000. Funds for such contracts shall be made available from funds available to the Public Health Service from appropriations for fiscal years beginning after fiscal year 1984.

"(b)(1) The Organ Procurement and Transplantation Network shall carry out the functions described in paragraph (2) and shall—

"(A) be a private nonprofit entity which is not engaged in any activity unrelated to organ procurement, and

"(B) have a board of directors which includes representatives of organ procurement organizations (including organizations which have received grants under section 371), transplant centers, voluntary health associations, and the general public.

"(2) The Organ Procurement and Transplantation Network shall—

"(A) establish in one location or through regional centers—

"(i) a national list of individuals who need organs, and

"(ii) a national system, through the use of computers and in accordance with established medical criteria, to match organs and individuals included in the list, especially individuals whose immune system makes it difficult for them to receive organs,

"(B) maintain a twenty-four hour telephone service to facilitate matching organs with individuals included in the list,

"(C) assist organ procurement organizations in the distribution of organs which cannot be placed within the service areas of the organizations,

"(D) adopt and use standards of quality for the acquisition and transportation of donated organs,

"(E) prepare and distribute, on a regionalized basis, samples of blood sera from individuals who are included on the list and whose immune system makes it difficult for them to receive organs, in order to facilitate matching the compatibility of such individuals with organ donors,

"(F) coordinate, as appropriate, the transportation of organs from organ procurement organizations to transplant centers,

"(G) provide information to physicians and other health professionals regarding organ donation, and

"(H) collect, analyze, and publish data concerning organ donation and transplants.

SCIENTIFIC REGISTRY

"Sec. 373. The Secretary shall, by grant or contract, develop and maintain a scientific registry of the recipients of organ transplants. The registry shall include such information respecting patients and transplant procedures as the Secretary deems necessary to an ongoing evaluation of the scientific and clinical status of organ transplantation. The Secretary shall prepare for inclusion in the report under section 376 an analysis of information derived from the registry.

GENERAL PROVISIONS RESPECTING GRANTS AND CONTRACTS

"Sec. 374. (a) No grant may be made under section 371 or 373 or contract entered into under section 372 or 373 unless an application therefore has been submitted to, and approved by, the Secretary. Such an application shall be in such form and shall be submitted in such manner as the Secretary shall by regulation prescribe.

"(b)(1) In considering applications for grants under section 371—

"(A) the Secretary shall give priority to any applicant which has a formal agreement of cooperation with all transplant centers in its proposed service area,

"(B) the Secretary shall give special consideration to organizations which met the requirements of section 371(b) before the date of the enactment of this section, and

"(C) the Secretary shall not discriminate against an applicant solely because it provides health care services other than those related to organ procurement.

The Secretary may not make a grant for more than one organ procurement organization which serves the same service area.

"(2) A grant for planning under section 371 may be made for one year with respect to any organ procurement organization and may not exceed $100,000.

"(3) Grants under section 371 for the establishment, initial operation, or expansion of organ procurement organizations may be made for two years. No such grant may exceed $500,000 for any year and no organ procurement organization may receive more than $800,000 for initial operation or expansion.

"(c)(1) The Secretary shall determine the amount of a grant made under section 371 or 373. Payments under such grants may be made in advance on the basis of estimates or by the way of reimbursement, with necessary adjustments on account of underpayments or overpayments, and in such installments and on such terms and conditions as the Secretary finds necessary to carry out the purposes of such grants.

"(2)(A) Each recipient of a grant under section 371 or 373 shall keep such records as the Secretary shall prescribe, including records which fully disclose the amount and disposition by such recipient of the proceeds of such grant, the total cost of the undertaking in connection with which such grant was made, and the amount of that portion of the cost of the undertaking supplied by other sources, and such other records as will facilitate an effective audit.

"(B) The Secretary and the Comptroller General of the United States, or any of their duly authorized representatives, shall have access for the purpose of audit and examination to any books, documents, papers, and records of the recipient of a grant under section 371 or 373 that are pertinent to such grant

"(d) For purposes of this part:

"(1) The term "transplant center" means a health care facility in which transplants of organs are performed.

"(2) The term "organ" means the human kidney, liver, heart, lung, pancreas, and any other human organ (other than corneas and eyes) specified by the Secretary by regulation and for purposes of section 373; such term includes bone marrow.

ADMINISTRATION

"Sec. 375. The Secretary shall, during fiscal years 1985, 1986, 1987, and 1988, designate and maintain an identifiable administrative unit in the Public Health Service to—

"(1) administer this part and coordinate with the organ procurement activities under title XVIII of the Social Security Act,

"(2) conduct a program of public information to inform the public of the need for organ donations,

"(3) Provide technical assistance to organ procurement organizations receiving funds under section 371, the Organ Procurement and Transplantation Network established under section 372, and other entities in the health care system involved in organ donations, procurement, and transplants, and

"(4) one year after the date on which the Task Force on Organ Transplantation transmits its final report under section 104(c) of the National Organ Transplant Act, and annually thereafter through fiscal year 1988, submit to Congress an annual report on the status of organ donation and coordination services and include in the report an analysis of the efficiency and effectiveness of the procurement and allocation of organs and a description of problems encountered in the procurement and allocation of organs.

REPORT

"Sec. 376. The Secretary shall annually publish a report on the scientific and clinical status of organ transplantation. The Secretary shall consult with the Director of the National Institutes of Health and the Commissioner of the Food and Drug Administration in the preparation of the report."

TITLE III—PROHIBITION OF ORGAN PURCHASES

Sec. 301. (a) It shall be unlawful for any person to knowingly acquire, receive, or otherwise transfer any human organ for valuable consideration for use in human transplantation if the transfer affects interstate commerce.

(b) Any person who violates subsection (a) shall be fined not more than $50,000 or imprisoned not more than five years, or both.

(c) For purposes of subsection (a):

(1) The term "human organ" means the human kidney, liver, heart, lung, pancreas, bone marrow, cornea, eye, bone, and skin, and any other human organ specified by the Secretary of Health and Human Services by regulation.

(2) The term "valuable consideration" does not include the reasonable payments associated with the removal, transportation, implantation, processing, preservation, quality control, and storage of a human organ or the expense of travel, housing and lost wages incurred by the donor of a human organ in connection with the donation of the organ.

(3) The term "interstate commerce" has the meaning prescribed for it by section 201(b) of the Federal Food, Drug and Cosmetic Act.

TITLE IV—MISCELLANEOUS

BONE MARROW REGISTRY DEMONSTRATION AND STUDY

Sec. 401. (a) Not later than nine months after the date of enactment of this Act, the Secretary of Health and Human Services shall hold a conference on the feasibility of establishing and the effectiveness of a national registry of voluntary bone marrow donors.

(b) If the conference held under subsection (a) finds that it is feasible to establish a national registry of voluntary donors of bone marrow and that such a registry is likely to be effective in matching donors with recipients, the Secretary of Health and Human Services, acting through the Assistant Secretary for Health, shall, for purposes of the study under subsection (c), establish a registry of voluntary donors of bone marrow. The Secretary shall assure that—

(1) donors of bone marrow listed in the registry have given an informed consent to the donation of bone marrow; and

(2) the names of the donors in the registry are kept confidential and access to the names and any other information in the registry is restricted to personnel who need the information to maintain and implement the registry, except that access to such other information shall be provided for purposes of the study under subsection (c).

If the conference held under subsection (a) makes the finding described in this subsection, the Secretary shall establish the registry not later than six months after the completion of the conference.

(c) The Secretary of Health and Human Services, acting through the Assistant Secretary for Health, shall study the establishment and implementation of the registry under subsection (b) to identify the issues presented by the establishment of such a registry, to evaluate participation of bone marrow donors, to assess the implementation of the informed consent and confidentiality requirements, and to determine if the establishment of a permanent bone marrow registry is needed and appropriate. The Secretary shall report the results of the study to the Committee on Energy and Commerce of the House of Representatives and the Committee on Labor and Human Resources of the Senate not later than two years after the date the registry is established under subsection (b).

Approved October 19, 1984.

CHAPTER 29 **The process of dying**

FREDERICK ADOLF PAOLA, M.D., J.D., F.C.L.M.*
JOHN A. ANDERSON, M.D., J.D., F.C.L.M.

WHEN DEATH OCCURS
THE DYING PATIENT
CONCLUSION

Perhaps one of the most difficult situations in the practice of medicine is the management of the dying patient; difficult because, in caring for the dying patient, the physician comes face to face not only with the limits of medical capabilities, not only with the mortality of the patient, but also with his or her own mortality:

And death means being no more. It cuts me off from all relation to the world and other human beings. It hurls me into non-being. Death teaches me that just as other things have ceased to be, so must I. Death tells me that all life is a flight to non-being. Human existence is a brief moment of light. . . . Death . . . is my supreme possibility (for it leads me to authentic concern about the things which really matter) but it is also the limit of all my possibilities. A man who realizes he is to die cannot give supreme concern to any other event. Man must face death every moment and every day.[1]

Traditionally physicians have been taught that their prime duties were the alleviation of pain and the prolongation of life. Success in achieving these goals has been variable at best, and often the physician is forced to choose between them.

Death has generally been defined as the cessation of life. Historically, the law has always accepted medicine's definition of death. Technological developments in medicine have precipitated the need for a legal reevaluation of the medical definition, since death has both a medical and a legal status. The interests of the deceased and family, health care providers, and society all require a reliable process of determining when death occurs.

WHEN DEATH OCCURS

As a first consideration it must be realized that there is no specific moment of dying. Humans die in stages.

During the ebbing of life there is a progression from clinical death to brain death, to biological death, to cellular death. Clinical death occurs when the body's vital functions—respiration and circulation—cease. When the brain is deprived of oxygen because of cessation of circulation, brain death is inevitable. Brain death follows clinical death almost immediately unless resuscitative procedures are started promptly, because the human brain under normal conditions cannot survive loss of oxygen for more than 6 to 10 minutes. If resuscitative measures are instituted at the moment of clinical death, brain death may be averted, and the patient may recover fully. On the other hand, brain death may follow despite reanimation efforts.

The brain also dies in steps. First the cerebral cortex, the site of the highest centers, ceases to function. Then successively, the cerebellum (the older part of the brain developmentally, having to do with equilibrium) and the so-called lower brain centers die. Ultimately the brain stem and the vital centers (controlling respiration, heart rate, and blood pressure) die. If there is irreversible destruction of the highest centers of the brain without damage to the vital centers, a permanent loss of consciousness results, but cardiorespiratory functions can continue. Sometimes these continue unaided, but most often only with artificial assistance. This is the so-called persistent vegetative state (PVS). When the lower areas of the brain are damaged in addition to the cerebrum, it still may be possible to maintain cardiovascular function for some time.

Ultimately, when all the components of the brain are dead, biological death, or permanent extinction of bodily life, occurs. Thereafter, the process of cellular death begins, and because of differences in cellular composition, the death of different parts of the body occurs at different times and stages. That is why viable organs such

*The authors gratefully acknowledge work from the previous contributor: Dorothy Rasinski Gregory, M.D., J.D., F.C.L.M.

as the heart or kidneys can be removed immediately after biological death and transplanted successfully. This also accounts for the fact that even after biological death, organs within the lifeless body can be maintained for a time by means of mechanical and chemical support.

The transfer from one state of viability to another may be slow or very rapid. This decline depends on age and physical, constitutional, and environmental factors, as well as on the life-extinguishing cause. There is a sequence of dying during which there comes a point of irreversibility, which physicians diagnose as death. When this point has been reached, nothing further can be done to restore life. In many instances, physicians can slow the process, but cannot prevent its ultimate conclusion.

Pronouncement of death

A formulation of death consists of (1) a definition of death, (2) criteria for determining that death has occurred, and (3) specific medical tests that show whether those criteria have been met.

Traditional formulation of death. A definition of death must "accurately show the quality so essentially significant to a living organism that its loss is termed death."[2] Traditionally, death was defined as the irreversible cessation of vital fluid (air and blood) flow. The corresponding ("heart-lung") criteria are the cessation of heart and lung function. Specific medical tests available to the physician to determine whether this criterion had been met included palpation for a pulse, auscultation for heart and breath sounds, use of a mirror held under the nares for evidence of condensation from exhaled breath, visualization of the optic fundus for vessel pulsation, and an electrocardiographic examination. If those examinations confirmed that vital functions had ceased, the physician would state that death had occurred. If the patient was young and the asystole or apnea promptly discovered, the physician might have delivered a precordial "thump" or injected intracardiac epinephrine in an attempt to stimulate the heart. If such methods were not employed or were unsuccessful, the physician pronounced the patient dead.

Impingement of technology. In the late 1950s and early 1960s, the medical community became aware of the fact that, in some cases of apparent cardiac arrest, the patient was actually in a ventricular tachyarrhythmia, and that prompt establishment of an airway, conversion of the cardiac rhythm, and reestablishment of an adequate cardiac output might sustain life. Efforts to perform cardiopulmonary resuscitation (CPR) began to be undertaken widely and became medically fashionable. About this same time, cardiac care units came into nationwide vogue, with a realization on the part of the medical community that, with proper monitoring, many of those patients who had suffered asystole or arrhyth-

mia following myocardial infarction, respiratory arrest, or other sudden catastrophe, and would otherwise have expired, might survive to leave the hospital.

With the great mushrooming of medical technology that was occurring—including the development of defibrillators, ventilators, newer and better antibiotics and chemotherapeutic agents, hemo- and peritoneal dialysis, and transplantation—medicine had new and expanded capabilities to support and sustain the lives of those who previously would have died. Driven by the twin duties of pain alleviation and prevention of death, the physician enthusiastically embraced these new advances with little attention given to ethical, sociological, or economic consequences.

"Brain death." With the development of modern resuscitation technology, it became possible to maintain heart and lung function for hours or days after all brain function had ceased. This created a troublesome dilemma for physicians. Discontinuing ventilatory support in such patients would cause the "death" of the patient, under the traditional formulation of death, and might be deemed the equivalent of a homicide.

The senselessness of maintaining patients in this hopeless condition and the increasing success of organ transplant programs led to a reexamination of the formulation of death.

This issue was first addressed by an ad hoc committee at the Harvard Medical School, convened to examine the definition of brain death. Its report appeared in an article entitled "A Definition of Irreversible Coma."[3] Using this term as synonymous with brain death, that article listed a series of criteria (the "Harvard criteria") to be employed in pronouncing brain death. These criteria included the following:

1. *Unreceptivity and unresponsivity:* a total unawareness of externally applied stimuli and inner need and complete unresponsiveness, despite application of intensely painful stimuli
2. *No spontaneous movements or breathing:* absence of all spontaneous muscular movement or breathing, as well as absence of response to stimuli such as pain, touch, sound, or light
3. *No reflexes:* fixed, dilated pupils; lack of eye movement despite turning the head or ice-water stimulus; lack of response to noxious stimuli; and generally lack of elicitable deep tendon reflexes

In addition, the committee recommended that the preceding observations be confirmed by two EEGs, taken at least 24 hours apart, documenting the absence of cortical electrical activity above baseline. It was also deemed necessary to exclude the presence of any metabolic states, hypothermia, or drug intoxication that might cause or contribute to a reversible loss of brain activity or function.[4]

These criteria proved to be extremely reliable, and provided a strong impetus for physicians, attorneys, and policymakers to examine the propriety of bringing the then-accepted legal definition of death into conformity with then-current medical knowledge.

President's commission recommendation. In 1978, Congress authorized the formation of a blue ribbon panel of medical researchers and practitioners, other health care specialists, ethicists, attorneys, and public representatives to investigate troublesome areas in medicine.[5] The following year, President Carter named individuals to that group, called the President's Commission for the Study of Ethical Problems in Medicine and Biomedical and Behavioral Research. One of the areas included in the commission's charge was the problem of the definitions of death.

In an elegantly researched and scholarly report, entitled "Defining Death," the commissioners urged the acceptance by all U.S. jurisdictions of a Uniform Determination of Death Act, which would establish the "irreversible cessation of all functions of the entire brain, including the brain stem . . ."[6] as the criterion of death so as to provide guidelines for physicians to determine that death had indeed occurred and to assist in its pronouncement. Toward that end, members of the commission, the American Bar Association (ABA), the American Medical Association (AMA), and the National Conference of Commissioners on Uniform State Laws met to propose such a model act.

1. *Determination of Death.* An individual who has sustained either (1) irreversible cessation of circulatory and respiratory functions, or (2) irreversible cessation of all functions of the entire brain, including the brain stem, is dead. A determination of death must be made in accordance with accepted medical standards.
2. *Uniformity of Construction and Application.* This act shall be applied and construed to effectuate its general purpose to make uniform the law with respect to the subject of this Act among states enacting it.

This model statute has since been approved by the AMA, the ABA, and the Uniform Law Commissioners, and endorsed by the American Academy of Neurology and the American Electroencephalographic Society. The President's commission has urged all states that have not yet adopted the use of brain death criteria in the determination of death to consider doing so.

With the development of newer technology, additional refinements in the physician's ability to demonstrate "irreversible cessation of all functions of the entire brain" are achievable. In cases where the Harvard criteria or similar guidelines have established brain death, angiographic techniques have been used to demonstrate absence of cerebral circulation. Similarly, absence of brain metabolism (lack of glucose uptake by the brain) has been verified by applying nuclear medicine techniques and positron emission tomography. Obviously, when the brain is receiving no circulation and is not metabolizing the only substrate it is capable of utilizing, the conclusion must be that there has been "irreversible cessation" of brain function and therefore brain death. These techniques have served to validate the concept of brain death, the determination of which is made "in accordance with accepted medical standards" as described in the Uniform Determination of Death Act. As newer modalities are developed to further enhance our capabilities, this determination will be made with greater scientific accuracy and reliability.

The formulation of death discussed by the President's commission is often referred to as "whole-brain" formulation. Under this formulation, death is defined as the irreversible loss of an organism's ability to "function as a whole (to integrate, regulate, and organize important organ systems)."[7] Whole-brain theorists posit that "the entire brain (cerebral hemispheres, brain stem, cerebellum, and diencephalon [thalamus and hypothalamus]) must be rendered permanently functionless to determine death."[8] Nevertheless, referring to this formulation as "whole-brain" is somewhat of a misnomer, because under the definition the essential quality (i.e., that quality the loss of which constitutes death) is the brain stem's ability for "noncognitive integration of vegetative functions."[9] Loss of the so-called higher brain functions of consciousness and cognition is irrelevant. Recently, New Jersey enacted a law with a conscience clause permitting competent adults with religious beliefs to designate in advance that the traditional, heart-oriented definition of death should be used applied to them.[10]

Consequences for the criminal law. The brain death criterion has been applied in unusual circumstances in criminal homicide cases. In one case in Arizona, the defendant argued that it was not his criminal actions that caused the death of the victim, but rather those of the physician who terminated the life-support systems.[11] Accordingly, he alleged, there was not enough evidence to warrant his conviction for murder. However, the court ruled that the murder conviction was justified, because brain death was also a valid test of death in Arizona, and because the victim's brain function had ceased as a result of the defendant's action and before life support was discontinued.

A comparable case arose in California, where the victim had been shot in the head during a robbery attempt.[12] There was evidence of brain death by EEG, although the victim's heart and lungs continued to function on a ventilator. In that case, the victim's family agreed to have him serve as a donor for cardiac transplantation surgery at Stanford University Hospital. The victim was pronounced dead using the Harvard criteria and then flown to Stanford where the heart was removed for transplantation. The defendant's attorney objected when the charge against his client was changed from assault with intent to murder to murder in the first degree. The defense attorney claimed that the surgeon who removed the heart actually "murdered" the victim by his surgical act. In this case again, the court disagreed. The patient (victim) had died and was considered brain dead as a result of the criminal act itself and nothing else. On the basis of this case, California judicially adopted the concept of brain death as had Arizona.[13] The brain-death formulation was subsequently adopted by statute in California and is now contained in Chapter 3.7, Section 7180 of California's Health and Safety Code.

Parenthetically, it should be noted that, in most cases, within 3 to 10 days after brain death per se occurs, total cardiovascular collapse usually ensues. There are only a few reported cases in which survival has been prolonged beyond that point in adults. In children, however, cardiac and circulatory functions may continue for a considerably longer period after electrocerebral silence occurs and the Harvard criteria for brain death have been met.[14] There have been few civil cases turning on the diagnosis of death by brain death criteria.

The higher brain formulation of death. Why is the definition of death important?

The definition of death debate is actually a debate over the moral status of human beings. . . . [While] humans are [still alive], full moral and legal human rights accrue. Saying people are alive is simply shorthand for saying that they are bearers of such rights. That is why the definition of death debate is so important.[15]

The traditional (heart-lung) definition of death measured the point at which clinical death occurred. The biological life of the human organism was taken as a sine qua non for personhood and, therefore, the traditional definition allowed one to identify specifically those cases in which humans ceased to be persons.

It has been suggested that the whole-brain formulation's definition of death is inadequate and should be replaced by one defining death as "the irreversible loss of consciousness and cognition."[16] Defining death to include irreversible PVS would merely require extending the definition to include situations where the brainstem is functioning but the neocortex is dead."[17] Under this formulation, permanent "failure of [those] brain areas responsible for consciousness and cognition" would be the criterion of death.[18] Although admittedly there remain practical obstacles to the implementation of this "higher brain"[19] formulation of death (including the subjective nature of consciousness[20] and the nonspeci-

ficity of confirmatory laboratory tests[21]), the consciousness formulation retains its theoretical appeal because consciousness and cognition, unlike the ability to integrate vegetative functions, are "irreplaceably spontaneous and innate," and thus "essential to the definition of human life."[22]

Although one criticism of the higher brain formulation of death has been the inability of clinicians to determine precisely the irreversible loss of higher brain functions, the AMA's Councils on Scientific Affairs and Ethical and Judicial Affairs have concluded that a diagnosis of PVS can be made with an error rate of less than one in a thousand.[23]

Veatch has recently suggested the following:

An individual who has sustained irreversible loss of consciousness is dead. A determination of death must be made in accordance with accepted medical standards. However, no individual shall be considered dead based on irreversible loss of consciousness if he or she, while competent, has explicitly asked to be pronounced dead based on irreversible cessation of all functions of the entire brain or based on irreversible cessation of circulatory and respiratory functions.

Unless an individual has, while competent, selected one of these definitions of death, the legal guardian or next of kin (in that order) may do so. The definition selected by the individual, legal guardian or next of kin shall serve as the definition of death for all legal purposes.[24]

Death certificate

After the patient has been pronounced dead, the attending physician should prepare the working copy of the death certificate, which includes most of the following data: name and address of the decedent, age, place and date of birth, names of parents (including mother's maiden name), birthplace of parents, race, and decedent's occupation. These data are included primarily for statistical and/or epidemiological purposes. The death certificate also provides space for the attending physician to indicate how long he or she has treated the patient, when he or she last saw the patient alive, and the immediate and contributing causes of death, together with their duration. Other conditions from which the patient may have suffered, which did not necessarily contribute to the cause of death, are also listed. Most states also provide for inclusion of data regarding surgery and/or biopsy and autopsy as indicative of the cause of death. It is important to note that the immediate cause of death is not always necessarily the mechanism of death, such as cardiac arrest or ventricular fibrillation, but rather the condition that eventually resulted in death, such as myocardial infarction with arrhythmia. Using this working document, the mortician will type the final death certificate, which is then presented to the physician for signature and dating. Burial or other disposition of the remains is not permitted in most states until the completed death certificate has been signed by the attending physician.

Cause of death

As noted previously, the cause of death listed on the death certificate should be the immediate cause, the condition that resulted in death rather than the mechanism of death.

In those situations in which the cause of death may be obscure, or the physician has not seen the patient in a specified period of time (which varies from state to state), state law usually requires the medical examiner or coroner to be contacted. The case then becomes a medical examiner's or coroner's case. The laws of the various states differ considerably with respect to circumstances under which the coroner or medical examiner must be notified regarding the death, and will determine whether or not autopsy is appropriate. Most states specify certain specific situations in which such notification is essential, including one or more of the following: dead-on-arrival cases; cases in which the cause of death cannot be determined because of inadequate stay in the hospital; cases in which death occurred following hospitalization for less than 24 hours; all cases of sudden, violent, suspicious, unexpected, unexplained, and medically unattended death; all intraoperative or perioperative deaths (including preoperative and immediate postoperative); death related to industrial employment; death resulting from therapeutic misadventure; death resulting from alleged, suspected, or known criminal activity; and death resulting from vehicular traffic accidents as well as train or airplane accidents.

The physician must understand the critical importance of contacting the medical examiner or coroner in his or her jurisdiction when there is any doubt about the circumstances surrounding the death. The physician should be willing to speak with the medical examiner or the staff to discuss the case with them at length. Requests for results or data on the medical examiner's autopsy or a copy of the autopsy protocol for the physician's records are usually honored.

Custody of body, authorization of autopsy, and disposal of remains

Although the individual may indicate before death that he or she wishes to have an autopsy performed, such a statement is advisory or directive only—not mandatory. As soon as death occurs, the next-of-kin are recognized by law to have a property interest in the body of the decedent. They are the ones, according to a schedule prescribed by state law, who may consent to an autopsy. The rank order of individuals who may grant such permission for autopsy or have custody of the remains is usually as follows: surviving spouse, eldest living child of the decedent (if of age), parent(s) of the decedent, legally appointed guardian, eldest living sibling of the deceased (if of age), aunt(s) and uncle(s) of the decedent, and other kin in order of consanguinity.

Obviously, before an autopsy can be requested, the patient must be pronounced dead by the physician, and appropriate family members or next-of-kin contacted. When death occurs in a hospital, the death pronouncement note must be written in the hospital record, and the autopsy request form completed and signed prior to the performance of that procedure. It is also appropriate to indicate on the permission form any restrictions on the extent of the examination, such as head excluded, chest only, abdomen only, and so on. Obviously, the more extensive the autopsy and the more tissues examined, the more accurate, valuable, and complete will be the information gathered for the benefit of the physicians, surviving family members, and society.

When there is controversy over consenting to an autopsy among members of a group of equal consanguinity, it is probably inadvisable or imprudent to accept the consent of only one member of the group who is willing to give it. Frequently the original permit may have been obtained from a low-priority relative only because that individual was the one first located following the death of the patient, and one of closer consanguinity subsequently objects. When there are no known relatives, custody of the body and responsibility for its disposition may be accepted by a friend, a lodge, or similar organization. However, such a casual custodian of a dead body may have no legal authority to grant permission for an autopsy.

Although it has occurred from time to time, it is considered unprofessional for a physician to use the threat of medical examiner contact as a tool to pry autopsy consent from a family in cases when the death is obviously due to natural causes, which would not otherwise require medical examiner involvement or investigation. Cooperation with the medical examiner, provision of appropriate information, access to physician and hospital records, and so on, allow as much knowledge as possible to be gained to help elicit the cause of death in confusing cases.

It is important to note that the medical examiner is not empowered to function as a watchdog over the clinical performance of physicians in the community. As is obvious by the nature of the work, however, the medical examiner or coroner may well become involved in cases of alleged professional negligence or incompetence. The investigations and examinations in such situations should be conducted in the same careful, thorough manner as would any other case. The final report should be prepared in a highly professional manner and should be available to all appropriate parties. A competent, careful, thorough, scientific, unbiased investigation and report serve the cause of justice in any medicolegal situation, whether civil or criminal.

Additional cases of death appropriate for medical examiner investigation are violent, accidental, and mysterious deaths, including suspected homicide or suicide. Those that may be due entirely or in part to any factor other than natural causes are also reportable. These include, but are not limited to, death associated with burns, chemicals, or electrical or radiation injury; death under suspicious circumstances; death of patients of public institutions not hospitalized primarily for organic disease; death of persons in the custody of law enforcement officers; all deaths that occur during, in association with, or as a result of diagnostic, therapeutic, or anesthetic procedures; any death due to neglect; and death of persons not disabled by recognizable disease.

Once the autopsy has been completed, or once death is pronounced when no autopsy is to be performed, the remains may be turned over to next-of-kin or surviving family members, a mortician, an embalmer, or a funeral director for burial, cremation, or other disposition. As noted previously, such final disposition cannot take place until the attending physician, the coroner, or the medical examiner has completed and signed the death certificate. It is critical that the physician's signature be added to the death certificate only after that certificate has been completed by a mortician or funeral director. Signing a blank death certificate or one that is incomplete may create serious problems for the attending physician.

THE DYING PATIENT
Traditional physician role

From the historical beginnings of medicine, the physician's goal was twofold: to preserve life and to relieve suffering. From the days of the Greek and Roman physicians through the early 1960s, these goals were not in conflict, but went hand-in-hand.

Admittedly, situations arose in which the physician might be tempted to hasten the patient's demise by giving an excessively large dose of morphine, possibly under the guise of pain relief, or to provide some other method of inducing the patient's death. However, the constraints of the Judeo-Christian religions, with their proscriptions against killing, the various ethical codes for physicians (Hippocrates, Maimonides), and the possibility of criminal prosecution for euthanasia frequently combined to prevent physicians from undertaking such activities. In the case of the dying patient, often there was little the physician could do other than provide psychological and emotional support, com-

plete pain relief was not possible without jeopardizing vital functions—which brings us to the double effect.

The double effect. Take, for example, a patient with widely metastatic cancer requiring narcotic analgesics for control of pain. As the patient's narcotic requirements escalate, it becomes increasingly difficult to control the pain without depressing the patient's respiratory drive. Because relieving pain and maintaining compromised function are both legitimate goals of medicine, what is the physician to do when these goals conflict?

Such situations are often analyzed in terms of the "double effect":

Some actions have several effects that are inextricably linked. One of those effects is intended by the agent and is ethically permissible (e.g., relief of pain); the other is not intended by the agent and is ethically questionable (e.g., respiratory depression). Proponents of this argument state that ethically permissible effect can be allowed, even if the ethically questionable one will inevitably follow, when the following conditions are present:
(a) The action itself is ethically good or at least indifferent, that is, neither good nor evil in itself (in this case, the action is the administration of a drug, a morally indifferent act).
(b) The agent must intend the good effects, not the evil effects, even though these are foreseen (in this case, the intention is to relieve pain, not to compromise respiration).
(c) The morally objectionable effect cannot be a means to the morally permissible one (in this case, respiratory compromise is not the means to relief of pain).[25]

The new Michigan ban against assisted suicide contains an exemption contemplating the double effect; it exempts the prescription, dispensing, or administration of medication designed "to relieve pain or discomfort and not to cause death, even if the medication or procedure may hasten or increase the risk of death."[26]

Effects of technology and a changing patient population

As has already been described in discussing the evolution of the concept of brain death, resuscitation techniques and technology began to be applied in the late 1960s, and their use was not limited to that group for whom resuscitation was originally recommended. As early as 1973, the American Heart Association (AHA) and the National Academy of Sciences (NAS) reinforced the original recommendations regarding CPR, urging that CPR be employed in the case of young individuals with sudden, unexpected arrest, or victims of drowning or electrocution. The 1973 AHA and NAS statements noted that "[CPR] is not indicated in certain clinical situations, i.e., terminal irreversible illness where death is not unexpected." CPR was also considered an innappropriate modality for the chronically ill individual with no hope of recovery.

Unfortunately, with the passage of time, resuscitation techniques and life-support measures were applied to a progressively sicker, older, more infirm population. CPR became a commonplace activity on the hospital scene whenever an arrest occurred. Its performance was straightforward and almost rote, frequently with no consideration given to patient selection or therapeutic aim.

In many cases, patients were resuscitated with no subsequent return of cognitive (higher brain) functions. Families and society were left with a burgeoning population of patients, maintained on ventilators, with no hope of return to a normal, sapient state. In those cases where brain death criteria were applicable, death might be pronounced using those criteria and the patient then withdrawn from the ventilator to "let nature take its course." In those cases where brain death criteria were not met and ventilator support could not be removed, the burden continued and the patient was maintained in his or her noncognitive, nonsapient state.

Not surprisingly, concerns arose that resuscitation was being innappropriately overutilized, in many cases on patients who were harmed by it rather than benefitted. The physician's goals of prolonging life and easing suffering had come into conflict.

Withholding and withdrawing treatment: the patient with capacity

There exists a legal consensus that the adult with capacity has a legally protected right to refuse life-sustaining[27] treatment. It has been pointed out that, historically, courts have grounded this right either in the common law right to self-determination, or the privacy and/or liberty guarantees of the federal or state constitutions, rather than in exceptions to homicide laws.[28]

Courts have characterized the termination of life support as a means of permissible "letting die,"[29] distinguishing it from impermissible "killing" (murder, suicide, or assisted suicide). Courts have generally given two reasons for this distinction: First, that the intention of the patient in refusing treatment is not self-destruction but rather control of their care; and second, that the cause of death in the patient who refuses life-sustaining treatment is the patient's illness, not the patient's refusal. A better explanation for this distinction is

[T]hat if liability is not to be imposed on physicians who withhold or withdraw life support, it is because they have no duty to provide it. The absence of a duty arises from the fact that the treatment has been declined by a competent patient or for an incompetent patient by a surrogate legally authorized to do so.[30]

The right of the patient with capacity to refuse unwanted medical treatment gained constitutional recognition in the majority's statement in *Cruzan v. Director*[31] to the effect that "[T]he principle that a competent patient has a constitutionally protected liberty interest in refusing unwanted medical treatment may be inferred from our prior decisions." The practical effect of the Court's characterization of the right to refuse unwanted medical treatment as a "liberty interest" rather than a fundamental right is that the state need not have a compelling countervailing interest in order to overcome a "liberty interest."

The rights of patients with the capacity to refuse life-sustaining treatment apply even to those who are not terminally ill.

In *Elizabeth Bouvia v. Riverside General Hosp.*,[32] Elizabeth Bouvia was a young woman with cerebral palsy and virtually no use of her voluntary muscles. As a result, she was unable to take her own life. She had hospitalized herself and "disclosed her intent to discontinue sufficient caloric intake so that she would eventually succumb to starvation." Bouvia asked the court to enjoin defendant hospital from administering artificial nutrition and hydration against her will, and from transferring or discharging her.

The Court, while stating that Bouvia "does have a fundamental right to terminate her own life and to terminate medical intervention," framed the issue differently. The issue was, according to the Court, "whether or not a severely handicapped, mentally competent person who is otherwise physically healthy and not terminally ill has the right to end her life *with the assistance of society*" (emphasis added).[32]

In a later case involving Ms. Bouvia, the California Court of Appeals held that she had a right to refuse nutrition and hydration in order to end her life.[33]

Withholding and withdrawing treatment: the patient who has lost capacity

There seems to be a legal consensus that, in theory, the right of a patient without capacity to refuse medical treatment should be coextensive with the corresponding right of a patient with capacity. The effective exercise of that right is, however, problematic. Thus some patients without capacity may be unable to express *any* preference with regard to treatment; other patients without capacity, although able to express treatment preferences, may be expressing preferences that are not authentic expressions of their will. Consequently, a decision concerning the treatment of the patient without capacity must be made by a surrogate decision-maker.

We pointed out earlier that the patient with capacity has the right to refuse life-sustaining treatment irrespective of that patient's medical condition or prognosis. Although the same is theoretically true regarding patients who have lost decision-making capacity,

[C]ourts . . . understandably look carefully at the patient's medical condition or prognosis before sanctioning surrogate decisions for nonautonomous patients who have not expressed a clear position of abating treatment. The clearest cases [have] involved patients who are terminally ill. . . . Courts have [also] upheld numerous decisions to abate treatment for patients in a persistent vegetative state. . . . Few courts have yet to grapple with the charged issue of abating treatment for nonvegetative, nonterminally ill patients [without capacity].[34]

Decision making for the patient without capacity/with an advance directive. Advance directives include "living wills, durable powers of attorney, appointment of health care proxies, . . . and other devices that allow a competent person to give directions concerning [his/]her medical treatment if [he/]she becomes incompetent."[35]

To better inform patients about their legal rights to execute advance directives and refuse treatment, Congress in 1990 enacted the Patient Self-Determination Act (PSDA).[36] This act, which took effect on December 1, 1991, mandated that health care institutions (including nursing homes, hospitals, home health agencies, hospices, clinics, and health maintenance organizations) in receipt of federal funds under Medicare and/or Medicaid provide each patient with written information regarding his or her rights under the laws of his or her state to participate in the medical decision-making process and to formulate an advance directive.

The PSDA encourages the use of advance directives by requiring hospitals to inform patients of their right to execute such directives.

LIVING WILL STATUTES. California was the first state to enact living will legislation, with its own Natural Death Act[37] in 1977. By 1992, all but three states had enacted living will laws providing a statutory mechanism for persons to exercise their legal right to refuse life-sustaining treatment in the event they lose decision-making capacity.[38]

Living will statutes are problematic:

Most of these statutes include fairly rigorous standards for preparing a binding directive. Many statutes provide, for example, that a directive becomes binding only if and when the patient is determined to be terminally ill—and typically that determination must be made by more than one physician. In some states, a directive is legally binding only if, after the onset of terminal illness but before the onset of incompetence (a fleeting moment for some patients), the patient reaffirms the directive. Increasingly, physicians and lawyers alike have criticized these statutory models both for their procedural obstacles and for failing to make clear which forms of care are to be foregone and [under] what circumstances.[39]

For these reasons, an increasingly attractive option for patients is to delegate the legal authority to make health care decisions to another person in the event that the patient becomes unable to make such decisions.

DURABLE POWER OF ATTORNEY AND HEALTH CARE PROXIES. Normally a power of attorney executed by an individual allows another, acting as his or her agent, to make decisions for him or her. In the event of the incompetence of the original declarant, the power of attorney lapses and becomes void. In other words, the agent can no longer act for the principal should the principal become incompetent after the original delegation of authority.

The *durable* power of attorney, on the other hand, permits decision-making by the agent in the event that the principal becomes incompetent. When extended to health care situations, it delegates to the agent the authority to make health care decisions for the principal, in the event of the latter's incapacity or incompetence.

As of 1987, all 50 states had general durable power of attorney statutes that were "probably adequate authority to empower a health care proxy decision-maker."[40] Further, as of 1992, all states except Alabama had enacted statutes that either explicitly authorized the delegation to a proxy of the legal authority to make health care decisions or that had been specifically interpreted as authorizing such a delegation (so-called "health care proxy" acts).[41] In *Cruzan,* the Supreme Court suggested that the Constitution might require that states give legal effect to the health care decisions of a duly appointed surrogate decision-maker.

Deciding for the patient without capacity/without a formal advance directive. There remains the problem of how to make medical decisions for patients who have lost capacity without ever having executed a formal advance directive. Under these circumstances, different states employ different procedures and different substantive criteria for surrogate decision making. In general, "[T]he consensus view is that there is a hierarchy of three standards to be applied in making decisions [under these circumstances] . . . : the subjective standard, the substituted judgment standard, and the best interests standard."[42] Thus, the decision-making process in such a case begins with an inquiry into whether or not the patient has executed an *informal* advance directive by expressing a desire either to accede to or decline treatment under the present circumstances.

THE SUBJECTIVE STANDARD. The strictest standard has been referred to as the subjective standard, under which the surrogate's decision is based on the patient's own preferences as expressed before loss of capacity. Under the subjective standard, the surrogate asks "What did the patient in fact decide before losing decision-making capacity?"[43] Expressions of those preferences are to be found, for example, in "oral directions to family members, friends, or health-care providers, reactions of the patient to medical treatment administered to others, the individual's religious beliefs, and the patient's previous pattern of behavior concerning his or her own medical care"[44] prior to the patient's loss of decision-making capacity.

New York State case law illustrates this approach. In the *Matter of Westchester County Medical Center,*[45] Mary O'Connor, a 78-year-old woman had, as a result of multi-infarct dementia, lost decision-making capacity as well as the ability to eat or drink normally. Mrs. O'Connor's doctors wanted to insert a nasogastric tube in order to feed and hydrate her artificially, but her families refused to consent, saying that this would be against their mother's wishes. Mrs. O'Connor had, while caring for several terminally ill relatives in the past, said that she would not want to be kept alive by artificial means were she unable to care for herself. The New York Court of Appeals held that there was no clear and convincing evidence that Mrs. O'Connor would decline artificial feeding/hydration when she was not terminally ill.

In *Cruzan v. Director, Missouri Dept. of Health,*[46] the U.S. Supreme Court held that the "liberty interest" protected by the Fourteenth Amendment's due process clause does not preclude states from requiring, as a prerequisite for forgoing life-sustaining treatment of patients without capacity, "that there be clear and convincing evidence that the patient herself decided prior to losing decision-making capacity that [life-sustaining] treatment should be stopped."[47] The state's adoption of this decision-making standard was justified by the state's interests in "preserving life and personal choice, preventing abuse by the surrogate, and ensuring accurate fact finding and reducing the risk of error."[48] It is important to understand that *Cruzan* permits, but does not require, states to adopt a "clear and convincing" evidentiary standard. Cruzan states that the "challenging task of creating appropriate procedures for safeguarding incompetents' liberty interests is entrusted to the 'laboratory' of the states . . . ."[49]

SUBSTITUTED JUDGMENT STANDARD. Under this standard, the surrogate asks "What would the patient decide if the patient were able to decide?"[50] New Jersey's famous *Quinlan*[51] case illustrates this approach.

Karen Quinlan was originally brought to a New Jersey hospital in a comatose state, where her consent to treatment was implied by the emergency doctrine. She was intubated and maintained on a respirator. Despite such treatment, she remained in a PVS[52] from which it became clear that she would not emerge. Because Karen would thus never have the capacity to assert her right to be free of unwanted physical intrusions, her father sought to assert this right for her, and asked that mechanical ventilation be stopped. Invoking the doctrine of "substituted judgment," the court held that "the only practical way to prevent destruction of [Karen Quinlan's] right [of privacy] is to permit the guardian and family of Karen to render their best judgment . . . as to whether she would exercise it in these circumstances."[53]

BEST INTERESTS STANDARD. Where it is unclear what the patient would decide if he or she were able to decide, most courts allow the surrogate to forgo life-sustaining treatment if doing so is in the patient's best interests. Meisel has pointed out that "no court that permits the use of the substituted judgment standard has rejected the application of a best interests standard if the evidence is insufficient to meet the former," although not all courts that permit the use of the substituted judgment standard have had to decide whether to permit the use of the best interests standard where the substituted judgment standard cannot be met.[54]

Note that it is well accepted that "continued [life-sustaining] treatment *per se* is not always in a patient's best interests, and forgoing [such] treatment is not always contrary to a patient's interests."[55]

Although the preceding three "standards" establish the facts that must be proven in order to enable a surrogate to forgo life-sustaining treatment, a separate consideration is "How convincingly must these facts be established?" In other words, what standard of proof must be met?

Most states, irrespective of which of the preceding three standards for surrogate decision-making they employ, require that those standards be met with "clear and convincing evidence." New York and Missouri, for example,

[r]equire clear and convincing evidence that *the patient himself or herself authorized* the forgoing of life-sustaining treatment before losing decision-making capacity. . . . [Other states require] clear and convincing evidence that the patient *would have* decided to forgo treatment—in effect, clear and convincing evidence of the substituted judgment standard. In other states what is required is clear and convincing evidence that it is not in the patient's best interests . . . that treatment be continued.[56] (Original emphasis.)

DECISION MAKING BY FAMILIES. Some 20 states have enacted so-called "family decision" acts, which codify the "age-old custom of turning to the next of kin for guidance about treatment when a patient is unable to make decisions personally."[57] Such acts are based on the twin assumptions that, first, when a patient's preferences are knowable, family members are the persons most likely to know them and, second, that where those preferences are not knowable, family members are the persons most likely to act in the patient's best interests. Recently, the New York State Task Force on Life and the Law made legislative recommendations regarding decision making by surrogates for incapacitated patients who have executed neither an advance directive nor a health care proxy.[58] According to the recommendations of the task force, such a patient

[S]hould be represented by a surrogate, chosen from a prioritized list [(court-appointed guardian; individual designated by others on the list; spouse; adult child; parent; adult sibling; close friend)]. . . . The surrogate should decide in accordance with the patient's wishes, to the extent that these wishes can be determined, and, failing that, in accordance with the patient's best interests. The surrogate has the same authority to make decisions . . . that the patient would have had, except . . . in the case of decisions to forgo life-sustaining treatment. . . . [While] "routine medical treatment may be provided on the decision of the attending physician . . . [and] "major medical treatment" may be administered on the decision of the attending physician in consultation with . . . a second physician appointed by the hospital . . . "decisions to withhold or withdraw life-sustaining treatment" entail . . . approval by a "bioethics review committee."[59]

Deciding for the patient who never had capacity.
Cruzan itself articulates no standards governing surrogate refusal of treatment on behalf of persons who have never been competent, and the Supreme Court has not yet been faced with this issue.

Massachusetts grappled with this issue in *Superintendent of Belchertown State School v. Saikewicz*.[60] Joseph Saikewicz was a 67-year-old mentally retarded man in urgent need of treatment for acute leukemia. Because of the severity of his mental retardation, however (he had an IQ of 10 and a mental age of about two years, eight months), he was unable to give informed consent to treatment. A court-appointed guardian ad litem recommended "that not treating Mr. Saikewicz would be in his best interests."[61] The probate judge agreed with the guardian ad litem.

The appeals court affirmed. The court used as the starting point of its analysis the principle that "a general right . . . to refuse medical treatment . . . must extend to the case of an incompetent, as well as a competent, patient because the value of human dignity extends to both . . . ."[62] The court reasoned, therefore, that in refusal of treatment cases involving never competent persons, courts should attempt

[T]o ascertain the incompetent person's actual interests and preferences. In short, the decision in cases such as this should be that which would be made by the incompetent person, if that person were competent, but taking into account the present and future incompetency of the individual as one of the factors which would necessarily enter into the decision-making process of the competent person.[63]

New York dealt differently with a similar case in the *Matter of Storar*.[64] John Storar was a 52-year-old mentally retarded man with a mental age of about five years. He had bladder cancer and a secondary anemia necessitating periodic blood transfusions, but was unable to give informed consent to the transfusions. His mother refused to give consent because the transfusion process distressed her son, and because he had an illness that was in any event terminal.

The New York Court of Appeals reasoned that since John Storar had never had capacity, he was in essence a child. Since, under New York law, "no parent can withhold a blood transfusion from a child when without it the child will die,"[65] the court ruled that the blood transfusions could not be withheld. The court reasoned that "it was unrealistic to try to determine what [John Storar] would want done under the circumstances . . . [, and] also rejected the substituted judgment test adopted by some [other] courts because [it] felt that no third party should be permitted to make a quality of life judgment for another."[66]

Do-not-resuscitate orders

In recent years, the concept of an individual's right to self-determination has taken center stage in the resuscitation decision. Both the legal and medical communities have recognized that this is no more than a corollary of the patient's right of informed consent. This right is considered to be weightier than the interests of the physician and/or hospital, and includes the right of informed refusal of resuscitation even in the ultimate care setting.

In those instances where patients did not wish to be resuscitated but were resuscitated anyway, physicians were considered to have violated the dictum enunciated by Justice Cardozo in the *Schloendorff* case[67] in 1914: "Every human being of adult years and sound mind has a right to determine what shall be done with his own body."

Constitutional support for the individual's right to refuse unwanted resuscitation was, like the right to refuse other unwanted medical treatment, derived from the "right to privacy," and from the liberty interest protected by the Fourteenth Amendment. Decisions not to resuscitate may be thought of as a subdivision of decisions to withhold medical treatment.

Although they have been perceived as a new development, do-not-resuscitate (DNR)[68] orders form part of the long-range picture in the evolution of our current awareness of mutual rights and responsibilities in the area of death and dying. In this context, it is relevant to consider the memorandum that appeared more than 20 years ago on the bulletin board of a large, respected teaching hospital: "The following patients are not to be resuscitated: those who are very elderly (over 65 years of age); those who are suffering from malignant disease; those with chronic chest disease; and those with chronic renal disease." This memo was posted at the Neasden Hospital in Britain in 1965. When it came to public notice, the news spread like wildfire through the British press. Great public hue and cry ensued. The hospital administration said that it did not intend the message the memo appeared to convey, or perhaps it was mistyped, or incorrectly interpreted; but regardless, hospital administration did not mean what was stated in the memo. This was apparently the first attempt to apply any type of protocol in nonresuscitation cases.

Today most hospitals have policies under which all patients will be resuscitated unless a written DNR order has been on their chart.

In addition, JCAHO required, effective January 1, 1988, that all facilities seeking accreditation must have a DNR policy, without defining the limits or criteria to be included within that policy.[69] There now seems to be a consensus that patients have the right, and should be afforded the opportunity, to exercise their autonomous decision not to be resuscitated. The "reflex resuscitation" of anyone experiencing an arrest is now disappearing in favor of antecedent decisions to forgo it or to have positive orders for resuscitation, if needed.

New York was the first state to regulate DNR orders comprehensively, in New York Public Health Law, Article 29-B, Sections 2960-2978. New York's DNR law presumes consent to resuscitation in the absence of an order not to resuscitate (ONTR). A physician may not write such an order without first obtaining the patient's consent, if the patient has decision-making capacity, or the consent of a duly appointed surrogate if the patient lacks decision-making capacity. The New York DNR law also provides a statutory list of acceptable surrogates where the patient is incompetent and has not, prior to losing capacity, appointed a surrogate. The surrogate must base his or her decision regarding CPR on the patient's wishes or, if the patient's wishes are unknown and unknowable, on the patient's best interests. Furthermore, a surrogate may consent to an ONTR only if it has been determined by an attending physician to a reasonable degree of medical certainty that the patient has a terminal condition, or that the patient is permanently unconscious, or that resuscitation would be medically futile, or that resuscitation would impose an extraordinary burden on the patient in light of the patient's medical condition.[70]

It should be emphasized that DNR laws such as New York's do not create a duty to resuscitate where previously none existed. Rather, they create a presumption that all patients who have not expressly consented to an ONTR would consent to resuscitative measures.

Futility

"Medical futility" is not easily defined, but "generally, the term means care that serves no useful purpose and provides no immediate or long-term benefit."[71] More specifically, futile care

[M]ay be that which does not address . . . the underlying illness . . . that in time will cause death, [or] . . . it may be care that does not achieve its immediate purpose. Whether . . . performing an appendectomy on a patient with incurable cancer would be futile depends on which of these two meanings one adopts.[72]

In discussing futility, then, one must be careful to distinguish between physiologically futile treatment (defined as treatment that is "clearly futile in achieving its physiologic objective and so [of] no physiologic benefit to the patient"[73]) and treatment with "important physiologic effects which medical judgment concludes [nonetheless] are *non-beneficial* to the patient as person."[74] Futility is an increasingly important issue in end-of-life medicine.

In re Wanglie. The case of Helga Wanglie was hailed in a *New England Journal of Medicine* editorial as "a new kind of right to die case."[75] While in earlier "right to die" cases it had been families and/or patients seeking to have life-sustaining treatment withheld or withdrawn over the objections of the health care providers, in the Wanglie case it was the patient's doctors who sought to withdraw life-sustaining treatment over the objections of the patient's family.

Helga Wanglie was an 86-year-old, ventilator-dependent Minneapolis woman in PVS. In November 1990, her physicians informed the Wanglie family that continued mechanical ventilation was nonbeneficial to Mrs. Wanglie as a person and that it should be discontinued.

Mrs. Wanglie's husband (a lawyer), daughter, and son rejected the idea of withdrawing ventilatory support, saying "that physicians should not play God, that the patient would not be better off dead, that removing life support showed moral decay in our civilization, and that a miracle could occur."[76] While the husband initially "told a physician that his wife had never stated her preferences concerning life-sustaining treatment" in the setting of PVS, he later "asserted that the patient had consistently said she wanted respirator support for such a condition."[77]

The hospital asked that the court appoint an independent conservator to decide whether continued use of the respirator was beneficial to the patient; and, in the event the conservator found its use was not beneficial, the hospital asked that a second hearing be held on the question of whether it was legally obliged to provide the respirator. On July 1, 1991, the court appointed the husband as conservator; and, noting that no request had yet been made for permission to stop treatment, declined to address the matter.[78] The hospital, unclear about its legal duty to continue to provide ventilatory support, announced that it would not discontinue such support. Three days later, Mrs. Wanglie died of sepsis-induced multisystem organ failure.

DNR orders and futility. Recently, it has been suggested that rather than automatically mandating or establishing hospital policies that CPR be applied in the event of every arrest, the decision regarding whether or not CPR will be employed should be raised before the fact. In those cases where CPR would be expected to benefit the patient, several authors have suggested that it should be ordered positively before the fact, as an order to be implemented if and when the patient experiences an arrest.[79]

Where resuscitation is considered futile therapy (it has been suggested that the use of CPR in patients who will not survive to be discharged from the hospital is futile[80]), advance decisions about CPR should be considered and DNR orders written.[81] If there is no reasonable expectation that the patient will benefit from resuscitation, it may then be considered an inappropriate (if not unethical) modality to employ, especially without having first consulted the patient to obtain consent.

It has even been argued that where the physician has determined that attempts at CPR would be futile in a particular patient, the physician has the authority to enter a DNR order without the consent of the patient or the patient's family. This follows from the principle that doctors have no duty to provide useless therapy to patients or to discuss useless therapy with them. Patients for whom CPR may be deemed futile include the following:

1. Patients who are brain dead.
2. Anencephalic newborns.
3. Patients with . . . metastatic cancer in [its] agonal stage.
4. Elderly patients with acute stroke, sepsis, or pneumonia.
5. Patients with severe cardiomyopathy.
6. Elderly patients with renal failure who are found pulseless and apneic.
7. Elderly patients with asystole, electro-mechanical dissociation, or agonal rhythms.
8. Very low birth weight newborns who suffer a cardiac arrest in the first 72 hours following birth.
9. Patients with severe chronic lung disease.[82]

Analysis of the relevant case law lends credence to the argument that a physician's liability for not providing futile CPR is remote, and that in fact a physician exposes himself or herself to greater liability by providing such treatment.[83] Where unilateral DNR orders are to be written, it would be prudent to do so under the auspices of hospital or medical staff guidelines for their issuance.[84]

Physician aid-in-dying

The legal controversy surrounding professional participation in the act of dying derives from the conflict between two competing traditions—the right to refuse medical treatment, on the one hand, versus the antisuicide tradition, on the other, as evidenced by society's discouragement of suicide and attempted suicide, and by the many criminal laws against assisted suicide.

Three levels of professional participation have been identified in the debate over physician-assisted dying: voluntary passive euthanasia (VPE), physician-assisted suicide (PAS), and physician-committed voluntary active euthanasia (VAE).

Passive euthanasia. VPE refers to the withdrawal or withholding of life-sustaining medical treatment, in accordance with the wishes of a competent patient or a duly appointed surrogate. "During the past two decades, passive euthanasia has been . . . accepted both legally and ethically in the United States."[85]

VPE was discussed extensively earlier, so here we limit our discussion to VPE as it concerns patient refusal of hydration and nutrition (PRHN).

Many health care providers are still reluctant to withhold or withdraw artificial hydration and nutrition, under any circumstances. This reluctance stems at least partly from "the social implications of withholding food and fluids, particularly because of its symbolism as communicating lack of caring."[86] This reluctance may also stem in part from their uncertainty about the medical/ethical/legal propriety of withholding/withdrawing food and fluids. Some state legislatures have compounded this problem by enacting living will statutes that exclude artificial hydration and nutrition from the life-sustaining treatments that may be withdrawn from terminally ill patients, or by describing artificial feeding as a necessary part of comfort care. Even New York's Health Care Agents and Proxies Law treats artificial hydration and nutrition as being somehow different from other life-sustaining treatments.[87]

Nevertheless, the Council on Ethical and Judicial Affairs of the AMA and the majority of courts as well—including the U.S. Supreme Court in *Cruzan*—treat artificial hydration and nutrition as just another form of medical treatment. The emerging consensus is to distinguish between artificially or technologically supplied hydration and nutrition (which is considered a form of medical treatment that may—indeed, must—be withheld or withdrawn when refused by the patient with capacity) and providing a patient with access to food and water (which is considered basic humane care that should always be provided).

It has recently been suggested that "educating chronically and terminally ill patients about the feasibility of patient refusal of hydration and nutrition (PRHN) [and helping them do so in a way that minimizes suffering] can empower them to control their own destiny without requiring physicians to reject the taboos on PAS and VAE that have existed for millenia."[88]

Despite these ancient taboos, there is evidence of a growing consensus in favor of the other two kinds of physician aid-in-dying. In 1991, Derek Humphry's book *Final Exit* reached the New York Times best seller list for nonfiction by urging terminally ill patients to commit suicide and urging physicians to assist them, or even engage in euthanasia.[89] Also in 1991, a public opinion poll revealed that nearly two-thirds of Americans supported both PAS and VAE for terminally ill patients.[90] Nevertheless, two relatively recent attempts to legalize "aid-in-dying" (a term that subsumes both physician-assisted suicide and voluntary active euthanasia) were unsuccessful.

In 1991, voters in Washington State defeated (by a 54% to 46% margin) Initiative 119, which would have sanctioned PAS or euthanasia by physicians when requested by competent patients with a terminal condition (i.e., patients with less than 6 months to live or patients in irreversible comas or PVS).[91] In November 1992, a similar initiative, Proposition 161,[92] was defeated by voters in California by an identical 54% to 46% margin.

Likewise, PAS and VAE remain legally problematic.

Physician-assisted suicide. PAS refers to the practice whereby the physician provides the patient with the medical know-how (e.g., discussing painless and effective pharmacologic means of committing suicide) and/or the means (e.g., writing a prescription) enabling that patient to end his or her own life.

Currently, although no state or federal law punishes an individual who commits or attempts suicide, some 30 states and two territories have enacted laws imposing criminal sanctions on individuals who assist in a suicide.[93] "States that specifically prohibit assisted suicide either classify it as a unique offense (e.g., CA, NY) or define it as a type of murder or manslaughter (e.g., AZ, OR, HI)."[94]

Jack Kevorkian gained notoriety in June 1990 when he assisted in the suicide of Janet Adkins, a woman with early Alzheimer's disease. Since then, he has assisted in the suicides of some 19 other persons whom he barely knew.[95] Largely in response to Kevorkian's activities, on February 15, 1993, the state of Michigan enacted a law making assisted suicide a felony punishable by up to 4 years in prison. The constitutionality of the law has been challenged by the Michigan ACLU, and has yet to be decided by the Michigan Courts of Appeals.

In 1991, the *New England Journal of Medicine* published Dr. Timothy Quill's account of his role in the suicide of Patricia Diane Trumbull, a long-standing patient of his with acute leukemia. In response to Diane's plans for assistance, Quill, prescribed barbiturates and told her how many to take to end her life. Despite the fact that assisted suicide has been criminalized by statute[96] for years in New York, a New York grand jury refused to return a criminal indictment against Dr. Quill, and the New York Board for Professional Medical Conduct ruled that no charge of professional misconduct was warranted.[97]

Physician-committed voluntary active euthanasia. Unlike PAS, where the final agent in the patient's death *is* the patient, in physician-committed VAE the final agent in the patient's death is the physician. VAE refers to the practice whereby the physician actively and directly (i.e., such as by administering a lethal injection of morphine or potassium) causes the death of a competent patient who voluntarily requests aid-in-dying.[98]

Currently, euthanasia is illegal in all states in the United States. Although no statutes specifically criminalize voluntary active euthanasia, case law has interpreted voluntary active euthanasia as a violation of criminal homicide statutes, so that perpetrators may be charged with murder, manslaughter, or criminal homicide. Because the criminal law exists to protect the public interest, as opposed to private interests, the patient's consent to, or even request for, the physician's lethal act is considered irrelevant.[99]

Nor does it matter that the physician's lethal act is motivated by mercy, since "in American criminal jurisprudence, the perpetrator's motive for killing is not an element of homicide."[100] Nor does the fact that the perpetrator was motivated by mercy necessarily vitiate the "malice aforethought" element required for murder, since courts have ruled that "the necessary malice consists of intentionally engaging in a legally proscribed killing."[101]

In 1988, *JAMA* published "It's Over, Debbie,"[102] an anonymous and possibly fictional account of an on-call gynecology resident who is paged in the middle of the night to the room of Debbie, a 20-year-old girl dying of ovarian cancer. The resident had had no prior contact with the patient, yet in response to an ambiguous request on Debbie's part—"Let's get this over with"—reportedly administered a lethal dose of morphine. Following the publication of this account, the authorities sought unsuccessfully to discover the identity of the author of "It's Over, Debbie" and no prosecution resulted.

Physician-assisted dying and criminal liability. It has been suggested that notwithstanding the existence of legal prohibitions against PAS and VAE, "in practice, the chances of a conviction are remote if the defendant is related to or knows the person well, performs the act openly at personal risk, has reason to believe the person is suffering, and there is no self-serving motive."[103] Indeed, in a recent search of reported decisions, no case could be found in which a physician was convicted of assisting in or causing the death of his patient.[104]

CONCLUSION

Currently accepted guidelines in this area are as follows:

1. Early communication between physician and patient (or patient's family or surrogate where appropriate) regarding diagnosis, prognosis, and therapeutic options together with reasonable expected goals is critical.
2. Patients should be encouraged to execute advance directives regarding their choices about treatment options or goals.[105] This would ensure that the proper locus of decision-making would be where it has been traditionally—at the bedside, between patient (family) and physician.
3. The patient's decision-making capacity should be carefully assessed.
4. An attempt should be made to seek unanimity among the members of the health care team.
5. It is a legal myth that "it is permissible to terminate extraordinary treatments, but not ordinary ones." Decisions about forgoing or discontinuing life-support measures on terminally ill patients must balance the benefit of the proposed therapy against the burden imposed on the patient. Such decisions must take into proper consideration the patient's constitutional liberty interests and common law right of informed consent. These rights must be juxtaposed against the state's interests as articulated in the U.S. Supreme Court decision in *Cruzan*.
6. Where families or surrogates must be involved, decisions should not be rushed. Time to deliberate must be provided, together with appropriate pastoral or social work support or psychological counseling as may be appropriate.

END NOTES

1. A. T. Padovano, *The Estranged God* 26 (Sheed and Ward, New York 1966).
2. S. J. Youngner, and E. T. Bartlett, *Human Death and High Technology: The Failure of the Whole-Brain Formulations,* 99 Annals Int. Med. 252 (1983).
3. A. Beecher, *Definition of Irreversible Coma: Report of the Ad Hoc Committee of the Harvard Medical School to Examine the Definition of Death,* 205 JAMA 337 (1968).
4. *Id.*
5. Pub. L. 95-622 (1978).
6. Report of the President's Commission for the Study of Ethical Problems in Medicine and Biomedical and Behavioral Research, *Defining Death: Medical, Legal and Ethical Issues in the Determination of Death* (1981).

7. Youngner, *supra* note 2, at 252.
8. J. L. Bernat, *How Much of the Brain Must Die in Brain Death?,* 3 J. Clinical Ethics 21-26 (1992).
9. Youngner, *supra* note 2, at 253.
10. R. M. Veatch, *The Impending Collapse of the Whole-Brain Definition of Death,* 23 Hastings Center Report 18-24, 22 (1993).
11. *State v. Fierro,* 124 Ariz. 182. 603 P.2d 74 (1979).
12. *People v. Saldana,* 47 Cal. App. 3d 954, 121 Cal. Rptr. 243 (1975).
13. *People v. Lyons,* Cal. Super. Ct., Oakland (May 21, 1974), *cited in* Friloux, *Death: When Does It Occur?,* 27 Baylor L. Rev. 10 (1975).
14. Korein, *Brain Death, Anesthesia and Neurosurgery,* 282, 284, 292-93 (J. Cottrell and H. Turndorf eds., C. V. Mosby Co., St. Louis 1980).
15. Veatch, *supra* note 10, at 22.
16. Youngner, *supra* note 2; *see also* R. M. Veatch, *The Whole-Brain Oriented Concept of Death: An Outmoded Philsophical Formulation,* 3 J. Thanatol. 13-30 (1975).
17. C. H. Baron, *Why Withdrawal of Life-Support for PVS Patients Is Not a Family Decision,* 19 Hastings Center Report 73-75 (1991).
18. Youngner, *supra* note 2, at 253.
19. R. M. Veatch, *Brain Death and Slippery Slopes,* 3 J. Clinical Ethics 187 (1992).
20. J. Miller, *Trouble in Mind,* Sci. Am. 180 (Sep. 1992).
21. J. L. Bernat, *The Boundaries of the Persistent Vegetative State,* 3 J. Clinical Ethics 176-180 (1992).
22. Youngner, *supra* note 2, at 257.
23. Council on Scientific Affairs and Council on Ethical and Judicial Affairs, *Persistent Vegetative State and the Decision to Withdraw or Withhold Life Support,* 263 JAMA 428 (1990).
24. Veatch, *supra* note 10, at 23.
25. A. R. Jonsen et al., *Clinical Ethics* 112-13 (3rd ed., McGraw-Hill, New York 1992).
26. Y. Kamisar, *Are Laws Against Assisted Suicide Unconstitutional?* 23 Hastings Center Report 32, at 33 (1993).
27. Life-sustaining treatment means "any medical intervention, technology, procedure, or medication that is administered . . . in order to forestall the moment of death, whether or not the treatment is intended to affect the underlying life-threatening disease(s) or biologic processes." *See* Hastings Center, *Guidelines on the Termination of Life-Sustaining Treatment and the Care of the Dying* 4 (1987).
28. D. W. Brock, *Voluntary Active Euthanasia,* 22 Hastings Center Report 19 (1992).
29. Forgoing life-sustaining treatment at the patient's behest is sometimes called "voluntary passive euthanasia" (VPE).
30. A. Meisel, *Legal Myths About Terminating Life Support,* 151 Archives Int. Med. 1497, at 1498 (1991).
31. *Cruzan v. Director,* 110 S.Ct. 2851 (1990).
32. *Elizabeth Bouvia v. Riverside General Hosp.,* No. 159780 Riverside Co., Cal. (Sup. Ct., Dec. 19, 1983).
33. *Bouvia v. Superior Court,* 225 Cal. Rptr. 287 (Cal. App. 1986).
34. L. Gostin and R. F. Weir, *Life and Death Choices after* Cruzan: *Case Law and Standards of Professional Conduct,* 69 The Milbank Q. 143, at 159-60 (1991).
35. J. A. Robertson, *Second Thoughts on Living Wills,* 21 Hastings Center Report 9 (1991).
36. Omnibus Reconciliation Act of 1990, Pub. L. 101-508 §§ 4206, 4751, 104 Stat. 1388, codified at 42 U.S.C. §§ 1395 cc(a)(1)(Q), 1395mm(c)(8), 1395cc(f), 1396a(a)(57), (58), 1396a(w). *See also* regulations at 57 Fed. Reg. 8194-8204 (Mar. 6, 1992).
37. *Note, The California Natural Death Act: An Empirical Study of Physicians' Practice,* 31 Stan. L. Rev. 913 (1979).
38. A. Meisel, *A Retrospective on Cruzan,* 20 L. Med. & Health Care 342, 344 (1992); *see also* J. Areen, *Advance Directives Under State*

Law and Judicial Decisions, 19 L. Med. & Health Care 91-100 (1991).

39. Areen, *supra* note 38, at 92; *see also* Robertson, *supra* note 35, at 6-9.
40. J. Areen, *The Legal Status of Consent Obtained from Families of Adult Patients to Withhold or Withdraw Treatment,* 258 JAMA 229 (1987).
41. Meisel, *supra* note 38, at 344.
42. Meisel, *supra* note 38, at 342.
43. *Id.*
44. Gostin and Weir, *supra* note 34, at 158.
45. *Matter of Westchester County Medical Center,* 72 N.Y.2d 517, 531 N.E.2d 607, 534 N.Y.S.2d 886 (N.Y. 1988).
46. *Cruzan, supra* note 31, at 2841.
47. Meisel, *supra* note 38, at 343.
48. Gostin and Weir, *supra* note 34, at 146.
49. *Cruzin, supra* note 31, at 2857.
50. Meisel, *supra* note 38, at 342.
51. *In the Matter of Karen Quinlan,* 70 N.J. 10, 335 A.2d 647, *cert. denied,* 429 U.S. 922 (1976).
52. Persistent vegetative state (PVS) is defined as "the irreversible loss of all neocortical functions [with] brainstem functions intact." It is an eyes-open unconsciousness." *See* R. E. Cranford, *Neurologic Syndromes and Prolonged Survival: When Can Artificial Nutrition and Hydration Be Forgone?* 19 L. Med. Health Care 13, at 14 (1991).
53. *Quinlan, supra* note 51; *see also Matter of Farrell,* 108 N.J. 335, 529 A.2d 404 (1987).
54. Meisel, *supra* note 38, at 343.
55. *Id.*
56. *Id.*
57. A. M. Capron, *Where Is the Sure Interpreter?* 22 Hastings Center Report 26-27 (Jul.-Aug. 1992).
58. The New York State Task Force on Life and the Law, *When Others Must Choose: Deciding for Patients Without Capacity* (New York State Task Force on Life and the Law, New York 1992).
59. J. D. Moreno, *Who's to Choose? Surrogate Decisionmaking in New York State,* 23 Hastings Center Report 6 (1993); *see also* The New York State Task Force, *supra* note 58.
60. *Superintendent of Belchertown State School v. Saikewicz,* 373 Mass. 728, 370 N.E.2d 417 (1977).
61. *Id.*
62. *Id.*
63. *Id.*
64. *Matter of Storar,* 52 N.Y.2d 363, 438 N.Y.S.2d 266, 420 N.E.2d 64, *cert. denied,* 454 U.S. 858, 102 S.Ct. 309, 70 L.Ed.2d 153.
65. S. Wachtler, *A Judge's Perspective: The New York Rulings,* 19 L. Med. & Health Care 60, at 61 (1991).
66. *Id.*
67. *Schloendorff v. Society of New York Hosp.,* 211 N.Y. 125, 105 N.E. 92 (1914).
68. DNR orders are sometimes referred to as "orders not to resuscitate."
69. *JCAHO 1989 Accreditation Manual,* M.A. 1.4.11, at 82 (1988).
70. *See also* Appendix 29-3.
71. F. H. Marsh and A. Staver, *Physician Authority for Unilateral DNR Orders,* 12 J. Legal Med. 115-165, at 117 (1991); *see also* Youngner, *Who Defines Futility?,* 260 JAMA 2094 (1988).
72. L. A. Albert, Cruzan v. Director, Missouri Department of Health: *Too Much Ado,* 12 J. Legal Med. 331-58, at 335 (1991).
73. Hastings Center, *Guidelines on the Termination of Life-Sustaining Treatment and the care of the Dying,* 32 (Indiana University Press, Bloomington 1987).
74. S. H. Miles, *Medical Futility,* 20 L. Med. & Health Care 310 (1992).
75. M. Angell, *The Case of Helga Wanglie: A New Kind of Right to Die Case,* 325 New Engl. J. Med. 511-12 (1991).
76. S. H. Miles, *Informed Demand for "Non-Beneficial" Medical Treatment,* 325 New Engl. J. Med. 513 (1991).
77. *Id.*
78. *In re Helga Wanglie,* Fourth Judicial District (Dist. Ct., Probate Ct. Div.) PX-91-283, Minn., Hennepin County.
79. Blackhall, *Must We Always Use CPR?,* 317 New Engl. J. Med. 1281-85 (1987).
80. Marsh and Staver, *supra* note 71, at 118.
81. Tomlinson and Brody, *Ethics and Communication in Do Not Resuscitate Orders,* 318 New Engl. J. Med. 43-46 (1988).
82. Marsh and Staver, *supra* note 71, at 119.
83. Marsh and Staver, *supra* note 71, at 144.
84. Marsh and Staver, *supra* note 71, at 119.
85. J. Persels, *Forcing the Issue of Physician-Assisted Suicide,* 14 J. Legal Med. 93 (1993).
86. J. L. Bernat et al., *Patient Refusal of Hydration and Nutrition: An Alternative to Physician-Assisted Suicide or Voluntary Active Euthanasia,* 153 Archives Int. Med. 2723-27, at 2725 (1993).
87. *See* Appendix 29-4, § 2982.
88. Bernat et al., *supra* note 86, at 2723; *see also* M. L. Cook, *The End of Life and the Goals of Medicine,* 153 Archives Int. Med 2718-19 (1993).
89. Derek Humphry, *Final Exit: The Practicalities of Self-Deliverance and Assisted Suicide for the Dying* (The Hemlock Society, Eugene, Ore. 1991).
90. Boston Globe, November 3, 1991, at 1.
91. R. Carson, *Washington's I-119,* 22 Hastings Center Report 7 (1992).
92. The California Death With Dignity Act, California Civil Code Title 10.5, Initiative; *see also* A. M. Capron, *Even in Defeat, Proposition 161 Sounds a Warning,* 23 Hastings Center Report 32-33 (1993).
93. M. T. CeloCruz, *Aid-in-Dying: Should We Decriminalize Physician-Assisted Suicide and Physician-Committed Euthanasia?,* 18 Am. J. L. & Med. 377 (1992).
94. L. O. Gostin, *Drawing a Line Between Killing and Letting Die: The Law, and Law Reform, on Medically Assisted Dying,* 21 J. L. Med. & Ethics 94-101, at 96 (1993).
95. New York Times, December 3, 1993, at A33, col. 1.
96. N.Y. Penal Law § 120.30
97. N.Y. Times, July 27, 1991, A1; *also* N.Y. Times, August 17, 1991, A25.
98. Involuntary euthanasia refers to the euthanasia of "a competent patient [who] explicitly refuses or opposes receiving euthanasia," while nonvoluntary euthanasia refers to the euthanasia of "a patient [who] is incompetent and unable to express his or her wishes about euthanasia." *See* D. W. Brock, *Voluntary Active Euthanasia,* 22 Hastings Center Report 10 (1992).
99. *State v. Fuller,* 203 Neb. 233, 241, 278 N.W.2d 756, 761 (1979); *State v. West,* 157 Mo. 309, 57 S.W. 1071 (1900).
100. CeloCruz, *supra* note 93, at 381.
101. *Id.*
102. Anonymous, *It's Over, Debbie,* 259 JAMA 272 (1988).
103. Gostin, *supra* note 94, at 97.
104. *Id.; see also* CeloCruz, *supra* note 93; *and* H. T. Engelhardt and M. Malloy, *Suicide and Assisting Suicide: A Critique of Legal Sanctions,* 36 Sw. L.J. 1003, 1029 (1982).
105. *But see* J. Lynn, *Why I Don't Have a Living Will,* 19 L. Med. & Health Care 101-04 (1991).

GENERAL REFERENCES

Albert, L. A., Cruzan v. Director, Missouri Department of Health: *Too Much Ado,* 12 J. Legal Med. 331 (1991).

Battin, M., *Voluntary Euthanasia and the Risks of Abuse: Can We Learn Anything from the Netherlands?* 20 L. Med. & Health Care 133-43 (1992).

Brock, D. W., *Voluntary Active Euthanasia,* 22 Hastings Center Report 10-22 (1992).

Brody, B., *Special Ethical Issues in the Management of PVS Patients,* 20 L. Med. & Health Care 104 (1992).

Cohen, C. B., and Cohen, P. J., *Required Reconsideration of DNR Orders in the Operating Room and Certain Other Treatment Settings,* 20 L. Med. & Health Care 354-63 (1992).

McKnight, D. K., and Bellis, M., *Foregoing Life-Sustaining Treatment for Adult, Developmentally Disabled Public Wards: A Proposed Standard,* 18 Am. J. L. & Med. 203-32 (1992).

Meisel, A., *A Retrospective on* Cruzan, 20 L. Med. & Health Care 340-53 (1992).

Miller, R. J., *Hospice Care as an Alternative to Euthanasia,* 20 L. Med. & Health Care 127-32 (1992).

Miller, T. E., *Public Policy in the Wake of* Cruzan: *A Case Study of New York's Health Care Proxy Law,* 18 L. Med. & Health Care 360-67 (1990).

S. G. Pollack, *Identifying Appropriate Decision-Makers and Standards for Decision,* 19 Hastings Center Report 63-65 (1989).

Rouse, F., *Advance Directives: Where Are We Heading After* Cruzan?, 18 L. Med. & Health Care 353-59 (1990).

Wachtler, S., *A Judge's Perspective: The New York Rulings,* 19 L. Med. & Health Care 60-62 (1991).

Weir, R. F., *The Morality of Physician-Assisted Suicide,* 20 L. Med. & Health Care 116-26 (1992).

Weir, R. F., and Gostin, L., *Decisions to Abate Life-Sustaining Treatment for Nonautonomous Patients,* 264 JAMA 1849-52 (1990).

Wolf, S. M., *Final Exit: The End of Argument,* 22 Hastings Center Report 30-33 (1992).

Youngner, S. J., and Bartlett, E. T., *Human Death and High Technology: The Failure of the Whole-Brain Formulations,* 99 Annals Int. Med. 252-58 (1983).

APPENDIX 29-1 Current Opinions of the Council on Ethical and Judicial Affairs of the American Medical Association, 1992

2.20 WITHHOLDING OR WITHDRAWING LIFE-PROLONGING MEDICAL TREATMENT

The social commitment of the physician is to sustain life and relieve suffering. Where the performance of one duty conflicts with the other, the preferences of the patient should prevail. If the patient is incompetent and did not previously indicate his or her preferences, the family or other surrogate decision-maker, in concert with the physician, must act in the best interest[s] of the patient.

For humane reasons, with informed consent, a physician may do what is medically necessary to alleviate severe pain, or cease or omit treatment to permit a terminally ill patient to die when death is imminent. However, the physician should not intentionally cause death. In deciding whether the administration of potentially life-prolonging treatment is in the best interest[s] of the patient who is incompetent, the surrogate decisionmaker and physician should consider several factors, including: the possibility for extending life under humane and comfortable conditions; the patient's values about life and the way it should be lived; and the patient's attitudes toward sickness, suffering, medical procedures, and death.

Even if death is not imminent but a patient is beyond doubt permanently unconscious, and there are adequate safeguards to confirm the accuracy of the diagnosis, it is not unethical to discontinue all means of life-prolonging medical treatment.

Life-prolonging medical treatment includes medication and artificially or technologically supplied respiration, nutrition or hydration. In treating a terminally ill or permanently unconscious patient, the dignity of the patient should be maintained at all times.

2.21 WITHHOLDING OR WITHDRAWING LIFE-PROLONGING MEDICAL TREATMENT — PATIENTS' PREFERENCES

A competent, adult patient may, in advance, formulate and provide a valid consent to the withholding or withdrawal of life-support systems in the event that injury or illness renders that individual incompetent to make such a decision. The preference of the individual should prevail when determining whether extraordinary life-prolonging measures should be undertaken in the event of terminal illness. Unless it is clearly established that the patient is terminally ill or permanently unconscious, a physician should not be deterred from appropriately aggressive treatment of a patient.

2.22 DO-NOT-RESUSCITATE ORDERS

Efforts should be made to resuscitate patients who suffer cardiac or respiratory arrest except when the circumstances indicate that cardiopulmonary resuscitation (CPR) would be futile or not in accord with the desires or best interests of the patient.

Patients at risk of cardiac or respiratory failure should be encouraged to express in advance their preferences regarding the use of CPR and this should be documented in the patient's medical record. These discussions should include a description of the procedures encompassed by CPR and, when possible, should occur in an outpatient setting when general treatment preferences are discussed, or as early as possible during hospitalization. The physician has an ethical obligation to honor the resuscitation preferences expressed by the patient.

Physicians should not permit their personal value judgments about quality of life to obstruct the implementation of a patient's preferences regarding the use of CPR.

If a patient is incapable of rendering a decision regarding the use of CPR, a decision may be made by a surrogate decisionmaker, based upon the previously expressed preferences of the patient or, if such preferences are unknown, in accordance with the patient's best interests.

If, in the judgment of the treating physician, CPR would be futile, the treating physician may enter a do-not-resuscitate order into the patient's record. Resuscitative efforts should be considered futile if they cannot be expected either to restore

cardiac or respiratory function to the patient or to achieve the expressed goals of the informed patient. When there is adequate time to do so, the physician must first inform the patient, or the incompetent patient's surrogate, of the content of the DNR order, as well as the basis of its implementation. The physician also should be prepared to discuss appropriate alternatives, such as obtaining a second opinion (e.g., consulting a bioethics committee) or arranging for transfer of care to another physician.

Do-not-resuscitate orders, as well as the basis for their implementation, should be entered by the attending physician in the patient's medical record.

DNR orders only preclude resuscitative efforts in the event of cardiopulmonary arrest and should not influence other therapeutic interventions that may be appropriate for the patient.

APPENDIX 29-2   ACP Ethics Manual*

DECISIONS NEAR THE END OF LIFE

Decisions near the end of life have a clinical and psychological intensity that distinguishes them from more routine clinical encounters.

Who should make the decision?

Patients who have decision making capacity and who are adequately informed of their clinical situation and options have the right to refuse any recommended medical treatment, including life-sustaining treatment, except in rare circumstances when the law forces a patient to accept treatment. The patient's right is based on the philosophical concept of autonomy, the common law right of self-determination, and the patient's liberty interest under the Constitution in refusing unwanted medical care. . . . [T]he patient's (rather than the physician's) assessment of the benefits and burdens of treatment should determine what treatment is administered or withheld.

Criteria for decisions

In order of priority, decisions should be based on advance directives, substituted judgments, and the best interests of the patient. . . .

Through *advance directives,* competent patients state what treatments they would accept or decline if they lost decision making capacity. . . .

Oral statements to family members, friends, and health care professionals are the most common form of advance directive . . . . [W]ritten advance directives have several advantages [and disadvantages]. . . .

The durable power of attorney for health care can be more comprehensive and flexible than the living will; the patient appoints a surrogate (also called an agent) to make decisions if the patient becomes unable to do so. . . .

Physicians should raise the issue of advance directives routinely with competent adult patients in outpatient visits and encourage them to provide advance directives and to discuss their preferences with their surrogate and family members. . . .

Two standards have been developed for surrogate decision making in cases where the patient has not left an advance directive. In a *substituted judgment,* the surrogate attempts to make the judgment that the patient, if competent, would have made. . . .

If the patient's values and preferences are unknown or unclear, decisions should be based on the patients *best interests.*

Dilemmas regarding life-sustaining treatments
Withdrawing or withholding treatment

The same reasons that justify not starting treatment also justify stopping treatment. Treatments should not be withheld solely for fear that if started they cannot be withdrawn, because patients may be denied potentially beneficial therapies. Court rulings and most ethicists have found no legal or ethical difference between withdrawing and withholding treatment. . . .

Do-not-resuscitate orders

Like other life-sustaining interventions, resuscitation may be withheld if informed patients or appropriate surrogates so choose.

In some cases, . . . a patient or surrogate continues to insist on resuscitation, even though the physician believes that it would be futile. Futility, as it pertains to resuscitation, has been defined to apply to either its initial failure to restore circulation and breathing or to the subsequent failure to discharge the patient alive from the hospital. It is appropriate for physicians to write a do-not-resuscitate (DNR) order when resuscitation would not restore circulation and breathing—for example, in

*Reprinted with permission from 117 *Annals Int. Med.* 947-60 (1992).

progressive multisystem organ failure. It is more controversial whether it is appropriate for physicians to write a unilateral DNR order in situations where discharge alive after resuscitation would be unprecedented. . . . If physicians write a unilateral DNR order, they must inform the patient or surrogate. If DNR orders are not written, it is unethical for physicians and nurses to perform half-hearted resuscitation efforts (so-called "slow codes").

Determination of death

Death of the entire brain, including the brain stem, is now an accepted standard in all the states for determining death when the use of cardiopulmonary life support precludes the use of traditional criteria. . . .

Irreversible loss of consciousness

Discontinuing life support for persons who are permanently unconscious or in a persistent vegetative state remains controversial when the patient's preferences are not known. . . . The current legal and ethical consensus is to make treatment decisions for such patients in the same manner as for other incompetent patients.

Intravenous fluids and artificial feedings

The majority position is to regard these as medical interventions with benefits and risks that must be assessed for each patient. Some physicians and families believe, however, that artificial feedings are basic care that may never be withheld or withdrawn. . . . When disagreements occur, physicians must appreciate that opinions on the benefits and burdens of these interventions involve value judgments and religious beliefs, as well as scientific expertise. . . . The physician may need to arrange transfer to another physician who is willing to follow the preferences of the patient or surrogate.

Physician-assisted suicide and euthanasia

Physician involvement in deliberately hastening a patient's death has long been prohibited in professional codes. . . . Despite ethical and legal prohibitions, some physicians report having provided medications to assist terminally ill patients in ending their lives. . . . [T]he ethics of such actions are in debate. . . .

Objections to assisted suicide and active euthanasia should not deter physicians from withholding or withdrawing medical interventions in appropriate situations. . . .

Some patients who suggest active euthanasia or assisted suicide have untreated depression or uncontrolled pain. The first response of the physician should be to ascertain the concerns and fears of the patient and to check for depression, uncontrolled pain, and other possibly reversible conditions. . . .

Physicians should make relief of suffering in the terminally ill patient their highest priority, as long as this accords with the patient's wishes. Ethically, strong support exists for gradually increasing medication in terminal illness to levels that relieve pain, even if a side effect is to shorten life.

APPENDIX 29-3   "Proportionality/disproportionality" of proposed treatment

The California Court of Appeal, in *Barber v. Superior Court,* offered the following analysis:

The question presented by this modern technology is, once undertaken, at what point does it cease to perform its intended function and who should have the authority to decide that any further prolongation of the dying process is of no benefit to either the patient or his family? A physician has no duty to continue treatment, once it has been proved to be ineffective. Although there may be a duty to provide life-sustaining machinery in the *immediate* aftermath of a cardio-respiratory arrest, there is no duty to continue its use once it has become futile in the opinion of qualified medical personnel. "A physician is authorized under the standards of medical practice to discontinue a form of therapy which in his medical judgment is useless. . . . If the treating physicians have determined that continued use of a respirator is useless, then they may decide to discontinue it without fear of civil or criminal liability. By useless is meant that the continued use of the therapy cannot and does not improve the prognosis for recovery." . . . Of course, the difficult determinations that must be made under these principles is the point at which further treatment will be of no reasonable benefit to the patient, who should have the power to make that decision and who should have the authority to direct termination of treatment. No precise guidelines as to when or how these decisions should be made can be provided by this court since this determination is essentially a medical one to be made at a time and on the basis of facts which will be unique to each case. . . .

However, we would be derelict in our duties if we did not provide some general guidelines for future conduct in the absence of . . . legislation. . . . [A] rational approach involves the determination of whether the proposed treatment is proportionate or disproportionate in terms of the benefits to be gained versus the burdens caused. Under this approach, proportionate treatment is that which, in the view of the patient, has at least a reasonable chance of providing benefits to the patient, which benefits outweigh the burdens attendant to the treatment. Thus, even if a proposed course of treatment might be extremely painful or intrusive, it would still be proportionate treatment if the prognosis was for complete cure or significant improvement in the patient's condition. On the other hand, a treatment course which is only minimally painful or intrusive may nonetheless be considered disproportionate to the potential benefits if the prognosis is virtually hopeless for any significant improvement in condition. . . . Thus, the determination as to whether the burdens of treatment are worth enduring for any individual patient depends on facts unique to each case, namely, how long the treatment is likely to extend life under what conditions. "[S]o long as a mere biological existence is not considered the *only* value, patients may want to take the nature of that additional life into account as well." . . . Of course, the patient's interests and desires are the key ingredients of the decision making process. When dealing with patients for whom the possibility of full recovery is virtually non-existent, and who are incapable of expressing their desires, there is also something of a consensus on the standard to be applied. "[T]he focal point of decision should be the prognosis as to the reasonable possibility of return of cognitive and sapient life, as distinguished from the forced continuance of the biological vegetative existence. . . ." "Prolongation of life . . . does not mean a mere suspension of the act of dying, but contemplates, at the very least, a remission of symptoms enabling a return toward a normal, functioning, integrated existence." . . . Clearly, the medical diagnoses and prognoses must be determined by the treating and consulting physicians under the generally accepted standards of medical practice in the community and, whenever possible, the patient himself should then be the ultimate decision-maker. (147 Cal. App. 3d 1017-1020).

APPENDIX 29-4 New York's Do-Not-Resuscitate Law*

Section 2961 Definitions

4. "Cardiopulmonary resuscitation" [hereinafter "CPR"] means measures . . . to restore cardiac function or to support ventilation in the event of a cardiac or respiratory arrest.

Section 2962 Presumption in favor of resuscitation . . .

1. Every person admitted to a hospital shall be presumed to consent to the administration of [CPR] in the event of cardiac or respiratory arrest, unless there is consent to the issuance of an "order not to resuscitate" [hereinafter ONTR] . . .

Section 2963 Determination of capacity . . .

1. Every adult shall be presumed to have the capacity to make a decision regarding [CPR] unless determined otherwise pursuant to this section or pursuant to a court order. . . .
2. A determination that an adult patient lacks capacity shall be made by the attending physician to a reasonable degree of medical certainty. . . .
3. (a) At least one other physician . . . must concur in the determination that an adult lacks capacity. . . .

Section 2964 Decision-making by an adult with capacity

1. (a) The consent of an adult with capacity must be obtained prior to issuing an order not to resuscitate. . . .

Section 2965 Surrogate decision-making

1. (a) The consent of a surrogate acting on behalf of an adult patient who lacks capacity . . . must be obtained prior to issuing an [ONTR]. . . .
   (b) The consent of a surrogate shall not be required where the adult had, prior to losing capacity, consented to an [ONTR]. . . .

4. (a) One person from the following list, to be chosen in order of priority listed, when persons in the prior subparagraphs are not reasonably available, . . . shall have the authority to act as surrogate on behalf of the patient:
   (i) a person designated by the adult . . .
   (ii) . . . a guardian . . .
   (iii) the spouse;
   (iv) a son or daughter eighteen years of age or older;
   (v) a parent;
   (vi) a brother or sister eighteen years of age or older; and
   (vii) a close friend.

5. (a) The surrogate shall make a decision regarding [CPR] on the basis of the adult patient's wishes including a consideration of the patient's religious and moral beliefs, or, if the patient's wishes are unknown and cannot be ascertained, on the basis of the patient's best interests.
   (c) A surrogate may consent to an [ONTR] on behalf of an adult patient only if there has been a determination by an attending physician . . . that, to a reasonable degree of medical certainty:
   (i) the patient has a terminal condition; or
   (ii) the patient is permanently unconscious; or
   (iii) resuscitation would be medically futile; or
   (iv) resuscitation would impose an extraordinary burden on the patient in light of the patient's medical condition and the expected outcome of resuscitation for the patient.

Section 2966 [P]atient without capacity for whom no surrogate is available

1. (a) If no surrogate is reasonably available . . . to make a decision regarding issuance of an [ONTR] on behalf of an adult patient who lacks capacity and who had not previously expressed a decision regarding [CPR], an attending physician may issue an [ONTR] the patient providing that the attending physician determines . . . that, to a reasonable degree of medical certainty, resuscitation would be medically futile. . . .

---

*From *McKinney's Consolidated Laws of New York Annotated,* Book 44, Public Health Law, Article 29-B, (West Publishing Co., St. Paul 1993).

APPENDIX 29-5 New York's Health Care Agents and Proxies Law*

Section 2980 Definitions

5. "Health care agent" . . . means an adult to whom authority to make health care decisions is delegated under a health care proxy.

8. "Health care proxy" means a document delegating the authority to make health care decisions. . . .

Section 2981 Appointment of health care agent

1. (a) A competent adult may appoint a health care agent. . . .
   (b) [E]very adult shall be presumed competent to appoint a health care agent unless such person has been adjudged incompetent or otherwise adjudged not competent to appoint a health care agent. . . .
2. (a) A competent adult may appoint a health care agent by a health care proxy, signed and dated by the adult in the presence of two adult witnesses who shall also sign the proxy. Another person may sign and date the health care proxy for the adult if the adult is unable to do so, at the adult's direction and in the adult's presence, and in the presence of two adult witnesses who shall sign the proxy. . . .
4. The agent's authority shall commence upon a determination . . . that the principal lacks capacity to make health care decisions.
5. (a) The health care proxy shall:
   (i) identify the principal and agent; and
   (ii) indicate that the principal intends the agent to have authority to make health care decisions on the principal's behalf.
   (b) The health care proxy may include the principal's wishes or instructions about health care decisions, and limitations upon the agent's authority.

Section 2982 Rights and duties of agent

1. Subject to any express limitations in the health care proxy, an agent shall have the authority to make any and all health care decisions on the principal's behalf that the principal could make.
2. [T]he agent shall make health care decisions: (a) in accordance with the principal's wishes, including the principal's religious and moral beliefs; or (b) if the principal's wishes are not reasonably known and cannot with reasonable diligence be ascertained, in accordance with the principal's best interests; provided, however, that if the principal's wishes regarding the administration of artificial nutrition and hydration are not reasonably known and cannot with reasonable diligence be ascertained, the agent shall not have the authority to make decisions regarding these measures.

Section 2983 Determinations of lack of capacity . . .

1. (a) A determination that a principal lacks capacity to make health care decisions shall be made by the attending physician to a reasonable degree of medical certainty. . . . For a decision to withdraw or withhold life-sustaining treatment, the attending physician who makes the determination that a principal lacks capacity to make health care decisions must consult with another physician to confirm such determination.

5. Notwithstanding a determination . . . that the principal lacks capacity to make health care decisions, where a principal objects to the determination of incapacity or to a health care decision made by an agent, the principal's objection or decision shall prevail unless the principal is determined by a court of competent jurisdiction to lack capacity to make health care decisions.

Section 2984 Provider's obligations

2. A health care provider shall comply with health care decisions made by an agent in good faith under a health care proxy to the same extent as if such decisions had been made by the principal.

Section 2986 Immunity

1. No health care provider . . . shall be subjected to criminal or civil liability, or deemed to have engaged in unprofessional conduct, for honoring in good faith a health care decision by an agent. . . .
2. No person acting as agent . . . shall be subjected to criminal or civil liability for making a health care decision in good faith. . . .

Section 2989 Effect on other rights

3. This article is not intended to permit or promote suicide, assisted suicide, or euthanasia; accordingly, nothing herein shall be construed to permit an agent to consent to any act or omission to which the principal could not consent under law.

Section 2992 Special proceeding authorized

The health care provider . . . may commence a special proceeding, in a court of competent jurisdiction, with respect to any dispute arising under this article, including, but not limited to, a proceeding to:
1. determine the validity of the health care proxy;
2. have the agent removed on the ground that the agent (a) is not reasonably available, willing and competent to fulfill his or her obligations . . . or (b) is acting in bad faith; or
3. override the agent's decision about health care treatment on the grounds that: (a) the decision was made in bad faith or (b) the decision is not in accordance with the standards set forth in . . . this article.

---

*From *McKinney's Consolidated Laws of New York Annotated,* Book 44, Public Health Law, Article 29-C (West Publishing Co., St. Paul 1993).

CHAPTER 30 Physician-assisted suicide

ARTHUR H. LESTER, M.D., J.D., F.A.C.O.G., F.C.L.M.

DEFINITION OF TERMS
PHYSICIAN AUTHORITY AND PATIENT AUTONOMY
PHYSICIAN-ASSISTED SUICIDE NOT LAWFUL
REQUEST FOR ASSISTANCE IN COMMITTING SUICIDE
CURRENT POSITIONS OF PROPONENTS
CONCLUSION

Physicians have been taught to treat disease and preserve the lives of all patients. Patients were taught to defer, in general, to the physician's treatment choices because of her or his superior education and commitment to act in the patient's best interest. This physician-patient relationship continues in some respects, and even where there is minimal expectation of survival, patients are subjected to painful procedures.

In the United States, we are taught that we alone are the master of our private affairs, including what shall and shall not be done with our bodies. We are now coming to believe that each of us is also entitled to select the time, place, and circumstances of death. However, death often does not occur in such a selected manner and many of us die in hospitals or nursing homes, alone and afraid, often subjected to unskilled, unwanted, painful treatment that diminishes autonomy and dignity.

Clearly, tensions may exist between patient desires and some traditional goals of medical care. Recent federal and state statutes have returned some control over the process of dying to the patient but a core problem still exists: how to *ensure* that death occurs with dignity, in comfortable surroundings without futile, painful treatment, without unjustified loss of life, *and without compromising the integrity of the medical profession.*

Some patients select the time, place, and manner of death and commit suicide and, increasingly, suffering patients are seeking assistance in committing suicide from physicians. Currently, for physicians who openly do so there are not only legal entanglements, but also professional and ethical conflicts. The current price for assisting in a patient's suicide may include loss of license, fines, incarceration, civil suits, and psychological stress.

Physicians' attitude that a patient's death signifies a medical failure often places his or her interest in opposition to that of the suffering patient who desires relief through death. Physicians are being asked to consider changing their goals from attempting to cure the incurable to "comfort care" with the goal of attaining a "good death." To some terminal patients a "good death" may be of more value than prolonging a life of misery. Physicians are also being asked to go farther and use the tools of healing to cause death through assistance at suicide.

Often, public policy directed at maintaining trust in the medical profession is cited as a reason physician-assisted suicide should not be allowed. Public policy also opposes assisted suicide for other reasons, which are set out later in this chapter.

The patient, physician, and state each have interests in medical care decisions made near the end of life that may come into conflict and must be balanced in order to optimize the patient's comfort and autonomy while attempting to comply with public policy and protect the rights of the physician.

This chapter introduces some of the legal and ethical concerns about assisted suicide in the United States and discusses the patient's absolute right to refuse care. Countervailing tensions are discussed such as state interests in preventing suicide, dilution of medical integrity, and adulteration of assisted suicide into euthanasia. A framework for conduct is proposed that may be employed if assistance at suicide is decriminalized, if the physician is ethically open to participation, and if the patient initiates suicide discussions.

No position is taken concerning the advisability of physician participation in patient suicide. There are sound philosophical, theological, and moral positions that prohibit such activities no matter what the degree of suffering. Experience in other countries where assisted death is recognized will not be cited but the reader is invited to explore this, most particularly as practiced in the Netherlands.

DEFINITION OF TERMS

Life-sustaining treatments or procedures merely replace physiologic functions that the patient's body is no longer able to perform. These are not intended to aid in recovery. Examples are some respirator care, pacemakers, and parenteral provision of nutrition and fluids. Some believe that intentional withholding or withdrawal of these is suicide or a step toward euthanasia.

Euthanasia is the deliberate killing of an innocent human being where the patient *does not* perform the final death-producing act. Euthanasia is generally discussed in the context of a patient who is deemed to be terminally ill and/or beyond productive life. No credible authority in the United States condones this activity and it is not lawful in any jurisdiction. *Active euthanasia* is accomplished through the medical administration of a lethal agent. This is the same act as homicide but it is said that the distinction is a matter of expected social role expressed through medical licensing, mental state, circumstances, and intent of the perpetrator. *Passive euthanasia* is accomplished through nontreatment or by withdrawal of life-sustaining treatment or procedures. The motivation for all euthanasia is said to be mercy for the patient.

Double effect treatment is the use of medication or treatment where the *primary intent* is to relieve suffering or to preserve life with the knowledge that such treatment may also cause death. In accepting treatment the *patient* balances its benefits against the burdens and risk of death. The intent is to control suffering while recognizing that death *may* occur. In euthanasia, the intent is to kill to relieve suffering. Examples of "double effect" treatment are toxic chemotherapy, heavy sedation and analgesia, and extensive cancer surgery.

Valid informed consent (informed consent) requires that the physician provide the patient with sufficient information about the medical condition, its expected course if left untreated, and treatment alternatives, including costs, risks, benefits, and chance of failure for each. Without such information the patient is subject to deception and manipulation and cannot be truly autonomous. Exactly *what* must be told varies with the patient's medical condition, psychological stability, and state statutory requirements ("prudent patient" or "prudent physician" standard).

Although some exceptions to these requirements for informed consent occur, such as where the patient is reasonably expected to become distraught on receiving bad news or where he may become a risk to himself or others, these elements of informed consent are universally recognized.

Physician-assisted suicide (assisted suicide) is defined, for the purposes of this chapter, as making medical information or the means to cause death available to the patient *with knowledge of the patient's intent to use it to commit suicide*. It also includes actual assistance in performing a final act. Physician-assisted suicide requires that the patient be given informed consent information and that she has the capacity to understand the medical condition, treatment alternatives, and prognosis in order to make a rational decision concerning this matter and to communicate the decision to the physician. As opposed to euthanasia, the autonomous patient performs or participates in the final act and can, therefore, change his mind at any time until then. In euthanasia, once the decision is transmitted to the agent, unless there is an understanding that the procedure will stop on demand, autonomy is lost. Physician-assisted suicide is not lawful in the United States and does not fall within the usual ethical boundaries of practice. An exception to this is administration of treatment where the double effect *may* occur.

PHYSICIAN AUTHORITY AND PATIENT AUTONOMY
The physician-patient relationship

Physicians have a duty fixed by choice and tradition to act in the best interests of their patients and, historically, with a few exceptions, have done so. Because of this caring behavior a bond of trust grew that allowed the patient to believe that the medical advice was in his best interests. On this basis patients often surrendered medical decision-making authority to the physician, who was expected to treat the patient with *beneficence*. (This held true even where the decision *appeared* to be harmful. For example, a patient who did not want surgery would submit because of the trust that what was being advised was for the patient's best interests.)

Opposing this paternalistic relationship is the principle of *patient autonomy* (self-governance), which states that the patient should not be treated (absent emergency) without her *actual* consent. Even where the patient selects what the physician believes to be a less advantageous program of treatment, autonomy dictates that that selection be honored. (Of course, if there is apparent failure to understand the medical facts or if the patient appears to lack decision-making capacity, a challenge to autonomy should be raised by the physician acting under the principles of paternalism and beneficence.) The autonomy concept of personal integrity, privacy, and liberty serves as the basis of well-recognized procedural elements of medical care such as the need to obtain informed consent for medical examination and treatment.

Also embodied in this concept of autonomy is the patient's absolute right to refuse medical care, the right to ask for withholding or withdrawal of treatment at any time, regardless of his condition, the right to die and the right to nominate another to make health care decisions. Note, though, that as reliance on the actual patient's decision becomes more attenuated (as in surrogate or proxy decisions), the importance of physician paternalism and beneficence increases.

The principle of patient autonomy requires that treatment be rendered only in accordance with patient consent and also applies to physician-assisted suicide and euthanasia. A patient considering these is entitled to the same type of information given to patients considering other medical alternatives.

Any treatment designed to cause death is currently considered by most physicians to be detrimental to the patient's well-being and, therefore, unsound and in violation of the physician's duties of paternalism, beneficence, and nonmalfeasance. As such, these types of treatments are not indicated and providing them violates current principles of medical ethics. Under these circumstances, or where there are other legal, moral, ethical, or personal objections, the physician has no obligation to provide assistance in suicide or to help the patient find someone who will.

The Hippocratic oath

The Hippocratic oath instructs that we do no harm to our patients. In considering what is harmful it is important to examine the *patient's* value system because, to some, death may not be viewed as harmful, whereas the prospect of survival with suffering or loss of dignity may be. In assisted suicide cases, conflict may exist between the physician's self concept and social role as healer, preserver of life, and reliever of suffering and the patient's desire for assistance in providing relief through death. Such conflicts should be openly discussed and the goals of future therapy determined under the principles of autonomy and its progeny, including informed consent. Physicians should adhere to their oath and attempt to deter deaths that are sought due to lack of information, lack of analgesia, family pressures, treatable depression, or due to pressure from any third party attempting to ration its resources.

Common law

Some of the autonomy principles requiring that the physicians follow acceptable patient directions are the grounds of several landmark court cases, but while deeply rooted in American tradition and law, it is not without limits. Often, unfortunately, no bright line can be found separating those items over which the patient retains complete control from those where it is shared, or where the patient lacks any control and judicial interpretation is required.

Common law standards of duty and ethical principles rooted in medicine's historical past generally act to protect the integrity of the physician where end-of-life decisions must be made. For example, a physician's liability for failing to offer or perform certain care depends on whether there is a duty to provide it. In keeping with this, judicial interpretation of the autonomy principle does not require that the physician provide items of care merely to satisfy a demand where it is not medically indicated or not thought to be helpful. Neither medical ethics nor legal duty requires provision of care that exceeds usual and customary standards. There is no requirement that a physician "do everything" in all circumstances, that she disclose or discuss procedures not accepted as feasible or appropriate, nor does she need to continue therapy that fails to provide an agreed-on goal.

There is, therefore, a legal and ethical distinction between the withdrawal or withholding of care that is not indicated or not desired from affirmative acts where the intent is to kill the patient. The former is not inherently contrary to the duty of beneficence or principle of patient autonomy, whereas the latter may be. Because there is no license to impose futile treatment on an unwilling patient, there is also no ethical or legal license to take a direct act that kills him.

State interests

State interests may be diametrically opposed to assisted suicide. States may allow assisted death to occur through removal of life-prolonging procedures when requested by the patient but no state approves of assisted suicide or active euthanasia. Summarized, the state interests are as follows:

1. Preservation of human life, in general.
2. Protecting the interests of innocent third parties.
3. Prevention of suicide.
4. Maintenance of ethical integrity of the medical profession.

Some analysts believe that as the patient's medical condition worsens, state interest in preserving life diminishes. Some also claim that state interests weaken and the patient's right to privacy increases as the degree of bodily invasion necessitated by treatment increases and the prognosis dims.

PHYSICIAN-ASSISTED SUICIDE NOT LAWFUL

In its framework, physician-assisted suicide as a treatment modality differs little from other acts of medical care. It is requested by the patient who believes it to be warranted, is subject to the doctrines of informed consent, must be indicated, lawful, and ethical, and must be a treatment the physician is willing to provide.

In a series of cases in the last part of this century, courts have, in a stepwise manner, come close to approval of physician-assisted suicide. This has been accomplished through recognition of the patient's inherent right to reject medical care and control certain aspects of that which is accepted. In these cases the limits of patient autonomy are examined over its range extending from complete autonomy to the right to demand that a third party assist in the killing. All courts who have considered the problem agree that there is no right to demand assistance in suicide from an unwilling physician, even if it becomes lawful. No court has approved of either physician-assisted suicide or active euthanasia.

In *Bouvia v. Superior Court*,[5] the California court stated that the right to die is "the ultimate expression of one's right to privacy" and includes the right to enlist medical assistance by removal of artificial life support. The patient making such a decision need *not* be in terminal condition and her considerations may include quality of life issues in addition to those of a purely medical nature. The court distinguishes between the refusal of treatment where death then occurs "naturally" due to the medical affliction and death due to an affirmative act.

Although some states found that the patient's right to decide whether to live or die is rooted in the common law, several U.S. Supreme Court decisions hold that it is a constitutionally protected "liberty interest." In addition, the Court found protection for third parties who withhold or withdraw artificial life-prolonging procedures pursuant to patient instructions because denial of such protection is, in effect, denial of the right.

Issues remaining to be more fully explored include evaluation of rights of the child and rights of the never competent. To date, courts have decided that the incompetent patient has the same rights as does the fully competent but among the practical problems of treating such patients is how to determine the desires of such patients, whether to apply the "substituted judgment" or "best interest" standards, and how to obtain informed consent.

Recent legislation, such as the federal Patient Self-Determination Act and similar state statutes, codifies the patient's right to make certain health care decisions. This indicates growing public recognition that the fear of continuing life far exceeds the fear of death in some and patients need not continue suffering. The medical profession must take an active role in shaping such

legislation by providing advice to representatives, state medical boards and jurists on matters involving principles of medical care, ethical codes, application of technology, and end-of-life care. This requires that physicians remain involved with the legal and social structures supporting our society and that we consider, with care, the changing needs of our patients.

REQUEST FOR ASSISTANCE IN COMMITTING SUICIDE
Analyzing the request

Located between allowing death to occur through withholding or withdrawing treatment and euthanasia, where death is caused by an affirmative act of a third person, is the concept of physician-assisted suicide. In physician-assisted suicide, death occurs by the patient's own hand but with the physician's knowing assistance.

When a patient requests help in committing suicide, it is important to explore the reasons to determine if that, in fact, is his or her intent. A threshold issue is the determination of the patient's rationality by examining the thought process and logic that took him or her from an understanding of the present clinical condition to the conclusion that death is desirable. Before doing this, the physician must first examine his or her own value system to discover any general objections to such a request to be as certain as possible that the request can be examined without bias.

Putting aside the important hypothesis that such a request is never rational or never moral as being beyond the scope of this chapter, issues to be explored in determining the rationality of such a request are the patient's understanding of the illness, treatment alternatives, prognosis, and information concerning treatment failures, costs, and risks. The physician should also determine whether the patient is able to communicate freely about the illness and treatment choices. A patient's reticence to communicate may reflect depression or uncertainty. Inability to communicate may have led to inadequate pain control, resulting in unnecessary misery. Overtreatment or ineffective care may have occurred or, even where the treatment is effective, its cost causes concern about family finances.

The patient requesting suicide may fear inadequate control of future pain, have *transient* yearnings to be done with the problem, or have the desire to not burden the family with the illness. A patient may also believe that suicide is expected, and this feeling may be reinforced by overbearing family members, health care providers, insurers, or the government.

Aside from the medical and financial aspects of terminal illness, the patient may be dealing with overwhelming feelings of isolation. By requesting suicide the patient may be actually seeking someone to listen to her fears of abandonment, isolation, and dying alone after having lost her personal and physical integrity. She may be seeking validation that she still has worth as an individual and will not be forgotten after death. Only after adequately addressing at least these issues can the rationality of the patient's decision to request assistance in suicide be examined.

In cases where the patient merely disagrees with advisers and selects suicide even though the advisers counseled against that solution, there is no basis on which to attempt to nullify that decision. Where, however, the patient's decision is so far out of a logical sequence that it indicates lack of rationality, and where that decision is not made according to a deeply held religious or ethical belief, it may be examined through court action.

After correction of those factors that can be changed, if the patient still requests death, the problem must be confronted.

Physician response

Physicians are poorly prepared to deal with a frank, earnest request by a patient for death. Such requests are rare and seem to defy the traditional seeking of relief through cure rather than death. The physician, on receiving such a request, should attempt to communicate frankly, with compassion and in a nonjudgmental manner, to determine the basis for the request. The patient's state of mind and decision-making ability should be explored and a determination should be made as to whether the patient suffers from treatable depression or is confused by medication side effects. The request also represents an opportunity to explore the adequacy of comfort care and if found wanting, to correct it (if possible). The request also offers the opportunity to discuss the patient's fears and provides a forum for guidance through the patient's final medical and personal needs.

Where the patient makes such a request, the physician should respond with empathy and, where requested, treatment goals may be changed from therapeutic to palliation despite an acknowledged double effect. The patient seeks, deserves, and should be given unconditional assurances from the physician that there will be no abandonment and that help will continue through death, within the bounds of medical ability, ethics, and the law. Where appropriate, referral of the patient to a hospice or for psychiatric care can be made.

Granting or denying the request

In opposition to physician-assisted suicide in support of the patient's right to die are economic and other considerations concerning the integrity of the medical profession. Among these are the following:

Economic arguments

1. Physician-assisted suicide will encourage rationing of health care. Those pointing to the cost of terminal care fear encouragement of suicide to save health dollars that can be "better used" for patients who have better expectations of recovery.
2. A physician who is paid more for acute than custodial care may wish that his or her chronically ill patient would die in order to increase time available to care for the better paying patients.

Both of these positions violate the fiduciary duty of a physician to his patient. No American court or legislature has suggested that the involuntary termination of an adult's life-sustaining treatment can be justified by the advantage that the death would bring to others.

Ethical arguments

1. The tools of healers should not be used to cause death. This position is taken because it is believed that to do so would undermine the patient's trust that the physician will protect her from harm. Hidden within this argument is the fear that the physician may use his or her position to unfairly influence the patient's choices when he or she or the family no longer deems the patient's life to have value or where there is the possibility of inheritance or other secondary gain. The depressed, ill, or medicated patient may not feel free to resist the suggestion of suicide.
2. Physician-assisted suicide represents the beginning of the "slippery slope" toward voluntary, involuntary, and, finally, nonvoluntary euthanasia. Physician assistance in suicide or performance of euthanasia are intentional killings and as such, are impermissible violent remedies to illness provided in the name of beneficence.
3. Physician involvement in causing death makes such activities appear acceptable. Abuses such as those that occurred in Nazi Germany where vulnerable poor, elderly, women, and minorities were executed could occur again.
4. The psychological effects on patients and doctors of the availability of assisted suicide are largely unknown. Available research is insufficient to determine whether the possibility of assisted suicide encourages the patient to give up sooner. It is also unknown whether the patient would try harder to cope with pain, knowing he can trust his physician to help find relief through death when palliation fails.

There is also little research on the effect that such availability would make on the physician. Will she give up attempts at a cure or palliation earlier? Will she substitute suicide for comfort care? Will she work harder with the patient to relieve the physical, social, or personal challenges of dying? Will the physician be able to deal with the distortion of the traditional healing role of medicine or with pressures brought by patients, families, or government that encourage the death of a given patient? Will the physician be able to wilfully and purposely assist in killing and then proceed to the subsequent patients and act in the traditional role of healer? Will the physician's career be attenuated by psychological burdens brought on by killing or assisting in the death of patients? What effect on career choice will follow if assisted suicide is allowed? When must a physician inform the patient the she is or is not willing to participate in assisted suicide? Will a new specialty of thanatology be required?

Practical problems

The practical problems of administrating a physician-assisted suicide program also require resolution. For example, where is the line to be drawn by medicine or society as to whose request should be honored and whose will not? What is the functional definition of "unbearable" pain and suffering? Is the definition objective or subjective, and what criteria apply to each? What level of proof of suffering shall be required? Even if generic criteria of eligibility are determined, who determines whether or not a given person qualifies for assisted suicide? Who should make decisions on borderline cases? Who should be the advocates?

How will patients who have no close relationship with a physician avail themselves of this right? How will patients who have no mobility or ability to communicate but who live with "unbearable" pain and suffering avail themselves of this? What due process should protect the patient while allowing proper patient autonomy? What effect will assisted suicide have on insurance coverage? What effect on a physician's civil and criminal liability? How shall the laws of medical malpractice be applied? For example, in cases of alleged negligence, how should damages be measured? What effect will assisted suicide have on the remaining family and loved ones or on their relationship with the physician who may also be their doctor? Who should be entitled to prevent assisted suicide? Will an injunction to prevent assisted suicide be available where the patient has knowingly waived all rights not to be killed?

CURRENT POSITIONS OF PROPONENTS

Proponents of physician-assisted suicide state that it is not a "slippery slope" but provides an acceptable plateau between medicine as it currently is practiced and euthanasia. Because it is, in essence, a passive medical activity, they claim, only a few cases of wrongful death are at risk. Further, it is argued that this is merely another tool on the continuum of care that includes aggressive pursuit of diagnosis, proper therapeutic care, and final comfort care. Physician-assisted suicide is claimed to be a way of ending life while preserving patient autonomy without jeopardizing the traditions of medicine.

Proponents of assisted suicide place great importance on assuring true patient autonomy and propose that criteria be developed to assure that there be as little as possible improper influence. Suggestions have been made that statutory guidelines should be created to prevent abuse and that adversarial review occur before the act.

Among more recently suggested medical approaches to assisted suicide are those of Timothy Quill, M.D., who has proposed "the good death" concept. Quill and others believe that where assisted suicide is performed only in the context of a meaningful doctor-patient relationship only after the primary physician has completed a full and fair investigation of the condition and has learned that it is, more likely than not, incurable, where all reasonable treatments have been discussed and offered, where there is severe, unrelenting suffering, no clouding of the patient's decision-making capacity through medication or treatable mental illness, and the patient, understanding the situation, has spontaneously and repeatedly raised the issue of assisted suicide, assistance represents a medical triumph rather than defeat.

Prior to physician-assisted suicide the patient should execute an informed consent form reflecting the circumstances, the discussions, and the method to be employed. Consultation with another physician is encouraged to be certain that each of these criteria has been met. In some cases, the family should be brought into the discussions but with the understanding that they have no power to stop the process if suicide is the patient's goal.

The advocates believe that physician-assisted suicide properly balances the ethical positions and legal rights of physicians and patients and that it does not offend the interests of the state. They believe its availability will help resolve the tensions between patient, physician, and state through negotiation and compromise. They believe that these discussions help reassure the patient that he will not be abandoned and that he will remain independent, maintain dignity, and be surrounded by his selected partners in life and in the place of his choice when death occurs.

These advocates point out that physician-assisted suicide is currently conducted in secret and that such concealment obstructs candor between the patient, family, and doctor. By permitting physician-assisted suicide, issues and treatments can be openly discussed and there will be less risk of abuse. Further, specialists in methods of producing death may be openly consulted to ensure that effective, humane methods are employed.

It is common for physicians to "disconnect" from patients who are dying and abandon them in a psychological, if not a physical, sense. Often this is to protect the physician from facing what he has been taught to be his own failure in care, from the pending loss of a patient and friend, or because the physician is uncomfortable, in general, confronting mortality. Permitting assisted suicide may help prevent such abandonment by allowing the physician to express his true feelings to the patient.

Where a patient's condition suggests that assisted suicide may be requested, a physician who is uncomfortable with that prospect will have the opportunity to resolve personal ambivalence and, if she cannot or will not provide this care, to help engage a physician in a timely manner who can form the proper relationship with the patient and then assist as requested. It has been said that abandonment of patients suffering from incurable pain and disease is "an immoral abrogation of medical power."

CONCLUSION

On being approached by a patient about assisted suicide, the physician should try to determine what is really being requested. Any shortfall in pain relief should be corrected and the patient should be assured of comfort and dignity.

Quill proposes that treatment to prevent death is appropriate until the patient has lived a natural life span in "biographical" terms. Afterwards, on patient request and with proper procedures, he proposes that assisted suicide may be conducted at the time and place of the patient's choice with spiritual support and in the presence of family and physician. According to Quill, this approach allows conversion to palliative care early enough in the suffering to actually help the patient.

Social and legal changes must be made before acceptance of physician-assisted suicide can occur. Criminal sanctions applied to those who assist in suicide must be removed and no civil cause of action should lie for such actions taken in good faith. Research is required to resolve the relevant philosophical and psychological issues as they affect patients, families, physicians, and public policy. Debate must occur so legislatures can establish proper criteria and due process. Physicians must acquire and share information on efficient, humane methods of causing death and specialists may be required to manage the physical aspects of suicide.

The role of the physician at the end of life has been traditionally limited to therapeutic and palliative care. Because patients now survive for greater periods of time with painful, terminal illnesses, they have begun to ask for assistance in dying. Within the medical profession, tensions exist between doing no harm, providing palliative care, preserving life, and honoring a patient's autonomous request. The common law and Constitution protect patient autonomy and privacy rights, including the right to refuse medical care. Many seek to expand this "right to die" to include physician-assisted suicide.

Just as patients examine their needs when afflicted with incurable suffering and determine what treatment to accept, so also must each physician examine her or his concepts of care and determine what she or he is willing to provide. If irreconcilable conflict exists between the patient and physician on goals or methods the physician may assist the patient in finding a substitute whose position is more acceptable.

Public policy issues concerning providing medical care to the terminally ill must also be resolved. The "slippery slope" from assisted suicide to euthanasia must be evaluated because this century has again witnessed the horror of adulterated medical procedures being used to kill the elderly, infirm, weak, and minorities. The public must remain confident that medical ethics continue to include the duty of beneficence while respecting patient autonomy. At this time, physician assistance in suicide is neither lawful nor generally accepted by medical ethicists.

Physicians must remember that there are limits to the ability to defeat disease and begin to consider *how* their patients die. Drs. Quill, Brody, Kevorkian, and others have reopened the debate over the limits on patient autonomy and have challenged the profession to expand the traditional role of physicians in end-of-life care.

This chapter has described some of the tensions that exist between the patient, the physician, and the state when assisted suicide is requested and provides a framework for dealing with such a request. For those whose personal code precludes such activity, this chapter provides further insight into the position of those who do choose to deal with such requests.

END NOTES

1. *Cruzan by Cruzan v. Harmon,* 760 S.W.2d 408 (Mo. 1988), *cert granted, Cruzan v. Director, Missouri Dept. of Health,* 109 S.Ct. 3240 (1989), 110 S.Ct. 2841 (1990).
2. Cundiff, D., *Euthanasia Is Not the Answer* (Humana Press, Totowa, N.J. 1992).
3. Albert, L.A., *Cruzan v. Director, Missouri Dept. of Health: Too Much Ado,* 12 J. Legal Med. 3 (Sep. 1991).
4. Annes, G.J., *Physician-Assisted Suicide — Michigan's Temporary Solution,* 328 New Eng. J. Med. 21 (May 27, 1993).
5. *Bouvia v. Superior Court,* 225 Cal. Rptr. 297, 179 Cal. App. 3d 1127 (Cal. App. 2 Dist. 1986).
6. Brock, D., *Life and Death: Philosophic Essays in Biomedical Ethics* (Cambridge University Press, New York 1993).
7. Brody, H., *Assisted Death — A Compassionate Response to a Medical Failure,* 327 New Eng. J. Med. 19 (Nov. 5, 1992).
8. Caine, E., and Conwell, Y., *Self Determined Death, the Physician,*

and Medical Priorities. Is There Time To Talk?, 270 JAMA 7 (Aug. 18, 1993).

9. Cloverdale, G.C., *Mercy Killing,* 85 J. So. Med. Assoc. Supp. 2 (Aug. 1992).

10. Conwell, Y., and Caine, E. *Rational Suicide and the Right to Die—Reality and Myth,* 325 New Eng. J. Med. 15 (Oct. 10, 1991).

11. *In re Conroy.* 486 A.2d 1209 (N.J. 1985).

12. Council on Ethical and Judicial Affairs, American Medical Association. *Decisions Near the End of Life,* 267 JAMA 16 (Apr. 22, 1992).

13. de Wachter, M.A.M., *Active Euthanasia in the Netherlands,* 262 JAMA 23 (1989).

14. Hall, M., and Ellman, I., *Health Care Law and Ethics* (West, St. Paul, Minn. 1990).

15. Hill, T.P., *The Right to Die, Legal and Ethical Considerations,* 85 J. So. Med. Assoc. Supp. 2 (Aug. 1992).

16. Marsh, F.H., and Staver, A., *Physician Authority for Unilateral DNR Orders,* 12 J. Legal Med. 2 (June 1991).

17. Paris, J., et al., *Beyond Autonomy—Physician's Refusal To Use Life-Prolonging Extracorporeal Membrane Oxygenation,* 329 New Eng. J. Med. 5 (July 29, 1993).

18. Pelligrino, E.D., *Compassion Needs Reason Too,* 270 JAMA 7 (Aug. 18, 1993).

19. Quill, T.E., et al., *Care of the Hopelessly Ill—Proposed Clinical Criteria for Physician-Assisted Suicide,* 327 New Eng. J. Med. 19 (Nov. 5, 1992).

20. Quill, T.E., *Doctor, I Want To Die. Will You Help Me?,* 270 JAMA 7 (Aug. 18, 1993).

21. *In re Quinlan.* 70 N.J. 10. 355 A.2d 647 (1976), *cert denied,* 429 U.S. 922 (1976).

22. *Satz v. Perlmutter,* 362 So. 2d 160 (Fla. App. 4 Dist. 1978), *aff'd,* 379 So. 2d 359 (1978).

23. Troug, R., and Brenner, T., *Participation of Physicians in Capital Punishment,* 329 New Eng. J. Med. 18 (Oct. 28, 1993).

CHAPTER 31   # Reproduction patients

MICHAEL S. CARDWELL, M.D., J.D., M.P.H., F.C.L.M.*

PRECONCEPTION ISSUES
CONCEPTION ISSUES
POSTCONCEPTION ISSUES
BIRTH-RELATED ISSUES
PERIPARTUM ISSUES

Patients with reproductive concerns are challenging both to the attorney and the physician. In addition to the inherent medical problems, these patients often have complex, intertwined family and social concerns that can muddle the medical aspects. The advances in obstetrical/neonatal medical technology during the past several decades have been amazing — almost miraculous in some instances. These seemingly medical miracles have raised unrealistically the expectation of laypersons. This chapter presents an overview of the medicolegal aspects of human reproduction.

PRECONCEPTION ISSUES
Genetic counseling

Approximately 3% to 5% of all infants are born with a congenital or hereditary disorder. More than one-quarter of all pediatric hospitalizations and deaths beyond the perinatal period are due to such disorders. More than 3000 genetic diseases have been described. Only in the past two decades has significant prenatal detection of congenital birth defects and genetic disease been possible.

Routine genetic screening has become the standard of care in many situations. Most states have enacted legislation requiring phenylketonuria (PKU) testing immediately after birth to allow effective treatment. The federal government has established voluntary screening centers for sickle cell trait.[1] Several states have also established blood screening as a prerequisite to marriage

or attendance at school. Screening may also occur at birth, or the states allow departments of health or school authorities to designate segments of the population for screening.[2] Prenatal screening for neural tube defects has been the subject of policy consideration. In the private sector some companies utilize genetic screening to detect hypersusceptibility to certain occupational exposures, although this is controversial because of the potential for discriminatory practice or abuse.[3] Donors of semen for artificial insemination are usually screened for genetic diseases (see the section on Conception Issues, later in this chapter).

Family practitioners and obstetricians may be liable if they fail to administer the prenatal care that is the standard practice within their medical community. This prenatal care might include testing for rubella titers or serum AFP indicating a risk of congenital defect. In *Monusco v. Postle,*[4] a physician was held liable to an infant for failure to test and immunize her mother for rubella before the child was conceived. Liability may also be found for failure to obtain a genetic history or to recognize a genetic disease in the parents or siblings that would suggest a risk of genetic disease in the fetus. Once a risk is identified, there is a duty to inform the prospective parent or pregnant patient that further workup or referral might be indicated, and possibly that termination of the pregnancy is an option. Further, recognition of a genetic disease requires counseling as to potential future offspring.

Two special types of medical malpractice claims, "wrongful birth" and "wrongful life," are each related to a physician's failure to properly assess or communicate risks of genetic defects to the patient, and a resulting denial to the patients of their option to decide whether

---

*The opinions or assertions contained herein are those of the author. The author acknowledges and appreciates work on this chapter from past contributors: Anne Campbell Liedtke, J.D.; Victor Walter Weedn, M.D., J.D., F.C.L.M.; William J. Winslade, Ph.D., J.D.

to terminate the pregnancy. The history and limited recognition of the wrongful birth/life causes of action are covered later in the section on Birth-Related Issues. Unrelated to the subject of genetic counseling are the "wrongful conception" or "wrongful pregnancy" claims (see Postconception Issues, later in this chapter), which are related to failed contraceptive measures. The terms *wrongful birth, wrongful life,* and *wrongful conception/pregnancy* are sometimes confused.

Wrongful birth/wrongful life cases have involved genetic counseling for known teratogens (such as rubella infections[5] and Dilantin administration[6]); autosomal dominant conditions that would be apparent in the parents (neurofibromatosis,[7] polyposis coli,[8] Larsen's syndrome[9]); autosomal recessive conditions (cystic fibrosis,[10] infantile polycystic kidney disease,[11] hereditary deafness,[12] Tay-Sachs disease,[13] thalassemia[14]), many of which could be discovered by carrier or prenatal testing; and x-linked conditions that could be discovered by prenatal testing (Duchenne muscular dystrophy,[15] hereditary blindness,[16] Down syndrome,[17] and hemophilia[18]). There might be a duty to refer a patient to a specialist in the field of genetic counseling if a case falls beyond the expertise of the attending physician. The American Medical Association (AMA) Council on Scientific Affairs' indications for such a referral are (1) genetic or congenital anomaly in a family member; (2) family history of an inherited disorder; (3) abnormal somatic or behavioral development in a child; (4) mental retardation of unknown etiology in a child; (5) pregnancy in a woman over the age of 35; (6) specific ethnic background suggestive of a high rate of genetic abnormality; (7) drug use or long-term exposure to possible teratogens or mutagens; (8) three or more spontaneous abortions, early infant deaths, or both; and (9) infertility.[19]

An important aspect of current genetic counseling is prenatal testing. Amniocentesis is the most commonly employed form of prenatal testing and is performed in the sixteenth week of gestation, although it can be performed from the thirteenth week up to term. The indications for genetic amniocentesis include advanced maternal age, abnormal alpha-fetoprotein levels, previously recognized genetic (disorders), and others.

Genetic amniocentesis is considered a low-risk procedure with a complication rate of about 0.5%, perhaps lower if performed under ultrasound guidance and after at least the sixteenth week of gestation. The mother risks uterine infection, intestinal perforation, and possible Rh sensitization. The fetus risks infection, hemorrhage, and trauma to the vital organs. Chorionic villus sampling (CVS) is a relatively new prenatal diagnostic technique that may replace amniocentesis. CVS can be performed in the first trimester, 7 to 10 weeks earlier than amniocentesis; the results are often known within a few days. This could allow decisions to abort to be made within the first trimester. However, interpretations using this technique are at present more difficult than with classical amniocentesis, and the first large collaborative study to compare the two procedures showed CVS to be associated with a slightly elevated but statistically insignificant risk of fetal loss compared with amniocentesis.[20]

Contraception

The U.S. Supreme Court has created a constitutional right of privacy that protects individuals' procreative choices from governmental intrusion. The right to use contraception was, in 1965, the earliest of these rights of privacy.[21] Specifically, neither laws nor regulations can abridge the access and use of contraceptives by married or single adults.[21,22] The Court struck down the federal Comstock Law and several state laws patterned after it that prohibited obscenity, contraception, and abortion. As early as 1970, congressional action, such as the Family Planning Services and Population Research Act,[23] indicated the shift toward governmental support of contraception and family planning.

Contraception-related litigation has also involved physician liability under theories of negligence in prescribing, negligence during a procedure, and inadequate or defective informed consent. A physician who fails to impress on the patient that the chosen contraceptive method is not foolproof may be liable for costs associated with an unwanted pregnancy (see the later section on Postconception Issues, where wrongful pregnancy is discussed). In a case in which personnel at a clinic misrepresented that an intrauterine device (IUD) had been recovered, the patient was allowed to bring an action alleging fraud.[24] Manufacturers have been found liable for inadequate warnings or defective products.

Contraception issues affect a significant proportion of our society: 78% of married couples and 69% of unmarried women aged 18 to 44 are exposed to the risk of unintended pregnancy.[25] One out of every 10 women age 15 to 19 becomes pregnant each year.[26] Even a contraceptive method with an annual failure rate of 1% that is used from age 30 to age 45 will leave one woman in seven with an unintended pregnancy.

Family planning: adults and adolescents. When the first birth control clinic in the United States opened in New York City in 1916, local authorities acted to shut it down within 10 days as a violation of obscenity laws.[27] Today, in contrast, the Social Security/Medicaid Act,[28] the federal Population Research and Voluntary Family Planning Programs Act,[29] and the related federal regulations along with state laws and regulations provide for federal and state funding for family planning services and programs. In 1987, the federal and state governments spent $386 million to provide family planning services.[30] Family planning has not yet, however, attained the status of an integrated component of comprehensive health care. Social, political, and economic pressures resulting from issues such as abortion, poverty, and sex education of teens continue to affect the status of family planning in the United States. For example, all federal family planning funds come with antiabortion strings attached.

Family planning involving teens has always been and is still a controversial issue. In 1981, Congress enacted the Adolescent Family Life Act and regulations[31] to fund innovative demonstration programs addressing the problems of teenage pregnancy and childbearing.[32] The availability and provision of contraceptives present slightly different issues when minors are involved, because the state has a more reasonable interest in controlling the behavior of minors. In several opinions, the Supreme Court cautioned that minors might not have rights equal to those of adults.[33] In *Doe v. Blum,*[34] a court held that minors to whom family planning and abortion information was not sent because they were not "heads of household," although they were eligible for AFDC benefits and Medicaid, did not state a cause of action. In *Bowen v. Kendrick,*[35] the U.S. Supreme Court found that the Adolescent Family Life Act of 1981 did not have the primary effect of advancing religion and did not create excessive entanglement of church and state, and so was found to be constitutional on its face, but not necessarily constitutional as applied. The act was designed to provide funding to various organizations, including and involving religious organizations, for services and research involving premarital adolescent sexuality and pregnancy. Grantees under the act were not allowed to use the funds for certain services, such as family planning services and abortion counseling. The Supreme Court in the past several years has shifted from a "strict scrutiny" test to "undue burden" test when reviewing abortion issues, especially in dealing with adolescents. In *Planned Parenthood v. Casey,*[36] the Court upheld the parental consent or judicial consent requirement for minors seeking an abortion.

Oral contraceptives. Most lawsuits involving oral contraceptive agents are product liability cases against the manufacturer for inadequate warning of adverse reactions. The reactions most likely to give rise to suits are stroke, pulmonary thromboembolism, heart attack, and ruptured hepatic adenoma. In a 1985 Massachusetts Supreme Court case,[37] the court, in contrast to some other jurisdictions, held that the duty to warn a consumer of adverse reactions goes beyond mere compliance with an FDA labeling requirement or reliance on a physician's warning. The court ruled in favor of the

plaintiff, declaring that the manufacturer must provide the patient directly with a written warning.

The physician must fully inform the patient of the possible side effects and alternatives. The presence of a contraceptive package insert does not absolve the physician of otherwise discussing with the patient in plain language the potential hazards. Documentation of these discussions is desirable. To conform with standard medical practice, a prescription must be based on accepted indications and contraindications. Before writing a prescription, the physician must perform an adequate physical exam and should perform relevant laboratory testing, including a Pap smear.

Physicians have been found liable for their negligent prescription of birth control pills. In *Klink v. G. D. Searle & Co.,*[38] a 19-year-old woman who had never had a normal menstrual period sought birth control. The physician explained the alternative methods but did not discuss possible side effects. Nearly a year and a half later, she suffered a stroke. The court ruled in the plaintiff's favor, because birth control pills were not a proper method of treatment for her primary amenorrhea and if used as a diagnostic method to establish uterine hormonal responsiveness should not have been continued longer than six months.

In *Hamilton v. Hardy,*[39] a woman moved, and her new physician saw no reason to discourage her from taking birth control pills but did change her prescription. She returned with migraine headaches and was told to continue the pills and not to worry. She then suffered a stroke. At no time did the physician discuss adverse side effects. The court held that this was a breach of the physician's duty to warn of possible hazards and that the physician was negligent in continuing therapy, as not even a "respectable minority" of physicians would have done so.

Intrauterine devices. Most lawsuits involving IUDs are product liability cases against the manufacturer for a product unreasonably dangerous because of a defective design. The complications most likely to give rise to lawsuits are uterine and pelvic infections, infertility, uterine perforation, and ectopic pregnancy.

The litigation over the Dalkon shield forced a recall of the product in 1984.[40] By mid-1985, the Dalkon shield manufacturer, A. H. Robins Company, had paid out $520 million to 9500 women for pelvic inflammatory disease, sterility, septic spontaneous abortion, and other injuries, with many other claims still outstanding and unfiled. Robins filed for bankruptcy; and in July 1988, the U.S. District Court for the Eastern District of Virginia confirmed a bankruptcy reorganization plan, overwhelmingly approved by the majority of Dalkon shield claimants, which provided for the establishment of a trust fund of at least $2.475 billion to pay the qualified outstanding claims, and allowed for consideration of some claims that did not originally meet the April 1986 filing deadline. Various attempts were made, via individual and class action lawsuits against third parties such as Robins's insurer, to circumvent the effects that the bankruptcy action might have on claimants. In November 1989, the U.S. Supreme Court denied review of a 4th Circuit opinion upholding an injunction in connection with Robins's bankruptcy reorganization plan that barred suits against such third parties.[41]

In 1986, Searle and Ortho withdrew from the IUD market in the United States due to the costs of litigation, although their products did not have the high complication rate of the Dalkon shield.[42] At the time of the decision to withdraw, 775 cases had been filed against Searle, of which 305 were pending; of the 10 that went to trial only 2 were successful.[43] In September 1988, a Minnesota jury awarded $8.75 million in damages against Searle in connection with its Copper-7 IUD. It has been generally noted that the resulting unavailability of the IUDs to American women was unfortunate, because the Dalkon shield was the only unreasonably unsafe product.[44]

For a few years, the Progestasert, a hormone-producing IUD by Alza Corporation with an effective lifetime of one year, was the only IUD marketed in the United States. In 1988, GynoPharma introduced the ParaGard T380A copper IUD in cooperation with The Population Council, effective for up to 10 years, according to ACOG. Marketing involves a 7-page patient informed consent form. Use of the device is limited; specifically, it is not to be used in women who have never been pregnant, who have a history of pelvic inflammatory disease (PID), or who engage in sex with multiple partners.

Manufacturers' defects notwithstanding, physicians have been found liable for negligent use and care of IUDs. As with birth control pills, the physician must fully inform the patient of risks and alternatives. The physician must prescribe in conformity with accepted medical indications and contraindications. A physical exam and pertinent lab tests before insertion must be performed and the patient monitored, initially within 3 months postinsertion, and then at least once a year.

In *Killebrew v. Johnson*,[45] the patient became pregnant despite insertion of an IUD. Her gynecologist was to perform an abortion, ligate the fallopian tubes, and remove the IUD. The IUD could not be found at the time of surgery and was not seen on postoperative X rays. The physician told her that the device was gone and that she should not worry. She developed abdominal pain, dysuria, and other complaints that progressed during the next two years. It was determined that the IUD was in the peritoneal cavity, and that it had been evident on the original postoperative films. The IUD was removed and her symptoms disappeared. The court held that the physician should have personally examined the X rays to determine the presence or absence of the IUD instead of relying on the radiologist's report.

Spermicidal jelly and subdermal implants. The U.S. Supreme Court refused to hear and thereby has let stand the case of *Wells v. Ortho Pharmaceutical Corp.*,[46] in which the manufacturer was found liable for the birth defects allegedly caused by its spermicidal jelly. Two studies since published in the *New England Journal of Medicine*[47] conclude that spermicides do not cause an increased risk of birth defects when used before, during, or after conception.

Norplant, a subdermal implant, is a long-acting contraceptive that uses flexible capsules of levonorgestrel. The capsules must be surgically inserted and is a minor office procedure. Contraception is effective for approximately five years. Side effects similar to progesterone-only contraception may occur. Up to this writing, no product liability cases at the appellate level have been litigated.

Sterilization

Surgical sterilization (bilateral tubal ligation, vasectomy, etc.) is usually thought to be an elective procedure to confer permanent contraception; however, it can also be a therapeutic, incidental, or involuntary procedure. When a woman's physical or mental health is threatened by pregnancy, and sterilization is medically indicated, the procedure is therapeutic. Sterilization is incidental when it is accomplished during therapy that is done for another purpose, such as by chemotherapy for cancer, hysterectomy for endometrial carcinoma, or bilateral orchiectomy for prostatic carcinoma. When involuntary sterilization is performed, it most often involves mentally retarded wards.

Voluntary sterilization. That contraceptive sterilization has become the most popular method of birth control in the United States may be a reflection of the fact that fewer birth control options are available in the United States than in other developed countries. Contraceptive sterilizations among young U.S. women (aged 20 to 29) is about 50% higher than comparable rates in Great Britain and the Netherlands.[48] Although success rates for sterilization reversals are still low, sterilization is responsible for two-fifths of the contraceptive practices among married U.S. women aged 25 to 34,[49] and an additional 16% are protected by sterilization of the male partner.[50] In 1987, federal and state governments spent $65 million to subsidize contraceptive sterilization services, 97% of which was federal funding (88% through Medicaid).[51]

The right of privacy, which protects an individual's procreative decisions from an unjustified intrusion of law and which has applied to contraception and abortion, logically extends to sterilization. In general, public hospitals cannot abridge choices of pregnancy, abortion, or sterilization, but private physicians and private hospitals can choose the procedures they perform. Specifically, public hospitals may not prohibit elective sterilization unless there is a state law to the contrary.[52] Public funding in a private hospital does not necessarily force it to perform abortion or sterilization. Private hospitals can even condition delivery of a pregnant woman on a subsequent sterilization. Individual practitioners and private hospitals may refuse to participate in abortion or sterilization procedures. Some state laws also contain "conscience clauses" that permit individual physicians and nurses to refuse participation because of religious or moral beliefs.

The general rules of informed consent apply to sterilization procedures. It is advisable to have a separate form for sterilization that, among other things, emphasizes (1) that the procedure intends a permanent condition and (2) that there is a small but real chance of failure, which may result in an unintended pregnancy.

Tubal ligation can be performed by a number of surgical techniques with different failure and complication rates. The failure rates range from 2% to fewer than 0.1%. Patients should normally be informed of failure rates and of alternative treatments. Faulty physician-patient communications are frequent sources of liability in this area. In cases such as *Sard v. Hardy*,[53] *Gowan v. Carpenter*,[54] and *Wilsman v. Sloniewicz*[55] in which physicians performed tubal ligations using the Madlener, Bleier clip, and Hulka hemoclip techniques associated with high failure rates, patients were allowed to sue, alleging that they were not informed of alternative sterilization procedures. In *Dohn v. Lovell*,[56] the Court of Appeals of Georgia elaborated on the Georgia Voluntary Sterility Act's description of a "full and reasonable medical explanation" in favor of a patient who told her physician that she wanted her tubes "cut, tied and burnt" when the doctor subsequently used clips without informing her and she became pregnant. At the same time, a heavy burden of proof will be encountered by a patient who subjectively claims at trial that she would not have had a tubal ligation, and would have opted instead for less effective oral contraceptives that made her sick, if she had been informed of the procedure's 1% failure rate.[57] An objective "reasonable person test" may be applied at trial.[58] Failure of sterilization procedures is the most common basis for the birth-related actions

called "wrongful conception" or "wrongful pregnancy" cases, as discussed later.

In addition to routine informed consent requirements, some states have statutory requirements that the procedure be performed only in a hospital or licensed facility.[59] Some states require that the physician consult with at least one other physician before the operation.[60] Courts have held that spousal consent cannot be required.[61] Because of the permanence of the operation, consent and notice provisions of the parents of unemancipated minors might withstand constitutional attack, unlike the situation with respect to abortion and contraception. Similarly, provisions that a minor must be at least 21 years old to consent to a sterilization procedure, in contrast to the usual age of majority (18), may or may not be valid.

If the elective sterilization procedure is to be paid by Medicaid, detailed regulations apply, to prevent poor and minority women from being pressured into the operation. Requirements for federal funding[62] include a medical indication and written consent using a special Department of Health and Human Service (DHHS) form signed 30 days (but not more than 180 days) prior to surgery, except in a certified emergency. Consent may not be obtained from anyone who is under 21 years of age, in labor, under the influence of alcohol or other drugs, mentally incompetent, or seeking an abortion. Patients must be informed that refusal will not affect future care funded by the federal government, that the sterilization is considered irreversible, and that alternate methods of birth control are possible. Failure to follow these regulations will result in nonpayment, not in criminal or civil liability. At least one state, California, has regulations similar to those of the federal government, including a mandatory waiting period between the time of consent and the performance of the sterilization.[63]

Where the sterilization is performed under the auspices of the government authority, the physician is viewed as an agent of the state and may be subject to constraints. In *Downs v. Sawtelle*,[64] a single, deaf-mute mother of two instituted a civil rights action alleging that physicians and several social service workers conspired to sterilize her against her will. State action was found in the functioning of the private community hospital because the town and the hospital were so intertwined.

Involuntary sterilization. In the early 1900s, involuntary sterilization was authorized and mandated by state legislation for imbeciles, idiots, sexual perverts, epileptics, the insane, and recidivist criminals.[65] The term *eugenic sterilization* has been applied to connote controlled procreation, in its negative sense, to prevent undesirable traits. Except for limited situations involving those mentally retarded who would be unable to appreciate the consequences of their acts or care for their children and who might pass on a hereditary form of retardation, the statutes have been found constitutionally invalid because they were considered cruel and unusual punishment, violative of the equal protection clause, or lacking due process. The constitutionality of compulsory sterilization for the mentally retarded was upheld in the landmark 1927 U.S. Supreme Court case of *Buck v. Bell*. Writing for the court, Justice Oliver Wendell Holmes stated:

It is better for all the world, if, instead of waiting to execute degenerate offspring for crime, or let them starve for their imbecility, society can prevent those who are manifestly unfit from continuing their kind. The principle that sustains compulsory vaccination is broad enough to cover cutting the Fallopian tubes . . . three generations of imbeciles are enough.[66]

More recent research has indicated that most forms of mental retardation are not hereditary. Many states legislatively authorize involuntary sterilization of wards who are genetically retarded.[67] The statutes generally require the following findings: the permanence of the condition; the sexual capacity of the ward; a high probability of transmission of the genetic disease; the inability of the ward to care for the offspring; the ward's inability to use less drastic forms of birth control; and minimal risk of personal injury to the ward.[68] Often the court must find that the sterilization is in the best interests of the ward.[69] In many jurisdictions, these findings must be based on clear and convincing proof rather than a mere preponderance of the evidence.[70] Most statutes include provisions that exculpate physicians and administrative officials from civil and criminal liability when acting in accordance with the law, although some allow civil liability in the case of a negligently performed procedure.[71] Many of the statutes fail to cover noninstitutionalized mentally retarded persons, and some courts have failed to grant the sterilization procedure because of the absence of legislative authority to do so; other courts have been willing to grant the sterilization so as not to discriminate against those who are cared for at home.[72]

Courts have recently begun to authorize involuntary sterilization on incompetent wards in the absence of any legislation on the subject.[73] This change has in part been due to the series of *Sparkman* decisions by lower federal courts and the Supreme Court in which it became clear, contrary to prior case law, that judges are protected by judicial immunity and that the private individuals instituting suit are not subject to liability for violation of federal civil rights law.[74] Some courts, when attempting to decide for the incompetent ward whether sterilization

is appropriate, will use a best interests test, focusing on the best interests of the individual irrespective of the choice he or she might have made.[75] The *Grady* court outlined nine factors to be considered when a court is determining what is in the best interest of the disabled person.[76] A minority of courts use a substituted judgment test,[77] an attempt to determine what the individual would decide if he or she were not incompetent.[78]

Several state supreme court decisions have found that the constitutional right to procreative choices protects a mentally retarded ward's right to compulsory sterilization and that to deny access would deny the equal protection guaranteed to other children. An excellent review of involuntary sterilization by Letterie and Fox[79] should be consulted by the interested reader.

Contraceptive deception

A recent series of cases, known as "contraceptive deception," have been reported in which one sexual partner deceives the other into a false belief of infertility or the taking of contraceptives. Typically, the issue is raised as a defense to a child support action by an unmarried male. In *Pamela P. v. Frank S.*,[80] a New York statute was upheld against a constitutional attack in which the defendant maintained that he should be allowed to prove the wrongful conduct of the mother. In *Stephen K. v. Roni L.*,[81] the father sued for fraud, negligent misrepresentation, and negligence. The court dismissed the case on public policy grounds: "The practice of birth control, if any, engaged by two partners in a consensual sexual relationship is best left to the individual involved, free from any governmental interference." The court noted that the father also could have taken precautions. However, in *Barbara A. v. John G.*,[82] a female was able to maintain a civil suit against a male who claimed to be sterile for bodily injury she received resulting from an ectopic pregnancy. In January 1990, the Superior Court of New Jersey affirmed a lower court decision denying relief on public policy grounds to a woman who alleged that the defendant's false representations to her about having had a vasectomy caused the birth of a healthy child.[83] The dissent agreed with public policies that prohibit court interference in private, consensual sexual relations and refuse to recognize the birth of a healthy child as an actionable wrong, but argued that the case is not distinguishable from cases in which defendants have been held liable for knowingly transmitting venereal diseases.

CONCEPTION ISSUES
Assisted conception and nontraditional parentage

Infertility is a common problem, occurring in about 15% of all U.S. couples. At the same time, there has been a significant drop in the number of adoptions owing to the legalization of abortion, the widespread use of contraceptives, and the increasing social tolerance of raising illegitimate children. New reproductive technologies can offer alternatives to adoption that are attractive in that they can provide parents with emotional, biological, and genetic involvement in the pregnancy.

These new technologies in a tolerant, pluralist society are giving rise to a host of nontraditional parentage situations and an entire new conceptual legal notion of "family." It is now possible for a child to have five "parents": the biological or genetic father (a sperm or testicle donor), the rearing or social father (the traditional father), the genetic mother (the ovum donor), the gestational or birthing mother (the surrogate mother), and the rearing or social mother (the traditional mother). The technologies central to these issues include artificial insemination by spouse or donor, *in vitro* fertilization (IVF), embryo transfer (ET), and cryopreservation of embryos. Gamete intrafallopian transfer (GIFT) is a variant of IVF except that the ova and sperm are placed into the fallopian tube of the host female for the fertilization to occur *in vivo* instead of into a petri dish. GIFT is considered the appropriate alternative for couples where certain factors interfere with the natural transport of gametes to the site of fertilization in the presence of healthy and patent tubes. Zygote intrafallopian transfer (ZIFT) allows the opportunity to observe and eliminate abnormally fertilized eggs. GIFT and ZIFT clinical pregnancy rates are approximately 30%.[84]

Surrogate motherhood is the use of artificial insemination into the womb of another female for gestation to term. It has most commonly been used when other reproductive technologies have failed, when the ovaries are absent or nonresponsive, when there is genetic disease, and to avoid pregnancy. The success rate is similar to that generally between couples, approximately 80%. Because of differing and sometimes misleading definitions of terms such as "success rate" and "pregnancy rate," it has been suggested that all clinical papers reporting results of the new reproductive technologies be required to include the statistic of "live births per 100 attempted oocyte retrievals," even though such a requirement would cause a nine-month delay between patient treatment and manuscript preparation.[85]

Legal issues of various nontraditional parenting arrangements include questions of lineage, inheritance, legitimacy, adultery, confidentiality, status of residual embryos, responsibility for diseases and defects, and the correlative rights of the different parties. There are also ethical and legal issues involved in the new area of preimplantation genetic screening.[86] Cytological analysis is now technically feasible prior to implanting the conceptus into the recipient.

In general, the laws governing these family and health issues are state laws, not federal laws, with the exception of federal constitutional provisions and federal fetal research regulations. Specific state legislation regarding the new reproductive possibilities is beginning to be promulgated. Nonspecific state laws that may affect this area include laws on adoption, paternity, legitimacy, inheritance, "baby-selling," child custody and support, homicide, feticide, abortion, fetal experimentation, and child abuse and neglect.

Artificial insemination. Artificial insemination (AI) is now relatively common. It consists of inoculation of the semen of the husband (AIH) or another donor (AID) into the reproductive tract of the woman. An estimated 40,000 cases of AID are performed each year in the United States. The process is so simple that women have performed the procedure on themselves.

AIH is most commonly used for oligospermia, ineffective coitus (i.e., premature ejaculation), hostile cervical mucus, endometriosis, and idiopathic infertility. The success rate is approximately 25%. In a few cases, men with vas obstructions have been able to have children by aspirating epididymal sperm.[87]

AID is most commonly used for aspermia, ejaculatory problems, endometriosis, oligospermia, hostile cervical mucus, and failed AIH. The success rate is approximately 25% per cycle for a pregnancy and approximately 17% for a viable infant (due to a high incidence of miscarriage).

Approximately half of the states have enacted legislation dealing with AI. Although AI has been used for decades, Georgia enacted the first statute in 1964.[88] This legislation attempted to respond to the problems arising from the use of sperm from an AID. In general, these statutes deal with the legal status of the resulting child, donor selection, practitioner licensing, and the confidentiality of records. In addition, most state legislation requires that AI be performed by a licensed physician. Even without specific legislation prohibiting insemination by nonphysicians, such an act might be considered to be the unauthorized practice of medicine.

In addition to statutes, many states have dealt judicially with questions of parental rights and obligations resulting from AIH and AID. Early court cases held that AID was adulterous and the child illegitimate, but the clear majority view today is to consider AID not to be adulterous (unless there has been actual sexual intercourse) and the children to be legitimate, based on public policy considerations and the desire not to stigmatize innocent children.[89] In *In re Baby Doe*,[90] the Supreme Court of South Carolina concluded that a husband who encourages and assists his wife in AI can be held liable for support of the resulting child even though the husband did not consent to the procedure in writing.

Most legislation codifies this judicial trend and creates a presumption of legitimacy *only* when the husband gives written permission for AID so that, in the absence of a written agreement, the AI donor will be considered the legal father and responsible for child support. In other jurisdictions, consent of the husband is presumed. A number of states expressly relieve the sperm donor of all obligations and rights to the child unless he is also the husband of the woman inseminated; as discussed later, these statutes can prove problematical when applied to cases in which the sperm donor actually intends to raise and be responsible for the child, as in surrogacy arrangements.

Some courts have imputed parentage rights and obligations on the biological father in times of conflict in an effort to preserve traditional family mores. In a 1968 California Supreme Court case, *People v. Sorenson,*[91] the court upheld a criminal prosecution of a man for failure to pay child support for the child born to his former wife after he had given his consent for AID. In *C.M. v. C.C.,*[92] the unmarried biological father sued for visitation rights after the mother refused visitation or any other parental role to him. Programs in governmental settings cannot abridge the constitutional rights of privacy and procreative choice. A single woman sued the Wayne State University artificial insemination clinic for restricting insemination to married couples; she argued that they had no right to so arbitrarily refuse her service.[93] The suit was settled on the condition that the restriction be dropped.

The confidentiality of donor records is a potential problem area. The child may claim the right to know his or her biological father. The sperm donor usually does not want responsibility for parentage and relies on the confidentiality of the physician's records. The mother and her spouse usually do not want the identity of the donor known to protect the family unit. At least eight states (California, Colorado, Hawaii, Minnesota, Montana, North Dakota, Washington, and Wyoming) have adopted the portion of the Model Uniform Parentage Act that allows the identity of a sperm donor to be obtained only on court order for "good cause."[94] Similarly, adopted children have no right to know their biological parents, although increasingly courts have allowed access to the information based on the showing of good cause.[95]

Infectious diseases such as HIV, hepatitis B, gonorrhea, herpes, syphilis, and chlamydia, among others, can be transmitted by the procedure. Screening procedures attempt to prevent the spread of sexually transmitted diseases. In the past, fresh semen was used in most cases because it is considered to be more effective; however, because artificial insemination has been associated with the transmission of HIV, which does not necessarily show

up on screening tests for up to six months or more, the Centers for Disease Control and the American Fertility Society now recommend that semen be routinely frozen and the donor submitted to repeat blood tests for HIV, once at the time of the donation and again six months later, before the specimen is used. In March 1990, the American Fertility and Sterility Society published *New Guidelines for the Use of Semen Donor Insemination,*[96] with specific and detailed guidelines on selection and screening of donors[97] and minimal genetic screening for gamete donors.[98] Genetic screening to prevent the transmission of genetic disease of semen donors other than the husband is mandated in New York and Oregon and is prudent and probably standard practice in most jurisdictions, despite the lack of binding laws and regulations so requiring.

In vitro fertilization. *In vitro* fertilization is now an alternative method of conception in which the sperm and ova are obtained and allowed to incubate outside the human body. The resulting embryo is then implanted back into the womb in which ideally it will be carried to term. Indications for IVF include absent or nonpatent fallopian tubes, inadequate motile sperm count, hostile cervical mucous, refractory endometriosis, and perhaps unexplained infertility. IVF has been called "the final common pathway of infertility therapy."[99] Approximately one-fourth of the attempts result in a pregnancy — with the successful implantation being the most critical step — and the live birth rate is in the range of 15%.

The first "test-tube baby" was Louise Brown, born in England in 1978. The first successful IVF program in the United States was established at the Eastern Virginia Medical School in Norfolk, which led to the first American IVF pregnancy in 1993. By 1993, there were more than 200 such programs in the United States.

If the sperm and the ova are supplied by the intended parents, and the natural mother is the woman who receives the embryos, then it is clear that traditional family legal principles would apply. If the sperm are not from the intended father, then new and existing family law principles concerning paternity and AID and perhaps adoption should apply. However, when an ovum is donated, or when a surrogate mother is utilized, whether or not she is also the source of the ovum, legal relationships are less clear (see the following section on Surrogate Motherhood).

Federal regulation of IVF to date has only applied to research. In 1973, the Department of Health Education and Welfare (DHEW — now DHHS) appointed a study group to recommend policies regarding biomedical research.[100] This group singled out IVF and ET, involving extracorporeal embryos, as deserving of special consideration and recommended the establishment of an ethical review board to establish guidelines and review the acceptability of research. The final DHEW regulations (1975) concerning the protection of fetuses, pregnant women, and products of IVF stated only that no IVF proposal be funded until reviewed and accepted by a federal Ethical Advisory Board (EAB) and an institutional review board (IRB). The first proposal was submitted in 1977. The EAB concluded in 1979 that "it is acceptable from an ethical standpoint to undertake research involving human *in vitro* fertilization and embryo transfer" provided certain general conditions are met. The EAB also recommended the drafting of model legislation to clarify the rights and responsibilities of the parties concerned before approval of any research. No research project ever received federal funding, and in 1980 the EAB was dismantled, creating a *de facto* moratorium on federally funded IVF and ET research. The National Institutes of Health (NIH), in 1988, declared that it would no longer fund research using fetal tissues until a study group reported its finding on the ethical and legal issues. The concern was that use of fetal tissue would promote abortions.

More than 25 states have passed antiabortion legislation that includes restrictions on fetal research. In many states the term "fetus" is specifically defined to include an embryo or product of conception. Most of these laws would not be applicable to IVF because they are expressly limited to research subsequent to or in anticipation of an abortion, or apply only when the fetus exhibits a heartbeat, umbilical cord pulse, spontaneous respiration, or spontaneous muscle movement. However, statutes that broadly proscribe fetal research may well be interpreted to restrict *in vitro* fertilization, especially the cryopreservation of embryos. State legislation on AI may also directly or implicitly apply to IVF. Physicians in many states have resorted to approaching their state or local district attorneys for their legal opinions—to ensure that they would not be prosecuted under state statutes—before proceeding with IVF programs.

Pennsylvania requires certain information to be filed with the state department of health by persons conducting or experimenting in IVF but imposes no direct regulations or limitations on the practice of *in vitro* fertilization. The child abuse and neglect laws of Illinois apply to physicians performing *in vitro* fertilization. The Illinois Abortion Act of 1977 includes the provision that "Any person who intentionally causes the fertilization of a human ovum by a sperm outside the body of a living human female shall with regard to the human being thereby produced be deemed to have the care and custody of a child for the purposes of Section 4 of the Act to Prevent and Punish Wrongs to Children."[101]

Section 4 provides that "It shall be unlawful for any person having the care or custody of any child, willfully to cause or permit the life of such child to be endangered, or the health of such child to be injured, or willfully cause or permit such child to be placed in such a situation that its life or health may be endangered."[102] The statute would seem to prohibit the destruction of unused embryos. In fact, the very process of placing an embryo in a petri dish and supplying adequate nutrients might be construed as a situation that may be so life endangering as to create liability. The constitutionality of these laws was unsuccessfully challenged in *Smith v. Hartigan*.[103] The statutes were interpreted such that the attorney general's office would not prosecute, allowing IVF programs to proceed. The position of the court was that the laws applied to the physicians only during the preimplantation stage when they had custody, and that if a conceptus was found to be defective, then destruction of the fetus would be considered a lawful pregnancy termination and not a willful injury. Then, in April 1990, the U.S. District Court of the Northern District of Illinois ruled that Section 6(7) of the law, prohibiting any experimentation using a human embryo that is not "therapeutic to the fetus," is unconstitutionally vague because it fails to define the terms "experimentation" and "therapeutic."

The risk of genetic defects from IVF is apparently no higher than in a conventional birth.[104] If a child is born defective, a program will not likely be found liable as long as the program followed accepted standards and did not have an above-normal rate of defective products. Nonetheless, it would seem prudent to perform some genetic screening, if only a history, on the husband and wife. The American Fertility Society published new *Minimal Standards for Program of Invitro Fertilization* in February 1990.[105] This report attempts to set standards for the skills required of personnel, the services offered, and the necessary facilities; these standards may be evidence of the standard of care in a malpractice suit. Preimplantation screening is now feasible and may allow the detection of cytogenic disorders and certain metabolic disorders. A single cell is removed from the blastomere and analyzed via the usual cytogenetic methods. Polymerase chain reaction assaying can be used for detection of single gene disorders.

Surrogate motherhood. When an individual is physically incapable of bearing a child, a surrogate mother or gestational mother may be desired as an alternative to adoption. The infertile client—usually a married couple, but it could be a single male or female—contracts for the services of a woman to bear a child and then relinquish her parental rights in favor of the contracting parents. Most often, the baby's biological father and his wife, the prospective adopting or "rearing" mother, are the contracting parents. Conception by artificial insemination of the surrogate mother is the usual procedure contemplated; recently, however, implantation after *in vitro* fertilization has been accomplished, which may or may not make use of the oocytes of the proposed rearing mother. Attorneys, physicians, or surrogate agencies often act as brokers in these arrangements. Although surrogacy has been practiced for centuries, open consideration of surrogate motherhood with the advent of medically sanctioned artificial procreative methods has become an option only in the last decade. Increasing public attention has prompted competing legislative proposals that would either sanction or outlaw these arrangements.

Public policy arguments against surrogate mothering, which may provide a basis for finding a surrogacy contract unenforceable, include arguments that it undermines traditional notions of family and threatens the sanctity of marriage, that it disregards and undervalues the strong attachment of the maternal bond, and that it is morally repugnant because children are treated like chattels. It is also argued that poor women would be economically exploited; indeed in one U.S. study,[106] 40% of volunteer surrogate mothers were found to be unemployed or on welfare. Some of the public policy arguments against this form of collaborative reproduction are reminiscent of public policy arguments originally made against artificial insemination.

Even if surrogacy contracts were not contrary to public policy, courts would not specifically enforce performance; that is, they would not force a woman to bear a child. In general, contracts are not enforceable when they are prohibited by law. State laws against baby bartering, paid adoption, or more recently, against surrogate arrangements might apply. The Thirteenth Amendment's prohibition against slavery and the sale of one person by another might also be applied to find a contract unlawful and therefore unenforceable. Despite unenforceability, suit may still be brought against the surrogate for emotional suffering by the contracting couple. Attempting the application of existing state laws to surrogacy situations can sometimes provide opportunities for judicial gymnastics. The sale of babies is illegal in all 50 states. Criminal penalties have been established for the offering, paying, or receiving of money or other consideration for the surrender of a child. However, it has been argued both successfully and unsuccessfully, in different states, that the baby bartering statutes should not apply to surrogacy because the parental relinquishment is voluntary and without the pressure of a preexisting pregnancy; payment is made by the natural father who presumably will act in the child's best interest; and the payment is not for the sale of the child but for the services rendered.[107] New state laws often limit the legitimacy of surrogacy arrangements depending on whether or not the surrogate earns a fee above and beyond the costs of pregnancy and delivery.

The perimeters of a constitutional right to procreate are indistinct. One author notes that although the U.S. Supreme Court has recognized a constitutional right to have sex without babies, constitutional protection of a right to have babies without sex is unclear.[108] Use of the privacy right to protect individual reproduction decisions might seem overly strained when applied to collaborative reproduction techniques that are, by definition, nonprivate; alternatives such as a privacy-related "constitutional right to procreate"[109] and a "right of intimate association" analysis[110] have been advocated.

The particular problem areas in which combinations of public policy arguments, contract law principles, state laws and constitutions, and federal constitutional doctrines are put to the test include situations where (1) the surrogate develops a maternal attachment and decides to keep the baby, (2) the surrogate decides not to go through with the contract and terminates her pregnancy by an abortion, (3) the surrogate inadvertently or wantonly exposes the child to noxious or teratogenic agents, or (4) the baby is defective and none of the potential parents wishes to take the baby. If the contract is upheld, then contractual provisions would be controlling; on the other hand, if the contract is unenforceable or void, then the courts would offer little or no help.

In view of the fact that close to 1000 babies have been born of surrogate mothers in the United States,[111] the incidence of court cases on the subject seems low. The majority of surrogacy arrangements proceed without judicial involvement, with few reported instances of parties reneging on their agreements.[112] Courts have uniformly refused to enforce surrogacy contracts, although custody is often awarded to the biological father and his wife under a "best interests of the child" analysis.

The Michigan case of *Malahoff v. Stiver*[113] illustrates how complex and entangled these situations can be. Surrogate mother Stiver gave birth to a microcephalic child. The Malahoffs, who contracted for the child, decided they no longer wanted the child and told the hospital to withhold treatment. The surrogate mother said she felt no maternal bond to the baby. Eventually the state became the guardian of the child. It was later determined that husband Malahoff was not the father, but rather husband Stiver, as the couple had not abstained from intercourse before the insemination. Malahoff brought suit against surrogate Stiver for not producing the child contracted for. The Stivers brought suit against the physician, attorney, and psychiatrist of the surrogate program for not advising them from refraining from intercourse before insemination. The Stivers also claimed that the child's defect was not passed on by his genetic parents, but by a virus transmitted by Malahoff's sperm. The case was not reported, but eventually the Stivers decided to keep the child, and the Malahoffs lost the money they had paid the attorney. The Michigan legislature dealt with surrogate parenting issues in 1988-1989 when it enacted a Surrogate Parenting Act, effective September 1, 1988,[114] which provided for temporary custody in case of disputes. The American Bar Association has approved a model Uniform Surrogacy Act.[115]

"Baby M." The most significant and publicized surrogate motherhood case to date is that of Baby M, decided by the New Jersey Supreme Court in 1988. The high court[116] reversed the lower appellate decision and declared the contract unenforceable because such contractual surrogate arrangements are otherwise against the public policy and interests. Nonetheless, custody was taken from Mary Beth Whitehead, the mother, and given to the Sterns, the contracting couple, on the basis of the best interests of the child.

Mary Beth Whitehead agreed to a surrogate motherhood arrangement with William Stern for $10,000 through Michigan attorney Noel P. Keane (the "father" of commercial surrogate motherhood) and the Infertility Center of New York (ICNY). Mrs. Whitehead was artificially inseminated with Mr. Stern's sperm in 1985. A child, "Baby M" ("Sarah Elizabeth" to the Whiteheads and "Melissa Elizabeth" to the Sterns), was born on March 27, 1986. The child was given to the Sterns by Mrs. Whitehead on March 30, but the child was handed back to Whitehead the next day after she expressed extreme emotional anxiety over the loss of the child, threatened suicide, and pled for a week's continuance. On May 5, Mr. Stern proceeded to the Whitehead residence with a court order calling for his temporary custody, but Richard Whitehead escaped with the child. Three months later the Whiteheads were located in Florida by a private detective. The child was returned to the Sterns on July 31. Mrs. Whitehead was allowed visitation rights for several hours a week pending the outcome of the trial.[117]

The judge of the trial court, which was the New Jersey Superior Court, focused on two issues: (1) the validity of the contract and (2) the custody of the child. The trial court dealt with arguments that the contract was void or unenforceable on the grounds that it was a contract of adhesion; was unconscionable, fraudulent, and illusory; and that the Whiteheads lacked legal capacity to contract. The validity of the contract was upheld in each case. The court proceeded to rule that contracts for surrogacy are valid. The contract was specifically enforced. Custody was awarded to the Sterns by the court on a best interests analysis. The judge terminated the parental rights of Mary Beth Whitehead and allowed Elizabeth Stern to adopt the child. No visitation was allowed.

The New Jersey Supreme Court largely reversed the holding of the trial court judge, ruling that the contract was invalid and unenforceable on two bases: (1) direct conflict with existing state statutes and (2) conflict with public policy.

The court held that the contract contravened the state baby bartering statute, because the contracted fee was determined to be for the delivery of a baby and not just a fee for a service. It did not reach the issue of violation of state and federal minimum wage regulations. The court held that the basis for the baby bartering law, public policy dictating against the sales of babies, also dictates against commercial surrogacy.

Next, the court noted that the contract provisions were contrary to state adoption law provisions. The court noted that the adoption laws, in contrast to the surrogacy arrangements, mandate safeguards such as counseling, evaluation, and legal advice for the protection of all concerned. The only legal advice that Mary Beth Whitehead received was a one-hour opportunity to have questions about the contract answered in an earlier surrogacy arrangement. The psychological evaluation was not for her benefit—she knew only that she had "passed." Furthermore, the court reasoned that in such a contract, the natural mother is irrevocably committed before she knows the strength of her bond with her child, before any amount of advice would satisfy her needs. She never makes a totally voluntary informed consent. The mandatory and irrevocable surrender of the child by contract was said to clearly conflict with New Jersey law on private adoption, because it is tantamount to termination of parental rights. The court cited *Sees v. Baber,*[118] in which the natural mother was entitled to have her child returned to her despite physical surrender of the child to the adopting parents four days after birth. Moreover, the court noted that the contract provides for custody decisions to be made without regard for the best interests of the child. Since the adoption of the child by Mrs. Stern in New Jersey required termination of the parental rights of the mother, the court held that the termination of Mrs. Whitehead's parental rights by the trial court had been improper and required that the adoption of the baby by Mrs. Stern be invalidated.

The court proceeded to hold the contract unenforceable as against public policy. It found that the public policy of the state protects children from the unnecessary separation of their natural parents, and that one parent should not be favored over the other; yet the whole purpose and effect of the surrogacy contract was to give the father exclusive rights to the child by destroying the rights of the mother.

Both parties asserted state and federal constitutional

claims. The Sterns argued that the right of procreation extends to the decision to choose to procreate through surrogacy. The court held otherwise.

The Sterns also contended that under the doctrine of equal protection, a surrogate mother should be treated the same as a sperm donor under the artificial insemination statute, but the court distinguished the two situations. Ms. Whitehead argued that a parent has a constitutional right to the companionship of a child and that the Thirteenth Amendment and the Parentage Act apply to commercial surrogate arrangements, but the court declined to review these issues.

The New Jersey Supreme Court reestablished parental rights in Ms. Whitehead, who was by that time Ms. Whitehead-Gould but, under the "best-interests-of-the-child" analysis, granted continuing custody of the child to the Sterns. Further proceedings at the trial court level granted extended visitation rights to Whitehead-Gould with overnight stays, including a two-week summer period. The Sterns did not appeal this decision.

Other surrogacy cases. Other reported cases of surrogacy indicate how surrogacy can distort traditional concepts of the family.[119] In California, Alejandro Munoz bore a child as a "favor" for her second cousin, Nattie Haro. Munoz had inseminated herself with a plastic syringe using sperm from Haro's husband. Later she sued for shared custody of the child, and her claim was upheld by the Supreme Court. In another California case, a lesbian woman bore a child after inseminating herself with sperm donated by the homosexual brother of her lover. After the lesbian couple broke up, a judge granted visitation rights to both women and the semen donor. In a midwestern state, two homosexual men have made arrangements through a surrogate agency to have someone else bear a child whom they will raise. The first reported case of surrogacy in South Africa involves a 48-year-old grandmother who delivered triplets for her daughter. She had been implanted with four embryos produced from her daughter's ova and her son-in-law's sperm, because the daughter had previously had a hysterectomy for uncontrolled hemorrhage during a delivery. In a case decided in late 1989, an Alaska court upheld the surrogacy arrangements that had been made between sisters when the biological mother changed her mind about giving the baby up for adoption after the maximum time period allowed by the Alaska adoption statute.[120]

As complications develop, the artificial nature of these arrangements will be tested. In Texas, a surrogate mother reportedly died in the eighth month of pregnancy due to pregnancy-related heart failure.[121] In Washington, D.C., an HIV-positive child was born, and both the contracting couple and the surrogate refused to claim the child. Future issues may include such topics as a female employee's decision to "moonlight" as a surrogate by making use of the health insurance benefits and pregnancy leave policy provided by her primary employer; violation of constitutional rights of the surrogate with respect to enforcement of contract provisions concerning her behavior during pregnancy and, conversely, the prospective rearing parents' rights to have those provisions enforced; and the possibility of physician liability for both the surrogate and the contracting couple when surrogacy arrangements do not turn out as planned. Three guiding sets of principles must always be addressed in considering surrogate arrangements: (1) contract law statutes and principles; (2) state statutes and principles related to family law, including criminal statutes; and (3) constitutional considerations. Before the Baby M case, most commentators suggested that courts would and should hold contracts for surrogacy void on grounds of public policy. On the other hand, courts may respond to the apparent and significant need filled by surrogate arrangements, as judged by their general and growing popularity, success, and public acceptance. In any event, it seems clear that, no matter how the validity of the contract or agreement is decided, the custody of the child will always be based on a "best interests" test.

Cryopreservation of embryos and gametes. The preservation of embryos and gametes by freezing is an integral part of IVF. The first successful births after freezing, thawing, and implantation of a human embryo were in 1984 by groups in Australia and the Netherlands. Cryopreservation has become routine for preserving multiple embryos for use in subsequent cycles. However, it poses special problems because the chances for exploitation are greatly increased. The possibility of embryo and gamete banks raises concerns over eugenic considerations and commercialism. Doctors are not uncommonly confronted with requests for postmortem sperm recovery in cases of sudden accidental death. The January/February 1990 *Hastings Center Report* comments that "no legislation exists to restrict or regulate sperm retrieval. Genetic manipulation becomes feasible on a widespread basis. The disruptive influence on the laws of inheritance by kindred born to later generations may also be significant. The disposal of embryos that are not used is morally repugnant to some groups who view it in the same way as they do abortion. From the same perspective, the legal culpability for the destruction of embryos might be viewed in light of the abortion laws. Few laws deal explicitly with the status and disposition of preimplantation embryos and, legally, embryos have no right to be implanted."[122]

Some special issues involved in cryopreservation have been exemplified in court cases. A wealthy couple died in an airplane crash, leaving millions of dollars and two frozen embryos in Australia.[123] Questions about whether the embryos belonged to the storage facility of the estate and about how the laws of inheritance should apply were resolved when a California superior court declared the wife's mother the sole heir to the estate, precluding any claim of the embryos if they should be thawed, implanted, and survive to childhood. In Virginia, another couple filed suit against a reproductive research institute in California when the institute refused to release the couple's cryopreserved embryos for transfer to another institute.[124] In a scenario that is likely to be repeated, a Tennessee couple who had cryopreserved seven embryos separated, and the husband filed a court action seeking to enjoin the wife from having the embryos implanted against his will. The Tennessee Supreme Court ruled that the biological father of the cryopreserved embryos had an absolute right not to become a birth father against his will.[125] The ethics committee of the American Fertility Society issued a statement identifying four primary areas of legal and ethical concern with cryopreservation: (1) the risk of cryo-injury, rendering the embryo useless after freezing and thawing; (2) the risk of birth defects in offspring produced by the freezing and storage of the embryo; (3) the possibility of failure in the mechanical support systems, either during the freezing process or during storage, with resultant loss of the embryo; and (4) the legal status of the embryo.[126] Cryopreservation of unfertilized oocytes would minimize the legal and ethical concerns. Unfortunately, that has proved to be a much more difficult procedure.

POSTCONCEPTION ISSUES
Prenatal injury issues

It is surprising how seldom traumatic injury to a pregnant woman causes injury to a fetus. The most common situation resulting in a liability for prenatal injury follows blunt abdominal trauma that is secondary to a motor vehicle collision.

Generally, there is no criminal liability for the prenatal injury of a stillborn infant; however, criminal liability is clear if the prenatal injury results in death or other injury in a child born alive. Most state penal codes, while statutorily prescribing criminal punishment for wrongful death of a person, define a "person" as a human being who has been born and is alive. This rule follows from Lord Coke's restatement of English law: "If a woman is quick with child and takes a potion, or if a man beats her, and the child is born alive and dies of the potion or battery, this is murder." However, approximately half of the states have specifically legislated a crime of feticide/homicide or involuntary manslaughter for the death of a fetus. The Supreme Judicial Court of Massachusetts decided 10 years ago in *Commonwealth v. Cass*[127] that a viable fetus is a "person" within the meaning of the Massachusetts vehicular homicide statute. For the first time, a state levied a criminal punishment, absent specific legislation, for the death of a fetus not born alive. In *State v. Wickstrom*,[128] the defendant, who beat his pregnant girlfriend, was convicted of first-degree criminal abortion, a violation of the criminal statute prohibiting the performance of abortions by nonphysicians.

There is a clear trend toward liberalizing civil liability for prenatal injury. The right to sue for damages for the death of another is based on wrongful death statutes that have been enacted in some form by all 50 states. The first decision on the applicability of these statutes to death from an intrauterine injury was *Dietrich v. Northampton*.[129] This decision was rendered by Justice Oliver Wendell Holmes and the Massachusetts Supreme Court in 1884. Justice Holmes stated that there was no compensable injury for an unborn child as the child was not yet "a being in existence" but was merely a part of its mother's body.

For the next 60 years, every court considering this issue followed this decision. The *Dietrich* rule was criticized by legal commentary, and by the mid-twentieth century decisions began to overrule this precedent. Although a few other cases had so held, *Bonbrest v. Katz*[130] was the key case overturning the Dietrich rule, and no case has since denied compensation for prenatal injuries of a fetus later born alive. This change is considered to be one of the most abrupt reversals of a well-settled rule in the history of tort law.

Most states have extended civil liability to persons causing intrauterine injury resulting in stillbirth. A few courts have limited liability for prenatal injury to those cases in which the fetus was viable (defined in the sense of *Roe v. Wade*[131] as a fetus so developed as to be capable of a separate existence) at the time of injury. In 1989, in *Cowe by Cowe v. Forum Group, Inc.*,[132] the Court of Appeals of Indiana established a cause of action for prenatal injury in a case where the defendant's negligent failure to diagnose the pregnancy of their retarded ward and their subsequent failure to render prenatal care resulted in injury to the child born. Although these cases have dealt with direct trauma to the infant, the rationale would appear to extend to toxic chemicals and even to teratogenic agents.

There is increasing interest in holding mothers responsible for the health of their offspring. At the same time, injunctive relief has usually been granted in emergency situations (see the later sections titled Birth-Related Issues and Court-ordered Obstetrical Interventions). In San Diego, a woman was charged for failing to summon medical help when she began to hemorrhage during her pregnancy. She delivered a son with severe brain damage later that day, who died approximately a month later. The municipal court judge dismissed criminal charges because the 1926 law with which she was charged was intended to force fathers to pay for the support of their children and did not apply to this situation. A woman in Toledo, Ohio, was charged with felony endangerment of her child for regularly using cocaine during her pregnancy. The grand jury returned an indictment when her daughter developed withdrawal symptoms a few days after birth. The mother tested positive for cocaine. The child was placed in a foster home, and the mother was placed in a drug rehabilitation program. The case was eventually dropped.

On the other hand, a child was allowed to maintain a civil action against its mother and her physician for prenatal negligence in *Grodin v. Grodin*[133] for the unreasonable exercise of parental discretion in the use of tetracycline, resulting in damage to her son's teeth. There has been much discussion concerning mandatory treatment of drug-addicted obstetrical patients. However, most commentators agree that such treatment is ineffective.[134]

Abortion

The history of legalized abortion is one of controversy. The first step toward legalization came in 1965, through the Supreme Court case of *Griswold v. Connecticut*.[135] In that case, the U.S. Supreme Court created a "zone of privacy" for married persons that prevented states from regulating their choice to use contraception. Then in *Roe v. Wade,* the Court declared that the right of privacy was broad enough to encompass a woman's decision to terminate her pregnancy.[136] In *Roe,* a Texas abortion statute, similar to those of 31 other states, was struck down in its entirety as unconstitutional. The Court reasoned that the state could invade the privacy of the mother to a limited extent when the state's interest in protecting the health of the mother or the life of the fetus became sufficiently strong. The court imposed these limitations:

1. Prior to the end of the first trimester, the decision to abort is strictly between the woman and her physician.
2. Beginning in the second trimester but before the fetus becomes viable, the state may impose regulations reasonably related to the mother's health.
3. During the period of fetal viability (roughly that of the third trimester), the state may regulate or prohibit all abortions except when necessary to preserve the health of the mother.

A wave of restrictive state and municipal abortion legislation was promulgated in reaction to *Roe.* Most were quickly struck down as unconstitutional. Gradually, in the wake of this activity, the Supreme Court seemed to retreat from its "strict scrutiny" standard toward the more lenient "rational basis" analysis to determine the constitutionality of legislation and regulations. This retreat led to a most significant trio of decisions that helped to define the outer limits of the right to abortion. In the *Maher v. Roe, Poelker v. Doe,* and *Harris v. McRae* decisions, the Court upheld government spending statutes that reimburse an indigent woman for the cost of childbirth but not for the cost of an abortion.[137]

Then, in *City of Akron v. Akron Center for Reproductive Health, Inc.,*[138] the Court—despite the urgings of the U.S. solicitor general to relax standards of review—reaffirmed its *Roe v. Wade* analysis of strictly scrutinizing abortion regulations in order to protect the fundamental right of privacy. In *Akron,* regulations requiring that all second trimester abortions be performed in a hospital were found to be invalid absent evidence that such routine hospitalization was medically necessary. Without a compelling state interest, the regulations were held to unconstitutionally decrease the availability of abortions by substantially increasing the cost. However, under the Reagan and Bush administrations, a partially new U.S. Supreme Court has become increasingly dissatisfied with the rationale of the *Roe v. Wade* opinion on abortion. In *Thornburgh v. American College of Obstetricians and Gynecologists,*[139] after the appointment of two Reagan-appointed justices and shortly before the appointment of a third, the Supreme Court granted review in a case that did not present substantially novel issues but rather was viewed as a chance to review the subject. In a close 5-to-4 decision, the Court struck down the Pennsylvania Abortion Control Act of 1982 and thereby affirmed its previous stance, with the dissent questioning the validity of *Roe v. Wade.*

In 1988, the pro-life administration was successful in pushing through regulations under Section 1008 of Title X of the Public Health Service Act that prohibit the counseling of clients concerning abortion or the referral of any patient to a physician for an abortion, even if requested, by any program receiving federal Title X funds. Further, the regulations require that if such a clinic provides for abortions or abortion counseling or referral from private funding sources, then those services must be financially and physically separate.

In 1991, the U.S. Supreme Court upheld the validity of the regulations in *Rust v. Sullivan.*[140] However, in January 1993, President Clinton, in an executive order, abrogated the so-called "Gag Rule." The restrictions on federal funding of abortions remain.

Webster. In 1989, the Supreme Court ruled on *Webster v. Reproductive Health Services.*[141] In *Webster,* the Court opened the door for greatly increased government regulation and restriction of abortions without actually overturning *Roe, Akron, Thornburgh,* or *Commonwealth.* Following the rationale of *Maher, Poelker,* and *McRae,* the Court upheld the constitutionality of a Missouri statute that, *inter alia,* forbids the use of state employees and of state facilities to perform or assist in any nontherapeutic abortions. Citing *McRae,* and relying on *Roe*'s philosophy that the states are free to make value judgments favoring childbirth over abortion, the Court reasoned that "the State's decision here to use public facilities and staff to encourage childbirth over abortion places no governmental obstacle in the path of a woman who chooses to terminate her pregnancy"; rather, "Missouri's refusal to allow public employees to perform abortions in public hospitals leaves a pregnant woman with the same choices as if the State had chosen not to operate any public hospitals at all." The Court declined to reassess the validity of *Roe* on the additional grounds that the Missouri statute was not a criminal statute forbidding all abortions. Unlike *Akron,* the Missouri statute was found to cause an insignificant increase in the cost of an abortion; furthermore, the statute did not contain any of the same flaws as the statute in *Thornburgh.*

The *Webster* decision upheld or declined to invalidate the Missouri statute on three further points. First, the statute's "pro-life" preamble was not addressed, on the grounds that the preamble did not regulate abortion. Second, the statute's determination-of-viability requirements, which create a presumption of viability at 20 weeks, which the physician must rebut, were upheld on the grounds that the provision can be interpreted, under the *Roe* analysis, as a constitutionally permissible exercise of state regulation concerning its compelling interest in protecting the life of a viable fetus. Finally, Missouri's prohibition of the use of public funds to counsel or refer women with respect to abortion was seen as a moot question by a unanimous Court, in view of the parties' agreement that the statute had been interpreted only to apply to state fiscal officers making budget decisions and had not been applied to the actions of individual health professionals, who were left free to counsel and refer.

Prior to *Webster,* the U.S. Supreme Court and lower federal courts disallowed a number of state and local statutory requirements that impermissibly restricted access to abortion: requirements for establishing a waiting period between the time of counseling and the performance of the abortion; the requirement that a physician must provide lengthy and detailed information specified by an ordinance; restrictive zoning ordinances[142] and building permits[143]; and requirements that fetal remains be disposed of in a humane and sanitary manner.[144] They have allowed requirements of the presence of a second physician during postviability abortions; requirements that physicians performing abortions maintain surgical privileges at an appropriate hospital[145]; and licensing criteria of medical facilities in

which abortions are performed that include licensure of outpatient facilities and that are consistent with accepted medical practice.[146] However, more recently the Supreme Court has upheld state statutes involving "pre-abortion" issues. In 1992 the Court decided *Planned Parenthood v. Casey.*[147] In *Casey* the court allowed the following issues to stand: state-required pre-abortion counseling, a wait of 24 hours prior to obtaining the abortion, parental or judicial consent for a minor, and state-required statistical reporting to public authorities.

Abortion and minors. Women under 21 years old account for a significant portion of all abortions in the United States.[148] In several opinions, the Supreme Court cautioned that minors might not have rights equal to those of adults.[149] The rationale for a more restrictive view of minors' rights is based on the states' more compelling interest in protecting the minors from their own uninformed or less-than-mature choices. Although no federal court has allowed parental consent or notice as a prerequisite to access to *contraceptives* by an unemancipated minor, the U.S. Supreme Court has, with increasingly well-defined restrictions, approved state parental notification and consent requirements for abortion.

The Court has not said that the failure to provide bypass alternatives in every instance is an undue burden.[150] These statutes can pose a significant hindrance to unemancipated minors who seek abortions, especially in rural areas, and so must be carefully and narrowly crafted to withstand strict judicial scrutiny. The Supreme Court has held that, for such a statute to be upheld, it "also must provide an alternative procedure whereby authorization for the abortion can be obtained."[151] Such a bypass mechanism provides that the minor's parent does not necessarily have a "right" to veto the abortion, and is most likely to be applied when, for example, (1) the minor is shown to be mature enough to give valid consent for the procedure; (2) when notification of the minor's parent or parents is shown to be in conflict with the minor's best interests, as in the case of the parents' abuse of the minor; or (3) despite the incapacity of the minor to give valid consent, the abortion is shown to be in the minor's best interests. Bypass procedures must also afford expedited appeals processes and ensure confidentiality throughout the process. A parental involvement statute must also have acceptable provisions concerning the burden of proof, waiting periods, and determination of court-appointed counsel.[152]

The practical differences between a statute requiring "consent" of a parent and a statute requiring "notice" to a parent are often insignificant. By requiring only that a minor notify a parent before receiving an abortion, a statute clearly does not give the parent veto power; however, parents may possess veto power independent of the existence of the statute because of their parental control over the minor. The same requirements generally apply to each type of parental involvement statute. The Council on Ethical and Judicial Affairs of the American Medical Association concluded that minors seeking abortions should not be required to involve their parents before the procedure.[153]

Paternity suits

Paternity suits are civil proceedings to establish paternity, usually for the purposes of child support, and have become significantly more common owing to the increased number of applicable situations and changes in policy considerations. Despite a declining birthrate, the percentage of illegitimate births in the United States has been accelerating; births out-of-wedlock account for 17% of all live births in the United States, and in some urban areas exceed 50%.[154] The Supreme Court, in a series of decisions since 1968, has declared unconstitutional laws that discriminate against illegitimate children, reversing the traditional common law view that an illegitimate child had no father.[155] Since 1975 federal law requires each state to develop guidelines for the determination of paternity and enforcement of child support and requires them to pay for the defense of indigents.[156] Nonetheless, only a very few of the many illegitimate children now achieve legal relationships with their fathers or receive child support.

Current paternity testing usually involves testing of red blood cell antigens (Landsteiner blood groupings) and often white blood cell antigens (histocompatibility leucocyte antigens, HLA), and may include isotype analysis of blood plasma proteins, such as haptoglobin. The standard six red cell antigen systems (ABO, Rh, MNSs, Kell, Duffy, Kidd) will exclude paternity of a falsely accused man in approximately 70% of the cases and, with the addition of HLA testing, will exclude 96% of the cases. Terasaki, analyzing 1000 disputed paternity cases where exclusion was not established by ABO blood typing, found that one-fourth of the cases were excluded by HLA testing and 80% of the remaining cases had a greater than 90% probability of paternity.[157] A new method of paternity testing that may replace current techniques is restriction fragment length polymorphism (RFLP) testing. It has the potential to be far more powerful because it is a direct reflection of differences in DNA sequences. Although more difficult and costly to perform, it is already being used in some centers. Most laboratories report approximately one-fourth of all alleged fathers will turn out to be excluded, that is, falsely accused.

Testing relies on the application of Mendelian genetic principles to genetic polymorphisms. A putative father can be "proved" not to be the true biological father (excluded) but can never be "proved" to be the true biological father, although the chances of paternity can be shown to be quite high (i.e., only one in one million individuals would have the same phenotype).

The appearance of a phenotypic character in the child not present in the putative parents is a first-order exclusion and can only rarely be negated by the presence of a suppressor gene, earlier enzymatic defect, chimerism, or mutation. The absence of a phenotypic character in the child, which should appear in the offspring of the putative parents, is a second-order exclusion, and is less convincing than a first-order exclusion. It can be negated by the action of a silent gene, by the presence of an unidentified allele, or by chimerism. Results are generally so clearly polarized for or against paternity that some district attorneys, after there has been an admission of sexual relations, have stipulated dismissal upon a finding of exclusion or an agreement of an admission of paternity where the results indicate a 90% or better probability of such.

Paternity suits are civil actions requiring proof by a preponderance of the evidence. The evidentiary laws on the admissibility of blood testing to determine paternity are of two types: inclusionary or exclusionary. Traditionally state laws have been exclusionary, in which they allow the admission of blood test results only when they conclusively exclude an accused man as the father. When paternity testing evidence is inadmissible, the courtroom proceeding focuses on the unsubstantiated allegation of the mother that a man is the father against his assertion that he is not.

Approximately half of the states have statutorily departed from admitting only exclusionary testing and have created an inclusionary rule that allows the admission of any serological tests, even when they indicate only a statistical likelihood of paternity. In many states this has been accomplished by the adoption of model legislation proposed by the Commission on Uniform State Laws: the Uniform Act on Blood Tests to Determine Paternity (1975), the Uniform Act on Paternity (1960), and the Uniform Parentage Act (1973). Additionally, case law in some states has created a judicial adoption of the inclusionary rule, often overcoming exclusionary status. In *Cramer v. Morrison*[158] the court found that the HLA test results were admissible as possible proof of paternity despite a statute that seemed to allow only exclusionary blood tests. The court reasoned that HLA testing is not the "blood test" contemplated by the statute; rather, the drafters had in mind the Landsteiner blood grouping tests available at the time the law was enacted.

Evidence of biological paternity is not necessarily

controlling. In the *Matter of the Marriage of Hodge and Hodge*,[159] the court determined the child's interests to be best served by the awarding of custody to the husband, who had been the primary parent. The wife's appeal was based on blood tests that excluded his paternity. This proof—that the husband was not the biological father—was irrelevant given the statutory presumption of legitimacy of a child born within wedlock. Many states would hold otherwise.

The constitutionality of a state statute that refuses men the opportunity, in some situations, to prove their paternity, has been upheld by the U.S. Supreme Court. In *Michael H. and Victoria D. v. Gerald D.*,[160] the Court explained that the state statute, which allowed only a husband or wife to dispute a husband's paternity, did not deny a putative father's due process rights, because the purpose of the statute was not to identify the true biological father of the child, but to support "overriding social policy that the husband should be held responsible for the child and that the integrity and privacy of the family unit should not be impugned."

Although the awarding of primary custody to fathers has become much more common in the past few decades, "paternity rights" have far to go before reaching the level of constitutional protection that is afforded maternity-related rights, such as the right to abortion. To date, the right to choose to end a pregnancy within statutory limits has been deemed to be exclusively that of the mother whose body is directly affected by the decision, despite a number of attempts by fathers to prevent the abortion.[161] The U.S. Supreme Court denied review of states' appellate court opinions, which state that a putative father may not prevent a pregnant woman from aborting his child.[162]

Recently, many state paternity statutes have been put to new uses that were not contemplated by the drafting legislators. Statutory presumptions that a man is the legal father of a child who is born during his marriage to the mother and artificial insemination statutes that provide for the legal paternity of a husband who consents to the insemination of his wife using the semen of a third-party donor can produce unexpected or untoward results when applied to surrogacy arrangements involving a married surrogate. For example, in an effort to obviate the state's automatic presumption of the husband's paternity in the New Jersey *Baby M* case, the contract between the Whiteheads and the Sterns required both the surrogate's husband's consent to the surrogacy arrangement and his explicit, written denial of consent to the insemination.[163]

Pregnancy discrimination

The U.S. Civil Rights Act of 1964 was amended by the Pregnancy Discrimination Act (PDA) to prohibit discrimination on the basis of pregnancy. This act was passed in response to the U.S. Supreme Court decision in *Gilbert v. General Electric Company*,[164] which held that employment disability insurance programs that excluded coverage of pregnancy and disability did not discriminate on the basis of sex and thus did not violate Title VII. Congress heard testimony on extensive discrimination against pregnant women and intended the PDA to provide relief for working women. In *California Savings and Loan Association v. Guerra*,[165] the court considered the case of Lillian Garland, who had taken pregnancy disability leave in 1982 but was not reinstated afterward because her position as a receptionist had been filled during her absence. The trial court held that the California employers were subject to reverse discrimination by the application of the state law requiring an employer to provide leave and reinstatement to a pregnant employee. The U.S. Supreme Court then held that the California statute was consistent with the PDA.

The final word as to whether employers could discriminate against pregnant women on the basis of fetal concerns was given by the U.S. Supreme Court in *International Union v. Johnson Controls*.[166] The "fetal protection policy" of Johnson Controls was found to be in direct violation of the PDA. Pregnant women may be discriminated against only if the pregnancy affected their ability to do their job. If pregnancy would affect the essence of the business then the employer could use "nonpregnancy" as a qualification.

"Wrongful conception" or "wrongful pregnancy"

Actions by parents against physicians for negligent contribution to unplanned pregnancies are termed "wrongful conception" or "wrongful pregnancy" cases. The injury in these specialized malpractice cases is the unplanned pregnancy, usually followed by the birth of a normal, healthy baby. The plaintiffs generally attempt to prove that the unplanned pregnancy is due to the negligence of the physician. There are primarily four situations that result in wrongful pregnancy cases: (1) a failed sterilization or failure to ascertain the success of a sterilization operation, (2) the ineffective prescription of contraceptives or counseling on contraception, (3) the failure to diagnose pregnancy in time for an elective abortion, and (4) an unsuccessful abortion.

Failure of sterilization procedures is the most common basis for a wrongful pregnancy action. It is well known that a certain small number of tubal ligations and vasectomy procedures will become recanalized and result in regained fertility. In the case of tubal ligation, the presence of fallopian tissue on histological sections as well as the length of the specimen taken will be important. Patients should normally be informed of alternative treatments. In the case of vasectomy, standard practice generally requires the use of contraception until the establishment of two aspermic postvasectomy specimens. The patient's noncompliance is often the reason for failure to obtain the specimens, but a physician may have the duty to warn the patient of the consequences of his noncompliance.

Initially, these cases met with little success.[167] The birth of a healthy baby was not considered to be a legal injury. As a matter of public policy, life was preferred over nonlife. Furthermore, the courts alluded to the inability to assess damages for the birth of a child. The first successful wrongful pregnancy case was the California case, *Custodio v. Bauer.*[168] This suit was brought by a woman who became pregnant soon after she underwent a tubal ligation. The award was considered the logical extension of a malpractice action; to deny the claim would be to allow the injury from a physician's negligent act to go uncompensated.

Wrongful pregnancy cases have also been brought under contract and warranty theories, based on declarations by the physician that the sterilization was irreversible, that the patient would have no more children, or that the sterilization was successful. In most cases these nonnegligence claims have been rejected, because the courts are reluctant to find such warranties without separate contracts for consideration other than the usual physician fees.[169]

Other wrongful pregnancy cases have been brought with some success under theories of informed consent based on the physician's failure to inform the patient that the sterilization procedure might not be successful. In *Sard v. Hardy,* a physician performed a cesarean section for the delivery of the plaintiff's third child and also a bilateral tubal ligation.[170] The patient and her husband were assured by the physician that she could not become pregnant again, although the Madlener technique used was associated with an unusually high failure rate. Two years later, after the patient again became pregnant, she successfully sued despite the signing of a consent form, alleging that the physician negligently failed to inform her that the procedure might not result in permanent sterility as intended and alleging that she was not informed of alternative sterilization procedures.

Surveys of state laws and court decisions recognizing or disallowing wrongful pregnancy actions are impeded by the fact that the "wrongful pregnancy" and "wrongful conception" labels have been used as synonyms for "wrongful birth" and "wrongful life" actions, which have since acquired distinct and separate meanings (see the section titled Birth-Related Issues). The vast majority of courts that have considered wrongful conception cases have viewed the case as being indistinguishable from an ordinary medical malpractice action where the plaintiff alleges a breach of duty on the part of a physician and resulting injury for failure to perform that duty. Although the cause of action now seems well established, the issue of damages is less well resolved. The first cases

allowing any recovery held that all prenatal and postnatal expenses related to the child's birth and all reasonable costs of support until the age of majority were recoverable, consistent with tort law that holds a wrongdoer liable for foreseeable injury resulting from his or her negligent act.[171] Such damages were a windfall to the parents and out of proportion to the defendant's negligence. Courts then began allowing the joy and pleasure of a child to mitigate these damages. In this so-called benefits rule, the jury must assess damages by offsetting the childbearing expenses against the tangible and the intangible benefits of having a child. The majority rule is to allow recovery for the pregnancy and the birth but not for the costs of rearing the child. This holding was first used in *Terrell v. Garcia* and is best articulated in *Cockrum v. Baumgartner.*[172] Justifications for rulings on this issue have included public policy, assessability of damages, lack of proximity to the cause, pure economic loss not suitable to tort law, and that the benefits outweigh the costs as a matter of law. In *Marciniak v. Lundborg,*[173] the Court of Appeals of Wisconsin barred recovery on the public policy grounds that allowance of recovery would "enter a field that has no sensible or just stopping point." Usually courts require plaintiffs to minimize their losses, but courts have been uniformly unwilling to require parents to abort a pregnancy or place the child for adoption to mitigate damages.[174]

In the unusual case in which a child is both conceived as a result of a physician's negligence and also born with a congenital deformity, disease, or mental impairment, then virtually all courts allow for the special costs pertinent to raising a handicapped child. Some courts in the past have allowed financial support to extend, not just until majority, but for the lifetime of the child. In these cases, both "wrongful pregnancy" and "wrongful birth/life" causes of action and related measurement of damages might be appropriate.

BIRTH-RELATED ISSUES
Wrongful birth

Claims of liability have been made for negligence that results in a defective child being born when that child is unwanted solely because of the defect. In such a claim, referred to as a "wrongful birth" claim, the negligence of the physician does not cause the defect itself. Rather, a physician may be liable when the defect is foreseeable or discoverable, and the physician fails to foresee or test for the defect. The plaintiff parents argue that they would have prevented the birth of the child, through the use of contraception or abortion, had they been properly informed and counseled.

When a child is born with a congenital defect, such as a hereditary disease or a physical or mental handicap, the physician might be found liable for wrongful birth for these reasons: failure to take a genetic history or otherwise screen for genetic disease, failure to correctly inform the parents of their chances of producing defective offspring, failure to recognize a genetic disease or teratogenic risk and so inform the parents of the possible consequences, failure to perform prenatal testing when indicated, failure to properly perform the testing or interpret the results, failure to inform the parents of possible prenatal testing or recommended amniocentesis, or failure to perform an abortion or refer to a willing physician.

The history of wrongful birth actions is parallel to but less well developed than that of wrongful pregnancy. The earliest cases were brought alleging illegitimacy as a compensable defect, but courts always rejected this as the basis for a claim.[175] The first cases involving an impaired infant were rejected based on the public policy preferring life over nonlife and the inability to assess damages.[176] Courts were also reluctant to find in the physician a duty to advise the parents of all possible genetic defects. Furthermore, they felt that the judicial proceedings themselves would engender a perception of the child as being unwanted and create a negative stigma in the child's mind.

The first successful case of recovery for wrongful birth was in the Texas case, *Jacobs v. Theimer.*[177] This case was brought by a woman who had contracted rubella during pregnancy and gave birth to a deformed child. The court found negligence in the physician's failure to warn of the potential harm of rubella to a fetus. Since the *Theimer* decision, wrongful birth claims have ultimately been recognized by every court that has considered the issue.

Most suits in the 1960s and 1970s resulted from inadequate counseling based on maternal risk factors, such as advanced maternal age, ethnic factors, or rubella exposure. Subsequent cases have focused on failure to recognize a genetic defect in the parent or older sibling.[178] Many cases involve naive or false reassurances offered by physicians to mothers that minimized the possible effects of a drug, illness, or disease on the pregnancy. The defense has largely centered on the facts of the case and, in particular, that (1) the parents failed to disclose all relevant facts that might have indicated the genetic predisposition or fetal risk, and (2) the mother would have given birth to the child anyway, especially if the defect is first discoverable after abortion is no longer an option.[179] Wrongful birth has been limited to legal actions against health care providers as opposed to employers.[180]

The doctrinal turning point allowing general acceptance of wrongful birth suits came in the *Roe v. Wade* decision, making clear that there was no public policy prohibiting abortions.[181] The *Roe* decision made clear that states were free to adopt policies preferring childbirth to abortion. Many states have passed or considered legislation prohibiting wrongful birth suits because it is feared that the wrongful birth cause of action will force physicians to identify defective fetuses and promote abortions. Dictum in the *Webster* case[182] indicated that such policies and legislation would be upheld as long as the state did not thereby create any affirmative barriers for a woman who is seeking an abortion. In *Hickman v. Group Health Plan, Inc.,*[183] the Minnesota Supreme Court in a 4-to-3 decision held that the state statute that prohibited the maintenance of an action for damages based on a wrongful birth theory does not contravene the right of a pregnant woman to choose an abortion. The court found no state action and no interference with the right to an abortion.

The controversy over damages in wrongful pregnancy cases extends to cases of wrongful births. The basis of the recoverable damages is similar except that, in the case of the "wrongful birth" of a defective child, unlike the case of a wrongful pregnancy, the parents want a baby and intend to support it, making recovery for ordinary childbearing expenses inappropriate. As in those unusual wrongful pregnancy suits that involve handicapped children, most courts have allowed the parents to recover the special costs of medical care and training of a handicapped child, often beyond majority.[184] Courts are also divided on whether a parent may recover for the emotional suffering of bearing a defective child. Some courts have allowed compensation for the parents' pain and suffering.[185]

Wrongful life

The main difference between a "wrongful birth" and a "wrongful life" claim is the identity of the plaintiff. Unlike a wrongful birth suit, in which the plaintiffs are the parents of the disabled child, a suit claiming wrongful life is brought by or on behalf of the disabled child, based on theories of physician negligence similar to the negligent actions alleged in wrongful birth cases. Essentially, the child argues that he or she should never have been born—that nonexistence is preferable to the life of an individual so handicapped by a congenital disability. These cases are in many ways quite similar to the "right to die" cases.

Only a small number of states recognize wrongful life as a valid cause of action. In most states, an inability to assess damages is perceived to exist as the result of an inability to place a value on nonlife, so that the various values of life and nonlife cannot be compared and contrasted. Furthermore, public policy generally favoring life over death is a barrier to wrongful life actions in many states. Overall, wrongful life has been an unpopular jurisprudential notion explicitly rejected in the majority of states that have considered it. Several states have passed legislation prohibiting wrongful life suits.

At the same time, there has been a clear precedential trend toward liberalizing recovery by infants for prenatal injuries. Quality of life issues (e.g., that death might be viewed as better than a lifetime of pain and suffering) continue to pervade the more traditional life and death decisions. In contrast to wrongful life cases, wrongful birth cases arising from virtually the same circumstances as wrongful life claims are now well accepted and courts do not have undue trouble assessing wrongful birth damages. Furthermore, fairness would dictate that awards be given to the child; by giving the award to the child, the judgment can be structured to ensure that he or she is benefitted, and that the money is not spent by the parents for their own gain. Like "wrongful conception/pregnancy" and "wrongful birth" actions, a survey of the acceptance of the wrongful life theory is hindered by conflicting or ambiguous application of those labels in a plethora of cases and attendant factual situations. Selecting appropriate causes of action may be challenging in complicated fact scenarios. Wrongful pregnancy, wrongful birth, wrongful life, and other related causes of action may all exist in the not-unthinkable hypothetical situation in which an unsuccessful sterilization procedure results in an unwanted pregnancy (wrongful pregnancy), the doctor is responsible for causing disabilities in the child because of the prescription of teratogenic medications prior to the diagnosis of pregnancy (standard obstetric malpractice), and then the parents are deprived of their right to choose to end the pregnancy when the physician fails to diagnose the pregnancy in a timely manner, or fails to perform prenatal tests that would have identified the child's disabilities (wrongful birth), which subjects the child to an unwanted existence (wrongful life).

PERIPARTUM ISSUES
Brain-damaged babies

Brain-damaged children are a frequent source of litigation arising from alleged negligence in perinatal care. The plaintiff attempts to show that an obstetrician's negligence, such as failure to monitor the fetus adequately or failure to perform a cesarean section when indicated, resulted in perinatal hypoxia that led to the damaged brain.

Current studies indicate that it is usually impossible to isolate a single cause of brain dysfunction in any given newborn. The conclusions of an NIH task force on causes of mental retardation (MR) and cerebral palsy (CP) indicate that the main causes of severe mental retardation are genetic, biochemical, viral, and developmental, but not birth trauma.[186] Severe MR is possibly associated with asphyxia only when accompanied by CP. Likewise, epilepsy is not thought to be related to birth

trauma unless accompanied by CP. Cerebral palsy is associated with perinatal asphyxia as well as other, often concurrent, conditions—such as prematurity or intra-uterine growth retardation. However, this association of CP to hypoxia is not strong, because most hypoxic newborns do not develop CP and most children with CP did not have documented perinatal hypoxia.

A recent review article gives the incidence of moderately severe or severe cerebral palsy as 1.5 to 2.5 per 1000 live births.[187] Periventricular leukomalacia was found to be a precursor of CP. Risk factors for CP were classified into three groups: factors occurring prior to pregnancy, such as a history of fetal wastage; factors occurring during pregnancy, i.e., poor fetal growth; and factors occurring in the perinatal period such as newborn encephalopathy. The review concluded that CP in term infants appears to be related to phenomena that preceded labor.

To arm themselves against future possible obstetric malpractice suits, many physicians are routinely obtaining cord gases at birth and ordering pathological examination of the placenta for all deliveries. Cord gases are valuable in determining whether the fetus was hypoxic or asphyxiated at birth. The cord gas values give a more objective assessment of the acid-base status than do the subjective Apgar scores. Placental examination may allow the determination of antenatal events such as infectious or inflammatory causes, which might have damaged the fetus's neurological system prior to labor and delivery.[188,189]

Litigation. The most common causes for litigation subsequent to the delivery of a "brain-damaged" baby are the following: (1) failure to perform a cesarean section in a timely manner, (2) failure to monitor fetal heart tones or to respond to monitored indicators of distress, (3) unavailability of the obstetrician, and (4) improper use of oxytocin (Pitocin). Rightly or wrongly, in screening cases, many attorneys use the presence of meconium staining as an indicator of culpability by the delivering physician. Other cases revolve around inadequate resuscitation of the newborn, improper anesthesia, and inappropriate evaluation of an ultrasound (particularly by obstetricians in their offices without proper training). Inadequate genetic counseling accounts for a relatively small but substantial and growing number of cases and is expected to become one of the most important areas of litigation (see section titled Wrongful Birth, *supra*).

Ironically, although most suits allege failure to perform or delay in performing a cesarean section, the cesarean rate in the United States far exceeds that of any other country and many claim it is excessive. Some claim the excess is a response to the obstetrical malpractice litigation. A few suits have been filed alleging that a cesarean section in a given case was unnecessary and performed for the obstetrician's convenience and pocketbook. Despite the current high rate of cesarean sections, there has been no fall in CP rates.

Trust funds. To ensure the availability of physicians to deliver babies, to stem the rising cost of obstetrical malpractice insurance premiums, and to more efficiently pay for the care of neurologically impaired newborns, the Virginia legislature in 1987 passed the Birth-Related Neurological Injury Compensation Act, popularly known as the "Bad Baby Bill."[190] The legislature established a workers' compensation-like no-fault program in which a neurologically damaged newborn requiring lifelong treatment and care would be accordingly compensated, if deemed appropriate by an administrative panel. The request and award would preclude a lawsuit against the obstetrician; however, the case would automatically trigger review by the state licensing board. Funding for the program would come from annual fees assessed against obstetricians, other physicians, hospitals, and insurance carriers. More recently, the U.S. Congress and Florida have modeled legislation based on this Virginia plan.

Florida has created a no-fault pool to provide unlimited lifetime medical expenses and limited wage loss replacement for infants who suffered serious birth-related neurological injuries as a result of a physician's negligence. The measure was modeled on the Virginia program. The plan would care for an estimated 60 babies each year and could cost more than $40 million. Florida's physicians would pay about half of it in 1989, and a state insurance fund would pay the rest. Obstetricians who sign up for the plan face a minimum annual fee of $5000; other doctors would pay at least $250, and private hospitals would pay at least $50 per birth. If the cost of the program exceeds the proposed fees, leaders say they will raise the fees.

Court-ordered obstetrical interventions. Medical advances in obstetricians' ability to monitor prepartum fetal conditions and increased knowledge about the effects of maternal behavior on infant health have provided new temptations of intervention for physicians and judges who perceive some preventable risk to an unborn child. One of the first cases involving court-ordered obstetrical intervention was *In re A.C.*[191] Although the court initially ordered a cesarean section on the dying mother in order to save the fetus, it eventually reversed itself afterward.

More recently in *Baby Boy Doe v. Mother Doe,*[192] the U.S. Supreme court refused to order a lower Illinois court to convene an emergency hearing on whether to order an emergency cesarean section. The mother refused on religious grounds to undergo the procedure. The ACOG and the ACLU, among others, have issued statements opposing court-ordered treatment for pregnant women on grounds of maternal rights, medical uncertainty, and the irregularity of the judicial proceedings involved.[193] In a *New England Journal of Medicine* article, Kolder reported the results of a national survey of the scope and circumstances of obstetrical procedures ordered by the court in the interest of fetuses over the objections of pregnant women in 21 cases during a five-year period.[194] Cesarean sections constituted the bulk (15) of the judicially mandated procedures, but hospital detentions and transfusions were also ordered. Court orders for cesarean sections had been obtained in 11 states and among the 21 cases in which court orders were sought, orders were obtained in 86%. One commentator has concluded that court-ordered intervention is ethical provided that it poses insignificant or no health risks to the woman or would promote her interests in life or health and there are compelling reasons to override her autonomy.[195]

END NOTES

1. National Sickle Cell Anemia Control Act, 86 Stat. 136 (1972).
2. *See* Reilly: *Genetics, Law, and Social Policy,* 50-52 (Harvard University Press, Cambridge 1977); *see also State Laws and Regulations Governing Newborn Screening* (Andrews, compiler, American Bar Foundation, Chicago 1985).
3. *See* Jecker, *Genetic Testimony and the Social Responsibility of Private Health Insurance Companies,* 21 J. L. Med. & Ethics 109-116 (1993).
4. *Monusco v. Postle,* 437 N.W.2d 367 (1989).
5. *Jacobs v. Theimer,* 519 S.W.2d 846 (Tex. 1975).
6. *Harbeson v. Parke-Davis,* 656 P.2d 483 (1983), 746 F.2d 517 (1984).
7. *Speck v. Finegold,* 439 A.2d 110 (1981).
8. *Brubaker v. Cavenaugh,* 542 F. Supp. 944 (1982).
9. *Moores v. Lucas,* 405 S.2d 1022 (1981).
10. *Schroeder v. Perkel,* 432 A.2d 834 (1981).
11. *Park v. Chessin,* 400 N.Y.S.2d 204 (1976), 440 N.Y.S.2d 110 (1977).
12. *Turpin v. Sortini,* 174 Cal. Rptr. 128 (1981), 643 P.2d 954 (1982).
13. *Curlender v. Bioscience Laboratories,* 165 Cal. Rptr. 477 (1980).
14. *Mellis v. Chicago Memorial Hosp.,* No. 70L-15177 (Ill Cir. Ct. Cook County, June 18, 1974).
15. *Nelson v. Krusen,* 635 S.W.2d 582 (1982).
16. *Lininger v. Eisenbaum,* 764 P.2d 1202 (Colo. 1988).
17. *Call v. Kezirian,* 185 Cal. Rptr. 103, 1982.
18. *Siemieniec v. Lutheran Gen. Hosp.,* 512 N.E.2d 691.
19. American Medical Association, Council on Scientific Affairs, *Genetic Counseling and Prevention of Birth Defects,* 248 JAMA 221-224 (1982).
20. 21 Fam. Plan. Perspect. 188 (1989).
21. *Griswold v. Connecticut,* 381 U.S. 479, 85 S. Ct. 1678 (1965).
22. *Eisenstadt v. Baird,* 405 U.S. 438, 92 S. Ct. 1029 (1972).
23. An act for the suppression of trade in and circulation of obscene literature and articles of immoral use: 17 Stat. Ch. 258 §148 (1873); The Family Planning Services & Population Research Act, Pub. Law No. 91-572 (Title X of the Public Health Services Act).
24. *Gaines v. Preterm-Cleveland, Inc.,* 514 N.E.2d 709 (Ohio, 1988).
25. 20 Fam. Plan. Perspect. 112 (1988).
26. 20 Fam. Plan. Perspect. 262 (1988).
27. 21 Fam. Plan. Perspect. 282 (1989).

28. Title XIX of the Public Health Service Act, 42 U.S.C. 1396a.
29. Title X of the Public Health Service Act, 42 U.S.C. 300 *et seq.*
30. 20 Fam. Plan. Perspect. 288 (1988).
31. Title XX of the Public Health Service Act, 42 U.S.C. 42 C.F.R. 59.5 *et seq.*
32. 21 Fam. Plan. Perspect. 123 (1989).
33. *E.G., Carey v. Population Services Internat'l,* 431 U.S. 678 (1977).
34. *Doe v. Blum,* 729 F.2d 186 (1984).
35. *Bowen v. Kendrick,* 108 S. Ct. 2562 (1988).
36. *Planned Parenthood v. Casey,* 112 S. Ct. 2791 (1992).
37. *MacDonald v. Ortho Pharmaceutical Corp.,* 475 N.E.2d 65 (Mass. 1985).
38. *Klink v. G. D. Searle & Co.,* 614 P.2d 701 (Wash. 1980).
39. *Hamilton v. Hardy,* 549 P.2d 1099 (Colo. 1976).
40. Peterson, *Women Face Birth Control Confusion,* USA Today, Feb. 5, 1986, at A1-2; Katz, *Dalkon Case Floods the Court,* USA Today, April 21, 1981, at A1; Middleton, *I.U.D. Discontinuation Seen as Unlikely to Affect Litigation,* 8 Nat. L. J. 13 (Feb. 17, 1986); *see also* Mintz, *At Any Cost: Corporate Greed, Women and the Dalkon Shield,* (Pantheon, New York 1985).
41. 58 U.S.L.W. 3307, and 21 Fam. Plan. Perspect. 246.
42. 20 Fam. Plan. Perspect. 288, 292 (1988).
43. *Searle Takes Two IUD's off U.S. Market,* Galveston Daily News, Feb. 1, 1986, at B7.
44. *E.g.,* Klitsch, 20 Fam. Plan. Perspect. 19 (1988).
45. *Killebrew v. Johnson,* 404 N.E.2d 1194 (Ind. 1980).
46. *Wells v. Ortho Pharmaceutical Corp.,* 788 F.2d 741 (1986) *writ denied,* 107 S. Ct. 437 (1986).
47. Louik et al., *Maternal Exposure to Spermicides in Relation to Certain Birth Defects,* 317 New Eng. J. Med. 474-78 (1987); Warburton et al., *Lack of Association Between Spermicide Use and Trisomy,* 317 New Eng. J. Med. 478-82 (1987); *also see New Studies Find No Link Between Spermicide Use and Heightened Risk of Congenital Malformations,* 20 Fam. Plan. Perspect. 42 (1988).
48. 20 Fam. Plan. Perspect. 288, 293 (1988).
49. *Id.*
50. 20 Fam. Plan. Perspect. 112, 116 (1988).
51. 20 Fam. Plan. Perspect. 288 (1988).
52. *Hathaway v. Worcester City Hosp.,* 475 F.2d 701 (CCA1 1973); *Padin v. Fordham Hospital,* 392, F. Supp. 447 (D.C. N.Y. 1975).
53. *Sard v. Hardy,* 379 A.2d 1014 (Md. 1977).
54. *Gowan v. Carpenter,* 376 S.E.2d 384.
55. *Wilsman v. Sloneiwicz,* 526 N.E.2d 645.
56. *Dohn v. Lovell,* 370 S.E.2d 789 (1988).
57. *Marshall v. Univ. of Chicago Hospitals and Clinics,* 520 N.E.2d 740 (1987).
58. *Ostergard v. United States,* 677 F. Supp. 1259 (D.C. Ma 1987).
59. Va. Code Ann. §§32-423 to 32-427; W. Va. Code Ann. §§16-11-1 to 16-11-2.
60. Ga. Code Ann. §§84-932, 84-934, 84-935.2; N.C. Gen. Stat. §§90-271.
61. *Ponter v. Ponter,* 342 A.2d 574 (N.J. Super. Ct. 1975).
62. 42 CFR §441.250-441.259 (1985).
63. 22 Cal. Admin. Code §§70707.1-70707.8 [tit 22,51305.1-51305.6 (1980)].
64. *Downs v. Sawtelle,* 574 F.2d 1 (1st Cir. 1978).
65. Reilly, *The Surgical Solution: The Writing of Activist Physicians in the Early Days of Eugenical Sterilization,* 26 Perspect. Biological Med. 637-56 (1983); *e.g.,* Idaho Code Ann. §§66-801 to 66-812, De. Code Ann. §§5701-5705.
66. *Buck v. Bell,* 274 U.S. 200, 47 S. Ct. 584 (1927).
67. Ala. Code Ann. 45 §243 (1958); Ark. Stat. Ann. §59-501 to 502 (1971); §82-301 (1973); Cal. Welfare & Instit. Code Ann. §7254 (1972); Conn. Gen. Stat. Ann. §17-19 (1973); Del. Code Ann. 16 §§5701-5705 (1953); Ga. Code Ann. §84-933 (1971); Idaho Code

Ann. §§39-3901 to 3910 (1961); Iowa Code Ann. §145.1 to 145.22 (1972); Me. Rev. Stat. Ann. 34 §2461-2468 (1965); Mich. Comp. Laws Ann. §§720.301 to 720.310 (1968); Minn. Stat. Ann. §§256.07-256.10 (1971); Miss. Code Ann. §§6957-6964, §41-45-1 to -19 (1972); Mont. Rev. Stat. Ann. §§69-6401 to 6406 (1970); N.C. Gen. Stat. §§35-36 to -56 (1973); N.D. Cent. Code §§25-04.1 to 25-04.1 -08 (1970); Okla. Stat. Ann. 43A §§341-346 (1954); Ore. Rev. Stat. §§436.010 to 436.150 (1973); S.C. Code Ann. §§32-671 to -680 (1968); Utah Code Ann. §§64-10-1 to -14 (1968); Vt. Stat. Ann. 18 §§8701-8704 (1986); Va. Code Ann. §§37.1-156 to -171 (1970); Wash. Rev. Code §9.92.100 (1956); Wis. Stat. Ann. §46.12 (1957).
68. *See, e.g.,* codes for Maine, Montana, North Carolina, and Utah.
69. Statutorily required in Michigan, Oklahoma, and Virginia.
70. *Motes v. Hall City Dept. of Family & Children Services,* 306 S.E.2d 260 (1983); *Matter of Truesdell,* 329 S.S.E.2d 630 (1985).
71. Miss. Code Ann. §41-45-1 to -19 (1972).
72. Courts failing to authorize in absence of statute include, among others, Alabama, *Hudson v. Hudson,* 373 S.2d 310 (1979); Missouri, Interest of MKR 515 S.W.2d 467 (1974); California, *Tulley v. Tulley,* 146 Cal. Rptr. 266 (1978), *cert. denied,* 440 US 967); Wisconsin, *Matter of Guardianship of Eberhardy,* 294 N.W.2d 540 (1980); Connecticut, *Ruby v. Massey,* 452 F. Supp. 361 (1978); Ohio, *Wade v. Bethesda Hosp.,* 337 F. Supp. 671 (1971); and Delaware, *Matter of SCE,* 378 A.2d 144 (1977). Courts authorizing sterilizations in absence of statute include *Stump v. Sparkman,* 436 US 951 (1978); New Jersey, *In re Grady,* 426 A.2d 567 (1981); New York, *In re Sallmaier,* 378 N.Y. A.2d 989 (1976); Pennsylvania, *In re Terwilliger,* 450 A.2d 1376 (1982); Colorado, *In re A.W.,* 637 P.2d 366 (1981); and California, *Conservatorship of Valerie N.,* 219 Cal. Rptr. 387 (1985). *See also* West, *Parens patriae judicial authority to order sterilization of mental incompetents,* 25 J. Legal Med. 523 (1981).
73. *E.g., In re Guardianship of Matejski,* 419 N.W.2d 576 (Iowa 1988).
74. *Sparkman v. McFarlin,* 6601 F.2d 261 (7th Cir. 1979).
75. *E.g., In re Grady,* 426 A.2d 467 (1981).
76. Vol. XV, Nos. 2-3, Am. J. L. & Med. 333, 356 (1989).
77. *Id.,* at 353.
78. *E.g., In re Moe,* 432 N.E.2d 712 (1982).
79. G. S. Letterie and W. F. Fox, *Legal Aspects of Involuntary Sterilization,* 53 Fertility and Sterility: 391-98 (1990).
80. *Pamela P. v. Frank S.,* 449 N.E.2d 713 (1983).
81. *Stephen K. v. Roni L.,* 164 Cal. Rptr. 618 (1980).
82. *Barbara A. v. John G.,* 193 Cal. Rptr. 422 (1983).
83. *C.A.M. v. R.A.W.,* 568 A.2d 556 (1990).
84. 50 Fertility and Sterility 519 (1988).
85. Letters-to-the-Editor, 52 Fertility and Sterility 384 (1989).
86. J. A. Robertson, *Ethical and Legal Issues in Preimplantation Genetic Screening,* 57 Fertility and Sterility 1-11 (1992).
87. Hasting Center Report (Jan./Feb. 1990).
88. Ga. Code §74-101.1 (1964).
89. Holding artificial insemination adulterous, *e.g., Gursky v. Gursky,* N.Y. S.2d 406 (1963); Modern view, *People v. Sorenson,* 437 P.2d 495 (1968).
90. *In re Baby Doe,* 353 S.E.2d 877 (1987).
91. *People v. Sorenson,* 437 P.2d 495 (Cal. 1968).
92. *C.M. v. C.C.,* 377 A.2d 821 (N.J. 1977).
93. *See* Quigley and Andrews, *Human In Vitro Fertilization and the Law,* 42 Fertility and Sterility 348-55, 353 (1984).
94. Uniform Laws Ann. 9A, Model Uniform Parentage Act, 1973. *See* 8 Family Law Quarterly 1 (1974).
95. Howe, *Adoption Practice, Issues, and Laws 1958-1983,* 17 Fam. L. Q. 173-97, 190-91 (1983); *Comment Breaking the Seal: Constitutional and Statutory Approaches to Adult Adoptees' Right to Identify,* 75 Nw. U. L. Rev. 316 (1980).

96. 53 Fertility and Sterility, Suppl. 1.

97. *Id.,* Appendix Z.

98. *Id.,* Appendix B.

99. Thatcher and DeCherney, 4 *Human Reproduction,* Suppl., 11-16 (1989).

100. 45 C.F.R. §46.201 (1981); §46.204(d) (1984).

101. Illinois Abortion Act of 1977.

102. *Id.*

103. *Smith v. Hartigan,* 82 Civ. 4324 (D.C. Ill. 1983).

104. Annas and Elias, *In Vitro Fertilization and Embryo Transfer: Medicological Aspects of a New Technique to Create a Family,* 17 Family Law Quarterly 199 (1983); *see also* Jones et al., *Three Years of In Vitro Fertilization at Norfolk,* 42 Fertility and Sterility 826 (1984).

105. 53 Fertility and Sterility 225 (1990).

106. Winslade, *Surrogate Mothers—Right or Wrong?* 7 J. Med. Ethics 153 (1981).

107. Ikemoto, *Providing Protection for Collaborative, Noncoital Reproduction . . .,* 40 Rutgers L. Rev. 1273, 1277 (1988).

108. *Id.,* at 1274.

109. Robertson, *Procreative Liberty and the Control of Conception, Pregnancy, and Childbirth,* 69 Va. L. Rev. 405 (1983).

110. Ikemoto, *supra* note 107, explaining Karst, *The Freedom of Intimate Association,* 89 Yale L.J. 624 (1980).

111. Office of Technology Assessment Report, *Infertility: Medical and Social Choices* 267 (1988).

112. *Id.,* at 268.

113. *Malahoff v. Stiver;* Newsweek, Feb. 14, 1983, at 76; N.Y. Times, Feb. 6, 1983.

114. Mich. Compiled Laws Secs. 722.853, 722.857, 722, 861.

115. 57 U.S.L.W. 2479 (Feb. 21, 1989).

116. *In re Baby M,* 537 A.2d 1227 (1988).

117. *In re Baby M,* 525 A.2d 1128 (1987).

118. *Sees v. Baber,* 74 N.J. 201 (1977).

119. Annas, *Protecting the Liberty of Pregnant Patients (Editorial),* 316 New Eng. J. Med. 1213-14 (1987).

120. *LJJ v. SAF and BFF,* 781 P.2d 973 (1989).

121. As reported in Sec. 7, Biolaw, U:747.

122. Robertson, Hastings Center Report 7 (Nov./Dec. 1989).

123. *"Australians Reject Bid to Destroy 2 Embryos,"* N.Y. Times, Oct. 24, 1984, at A18; Smith, *Australia's Frozen "Orphan" Embryos: A Medical, Legal, and Ethical Dilemma,* 24 J. Fam. L. 27 (1985-1986).

124. *York v. Jones,* 89-373-N. U.S. Dist. Ct. Eastern District Va., July 11, 1989; 17 Health Law Digest 85.

125. *Davis v. Davis,* No. E-14496 (Sep. 21, 1989); *citing* 2 Lancet 790 (1988).

126. 53 Fertility & Sterility 203 (1990); *citing* 2 Lancet 790 (1988).

127. *Commonwealth v. Cass,* 467 N.E.2d 1324 (Mass. 1984).

128. *State v. Wickstrom,* 405 N.W.2d 1 (Mn A. 1987).

129. *Dietrich v. Northampton,* 138 Mass. 14 (1884).

130. *Bonbrest v. Katz,* 65 F. Supp. 138 (D.C. 1946).

131. *Roe v. Wade,* 410 U.S. 113, 93 S. Ct. 705 (1973).

132. *Cowe by Cowe v. Forum Group, Inc.,* 541 N.E.2d 962 (1989).

133. *Grodin v. Grodin,* 301 N.W.2d 869 (1987).

134. W. Chavkin, *Mandatory Treatment for Drug Use During Pregnancy,* 266 JAMA 1556-61 (1991).

135. *Griswold, supra* note 21.

136. *Dohn, supra* note 56.

137. *Maher v. Roe,* 432 U.S. 464, 97 S. Ct. 2376 (1977); *Poelker v. Doe,* 432 U.S. 519, 97 S. Ct. 2391 (1977); and *Harris v. McRae,* 448 U.S. 297, 100 S. Ct. 2671 (1980).

138. *City of Akron v. Akron Center for Reproductive Health, Inc.,* 462 U.S. 416, 103 S. Ct. 2481 (1983).

139. *Thornburgh v. American College of Obstetricians and Gynecologists,* 471 U.S. 1014 (1986).

140. *Rust v. Sullivan,* 111 S.Ct. 1759 (1991).

141. *Webster v. Reproductive Health Services,* 109 S.Ct. 3040 (1989).

142. *Haskell v. Washington Township,* No. 87-3927, CA 6, 12/20/88.

143. *P.L.S. Partners v. City of Cranston,* 696 F. Supp. 788, D RI (1988).

144. Disallowed waiting period: *Akron Center for Reproductive Health, Inc. v. City of Akron,* 102 S. Ct. 2266 (1982); detailed counseling: *Akron Center for Reproductive Health, Inc. v. City of Akron,* 102 S. Ct. 2266 (1982); and humane disposal: *Akron Center for Reproductive Health, Inc. v. City of Akron,* 102 S. Ct. 2266 (1982).

145. *Women's Health Center of West County v. Webster,* CA 8, No. 88-1663 (Mar. 31, 1989).

146. Parental consent with judicial bypass option: *Belloti v. Baird,* 443 U.S. 622 (1979); performance in licensed facilities including outpatient clinics: *Baird v. Dept. of Public Health,* 599 F.2d 1098 (1979); presence of second physician: *Planned Parenthood v. Ashcroft,* 51 USLW 4783 (June 15, 1983).

147. *Planned Parenthood, supra* note 36.

148. 21 Family Planning Perspectives 85 (1989).

149. *Supra* note 33.

150. *MacDonald, supra* note 37.

151. *Bellotti v. Baird,* 443 U.S. 622 (1989).

152. *E.g., Jacksonville Clergy Consultation Service, Inc. v. Marinez,* 707 F. Supp. 1301 (M.D. Fla. 1989).

153. *Mandatory Prenatal Consent to Abortion,* 269 JAMA 82-86 (1993).

154. Persyn, *A Survey of the Admissibility of Blood Test Results in Paternity Actions in the Fifty States and the District of Columbia,* 8 J. Legis. 301-21, 301 (1981).

155. Page-Bright, *Providing Paternity—Human Leukocyte Antigen Test,* 27 J. Forensic Sci. 135-53 (1982); Joint AMA-ABA Guidelines, *Present Status of Serologic Testing in Problems of Disputed Parentage,* 10 Fam. L. Q. 247-85 (1976).

156. Pub. L. 93-647 (1975).

157. Terasaki, *Resolution by HLA Testing of 1000 Paternity Cases Not Excluded by ABO Testing,* 16 J. Fam. L. 543-57 (1977-78).

158. *Cramer v. Morrison,* 143 Cal. Rptr. 865 (1979).

159. *Matter of the Marriage of Hodge and Hodge,* 713 P.2d 1071 (Ore. 1986).

160. *Michael H. and Victoria D. v. Gerald D.,* No. 87-746, *decided* June 15, 1989; *see* 57 U.S.L.W. 4691.

161. *E.g., Conn v. Conn,* 525 N.E.2d 612 (In App. 1988); *Doe v. Smith,* 108 S. Ct. 2136 (1988).

162. *E.g., Smith v. Doe,* 109 S. Ct. 3264 (1989), 57 U.S.L.W. 3855, as reported by 17 Health L. Dig. 90; *Lewis v. Lewis* and *Myers v. Lewis,* U.S. Sup. Ct. Nos. 88-555 and 88-683, 57 U.S.L.W. 3373.

163. Office of Technology Assessment Report *Infertility: Medical and Social Choices* (1988).

164. *Gilbert v. General Electric Co.,* 429 U.S. 125 (1976).

165. *California Savings and Loan Ass'n. v. Guerra,* 55 L.W. 4077 (1987).

166. *International Union v. Johnson Controls,* 111 S.Ct. 1196 (1991).

167. *Hays v. Hall,* 477 S.W.2d 402, 1972, 488 S.W.2d 412 (1973); *Christiansen v. Thornby,* 255 N.W. 1620 (1934).

168. *Custodio v. Bauer,* 59 Cal. Rptr. 463 (Cal. 1967).

169. *Murray v. Univ. of Pennsylvania Hosp.,* 490 A.2d 839 (1985); and *Szekeres v. Robinson,* 715 P.2d 1076 (1986).

170. *Supra* note 53.

171. *Supra* note 100.

172. *Terrell v. Garcia,* 496 S.W. 124 (Tex. 1973); *Cockrum v. Baumgartner,* 425 N.E.2d 968 (Ill. 1981).

173. *Marciniak v. Lundborg,* 433 N.W.2d 617 (1988).

174. *E.g., Johnson v. Univ. Hospitals of Cleveland,* 540 N.E.2d 1370 (1989).

175. *Zepeda v. Zepeda,* 190 N.E.2d 849 (1963).

176. *Gleitman v. Cosgrove,* 227 A.2d 689 (1967).

177. *Jacobs, supra* note 5.

178. *E.g., Lininger v. Eisenbaum,* 764 P.2d 1202 (Colo. 1988).

179. *Spencer v. Seikerl,* 742 P.2d 1126 (Ok. 1987).

180. *Coley v. Commonwealth Edison Co.,* 703 F. Supp. 748 (ND ILL. 1989).

181. *Supra* note 131.

182. *Webster,* 109 S.Ct. 3040, No. 88-605, *decided* July 3, 1989.

183. *Hickman v. Group Health Plan, Inc.,* 396 N.W.2d 10 (1986).

184. *James G. v. Casserta,* 332 S.E.2d 872 (1985).

185. *Blake v. Cruz,* 698 P.2d 315 (1984); *but see Spock v. Finegold,* 408 A.2d 496 (1979).

186. Freeman, ed., *Prenatal and Perinatal Factors Associated with Brain Disorders,* NIH, Publication No. 85-1149 (Apr. 1985).

187. K. C. K. Kuban and A. Leviton, *Cerebral Palsy,* 330 New Eng. J. Med. 188-95 (1994).

188. K. Benirschke, *The Placenta in the Litigation Process,* 162 Am. J. Obstet. Gynecol. 1445-50 (1990).

189. C. M. Salafia and A. M. Vintzileos, *Why All Placentas Should be Examined by a Pathologist in 1990,* 163 Am. J. Obstet. Gynecol. 1282-93 (1990).

190. Va. Art. 38.2-5000 to 38.2-5021 (1987).

191. *In re A.C.,* No. 87-609 (Apr. 26, 1990); *see also* 58 U.S.L.W. 2644.

192. *Baby Boy Doe v. Mother Doe,* No A-502, U.S. S. Ct., 62 U.S.L.W. 3428 (Dec. 18, 1993).

193. ABA J. 84-88 (Apr. 1989).

194. Kolder, Gallagher, and Parsons, *Court-Ordered Obstetrical Interventions,* 316 New Eng. J. Med. 1192-96 (1987).

195. C. Strong, *Court-Ordered Treatment in Obstetrics: The Ethical Views and Legal Framework,* 78 Obstet. Gynecol. 861-68 (1991).

GENERAL REFERENCES

Borten and Friedman, I, II, *Legal Principles and Practice In Obstetrics and Gynecology* (1989, 1990).

Curran, *Law-Medicine Notes* (1989).

Elias and Annas, *Reproductive Genetics & the Law* (1987).

Institute of Medicine, *Medical Professional Liability and the Delivery of Obstetrical Care* (1989).

Schwartz and Tucker, *Handling Birth Trauma Cases* (1985), updated annually.

Volk and Morgan, *Medical Malpractice: Handling Obstetric and Neonatal Cases* (1986), updated annually.

CHAPTER 32

Children as patients

JOSEPH P. McMENAMIN, M.D., J.D., F.C.L.M.*

GARLAND L. BIGLEY, R.N., J.D.

INFORMED CONSENT

MINORS' RIGHTS

STATE INTERVENTION

STERILIZATION

CONTRACEPTION

ABORTION

INVOLUNTARY CIVIL COMMITMENT OF MINORS

CHILD ABUSE

Although much of the law governing medical care of children is indistinguishable from that governing medical care of adults, certain features of the former are unique. These features arise in large part because minors are seen to need special protection from others and from themselves, and are generally deemed incompetent (except in specific circumstances) to grant valid consent for their own treatment. The law's solicitude for the special needs of minors sometimes gives rise to poignant conflicts between the desires and values of parents — often inviolable in other settings — and those of the child or those of the state as *parens patriae*. Resolution of these conflicts often falls to the courts. In this chapter, some of the legal issues peculiar to the care of children are explored.

INFORMED CONSENT

In general, a doctor is obliged to secure the informed consent of a patient before treatment. That a child is too young and immature to give consent in his or her own right does not relieve the physician from the responsibility to obtain informed consent.

Under the early common law doctrine of medical consent. . . [a] physician was obliged to obtain the consent of the child's parents, guardian, or someone standing in loco parentis, before performing any surgery, administering any medicine, or, for that matter, touching the child's body for an examination. . . . A minor was anyone under twenty-one, and the rule

*The authors gratefully acknowledge work from the previous contributor: William B. Tiller, J.D.

was absolute. . . . There was only one source for the consent for the treatment of a minor — the minor's parent or guardian — and the consent was valid for all purposes so long as no fraud or deception was involved in the physician's description of the treatment.[1]

The parents had the right to give or withhold consent because "the custody, care and nurture of the child reside first in the parents."[2] The basis for the right of parents to grant or withhold consent is that their "liability for support and maintenance of their child may be greatly increased by an unfavorable result from the operational procedures upon the part of a surgeon."[3] The failure to secure such informed consent may render the physician liable to the parents.[4] The parents' power to consent may extend to withdrawal of life-support systems from the child,[5] and in proper circumstances to compelling the child to submit to treatment.[6]

One parent is generally sufficient to furnish consent.[7] A caretaker, however, even an adult sibling temporarily entrusted with care of the child, is generally not empowered to grant consent to treatment.[8] Where, however, a person *in loco parentis*[9] is given a written authorization executed by a parent (as is commonly done for the supervisors of summer camps, for example), he or she may be in a position to consent more broadly to medical care.

Although informed consent is generally governed by state law and each state's law is different, a physician is ordinarily not obliged to disclose risks so improbable that they are not reasonably foreseeable or so minor as to be of no consequence to the patient.[10] The extent of consent granted is a question of fact for the jury.[11] Where a parent lacks mental capacity to consent to an operation on a child, the doctor has in some circumstances been held liable for failing to recognize such incapacity.[12] Whether a physician failed to explain to the mother the material risks of the operation, the risks of not operating, and alternatives, if any, to surgery are jury questions.[13]

A cause of action grounded in a lack of informed consent will not succeed unless the plaintiff can show that, had the consent of the parent been asked, it would not have been freely given.[14] Thus, a "but for" test of causation is imposed and applied objectively rather than subjectively.[15] Where there is evidence that the parents, if consulted, would have declined consent, liability may be found.[16] On the other hand, a parent who has not given consent may tacitly do so retroactively by permitting the child to return for follow-up procedures or by accepting contributions for the child's education from a public responding to press reports describing the procedure and the child's heroism in submitting to it.[17]

Surgery on a minor to benefit another

In the consent context, a particularly thorny issue arises when surgery on a minor is proposed for the benefit of another person. In general, consent will not be inferred without parental permission, as illustrated in the case of *Bonner v. Moran*.[18] There, skin grafting from a 15-year-old boy to his burned cousin, done in 1941 when skin homografting was relatively new and risky, was not permissible without the consent of the parents. The court held that the principal criterion in assessing the adequacy of consent by the minor himself is "whether the proposed operation is for the benefit of the child and is done with a purpose of saving his life or limb."[19] Finding no such benefit or purpose in *Bonner,* the court held that consent was required not only of the boy donor but also of his parents.

Even with parental consent, however, there is considerable disagreement among the courts as to whether surgery may be performed where the minor patient is unable to consent in a fully informed way and the proposed procedure is to benefit another. This controversy is best illustrated by cases in which the parents seek authority to permit surgery on their mentally retarded child to benefit an intellectually normal sibling.

In *In re Richardson*,[20] the court held that neither the child's parents nor the courts could authorize donation of a mentally retarded minor's kidney to his sister because doing so was not in his best interest. The court noted that the transplant was not "an absolute immediate necessity" to preserve the donee's life. The court also concluded that it was highly unlikely that, assuming a successful transplant, the donee would be able to care for the donor after the parents' deaths.[21] The plaintiffs argued that (1) the etiology of the donee's renal failure was systemic lupus erythematosus (SLE) that could not be treated because doing so would conflict with treatment for the donee's coexisting hypertension; (2) if the transplant were done, "drugs used to counteract rejection of the transplanted kidney could also be useful in treating SLE"; and (3) the hypertension might be "alleviated with a successful transplant."[22] None of these arguments was sufficient, however, to dissuade the court from its conclusion that transplantation was not in the best interest of the donor and that it should not be performed despite the wishes of the parents.

Similarly, in *In re Guardianship of Pescinski*,[23] the Supreme Court of Wisconsin held that a county court lacked the power to order a nephrectomy on an incompetent adult schizophrenic or to order transfer of the kidney so harvested to his sister.

Numerous courts have held to the contrary, however. In the case of *Strunk v. Strunk*,[24] an adult with a mental age of 6, an IQ of 35, and a speech defect was allowed to donate a kidney to his mentally normal brother, who was on dialysis and dying of chronic glomerulonephritis. The court concluded that the donor would feel guilty if his brother died and that his brother's survival was necessary for treatment and rehabilitation of the mentally retarded donor at least in part because the brother's parents were both in their fifties.[25] "The court relied on the inherent rule . . . that the chancellor has the power to deal with the estate of the incompetent in the same manner as the incompetent would if he had his faculties."[26] The court concluded that, were the donor possessed of full faculties, he would consent to the operation, and because it believed that a court of equity had the power to permit the natural parent to consent to such surgery, it authorized the kidney transplant.

The court in *Hart v. Brown*[27] permitted the parents of 7-year-old identical twins to consent to a kidney transplant from one twin to the other. The recipient had hemolytic-uremic syndrome and malignant hypertension, and her condition was deemed fatal without transplant. The court found (1) virtually no long-range risk absent significant trauma, (2) the short-range risk to the donor also was negligible, (3) the alternative to transplantation (immunosuppression) was risky, (4) the donor strongly identified with her sister, and (5) she would experience great loss if her sister died. Furthermore, the donor had been informed of the operation and "insofar as she [was] capable of understanding, she desire[d] to donate her kidney so that her sister [could] return to her."[28] Balancing the rights of the parents and the rights of the donor child, the court concluded that "the natural parents [could] substitute their consent for that of their minor children after a close, independent and objective investigation of their motivation and reasoning."[29] In *Hart,* the court found that such investigation had been accomplished by virtue of the partici-pation of (1) a clergyman who testified that the "parents are making a morally sound decision"; (2) the defendant physicians; (3) guardians ad litem for the donor and for the donee; and (4) the court itself."[30] The court went so far as to say that prohibition of consent would be "most unjust, inequitable and injudicious."[31]

Similarly, the Texas court in *Little v. Little*[32] held that the mother of a 14-year-old, mentally incompetent daughter with Down syndrome could consent to trans-planting a kidney from her daughter to her son, who suffered from end-stage renal disease. The proposed nephrectomy would not constitute "medical treatment" for the donor daughter—so as to give the guardian authority to consent under the statute empowering a guardian to consent to medical treatment for the daughter. Nevertheless, although no Texas statute spe-cifically recognized any right of a minor or nonresident medical incompetent to participate as a donor in organ transplantation, the court concluded that the donor would enjoy substantial psychological benefit from participation. The court did not believe that the donor was capable of genuine informed consent, but it found a close relationship between donor and donee, as well as "a genuine concern by each for the welfare of the other, an awareness by [the donor] of the nature of [the donee's] plight and an awareness of the fact that she [was] in a position to ameliorate [the latter's] burden."[33]

Tests of consent

Several doctrines have evolved in cases examining the validity of consent to treatment of a child. The bound-aries between these doctrines are often indistinct. For example, where courts grant a parent permission to consent to surgery on a minor for the benefit of another person, they sometimes use the so-called *substituted judgment* standard.[34] The goal of the doctrine is to leave to the individual, to the greatest possible extent, the right to decide his or her own course. The purpose is to recognize "the free choice and moral dignity of the incompetent person."[35] Nonetheless, some courts have held the substituted judgment test to be of "limited relevance" in cases involving immature minors or those who have always been incompetent because of their inability to articulate an opinion about their own preferences.[36] The substituted judgment test is different from the widely used *best interest of the child* test because, in the latter, the inquiry is "essentially objective in nature, and the decisions are made not by, but on behalf of the child."[37] Nevertheless, "the criteria to be exam-ined and the basic applicable reasoning are the same."[38]

Under the best interest rule, treatment over parental objection can generally be required if one of three criteria can be met: (1) the child would be harmed by withholding the treatment; (2) treatment is appropriate in the substituted judgment of the doctor, that is, the child would have agreed to therapy had he the same knowledge as the physician, who is acting on the same motives and considerations as would have moved the child; and (3) under risk-benefit analysis therapy is indicated.[39]

In some jurisdictions, the courts attempt to *balance the interests* of the parties in deciding whether therapy without parental consent is appropriate. These courts examine some or all of the following: (1) the harm to the child and others from nonintervention, (2) the probabil-ity that the procedure will improve the child's condition, (3) the reasonableness of the parent's choice, (4) the risk of the treatment or procedure, (5) the need for and availability of the cooperation of the child, and (6) the proposed treatment. Among the jurisdictions invoking the interest balancing doctrine, there is some variability in the emphasis placed on each of these factors. There is plainly some degree of overlap between the best interest test and the interest balancing test, each of which was developed independent of the other. Al-though there is clearly tension between these theories and the autonomy and liberty interests of the parents, in those jurisdictions where these tests are applied, a judgment has been made that the state must intervene on behalf of those of its citizens who are unable to seek for themselves treatment that the law deems necessary and appropriate.

Where interest balancing is carried out, it may be done in a best interest context:

[T]he issue of [state ordered therapy over parental objec-tion] places three sets of interest in competition: (1) the "natural rights" of parents; (2) the responsibility of the State; and (3) the personal needs of the child. . . . Courts which have considered the question, after balancing these three interests, uniformly have decided that state intervention is appropriate where the medical treatment sought is necessary to save the child's life.[40]

Exceptions to required parental consent

Several exceptions exist to the basic rule that parental consent is required before medical intervention can be undertaken. The most commonly recognized situations involve emergencies, mature minors, and medical eman-cipation. A fourth exception is sometimes allowed when the parents are unavailable, making it impracticable to obtain consent in time to accomplish proper results, but the distinction between this and emergencies appears somewhat vague.[41] Exceptions to the requirement of parental consent are not applicable where the proposed intervention is done for the benefit of another and involves sacrifice on the part of the minor.[42] Institution-alized minors may be able to consent to an additional period of supervision beyond the age of majority, despite delaying their own liberty, depending on (1) age and level of maturity, (2) whether they have the advice of counsel, (3) their capacity to understand the decision to consent to an extra year of treatment, (4) the existence of guardians ad litem, and (5) the opportunity to confer with their parents.[43] Even unemancipated minors may be permitted to consent to procedures such as blood donations or to diagnosis and treatment for sexually transmitted diseases.[44]

Emergencies. The *emergency exception* may be the best known departure from the standard rule. Courts have often ruled that when a child's health was immediately endangered, the law implied the consent of the parents on the theory that had they known of the situation they would have authorized treatment.[45] Emergencies are variously defined in different jurisdictions. One of the best definitions may be found in an Arkansas statute:

[A] situation wherein, in competent medical judgment, the proposed surgical or medical treatment or procedures are immediately or imminently necessary and any delay occasioned by an attempt to obtain consent would reasonably be expected to jeopardize the life, health, or safety of the person affected or would reasonably be expected to result in disfigurement or impaired faculties. . . .[46]

A defendant invoking the emergency exception must establish it by a preponderance of the evidence.[47]

The rationale for the emergency exception is articulated poignantly in *Luka v. Lowrie:*

Many small children are injured upon the streets in large cities. To hold that a surgeon must wait until perhaps he may be able to secure the consent of the parents before giving to the injured one the benefit of his skill and learning, to the end that life may be preserved, would . . . result in the loss of many lives which might otherwise be saved. It is not to be presumed that competent surgeons will wantonly operate nor that they will fail to obtain the consent of parents to operations where such consent may be reasonably obtained in view of the exigency. Their work is, however, highly humane and very largely charitable in character, and no rule should be announced which would tend in the sufferers of the benefit of their services.[48]

A surgeon need not seek parental consent when threatened with an emergency; in fact, doing so may give rise to accusations of malpractice if seeking such consent would consume time critical to proper management of the case.[49] The emergency exception defense is enhanced when the defendant can show that he or she consulted with other physicians before doing the procedure.[50] This is so because the existence of one or more second opinions confirming the first make it less likely that consent would be withheld.[51]

Injuries need not be life-threatening to be severe enough to justify the emergency exception.[52] Before the exception is recognized, however, an existing emergency, not merely a potential one, may be required.[53]

Mature minors. The second major exception to the general rule requiring parental consent is the *mature minor* rule. Simply stated, a mature minor is one who can appreciate and understand the nature of a proposed procedure and its consequences. Usually, a minor will not be deemed mature until the age of at least 15 years. The likelihood that a health care professional may successfully invoke this exception increases where the proposed procedure is clearly beneficial and uncomplicated, where obtaining parental consent is impracticable, where the risk of harm to the minor is insubstantial, and where the information provided by the physician to the child is sufficiently detailed and couched in language sufficiently simple for the minor to grant consent that may be deemed to be informed.

An example of a mature minor is found in the case of *Younts v. St. Francis Hosp. and School of Nursing.*[54] In *Younts,* an intelligent 17-year-old patient suffered a tuft fracture and skin avulsion of the distal phalanx of her ring finger when a door was accidentally closed on it. Her mother was semiconscious at the time under anesthesia. The patient's father, divorced from her mother, lived some 200 miles away, and his address was neither known nor immediately available. The patient was awake throughout the procedure and aware of what was done. She made no objection to the procedure; the repair was necessary and customary; the result was good; the family's private doctor had been consulted and had consented to the procedure; and the mother conceded that she would have followed the advice of the family doctor had she had it. The court held that the minor was sufficiently mature that the mother's consent was not necessary for the surgery performed.[55] The court wrote that the "sufficiency of a minor's consent depends on his ability to understand and comprehend the nature of the surgical procedure, the risks involved and the probability of attaining the desired results in the light of the circumstances which attend."[56]

Similarly, plastic surgery on the nose of an 18-year-old woman with her consent has been found to be within the scope of the mature minor exception.[57] Likewise, a 17-year-old may be sufficiently mature to consent to smallpox vaccination.[58]

The criteria by which a minor's maturity is judged vary somewhat with the jurisdiction. Among the frequently invoked considerations are marital status, age, education (particularly whether high school has been completed), status as head of family, and financial independence.[59]

Just as a physician should obtain a mature minor's consent before rendering treatment, he or she should similarly obtain a mature minor's consent before withholding life-saving treatment. The Supreme Court of

West Virginia found error where a trial court failed to instruct a jury that it could consider a minor's maturity level in deciding whether a 17½-year-old, suffering from muscular dystrophy and a viral infection, was mature enough to require his consent before placing a "do not resuscitate" order in his chart.[60]

A court may find a minor who seeks medical care to be too immature to give valid consent, of course, thus requiring parental involvement. In *H.B. v. Wilkinson*,[61] the court ruled that a minor seeking an abortion was immature, listing among the criteria it considered the minor's experience, perspective, and judgment. Experience, said the court, related to work, living away from home, and handling of personal finances. Perspective called for appreciation and understanding of the gravity and consequences of abortion. Judgment required full information and the ability to weigh alternatives independently and realistically and was related to freedom from stress. Finding the minor immature, the court made the following observations: (1) there was stress and nervousness in the minor's hesitancy and uncertainty in her demeanor and testimony, (2) the minor had never lived away from home nor been regularly employed, (3) she had relied on advice from other teenagers and had expected to keep secret from her parents any possible complication from the abortion she sought, (4) she had dismissed without due consideration the possibility of postabortion depression, and (5) she had purposefully failed to use contraceptives in the cavalier belief that abortion would be readily available. Accordingly, the court concluded that her doctor was obliged under state law to notify the minor's parents that she was seeking an abortion.

Although a minor is generally permitted to escape from any contract made before reaching the age of majority, in many jurisdictions a minor has traditionally been able to bind others and to be bound by a contract for "necessaries." Where a medical procedure can be deemed covered by the term *necessaries,* this same ability to make a binding contract may be found.[62] In those jurisdictions where the mature minor rule is accepted, it may be invoked to justify a decision not to notify parents of a minor's desired therapy where to notify them would not be in the minor's best interest.[63]

A mature minor may consent to therapy or decline it. A minor as young as 14 may be granted rights by statute that "may not be waived by the parent or guardian."[64] These include a right to refuse confinement for treatment, at least in cases involving mental therapy calling for isolation and confinement.[65] If therapy is refused on religious grounds, the minor's wishes may be honored as long as life is not threatened and contagion is unlikely.[66]

Emancipation. The third exception to the parental consent rule is the *emancipation* exception. This excep-

tion tends to overlap that of the mature minor. A court may deem to be emancipated a minor who is married or economically independent, is abandoned by the parent, maintains a separate home, or is in the military. Statutes may define the age of medical emancipation.[67] Some courts may find emancipation even without a statute:

> A married minor, 18 years of age, who has successfully completed high school and is the head of his own family, who earns his own living and maintains his own home, is emancipated for the purpose of giving a valid consent to surgery if a full disclosure of the ramifications, implications and probable consequences of the surgery has been made by the doctor in terms . . . fully comprehensible to the minor.[68]

Even in those jurisdictions that recognize the mature minor rule, however, a physician who offers to treat a minor who appears to satisfy the law's criteria for maturity should do so only with great caution. A doctor's determination of a child's legal capacity to give consent may be neither authoritative nor binding.[69] "Whether a minor is 'emancipated' is a legal question, ultimately answerable by a court of law. A doctor may, like anyone else, make a reasoned judgment based upon relevant factors, but gives treatment to a minor believed to be emancipated at his own risk."[70] In some jurisdictions, the fear of second-guessing by a jury has been largely obviated by legislation that specifically entitles a doctor to rely in good faith upon a child's assertion of emancipation.[71]

A minor may be "partially emancipated," that is, emancipated for some purposes but not others. In *In Interest of E.G.*,[72] a 17-year-old leukemic was held medically neglected after her parents, Jehovah's Witnesses, refused to consent to a transfusion that was necessary to save her life. Nonetheless, noting that she had studied her religion for several years and had been baptized, which rendered her an adult in the eyes of her church, the Illinois Supreme Court ruled that the trial court should have considered her partially emancipated after finding her neglected, so she could, in the exercise of her First Amendment rights, decline the transfusion in her own behalf.[73]

Remote parents. Finally, parental consent may be unnecessary where the parents are so remote that securing their consent would consume too much time to permit optimal management of the patient's medical problems. Just as the emancipated minor exception overlaps the mature minor exception, the remote parents exception tends to overlap the emergency exception. Sufficient "remoteness" was found where the parents lived only 8 miles away but lacked a phone,[74] where the parent was not to be found at the place of work indicated in school records,[75] and where the mother was anesthetized and the divorced father was at an unknown address 200 miles distant.[76]

Treatment against parental wishes

Under either of two theories, parents have often been held to be obliged to provide medical care for their children. First, there may simply be a statute requiring it.[77] Absent a statute, some courts have held that the right of parents to control the nurturing and upbringing of their children "is in the nature of a trust reposed in them, and is subject to their correlative duty to care for and protect the child; and the law secures their right only so long as they shall discharge their obligation."[78] Whether legal justification for intervention is provided by statute or not, the rationale is clear: "[W]here a child's well-being is placed in issue, it is not the right of parents that are chiefly to be considered. The first and paramount duty is to consult the welfare of the child."[79] Where medication is "as necessary for the child's survival as [is] food," the state may act to preserve the child's life and health.[80]

Religious convictions and treatment of minors

Normally, of course, the state's interest in preserving the health and safety of the children within its jurisdiction coincides with that of the parents. In some circumstances, however, this is not the case. Where conflict between the desires of the parents and the rights of the state arise, the law must choose between the two. Controversies created by religious beliefs are among the most difficult to resolve. Under the First Amendment, of course, Americans are guaranteed the free exercise of religion, and the government is forbidden to take steps to establish any religion. Parents who are entirely sincere in their religious beliefs may invoke the First Amendment in support of attempts to withhold treatment from their children. The courts, however, in a variety of circumstances, have held that parental rights may be subordinate to the state's interest in the care of children. "Parents may be free to become martyrs themselves. But it does not follow that they are free, in identical circumstances, to make martyrs of their children before they have reached the age of full and legal discretion when they can make that choice for themselves."[81] The courts have distinguished two concepts within the First Amendment: the freedom to believe and the freedom to act. "The first is absolute but, in the nature of things, the second cannot be."[82] Among the most notable court decisions where public policy overrode religious practices are cases involving polygamy permitted under the laws of the Church of Jesus Christ of Latter Day Saints[83]; the sale of religious publications by a minor Jehovah's Witness in the belief she was discharging a religious duty[84]; compulsory military instruction at a state university[85]; and use of poisonous snakes in religious ceremonies in accordance with the teachings of the Zion Tabernacle Church.[86]

In the first verdict of its kind, in a 1993 civil suit, a Minnesota jury awarded a boy's biological father and sister $5.2 million in compensatory damages and $9 million in punitive damages for the minor's death attributable to the withholding of medical treatment by the child's mother, stepfather, and various officials of the First Church of Christ, Scientist.[87] The child had died from untreated diabetes while the defendants engaged in Christian Science prayer rather than provide conventional medical treatment.[88] Seven defendants were ordered to share in paying the compensatory damages, which were later reduced to $1.5 million, but only the Christian Science Church was ordered to pay the $9 million in punitive damages.[89]

This is not to suggest that parental rights are invariably subordinated to public policy. A statute requiring parents to send their children between the ages of 8 and 16 years of age to public schools was held unconstitutional because it interfered with the liberty of parents and guardians to direct the upbringing and education of their children.[90] Forbidding the teaching of any but the English language in school violated the guarantees of liberty of the Fourteenth Amendment; the law could not be upheld, absent a sudden emergency rendering knowledge of foreign languages clearly harmful.[91] Finally, compulsory education beyond the eighth grade that would endanger or possibly destroy the free exercise of the religious beliefs of members of the Old Order Amish religion and the Conservative Amish Mennonite Church was held unconstitutional, particularly given the continuing informal and vocational education the Amish provided their children.[92]

MINORS' RIGHTS

Not only do the courts weigh the conflicting interests of the state and of parents, but they also are obliged to consider the interests of the children themselves.[93]

The Supreme Court has written that "constitutional rights do not mature and come into being magically only when one attains the state-defined age of majority."[94] To an extent not fully delineated, it appears that minors may refuse at least highly intrusive interventions made in their behalf despite their parents' approval:

Children, as well as adults, have substantial liberty interests that are protected from state action by the fourteenth amendment. . . . These liberty interests include the right not to be confined unnecessarily for medical treatment. . . . [In common] with this right is the right to be free of unnecessary restrictions of other fundamental rights once confined to a state institution.[95]

This solicitude for the rights of children has also been applied to a "no code" situation where, in the substituted judgment of the court, the minor would have declined resuscitation. In *Custody of a Minor,*[96] an infant with cardiac defects, including pulmonary atresia, a hypoplastic right ventricle, a hypoplastic pulmonary artery, and a patent ductus arteriosus, underwent palliative surgery in the form of a modified Blalock-Taussig shunt. The child developed significant bacterial infection and was put on a ventilator after the shunt failed. Under the relevant statutes, the juvenile court had jurisdiction of the case and the power and means necessary to exercise its jurisdiction. The court held itself able to determine that, under certain circumstances, treatment could be withheld. Distinguishing the case before it from *In re Dinnerstein,*[97] the factors the court reviewed were those previously enumerated in *Matter of Spring*[98]:

(1) The child is a ward of the State in the custody of the [department of social services]; (2) the child's mental faculties have not developed to the point where he is competent to make the decision; (3) the parents have failed to exercise their parental responsibilities toward the child; (4) the child's condition is incurable and the prognosis for successful treatment is negative; (5) medical opinion on diagnosis and prognosis was clear and unanimous as to the child's condition and future; (6) attempts to rescue would be painful and intrusive. We add that the child already was within the jurisdiction of the court before the question whether a "no code" order should be made — and continued — arose. In these circumstances, we think the language of the court in *Spring* is particularly apt: "When a court is properly presented with the legal question, whether treatment may be withheld, it must decide the question and not delegate it to some private person or group."[99]

The court noted that the parties all agreed that a no code order was appropriate but concluded that, although such agreement was "given deference, [it] neither defeats the jurisdiction of the court in a case such as this nor binds it to accept their position."[100] Invoking *Superintendent of Belchertown State School v. Saikewicz,*[101] the court applied the substituted judgment test and concluded that a no code order was appropriate. It wrote:

Contrary to what some of the parties to this case suggest, the issue presented here is not one of "right to life." In a "no code" case, the question is not of life or death but the manner of dying and what "measures are appropriate to ease the imminent passing of an irreversibly, terminally ill patient in light of the patient's history and condition." [citation omitted] While this manner of dying may be "a question peculiarly within the competence of the medical profession," [citation omitted] the possibilities of private decision making present in *Dinnerstein* are not present here.[102]

The court rejected the argument that the burden of proof necessary to sustain a no code order was extremely high:

To require judges in reviewing medical judgments to reach a level of moral certainty . . . not only makes judicial approval of "no code" orders highly unlikely, but would cause those terminally ill patients involved to suffer unnecessary pain and loss of dignity. . . . We refuse to lay down a rule requiring a physician to testify that he . . . has personal knowledge, to a moral certainty, that the ward's future is hopeless. Such a rule would not only be unworkable but hardly realistic. We require no more than the procedure followed by the Juvenile Court judge in this case; the entering of detailed findings, supported by the evidence, "indicating those persuasive factors that determine[d] the outcome." The court concluded that a child capable of understanding the situation would have declined therapy and, hence, the court was justified in authorizing the no code order.[103]

STATE INTERVENTION

The standard of care applicable to parents obliged to provide medical attention for their children is analogous to the standard of care for physicians confronting malpractice actions. As the New York Court of Appeals wrote when constructing a state statute, "[T]he standard is at what time an ordinarily prudent person, solicitous for the welfare of his child and anxious to promote its [sic] recovery, deems it necessary to call in the services of a physician."[104]

In many jurisdictions, statutes permit the state to take custody of a *neglected* or *dependent child,* terms that are variously defined[105] but which have been construed to include a child deprived of medical services by the parents.[106] Examples of such deprivation included the denial of smallpox vaccination viewed by the parents as "harmful and injurious,"[107] refusal to submit to surgery necessary to save the life of a fetus,[108] refusal to permit blood transfusion required for surgery to correct congenital heart disease,[109] and withholding chemotherapy from a child suffering from malignancy.[110] Statutes finding neglect under such circumstances have been upheld against attacks under the freedom of religion clauses of federal and state constitutions and under the due process clause of the U.S. Constitution.[111] However, courts may in such circumstances instruct state authorities to respect the religious beliefs of the parents and to accede as much as possible to their wishes without interfering with the court-ordered medical care.[112]

Although the precise limits of the requirement for the provision of medical care by parents are difficult to set, the Illinois statute construed in *Wallace v. Labrenz*[113] may be fairly typical:

[T]he statute defines a dependent or neglected child as one which [sic] "has not proper parental care." . . . Neglect, however, is the failure to exercise the care that the circumstances justly demand. It embraces willful as well as unintentional disregard of duty. It is not a term of fixed and measured meaning. It takes its context always from specific circumstances, and its meaning varies as the context of surrounding circumstances changes. . . . [I]t is of no consequence that the parents have not failed in their duty in other respects.[114]

Many jurisdictions provide exemption from the definition of a neglected child one treated in good faith solely by spiritual means in accordance with the tenets of a recognized religious body.[115] Such statutes do not necessarily prevent a court from concluding in a proper case that spiritual treatment alone is insufficient, or from ordering conventional medical therapy where needed, including, if necessary, ongoing monitoring in follow-up after the acute problem is rectified.[116] When the statute authorizes "other remedial care" as an alternative to medicine, while penalizing willful failure to provide a minor with necessary medical attention, unorthodox substitutions for medical attendance may not necessarily be permissible.[117] Such statutes may raise thorny equal protection, First Amendment, and other constitutional issues, because they may give preference to one group of potential offenders over others based on that group's self-proclaimed religious tenets, and because they may involve the state in excessive entanglement with such questions as "What is a recognized religious body?," "What are its tenets?," and whether the accused acted in accord with such tenets.[118] Some courts, however, have no trouble finding that a parent's decision to "let God decide if the child will live or die" is not the kind of religious belief protected under such statutes.[119]

Where medical intervention may be deemed elective, parental refusal of such intervention may be permitted if the court does not find neglect or dependency.[120] In some instances, courts have refused to intervene despite medically compelling circumstances. The Illinois Appeals Court, for example, declined to find a child neglected whose sibling had been sexually abused at home, who herself had twice gone into diabetic ketoacidosis probably because of "misuse of insulin at home," and whose mother—suffering from a psychiatric disorder exacerbated by the stresses of child care—had a history of suicide attempts, sexual promiscuity, and placing the diabetic child in a foster home.[121]

Where, however, a parent's refusal to provide medical care is deemed egregious, criminal liability may be found.[122] Religious beliefs are no defense to neglect of this magnitude.[123] Significant neglect, however, even including neglect sufficient to cause death, may not necessarily be sufficient to sustain a charge of manslaughter.[124] This appears to be particularly true where the neglect is not shown to be willful.[125]

Parens patriae

The power that permits courts to intervene to mandate medical care for children whose parents fail to provide it is known as *parens patriae*[126]; this is distinct from the police power that justifies, for example, fluoridation of water:

The rationale of parens patriae is that the State must intervene . . . to protect an individual who is not able to make decisions in his own best interest. The decision to exercise the power of parens patriae must reflect the welfare of society as a whole, but mainly it must balance the individual's right to be free from interference against the individual's need to be treated, if treatment would in fact be in his best interest.[127]

The *parens patriae* power allows the state constitutionally to act as the "general guardian of all infants."[128] Its origins are found in antiquity:

[I]n ancient times the King was regarded as "Parens Patriae" of orphaned or dependent infants. . . . Under our system of government the state succeeds to the position and power of the king. Both King and State exercise this power in the interests of the people. Society has a deep interest in the preservation of the race itself. It is a natural instinct that lives of infants be preserved.[129]

Under the doctrine of *parens patriae*, courts are empowered to consent to treatment when the parents are unavailable to do so. This is seen where the parents have abandoned the child[130] or where they are just temporarily unavailable.[131] Court intervention in mandating therapy need not be predicated on an immediate threat to life or limb.[132] Although the criteria vary, one frequently invoked standard is the substituted judgment test: "In this case, the court must decide what its ward would choose, if he were in a position to make a sound judgment. Certainly, he would pick the chance for a fuller participation in life rather than a rejection of his potential as a more fully endowed human being."[133] Not only can the court overrule objections of both parent and child, under the right circumstances, it can overrule the objection of the surgeon who is to do the procedure.[134]

A serious threat to life, however, is not per se grounds for the intervention of the court under the *parens patriae* doctrine. If, for example, an infant is born with myelomeningocele, microcephaly, and hydrocephalus, and failure to operate would not place the infant in imminent danger of death, surgery may not be ordered over parental objection despite its efficacy in significantly reducing the risk of infection. In *Weber v. Stoney Brook Hosp.*, the court noted:

[S]uccessful results could also be achieved with antibiotic therapy. Further, while the mortality rate is higher where conservative medical treatment is used, in this particular case the surgical procedures also involved a great risk of depriving the infant of what little function remains in her legs, and would also result in recurring urinary tract and possible kidney infections, skin infections, and edemas [sic] of the limbs.[135]

The court concluded that the child was not neglected even though the parents had chosen the arguably riskier of two alternatives, both of which were considered valid choices by the available expert medical testimony.

The most commonly accepted situation in which medical therapy may be ordered for children over the wishes of their parents is where the life of the child is at stake.[136] Such intervention may be ordered even when the likelihood of success is only 50%.[137] State intervention, however, may be predicated on less critical medical need. Parental objection is insufficient in most states to overcome state requirements for prophylaxis against gonococcal ophthalmia neonatorum.[138] Surgery has been ordered where necessary to stabilize and prevent aggravation of a deformed foot when the surgery was deemed to be in the best interest of the child and despite opposition by the patient's father.[139] Even a tonsillectomy may be ordered over the objections of parents with religious reservations about the procedure, at least where the child is in the hands of a state department of social service.[140] Plastic surgery for treatment of harelip and cleft palate may be ordered by a court over parental objection.[141] Surgery may also be ordered if the court considers it necessary for the psychological well-being of the child despite the absence of a present threat to physical health. Accordingly, surgery has been ordered even though it was dangerous and offered only partial correction without cure of a facial deformity.[142] In addition, an autopsy may be ordered, notwithstanding religious proscription, where state law requires the authorities to determine the cause of death.[143]

Parental refusals of medical intervention are most likely to be upheld where the child's condition is not life-threatening, and where the treatment itself would expose the child to great risk.[144] Such refusals are sometimes upheld even when the "proposed therapy would offer great benefit to the child."[145] The court may also stay its hand if it is persuaded that the child is antagonistic to the proposed therapy and that his or her cooperation would be necessary to derive any benefit from the treatment.[146]

Most of the time, a court will avoid intervening when the malady sought to be treated is not life-threatening.[147] Tragically, courts sometimes fail to intervene even in the presence of disorders that are clearly life-threatening. In *In re Hofbauer,*[148] the parents of a 7-year-old boy with Hodgkin's disease treated him, not with radiotherapy and chemotherapy, but with "nutritional or metabolic therapy" including laetrile. There was "expert" testimony that laetrile is effective; the father indicated he would agree to conventional therapy if the "doctor" prescribing the placebos advised it. The court was persuaded that the parents were concerned and loving— that the child was not neglected—and ruled "[G]reat deference must be accorded a parent's choice as to the mode of medical treatment to be undertaken and the physician selected to administer the same."[149] The statute at issue in *Hofbauer* allowed the following interpretation:

"Adequate medical care" does not require a parent to beckon the assistance of a physician for every trifling affliction which a child may suffer. . . . We believe, however, that the statute does require a parent to entrust [the child's] care to that of a physician when such course would be undertaken by an ordinarily prudent and loving parent, "solicitous for the welfare of his child and anxious to promote the child's recovery."[150]

The court refused to find as a matter of law that the boy's parents had undertaken no reasonable efforts to ensure that acceptable medical treatment was being provided him, given the parents' concern about side effects from medical management, the alleged efficacy of the nutritional therapy and its relative lack of toxicity, and the parents' agreement that conventional treatment would be administered to the child if his condition so warranted. The parents' position would be upheld as long as they had provided for their child a form of treatment "recommended by their physician and which has not been totally rejected by all responsible medical authority" as, implied the court, treatment with laetrile had been.[151]

A different approach was taken in *Custody of a Minor.*[152] Applying the best interest of the child rule, the court decided that the trial court was justified in concluding that "metabolic therapy" was not only medically ineffective in the management of leukemia but was toxic to the child and contrary to the child's best interests. This conclusion, in the court's opinion, justified the finding that the child was without necessary and proper medical care, and that the parents were unwilling to provide the care required of them by the parental neglect statute.

The best interest of the child may justify intervention even when life itself is not threatened as was held in *In re Karwath.*[153] There, the parents had given their child up for adoption because of the mother's emotional illness and the father's unemployment and financial distress. Concern about possible hearing loss and rheumatic fever prompted the child's physician to recommend a tonsillectomy, and the father demanded that it not be done unless necessary "beyond the shadow of a doubt."[154] This position was based on the father's religious faith, although the court's opinion does not elaborate on the point. The father wanted chiropractic, medicine, and surgery attempted, in that order, and second and third opinions secured finding the procedure "necessary with reasonable medical certainty to restore and preserve the health of these wards of the state" before surgery could be undertaken. The court ordered that the surgery be done.[155] That the parents' objection was religiously based made no difference.

Our paramount concern for the best interest and welfare of the children overrides the father's contention that absolute medical certitude of necessity and success should precede surgery. Nor is it required that a medical crisis be shown constituting an immediate threat to life and limb.[156]

The police power

Certain public health measures are enacted pursuant to police power and upheld by the courts despite parental objection on a variety of grounds. The two best examples of this in the health care area are the vaccination of school children and fluoridation of water supplies, performed primarily for the benefit of children. Police power is an umbrella term not readily susceptible to precise definition:

While it is perhaps, almost impossible to frame a definition of the police power which shall accurately indicate its precise limits, so far as we are aware, all courts that have considered the subject have recognized and sanctioned the doctrine that under the police power there is general legislative authority to pass such laws as it is believed will promote the common good, or will protect or preserve the public health; and the power to promote or secure those objects rests primarily with the [legislature] subject to the power of the courts to decide, whether a particular enactment is adapted to that end.[157]

Often, promulgation of regulations is done not by the legislature but rather by a municipality, a board of public health, or some other arm of the state. In general, the courts will give deference to determinations made by these bodies:

[A] determination by the legislative body that a particular regulation is necessary for the protection or preservation of health is conclusive on the courts subject only to the limitation that it must be a reasonable determination, not an abuse of discretion, and must not infringe rights secured by the Constitution.[158]

Under this standard, most such regulations will be upheld, because "abuse of discretion" is seldom found.

Vaccination. Some health professionals today may be surprised to learn that there is a long history of disputes, continuing to recent times, concerning the validity of state and local regulations that require vaccination of school children as a prerequisite for attendance in public schools.[159] A number of early decisions upheld these regulations only because epidemics of smallpox in some communities warranted vaccination as an emergency measure.[160] In some cases, the constitutionality of the vaccination requirement was upheld only because the court construed it to mean, not that vaccination was mandated, but rather that school attendance without vaccination was not permitted.[161] More recently, it has been held that a child has no absolute right to enter school without immunization, and the school board has full authority to compel it.[162]

Questions of federal constitutionality, at least, were essentially laid to rest in the case of *Jacobson v. Massachusetts*.[163] In *Jacobson,* an adult who apparently feared side effects as a consequence of a bad experience with immunization as a child refused to submit to vaccination under a compulsory vaccination law. The court upheld his conviction:

There is, of course, a sphere in which the individual may assert the supremacy of his own will, and rightfully dispute the authority of any human government . . . to interfere with the exercise of that will. But it is equally true that in every well-ordered society charged with the duty of conserving the safety of its members the rights of the individual in respect of his liberty may at times, under the pressure of great dangers, be subjected to such restraint, to be enforced by reasonable regulations as the safety of the general public may demand.[164]

The court found no violation of equal protection in the statute's exception favoring children who are medically unfit to be vaccinated, despite the absence of such an exception for adults in like condition, both because there was no reason to suspect that an unfit adult would be required to submit to vaccination and because regulations appropriate for adults are not always safely applied to children.[165] Few cases before, and apparently, no cases after *Jacobson* have found vaccination requirements to be unconstitutional.[166] The courts have rejected constitutional attacks on both equal protection and due process grounds.[167]

Despite the special solicitude of the courts for First Amendment rights, compulsory vaccination has been upheld even when it conflicts with the religious beliefs of citizens.[168] This is true even where, under state law, a board of education was empowered, although not required, to exempt a child whose parents object to immunization on religious grounds.[169] Personal liberty, including freedom of religion, is a relative and not an absolute right, which must be "considered in the light of the general public welfare."[170] The right to practice religion freely does not include liberty to expose the community or the child to communicable diseases or the latter to ill health or death.[171] Nevertheless, some courts, generally in earlier cases only, have found it necessary to point out that vaccination requirements do not prevent children from attending schools, and children who are thereby excluded are excluded by their own consciences.[172] In other cases, the courts have questioned whether the plaintiff's religious beliefs really did compel the conclusion that vaccination was immoral.[173]

Where, however, a statute provides an exemption for members of a recognized church or religious denomination whose tenets conflict with the practice of vaccination, a mother's opposition based on her personal belief in the Bible and its teachings was sufficient to entitle her and her children to the exemption.[174] A similar statute was held not applicable to a man objecting to immunization because one of his children had earlier contracted hepatitis secondary to a diphtheria shot. In so holding, the court found no violation of equal protection or due process.[175] Where exemptions are enacted for persons religiously opposed to vaccination, a local school board may not be given discretion to determine who can qualify.[176]

The vaccination regulations have been repeatedly upheld as a reasonable exercise of the police power.[177] There need no longer be evidence of an epidemic,[178] nor even of a single case,[179] to warrant imposition of the regulation. The regulation does not involve the state in the practice of medicine.[180] Evidence impugning the value of vaccination need not even be considered by the courts, because such evidence is more appropriately presented to the legislature or its duly constituted agencies, such as the state board of health.[181]

Finally, there is no violation of the right to a free public education, nor is it a violation of state compulsory education laws to make vaccination a prerequisite to school attendance: "[H]ealth measures prescribed by local authorities as a condition of school attendance do not conflict with statutory provisions conferring on children of proper age the privilege of attending school nor with compulsory education laws."[182] This is true even though it leads to the exclusion of children whose physical condition precludes vaccination.[183] It has been held that, where a father did nothing to prevent the vaccination of his son, the child was not neglected under a regulation that barred him from school because he was unvaccinated.[184] More often, however, failure to provide for vaccination of a child may warrant a finding of parental neglect, and the resultant appointment of a guardian to consent to and arrange vaccination.[185]

Transfusions

Only flesh with its soul—its blood—YOU must not eat. And, besides that YOUR blood of YOUR souls shall I ask back. From the hand of every living creature shall I ask it back; and from the hand of man, from the hand of each one who is his brother, shall I ask back the soul of man.[186]

If anyone at all belonging to the house of Israel or the proselytes who reside among them eats any blood at all, against the person who eats blood I will set my face, and I will cut him off from his people; the life of every creature is identical with its blood.[187]

These and other scriptural passages[188] provide the the-

ological underpinning for the belief of certain religious groups, notably the Jehovah's Witnesses, that blood transfusions are contrary to the law of God. Since transfusions are a well-accepted component of the therapeutic armamentarium, many cases have examined the right of the state as *parens patriae* to protect the health of children within its jurisdiction as against the right of parents to raise their children according to their religious beliefs. *Parens patriae,* defined in this context as "a sovereign right and duty to care for a child and protect him from neglect, abuse and fraud during his minority" has been the basis in a number of cases for compelling transfusion of a child whose parents objected on religious grounds.[189] As we have seen in other instances, the courts distinguish between religious beliefs and opinions, which are held inviolable, and "religious practices inconsistent with the peace and safety of the state."[190] One court, in justifying such a decision, wrote:

[I]t was not ordered that he [the child's father] eat blood, or that he cease to believe [a transfusion] is equivalent to the eating of blood. It is only ordered that he may not prevent another person, a citizen of our country, from receiving the medical attention necessary to preserve her life.[191]

A party seeking court intervention to authorize transfusion over parental objection is not exposed to civil liability.[192]

As in other areas where religious beliefs and children's welfare may conflict, a court may stay its hand "[w]here the proposed treatment is dangerous to life, or there is a difference of medical opinion as to the efficacy of a proposed treatment, or where medical opinion differs as to which of two or more suggested remedies should be followed."[193] At least one court refused to order transfusions where the patient had no minor children; the patient had notified the doctor and hospital of his belief that acceptance of transfusion violated the laws of God; the patient had executed documents releasing the doctor and hospital from civil liability; and there appeared to be no clear and present danger to society.[194] Even where a child is involved, a court may refuse to order transfusions if the child is not faced with a threat to his life.

If we were to describe the surgery as "required" like the [New York] Court of Appeals, our decisions would conflict with the mother's religious beliefs. Aside from religious considerations, one can also question the use of that adjective on medical grounds since an orthopedic specialist testified that the operation itself was dangerous. Indeed, one can question who, other than the Creator, has the right to term certain surgery as "required." The fatal/nonfatal distinction also steers the courts of this Commonwealth away from a medical and philosophical morass: If spinal surgery can be ordered, what about a hernia or gall bladder operation or a hysterectomy?. . . [A]s between a parent and the state, the state does not have an interest of sufficient magnitude outweighing religious beliefs when the child's life is *not immediately imperiled* by his physical condition.[195]

A court is most inclined to order a transfusion when life is threatened. In some situations, this has been done even when the patient was an adult.[196] As a general matter, the willingness of the court to intervene increases in the case of a minor,[197] notwithstanding parents' arguments on due process[198] and free exercise grounds.[199] Although, in general, courts are more reluctant to order the transfusion of adults, when the adult is an expectant mother, the court may well ignore the question of the right to transfuse and proceed with the transfusion order on the basis of the right to treat the child.[200]

Where a child's life is in danger, the court may adopt streamlined procedures to preserve life that would not be followed or tolerated under other circumstances. For example, a transfusion can be ordered first, and the hearing over the propriety of the order may be held later.[201] A hearing may be held in advance of the need for transfusion, for instance, where a mother near term has a history of Rh incompatibility and has given birth in the past to other children with erythroblastosis fetalis requiring transfusion.[202] Even in a state where a statute provides immunity from criminal prosecution for parents treating their children in accordance with their religious beliefs, the state may nevertheless appoint a guardian to approve transfusions when necessary to save the life of the child.[203] This is the mechanism by which most courts enter transfusion orders.

While courts ordinarily find "neglect" only where parents abandon their children or otherwise fail to provide for their basic needs, such a term can be and often is applied where transfusion is required over the religious objections of parents, notwithstanding the sincerity and depth of the parents' beliefs. In *State v. Perricone,*[204] a child was afflicted with congenital heart disease that, from the court's description, suggests tetralogy of Fallot. Transfusions were required for proper management of his condition. The parents, who were Jehovah's Witnesses, refused to permit such transfusions, and they were found guilty of neglect of their son even though the court found them to have "sincere parental concern and affection for the child."[205]

A group of Jehovah's Witnesses in the state of Washington brought a class action suit to have declared unconstitutional a state statute that declared a child "dependent" — and, hence, eligible for appointment of a guardian — where transfusion "was or could be vital to save the patient" and the parents refused to permit it.[206] The court held the statute constitutional, and the Supreme Court of the United States affirmed per curiam.[207] That parents "have not failed in their duty to the child in other respects" provides them no more shelter under such a statute than does the sincerity of their religious beliefs.[208] In analyzing the tension between the free exercise clause and statutes of this type, the court in *People v. Pierson*[209] wrote, "We place no limits on the power of the mind over the body, the power of faith to dispel disease or the power of the Supreme Being to heal the sick. We merely declare the law as given us by the legislature."

A threat to the very life of a child is not always deemed necessary for a court to order transfusion over parental objection. Where brain damage was threatened by rising bilirubin in a child with erythroblastosis fetalis, the court found sufficient grounds to order transfusion, even though no mention was made of an actual threat to life.[210] In *In re Sampson*,[211] the parents did not oppose plastic surgery required for palliation of massive disfigurement of the right face and neck secondary to von Recklinghausen's disease (neurofibromatosis) in a 15-year-old boy; they did, however, object to the transfusions that such extensive surgery would require. Although there was no threat to life, and although the physicians advised delay until the boy was old enough to consent — because doing so would diminish the risks of the surgery — the trial court ordered surgery and was upheld on appeal. The court rejected as too restrictive the argument that it could intervene only where the life of the child is endangered by a failure to act. The Court of Appeals distinguished its earlier opinion in *In re Seiferth*,[212] writing that *Seiferth* turned on the question of a court's discretion and not the existence of its power to order surgery in a case where life itself was not at stake. The court had no trouble finding that religious objection to transfusion does not "present a bar at least where the transfusion is necessary to the success of the required surgery."[213]

Where a child is approaching the age of maturity, and where his or her life is not in imminent danger, the minor patient may have the right to express an opinion about the morality of transfusions and his or her willingness to submit to them. In *In re Green*,[214] a 16-year-old boy with scoliosis required surgery to prevent his eventually becoming bedridden. His parents, Jehovah's Witnesses, opposed the use of transfusions that the surgery would necessitate. The record did not disclose whether the patient himself was a Jehovah's Witness or planned to become one. The court wrote:

[U]nlike *Yoder* and *Sampson,* our inquiry does not end at this point, since we believe that the wishes of the sixteen-year-old boy should be ascertained; the ultimate question, in our view, is whether a parent's religious beliefs are paramount to the possibly adverse decision of the child. While the record before us gives us no indication of [the child's] thinking, it is the child rather than the parent in this appeal who is directly involved which thereby distinguishes *Yoder*'s decision not to discuss the beliefs of the parents vis-a-vis the children. In *Sampson,* the family court judge decided not to "evade the responsibility for a decision now by the simple expedient of foisting upon this boy the responsibility for making a decision at some later date...." [citation omitted] While we are cognizant of the ... problems of this approach ... we believe that [the boy] should be heard.[215]

Recently, however, both the Illinois and the U.S. Supreme Courts stopped short of imposing their authority when an unborn child's life was endangered because the mother refused, on religious grounds, to undergo a cesarean section. The Illinois Supreme Court declined to review an appellate court decision that upheld a Pentacostal's right to refuse a cesarean section delivery, even though doctors deemed it essential for her unborn child's survival, and the U.S. Supreme Court, in *Baby Boy Doe v. Mother Doe,*[216] followed suit by declining to order the lower court to convene an emergency hearing in the case.

STERILIZATION

The right to procreate is fundamental.[217] The U.S. Supreme Court has not addressed the question of whether there is a comparably fundamental right to be sterilized, but many states and lower federal courts have so concluded.[218]

Voluntary sterilization

Competent emancipated minors have been held entitled to consent to sterilization following a full explanation of the procedure and its consequences.[219]

Involuntary sterilization

Because developmentally disabled minors are so often incapable of informed consent, however, the courts have frequently been asked to decide whether such minors may be sterilized nonconsensually. These requests are often sought by the parents or guardians of a developmentally disabled child as the latter approaches childbearing age and the former begin to worry about the child's welfare after their deaths.[220]

Courts' power. A threshold issue for a court confronting a petition seeking sterilization of a developmentally disabled minor is often whether, absent a specific legislative grant of authority, the court has jurisdiction to rule. There is a rather sharp split of authority in the reported cases.[221] A substantial number of courts have concluded that specific statutory authorization was necessary to permit them to grant sterilization petitions for incompetent minors,[222] particularly where the court petitioned was of limited jurisdiction.[223] A roughly equal number of cases have held that specific enabling legislation is not necessary, often finding jurisdiction in the inherent *parens patriae* power of the court.[224] Although all courts recognize the importance of the sterilization decision, some find in that importance an argument against jurisdiction,[225] whereas others see the opposite.[226] The trend toward repeal of sterilization laws has brought this issue into sharper focus.[227] Perhaps all that can be said in jurisdictions without such laws is that the practitioner should determine how the local courts have resolved the issue.

Judicial immunity. Courts enjoy broad discretion to render decisions free from any fear of civil liability. This is known as *judicial immunity.* Sterilization, however, impinges on rights deemed so sacred that even the sacrosanct position of the judiciary may sometimes be open to attack for authorizing such procedures. In *Sparkman v. McFarlin,*[228] a state court ordered the sterilization of a 15-year-old girl. The 7th Circuit held the trial judge vulnerable to suit, ruling that judicial immunity was inapplicable because the judge lacked jurisdiction to hear the petition. The court based its decision on the following factors: (1) no statutory predicate for the procedure existed at the time, (2) no guardian ad litem or hearing had been arranged, (3) the judge issued the order on the mother's petition supported solely by her affidavit of the girl's retardation and promiscuity, and (4) the patient had been told that the purpose of the surgery was to perform an appendectomy rather than a tubal ligation. The Circuit Court concluded that in the "clear absence of jurisdiction," immunity did not exist.[229]

Nonetheless, reversing the 7th Circuit, the U.S. Supreme Court wrote:

Judge Stump had "original exclusive jurisdiction in all cases at law and equity whatsoever" ... [T]here was no Indiana ... case law in 1971 prohibiting a circuit court, a court of general jurisdiction, from considering a petition of the type presented to Judge Stump. The statutory authority for the sterilization of institutionalized persons in the custody of the State does not warrant the inference that the court ... has no power to act on a petition for sterilization of a minor in the custody of her parents, particularly where the parents have authority under the statutes to "consent and contract for medical care ... or treatment of [the minor] including surgery."[230]

In *Wade v. Bethesda Hosp.,*[231] the same judge who had granted an order for sterilization in *In Re Simpson*[232] ordered sterilization on the basis of a statute entrusting to the probate court the care and supervision of mentally retarded persons. The judge was sued for damages in a civil action. The federal district court denied his motion for summary judgment based on judicial immunity, ruling that without specific statutory authority the judge was without jurisdiction to order the operation.[233] Hence, according to the court, the judge could not invoke judicial immunity as a shield.

The *Wade* court also rejected the argument of a codefendant physician and hospital that they enjoyed immunity from suit because they had acted pursuant to a court order. The court reasoned that although the probate court had ordered sterilization, it had not ordered that these individuals perform it:

Nor are the defendants [Dr.] Daw and Bethesda [Hospital] correct in their contention that they could rely upon [Judge] Gary's order and act pursuant to it with immunities from civil suit. The law granting immunity to judicial and quasi-judicial officers is basically clear. Such immunity has been extended to other public officials acting pursuant to expressed court order [citations omitted] . . . The defendants Daw and Bethesda are clearly not public officials, nor [sic] were not expressly directed by Gary to take any action. Therefore, neither of these defendants can claim immunity for their [sic] part in their sterilization of the plaintiff.[234]

In view of the Supreme Court's decision in *Sparkman*, the validity of this holding may be questionable; certainly the imposition of liability on a physician and hospital acting on a court order seems unreasonable. No other decision seems to have agreed with *Wade* on this issue.

Procedure. Assuming the court deems itself authorized to entertain a petition for sterilization of a developmentally disabled minor, it may well impose elaborate, often rigid procedural and substantive safeguards to protect against perceived past sterilization abuses. One of the earliest and most comprehensive discussions of such safeguards appears in *In re Guardianship of Hayes*[235]:

The decision [to sterilize] can only be made in a superior court proceeding in which (1) the incompetent individual is represented by a disinterested guardian ad litem, (2) the court has received independent advice based upon a comprehensive medical, psychological and social evaluation of the individual, and (3) to the greatest extent possible, the court has elicited and taken into account the view of the incompetent individual.

Within this framework, the judge must find by clear, cogent and convincing evidence that the individual is (1) incapable of making his or her own decision about sterilization, and (2) unlikely to develop sufficiently to make an informed judgment about sterilization in the foreseeable future.

Next, it must be proved by clear, cogent and convincing evidence that there is a need for contraception. The judge must find that the individual is (1) physically capable of procreation, and (2) likely to engage in sexual activity at the present or in the near future under circumstances likely to result in pregnancy, and must find in addition that (3) the nature and extent of the individual's disability, as determined by empirical evidence and not solely on the basis of standardized tests, renders him or her permanently incapable of caring for a child, even with reasonable assistance.

Finally, there must be no alternatives to sterilization. The judge must find that by clear, cogent and convincing evidence (1) all less drastic contraceptive methods, including supervision, education and training, have been proved unworkable or inapplicable, and (2) the proposed method of sterilization entails the least invasion of the body of the individual. In addition, it must be shown by clear, cogent and convincing evidence that (3) the current state of scientific and medical knowledge does not suggest either (a) that a reversible sterilization procedure or other less drastic contraceptive method will shortly be available or (b) that science is on the threshold of an advance in the treatment of the individual's disability.[236]

Sterilization may be authorized only if it is determined to be in the best interest of the disabled person, with due consideration of age and educability, potential as a parent, medical indications for the procedure, and availability of contraceptive alternatives.[237] Other courts have required consideration of such issues as the possibility of trauma or of psychological damage from pregnancy, childbirth, or sterilization; the advisability of delay; and the patient's present or future ability to care for a child with or without the help of a spouse.[238] The extent to which the availability and use of new long-term, implantable, subdermal contraceptive devices such as Norplant will affect future decisions on the issue of sterilization of the developmentally disabled is not yet known.

Some courts have specifically required a finding that the petitioner is acting in good faith,[239] as "the interests of the parents of a retarded person cannot be presumed to be identical to those of the child" in sterilization proceedings.[240] In considering the best interests of the developmentally disabled, the court is to consider neither the convenience of the parents or guardians nor the interests of society at large.[241]

Where a guardian is appointed, he or she "must have full opportunity to meet with the incompetent person, to present proofs and cross-examine witnesses at the hearing, and to represent zealously the interests of his or her ward in other appropriate ways."[242] One court ruled that a guardian ad litem must assume an adversary position on behalf of the incompetent and if not, independent counsel must be appointed "to ensure a thorough adversary exploration of the issues."[243] The developmentally disabled person generally need not be present at the hearing.[244] Many courts, however, have required the judge to meet the individual personally to formulate his or her own impressions of the individual's competence,[245] elicit when possible the individual's views on the sterilization question, and to afford great deference to those views.[246]

The "clear and convincing" evidence generally required before sterilization can be authorized more rigorously protects the minor incompetent's procreative rights than does the customery civil "preponderance of the evidence" standard.[247]

[The] "clear and convincing" standard of proof should apply in this kind of case. Preponderance of the evidence does not sufficiently protect [the incompetent's] interest in preserving her physical integrity. On the other hand, "beyond reasonable doubt" is overprotective . . . [and] inappropriate in a proceeding in which the overriding consideration is the incapacitated person's best interest. . . .[248]

The basis for the sterilization decision is generally to be the substituted judgment of the court; that is, the court is to reach that conclusion that the disabled person would reach, were he or she able to do so, considering all factors relevant to the decision, including the very fact of the minor's incompetency.[249] This approach is somewhat problematic, because for someone who has been developmentally disabled since birth a subjective inquiry is pointless and an objective analysis must be substituted.[250]

Institutionalized developmentally disabled minors.
The law's vigilance against inappropriate sterilization is even greater for developmentally disabled minors who are institutionalized. A court may specifically require a finding of "medical necessity" before it will authorize sterilization of a developmentally disabled minor inhabitant of a state institution.[251] A sterilization is "medically necessary" when it is needed to protect the life or mental or physical health of the patient.[252] In *Ruby v. Massey*,[253] the court ruled that where statutory authorization for sterilization of minor incompetents is restricted to those enrolled in state schools for the mentally retarded, the state cannot refuse the request of parents seeking sterilization for their children who were denied admission for want of space. In *Ruby*, three sets of parents of blind, deaf, and severely retarded girls sought hysterectomies for the girls from named physicians and from the University of Connecticut Health Center, all of whom had refused for lack of "legislative authority authorizing parental consent for such operation[s] in Connecticut."[254] The health care providers were frank to admit that their fear of civil liability was the sole reason for their refusal.[255] The court reasoned that because the children were themselves incapable of consent, and because the right of plaintiffs' children to be sterilized is rooted in the Constitution, the state was obliged to make sterilization available to these children just as it did for those who had been admitted to the institution.[256]

A hospital's refusal to sterilize

Many hospitals, particularly those established and supported by various religious groups, refuse to perform sterilizations for reasons of conscience. The Hill-Burton Act, through which many hospitals receive federal funds, was amended in 1973 to provide that receipt of such funds could not be used as a basis to compel a hospital to perform sterilizations against the dictates of its religious or moral beliefs.[257] This amendment has been held constitutionally sound; it does not violate the establishment clause[258]; and to the extent, if any, that it infringes on any constitutionally cognizable right to privacy, such infringement is outweighed by the need to protect the religious freedom of denominational hospitals.[259]

CONTRACEPTION

The right of adults to obtain and use contraceptives is well established.[260] The states, however, seek to protect minor females "from the evil effects and unsuspected harms of actions which go against the mores of society," and from physical harms that may ensue from contraception; they are also astute to enforce the rights of parents to control the family.[261] Despite these state aspirations, and despite the moral anguish their decisions cause many Americans, the courts have held that minors have the right to use contraceptives just as adults do:

[W]e perceive no developmental differences between minors and adults that may affect the gravity of the right asserted by sexually active minors to family planning services and materials. The interest of minors in access to contraceptives is one of fundamental importance. The financial, psychological and social problems arising from teenage pregnancy and motherhood argue for our recognition of the right of minors to privacy as being equal to that of adults.[262]

A leading case examining the power of states to prohibit minors' access to contraception is *Carey v. Population Services International*.[263] In *Carey*, the Supreme Court decided that a New York statute prohibiting the sale or distribution of nonprescription contraceptives to persons under 16, and prohibiting distribution of nonmedical contraceptives to persons over 15 except through a licensed pharmacist, violated the right to privacy of affected purchasers under the Fourteenth Amendment.[264] The Court reasoned that the goal of deterring teenage sexuality was insufficient justification for the statute because the state could not reasonably prescribe an unwanted child or an abortion as punishment for fornication, and noted that the state had adduced no evidence that teens would restrain or cease sexual activity for want of contraceptives.[265] The *Carey* Court also held that statutory provisions prohibiting advertisement and displays of contraceptives violated the First Amendment right to free speech.[266] The Court did not, however, address the issue of whether a minor could be required to obtain parental consent before acquiring contraceptives; lower courts have ruled in the negative on this question *(vide infra)*.

In 1970, Congress passed the Family Planning Services and Population Research Act (Title X of the Public Health Services Act)[267] establishing a system of federally funded public and nonprivate family planning projects, and authorizing grants and contracts for family planning services, including services to sexually active minors requesting them.[268] Under the Aid to Families with Dependent Children (AFDC)[269] and Medicaid programs of the Social Security Act,[270] state and local welfare agencies must provide contraceptive services to those eligible for them, including "minors who can be considered to be sexually active."[271] Regulations promulgated pursuant to Title X require that such services be made available without regard to age or marital status.[272] Minors may be given contraceptives under circumstances where an adult similarly situated would receive them, state parental consent statutes notwithstanding.[273]

Parental consent

Statutes or regulations purporting to require parental consent before minors can obtain contraceptive services have generally been disfavored. In *T. H. v. Jones,*[274] for example, the court struck down a parental consent requirement on grounds it conflicted with the goals of the AFDC and Medicaid programs. Similarly, the court in *Doe v. Pickett*[275] held that such a requirement violates the rights of applicants under Title X and inhibits fulfillment of the congressional goal of providing family planning services to all desiring them. A state court in Washington has ruled that Planned Parenthood could provide family planning information and contraceptives to minors without parental consent without violating their parents' "Fourteenth Amendment right to care, custody, and nurture of their children."[276] States may, however, require consent in programs not funded under Title X.[277] When schools offer contraceptive information, either parental consent or an opt-out option is almost always required.[278]

Parental consent requirements that potentially restrict condom distribution in New York City's public high schools have continued to come under attack, however.[279] In early 1994, the New York Civil Liberties Union sought to set aside a 1993 state court ruling that forbade condom distribution without parental consent.[280] Some apparently fear that parental opt-out policies will stymie efforts, supported by the Clinton administration, to expand school-based health clinics.[281] Clinton's commitment to the expansion of the clinics was enthusiastically echoed by former Surgeon General Joycelyn Elders on whose desk purportedly "sat an arrangement of faux roses fashioned from the red wrappers of several Lifestyles condoms."[282]

Parental notification

A 1981 amendment to Title X required that "to the extent practical, entities which receive grants or contracts under this subsection shall encourage family participation in projects assisted under this subsection" (the "squeal rule").[283] The Department of Health and Human Services then proposed and adopted a regulation requiring Title X grantees to notify parents when contraceptives were prescribed for unemancipated minors.[284] Exceptions to this requirement were granted only where the project director or designated clinic head determined that notification would result in physical harm to the minor at the hands of her parent or guardian[285] or when the services provided were for treatment of sexually transmitted disease.[286] These new regulations were promptly challenged in the courts.

In *Planned Parenthood Federation, Inc. v. Heckler,*[287] the D.C. circuit court upheld a district court injunction granted on behalf of private family planning services, barring enforcement of regulations requiring any federally funded agency (1) to give parental notification,[288] (2) to comply with state laws requiring parental notice of or consent to provision of such services,[289] and (3) to ascribe to minors their parents' financial resources in evaluating the minors' eligibility for services. The court found these regulations to be inconsistent with congressional intent in enacting Title X and therefore beyond the limits of authority of the Secretary of Health and Human Services. Finding that the amendments encouraging family participation in the minor's decision-making were subordinate to the minor's right to confidentiality, the court concluded that Congress had not authorized the secretary to require compliance with state parental consent or notification requirements.[290] Parental notification, said the court, "undermine[d] both Congress' specific policy of confidentiality and its overriding concern about the escalating pregnancy rate.[291] Finally, ascribing to the minor the financial resources of the parents was deemed tantamount to a parental notification requirement and so was similarly held invalid.[292] Because family planning services dispensed on the basis of need would obviously be more difficult for a minor to obtain if her family's financial resources were ascribed to her, this decision expands the number of minors eligible to receive family planning services under Title X.[293]

The Sixth Circuit has specifically ruled that a clinic's practice of distributing contraceptives to minors without parental notification did not violate the parents' constitutional right to participate in the decisions of their minor children regarding sexuality and contraception, since attendance at the clinic was voluntary and there was no bar to parental involvement.[294] Existing law, then, would appear to hold that federally funded family planning services may provide contraceptives to minors on request without parental notice and certainly without parental consent. This may or may not remain true in the future, as discussed in the following section.

ABORTION

Despite the state's interest in preventing illicit sex among minors, protecting minors from their own improvidence, fostering parental control, and supporting the family as a social unit, minors have been held to have a right to an abortion just as adults do and for many of the same reasons.[295] According to the U.S. Supreme Court,

> [t]he potentially severe detriment facing a pregnant woman, see *Roe v. Wade*, 410 U.S. at 153, is not mitigated by her minority. Indeed, considering her probable education, employment skills, financial resources, and emotional maturity, unwanted motherhood may be exceptionally burdensome for a minor. In addition, the fact of having a child brings with it adult legal responsibility, for parenthood, like attainment of the age of majority, is one of the traditional criteria for the termination of the legal disabilities of minority. In sum, there are few situations in which denying a minor the right to make an important decision will have consequences so grave and indelible.[296]

Nevertheless, state regulation of abortion, even for adults, is permissible to foster "compelling state interest[s]" by "narrowly drawn" legislation.[297] In *Planned Parenthood of Southeastern Pennsylvania v. Casey*, the U.S. Supreme Court held that a state may regulate the abortion process even during the first trimester, so long as it does not place an "undue burden" on the mother's ability to decide whether to terminate her pregnancy.[298]

The state interests as just recited justify a greater degree of state control in a minor's abortion decision than the courts permit in adult abortion cases, or in cases where minors face decisions related to reproduction other than abortion, such as contraception.[299] Given "the peculiar vulnerability of children; their inability to make critical decisions in an informed, mature manner; and the importance of the parental role in child rearing," states have a significant interest in promoting parental involvement in a child's abortion dilemma.[300]

Parental consent

A state may not condition a minor's abortion on parental consent alone.[301] The Supreme Court has held that "the State does not have the constitutional authority to give a third party an absolute, and possibly arbitrary, veto over the decision of the physician and his patient to terminate the patient's pregnancy, regardless of the reason for withholding the consent."[302] A private

hospital may not suffer the same constraints, however, because a private facility is not a "state actor," to which the Fourteenth Amendment's guarantees of liberty and due process apply.[303]

A minor may not be compelled against her wishes to submit to abortion merely because her own mother wants her to,[304] and coercing a minor to abort violates her constitutionally protected freedom to choose to carry the pregnancy to term.[305]

Where a state desires to impose a parental consent requirement, it must also provide an alternate authorization procedure. In this so-called "bypass" procedure, the minor is entitled to show either:

> (1) that she is mature enough and well enough informed to make her abortion decision, in consultation with her physician, independently of her parent's wishes; or (2) that even if she is not able to make this decision independently, the desired abortion would be in her best interests. The proceeding in which this showing is made must assure that a resolution of the issue, and any appeals that may follow, will be completed with anonymity and sufficient expedition to provide an effective opportunity for an abortion to be obtained. In sum, the procedure must ensure that the provision requiring parental consent does not in fact amount to the "absolute, and possibly arbitrary, veto" that was found impermissible in *[Planned Parenthood of Central Missouri v.] Danforth*.[306]

Bypass: procedural features

The state's bypass procedure may not require advance notification of the minor's parents that she has applied for judicial authorization.[307] Nor may the state require notification after a court denies such an application.[308] The court must grant the minor's request upon determining that she is mature, whether it believes an abortion is in her best interests or not, or upon determining that, despite her immaturity, granting her petition is in her best interests.[309] The state may not require the minor to decide whether to base her petition upon her maturity, her best interests, or both.[310] Nor may it require that the petitioner prove her case by clear and convincing evidence.[311]

In a bypass procedure, the trial court may question the minor concerning her understanding of her alternatives and the judgment she used to weigh them, and may consider her conduct in assessing her maturity.[312] In *In re T.H.*,[313] the Indiana Supreme Court upheld a trial court's denial of a petition for waiver of parental consent, because the trial court, uncertain about the fetal age (18 to 23 weeks), was consequently uncertain about the magnitude of the risk to T.H.; because the court deemed the minor immature despite testimony to the contrary; and because the minor's legal guardian, the Department of Public Welfare, would not consent to the abortion, but had agreed to provide all care T.H. would need during pregnancy and childbirth, including placing the baby for adoption. If the minor was not or did not claim to be mature enough or competent to give informed consent, the same court ruled it would determine whether abortion was in the minor's best interests only after parental consultation, under a statute requiring only such consultation, and not parental approval.[314]

A bypass proceeding must be held with "sufficient expedition to provide an effective opportunity for an abortion to be obtained."[315] A bypass procedure that could take up to 22 days failed to meet this criterion, even though an appellate court was empowered by the statute to increase or decrease the time needed for various steps in the proceedings.[316] Statutory silence on the time frame for a court decision may render the statute unconstitutional,[317] although in 1992 that issue was not raised when the U.S. Supreme Court considered the constitutionality of a Pennsylvania statute's bypass provision that contained no specified time frame for judicial action.[318] A bypass proceeding should also provide for anonymity of the minor,[319] although an opportunity to change venue is apparently not constitutionally mandated.[320]

Some courts have held that the bypass statute must provide for appointment of counsel to represent the minor.[321] Procedure must be spelled out in detail because abortion has been deemed a fundamental right, which, if not exercised in a timely manner, may be irrevocably lost, and because the minors for whom bypass is established are legally unsophisticated.[322] "Pocket approval," for example, whereby a court may grant a petition for a minor's abortion by mere silence, unduly burdens the minor's decision.[323] Such approval

[p]uts the physician in a difficult position. If the [state] district court does nothing, authorization for the physician to perform the abortion is deemed to have been granted. The physician is subjected to liability if the abortion is performed without authorization, but the physician has nothing tangible to rely upon to prove compliance with the law. In the case of "pocket approval," no record is made of the authorization.[324]

The statute creating the bypass mechanism should also specify appellate procedure, which, like that in the trial court, must be handled on an expedited basis.[325]

Because parental consent requirements, in the absence of a bypass provision, have been held unconstitutional, it is not surprising that statutes purporting to impose criminal sanctions on physicians failing to comply with such statutes have generally been struck down. For example, in *State v. Koome,*[326] the Washington Supreme Court reversed the conviction of a doctor who had aborted a minor's fetus without consent of the minor's parents.

Parental notification

Whether, how, and when a state may require parental notification of—as opposed to consent to—a minor's abortion decision remains somewhat uncertain. In *H.L. v. Matheson,*[327] the Supreme Court upheld a Utah statute requiring parental notice where the minor seeking abortion was immature, unemancipated, and dependent. In *Matheson,* the Court recognized parental authority to direct the rearing of their children as basic to the structure of our society.[328]

Noting that "abortion is associated with increased risk of complications in subsequent pregnancies" and that the emotional and psychological effects of the pregnancy and abortion experience are markedly more severe in girls under 18 than in adults, the *Matheson* Court found that the Utah statute served important considerations of family integrity in protecting adolescents by giving parents an opportunity to provide information to the physician that the minor herself may be unable to furnish.[329] The court also recognized a "significant state interest" in the better medical care that such notice affords "by providing an opportunity for parents to supply essential medical and other information to a physician."[330] The statute was constitutionally sound despite its failure to specify what such information might be and to provide a mandatory delay period after the doctor notified the parents, and even though it could inhibit some abortions[331]:

That the requirement of notice to parents may inhibit some minors from seeking abortions is not a valid basis to void the statute. . . . The Constitution does not compel a state to fine-tune its statutes so as to encourage or facilitate abortions. To the contrary, state action "encouraging childbirth except in the most urgent circumstances" is "rationally related to the legitimate governmental objective of protecting potential life."[332]

In *Hodgson v. Minn.,*[333] the U.S. Supreme Court affirmed a decision of the Eighth Circuit,[334] construing a notice/bypass statute held to be unconstitutional in the trial court. The statute provided that, subject to certain exceptions, no abortion could be performed on an expectant mother under 18 years of age until at least 48 hours after both of her parents were notified, even if the parents were separated or divorced. The statute also provided that, if a court enjoined enforcement of the two-parent notification requirement, the same two-parent notification requirement remained effective unless a court of competent jurisdiction ordered the abortion to proceed without notice on proof by the minor that she was "mature and capable of giving informed consent" or that an abortion without notice to both parents would be in her best interests. The Supreme Court held that the two-parent notification requirement reasonably furthered no legitimate state interest, and could actually disserve the state's interest in protecting and assisting the minor child of a dysfunctional family; the Court found this provision unconstitutional. A different majority of the Court, however, approved the bypass procedure.

In *Ind. Planned Parenthood v. Pearson,*[335] the Seventh Circuit, reversing the district court, ruled that notification of parents after denial of an unemancipated minor's petition for waiver of parental notification unconstitutionally burdened the minor's abortion decision. Further defining notification requirements, in *Ohio v. Akron Center for Reproductive Health,*[336] the Supreme Court reversed the Sixth Circuit, which had ruled that a notification requirement was constitutionally impermissible in the case of a mature minor, or one whose best interests do not include parental notification of the abortion decision. The statute under scrutiny made it a crime for anyone to abort the fetus of a single, unemancipated minor unless the abortionist provided timely notice to *one* of the minor's parents, or a juvenile court authorized the minor to consent. Bypass would not be authorized unless (1) the minor, by clear and convincing proof, showed that she was sufficiently mature and informed to make the abortion decision herself; (2) one of her parents had habitually abused her; or (3) parental notification was not in her best interests. The Supreme Court found the statute to be constitutionally sound, because it permitted the minor to obtain an abortion where she was mature enough to choose it irrespective of her parents' wishes, or where she could show it was in her best interests to abort; it protected the minor's confidentiality adequately; and its time limits on judicial action were tight enough to permit expedition of the process.[337]

Applying such a bypass provision in 1993, an Ohio Appeals Court reversed a trial judge's decision that a minor had failed to establish her maturity adequately, thereby preventing her from bypassing a statutory parental notification requirement. The trial court had found the minor immature despite the following facts: (1) She was almost 18 years old; (2) she worked 13 hours per week; (3) she was an honor student; and (4) she saved her money for college.[338] Considering the factual record, the appeals court found that the trial judge had abused his discretion.

Since *Webster v. Reproductive Health Services,*[339] the power of the states to regulate abortion has increased significantly, although in 1992, in *Planned Parenthood of Southeastern Pennsylvania v. Casey,*[340] the Supreme Court reaffirmed the basic tenets of *Roe v. Wade.* Given the current makeup of the court, it appears that *Casey* will allow the states to circumscribe, but not abolish, a minor's right to abort her fetus.

INVOLUNTARY CIVIL COMMITMENT OF MINORS

Involuntary civil commitment is generally governed by state statutes. These statutes vary widely from state to state. Most of them provide that commitment must be justified by five findings: (1) the patient is mentally ill, (2) the patient is dangerous to self or others, (3) the patient needs care and treatment, (4) the proposed commitment is the least intrusive means necessary to protect the patient or the community, and (5) if the commitment is solely to protect the patient, he or she lacks the ability to decide if taking such action is desirable.[341]

Individuals of any age committed involuntarily to state institutions for treatment of mental illness, mental retardation, or for any other reason retain their due process rights. A child so committed, like an adult, "has a substantial liberty interest in not being confined unnecessarily for medical treatment and . . . the state's involvement in the commitment decision constitutes state action under the Fourteenth Amendment."[342]

When at the request of the child's natural parents the child is evaluated for admission to a state mental institution, the decision must be made by a neutral fact-finder. Such a fact-finder need not be law-trained or a judicial or administrative officer for the procedure to pass federal constitutional muster. Nor is it constitutionally necessary for an admitting psychiatrist to conduct a formal or quasi-formal adversarial hearing; the psychiatrist can make the admission decision.[343] For children without natural parents, the state custodial agency may "constitutionally . . . speak for the child."[344]

Where indefinite commitment is sought, its proponent must prove the case by "clear and convincing" evidence.[345] In commitment proceedings, the U.S. Constitution does not require proof "beyond reasonable doubt" as it does in criminal prosecutions.[346] The states, however, may impose such a rigorous procedural safeguard if they wish[347] or may provide an array of other protections as well. In California, for example, a minor 14 years of age or older may not be committed to a state institution, even upon application by his parents, until after notice and hearing.[348] The proponent must show that the treatment proposed is likely to be beneficial to the minor.[349] However, the proponent need not show the minor is "gravely disabled" or "dangerous," even though this standard must be applied to minor wards of the court.[350] The minor must be afforded the opportunity to appear in person, to present evidence in his or her own behalf, and to confront and cross-examine adverse witnesses.[351] The minor must also be provided counsel.[352] A record of the proceedings adequate for meaningful judicial or appellate review must be maintained.[353] Any commitment ordered must "bear some reasonable relation to the purpose for which the individual is committed."[354] In California, a postadmission evaluation by hospital staff has been held insufficient to avoid misdiagnosis.[355]

California does not, however, require a jury trial or a judicial hearing before committing a minor at the parents' request; an administrative hearing is sufficient for due process purposes.[356] Nor does it require provision for judicial oversight where parents detain their child in a private mental hospital, because such commitment entails no state action.[357]

The contrast between California's procedural requirements for commitment of minors and those mandated by the U.S. Constitution are mirrored in numerous procedural differences among the states. These differences are seen in such issues as the timing of preadmission review, if any; whether such review is mandatory; whether the minor has the right to counsel; the substantive standard of review; the weight, if any, given the minor's preferences; and the extent to which admissions to private facilities are governed by the state's commitment statute.[358] The courts, however, have generally been rigorous in application of whatever procedural rules govern commitment in their own jurisdictions.[359] The jurisdiction of courts of equity over minors and others under a disability is deemed plenary to afford whatever relief may be necessary to protect the individual's best interests.[360] A court may strike down a commitment statute that fails to afford meaningful judicial review[361] or that sets overly broad or impermissibly vague criteria for commitment.[362]

For instance, Massachusetts permits commitment of a mentally ill ward to a mental health facility only if the court finds the commitment to be in the ward's best interests and if, beyond reasonable doubt, failure to commit would create "a likelihood of serious harm."[363] Massachusetts requires[364] the same level of proof when extending a minor's commitment beyond the age of 18.

Before commitment, Alabama requires a showing, by substantial evidence, that the minor's "mental illness or mental retardation poses a real and present threat of substantial harm to himself or to others."[365] North Carolina has held that, although a precommitment hearing was not necessary to afford due process to a minor committed at his parent's behest, a medical examination within 24 hours after admission to determine whether treatment was necessary, and a provision permitting release of the minor upon request within 72 hours, were insufficiently protective of the minor's due process rights to survive constitutional scrutiny.[366]

Under certain circumstances, a minor involuntarily committed has the right to refuse treatment,[367] especially treatment with major tranquilizers, electroshock, psychosurgery, and the like, at least in nonemergency situations.[368]

Like so many other facets of commitment, the permissible duration of the minor's detention may vary greatly from state to state. In Connecticut, for example, a parent was not permitted to continue "voluntary" confinement of her 17-year-old son in a psychiatric ward against his wishes.[369] Yet detaining a child in a private mental hospital for treatment without the child's consent may be permissible under California law and, because such detention is not a state action, violates neither due process nor equal protection rights.[370] A mother may be entitled to withdraw her child from a treatment center if she is dissatisfied with the treatment or the attitudes of staff members, even if the reasons for her dissatisfaction are incorrect and despite her poverty, so long as she intends to provide appropriate care in some manner.[371]

Conditions in the institution

Conditions inside state institutions must meet the standards set forth in *Youngberg v. Romeo*.[372] In *Youngberg*, a 33-year-old man with an IQ of 10 or 11 and a history of violent behavior was admitted to a state hospital at the behest of his mother, who was unable to care for him. At the hospital, he was injured by his own violence and by the reaction of the other residents to him. The Court held that keeping the patient in unsafe conditions violated his constitutionally protected liberty interest (under the due process clause of the Fourteenth Amendment) in having reasonably safe conditions of confinement and freedom from unreasonable bodily restraints. Such confinement also infringed his right to such minimally adequate training as reasonably may be required by these interests. "Minimally adequate training required by the Constitution" is presumptively that recommended by a trained professional.[373] Although Romeo was chronologically an adult, he was a child intellectually, so the Court's holding may be held applicable to minors; and since, of course, the Supreme Court was construing the U.S. Constitution, its holding governs all state institutions.

CHILD ABUSE

The prevalence of child abuse in the United States is alarming, and the harm it causes is enormous.[374] Estimates have ranged from more than one million to as many as four million incidents per year and by one estimate have increased 50-fold in the past 20 years.[375] Although reports of child abuse are twice as high as the number of substantiated cases, estimates are that "about 1.16 million children were victims of child abuse and neglect in 1992, a 10 percent increase from 1991."[376]

Child abuse is the most common cause of death of small children in this country.[377] In fact, "[s]tatistics show that 90 percent of all children who are murdered are under age six."[378] According to another estimate, the victims in 25% to 50% of these incidents may be permanently injured or killed within a matter of months in repeated abusive episodes.[379] Repeated beatings are the rule rather than the exception.[380] The problem has reached these epidemic proportions despite the fact that abusers can be convicted of such serious crimes as assault and battery or manslaughter.[381] Perhaps most tragically, the perpetrators of child abuse have often been victims of child abuse themselves; the problem poses the very grave threat of self-perpetuation.[382]

Perpetrators of child abuse have been characterized as prone to alcoholism, sexual promiscuity, unstable marriages, and criminal activity. Often psychopathic or sociopathic, "[t]hey are quick to react with poorly controlled aggression."[383] Perpetrators also tend to abuse their spouses.[384] Abuse can occur at the hands of foster or adoptive parents, other relatives, or family friends.[385] It is common for physicians to treat abused children whose siblings appear to be unabused.[386]

Some data link child abuse to socioeconomic status: in 40% of the reported cases, no parent or caretaker was employed, and 43% of the families received some sort of public assistance compared with 11% nationwide. Forty-three percent of the reports occurred in single-mother families, compared with 14% of all U.S. families, leading to the inescapable conclusion that stress and poverty are related to abuse and neglect.[387]

Caffey, however, whose pioneering work in 1946 was in large measure responsible for the now widespread recognition of the battered child syndrome, takes an apparently contrary position:

Perpetrators . . . are characteristically of normal intelligence and represent all races, creeds in all cultural, economic, social, and educational levels and are distributed proportionately in all parts of the country. As a group, with a few exceptions, they suffer from the same neuroses, the same emotional and character problems in the same range and degree as any randomly selected group of same milieu and size. Less than 10% are psychopaths.[388]

It may be that these authors base their conflicting conclusions on their experiences with patient populations of different socioeconomic classes. Alternatively, underreporting may be even more common in middle and upper class families than it is among the poor.[389]

Battered child syndrome

In their classic article on child abuse, Hefler and Kempe wrote that "[t]he syndrome should be considered in any child exhibiting evidence of fracture of any bone, failure to thrive, soft tissue swellings or skin bruising, in any child who dies suddenly, or where the degree and type of injury is at variance with the history given regarding the occurrence of the trauma."[390] The authors supply additional details:

The battered-child syndrome may occur at any age but, in general, the affected children are younger than three years. [Usually] the child's general health is below par, and he shows evidence of neglect including poor skin hygiene, multiple soft tissue injuries, and malnutrition. One often obtains a history of previous episodes suggestive of parental neglect or trauma. A marked discrepancy between clinical findings and historical data as supplied by the parents is a major diagnostic feature. . . . The fact that no new lesions . . . occur while the child is in the hospital . . . lends added weight to the diagnosis. . . . Subdural hematoma, with or without fracture of the skull, is . . . an extremely frequent finding. . . . The characteristic distribution of these multiple fractures and the observation that the lesions are in different stages of healing are of additional value in making the diagnosis.[391]

Pattern scars or bruises, such as cigarette or immersion burns, lacerations or abrasions of areas not normally so injured, such as the palate or external genitalia, and behavior changes (noncompliance, anger, isolation, destructiveness, developmental delays, excessive attention-seeking, and lack of separation anxiety) are also characteristic.[392] It would seem, then, that a physician confronted with this clinical picture would be justified in entertaining a diagnosis of child abuse.[393]

Neglect, in contrast to physical abuse, is more apt to present as malnutrition, recurrent pica, chronic fatigue or listlessness, poor hygiene, inadequate clothing for the circumstances, or lack of appropriate medical care such as immunizations, dental care, and eyeglasses.[394] Behavioral signs may also be present, including poor school attendance, age-inappropriate responsibility for tasks such as housework, drug or alcohol abuse, and a history of repeated toxic ingestions.[395]

Sexually abused children may have difficulty in walking or sitting; thickened and/or hyperpigmented labial skin; torn, stained, or bloody underclothing; bruised or bleeding private parts; vaginal discharge and/or pruritus; recurrent urinary tract infections; venereal disease; pregnancy; and lax rectal tone. It is reasonable to expect that these unfortunate children may be at increased risk for AIDS, although the commonest cause of this syndrome in children is undoubtedly maternal-fetal infection.[396] A vaginal opening greater than 4 mm in horizontal diameter is said to be characteristic of the sexual abuse of prepubescent girls.[397] Victims of sexual abuse may also have poor self-esteem, attempt suicide, display regressive behavior such as enuresis, masturbate excessively, be sexually promiscuous, withdraw from reality, express shame or guilt, and experience distortion of body image.[398]

Not all cases, of course, will present in classic fashion, nor will typical findings always be caused by child abuse. "[A]t any one time [children] may coincidentally show a variety of types of physical marks (e.g., a black eye, cut lip, bruised ears, scratches, and diaper rash burns), even though their parents may be loving, concerned and reasonably careful."[399] Hence, diagnosis may not be straightforward, particularly since the history is unlikely to be easily obtained from intimidated young patients or from their guilt-ridden parents.

Reporting child abuse

In every American jurisdiction, it is now the legal obligation of the examining physician to report suspected cases of child abuse to authorities designated by statute.[400] Significantly, all the statutes provide immunity from civil liability for doctors reporting suspected child abuse in good faith (vide infra). Some statutes, such as North Dakota's, extend this protection to any reporter, other than the alleged child abuser, whether acting under statutory compulsion or not.[401] Typically, the immunity extends to suits for slander, libel, breach of confidence, or invasion of privacy.[402] Almost all states now require professionals in other fields to report as well, including those in education, social work, child care, and law enforcement.[403]

Abusing parents have attacked these laws on a variety of grounds. In several cases, the constitutionality of interrogating the suspected abusers without first issuing Miranda warnings was challenged. In all cases, this argument was rejected.[404] An alleged abuser attacked as unconstitutionally vague a statute permitting an inference of neglect to be drawn where there is evidence of illness or injury to a child in the custody of a parent, guardian, or custodian who is unable to give satisfactory explanation for the illness or injury. Here, too, the statute was upheld.[405] A reporting statute was also upheld under a father's claim that it unconstitutionally infringed on his interest in seeking psychiatric help; there was no violation of his privilege against self-incrimination where the statute did not impose investigative duties on the psychiatrist and did not compel him to reveal details given by the patient.[406]

Some parents have tried to invoke the physician-patient privilege to shield themselves from the effects of disclosure. This argument has been rejected on grounds that the policy considerations underlying the reporting statutes trump those justifying the doctor-patient privilege.[407] In Alaska, however, a clinical psychologist successfully invoked the privilege between himself and his child-molesting client, despite a reporting law abrogating the privilege, because the abrogation applied only to child protection proceedings instituted to identify and protect victims, and not to criminal proceedings resulting from a report of abuse. (The decision did not require any answer to the question whether the psychologist's client could have invoked the privilege.)[408] In California, communication between psychotherapist and defendant-patient was privileged, where the information that could be gleaned was mere repeated data already obtained from the victim.[409] With few exceptions, then, the courts have upheld reporting statutes.

Notwithstanding the existence and validity of these laws, many cases of child abuse are believed to go unreported, as noted earlier. Numerous reasons have been proffered to explain this phenomenon.

Until relatively recent times, of course, the battered child syndrome was not recognized even by medical specialists.[410] The common law imposed no duty to report, even when the syndrome was recognized[411] and, as noted, the diagnosis is not always clear to the clinician[412] and the legal definition may vary with the jurisdiction.[413]

Physicians knowledgeable about child abuse suspect that reporting may make the parents both more abusive and more reluctant to seek further medical care for their child in the future.[414] Hence, unless it is possible to hospitalize the patient long enough to ensure that a satisfactory foster home for the victim or effective counseling for the parents can be secured, the doctor might be justified in concluding it is in the child's best interest not to report. The physician may anticipate that the child will remain in the parents' care, despite their abuse, as often happens in all but the most egregious cases. The doctor may conclude that the best hope for serving the child is to maintain good rapport with the parents and work to prevent recurrences privately without the intervention of the authorities. The physician may also hesitate to report questionable cases so as not to contribute to the undeserved but heartfelt guilt of blameless parents whose children's injuries are unrelated to abuse.[415]

Some doctors may be unwilling to believe that parents could willfully injure their own child.[416] Other practitioners may remain silent from a misplaced loyalty to confidentiality, failing to recognize that the patient is not the parent but the child. Some may simply not know correct reporting procedure.[417] Some doctors may fear the economic consequences of antagonizing the patient's parents who, if not patients themselves, are at least the minor patient's financial guarantors. Parents may also be willing and able to harm the doctor's reputation in the community by claiming that he or she has made terrible and unwarranted accusations about them.[418]

One powerful reason physicians fail to report cases of abuse may be a fear of civil liability for doing so. Many may be unaware that, as noted above, under the reporting statutes in effect at the time of this printing in all U.S. jurisdictions, they enjoy immunity from suit even if they misdiagnose child abuse.[419] This immunity has been upheld under state constitutional due process attack.[420] A physician may not be able to rely on such a statutory grant of immunity, however, if he or she informs some person or agency of his or her suspicions, but fails to report the suspected child abuse in the manner required by law. In a 1992 California case, *Searcy v. Auerbach*,[421] a child's mother was allowed to sue a psychologist for libel, professional negligence, and intentional, as well as negligent, infliction of emotional distress after he told her ex-husband in writing that he suspected her child was abused while in her custody. Merely telling the father, who related the suspicions to Texas authorities, did not comply with the California statute and, therefore, no immunity attached.

Similarly, in Missouri a physician could not rely on the immunity granted under a child abuse reporting statute because he reported the abuse he erroneously suspected to the police, not to the Division of Family Services as required by the statute.[422]

Even where a doctor is quite confident of a diagnosis of child abuse, he or she may fail to report because of the "threat of mere possibility of legal entanglement."[423] It has been argued that immunity provisions are unnecessary because such causes of action as defamation, malicious prosecution, or breach of confidence are all defeated by a showing of good faith.[424] The weakness of this argument is apparent, however, because physicians are unlikely to be aware of the effectiveness and availability of this defense and because, even if they were so aware, they might still dread the possible need to mount a defense at all.[425]

In general, doctors are probably also unaware that in at least 42 states, a failure to report child abuse can result in criminal prosecution.[426] As a rule, such failures are classified as misdemeanors,[427] and criminal penalties have been criticized because the symptoms of battered child syndrome may be subtle.[428] A search of state cases reveals no criminal prosecutions for failure to report, however.[429] It is unlikely that misprision of a felony remains viable as a theory on which to ground criminal prosecution for nonreporting.[430]

On the other hand, some commentators have claimed that mandatory reporting laws are meaningless if toothless, that sanctions make it easier for the physician to placate parents irate about mistaken reporting, and that even small penalties create a stigma doctors would seek to avoid.[431] Considering the rarity of criminal actions against nonreporting doctors, however, these arguments seem, at least at present, to have more theoretical appeal than practical value.

Allegedly negligent failure to report. Rarely have malpractice claims been reported in which the theory of liability was negligent failure to report child abuse (as opposed to negligent diagnosis and/or reporting as was alleged in *Searcy v. Auerbach*[432]). In *Landeros v. Flood*,[433] however, the California Supreme Court held that such a theory stated a cause of action under California law. In *Landeros*, an 11-month-old girl was brought to codefendant hospital for diagnosis and treatment of a comminuted spiral fracture of her right tibia and fibula, for which the mother could offer no explanation. The child demonstrated numerous bruises and abrasions and, unbeknownst to the defendant examining doctor, a nondepressed linear skull fracture as well. Although the physician properly set the child's leg, he failed to diagnose and report child abuse. The patient was released to the care of her parents, who inflicted multiple subsequent injuries, including human bites and second- and third-degree burns sufficient to render likely the loss of use or the amputation of her left hand. Later, the child's new foster parents sued both doctor and hospital for negligence for failing to report the case on initial presentation, on theories of common law negligence, noncompliance with the penal code section requiring reports of injuries related to any violation of state law, and noncompliance with the child abuse reporting statutes.[434]

The Supreme Court of California held that plaintiff was entitled—although because of the reporting statute, not required[435]—to show by expert testimony that the standard of care at the time of the events in the case included reporting and that, therefore, the trial court was in error in sustaining defendant's demurrer on this issue.[436] The court rejected defendant's theory that the parents' later beating of the patient was a superseding cause absolving defendant of responsibility because, if such beatings were reasonably foreseeable they would not give rise to a defense.[437] The court held further that plaintiff was entitled to show noncompliance with the reporting statutes to raise a presumption of failure to exercise due care as an alternative legal theory to common law negligence.[438] Hence, in California, a doctor who negligently fails to report a suspected case of child abuse may be found liable in a civil action. The California court did indicate, however, that to establish criminal liability, one must show that the physician was actually aware of the child abuse, so that the failure to report is not merely negligent, but willful.[439] There is at least one other unreported California case in which negligence per se was alleged against the defendant physician for breach of statutory duty to report, but the $5 million suit was settled out of court for $600,000.[440]

The few reported cases since *Landeros* have adopted a different position on the issue of civil liability for failure to report child abuse. The Georgia and Minnesota courts of appeals have held that no private right of action is created by their respective child abuse reporting statutes. Accordingly, they have refused to allow civil suits against doctors. In *Cechman v. Travis,*[441] an administratrix sued a hospital and treating physicians on behalf of a deceased child who was killed by her abusive father after being treated at the defendant institution. Although a criminal statute required that a licensed physician report suspected cases of child abuse, the court held that the statute created no private right of action in tort, in favor of an abused victim.[442] Furthermore, the doctor had no common law legal duty to protect the child from the father, thus no common law medical malpractice claim would lie.[443]

Likewise, in *Valtakis v. Putnam,*[444] the Minnesota Court of Appeals held that Minnesota's Child Abuse Reporting Act did not create a private right of action. The case involved a suit against a psychologist and others for failure to make a proper report of a child's sexual abuse. The victim alleged that Minnesota Statute Section 626.556 created two penalties—a misdemeanor sanction as well as a civil suit.[445] The court disagreed. The court found that (1) the defendants had complied with the statute; (2) "no common law duty existed before the statute was enacted"; and (3) a reading of the statutory language revealed that no such right of action was either expressly or impliedly created.[446]

In *Marcelletti v. Bathani,*[447] the Michigan Court of Appeals likewise declined to extend a private right of action to an injured infant, despite clear statutory language creating civil liability for failure to report suspected child abuse. In *Marcelletti,* the injured infant sued a physician, Dr. Bathani, for failing to report the abuse of another unrelated child by a babysitter common to both children. The court refused to extend a right of action to the plaintiff because the statute provided an action for civil liability only to a child whose harm was proximately caused by a failure to report. The court found that the Marcelletti infant's injury was not proximately caused by failure of the defendant to report the abuse of another unrelated child.[448] Moreover, ruled the court, no common law duty existed in Michigan that would support a civil action against Dr. Bathani.[449] The ability to sue, where otherwise appropriate, was a creature of statute only.

Despite *Landeros,* the more recent decisions suggest that in the absence of explicit statutory authorization, the courts may be reluctant to extend a private right of action to plaintiffs alleging harm from failure to comply with reporting statutes.

State liability

Agencies charged with responsibility for placement of foster children have in some cases been held liable under the reporting statutes for abuse by the foster parents they have selected, where the agencies knew or should have known of the abuse.[450] Some courts have found an affirmative obligation under the Fourteenth Amendment to protect or to intervene on behalf of a known or suspected child abuse victim where a special custodial relationship is created or assumed by governmental agencies.[451] Another court, ruling that a child confined to a state mental health facility has a substantive due process liberty interest in reasonably safe living conditions, found a violation of that interest where foster parents with whom the state had placed the child severely injured him and the state failed to intervene.[452] Where, however, a child is abused by his father while in the father's custody, a county agency is under no duty to protect the child, even though it knew of the abuse, as the state had played no part in the creation of the dangers the child faced, nor had it done anything to render the child any more vulnerable to such dangers.[453] That the state had once taken temporary custody of the child did not alter this conclusion, since in returning the child to his father's custody it placed him in a position no worse than that in which he would have been had it not acted at all.[454]

The writers wish to acknowledge the assistance of the following individuals at McGuire, Woods, Battle & Boothe, L.L.P., all of whom helped in various ways to prepare the manuscript: Thomas E. Spahn, Esq., Linda B. Hallion, Dolores J. Marshall, Paulette M. Johnson, and Patricia B. Holland.

END NOTES

1. Office of the Attorney General of the State of Utah, No. 84-77, Slip Opinion (Dec. 28, 1984); *see also People ex rel. O'Connel v. Turner,* 55 Ill. 280 (1870).
2. *Prince v. Massachusetts,* 321 U.S. 158, 166, *reh'g denied,* 321 U.S. 804 (1944).
3. *Lacey v. Laird,* 139 N.E.2d 25, 30 (Ohio 1956); *see also Potter v. Thomas,* 164 N.Y.S. 923 (1917).
4. *Burton v. Brooklyn Doctors' Hosp.,* 88 A.D.2d 217, 452 N.Y.S.2d 857 (N.Y.A.D. 1st Dept. 1982).
5. *E.g., In re Guardianship of Barry,* 445 So.2d 365 (Fla. App. 1984).
6. *Friedrichsen v. Niemotka,* 177 A.2d 58 (N.J. Super. 1962).
7. *See, e.g.,* Ga. Code Ann. §31-9-6 (Supp. 1979); *see also* Section on Abortion, *infra; see also, Zimmerman v. N.Y.C. Health and Hosp. Corp.,* 458 N.Y.S.2d 552 (N.Y.A.D. 1983).
8. *Rishworth v. Moss,* 191 S.W. 843 Tex. Civ. App. 1917), *aff'd,* 222 S.W. 225 (Tex. Comm. App. 1920).
9. The term 'in loco parentis' is a common law phrase, determined by courts of equity to cover various situations where . . . parental rights and duties should attach to a person not a blood relative of the child." Utah Attorney General Opinion Nos. 84-77, *supra* note 1.
10. *Reiser v. Lohner,* 641 P.2d 93 (Utah 1982), *rev'd on other grounds, Johnson v. Rogers,* 763 P.2d 771 (Utah 1988); *see also Haven v. Randolph,* 342 F. Supp. 538 (D.D.C. 1992), *aff'd,* 494 F.2d 1069 (D.C. Cir. 1974).
11. *Wells v. Van Nort,* 125 N.E. 910 (Ohio 1919); *accord Estate of Leach v. Shapiro,* 469 N.E.2d 1047 (Ohio Ct. App. 1984).
12. *Zimmerman, supra* note 7, at 553.
13. *Id.*

14. *Bakker v. Welsh,* 108 N.W. 94 (Mich. 1906); *accord Younts v. St. Francis Hosp. & School of Nursing, Inc.,* 469 P.2d 330 (Kan. 1970).

15. *Flores v. Flushing Hosp. & Medical Ctr.,* 490 N.Y.S.2d 770, 772 (App. Div. 1985).

16. *Zoski v. Gaines,* 260 N.W. 99 (Mich. 1935).

17. *Bonner v. Moran,* 126 F.2d 121, (D.C. Cir. 1941).

18. *Id.*

19. *Id.* at 123.

20. *In re Richardson,* 284 So.2d 185 (La. App. 4 Cir. 1973).

21. *Id.* at 187.

22. *Id.* at 186.

23. *In re Guardianship of Pescinski,* 226 N.W.2d 180 (Wis. 1975).

24. *Strunk v. Strunk,* 445 S.W.2d 145 (Ky. App. 1969); *see also* M. Anderson, *Encouraging Bone Marrow Transplants from Unrelated Donors: Some Proposed Solutions to a Pressing Social Problem,* 54 U. Pitt. L. Rev. 477 at n. 149 (Winter 1993).

25. Compare *In re Richardson, supra* note 20.

26. *Strunk, supra* note 24.

27. *Hart v. Brown,* 368, 289 A.2d 386 (Conn. Super. Ct. 1972); *but see Curran v. Bosze,* 566 N.E.2d 1319 (Ill. 1990).

28. *Id.* at 389.

29. *Id.* at 390.

30. *Id.*

31. *Id.* at 391.

32. *Little v. Little,* 576 S.W.2d 493 (Tex. Civ. App. 1979).

33. *Id.* at 498.

34. *See, e.g., Care & Protection of Beth,* 587 N.E.2d 1377 (Mass. 1992).

35. *Custody of a Minor,* 379 N.E.2d 1053, 1065 (Mass. 1978); *see also City Bank Farmer's Trust Co. v. McGowan,* 323 U.S. 594 (1945).

36. *In re C.A.,* 603 N.E.2d 1171, 1180 (Ill. Ct. App. 1993).

37. *Rosebush v. Oakland County Prosecution,* 491 N.W.2d 633, 639 (Mich. App. 1992); *see also Custody of a Minor,* 393 N.E.2d 836 (1979).

38. *Custody of a Minor, supra* note 35, at 1065; *but see* Robertson, *Is 'Substituted Judgment' a Valid Legal Concept?,* 5 Issues in L. & Med. 197 (1989).

39. *Custody of a Minor, supra* note 35.

40. *Custody of a Minor, supra* note 35, at 1061, 1062.

41. *Bonner, supra* note 17; *Younts, supra* note 14. *See* Uniform Law Commissioners' Model Health-Care Consent Act §2.

42. *Bonner, supra* note 17, at 123.

43. *State v. F.L.A.,* 608 P.2d 12 (Alaska 1980).

44. *See, e.g.,* Utah Code Ann. §15-2-5 and §26-6-18 (1953), (1986 vol.); Ark. Stat. Ann. §20-16-508 (1993).

45. Office of the Attorney General of the State of Utah, *supra* note 1.

46. Ark. Stat. Ann. §20-9-603 (1993).

47. *Rogers v. Sells,* 61 P.2d 1018 (Okla. 1936); *see also Miller v. Rhode Island Hosp.,* 625 A.2d 778, 782 (R.I. 1993).

48. *Luka v. Lowrie,* 136 N.W. 1106, 1110-11 (Mich. 1912).

49. *Jackovach v. Yocom,* 237 N.W. 444, 449 (Iowa 1931); *accord Wells v. McGehee,* 39 So.2d 196 (La. App. 1949).

50. *See, e.g., Jackovach,* 237 N.W. 444; *see also Luka, supra* note 48.

51. *Luka, supra* note 48, at 1110.

52. *Sullivan v. Montgomery,* 279 N.Y.S. 575, 578 (N.Y. 1935); *Wells, supra* note 49.

53. *Tabor v. Scobee,* 254 S.W.2d 474 (Ky. 1951); *see also Dewes v. Indian Health Serv., Public Health Serv.,* 504 F. Supp. 203 (D.S.D. 1980).

54. *Younts v. St. Francis Hosp. and School of Nursing,* 469 P.2d 330 (Kan. 1970).

55. *Id.* at 338.

56. *Id.* at 337.

57. *Lacey v. Laird,* 139 N.E.2d 25 (Ohio 1956).

58. *Gulf & S.I.R. Co. v. Sullivan,* 119 So. 501 (Miss. 1928).

59. *Smith v. Seibly,* 431 P.2d 719 (Wash. 1967); *see also Bach v. Long Island Jewish Hosp.* 267 N.Y.S.2d 289 (1966).

60. *Belcher v. Charleston Area Med. Center,* 422 S.E.2d 827 (W.Va. 1992).

61. *H.B. v. Wilkinson,* 639 F. Supp. 952 (D. Utah 1986) (Utah law); *see also* Section on Abortion, *infra.*

62. *E.g., Michaelis v. Schori,* 24 Cal. Rptr. 2d 380 (Ct. App. 2nd Dist. 1993); *see also Bishop v. Shurley,* 211 N.W. 75 (Mich. 1926); *see also Greenspan v. Slate,* 97 A.2d 390 (N.J. 1953); *Osborn v. Weatherford,* 170 So. 95 (Ala. App. 1936).

63. *Baird v. Attorney General,* 360 N.E.2d 288 (Mass. 1977).

64. *In re Roger S.,* 569 P.2d 1286, 1288 (Cal. 1977).

65. *Id.*

66. *Osgood v. District of Columbia,* 567 F. Supp. 1026 (D.D.C. 1983); *see also Cruz v. Bento,* 405 U.S. 319 (1972) (adult case). *In re E.G.,* 549 N.E.2d 322 (Ill. 1989).

67. *See, e.g.,* Or. Rev. Stat. §109.640 (1992); *see also* Idaho Code §39-4304 (Supp. 1976), Ala. Code §22-8-3 (1975).

68. *Smith, supra* note 59, at 723. *See also L.R. v. Hansen,* Civ. No. C-80-0078J (2880) (Dist. Ct. of Utah, unpublished).

69. Opinion of the Attorney General of Utah, *supra* note 1.

70. *Id.*

71. *See, e.g.,* Ala. Code §22-8-7 (1993).

72. *In Interest of E.G.,* 549 N.E.2d 322 (1989).

73. *Id.*

74. *Jackovach,* 237 N.W. 444.

75. *Wells, supra* note 49.

76. *Younts, supra* note 54.

77. *See, e.g., People v. Pierson,* 68 N.E. 243 (1903); *but see Justice v. State,* 42 S.E. 1013 (Ga. 1902).

78. *In re Jensen,* 633 P.2d 1302 (Or. App.), *review denied,* 639 P.2d 1280 (Or. 1981).

79. *Custody of a Minor,* N.E.2d at 843. *See also Belcher v. Charleston Med. Center,* 422 S.E.2d 827 (W. Va. 1992).

80. *Morrison v. State,* 252 S.W.2d 97, 103 (Mo. App. 1952).

81. *Prince, supra* note 2.

82. *Cantwell v. Connecticut,* 310 U.S. 296, 303-304 (1940).

83. *Reynolds v. U.S.,* 98 U.S. 145, 166 (1878); *see also Davis v. Beason,* 133 U.S. 333, 342-343, (1890).

84. *Prince, supra* note 2.

85. *Hamilton v. Regents of the Univ. of Calif.,* 293 U.S. 245 (1934), *reh'g denied,* 293 U.S. 633 (1935).

86. *State v. Massey,* 51 S.E.2d 179 (N.C.), *appeal dismissed for want of a substantial federal question, sub. nom., Bunn v. North Carolina,* 336 U.S. 942 (1949).

87. *Christian Science Church Loses First Civil Suit on Wrongful Death of a Child,* 270 JAMA 1781 (Oct. 20, 1993).

88. *Id.*

89. *Id.; Christian Science Church Wins Judgment Reduction,* St. Louis Post Dispatch, March 19, 1994, § News, at 05A; *see also Christian Scientists Sued in Death Child's Mother Says Son Would Have Lived With Treatment,* St. Paul Pioneer Press (ST), Dec. 17, 1993, § Metro, at 8C.

90. *Pierce v. Society of Sisters,* 268 U.S. 510, 535 (1925).

91. *Meyer v. Nebraska,* 262 U.S. 390 (1923).

92. *Wisconsin v. Yoder,* 406 U.S. 205 (1972).

93. *State v. Koome,* 530 P.2d 260, 263 (Wash. 1975); *but see Bellotti v. Baird,* 443 U.S. 622, *reh'g denied,* 444 U.S. 887 (1979).

94. *Planned Parenthood v. Danforth,* 428 U.S. 52, 74 S. Ct. 2831 49 L.Ed.2d (1976).

95. *Milonas v. Williams,* 691 F.2d 931, 943 (10th Cir. 1982), *cert. denied,* 460 U.S. 1069 (1983); *see also Parham v. J.R.,* 442 U.S. 584 (1979).

96. *Custody of a Minor,* 434 N.E.2d 601 (Mass. 1982).

97. 380 N.E.2d 134 (Mass. Ct. App. 1978).

98. *In re Dinnerstein, Matter of Spring*, 405 N.E.2d 115 (Mass. 1980).

99. *Custody of a Minor, supra* note 96, at 608.

100. *Id.*

101. *Superintendent of Belchertown State School v. Saikewicz*, 370 N.E.2d 417 (Mass. 1977).

102. *Custody of a Minor, supra* note 96, at 609 (citing *In re Dinnerstein*, 380 N.E.2d 134 (Mass. App. 1980)). *Compare In re Baby K*, 1994 WL 38674 (4th Cir. 1994).

103. *Id.* at 610.

104. *People v. Pierson*, 68 N.E. 243, 244 (N.Y. 1903); *see also Owens v. State*, 116 P. 345 (Okla. Cr. 1911); *see also People v. Edwards*, 249 N.Y.S.2d 325 (N.Y. Co. Ct. 1964); *see, e.g., In re Carstairs*, 115 N.Y.S.2d 314 (N.Y. Dom. Rel. Ct. 1952).

105. *See, e.g.,* Ala. Code §12-15-1(10) (1993); *see also Jehovah's Witnesses v. King Co. Hosp. Unit No. 1*, 278 F. Supp. 488 (W.D. Wash. 1967), *aff'd*, 390 U.S. 598, *reh'g denied*, 391 U.S. 961 (1968).

106. *See, e.g., Heinemann's Appeal*, 96 Pa. 112, 42 Am. Rep. 532 (Ct. App. 1880); *see also Mitchell v. Davis*, 205 S.W.2d 812 (Tex. Civ. App. 1947).

107. *In re Marsh*, 14 A.2d 368 (Pa. Super. Ct. 1940).

108. *Jefferson v. Griffin Spalding County Hosp. Auth.*, 274 S.E.2d 457 (Ga. 1981).

109. *State v. Perricone*, 181 A.2d 751 (N.J.), *cert. denied*, 371 U.S. 890 (1962); *In re Santos*, 227 N.Y.S.2d 450 (N.Y.A.D. 1 Dept.), *appeal dismissed*, 185 N.E.2d 552 (N.Y. 1962).

110. *Custody of a Minor*, 393 N.E.2d 836, 846 (Mass. 1979); *but see Newmark v. Williams*, 588 A.2d 1108 (Del. 1991).

111. *Perricone, supra* note 109, at 757; *see also Levitsky v. Levitsky*, 190 A.2d 621 (Md. 1963); *but see Osier v. Osier*, 410 A.2d 1027 (Me. 1980).

112. *Matter of Hamilton*, 657 S.W.2d 425 (Tenn. App. 1983).

113. *Wallace v. Labrenz*, 104 N.E.2d 769 (Ill. 1952).

114. *Id.* at 773.

115. *See, e.g., In re Eric B.*, 235 Cal. Rptr. 22 (Cal. App. 1987), *review denied*.

116. *Id.* The court need not "hold its protective power in abeyance until harm to a minor child is not only threatened but actual. The purpose of dependency proceedings is to prevent risk, not ignore it." *Id.* at 26. *See also In re Ivey*, 319 So. 2d 53 (Fla. App. 1975); *see also Matter of Jensen*, 633 P.2d 1302 (Or. App.), *review denied*, 639 P.2d 1280 (Or. 1981).

117. *People v. Arnold*, 426 P.2d 515 (Cal. 1967).

118. *State v. Miskimens*, 490 N.E.2d 931 (Ohio Com. Pl. 1984).

119. *E.g., In re Application of Cicero*, 421 N.Y.S.2d 965 (N.Y. Sup. 1979).

120. *See, e.g., Newmark*, 588 A.2d 1108; *In re Frank*, 248 P.2d 553 (Wash. 1952).

121. *In re Gonzales*, 323, N.E.2d 42, 46-47 (Ill. App. 1974); *see also People in the Interest of D.L.E.*, 614 P.2d 873 (Colo. 1980).

122. *State v. Chenoweth*, 71 N.E. 197 (Ind. 1904); *see also Stehr v. State*, 139 N.W. 676 (Neb. 1913), *aff'd*, 142 N.W. 670 (1913); *see also Beck v. State*, 233 P. 495 (Okla. Cr. 1925); *see also People v. Vogel*, 242 P.2d 969 (Cal. App. 4th Dist. 1952); *see also State v. Dumlao*, 491 A.2d 404 (Conn. App. 1985); *see also State v. Clark*, 261 A.2d 294 (Conn. Cir. A.D. 1969); *see also State v. Staples*, 148 N.W. 283 (Minn. 1914); *see also State v. Beach*, 329 S.W.2d 712 (Mo. 1959); *see also State v. Watson*, 71 A. 1113 (N.J. Sup. 1909); *see also Commonwealth v. Barnhart*, 497 A.2d 616 (Pa. Super. 1985), *appeal denied*, 538 A.2d 874 (Pa.), *cert. denied*, 488 U.S. 817, (1988); *see also People v. Edwards*, 249 N.Y.S.2d 325 (N.Y. Co. Ct. 1964); *see also State v. Barnes*, 212 S.W. 100 (Tenn. 1918); *see also Oakley v. Jackson*, 1 K.B. 216 (1914); *see also Rex. v. Lewis*, 6 Ont.

L. 132 1BRC 732-CA (1903). *See Nozza v. State*, 288 So. 2d 560 (Fla. App.), variously designated "involuntary," *Barnhart*, 497 A.2d 616; *Faunteroy v. U.S.*, 413 A.2d 1294 (D.C. App. 1980); *State v. Zobel*, 134 N.W.2d 101 (S.D. 1965), *cert. denied*, 382 U.S. 833, (1965), *overruled on other grounds, State v. Waff*, 373 N.W.2d 18 (S.D. 1985).

123. *See* cases cited *supra* n. 122.

124. *Bradley v. State*, 84 So. 677, 679 (Fla. 1920); *see also Singleton v. State*, 35 So. 2d 375 (Ala. 1948); *see also Craig v. State*, 155 A.2d 684 (Md. 1959); *see also People v. Osborn*, 508 N.Y.S.2d 746 (N.Y. 1986); *see also People v. Northrup*, 442 N.Y.S.2d 658 (N.Y. 1981).

125. *State v. Watson*, 71 A. 1113, 1114 (N.J. 1909); *see also State v. Osmus*, 276 P.2d 469 (Wyo. 1954); *but see Eaglen v. State*, 231 N.E.2d 147 (Ind. 1967) and *State v. Williams*, 484 P.2d 1167 (Wash. App. 1971); *see also Howell v. State*, 350 S.E.2d 473 (Ga. App. 1986); *see also Justice v. State*, 42 S.E. 1013 (Ga. 1902); *see also People v. Markel*, 129 N.W.2d 894 (Mich. 1964); *see also State v. Shouse*, 186 S.W. 1064 (Mo. 1916). *See also Matter of Appeal in Chochise County*, Juvenile Action No. 5666-J, 650 P.2d 459 (Ariz. 1981). *But see State v. Clark*, 261 A.2d 294 (Conn. 1969). Occasionally, a causation defense succeeds, *Bradley*, 84 So. 677, as may a procedural defense. *People v. Arnold*, 426 P.2d 515 (Cal. 1967).

126. *Parens patriae* empowers the state to "care for infants within its jurisdiction and to protect them from neglect, abuse, and fraud . . . That ancient, equitable jurisdiction was codified in our Juvenile Court Act, which expressly authorized the court, if circumstances warrant, to remove the child from the custody of its [sic] parents and awards its [sic] custody to an appointed guardian." *Wallace*, 104 N.E.2d at 773.

127. *In re Weberlist*, 360 N.Y.S.2d 783, 786 (N.Y. 1974).

128. *Hawaii v. Standard Oil Co.*, 405 U.S. 251, 257 (1972).

129. *Morrison v. State*, 252 S.W.2d 97, 102 (Mo. App. 1952).

130. *In re Commissioner of Social Servs.*, 339 N.Y.S.2d 89 (N.Y. Fam. Ct. 1972); *see also Weberlist*, 360 N.Y.S.2d 783; *In re Taner*, 549 P.2d 702 (Utah 1976). *See, e.g., People v. Sorensen*, 437 P.2d 495 (Cal. 1968); *see also Karen T. v. Michael T.*, 484 N.Y.S.2d 780 (N.Y. 1985); *see also Wener v. Wener*, 312 N.Y.S.2d 815 (N.Y. 1970). *But see, Pamela P. v. Frank S.*, 443 N.Y.S.2d 343 (N.Y. 1981).

131. *Browning v. Hoffman*, 111 S.E. 492 (W. Va. 1922).

132. *See, e.g., Commissioner of Social Serv., supra* note 130; *Weberlist, supra* note 127; and *Taner, supra* note 130.

133. *Weberlist*, 360 N.Y.S.2d 783. *See generally* n. 36, *supra*, and associated text.

134. *In re Sampson*, 317 N.Y.S.2d 641, 658 (N.Y. Ct. 1970), *aff'd*, 323 N.Y.S.2d 253 (N.Y.A.D. 3 Dept.), *appeal denied*, 275 N.E.2d 339 (N.Y. 1971).

135. *Weber v. Stoney Brook Hosp.*, 467 N.Y.S.2d 685, 686-687 (N.Y. 1983).

136. *Custody of a Minor (No. 3)*, 393 N.E.2d 836; *see also In re Clark*, 185 N.E.2d 128 (Ohio Ct. Com. Pleas 1962); *Wallace, supra* note 113; *Morrison*, 252 S.W.2d 97; *In re Eric B.*, 189 Cal. App. 3d 996.

137. *Matter of Vasko*, 263 N.Y.S. 552 (N.Y. 1933).

138. *Office of Attorney General of St. of Utah. No. 81-57, Slip Opinion (Dec. 14, 1981)*.

139. *Matter of Rotkowitz*, 25 N.Y.S.2d 624 (N.Y. Dom. Rel. Ct. 1941).

140. *In re Karwath*, 199 N.W.2d 147, 150 (Iowa 1972).

141. *In re Seiferth*, 127 N.E.2d 820 (N.Y. 1955); *see also In re Gregory S.*, 380 N.Y.S.2d 620 (1976); *In re Gregory S.*, 245 N.W.2d 183 (N.Y. Fam. Ct. 1976); *In re Welfare of Price*, 535 P.2d 475 (Wash. App. 1975); *In re Ray*, 408 N.Y.S.2d 737 (N.Y. Fam. Ct. 1978); *In re J.M.P.*, 669 S.W.2d 298 (Mo. App. 1984).

142. *Sampson*, 317 N.Y.S.2d 641.

143. *Snyder v. Holy Cross Hosp.*, 352 A.2d 334 (Md. App. 1976).

144. *In re Hudson*, 126 P.2d 765 (Wash. 1942); *accord Custody of a Minor*, 379 N.E.2d 1053 (Mass. 1978).

145. *Custody of a Minor*, 379 N.E.2d at 1062.

146. *Seiferth, supra* note 141, at 822.

147. *In re Hudson*, 126 P.2d at 778; *see also* Wash. Rev. Code Ann. §26.440.020 (West Supp. 1982). *See* Comment, *Relief for the Neglected Child: Court-Ordered Medical Treatment in Non-Emergency Situations*, 22 Santa Clara L. Rev. 471 (1982).

148. *In re Hofbauer*, 393 N.E.2d 1009 (1979).

149. *Id.* at 1013.

150. *Id.*

151. *Id.* at 1014.

152. *Custody of a Minor*, 393 N.E.2d 836.

153. *In re Karwath*, 199 N.W.2d 147.

154. *Id.* at 149.

155. *Id.* at 150.

156. *Id.*

157. *State v. Board*, 81 N.E. 568, 569 (Ohio 1907).

158. *De Aryan v. Butler*, 260 P.2d 98, 102, (Cal. App.), *cert. denied*, 347 U.S. 1012 (1953).

159. *See, e.g., McCartney v. Austin*, 293 N.Y.S.2d 188 (N.Y. Sup. 1969), *aff'd*, 298 N.Y.S.2d 26 (N.Y.A.D. 1969); *In re Elwell*, 284 N.Y.S.2d 924 (N.Y. Fam. Ct. 1967); *State v. Board of Educ.*, 204 N.E.2d 86 (Ohio Ct. App. 1963); *State ex. rel. Dunham v. Board of Educ.*, 96 N.E.2d 413 (Ohio 1951).

160. *Hagler v. Larner*, 120 N.E. 575 (Ill. 1918); *Hill v. Bickers*, 188 S.W. 766 (Ky. 1916); *State ex rel. Freeman v. Zimmerman*, 90 N.W. 783 (Minn. 1902); *City of New Braunfels v. Waldschmidt*, 207 S.W. 303 (Tex. 1918); *see also Rhea v. Board of Educ.*, 171 N.W. 103 (N.D. 1919).

161. *McSween v. Board of School Trustees*, 129 S.W. 206 (Tex. Civ. App. 1910).

162. *State ex rel. Mack v. Board of Educ.*, 204 N.E.2d 86 (Ohio App. 1963).

163. *Jacobson v. Massachusetts*, 197 U.S. 11 (1905).

164. *Id.* at 29.

165. *Id.* at 30, 39.

166. *See, e.g., French v. Davidson*, 77 P. 663 (Cal. 1904); *Abeel v. Clarke*, 24 P. 383 (Cal. 1890); *Bissell v. Davison*, 32 A. 348 (Conn. 1894); *Hagler v. Larner*, 120 N.E. 575 (Ill. 1918); *Board of Ed. v. Maas*, 152 A.2d 394 (N.J. Super. 1959), *aff'd*, 158 A.2d 330 (N.J. 1960); *Sadlock v. Board of Ed.*, 58 A.2d 218 (N.J. 1948); *State v. Board of Ed.*, 81 N.E. 568 (Ohio 1907); *Field v. Robinson*, 48 A. 873 (Pa. 1901); *Commonwealth v. Pear*, 66 N.E.2d 719 (Mass. 1903); *State ex. rel. Cox v. Board of Ed.*, 60 P. 1013 (Utah 1900); *see also Application of Ritterbaud*, 562 N.Y.S.2d 605 (N.Y. Sup. 1990).

167. *Maas, supra* note 166.

168. Examples include chiropractors (*Mosier v. Barren County Bd. of Health*, 215 S.W.2d 967 (Ky. 1948)) and members of the General Assembly and Church of the First Born (*Mannis v. State ex. rel. Dewitt School Dist. No. 1*, 398 S.W.2d 206 (Ark. 1966)); *see also Wright v. Dewitt School Dist.*, 385 S.W.2d 644 (Ark. 1965); *State ex. rel. Dunham v. Board of Ed.*, 96 N.E.2d 413 (Ohio 1951). *See also Mannis v. State*, 398 S.W.2d 206 (Ark. 1960).

169. *Maas, supra* note 166, at 407-408.

170. *Sadlock, supra* note 159.

171. *People v. Pierson*, 68 N.E.243 (N.Y. 1903); *accord In re Whittmore*, 47 N.Y.S.2d 143 (N.Y. 1944); *Wright, supra* note 168; *Cude v. State*, 377 S.W.2d 816 (Ark. 1964).

172. *Staffle v. San Antonio*, 201 S.W. 413, 415 (Tex. Civ. App. 1918).

173. *Maas, supra* note 166; *see also McCartney*, 293 N.Y.S.2d 188; *Elwell, supra* note 159.

174. *Dalli v. Board of Educ.*, 267 N.E.2d 219, 223 (Mass. 1971); *accord Maier v. Besser*, 341 N.Y.S.2d 411 (N.Y. Sup. 1972); *see also Kolbeck v. Kramer*, 202 A.2d 889 (N.J. Super. Ct. 1964); *see also*

175. *Davis v. State*, 451 A.2d 107 (Md. 1982); *accord Campain v. Marlboro Cent. School Dist. Bd. of Educ.*, 526 N.Y.S.2d 658 (N.Y.A.D. 3 Dept. 1988).

176. *Itz v. Penick*, 493 S.W.2d 506 (Tex. 1973).

177. *Avard v. Dupuis*, 376 F. Supp. 479 (D.N.H. 1974).

178. *See, e.g., Zucht v. King*, 260 U.S. 174 (1922); *Duffield v. Williamsport School Dist.*, 29 A. 742 (Pa. 1894); *Hartman v. May*, 151 So. 737 (Miss. 1934); *State v. Hay*, 35 S.E. 459 (N.C. 1900); *McSween, supra* note 161.

179. *Maas, supra* note 166; *Mosier, supra* note 168; *Hartman, supra* note 177.

180. *Maas, supra* note 166, at 405; *Pierce v. Board of Educ.*, 219 N.Y.S.2d 519 (N.Y. Sup. 1961).

181. *State v. Drew*, 192 A. 629 (N.H. 1937).

182. *Seubold v. Ft. Smith Special School Dist.*, 237 S.W.2d 884 (Ark. 1961); *Wright*, 385 S.W.2d 644.

183. *Maas, supra* note 166, at 408; *accord Viemeister v. White*, 72 N.E. 97 (N.Y. 1904); *Blue v. Beach*, 56 N.E. 78 (Ind. 1900); *Hartman, supra* note 177; *McSween*, 129 S.W. 206 (Tex. Cir. App.); *Staffle*, 201 S.W. 413; *Zucht, supra* note 177; *City of New Braunfels v. Waldschmidt*, 207 S.W. 303 (Tex. 1918); *Freeman v. Zimmerman*, 90 N.W. 783 (Minn. 1902); *State v. Hay*, 35 S.E. 459 (N.C. 1900); *Bissel v. Davison*, 32 A. 348 (Conn. 1894); *Morris v. Columbus*, 30 S.E. 850 (Ga. 1898); *Duffield*, 29 A. 472 (Pa.).

184. *Hutchins v. Durham*, 49 S.E. 46 (N.C. 1904).

185. *State v. Dunham*, 93 N.E.2d 286 (Ohio 1950).

186. *Elwell, supra* note 159; *Cude*, 377 S.W.2d 816 (Ark.); *In re Marsh's Case*, 14 A.2d 368, 371 (Pa. Super. Ct. 1940); *Mannis*, 398 S.W.2d 206 (Ark.).

187. *Genesis* 9:4-5 (*quoted in Perricone, supra* note 109, at 756).

188. *Leviticus* 17:10-14 (*quoted in Morrison v. State*, 252 S.W.2d 97, 99 (Mo. App. 1952)).

189. *Leviticus* 3:17, 7:26, 27; *Deuteronomy* 12:23; 1*Chronicles* 11:16-19; 2 *Samuel* 23:15-17; *Acts* 15:28, 29, 21:25; 1 *Samuel* 14:32, 33 (*cited in Sampson*, 317 N.Y.S.2d at 646 (N.Y. Fam. Ct. 1970)).

190. *Perricone, supra* note 109; *Hoener v. Bertinato*, 171 A.2d 140 (N.J. Juv. & Dom. Rel. Ct. 1961).

191. *Hoener, supra* note 189, at 143.

192. *Morrison, supra* note 129, at 100.

193. *Harley v. Oliver*, 404 F. Supp. 450 (W.D. Ark. 1975); *see also Staelens v. Yake*, 432 F. Supp. 834 (N.D. Ill. 1977).

194. *Morrison, supra* note 129, at 102.

195. *In re Brooks' Estate*, 205 N.E.2d 435 (Ill. 1965).

196. *In re Green*, 292 A.2d 387, 392 (Pa. 1972), *aff'd*, 307 A.2d 279 (Pa. 1973).

197. *Application of President & Directors of Georgetown College Inc.*, 331 F.2d 1000, *reh'g denied*, 331 F.2d 1010 (D.C. Cir. 1964), *cert. denied*, 377 U.S. (918); *John F. Kennedy Memorial Hosp. v. Heston*, 279 A.2d 670 (N.J. 1971).

198. *Wallace, supra* note 113; *see also Application of Brooklyn Hosp.*, 258 N.Y.S.2d 621 (N.Y. Sup. 1965); *In re Clark*, 185 N.E.2d 128 (Ohio Ct. Com. Pleas 1962); *see also Perricone, supra* note 109.

199. *Clark, supra* note 197.

200. *Id.*

201. *Raleigh Fitkin-Paul Morgan Memorial Hosp. v. Anderson*, 201 A.2d 537 (N.J.), *cert. denied*, 377 U.S. 985 (1964).

202. *Clark, supra* note 197.

203. *Hoener, supra* note 189, at 143-144.

204. *Perricone, supra* note 109, at 759. *See also* notes 112-116, *supra*, and associated text.

205. *Perricone, supra* note 109.

206. *Id.* at 759.

207. *Jehovah's Witnesses v. King Co. Hosp. Unit No. 1*, 278 F. Supp. 488 (W.D. Wash. 1967), *aff'd* 390 U.S. 598, *reh'g denied*, 391 U.S. 961 (1968).

207. *Id.*

208. *Hoener, supra* note 189, at 143.

209. *People v. Pierson,* 68 N.E. 243 (N.Y. 1903).

210. *Muhlenberg Hosp. v. Patterson,* 320 A.2d 518 (N.J. Super. Ct. Law Div. 1974).

211. *In re Sampson,* 317 N.Y.S.2d 641 (N.Y. Fam. Ct. 1970), *aff'd,* 323 N.Y.S.2d 253 (N.Y.A.D. 3 Dept.), *app. denied,* 275 N.E.2d 339 (N.Y. 1971).

212. *Seiferth, supra* note 141.

213. *In re Sampson,* 278 N.E.2d 918 (N.Y. 1972); *see also Santos v. Goldstein,* 227 N.Y.S.2d 450 (N.Y.A.D. 1 Dept. 1962), *appeal dismissed,* 232 N.Y.S.2d 1026 (N.Y. 1962).

214. *In re Green,* 292 A.2d 387 (Pa. 1972), *appeal after remand,* 307 A.2d 279 (Pa. 1973).

215. *Id.* at 392. *Perricone, supra* note 109; *In re Hudson,* 126 P.2d 765 (Wash. 1942).

216. *Baby Boy Doe v. Mother Doe,* _____ U.S. _____, 114 S. Ct. 652 (1993).

217. *Skinner v. Oklahoma,* 316 U.S. 535, 541-543 (1942); *see also Loving v. Va.,* 388 U.S. 1 (1966); *Griswold v. Connecticut,* 381 U.S. 479 (1965); *but see City of Dallas v. Stanglin,* 159 109 S.Ct. (1989).

218. *Ruby v. Massey,* 452 F. Supp. 361, 368 (D. Conn. 1978); *Relf v. Weinberger,* 372 F. Supp. 1196 (D.D.C. 1974); *Conservatorship of Valerie N.,* 707 P.2d 760, 773, 774 (Cal. 1985); *In re A. W.,* 637 P.2d 366, 369-70 (Colo. 1981); *In re Grady,* 426 A.2d 467, 473, 474 (N.J. 1981).

219. *Smith v. Seibly,* 431 P.2d 719 (Wash. 1967). See n. 61, *supra,* and accompanying text. *But see Tabor v. Scobee,* 254 S.W.2d 474 (Ky. 1951). *See also Relf,* 372 F. Supp. 1196.

220. *See, e.g., In re Guardianship of Hayes,* 608 P.2d 635, 637 (Wash. 1980).

221. *See generally,* R. Cepko, *Involuntary Sterilization of Mentally Disabled Women,* 8 Berkeley Women's L.J. 122 (1993).

222. *Wade v. Bethesda Hosp.,* 337 F. Supp. 671, 673-4 (S.D. Ohio 1971), *motion denied,* 356 F. Supp. 380 (S.D. Ohio 1973); *Hudson v. Hudson,* 373 So.2d 310, 312 (Ala. 1979); *Guardianship of Tulley,* 146 Cal. Rptr. 266 (Cal. Ct. App. 1978), *cert. denied,* 440 U.S. 967 (1979); *Guardianship of Kemp,* 118 Cal. Rptr. 64, 66-67 (Cal. App. 1974); *Matter of S.C.E.,* 378 A.2d 144 (Del. Ch. 1977); *Holmes v. Powers,* 439 S.W.2d 579, 580 (Ky. Ct. App. 1968); *In re M.K.R.,* 515 S.W.2d 467, 470 (Mo. 1974); *Application of A.D.,* 394 N.Y.S.2d 139 (N.Y. Sur. 1977); *aff'd on other grds; In re Lambert,* No. 61-156 (Tenn. Ct. App. Oct. 29, 1976), *noted in* 44 Tenn. L. Rev. 879 (1977); *Frazier v. Levi,* 440 S.W.2d 393, 394 (Tex. Civ. App. 1969).

223. *See In re A. W.,* 637 P.2d 366, 374 n.18, citing *Wade v. Bethesda Hosp., supra* note 222; *Kemp, supra* note 222; *M.K.R., supra* note 222; and *Frazier, supra* note 222.

224. *In re C.D.M.,* 627 P.2d 607 (Alaska 1981); *In re A.W.,* 637 P.2d 607; *P.S. by Harbin v. W.S.,* 452 N.E.2d 969 (Ind. 1983), *vacating A.L. v. G.R.H.,* 325 N.E.2d 501 (Ind. Ct. App. 1975), *cert. denied,* 425 U.S. 936 (1976); *In re Penny N.,* 414 A.2d 541 (N.H. 1980); *In re Grady,* 426 A.2d 467; *In re Sallmaier,* 378 N.Y.S.2d 989, 991 (N.Y. Sup. Ct. 1976); *In re Simpson,* 180 N.E.2d 206, 208 (Ohio Prob. Ct. 1962); *In re Guardianship of Hayes,* 608 P.2d 635 (Wash.); *In re Guardianship of Eberhardy,* 307 N.W.2d 881 (Wis. 1981).

225. *See Hudson, supra* note 222, at 311, 312; *Tulley, supra* note 222, at 268; *S.C.E.,* 378 A.2d at 145; *M.K.R., supra* note 222, at 470-471; *Eberhardy, supra* note 224, at 885.

226. *See A.W., supra* note 224, at 369; *In re Moe,* 432 N.E.2d 712, 718-20 (Mass. 1982) (adult case); *Grady, supra* note 224, at 471; *In re Terwilliger,* 450 A.2d 1376, 1381 (Pa. Supr. Ct. 1982).

227. Following *Buck v. Bell,* 274 U.S. 200 (1927), "twenty states passed eugenical sterilization statutes in the ensuing ten years,

most of them clearly patterned after the Virginia law [upheld in *Buck*].

228. *Sparkman v. McFarlin,* 552 F.2d 172 (7th Cir. 1977), *rev'd, sub nom. Stump v. Sparkman,* 435 U.S. 349, *reh'g. denied,* 436 U.S. 951 (1978).

229. *Id.,* 552 F.2d at 174. In *S.C.E.,* 378 A.2d 144 (the court declined a petition for a sterilization found to be in the minor's best interests and recommended by her doctors largely because of the 7th Circuit's holding in *Sparkman*).

230. *Stump, supra* note 228, at 357, 358 (the Court was not persuaded by *A.L. v. G.R.H.,* 325 N.E.2d 501, in which the Indiana Court of Appeals held that parents lack the right at common law to have their minor children sterilized because [that opinion].).

231. *Wade v. Bethesda Hosp.,* 356 F. Supp. at 383.

232. *In Re Simpson,* 180 N.E.2d 206 (Ohio Prob. 1962).

233. *Wade, supra* note 222, at 674 (motion for reconsideration).

234. *Wade, supra* note 231, at 383, 384.

235. *Hayes, supra* note 224.

236. *Id.* at 641.

237. *Id.* Similar requirements were imposed in *C.D.M., supra* note 224; *Valerie N.,* 40 Cal. 3d at 165, 166; *A.W., supra* note 224, at 375, 376; *Wentzel v. Montgomery Gen. Hosp., Inc.,* 447 A.2d 1244, 1253-4 (Md. 1982), *cert. denied,* 459 U.S. 1147 (1983); *Moe, supra* note 226, at 721; *Grady, supra* note 224; *In re Application of Nilsson,* 471 N.Y.S.2d 439 (N.C. 1983), *In re Truesdell,* 329 S.E.2d 630, 634-36 (N.C. 1985); *Terwilliger, supra* note 226, at 1383, 1384. A number of states have codified these requirements.

238. *Grady, supra* note 224, at 483; *Terwilliger, supra* note 226, at 1382; *Wentzel, supra* note 237 at 1254.

239. *See, e.g., In re Penny N., supra* note 224, at 543; *In re Nilsson, supra* note 237.

240. *Hayes, supra* note 224, at 640; *C.D.M., supra* note 224, at 614.

241. *Terwilliger, supra* note 226, at 1382; *Penny N., supra* note 224, at 543.

242. *Grady, supra* note 238, at 482; *accord In re C.D.M., supra* note 224, at 612.

243. *In re Guardianship of K.M.,* 816 P.2d 71, 75 (Wash. Ct. App. 1991); *accord In re Moe,* 432 N.E.2d 712.

244. *Grady, supra* note 224, at 482.

245. *Grady, supra* note 224, *accord In re C.D.M., supra* note 224, at 614; *A.W., supra* note 224, at 375; *Wentzel, supra* note 237 at 1253; *Terwilliger, supra* note 226, at 1383.

246. *A.W., supra* note 224, at 375, *Terwilliger, supra* note 226, at 1383.

247. *Hayes, supra* note 224, at 641; *cf., Addington v. Texas,* 441 U.S. 418, 424 (1979).

248. *Penny N., supra* note 224, at 543.

249. *See In re A.W., supra* note 224, at 375-76; *In re Moe, supra* note 226, at 719; *Grady, supra* note 224, at 475; *Hayes, supra* note 224, at 640-641.

250. *See Moe, supra* note 226, at 720; *cf. Saikewicz, supra* note 101, at 431.

251. *See Wyatt v. Aderholt,* 368 F. Supp. 1384, 1388 (M.D.Ala. 1974).

252. *In re A.D.,* 408 N.Y. S.2d 104; *Hudson, supra* note 222.

253. *Ruby v. Massey,* 452 F. Supp. 361, 367-69 (D. Conn. 1978).

254. *Id.* at 364.

255. *Id., cf., S.C.E.,* 627 P.2d 607, wherein a trial judge reached a similar conclusion for similar reasons.

256. *Id.* at 368, 369.

257. 42 U.S.C.S. §300a-7.

258. *Chrisma v. Sisters of St. Joseph of Peace,* 506 F.2d 308 (9th Cir. 1974).

259. *Taylor v. St. Vincent's Hosp.,* 523 F.2d 75 (9th Cir. 1975), *cert. denied,* 424 U.S. 948 (1975).

260. *Eisenstadt v. Baird,* 405 U.S. 438 (1971); *Griswold v. Conn.,* 381 U.S. 479 (1964); *T.H. v. Jones,* 425 F. Supp. 873 (D. Utah 1975), *aff'd on statutory grounds,* 425 U.S. 986 (1976).

261. *T.H., supra* note 260, at 881.
262. *Id.; accord Planned Parenthood Fed'n of America, Inc. v. Heckler,* 712 F.2d 650 (D.C. Cir 1983).
263. *Carey v. Population Services International,* 431 U.S. 678 (1977).
264. *Id.*
265. *Id.* at 694-96.
266. *Id.* at 700-02.
267. 42 U.S.C. §300-300a-6.
268. *Id.; see also* S. Rep. No. 822, 95th Cong., 2d Sess. 24 (1978), H.R.Rep. No 1191, 95th Cong., 2d Sess. 31 (1978); *New York v. Heckler,* 719 F.2d 1191, 1192 (2d Cir. 1983).
269. 42 U.S.C. §602(a)(15)(West Supp. 1993).
270. 42 U.S.C. 1396 d(a)(4)(c)(West Supp. 1993).
271. *Id.*
272. 42 C.F.R. §59.5(a)(4)(1993).
273. *Planned Parenthood Association of Utah v. Schweiker,* 700 F.2d 710, 721 (D.C. Cir. 1983).
274. *T.H. v. Jones,* 425 F. Supp. 873; *contra Doe v. Planned Parenthood Ass'n of Utah,* 510 P.2d 75 (Utah), *stay denied,* 413 U.S.917, *appeal dismissed, cert. denied,* 414 U.S. 805 (1973); *Doe v. Irwin,* 428 F. Supp. 1198 (W.D. Mich.), *vacated and remanded,* 559 F.2d 1219 (6th Cir. 1977), *rev'd,* 615 F.2d 1162 (1980), *cert. denied,* 449 U.S. 829 (6th Cir. 1980).
275. *Doe v. Pickett,* 480 F. Supp. 1218 (S.D. W. Va. 1979).
276. *Stone v. Mead School Dist.* No. 81-2-02990-1 (Wash. Super. Ct. 1983), *cited in* Paul and Klassel, *Minors' Rights to Confidential Contraception Services: The Limits of State Power,* 10 Wom. R.L.Rev. 45, 50 n. 68 (1987) [hereinafter cited as *Minors' Rights*].
277. *See, e.g.,* Opinion of the Attorney General of Oklahoma, No. 85-73 (Jan. 24, 1986), discussing Okla. Stat. Ann. tit. 673, §§2601-2604 (West 1973 & Supp. 1978), *cited in Minors Rights, supra* note 273, at 50, n. 272.
278. *See, e.g., Alfonso v. Fernandez,* 1993 WL 540636 (N.Y.A.D. 2nd Dept.) (unpublished opinion).
279. Edna Negron, *School Condom Rule Challenged,* Newsday, Jan. 29, 1994, §News, at 13.
280. *Id.* (Civil Liberties Union seeks a set aside of the ruling in *Alfonso, supra* note 278.
281. *Id.*
282. Claudia Dreifus, *Joycelyn Elders,* The New York Times, Jan. 30, 1944, §6, at 16.
283. 42 U.S.C. §300(a)(1981); *Heckler, supra* note 268.
284. 42 C.F.R. §59.5(a)(12)(1981); *see also* 48 Fed. Reg. 3600, 3614 (1983); *Heckler, supra* note 268.
285. 42 C.F.R. §59.5(a)(12)(i)(B)(1981); *Heckler, supra* note 268, at 1193.
286. 42 C.F.R. §59.5(a)(12)(i)(E)(1981); *Heckler, supra* note 268, at 1193.
287. *Planned Parenthood Federation, Inc. v. Heckler,* 712 F.2d 650 (D.C. Cir. 1983).
288. 42 C.F.R. §59.5 (a)(12)(i)(A)(1981).
289. *Id.* at §59.5(a)(12)(ii).
290. "The Secretary's requirement that Title X grantees comply with prevailing state law on parental notification or consent constitutes an invalid delegation of authority to the states. . . in the absence of Congress' express authorization to HHS to empower the states to set eligibility criteria, the Secretary has no power to do so." *Planned Parenthood, supra* note 262, at 663.
291. *Id.* at 660, 661.
292. *Id.; accord New York v. Heckler, supra* note 268, at 1197, *Planned Parenthood Ass'n of Utah v. Matheson,* 582 F. Supp. 1001, 1009 (D.Utah 1983); *State of New York v. Schweiker,* 557 F. Supp. 354 (S.D.N.Y. 1983).
293. Current regulations still give priority to "persons from low income families," 42 C.F.R. §59.5(a)(5)(1993), but such preference has

been held not to justify ascribing to the minor her family's resources. *Heckler, supra* note 268, at 1197.
294. *Doe v. Irwin,* 615 F.2d 1162, 1168 (6th Cir.), *cert. denied,* 449 U.S. 829 (1980).
295. *Planned Parenthood of Cent. Missouri v. Danforth,* 428 U.S. 52 (1976); *Poe v. Gerstein,* 517 F.2d 787, 792 (5th Cir. 1975), *aff'd,* 428 U.S. 901 (1976). *See also Juvenile H. v. Crabtree,* 833 S.W.2d 766 (Ark. 1993).
296. *Bellotti v. Baird,* 443 U.S. 622, 642 (1979), *reh'g denied,* 444 U.S. 887 (1979), ("Bellotti II") (plurality opinion). *See also City of Akron v. Akron Center for Reprod. Health,* 462 U.S. 416 (1983).
297. *Roe v. Wade,* 410 U.S. 113, 155, *reh'g denied,* 410 U.S. 959 (1973), *holding limited by Webster v. Reproductive Health Services,* 492 U.S. 490 (1989), *holding modified by Planned Parenthood of Southeastern Pennsylvania v. Casey,* _____ U.S. _____, 112 S.Ct. 2791 (1992).
298. _____ U.S. _____, 112 S.Ct. 2791 (1992). *But see* Comment, E. Schneider, *Workability of the Undue Burden Test,* 66 Temple L. Rev. 1003 (Fall 1993) for a critique of *Casey's* "undue burden test"; *see also* J. Horan, *A Jurisprudence of Doubt: Planned Parenthood v. Casey,* 26 Creighton L. Rev. 479 (Feb. 1993) (explaining the *Casey* Court's rationale).
299. *H.L. v. Matheson,* 450 U.S. 398, 412, 413 (1981), *Danforth, supra* note 295, at 74, *Bellotti, supra* note 296, at 642.
300. *Bellotti, supra* note 296, at 634; *see also H.L., supra* note 299.
301. *Danforth, supra* note 295, at 74; *accord Casey, supra* note 297; *see also Gary-Northwest Indiana Women's Servs., Inc. v. Bowen,* 421 F. Supp. 734 (N.D. Ind. 1976), *aff'd* 429 U.S. 1067 (1977); *Wynn v. Scott,* 448 F. Supp. 997 (N.D. Ill. 1978), *aff'd sub nom. Wynn v. Carey,* 582 F.2d 1375 (7th Cir. 1978); *Wolfe v. Schroering,* 541 F.2d 523 (6th Cir. 1976); *Jones v. Smith,* 474 F. Supp. 1160 (S.D. Fla. 1979); *Abortion Coalition of Mich., Inc. v. Mich. Dept. Pub. Health,* 426 F. Supp. 471, 477 (E.D. Mich. 1977); *State v. Koome,* 530 P.2d 260 (Wash. 1975).
302. *Danforth, supra* note 294, at 74; *see also Wynn v. Carey, supra* note 301, at 1386.
303. *See, e.g., Simopoulos v. Commonwealth,* 227 S.E.2d 194, 204 (Va. 1981).
304. *In re Smith,* 295 A.2d 238 (Md. Ct. App. 1972).
305. *Planned Parenthood of Southeastern Pa. v. Casey,* _____U.S. _____, 112 S.Ct. 2791 (1992) (citing *Arnold v. Board of Educ. of Escambia County, Ala.,* 880 F.2d 305 (11th Cir. 1989)).
306. *Bellotti, supra* note 296, at 643-44 (footnotes omitted) (citing *Danforth,* 428 U.S. 52). *See also Planned Parenthood Ass'n of Kansas City, Mo., Inc. v. Ashcroft,* 462 U.S. 476 (1983); *Margaret S. v. Treen,* 597 F. Supp. 636 (E.D. La. 1984), *aff'd, sub nom. Margaret S. v. Edwards,* 794 F.2d 994 (5th cir. 1986); *In re Application of Doe,* 407 So.2d 1190 (La. 1981).
307. *Bellotti, supra* note 296, at 644; *Wynn, supra* note 301, at 1388.
308. *Indiana Planned Parenthood Affiliates Ass'n, Inc. v. Pearson,* 716 F.2d 1127, 1141 (7th Cir. 1983).
309. *Bellotti, supra* note 296, at 647, 648. *See, e.g., Scheinberg v. Smith,* 659 F.2d 476, 481 (5th Cir.), *reh'g. denied,* 667 F.2d 93 (5th Cir. 1981), *on remand,* 550 F. Supp. 1112 (S.D. Fla. 1982); *Jones v. Smith,* 474 F. Supp. 1160, 1166 (S.D. Fla. 1979).
310. *Akron Center for Reprod. Health v. Slaby,* 854 F.2d 852, 863 (6th Cir. 1988), *rev'd on other grounds, Ohio v. Akron Center for Reprod. Health,* 497 U.S. 502 (1990).
311. *Id.* at 864.
312. *H.B. v. Wilkinson,* 639 F. Supp. 952 (D. Utah 1986).
313. *In re T.H.,* 484 N.E.2d 568 (Ind. 1985); *but see In re Moe,* 423 N.E.2d 1038 (Mass. App. Ct. 1981).
314. *In re T.P.,* 475 N.E.2d 312 (Ind. 1985).
315. *Bellotti, supra* note 296, at 644.
316. *Slaby, supra* note 310, at 868.

317. *Glick v. McKay,* 616 F. Supp. 322 (D. Nev. 1985), *aff'd* 937 F.2d 434 (9th Cir. 1991).

318. *Casey, supra* note 305, 112 S.Ct. at 2832 and Appendix at 2833-35.

319. *Bellotti, supra* note 296, at 644; *see also The Cincinnati Post v. Court of Appeals, 2nd Appellate Jud. Dist. of Ohio,* 604 N.E.2d 153 (Ohio 1992). *See also Eubanks v. Brown,* 604 F. Supp. 141 (W.D. Ky. 1984).

320. *Planned Parenthood Ass'n of Atlanta Area, Inc. v. Harris,* 670 F. Supp. 971, 992 (N.D. Ga. 1987), later proceeding 691 F. Supp. 1419 (N.D. Ga. 1988). *See also Margaret S., supra* note 306, at 652; *Slaby, supra* note 310, at 866.

321. *Wynn, supra* note 301, at 1389; *Pearson, supra* note 308 at 1137, 1138; *but see Foe v. Vanderhoof,* 389 F. Supp. 947 (D. Colo. 1975); *but see Ohio v. Akron Center for Reprod. Health,* 497 U.S. 502 (1990).

322. *Wynn, supra* note 301, at 1389; *Bellotti, supra* note 296, at 642.

323. *Slaby, supra* note 310, at 868, 869, *citing Glick v. McKay, supra* note 317, at 325.

324. *Glick, supra* note 317, at 325, *quoted in Slaby, supra* note 310, at 868.

325. *Pearson, supra* note 308 at 1135-6; *see also Glick, supra* note 317, at 326-27; *but see T.L.J. v. Webster,* 792 F.2d 734 (8th Cir. 1986).

326. *State v. Koome,* 530 P.2d at 262. *Accord Hoe v. Brown,* 446 F. Supp. 329 (N.D. Ohio 1976); *Harris,* 670 F. Supp. 971.

327. *H.L. v. Matheson,* 450 U.S. 398 (1981); *see also Akron Center, supra* note 296, at 440.

328. *H.L., supra* note 327, at 410.

329. *Id.* at 411.

330. *Id.*

331. *Id.* at 412, 413. *Casey,* _____U.S. at _____, 112 S.Ct. at 2825; *Hodgson v. Minn.,* 853 F.2d 1452, 1465 (8th Cir. 1988), *cert. granted,* 492 U.S. 917 (1989), *aff'd,* 497 U.S. 417 (1990). *But see Zbaraz v. Hartigan,* 763 F.2d 1532 (7th Cir. 1985), *aff'd without op.,* 484 U.S. 171 (1987) (24 hours), *reh'g denied,* 484 U.S. 1082; *Pearson, supra* note 308 at 1142, 1143; *Accord.*

332. *H.L., supra* note 327, at 413 (footnotes omitted).

333. *Hodgson v. Minn.,* 497 U.S. 417 (1988).

334. *Hodgson v. Minn.,* 648 F. Supp. 756 (D. Minn. 1986), *cert. denied,* 479 U.S. 1102 (1987), *rev'd,* 853 F.2d 1452 (8th Cir. 1988), *aff'd,* 497 U.S. 417.

335. *Pearson, supra* note 308 at 1132.

336. *Akron Center, supra* note 310; *Slaby, supra* note 310, at 861.

337. *Id.; but see Casey, supra* note 305.

338. *In re Complaint of Jane Doe,* 613 N.E.2d 1112 (Ohio Ct. App. 1993); *see also In re Jane Doe 1,* 566 N.E.2d 1181 (Ohio 1991).

339. *Webster v. Reproductive Health Services,* 492 U.S. 490 (1989).

340. *Casey, supra* note 305.

341. Krauskopf and Burnett, *The Elderly Person: When Protection Becomes Abuse,* 18 Trial 60 (Dec. 1983).

342. *Parham v. J.R.,* 442 U.S. 584, 600 (1979); *see also* R. Redding, *Children's Competence To Provide Informed Consent for Mental Health Treatment,* 50 Wash. and Lee L. Rev. 695 (Spring 1993).

343. *Id.* at 607; *but see P.F. v. Walsh,* 648 P.2d 1067 (Colo. 1982).

344. *Parham, supra* note 342 at 619; *see also Application of Gault,* 387 U.S. 1 (1967).

345. *Addington v. Texas,* 441 U.S. 418 (1979) (in most civil litigation, of course, the plaintiff need but present a "preponderance of the evidence" to prevail).

346. *Id.*

347. *See* Annotation, *Modern Status of Rules as to Standard of Proof Required in Civil Commitment Proceedings,* 97 A.L.R. 3d 780; *see also,* Note, *The Supreme Court, 1978 Term,* 93 Harv. L. Rev. 60, 98 (1979).

348. *In re Roger S.,* 569 P.2d 1286 (Cal. 1977). *See* Comment, *In re Roger S.: The Impact of a Child's Due Process Victory on the California Mental Health System,* 70 Cal. L. Rev. 375 (1982).

349. *In re Roger S., supra* note 348, at 1288. *Compare In re Michael E.,* 538 P.2d 231 (Cal. 1975). *See also In re Aline D.,* 536 P.2d 65 (Cal. 1975).

350. *In re Roger S., supra* note 348, at 1296.

351. *Id.*

352. *Id. See also In re Antoine C.,* 230 Cal. Rptr. 738 (Cal. App. 4 Dist. 1986).

353. *In re Roger S., supra* note 348, at 1296.

354. *Id.* at 1295 (quoting *Jackson v. Indiana,* 406 U.S. 715, 738 (1972)).

355. *Id.; compare Bartley v. Kremens,* 402 F. Supp. 1039 (E.D. Pa. 1975), *vacated,* 431 U.S. 119 (1977).

356. *In re Roger S., supra* note 348, at 1297. For a criticism of *Roger S.,* see Hoffman, *The 'Due Process' Rights of Minors in Mental Hospitals,* 13 U.S.F.L. Rev. 63 (1979).

357. *In re S.,* 135 Cal. Rptr. 893 (Cal. App.), *appeal dismissed,* (1977).

358. Weithorn, *Mental Hospitalization of Troublesome Youth: An Analysis of Skyrocketing Admission Rates,* 40 Stan. L. Rev. 773, 781, 782, nn. 54-62 and accompanying text (Feb. 1988).

359. *See, e.g., Eilers v. Coy,* 582 F. Supp. 1093 (D. Minn. 1984); *In re Katic,* 439 A.2d 1235 (Pa. Super. 1982); *Matter of Gardner,* 459 N.E.2d 17 (Ill. App. 1984).

360. *Wentzel v. Montgomery Gen. Hosp., Inc.,* 447 A.2d 1244 (Md. 1982), *cert. denied,* 459 U.S. 1147 (1983).

361. *See, e.g., Johnson v. Solomon,* 484 F. Supp. 278 (D. Md. 1979).

362. *Colyar v. Third Judicial Dist. Court,* 469 F. Supp. 424 (D. Utah 1979).

363. *Doe v. Doe,* 385 N.E.2d 995, 999 (Mass. 1979).

364. *See Commonwealth v. Rosenberg,* 573 N.E.2d 949, 955, 958 (Mass. 1991).

365. *In re Y.P.,* 603 So.2d 1050, 1051 (Ala. Civ. App. 1992).

366. *In re Long,* 214 S.E.2d 626 (N.C. 1975), *cert. denied,* 217 S.E.2d 665 (N.C. 1975).

367. *Nelson v. Heyne,* 491 F.2d 352 (7th Cir. 1974), *cert. denied,* 417 U.S. 976 (1974).

368. *In re The Mental Health of K.K.B.,* 609 P.2d 747 (Okla. 1980) (adult case). *See also Rennie v. Klein,* 653 F.2d 836 (3d Cir. 1981), *vacated and remanded for further consideration in light of Youngberg v. Romeo,* 458 U.S. 1119 (1982).

369. *Melville v. Sabbatino,* 313 A.2d 886 (Conn. Super. 1973).

370. *In re John S.,* 35 Cal. Rptr. 893 (Cal. 1977).

371. *In re B.,* 497 S.W.2d 831 (Mo. App. 1973).

372. *Youngberg v. Romeo,* 457 U.S. 307 (1982), *on remand,* 687 F.2d 33 (3d Cir. 1982) This principle has also been applied to persons voluntarily admitted to governmental institutions. *See also LaShawn v. Dixon,* 762 F. Supp. 959, 992 (D.D.C. 1991) (citing *Youngberg); Flowers v. Webb,* 575 F. Supp. 1450 (E.D.N.Y. 1983).

373. *Youngberg, supra* note 372, at 323. *Compare Association of Retarded Citizens of N.D. v. Olson,* 561 F. Supp. 473 (D.N.D. 1982).

374. N.J. Mitrichen, *Child Abuse: An Annotated Bibliography* (1982), cited in Heins, *"The Battered Child" Revisited,* 251 JAMA 3295, 3298 n. 19 (1984).

375. *National Briefs,* The Houston Chronicle, Oct. 28, 1993, at A4; *The Child Abuse Epidemic,* 1974 U. Ill. L. Rev 403, 404 (1974).

376. *Reported Cases of Child Abuse Still on Rise, Committee Says,* St. Petersburg Times, April 28, 1993, § National; Health & Medicine, at 8A; *see also* R. Lowry & R. Samuelson, *How Many Battered Children; Finding Real Statistics on Child Abuse,* National Rev. 46 (Apr. 12, 1993); Council on Scientific Affairs, American Medical Association, *AMA Diagnostic and Treatment Guidelines Concerning Child Abuse and Neglect,* 254 JAMA 796 (1985) [hereinafter cited *Council Report*]; Study Findings—National Study of the Incidence and Severity of Child Abuse and Neglect, U.S. Dept. Health and Human Services (DHHS Pub. No. [OHDS] 81-30325 (1981) (more than 1 million reports of abuse or neglect each year).

377. *The Child Abuse Epidemic, supra* note 375, at 403.

378. *House, Senate Pass Death Penalty for Child Killers,* United Press International, May 28, 1993, § Regional News (Texas Legislature); *see also* Karen Peterson, *Abuse of Children Is on the Rise,* USA Today, April 7, 1993, § Life, at 1D.

379. R.E. Helfer and C.H. Kempe, *The Battered Child* at 51 (1968).

380. Johnson and Morse, *Injured Children and Their Parents,* 15 Children 147-152 (1968). *See also Krikorian v. Barry,* 242 Cal. Rptr. 312, 315 (Cal. App. 2 Dist. 1987).

381. *Commonwealth v. Gallison,* 421 N.E.2d 757 (Mass. 1981). Abusers may also be convicted for criminal negligence, *see Brewer v. State,* 274 S.E.2d 817 (Ga. App. 1980); *State v. Fabritz,* 348 A.2d 275 (Md. 1975), *followed on remand,* 351 A.2d 477 (Md. App.), *cert. denied,* 425 U.S. 942 (1976); *Commonwealth v. Humphreys,* 406 A.2d 1060 (Pa. Super. 1979), *overruled on other grounds, Commonwealth v. Burchard,* 503 A.2d 936 (Pa. Super. 1986); *Commonwealth v. Morrison,* 401 A.2d 1348 (Pa. Super. 1979); *Williams v. State,* 680 S.W.2d 570 (Tex. App. 1984), *review referred, en banc,* 692 S.W.2d 100 (Tex. Crim. 1985). In homicide prosecutions, physician testimony has been held admissible to show death was caused by child-battering, *Utah v. Morgan,* 1993 WL 532410 (Utah Ct. App.); *People v. Sexton,* 334 N.E.2d 107 (Ill. App. 1975); *Commonwealth v. Boudreau,* 285 N.E.2d 915 (Mass. 1972); *State v. Durfee,* 322 N.W.2d 778 (Minn. 1982); *State v. Wilkerson,* 247 S.E.2d 905, (N.C. 1978); *Martin v. State,* 547 P.2d 396 (Okla. Crim. 1976), or by nontreatment after battering, *Bergmann v. State,* 486 N.E.2d 653 (Ind. App. 1985). In prosecutions for child abuse, courts may similarly receive expert physician testimony to establish that the child was battered. *People v. Jackson,* 95 Cal. Rptr. 919 (Cal. App. 4 Dist. 1971); *People v. Ewing,* 140 Cal. Rptr. 299 (Cal. App. 3 Dist. 1977); *Cahoon v. U.S.,* 387 A.2d 1098 (D.C. App. 1978); *State v. Muniz,* 375 A.2d 1234 (N.J. N.J. Super. A.D. 1977); *State v. Mapp,* 264 S.E.2d 348 (N.C. App. 1988), *State v. Fredell,* 193 S.E.2d 587 (N.C. App. 1972), *aff'd,* 195 S.E.2d 300 (N.C. 1973). *See generally,* Annotation, *Validity and Construction of Penal Statute Prohibiting Child Abuse,* 1 A.L.R. 4th 38.

382. Kempe, *The Battered Child Syndrome,* 181 JAMA 17 (1962).

383. *Id.*

384. *Council Report, supra* note 376, at 797.

385. Helfer and Kempe, *supra* note 379.

386. Wecht, *Child Abuse: Societal Dilemma & Medicolegal Problem,* 12 Legal Aspects of Medical Practice 9, at 3 (Sep. 1984).

387. Heins, *supra* note 374, at 3298, citing American Humane Association, *Highlights of Official Child Neglect and Abuse Reporting, Annual Report 1981* (1983); *see also* Brown, *Medical and Legal Aspects of the Battered Child Syndrome,* 50 Chi. Kent L. Rev. 45, 50 (1973) (hereinafter cited as Brown).

388. Caffey, *The Parent-Infant Traumatic Stress Syndrome; (Caffey-Kempe Syndrome), (Battered Babe Syndrome),* 114 Am. J. Roentgenology, Radiation Therapeutics, and Nucl. Med. 218, 227 (1972).

389. *Council Report, supra* note 376 at 7978.

390. Helfer and Kempe, *supra* note 379, at 105.

391. *Id.* at 106.

392. *Council Report, supra* note 376, at 797, 798.

393. Most courts have held admissible expert testimony on the diagnosis and manifestations of child abuse. *See generally,* Annotation, *Admissibility of Expert Medical Testimony in Battered Child Syndrome,* 98 A.L.R. 3d 306. *See also supra* note 381, *Compare* Annotation, *Admissibility at Criminal Prosecution of Expert Testimony in Battering Parent Syndrome,* 43 A.L.R. 4th 1203.

394. *Council Report, supra* note 376, at 798.

395. *Id.*

396. *Id.*

397. Cantwell, *Vaginal Inspection as it Relates to Child Sexual Abuse in Girls under Thirteen,* 7 Child Abuse and Neglect 171 (1983).

398. *Id.*

399. Ganley, *The Battered Child: Logic in Search of Law,* 8 San Diego L. Rev. 364, 365, n. 2 (1971); *see also* Silver, *Child Abuse Syndrome: The "Grey Areas" in Establishing Diagnosis,* 44 Pediatrics 595 (1969); *In re Jertrude O.,* 466 A.2d 885 (Md. App. 1983).

400. These laws are compiled and compared in, *e.g.,* Note, *Physician's Liability for Noncompliance with Child Abuse Reporting Statutes,* 52 N. Dak. L. Rev. 736 (1976) (hereinafter cited as *Physician's Liability);* Fraser, *A Pragmatic Alternative to Current Legislative Approaches to Child Abuse,* 12 Am. Crim. L. Rev. 103 (1974); Donovan, *The Legal Response to Child Abuse,* 11 Wm. & Mary L. Rev. 960 (1970). In California, the reporting statute lodges substantiated reports in a statewide data bank. The law does not require a professional, with no knowledge or suspicion of actual abuse, to report a minor as a victim solely because the child is under 14 years old and indicates that he engages in voluntary consensual sexual activity with another minor the same age. *Planned Parenthood Affiliates v. Van de Kamp,* 226 Cal. Rptr. 361 (Cal. App. 1 Dist. 1986). In Florida, a psychiatrist treating an abusing father for emotional difficulties was not required to report the abuse under the reporting statute's mandate, which was limited to "any person . . . servicing *children,*" since the psychiatrist had never cared for the abused child but only for the father. *Groff v. State,* 390 So.2d 361 (Fla. Dist. Ct. App. 1980), *aff'd after remand,* 409 So.2d 44 (Fla. Dist. Ct. App. 1981). In Minnesota, however, a man convicted of criminal sexual conduct with a 13-year-old boy was held properly convicted when the state acted on information from a crisis intake worker whom the defendant had phoned to discuss the incident; no privilege attached to the relationship between the worker and the defendant. *State v. Sandberg,* 392 N.W.2d 298 (Minn. App. 1986), *modified on other grounds,* 406 N.W.2d 506 (Minn. 1987). For a discussion of the consequences of reporting on parental rights, *see* Annotation, *Physical Abuse of Child by Parent as Ground for Termination of Parent's Right to Child,* 53 A.L.R. 3d 605, and Annotation, *Sexual Abuse of Child by Parent as Ground for Termination of Parent's Right to Child,* 58 A.L.R. 3d 1074. *See also* Annotation, *Validity of State Statute Providing for Termination of Parental Rights,* 22 A.L.R. 4th 774, and Annotation, *Validity and Application of Statute Allowing Endangered Child to Be Temporarily Removed from Parental Custody,* 38 A.L.R. 4th 756. For a discussion of the consequences when the authorities fail to intervene on behalf of abused children, *see generally* Annotation, *Tort Liability of Public Authority for Failure to Remove Parentally Abused or Neglected Children from Parents' Custody,* 60 A.L.R. 4th 942.

401. *Physician's Liability, supra* note 400, at 740; *see also* N.D. Cert. Code § 50-25.1-09.

402. *Malpractice—Physician's Liability for Failure to Diagnose and Report Child Abuse,* 23 Wayne L. Rev. 1187, 1191 (1977) (hereinafter cited as *"Malpractice—Physician's Liability").*

403. Besharov, *'Doing Something' About Child Abuse: The Need to Narrow the Grounds for State Intervention,* 8 Harv. J.L. and Pub. Policy 539 (1988). Such laws have been criticized as too vague and hence conducive to both overreporting and underreporting, Weisberg and Wald, *Confidentiality Laws and State Efforts to Protect Abused or Neglected Children: The Need for Statutory Reform,* 18 Fam. L.Q. 143 (1984), and as self-defeating, Paulsen, *The Legal Framework for Child Protection,* 66 Colum. L. Rev. 679 (1966) ("Everyone's duty may easily become nobody's duty," *id.* at 713). The Attorney General of Texas has read his state's reporting requirements to apply even to clerics learning of abuse in their professional capacities. Op. Tex. Atty. Gen. No. JM-342

(Aug. 5, 1985). For an analysis of this position, *see* Note, *The Clergy—Penitent Privilege and the Child Abuse Reporting Statute—Is the Secret Sacred?*, 19 John Marshall L. Rev. 1031 (1986). *See also Mullen v. United States*, 263 F.2d 275 (D.C. Cir. 1958).

404. *See, e.g., People v. Battaglia*, 203 Cal. Rptr. 370 (Cal. App. 2 Dist. 1984); *People v. Salinas*, 182 Cal. Rptr. 683 (Cal. App. 5 Dist. 1981); *Commonwealth v. Anderson*, 385 A.2d 365 (Pa. Super. 1978).

405. *In re L.E.J.*, 465 A.2d 374 (D.C. Ct. App. 1983); *see also People v. Ewing, supra* note 381; and *Hunter v. State*, 360 N.E.2d 588 (Ind. App.), *cert. denied*, 434 U.S. 906, (1977).

406. *People v. Younghanz*, 202 Cal. Rptr. 907 (Cal. App. 4 Dist. 1984). However, said the court, to protect the patient's expectation of privacy, the therapist should warn the patient of his statutory duty to testify against the patient concerning instances of child abuse; if the patient then continues therapy, he waives any right to challenge admissibility of the evidence later. Once a psychotherapist advised the defendant of this duty at their first psychotherapeutic session, however, she was not required to warn him of her duty to report or to testify to admissions made in subsequent sessions. *People v. John B.*, 237 Cal. Rptr. 659 (Cal. App. 2 Dist. 1987).

407. *See, e.g., State v. Fagalde*, 539 P.2d 86 (Wash. 1975): *State v. Jacobus*, 348 N.Y.S.2d 907 (N.Y. Sup. 1973). *See, e.g., Battaglia, supra* note 404; *Hunter, supra* note 405; *State v. Odenbrett*, 349 N.W.2d 265 (Minn. 1984); *Alexander v. State*, 534 P.2d 1313 (Okla. Crim. 1975); *State v. Anderson*, 616 P.2d 612 (Wash. 1980) *appeal after remand*, 538 P.2d 1205 (Wash.); *cert denied*, 459 U.S. 842 (1982); *State v. Fagalde*, 539 P.2d 86. *But see State v. Andring*, 342 N.W.2d 128 (Minn. 1984).

408. *State v. R.H.*, 683 P.2d 269 (Alaska App. 1984). *See also Daymude v. State*, 540 N.E.2d 1263 (Ind. App. 1989).

409. *People v. Stritzinger*, 668 P.2d 738 (Cal. 1983).

410. *Landeros v. Flood*, 123 Cal. Rptr. 713 (Cal. App. 1975) (dicta), *vacated on other grounds*, 551 P.2d 389 (Cal. 1976).

411. *Id.* at 720.

412. *Silver, supra* note 399.

413. 2 Am Jur *Proof of Facts* 2d 365, 390.

414. Brown, *supra* note 387, at 64.

415. Karelitz, *Maltreatment of Children*, 37 Pediatrics 377, 379 (1966).

416. Goodpasture and Angel, *Child Abuse and the Law: The California System*, 26 Hastings L.J. 1081, 1094 (1975).

417. Silver, *Child Abuse Laws—Are They Enough?*, 199 JAMA 65 (1967).

418. Wolff, *Are Doctors Too Soft on Child Beaters?*, 43 Med. Econ. 84, 85 (1966).

419. *See, e.g., Harris v. City of Montgomery*, 435 So.2d 1207, 1213 (Ala. 1983); *Brown v. Scott*, 259 S.E.2d 642 (Ga. App. 1979). In California, a mandatory reporter enjoys immunity from liability even for knowingly false reports—although a voluntary reporter can be liable for a false report if he or she knew the report was false or if it was made with reckless disregard for the truth or falsity of the report. Legislation also provides state reimbursement for legal expenses incurred by mandatory reporters who successfully defend against claims resulting from reporting. *Krikorian v. Barry, supra* note 380, at 316. *See also Storch v. Silverman*, 231 Cal Rptr. 27 (Cal. App. 2 Dist. 1986) (physician reporting sexual abuse of child immune from suit for negligent infliction of emotional distress brought by parents alleging defendant lacked reasonable suspicion of existence of abuse).

420. *E.g., Harris, supra* note 419, at 1213.

421. *Searcy v. Auerbach*, 980 F.2d 609 (9th Cir. 1992).

422. *Comstock v. Walsh*, 848 S.W.2d 7 (Mo. 1993).

423. Sussman, *Reporting Child Abuse: A Review of the Literature*, 8 Fam. L.Q. 245, 293 (1974).

424. *Id.* at 293, 294.

425. *See generally* Hansen, *Doctors, Lawyers and the Battered Child Law*, 5 J. Trauma 826, 827 (1965).

426. Besharov, *The Vulnerable Social Worker: Liability for Serving Children and Families* (National Association of Social Workers, 1985). (Hereinafter cited as Besharov.)

427. *See, e.g., Cechman v. Travis*, 414 S.E.2d 282, 284 (Ga. Ct. App. 1991) (in dicta), *cert. denied*, (1992); *see also* Sussman, *supra* note 423.

428. Shepherd, *The Abused Child and the Law*, 22 Wash. & Lee L. Rev. 182, 192 (1968).

429. *See, e.g.,* Kohlman, *Malpractice Liability for Failure to Report Child Abuse*, 49 Cal. St. B. J. 118, 121 (1974). A search of cases since 1974 also reveals no criminal prosecutions for failure to report.

430. *Pope v. State*, 396 A.2d 1054 (Md. 1978).

431. Sussman, *supra* note 423.

432. *Searcy, supra* note 421.

433. *Landeros v. Flood*, 551 P.2d 389 (Cal. 1976).

434. *Id.* at 391-92.

435. *Id.* at 394, n. 8.

436. *Id.* at 394.

437. *Id.* at 395.

438. *Id.* at 396-97.

439. *Id.* at 397.

440. *Robinson v. Wical*, C.A. No. 37607 (Cal. Super Ct. San Luis Obispo, filed Sept. 4, 1970), *cited in* Note, *Torts: Civil Action Against Physician for Failure to Report Cases of Suspected Child Abuse*, 30 Okla. L. Rev., 482, 485 n. 21 (1977).

441. *Cechman v. Travis*, 414 S.E.2d 282.

442. *Id.*

443. *Id.*

444. *Valtakis v. Putnam*, 504 N.W.2d 264 (Minn. Ct. App. 1993).

445. *Id.* at 266.

446. *Id.*

447. *Marcelletti v. Bathani*, 500 N.W.2d 124 (Mich. Ct. App. 1993) (citing Michigan's Child Protection Law, M.C.L. § 722.621 *et seq.;* M.S.A. § 25.248(3)(1)).

448. *Id.* at 126.

449. *Id.* at 129-30.

450. *Doe v. New York City Dept. of Social Services*, 649 F.2d 134 (2d Cir. 1981), *cert. denied sub nom. Catholic Home Bureau v. Doe*, 446 U.S. 864 (1983); *see also Bartels v. Westchester County*, 429 N.Y.S.2d 906 (N.Y.A.D. 1980); *but see Blanca C. v. Nassau County*, 480 N.Y.S.2d 747 (N.Y.A.D. 1984), *aff'd*, 481 N.W.2d 545 (N.Y. 1985).

451. *Jensen v. Conrad*, 747 F.2d 185 (4th Cir. 1984), *cert. denied*, 470 U.S. 1052, (1985).

452. *Taylor ex rel Walker v. Ledbetter*, 818 F.2d 791 (11th Cir. 1987) *(en banc), cert. denied*, 489 U.S. 1065.

453. *DeShaney v. Winnebago County Dept. of Soc. Servs.*, 489 U.S. 189 (1989).

454. *Id; cf.* Estate of Bailey by *Oare v. County of York*, 768 F.2d 503 (3d Cir. 1985). *See also Doe v. Bobbitt*, 665 F. Supp. 691 (N.D. Ill. 1987), *motion granted in part & denied in part*, 682 F. Supp. 388 (N.D. Ill. 1988).

CHAPTER 33 Geriatric patients

MARSHALL B. KAPP, J.D., M.P.H.*

TRANSFER TRAUMA
FALSE IMPRISONMENT
ELDER ABUSE AND NEGLECT
ALZHEIMER'S DISEASE
OTHER PSYCHOLOGICAL PROBLEMS
PROBLEMS WITH DECISION MAKING AND CASE MANAGEMENT IN HOSPITALS AND LONG-TERM
    CARE FACILITIES
CONCLUSION

Medical advances are enabling average Americans to live longer than their predecessors. In recent years, the segment of our population that is over 65 years old has increased astronomically. This growth may be summarized as follows.[1] In 1776, about 50,000 people or 2% of the U.S. population was 65 or older. By 1900 the percentage had risen to 4%, by 1975 to 10.5%. The proportion is estimated to be 13% by the year 2000 and 21% in 2030. In 1900 the life expectancy was 49 years, and only 40% of the total population reached age 65. In 1986 the life expectancy was 75 years, and 80% of persons in their thirties are expected to be alive in 2020.[2] At every age level over 65, more females than males survive.[3]

The fastest growing segment of the population is the "oldest old." In 1900, fewer than 1 million Americans were 75 years of age and older, and only 100,000 were 85 years of age and older. By 1980, 9.5 million persons were 75 and older, and 2.3 million were 85 and older. By the year 2000, it is projected that the number of persons aged 75 and older will have risen to about 12.3 million. The increase in numbers of the 85 + population is even more dramatic: from 123,000 in 1900 to almost 5 million by the year 2000.

Approximately 1.5 million people currently live in more than 20,000 nursing homes in the United States. The vast majority of nursing home residents are elderly, with an average age of 82, and projections from current trends suggest that one of every four persons who reaches the age of 65 can expect to spend some portion of his or her life in a nursing home. According to the federal Agency for Health Care Policy and Research, one of every 11 Americans who turned 65 in 1990 will spend at least five years in a nursing home. Nursing home residents comprise about 5% of the nation's over-65 population.

The likelihood of developing chronic health conditions increases sharply with age. Most older people have at least one chronic condition and multiple conditions are not uncommon. The most common chronic conditions in persons age 65 and older are arthritis, hypertension, hearing impairment, heart conditions, visual impairments, and diabetes. Other problems include severe cognitive dysfunction, serious memory loss, dementia, and depression. Physical illness often creates mental stress, which can create serious physical complications in the aged. The major causes of death for people aged 65 and older are heart disease, stroke, and cancer.

The elderly are politically active. Among the major self-advocacy groups of the elderly are the Gray Panthers and the American Association of Retired Persons. Examples of the political might of the elderly lobby are Congress's repeal in 1989 of the unpopular Medicare Catastrophic Coverage Act[4] and passage of the 1987 Nursing Home Quality Reform Act.[5]

This chapter focuses on selected problems of transfer trauma, false imprisonment, elder abuse, Alzheimer's disease, and the difficulties of decision-making and case management in hospitals and long-term care facilities. Problems involving end-of-life decision-making are discussed elsewhere.

*The author gratefully acknowledges work from previous contributors: Herbert F. Gretz, M.D., J.D., F.C.L.M., and Colette I. Hughes, J.D.

488

TRANSFER TRAUMA

Transfer trauma, also called "transplantation shock" or "relocation effect," is defined by Hughes:

Transfer trauma is the medically accepted term of art used to describe the dangerous effects of involuntary relocation on nursing home patients. The basic principle of this phenomenon . . . is the recognition that the transfer of geriatric patients to any unfamiliar surroundings produces an increased rate of morbidity and mortality.[6]

Transfer trauma involves both physiological and psychological stresses in the elderly.

Transfer trauma is most apparent when the residents are suddenly transferred. The shock caused by a rapid change in surroundings can cause death, illness, depression, or some forms of regressive behavior. The key factor in determining the effects of a transfer is the degree of control a resident believes he or she possesses, combined with the extent of the change in environment and with the patient's cognitive level of disorientation. Transfer trauma does not occur in all instances, of course, and some studies have failed to find increases in mortality rates.

Psychologically, many nursing home residents feel an attachment to the facility. They develop friendships with peers, rapport with the staff, and feelings of security. Even when they are unhappy with aspects of the facility, they may fear moving to a new location. Hughes quotes an elderly nursing home resident who was informed that he must involuntarily relocate:

I could tell you a lot; there is so much happening. We are treated as if we were in Nazi Germany or Russia. The food is slop; the residents are pushed, prodded and mishandled. We are told nothing. Then we are told this place is closing and we must move. . . . I want to stay here — I won't leave. Where would I go? As bad as it is, there are no better. I would again be separated from my friends; *they would ship us out of here like freight.*[7]

The feelings of dependency and vulnerability experienced by severely ill residents add to the shock of being informed they must move.

The first observed cases of transfer trauma occurred in elderly patients hospitalized for the first time. These patients had increased morbidity over patients who were younger or who had experienced multiple hospitalizations.[8] The earliest studies found death rates among elderly hospitalized mental patients to be approximated at 50% to 60% the first year; half of the deaths occurred within the first 3 months. One study showed increased morbidity after the closing of a chronic disease home.[9] Other studies showed premature morbidity following a fire in the geriatric ward of a Kansas state hospital[10] and following the transfer of aged women from one Illinois state home to another.[11] Elderly men suffered more

frequently than elderly women. Also, although transfer trauma is not limited to psychiatric patients, Kral found psychotic elderly persons suffered more than nonpsychiatric patients of the same age.[12]

Any involuntary relocation can precipitate transfer trauma. Relocations from one home to another, from home to facility, from facility to facility, from facility to home, and from one ward to another within the same facility can traumatize patients of any age. Among the elderly, there is a correlation between the severity of transfer trauma and the type of relocation.

Elderly persons with organic brain syndromes (brain tissue impairment) are more likely to develop transfer trauma than those with purely psychogenic mental disorders. Patients with left cerebral damage have a better prognosis than those with right cerebral damage, and both groups do better than those with bilateral cerebral damage.[13] On the positive side, an elderly person who survives the first post-transfer year will be no worse off than persons who were not involuntarily relocated.[14]

There is a direct correlation with longevity and the enthusiasm the patient has for the relocation. A direct correlation also exists with the improved quality of the new facility. An 8-year follow-up of applicants seeking voluntary relocation to a higher quality apartment facility for the elderly showed a significantly lower death rate in successful, as compared with unsuccessful, applicants.[15]

Preventive medicine is the most effective means to reduce transfer trauma. The medical profession should consider all elderly persons subject to abrupt relocation as being at risk. The quality of living at the new facility should be assessed in terms of emotional, social, and medical support. With preventive measures taken before, during, and after relocation, transfer trauma can be eliminated. Severe anxiety and depression over relocation may require psychiatric desensitization techniques. The Wolpe method of progressive phobic desensitization, for example, teaches the patient progressive muscular relaxation.[16] Once relaxed, the patient is instructed to visualize the new location. Under the principle of reciprocal inhibition, anxiety and relaxation cannot coexist. After a series of sessions, the elderly patient loses apprehension about relocation.

Legal implications of transfer trauma

The Nursing Home Quality Reform Act, passed as part of the Omnibus Budget Reconciliation Act (OBRA) of 1987[17] and based on a 1986 landmark Institute of Medicine report,[18] addresses many problems, including the problem of transfer of facility residents. The act abolishes the previous distinctions between skilled nursing and intermediate levels of care, so involuntary transfer between these two levels will no longer occur. There is a new statement of patient rights, and the facility may not transfer a resident except under specified circumstances: (1) situations in which the resident agrees to the proposed transfer; (2) medical necessity (e.g., the patient requires acute care that can be provided only in a hospital environment); (3) failure to pay the nursing home for services provided; and (4) for the resident's "welfare or that of other patients." A physician must document the reason and, except in an emergency, the facility must provide advance notice to the resident and family members. These transfer restrictions are consistent with those imposed by most state nursing home regulations and statutes, as well as standards of the Joint Commission on Accreditation of Healthcare Organizations (JCAHO).[19]

The Nursing Home Quality Reform Act, which is binding on all nursing homes participating in the Medicare or Medicaid reimbursement programs, also contains provisions requiring nursing homes to engage in preadmission screening and annual resident review (PASSAR) to assure that individuals whose primary needs concern mental health are not confined in nursing homes without appropriate treatment.[20] The unintended result may be the refusal of nursing home admission for, or the involuntary transfer from nursing homes of, mentally compromised older persons, who end up committed to public mental institutions where, at least theoretically, proper mental health services are available.

A number of attorneys have relied on the concept of transfer trauma in challenging attempted involuntary transfers. In the *Town Court* case,[21] legal advocates unsuccessfully tried to have the U.S. Supreme Court accept transfer trauma as the basis for holding that nursing home residents possess a constitutional right to challenge a state agency's decision to terminate a substandard nursing home from participation in the Medicaid program. Instead, the Court's 7 to 1 decision found the residents' substantive due process (Fourteenth Amendment) liberty interests in this situation insubstantial either because the transfer trauma effect had not been conclusively proved by medical evidence or, if it does exist, its deleterious results are only incidentally or indirectly caused by the government's action in decertifying the nursing home.

The *Town Court* case does not, however, mean that transfer trauma in the judicial forum is dead. On the contrary, the door has been left open, at least by implication, for health care professionals to join with legal advocates in compiling and presenting data that the courts would accept as conclusive proof of transfer trauma.[22] Even if the courts exact too demanding a standard of proof to make the general concept of

transfer trauma a viable argument for entitling residents to a voice in the way the government deals with their nursing home, the transfer trauma argument may be used, where supported by sufficient health care professional testimony about the probable effects of forced relocation on a particular resident, to prevent the nursing home itself from initiating the transfer.

FALSE IMPRISONMENT

Persons who have been committed to a psychiatric hospital and persons subjected to guardianship have the protection of the courts in terms of due process prior to deprivations of liberty and continued judicial jurisdiction while liberty is being restricted. Although federal and state regulations, as well as common law tort actions or their threat, protect the rights of residents within nursing homes, there are scant legal safeguards in the nursing home admission process to assure a voluntary and informed choice about initial entry on the entering individual's part.

False imprisonment is an intentional tort, and there is a question whether a plaintiff must prove an actual physical barrier or a perceived barrier to the escape.[23] Few causes of action based on this theory have been utilized because nursing home residents usually lack political and economic power and the physical and mental wherewithal to bring claims. In addition, there is low expected remuneration in such cases, caused by the short life expectancy and the lack of earning power of the resident—those factors being the standard measure of damages.

ELDER ABUSE AND NEGLECT

Mistreatment of older persons may take a number of forms. Palincsar and Cobb[24] subclassify elder mistreatment into five types: (1) "passive neglect," wherein a well-intentioned caretaker simply is incapable of meeting the elder's needs; (2) "active neglect," wherein the caretaker maliciously overmedicates or undermedicates and/or withholds basic life necessities; (3) "psychological abuse," including profanity and intimidating verbal conduct; (4) "financial abuse," wherein a caretaker squanders the patient's funds or refuses to make expenditures essential to the medical or general well-being of the patient; (5) "physical abuse," which ranges from sexual improprieties to battery, and offends the dignity of the patient. Elder mistreatment may vary in its effects, frequency, severity, duration, and intention.[25]

Using the *parens patriae* power—the authority of a society to protect people who cannot protect themselves—more than 40 states have now passed laws mandating that health personnel report suspected abuse cases to designated law enforcement or public health officials; the remaining states (Colorado, Illinois, New

Jersey, New York, North Dakota, Pennsylvania, South Dakota, and Wisconsin) provide for voluntary reporting. Most states coordinate these reporting requirements or permissions with their adult protective services systems for providing indicated health and social interventions to elders, over objection if necessary.[26] The trigger for the reporting requirement or permission is the presence of evidence justifying reasonable suspicion of mistreatment; an actual finding (or nonfinding) of mistreatment does not occur until the adult protective services agency completes its investigation based on the initial report.

Although various state statutes differ in minor particulars, they all mandate or permit reporting by physicians[27] as well as other professionals who, because of their positions and relationships, are uniquely situated to observe situations of suspected elder mistreatment. All of the mandatory statutes impose criminal and/or civil penalties for noncompliance with reporting requirements. The statutes uniformly provide for immunity from civil or criminal liability on account of such reports as long as they were made in good faith and without malicious intent. Normal rules relating to confidentiality are also waived in the context of court testimony about the facts of the clinician's report.

In addition to their generic elder mistreatment legislation, a number of states have enacted special statutes dealing with institutional abuse and neglect of the elderly. The 1987 Nursing Home Quality Reform Act tries to mitigate the problem of institutional mistreatment by, among other things, requiring a minimum amount of nurse aide training and a central registry of nursing home staff members who have been found to abuse residents.

It has been estimated that between 1.5 and 2 million older adults are abused or neglected annually in the United States. In one community-based cross-sectional survey, 32 of 1000 older adults reported that they had experienced some form of mistreatment at least once since reaching the age of 65. This same population sample was asked whether they had been mistreated in the past year, yielding an estimated incidence rate of 26 new cases per 1000 older persons.[28] It is estimated that only 1 in 14 elder mistreatment cases is reported to a public agency.[29]

The abused older person may not wish to report an incident of abuse by a family member because the only solution would be placement of the elder person in a nursing home, which may be less desirable than the present situation. The elder may not want an abusing family member to be punished. Many victims fear retaliation if they file a report. Other victims are dependent on the abusive caretaker. Victims with impaired mental functioning may be unaware that they have been abused.

The primary care physician should be able to identify high-risk families and provide guidance so the family can seek the help of the proper community-based services.[30] The family unit should be maintained and the least restrictive alternatives used to prevent or solve the problem.

A second opportunity for the discovery of elder abuse is the emergency room (ER). The ER physician should always keep in mind the possibility of abuse when examining the elderly for injuries. The physician should try to interview the patient alone without the influence of a family member or a nursing home attendant. The physician should be aware of any inconsistency between the type of injury and the description as to how it occurred. If the patient tells of abuse, then the chart should be documented with a complete history of the circumstances, including how long, how frequently, why, and by whom. The physician must be aware of the applicable state law as to the mandatory or voluntary reporting of elder abuse and also what social services or community services are available to assist the abused patient.[31]

What remedies exist for elder abuse? Abusers are often frustrated persons who project and displace anger onto old people. Often, too, they are alcohol and drug abusers. Many, however, are family members or close friends who have genuine concerns for the elder. Where the abuse is marginal, the abuser may be amenable to psychotherapy, where he or she can explore the tensions that underlie the abuse. In many cases, the abused elder may participate in therapy in order to resolve negative feelings toward the abuser. Some abusers may be rehabilitated to the point where they may resume care of the elder. This remedy assumes that the abuser is amenable to therapy, was not conscious of or deliberative in committing the abuse, and is someone with whom the elder would wish to develop an ongoing relationship. The loyal son or daughter who subconsciously allowed nonfamily stresses to build up and who lost control in an isolated instance would be a good therapy candidate.

Family counseling and group therapy are other methods. A skilled psychotherapist would be invaluable in a therapy session where both the abused and the abuser could explore their feelings toward one another and resolve the negative issues that originally triggered the abuse.

Physicians and other health professionals have an ethical duty to report abuses toward patients, as well as a legal obligation in most states. Nonetheless, the effectiveness of reporting laws in this arena is quite poor.[32] Many professionals fear being sued by the accused if they report, despite universal statutory immunity provisions and the fact that some courts have held them liable for failure to report. Often, reluctance to report is based on despair (too frequently well founded) that limited resources mean that no good intervention strategy will be available to improve the elder's quality of life as a consequence of the professional's report. Put differently, the professional may believe that a report of mistreatment carries the risk of making the situation worse instead of better.

ALZHEIMER'S DISEASE

In 1907 Alois Alzheimer published his work describing a disease with "neurofibrillary tangles." It has been estimated that 4 million people are affected, and it is projected that 14 million will be affected by the year 2050.[33] Experts project that 10% of individuals over 65 are affected by Alzheimer's. An age breakdown indicates that 3% of those between 65 and 74 years are affected; 18.7% between 75 and 85, and 47.2% over 85 years.

The course of the disease is irreversible and always fatal with a duration of 6 to 20 years, averaging 10 years. Ten percent to 30% of the cases are in family groups, pointing to a genetic factor. Also pointing to a genetic factor is the fact that individuals with Down syndrome, if they live past age 40, almost always acquire Alzheimer's disease. The disease appears to be a breakdown of the neurotransmitter acetylcholine. There is an accumulation of amyloid precursor protein, causing disruption of the neurons. At present there is no cure. The federal Food and Drug Administration (FDA) in 1993 approved the drug Cognex as a treatment, although the experimental results have been modest. Several other drugs are undergoing trials, funded by the federal government and private pharmaceutical firms. Most of the afflicted remain in the home care environment out of patient and family preference and because nursing homes are reluctant to accept disruptive patients.

Depression in these patients may respond to tricyclic antidepressants or monamine oxidase inhibitors. Agitation or psychotic signs may be treated with neuroleptics such as haloperidol or fluphenazine. If the patient has preexisting parkinsonism, a low dose of thioridazine may be tried instead.[34]

In Alzheimer's early stages, the patient usually lives at home. Families should maintain a structured, protective living environment to avoid stressing the patient.[35] The family should watch for insidious signs of deterioration. At first, the patient may seem mildly forgetful, but have no social or employment problems. In later stages, the patient may complain of poor work performance, visuospatial defects, poor speech, or inability to travel without losing the way. Legal consultation should be secured early to assist the patient and family in planning ahead and making appropriate financial and personal arrangements for the patient's future decisional incapacity.[36]

The Alzheimer's Disease and Related Disorders Association (ADRDA) (now known as the Alzheimer's Association) in Chicago helps families to cope with this tragic situation. ADRDA publishes a newsletter, lay information books, and lists of local service organizations. ADRDA has local affiliates throughout the United States.

OTHER PSYCHOLOGICAL PROBLEMS

The elderly are afflicted not only with organic senile/presenile disorders, but also with the panoply of psychiatric disorders common in younger age groups. For example, "major depressive episode" (MDE) affects all ages. In the elderly, clinicians often refer to MDE as "pseudodementia"—depression, to delineate it from the true organic dementias previously discussed. Also, the memory loss and normal psychological impairment in the elderly can increase attributes, traits, or eccentricities that were more subdued when the person was younger.

One symptom, often dismissed or misdiagnosed by physicians, that statistically affects the elderly more is pain, such as that arising from "myofascial pain syndrome"—a disorder of striated muscle characterized by tender, indurated bands or nodules called trigger points, hyperirritability of pain-mediating sensory nerves, and frequent referral of pain to distant sites, including visceral organs.

PROBLEMS WITH DECISION MAKING AND CASE MANAGEMENT IN HOSPITALS AND LONG-TERM CARE FACILITIES

Quality medical care requires consideration of the elder's physical and mental health, socioeconomic status, environmental circumstances, and functional status.[37] The goal is to preserve function and independence in the elderly. Medical problems result from the interaction of five factors: impaired mobility, impaired cognition, incontinence, impaired homeostasis, and iatrogenic disease.[38]

The physician usually is viewed as the coordinator of every aspect of the patient's therapy. In practice, however, decision-making can be a fragmented process. A hospital or nursing home stay sets up a complex interaction between parties with different, sometimes even inconsistent, goals. Private health insurers, Medicaid utilization reviewers, social workers, discharge planners, friends, family, conservators, outside agencies, and the elder all may have input into the decision-making process. Provider overhead, the purpose of the stay, and the elder's resource structure also influence care decisions. Decentralized decision-making can create confusion or worse.

For example, social workers are often ignored by other staff, even though they can provide valuable information about the elder's living context and access to community resources. Medicaid utilization reviewers are timekeepers who safeguard public funds by ensuring that hospital stays are as brief as necessary. Family members may pressure a physician into prolonging the elder's hospital stay in order to avoid having to provide home care. The case management "team" may not function as a team at all.

Some progress has been made during the past decade in creating and refining a more coordinated long-term care system for the elderly, encompassing a broad continuity of services in a variety of settings. Improving on the quality and availability of these comprehensive, coordinated services should be a primary goal for gerontological professionals in the next several years. Any health care financing and delivery reform initiatives emanating from Washington or the states must be consistent with, and supportive of, this goal.

CONCLUSION

The older population in the United States will continue to grow in size and heterogeneity and will continue to present society with a panoply of interesting medical and legal challenges. It is incumbent on health and legal professionals to address these emerging issues thoughtfully and to embrace the people they concern enthusiastically.

END NOTES

1. Kapp, *Geriatrics and the Law: Patient Rights and Professional Responsibilities* 2 (2nd ed. 1992).
2. *Id.* at 4.
3. *Id.*
4. The Medicare Catastrophic Coverage Act was passed in 1988 as Public Law No. 100-360 and repealed in 1989 as Public Law No. 101-234.
5. 42 U.S.C. §§1395i-3(a)-(h) and 1396r(a)-(h).
6. Hughes, *Liberty from Transfer Trauma: A Fundamental Life and Liberty Interest,* 9 Hastings Const. L. Q. 429-30 (1982).
7. *Id.* at 429.
8. Camargo and Preston, *What Happens to Patients Who Are Hospitalized for the First Time Over Sixty-Five?,* 102 Am. J. Psychiatry 168-73 (1945).
9. Aldrich and Mendkoff, *Relocation of the Aged and Disabled: A Mortality Study,* 11 *J. Am. Geriatrics Society* 185-94 (1963).
10. Aleksandrowicz, *Fire and Its Aftermath on a Geriatric Ward,* 25 Bull. Menninger Clinic 23-32 (1961).
11. Miller and Lieberman, *The Relationships of Affect State and Adoptive Capacity to Reactions to Stress,* 20 J. Gerontology 492-97 (1965).
12. Kral, *Stress Reactions Resulting from the Relocation of an Aged Population,* 13 Canadian Psychiatric Assn. J. 201-09 (1968).
13. Pino, *The Differential Effects of Relocation on Nursing Home Patients,* 18 Gerontologist 167-72 (1978).
14. Pablo, *Intra-Institutional Relocation: Its Impact on Long-Term Care Patients,* 17 Gerontologist 426-35 (1977).
15. Carp, *Impact of Improved Living Environment on Health and Life Expectancy,* 17 Gerontologist 242-49 (1977).
16. Lazare, *Outpatient Psychiatry* 633-34 (1979).
17. Pub. L. 100-203 (1987).
18. Institute of Medicine, *Improving the Quality of Care in Nursing Homes* (National Academy Press, Washington, D.C. 1986).
19. Joint Commission on Accreditation of Health Care Organizations, *Accreditation Manual for Long Term Care Facilities* (1993).
20. Mental Health Law Project and Legal Counsel for the Elderly, *Enforcing the Rights of Older People With Mental Disabilities, Volume II — Preadmission Screening and Annual Resident Review: A Manual for Advocates* (1993).
21. *O'Bannon v. Town Court,* 447 U.S. 773 (1980).
22. Annas, *Transfer Trauma and the Right to a Hearing,* 10 Hastings Center Report 23-24 (1980).
23. Prosser, *The Law of Torts* 44 (5th ed., West Publishing 1984).
24. Palinscar and Cobb, *The Physician's Role in Detecting and Reporting Elder Abuse,* 3 J. Legal Med. 413-41 (1982).
25. Stein, *Elder Abuse and Neglect: A National Research Agenda,* (National Aging Resource Center on Elder Abuse, Washington, D.C. 1991).
26. Strauss, Wolf, and Shilling, *Aging and the Law* 349-72 (1990).
27. American Medical Association, *Diagnostic and Treatment Guidelines on Elder Abuse and Neglect* (1992).
28. Pillemer and Finkelhor, *The Prevalence of Elder Abuse: A Random Sample Survey,* 28 Gerontologist 51-57 (1988).
29. American Medical Association, *supra* note 27, at 6.
30. Obrien, *Elder Abuse and the Primary Care Physician,* 114 Med. Times 60 (Dec. 1986).
31. Bloom et al., *Detecting Elder Abuse,* 44 Geriatrics 40 (June 1989).
32. U.S. General Accounting Office, *Elder Abuse: Effectiveness of Reporting Laws and Other Factors* (GAO/HRD-91-74 Apr. 1991).
33. U.S. Congressional Office of Technology Assessment, *Losing a Million Minds: Confronting the Tragedy of Alzheimer's Disease and Other Dementias* (OTA-BA-323 Apr. 1987).
34. Jenike, *Alzheimer's Disease: Clinical Care and Management,* 27 Psychosomatics 407-16 (1986).
35. *Id.* at 413.
36. Frolik and Brown, *Advising the Elderly or Disabled Client* (Rosenfeld Launer Publications Englewood Cliffs, NJ 1992).
37. Hazard and Burton, *Health Problems of the Elderly, in Harrison's Principles of Internal Medicine* 450-54 (Braunwald, ed., 11th ed. 1987).
38. *Id.* at 452.

CHAPTER 34 Oncology patients

MELVIN A. SHIFFMAN, M.D., J.D., F.C.L.M.*

STANDARD OF CARE
INFORMED CONSENT
MISDIAGNOSIS AND DELAY IN DIAGNOSIS OF CANCER
RADIATION THERAPY
CHEMOTHERAPY
UNORTHODOX CANCER TREATMENTS
CONCLUSION

The oncology patient presents particular medical and surgical problems for the physician. Most lawsuits involve misdiagnosis or, in reality, late diagnosis. There are also legal actions that involve proper treatment and, invariably, the question of the statute of limitations.

Patients alleging misdiagnosis are basically complaining of a "loss of chance." Almost always there is the question of whether the misdiagnosis caused the patient's injury to a reasonable medical certainty or probability, or whether the natural course of events was unchanged.

Lesser legal problems involve patients' failure to comply. It often becomes necessary to invoke as a defense the patients' contributing or comparative negligence. Chemotherapy is fraught with complications. For oncology patients, informed consent, or informed refusal if care and management are refused, is very important. The physician may choose to use therapeutic professional discretion to keep medical facts from the patient when the physician believes disclosure would be harmful, dangerous, or injurious to the patient.

Because patients with cancer are often desperate, a physician must address the legal consequences of administering unorthodox treatment, particularly if the patient insists on it. The use of radiation therapy is frequently the source of medicolegal problems. The resolution of these problems involves invoking risk-benefit judgment, comparing the anticipated benefits from therapy with its risks, and weighing the consequences of no treatment.

STANDARD OF CARE

There are now recognized specialties in medical and surgical oncology. Consequently, any physician treating a patient with cancer would be advised to review his or her care of a cancer patient with someone practicing in the recognized specialty of medical and/or surgical oncology for the simple reason that once a lawsuit is filed, the treating physician, in most jurisdictions, will be held to the standard of care/standard of practice exercised by the reasonably prudent medical oncologist and/or surgical oncologist, depending on the medical care that is at issue.

In most states the "locality rule" in determining standard of care has been abandoned. This is particularly true in areas of medical specialty (cancer, heart disease, etc.) such that a physician's care will not be compared only to other physicians in the immediate community. Rather, the standard of care will be that standard practiced by the reasonably prudent physician practicing in a similar community for a patient of like or similar circumstances.[1]

Consequently, it is critical that a physician be mindful of the need to confer with cancer specialists when taking on the primary care of a cancer patient in order to assure that the patient receives treatment consistent with the standard of care. This is especially necessary when diagnosis and treatment regarding the cancer patient are evolving at a rapid rate. There are recognized tumor forums/tumor boards associated with hospitals or cancer centers as well as many teaching institutions with

*The author gratefully acknowledges work from previous contributors: Bridget Baynes, R.N., J.D., Martin B. Flamm, M.D., J.D., F.C.L.M., and Kenneth M. Sigelman, M.D., J.D., F.C.L.M.

specialty areas in various aspects of cancer care. These centers will not only be consulted at the time litigation is initiated, but they can advise the treating physician and safeguard against a medical negligence action based on the allegation that a physician's care fell below the acceptable standard of practice. In the long run, consultation with a physician or surgeon specializing in a given field will be much more cost-effective than defending against a lawsuit for failure to consult.

Physicians, however, should also be aware that university centers may treat cancer patients as part of a study. Such treatment will not necessarily coincide with that which is recognized and accepted for cancer patients outside of the study basis for standard of care. Rather, standard of care is best defined as that care exercised by the reasonably prudent medical specialists treating cancer patients with the same or similar type of cancer.

There is also greater concern today that corporate medicine, such as health maintenance organizations and preferred provider organizations, may, in fact, impinge on the quality of care given the cancer patient because of an underlying motivation to reduce costs, which such organizations accomplish by limiting physician's fees and hospital fees, thereby prompting the physicians and hospitals to increase their patient volume. In so doing, less actual time is spent with the patient and so there is greater likelihood of medical error. Therefore, it is unlikely that the standard of care delivered by the health maintenance organization will be held as the applicable standard of reasonably prudent medical care for purposes of a professional negligence or medical malpractice question, but the health maintenance organization will have to comply with the accepted community standard of care.

INFORMED CONSENT

Generally speaking, the law in all states requires a physician to obtain the consent of a patient before treating or operating on that patient. In the absence of that consent, the physician may be held liable in a civil lawsuit for battery, assault, and professional negligence or medical malpractice. In California, as well as other states, it has been held that a person of adult years has the right, in the exercise of control over his or her own body, to decide whether or not to submit to lawful medical treatment.[2] The problem arises, however, when the issue is raised as to whether or not that adult person understood to what he or she was consenting. In the absence of a knowing consent, any consent given is deemed vitiated or null and void as a matter of law.

The cancer patient presents a special set of circumstances, which, in many states, has prompted the passage of legislation that codifies additional legal obligations for a physician treating a cancer patient in order to obtain an informed consent to treat. An adequately informed patient will help to prevent charges of lack of informed consent or assault and battery, and will assure that the physician meets the duty of due care in advising the patient of all available options to assure that the consent given is one based on adequate information.

More important, time and experience have proven that when a knowing and consensual participation in treatment is obtained from a patient, when there is good communication between physician and patient, there is much lower incidence of malpractice litigation even when physician error is present. To avoid informed consent problems, a physician should consider and be familiar with the following:

1. The controlling state laws of the jurisdiction, which may provide specific requirements for a physician to inform the patient of alternative treatment modalities, should be considered.

2. The physician should consider the need to offer a patient referral, depending on the expertise of the treating physician; that is, if surgery is the recommended treatment, the patient should be offered a referral to a medical practitioner to review medical management versus surgery even when there is no legislative requirement for this. Conversely, if chemotherapy or radiotherapy is proposed, the patient should be offered the benefit of a consultation with a surgeon to assure adequate exposure to alternative modalities. This is one of the most effective ways to avoid a later allegation of undue influence or pressure. Once the offer of a consultation or second opinion is recorded in the chart, there is much less chance for a patient to allege he or she was railroaded into a particular course of treatment without an adequately informed consent.

3. The physician must determine whether there has been a sufficient cooling-off period or a lapse of time between telling a patient of his or her cancer and obtaining the consent to treat. Does the patient understand the therapy proposed versus a scenario in which the patient is still in a shock/fear syndrome and thus agrees to treatment in desperation, fear, and confusion?

4. In the particular case considered, should the condition and/or proposed treatment be discussed with close family members, not only to answer their questions concerning the method of care/treatment proposed, but particularly when there is any question that the patient is not capable/competent to assure an informed consent?

When the question is raised as to whether a patient's consent was an informed one, it is generally the testimony from medical practitioners who treat patients of similar circumstances with a similar illness that will determine what information should have been conveyed to the patient in order to assure that the patient's consent was informed. In a few states, however, there is also a legislative standard or state statute that articulates what the physician needs to tell a patient. In California, for example, Health & Safety Code Section 1704.5 mandates that a physician inform any woman with breast cancer, in writing, of the various viable treatment modalities available for her particular type of cancer.

Also, in a state such as California, it has been determined that the physician's duty to inform can be measured by a jury's finding as to what a reasonably prudent patient would want to know. Some states require a finding that the physician's failure to obtain an informed consent prior to treatment was conscious or willful before the patient can successfully start an action for battery or assault. In almost all states, however, a failure to obtain the patient's informed consent prior to treatment or surgery constitutes professional negligence or medical malpractice that can be successfully plead and proven on showing (1) that the consent given was insufficient and thus vitiated and (2) that the physician's failure to provide necessary information was a cause of the harm or injury that the patient sustained.

Thus, it is necessary that the injury or damage complained of by the patient be a direct or legal consequence of insufficient information, the lack of informed consent, before a patient will prevail in a medical negligence action premised on a theory of insufficient or nonexistent informed consent.

As many as 17 states have statutes that deal directly with informed consent to medical treatment. These states seem to have passed such legislation to control expansion of the doctrine. Consequently, if a physician provides a patient with the type of information that the statute requires, and records this fact in the medical records at the time the patient consent is obtained, the physician overcomes any informed consent problem as a matter of law.[3]

Illustrative of the measures that can be taken to itemize the information that must be given to the patient is the disclosure list formulated by the Texas Medical Disclosure Panel.[4] Box 34-1 lists those treatments and procedures that require full disclosure by the physician or health care provider to the patient or person authorized to consent for the patient.

Unfortunately, most statutes, unlike court decisions, do not emphasize that the patient must comprehend the information conveyed. In brief, the physician and/or surgeon would be most protected if the consent obtained from the patient not only met the statutory requirements, but was also obtained after the patient had an opportunity to overcome the fear and shock initially associated with learning of the cancer. Another safeguard would be to discuss the patient's treatment with immediate family members and record this fact in the medical record. There is one instance, however, that applies in all states, when an informed consent is not necessary: in an emergency when the patient's life or limb is at serious risk. In such situations, the patient's consent is not a necessary prerequisite to treatment.

The foregoing is not intended as an exhaustive discussion of the laws in all states, but the major considerations have been identified. Again, to safeguard against lawsuits based on lack of informed consent, the physician should:

1. Assure a sufficient cooling-off period so that the patient has an opportunity to comprehend proposed treatment without the influence of the immediate fear and shock associated with the diagnosis of cancer.
2. Provide information of alternative treatment modalities and even recommend consultation with a physician who might propose an alternative form of treatment.
3. Discuss the proposed treatment with other family members and record the fact of all discussions with the patient or family members, noting the subject matter of the discussion and family responses, if any.
4. Review the applicable legislation of a given jurisdiction to make certain that, as a physician, any information required by statute is communicated to the patient.

The laws in most states require a physician and/or surgeon to disclose and provide the patient with all the information to which he or she is entitled under material standard. More simply put, the patient is entitled to be informed of all material facts concerning the risks or the proposed or alternative methods of treatment and their rate of effectiveness such as would objectively inform a reasonable person of the possible consequences of the proposed course of treatment.[5]

MISDIAGNOSIS AND DELAY IN DIAGNOSIS OF CANCER

Failure or delay in the diagnosis of cancer is the leading allegation in physician malpractice cases, comprising more than 10% of all physician malpractice suits. Lawsuits that claim a failure to diagnose cancer are more than twice as common as cases based on failure to diagnose fractures or dislocations, failure to diagnose pregnancy problems, or postoperative surgical complications, and are three times more common than cases based on alleged improper treatment or incorrect drug therapy, failure to diagnose infection, improper treat-

BOX 34-1
FULL DISCLOSURE LIST OF THE TEXAS MEDICAL DISCLOSURE PANEL

1. Endocrine system treatments and procedures.
   a. Thyroidectomy
      (1) Injury to nerves resulting in hoarseness or impairment of speech.
      (2) Injury to parathyroid glands resulting in low blood calcium levels that require extensive medication to avoid serious degenerative conditions, such as cataracts, brittle bones, muscle weakness, and muscle irritability.
      (3) Lifelong requirement of thyroid medication.
2. Eye treatments and procedures.
   a. Reconstructive and/or plastic surgical procedures of the eye and eye region, such as blepharoplasty, tumor, fracture, lacrimal surgery, foreign body, abscess, or trauma.
      (1) Worsening or unsatisfactory appearance.
      (2) Creation of additional problems such as:
         1. Poor healing or skin loss.
         2. Nerve damage.
         3. Painful or unattractive scarring.
         4. Impairment of regional organs, such as eye or lip function.
      (3) Recurrence of the original condition.
3. Hematic and lymphatic system.
   a. Transfusion of blood and blood components.
      (1) Fever.
      (2) Transfusion reaction, which may include kidney failure or anemia.
      (3) Heart failure.
      (4) Hepatitis.
      (5) AIDS (acquired immune deficiency syndrome).
      (6) Other infections.
4. Integumentary system treatments and procedures.
   a. Radical or modified radical mastectomy. (Simple mastectomy excluded.)
      (1) Limitation of movement of shoulder and arm.
      (2) Swelling of the arm.
      (3) Loss of the skin of the chest, requiring skin graft.
      (4) Recurrence of malignancy, if present.
      (5) Decreased sensation or numbness of the inner aspect of the arm and chest wall.
   b. Reconstruction and/or plastic surgical operations of the face and neck.
      (1) Worsening or unsatisfactory appearance.
      (2) Creation of several additional problems such as:
         1. Poor healing or skin loss.
         2. Nerve damage.
         3. Painful or unattractive scarring.
         4. Impairment of regional organs, such as eye or lip function.
      (3) Recurrence of the original condition.
5. Nervous system treatments and procedures.
   a. Craniotomy (craniectomy) for excision of brain tissue, tumor, vascular malformation, and cerebral revascularization.
      (1) Additional loss of brain function, including memory.
      (2) Recurrence or continuation of the condition that required this operation.
      (3) Stroke.
      (4) Blindness, deafness, inability to smell, double vision, coordination loss, seizures, pain, numbness, and paralysis.
   b. Craniotomy (craniectomy) for cranial nerve operation, including neurectomy, avulsion, rhizotomy, or neurolysis.
      (1) Numbness, impaired muscle function, or paralysis.
      (2) Recurrence or continuation of the condition that required this operation.
      (3) Seizures.
   c. Spine operation. Including laminectomy, decompression, fusion, internal fixation or procedures for nerve root or spinal cord compression; diagnosis; pain; deformity; mechanical instability; injury; removal of tumor; abscess or hematoma. (Excluding coccygeal operations.)
      (1) Pain, numbeness, or clumsiness.
      (2) Impaired muscle function.
      (3) Incontinence or impotence.
      (4) Unstable spine.

Continued.

BOX 34-1
FULL DISCLOSURE LIST OF THE TEXAS MEDICAL DISCLOSURE PANEL—cont'd

    (5) Recurrence or continuation of the condition that required the operation.
    (6) Injury to major blood vessels.
  d. Peripheral nerve operation; nerve grafts, decompression, transposition or tumor removal; neurorrhaphy, neurectomy, or neurolysis.
    (1) Numbness.
    (2) Impaired muscle function.
    (3) Recurrence or persistence of the condition that required the operation.
    (4) Continued increased or different pain.
6. Urinary system.
  a. Partial nephrectomy (removal of part of the kidney).
    (1) Incomplete removal of stone(s) or tumors if present.
    (2) Obstruction of urinary flow.
    (3) Leakage of urine at surgical site.
    (4) Injury to or loss of kidney.
    (5) Damage to adjacent organs.
  b. Radical nephrectomy (removal of kidney and adrenal gland for cancer).
    (1) Loss of the adrenal gland.
    (2) Incomplete removal of tumor.
    (3) Damage to adjacent organs.
  c. Nephrectomy (removal of kidney).
    (1) Incomplete removal of tumor if present.
    (2) Damage to adjacent organs.
    (3) Injury to or loss of kidney.
  d. Prostatectomy (partial or total removal of prostrate).
    (1) Leakage of urine at surgical site.
    (2) Obstruction of urine flow.
    (3) Incontinence (difficulty with urinary control).
    (4) Semen passing backward into bladder.
    (5) Difficulty with penile erection (possible with partial and probable with total prostratectomy).
  e. Total cystectomy (removal of urinary bladder).
    (1) Probable loss of penile erection and ejaculation in the male.
    (2) Damage to other adjacent organs.
    (3) This procedure will require an alternate method or urinary drainage.
  f. Partial cystectomy (partial removal of urinary bladder).
    (1) Leakage of urine at surgical site.
    (2) Incontinence (difficulty with urinary control).
    (3) Backward flow of urine from bladder into ureter (tube between kidney and bladder).
    (4) Obstruction of urine flow.
    (5) Damage to other adjacent organs.
  g. Urinary diversion (ileal conduit, colon conduit).
    (1) Blood chemistry abnormalities requiring medication.
    (2) Development of stones, strictures, or infection.
    (3) Routine lifelong medical evaluation.
    (4) Leakage of urine at surgical site.
    (5) Requires wearing a bag for urine collection.
  h. Ureterosigmoidostomy (placement of kidney drainage tubes into the large bowel).
    (1) Blood chemistry abnormalities requiring medication.
    (2) Development of stones, strictures, or infection.
    (3) Routine lifelong medical evaluation.
    (4) Leakage of urine at surgical site.
    (5) Difficulty in holding urine in the rectum.
  i. Urethroplasty (construction/reconstruction of drainage tube from bladder).
    (1) Leakage of urine at surgical site.
    (2) Stricture formation.
    (3) Additional operation(s).

ment of a fracture or dislocation, improper treatment for lack of supervision, or improper treatment for an infection.

Failure to diagnose cancer or delay in the diagnosis of cancer can be devastating to a patient and to the patient's family. It may result in a patient having to undergo more extensive treatment, reduce the chances of survival, lead to unnecessary death, and cause physical and emotional burdens that an earlier diagnosis could have averted.

Liability may be based on a physician's own negligent action or inaction, or both. A pathologist in the *Long v. Patterson* case[6] reported a skin mole biopsy as benign. Later review by another pathologist found malignant melanoma. A jury awarded $1,286,000 for the death of the 17-year-old patient due to the pathologist's own negligent action.

In 1982, in *Sygman v. Kahn,*[7] a 40-year-old teacher complained of a breast lump, and was sent by her doctor for a mammogram, which was reported as negative. A cancer was found on a biopsy seven months later. The jury awarded $900,000, finding the doctor liable for failure to perform a follow-up testing, including a biopsy, but only 60% at fault for his negligent inaction.

The case of *Davis v. U.S.*[8] concerned a physician performing a proctoscopy on an 18-year-old patient with rectal bleeding, who saw a "venous lake" where a fatal cancer was later found. A jury awarded $660,000 because the error of diagnosis was compounded by the error of not following up the abnormality even though the bleeding persisted. The negligence was both the physician's own negligent action of misdiagnosis and his own negligent inaction of not ordering additional follow-up.

Liability may be based also on the acts or inactions of others, under the fundamental principles of agency law. This rule applies whether the acts or omissions were in the doctor's presence or absence, and whether or not the doctor had the actual ability to control the employee's conduct.

The standard of care to which a physician specialist will be held may then depend on in which state or jurisdiction the physician has his or her practice, degree of specialization, whether the physician is certified by a national specialty board, what procedures or treatments may be utilized in the practice, and the nature of the patient's complaints.

For this reason, a rule regarding the standard of care in diagnosis of cancer valid for all physicians in all states, and encompassing all specialties and procedures in all clinical circumstances, is impossible to formulate. Each physician must make an effort to learn the current standards in his or her own geographical area or similar locality, the standards of the national certifying board if the physician practices a recognized specialty, and

should also be aware of current trends (if his or her state uses the old locality rule, in particular).

An example is the problem of defining the standard of due care in diagnosing cancer. Many suits now being filed involve failure to diagnose breast cancer. Approximately 50% of suits for failure to diagnose breast cancer named physicians in four areas of medical practice. Approximately 38% of suits for failure to diagnose breast cancer were filed against specialists in obstetrics and gynecology (18.3%), internal medicine (10.8%), and pathology (9.1%). However, 22.5% were against general practitioners and family practitioners. Suits against radiologists and other specialists were less common.[9] Currently, the standard of care owed by the general practitioner in diagnosing breast cancer is not the same as the standard of care owed the same patient by a national board–certified obstetrician or gynecologist practicing in the same geographical area in many jurisdictions. An obstetrician or gynecologist is more likely to be successfully sued than is a family practitioner who has negligently missed a breast cancer in a similar patient under similar circumstances, for example, in those jurisdictions that hold specialists to a higher standard of care than generalists, even though a family practitioner is more likely to be sued at the outset.

Causation and damages

Although a physician may have acted or failed to act negligently, and has failed to fulfill the standard of care owed the patient, a successful lawsuit cannot be maintained unless the misdiagnosis in cancer diagnosis caused some calculable harm to the patient.

In failure to diagnose cancer cases, damages are meant to compensate a patient for physical pain and suffering and emotional distress due to the requirement for additional treatment, loss of life, or loss of chance of survival due to the delay in diagnosis and treatment. Monetary damages may also be awarded to the patient's family for harm done to them.

Delay in diagnosis and treatment of cancer, however, are generally not compensable if the delay did not materially affect the ultimate treatment and outcome of the disease. A long delay in the diagnosis of a uniformly fatal type of cancer or a very short delay in a potentially curable cancer may result in a judgment against a physician, especially if the patient presents with a later stage of that cancer at the time of the delayed diagnosis and treatment.

An example is the case of *Kremer v. Kaiser Foundation Hosp.*[10] A 22-year-old man had a fatal testicular cancer, but his family claimed he would have survived had a scrotal exam been done two years earlier, when he was examined for abdominal pain, diarrhea, vomiting, and blood in the stool. The jury agreed with the defendant physician and clinic, which argued that testicular cancer is a very fast-moving disease and that it was doubtful earlier examination would have identified the cancer or affected the outcome of the disease.

In the case of *Brown v. Nash,*[11] a woman in her fifties was referred to a general surgeon when she noted a thickening in her breast. A biopsy was not performed for two years, and the woman died of metastatic breast cancer. A Boston jury in 1985 awarded the plaintiff family $3 million. The long delay in her diagnosis and treatment was held to be the cause of her death.

In the *Nathanson v. Yarvis* case,[12] a 63-year-old woman was seen by her doctor over a five-month period for vague pain in the lower left quadrant of her abdomen. A rectal exam revealed a tender area, and a barium enema was scheduled but not performed. Three months later she had a colon resection, hysterectomy, and salpingo-oophorectomy for metastatic adenocarcinoma of the colon. The jury verdict was for the defense. Because the tumor was so slow growing, it may have been present for as long as 2½ years, and the delay in diagnosis was held not to be the predominant cause of her injuries.

There has been a recent trend to go beyond traditional causation principles to allow recovery for loss of a chance of a cure. In some jurisdictions it is no longer necessary for a plaintiff to have to show that he or she has already suffered an actual loss because of a delay in diagnosis and treatment, but only some potential loss.[13]

In *Morrison v. Stallworth,*[14] a 45-year-old woman had two negative examinations by her OB/GYN doctor despite her complaint of a breast lump. Subsequently, biopsy revealed malignancy. The court of appeals held that evidence regarding shortened life expectancy as a compensable element of damages was wrongfully excluded by the trial court, although the trial court had found no liability, and ordered a new trial.

Contributory negligence in cancer patients

Contributory negligence is conduct on the part of the patient that is a contributory cause to his or her own injuries, which falls below the standard one owes oneself to avoid one's own injury at the hands of another. There is no requirement to act; the duty of self-protection always exists and is violated by unreasonable inaction in the face of danger.

At common law, a patient-plaintiff's contributory negligence is an absolute and complete bar to any recovery for the negligence of the patient as compared to the negligence of the physician.

An example is the *Robbins v. Geller* case.[15] A 51-year-old engineer complained of a changing skin mole. He was told not to worry by his first physician, but was offered the option of a biopsy by a second physician defendant, who thought the lesion was benign. The plaintiff never kept the appointment to have the biopsy

done by a dermatologist and died of malignant melanoma two years later. The jury held for the defendants, because the patient-plaintiff was referred to a specialist and chose himself not to keep the appointment.

Comparative negligence

Because contributory negligence acts as a complete bar to a patient-plaintiff's recovery, causing many harsh results, the majority of states by statute or judicially have adopted the doctrine of comparative negligence.

Under comparative negligence, malpractice recovery places the economic loss on the parties in proportion to their fault. In pure comparative negligence states, the plaintiffs can recover a percentage of their damages where their own negligence exceeds that of the defendant. For example, if the patient is 90% at fault, he or she can still recover 10% of the damages. Other states have a partial comparative negligence scheme, which denies recovery to any plaintiff who is one half or more at fault.

In the case of *Moore v. Preventive Medical Group,*[16] a 40-year-old part-time actor/model, during a regular checkup, asked about a black spot on his ear and was told not to worry about it; however, he was referred to a dermatologist for biopsy. A malignant melanoma was discovered six months later, and he ultimately lost half of his ear. The jury awarded $733,000 but reduced the judgment 24% due to the patient's comparative negligence for the delay in following up the recommendation to have a biopsy.

Loss of enjoyment of life

A category of damages consisting of the loss of enjoyment of life, which flows from physical impairments that limit the plaintiff's capacity to share in the amenities of life,[17] is sometimes termed *hedonistic* (hedonism is the doctrine that regards pleasure and happiness as the highest good) *damages.* A minority of jurisdictions do not allow any recovery for loss of enjoyment of life[18] arguing that it would encourage excessive damage awards and result in double compensation for the plaintiff. Most jurisdictions allow consideration of loss of enjoyment of life as one of the factors in an award for pain and suffering.[19] Some jurisdictions, however, have found loss of enjoyment of life to be an element of damages that is separate and distinct from pain and suffering.[20]

Loss of enjoyment of life can be clearly distinguished from other forms of compensable injury. The activities and functions in this category of damages are generally of a nonremunerative nature.[21] These include loss of smell and taste, and loss of the ability to dance, take walks, bowl, engage in sports, play musical instruments, perform household chores, and engage in sexual activity.

In *Ferguson v. Vest,*[22] the 63-year-old plaintiff was given radiation therapy to the vagina based on a Class V

Pap smear without the benefit of a biopsy. It was later discovered that she was cancer-free before radiation therapy was begun. The plaintiff claimed that defendants knew she had previously received a curative dosage of radiation to the vagina. She developed vaginal necrosis and stenosis, bladder and bowel dysfunction, and mental and emotional distress. She had temporary colostomies twice and had to have the vagina removed. She requires dilations of the urethra every three weeks. The verdict was for $2,332,000 including $1,200,000 for hedonic damages, or loss of ability to enjoy life's simple pleasures.

In *Nussbaum v. Gibstein,*[23] the plaintiff had a 1-centimeter mass noted in the breast in September 1982 by the defendant, and no tests were performed. Ten months later she had a painful lump in her left breast and a swelling under her left arm, which was diagnosed as cancer that had metastasized to bone. She died of the cancer 2 years later. The court held that loss of enjoyment of life was a compensable element of damages apart from specific award of damages for pain and suffering encountered by the patient during the 2-year battle with breast cancer. Loss of enjoyment of life damages require evidence of the nature and extent of the injured plaintiff's life-style prior to being injured and the limitations of his or her enjoyment of the pursuits of life following the injury.

In *Savelle v. Heilbrunn,*[24] the plaintiff had a hysterectomy and bilateral salpingo-oophorectomy for fibroids. The pathology was reported as showing no evidence of malignancy. Approximately 1 year later she had back pain, which was diagnosed as metastatic uterine leiomyosarcoma. Chemotherapy was started and the response was excellent. Following the discontinuation of chemotherapy because of the possibility of accumulative adverse effect, the tumor began to grow. Despite radiation therapy, the plaintiff had severe pain, is confined to home, and needs 24-hour-a-day nursing assistance. The defendant settled for $100,000, the limit of liability under Louisiana law. The court found the Louisiana Patient's Compensation fund liable for $400,000 additional damages for the physician's failure to diagnose the patient's uterine cancer and for loss of opportunity to receive earlier treatment with an increased chance of survival and better quality of life.

Recurrent problems in lawsuits resulting from a failure to diagnose cancer

Although variations in the standard of care and damage awards make generalizations imprecise, there are circumstances under which successful actions for failure to diagnose cancer have repeatedly arisen.

These recurrent themes are presented here in a manner to help prevent lawsuits from failure to diagnose

cancer while improving patient care, and should be of value to all those physicians who treat or examine patients in various clinical settings.

Medical history. The medical history is an important part of the diagnostic workup of cancer, as well as other diseases, and is stressed in the introductory course in physical diagnosis in most medical schools.

Unfortunately, many physicians neglect this important aspect of medical practice once out of medical school and either take no history at all or fail to go into depth in their patient interviews. Failure to take a medical history, or obtaining an incomplete medical history, may be a significant factor in failure to diagnose a cancer case.

As a result of a failure to obtain an adequate history, a physician may not include the diagnosis of certain cancers in the differential diagnoses or may not give proper weight to a diagnosis of possible cancer when evaluating certain clinical signs and symptoms. This inappropriately low suspicion of cancer may at times be negligent.

EXAMPLE 1. Family history or racial history of certain cancers is an important factor in evaluating asymptomatic patients for cancer screening, as well as for obtaining the proper, indicated tests in certain symptomatic patients.[25]

EXAMPLE 2. Occupational exposure, such as asbestos-related occupations, or social habits, such as alcoholism or smoking, may be important factors in the medical history in evaluating a patient for pulmonary neoplasm, liver cancer, or other malignancies and, if not elicited, could be important in establishing negligence in failure to diagnose certain cancers.

EXAMPLE 3. Significant X-ray exposure (e.g., breast neoplasia following tuberculosis pneumothorax collapse therapy, or thyroid cancer as a sequel to childhood radiation of benign head and neck problems), other radiation exposures (e.g., Thoratrast-induced liver cancer), or chemical exposure (e.g., benzene-induced malignancy) may be significant.

EXAMPLE 4. Exposure of a patient's forebears to certain drugs or carcinogens may increase the patient's own cancer risk (e.g., vaginal clear-cell carcinoma in DES daughters). Failure to inquire of this history, warn of dangers, and give guidelines to the patient herself may be considered negligent.[26]

Overreliance on certain facts obtained in taking the medical history may be just as significant in certain cases as failure to take an adequate history. Failure to detect the clues of certain symptoms as related by the patient because of a history of "cancerophobia" has been a factor in certain failures to diagnose cancer cases.[27]

Physical examination. Failure to perform a physical examination, performing an inadequate examination, overreliance on a negative examination, or failure to perform a follow-up examination may contribute to suits for failure to diagnose cancer.

Failure to perform an examination, especially after a presenting complaint referable to an organ later found cancerous, figures prominently in many failures to diagnose cancer cases, as does failure to perform follow-up examinations. In the 1985 case of *Gorman v. LaSasso,*[28] a Colorado jury awarded $1 million to a woman in her thirties who complained about the presence of a lump in her breast for six months, which was not investigated until the fourth time she complained about it.

Ordering a test in lieu of a physical examination will not necessarily protect a physician. A California jury in 1982 held for the plaintiff, who was dying of metastatic breast cancer, when her cancer was not diagnosed after her internist relied on a falsely negative mammogram report, prescribed pain medication for her breast lump, and told her to return only if the lump enlarged. An appellate court added $55,368 to the award for what the court called a frivolous appeal.[29]

Referral and testing. A physician has an affirmative duty to obtain or perform appropriate tests in the diagnosis of a suspected cancer. In *Barenbrugge v. Rich,*[30] a gynecologist did not order a mammogram on his 28-year-old patient after she presented with a breast lump later proven cancerous. He contended the test was dangerous for women under 30. His consultation with a general surgeon, who also did not order the test, did not exonerate him from blame. A jury verdict for $3 million was returned by a 1985 Illinois jury.

Failure of a physician to refer to another physician or specialist for a suspected cancer may also be a negligent act of omission. In the case of *O'Dell v. Chesney,*[31] a doctor of chiropractic treated a 63-year-old man for rectal bleeding and diabetes for two years. He was held negligent for failing to refer the patient to a medical doctor. The plaintiff died from colorectal cancer. The jury verdict of $125,000 was reduced by 40% because of the plaintiff's comparative negligence.

Failure of a physician to read the test report or consultant's recommendations or to communicate the report or recommendations to the patient may be negligent. In *Mehalik v. Morvant,*[32] a 42-year-old Louisiana woman was referred by her doctor for a mammogram to evaluate a breast lump. She was told by her doctor the mammogram report was negative, although the radiologist reported a suspicious mass and recommended follow-up. Relying on this report, she did not return for follow-up. A large breast cancer was confirmed later at biopsy, and the patient sued her physician for damages, with a resultant settlement.

Failure to repeat a test, perform additional studies, such as monoclonal antibody studies, or refer for biopsy when an initial test is negative may be negligent when clinical suspicion is (or should be) high that cancer may still be present.

A Massachusetts jury in the 1985 case of *Brown v. Nash,*[33] awarded $3 million to a woman because a surgeon failed to diagnose her breast cancer when he relied on a negative mammogram report, despite a changing physical abnormality noted in her breast. He elected, relying on the false-negative report, not to do a biopsy of an area later shown to be cancerous. The changing mass should have alerted him that a cancer was present, despite the negative report.

In *Glicklich v. Spievack,*[34] another Massachusetts court awarded $578,000 to a woman who was not referred by her primary care doctor to a surgeon for a biopsy, even though he relied on a false-negative mammogram report and a negative needle biopsy of a breast lump later diagnosed as malignant.

Even where a biopsy report is negative, overreliance on that report may be negligent when clinical suspicion should be high.

A federal judge in 1985, in the case of *Burke v. United States,*[35] awarded $1 million to a Maryland woman whose breast biopsy was erroneously interpreted as benign by a pathologist. Relying on this biopsy report, her surgeon dismissed her complaints of further change in her breast and did not order additional testing or perform another biopsy of the area, which later proved cancerous.

Mere reliance on a test performed by a consultant does not always mean negligence, however. A Louisiana court in *Lauro v. Travelers Insurance Co.*[36] held that it was not negligent for a surgeon to have removed a breast for cancer when a frozen section revealed a malignancy, even though later study revealed that a nonmalignant myeloblastoma (a very rare tumor) was found on final review.

Failure to follow recommended protocol. The American Cancer Society and various professional specialty organizations have for a number of years published guidelines for physicians, suggesting schedules or protocols for early cancer detection.

Although not binding in any way, these recommendations are widely disseminated via the mass media and are common public knowledge.

Failure to follow these protocols is not necessarily evidence of negligent failure to diagnose cancer. In fact, many physicians in practice do not follow these guidelines,[37,38] either because of ignorance or because they disagree with the society's educational program, which emphasizes the importance of early cancer detection.

However, it is common in litigation involving cancer diagnosis for attorneys to use compliance or noncompliance with published guidelines for health care,

1. Health counseling and cancer checkup to include examination for cancers of the thyroid, testicles, prostate, ovaries, lymph nodes, and skin every 3 years over the age of 20 and every year over the age of 40.
2. Sigmoidoscopy over the age of 50 to include two negative exams 1 year apart and then every 3 to 5 years.
3. Stool guaiac slide test every year over the age of 50.
4. Digital rectal examination every year over the age of 40.
5. In females:
   a. Pap test 1 year apart from age 18 and under age 18 if sexually active. After three consecutive negative exams, Pap test may be performed less frequently at physician's discretion.
   b. Pelvic examination every year from age 18 or under age 18 if sexually active.
   c. Endometrial tissue sample at menopause in women at high risk with a history of infertility, obesity, failure to ovulate, abnormal uterine bleeding, or estrogen therapy.
   d. Breast self-examination monthly over the age of 20.
   e. Breast examination every 3 years from age 20 to 40 and every year over the age of 40.
   f. Mammography every 1 to 2 years from age 40 to 49, and every year over the age of 50.

whether called "standards" or not, as evidence of satisfaction of the standard of care required.

Box 34-2 shows the guidelines for cancer-related checkups recommended by the American Cancer Society.[39]

RADIATION THERAPY

More than half of all cancer patients will ultimately need radiation therapy. The benefits of therapy must be weighed against the possible complications by the physician and the patient. Newer techniques have been developed with the use of the electron and proton beams to allow more accurate placement of the treatment with less damage to surrounding tissues.

Principles

Ionizing radiation may be used in the treatment and palliation of malignant tumors. Radiation sources include the cobalt-60 teletherapy unit, linear accelerator, and radioactive isotopes such as iridium-192, iodine-125, and phosphorus-32.[40]

The biological effects of radiation are directly pro-

portional to the dose. Cell death occurs from inability to reproduce, metabolic cell failure, or degeneration of the cell structure. Malignancies and normal body organs vary in their sensitivity to radiation, and therefore the dosage must be regulated in accordance with the desired results. It is possible to sensitize tissues to increase the response to radiation by the use of oxygen, nitric oxide, metronidazole, or through the use of hyperthermia.

Complications

Proper radiation may result in skin burns consisting of erythema (redness) or desquamation (dry or wet).[41] Ulceration with necrosis may be seen with prolonged healing time and scar deformity. Permanent pulmonary fibrosis in the treatment field for cancer of the breast does occur at times. Radiation enteritis following treatment of intra-abdominal malignancies is not unknown. Excessive radiation has been one source of litigation.

In *Duke v. Morphis,*[42] radon seeds were implanted in the supraclavicular area for treatment of a malignancy. The patient suffered myelopathy and paralysis, blaming the radiation treatment plan and the manner of supervision. The plaintiff was awarded $266,700.

In *Rudman v. Beth Israel Medical Center,*[43] a similar problem of paralysis following radiation treatment of a head and neck cancer brought a $2 million settlement.

In *Barnes & Powers v. Hahnemann Medical College and Hospital,*[44] a patient with cervical cancer was treated with radiation therapy and radium implants. Following a radical hysterectomy she suffered radiation cystitis, vesicovaginal fistula, radiation fibrosis of the ileum, and radiation fibrosis of the vagina. Multiple further surgeries were necessary to correct these problems. The case was settled for an undisclosed amount.

CHEMOTHERAPY

Medical oncology is a changing field with new chemotherapeutic agents and new combinations of agents being experimented with at a rapid pace. No other medical specialty handles extremely dangerous drugs almost on a daily basis. The potential side effects of these medications can affect every organ system, and yet these drugs are helping to save or prolong more lives.

Many of the antineoplastic drugs are mutagenic, teratogenic, and carcinogenic in animals.[45] Exposure to these agents can result in the appearance of mutagenic substances in the urine.[46] There have been reports of an increased incidence of acute myelogenous leukemia in patients treated with alkylating agents,[47] and bladder cancer has been associated with the use of cyclophosphamide, especially in low doses over prolonged periods of time.[48]

Chemotherapeutic agents can be fetotoxic and, therefore, potentially dangerous to health care personnel. Drugs that have been associated with fetal malformations include folate antagonists, 6-mercaptopurine, and alkylating agents,[49] and the MOPP (nitrogen mustard, vincristine, procarbazine, prednisone) treatment for Hodgkin's disease.[50] Personnel safety guidelines have been established to protect personnel who are mixing and administering antineoplastic drugs.[51]

Many patients are already aware of some of the possible physical effects of chemotherapy and are fearful of feeling sicker than they already are. This makes the job of the oncologist more difficult when trying to convince patients of the potential favorable effect on their malignancy and at the same time playing down the potential dangers. Patients, however, require knowledge of the possible benefits and the possible complications as well as any viable alternative of treatment and their potential complications.

Principles

Chemotherapeutic agents are used to kill malignant cells. Because cellular destruction occurs by the effect on reproducing cells, those cells dividing frequently are more susceptible. The drugs, however, do not discriminate between normal and malignant tissues. Therefore, normal organ systems may be adversely affected.

Complications

Hypersensitive reactions may occur with edema, rash, bronchospasm, diarrhea, and hypotension.[52] Some drugs such as Doxrubicin or Mitoxantrone are cardiotoxic. Bleomycin may cause pulmonary fibrosis. Hair loss (alopecia), leukopenia, and anemia are accepted side effects.

When there is extravasation with these highly toxic agents, tissue damage and necrosis can occur.

In *Lefler v. Yardumian,*[53] there was a leak of intravenous chemotherapy agents into the subcutaneous area of the arm. Tissue ulceration and damage to the tendons of the left hand occurred. The defense claim that the plaintiff was negligent in causing her own injuries resulted in a defense verdict.

Inadvertent overdose has been a source of litigation. In *Newman v. Geschke,*[54] a patient with throat cancer was given 12 to 15 mg of vincristine by the office nurse. This was 9 to 10 times the normal prescribed dosage. He developed neuropathies, bowel and bladder incontinence, weight loss, and alopecia, and required 3 weeks of hospitalization. The case was settled for $450,000.

UNORTHODOX CANCER TREATMENTS

Despite persistent efforts to achieve early detection, and exhaustive research aimed at developing effective treatment modalities, cancer continues to be a leading cause of death in the United States. Conventional cancer therapy includes surgery, chemotherapy, and radiation therapy in various combinations, depending on the nature and extent of disease involved in each particular case. Elaborate treatment protocols have been developed for virtually every stage of every type of cancer. These medical advances have undoubtedly resulted in increased survival or improved quality of life for some cancer patients. For many others, however, conventional cancer therapy has simply come to mean a sequence of painful, even disabling, experiences that do not in any way alter the inexorable course of the disease, and do not make them more comfortable, productive, or fulfilled during the time that remains.

For many years, cancer victims have attempted to seek out whatever ray of hope may be offered, even in the form of treatment that the medical establishment finds to be unproven, ineffective, or even fraudulent. These include metabolic therapy, diet therapies, megavitamins, mental imagery applied for antitumor effect, and spiritual or faith healing.[55] Despite recent technological advances in orthodox medical care, unorthodox cancer treatments are increasing in popularity.[56]

Cancer victims, particularly those who are terminally ill, are vulnerable to exploitation because of their predicament. Desperate for any glimmer of hope, they are easy prey for charlatans intent on financial gain. Traditionally, the law has protected those unable to protect themselves on the basis of *parens patriae.* This rationale has most frequently been applied to juveniles and the developmentally disabled.

However, the state's interest in protecting its citizens must be balanced against an individual's right to have control over his or her own body and to make decisions regarding his or her own medical care. Most cancer patients are adults in full control of their mental faculties, which distinguishes them from other citizens the state seeks to protect under the *parens patriae* rationale.

It is this basic conflict between the state's interest in the health and welfare of its citizens and the right of the individual to make decisions affecting his or her health that has confronted legislatures and courts attempting to deal with the problem of unorthodox cancer treatments.

To date, this conflict has not been resolved uniformly. Considerable variation currently exists among the various states with regard to regulation of unorthodox cancer treatment. Interestingly, where there has been legislative action, most legislatures have granted the individual some measure of freedom in selecting cancer treatment that is unproven. In most states that have acted legislatively, however, this freedom is not unlimited. When courts have considered the subject of unorthodox cancer treatment, they have focused more on the state's right to regulate the lives of its citizens under the police power.

Legislative approaches

The overwhelming majority of legislation dealing with unorthodox cancer treatment has concerned Laetrile (amygdalin). Nineteen states have enacted legislation authorizing the manufacture, sale, and distribution of Laetrile.[57] Other unorthodox cancer treatments that have received legislative protection include DMSO (dimethyl sulfoxide),[58] Gerovital H3 (procainamide hydrochloride with preservatives and stabilizers),[59] lily plant extract,[60] and prayer.[61]

Most states that have legislatively authorized the use of Laetrile have placed concurrent restrictions on its accessibility. Twelve states require that the treatment be prescribed by a licensed physician.[62] Three states allow the use of Laetrile only as an adjunct to conventional medical therapy.[63] Many of the states that require a licensed physician's prescription of the unorthodox treatment also require that the patient first sign a consent form indicating that the physician has explained that Laetrile or DMSO has not been proved to be effective in the treatment of cancer or other human diseases, that it has not been approved by the Food and Drug Administration for the treatment of cancer, that alternative therapies exist, and that the patient requests treatment with Laetrile or DMSO.[64]

Several states have attempted to maintain a precarious balance between police power and individual rights by reserving the right to prohibit unconventional cancer treatment when it is found to be harmful as prescribed or administered in a formal hearing before the appropriate state board.[65]

The most sweeping exercise of police power has been enacted in California, where it is a crime to sell, deliver, prescribe, or administer any drug or device to be used in the diagnosis, treatment, alleviation, or cure of cancer that has not been approved by the designated federal agency or by the state board.[66] As discussed later, the statute has been upheld by the California Supreme Court against a constitutional challenge based on the right of privacy.[67]

Judicial determination regarding unorthodox cancer therapy

The lack of uniformity among the states in regulating the use of unorthodox cancer treatments has created an environment in which patients who reside in states that do not authorize the manufacture, sale, or distribution of Laetrile or other unconventional therapies have attempted to obtain those substances from other states, or even from neighboring countries.[68] In several instances, patients have resorted to legal action in attempting to obtain Laetrile.

The most extensively litigated case has been *Rutherford v. United States,* which has generated eight federal court opinions,[69] including one from the U.S. Supreme Court.[70] *Rutherford* was a class action suit brought on behalf of terminally ill cancer patients who sought to enjoin the federal government from interfering with the interstate shipment and sale of Laetrile. The district court granted the injunction and ordered the government to permit Mr. Rutherford to purchase Laetrile. The basis for the ruling was that Laetrile, in proper doses, was nontoxic and effective in curing Mr. Rutherford's cancer.[71]

On appeal, the Court of Appeals for the Tenth Circuit instructed the district court to remand the case to the Food and Drug Administration in order to determine whether Laetrile was a new drug as defined in the federal Food, Drug, and Cosmetic Act,[72] and whether it was exempt from premarketing approval by the Food and Drug Administration (FDA) under either of the act's grandfather clauses.[73]

The FDA found that Laetrile did constitute a new drug under the applicable statutory definition because it was not generally recognized among experts as safe and effective for its prescribed use.[74] The FDA further determined that Laetrile was not exempt from premarketing approval under the applicable statute criteria.[75]

The case was then sent back to the district court, which reversed the FDA's determination and held that Laetrile was entitled to an exemption from premarketing approval, and further held that denial of cancer patients' rights to use a nontoxic substance in connection with their personal health violated their constitutional right of privacy.[76]

The Court of Appeals for the Tenth Circuit subsequently approved the lower court decision allowing the plaintiffs to obtain Laetrile, but did not address the constitutional issue.[77]

The U.S. Supreme Court granted *certiorari,* and reversed the Tenth Circuit's ruling.[78] The Supreme Court did not consider the right of privacy issue. It held that, under applicable statutory law, Laetrile was not a "safe and effective" drug, and therefore FDA approval was required prior to interstate distribution. The Court felt that, if an exception were to be made in the case of terminally ill cancer patients, that decision was for the legislature rather than the courts to make.[79]

On remand, the Tenth Circuit touched only briefly on the constitutional right of privacy issue.[80] The court simply stated that, within the context of the facts before it, a patient's selection of a particular treatment, or at least a medication, is within the area of governmental interest in protecting public health.[81]

Unfortunately, five years of litigation in the *Rutherford* case failed to yield a thorough analysis of the critical issue of whether the constitutional right of privacy affords cancer patients the right to select the treatment of their choice.

While *Rutherford* was being litigated, the California Supreme Court had occasion to consider the question of whether the state's police power could be used to restrict an individual's right of access to drugs of unproven effectiveness. *People v. Privitera*[82] involved prosecution of a physician and other individuals for conspiracy to sell and to prescribe an unapproved drug—Laetrile—intended for the alleviation or cure of cancer, in violation of applicable California statutory law.[83] The defendants appealed on the ground that the statute was unconstitutional, and that the state and federal constitutional rights of privacy encompassed a right to obtain Laetrile.

The court, by a 5-to-2 majority, held that Laetrile was a drug of unproven efficacy and is not included in either the federal or state constitutional rights of privacy. The court further held that the statute prohibiting the prescription or administration of any drug not approved by the FDA or state board was a permissible exercise of the state's police power, because it bore a reasonable relationship to the achievement of the legitimate state interest in the health and safety of its citizens.[84] The court distinguished previous cases recognizing various personal determinations as falling within the right of privacy on the ground that the prior cases were limited to such matters as marriage, procreation, contraception, family relationships, child rearing, and education, but did not include medical treatment.[85] This somewhat narrow interpretation was vigorously attacked by the dissent, which noted that the right to continue or terminate a pregnancy certainly involved medical treatment.[86] The dissent further noted that "the right to control one's own body is not restricted to the wise; it includes the foolish refusal of medical treatment."[87]

It is significant to note that none of the parties to the *Privitera* case was a cancer patient. The defendants in *Privitera* were individuals who had represented to the public that Laetrile was an effective cure for cancer and who had distributed Laetrile for profit. In some cases, the defendants neither obtained a medical history nor performed a physical examination on the patients to whom Laetrile was prescribed.[88] It is unfortunate that the court ruled on the right of privacy issue in a case in which those raising it had questionable standing to do so.

CONCLUSION

Despite a massive resource outlay directed at early detection and effective treatment of cancer, millions of cancer-related deaths are reported each year. Virtually none of the treatments labeled by orthodox medicine as ineffective has been the subject of well-controlled scientific studies.[89] The scope of research must be broadened to include all modalities in which there appears to be substantial public interest.[90] As a broader range of information becomes available, patients will be able to make more informed decisions regarding treatment.

Although some states have enacted legislation allowing patients to obtain certain types of alternative cancer therapies, the majority of state legislatures remain silent on this issue. The courts have been reluctant to affirm a cancer patient's right to select his or her own treatment as encompassed by the constitutional right of privacy. There appear to be several reasons for this: (1) An ideal fact situation, clearly defining the issue, has not yet been presented to the courts; (2) because of the rapid progression of many types of cancer, the slow justice often afforded by the court system may not be a practicable forum for terminally ill cancer patients; and (3) the courts seem disposed to defer to the state of orthodox medical knowledge as set forth in the legislative histories usually quoted in the court opinions.

Certain individual decisions regarding health care have already been recognized as falling within the constitutionally protected right of privacy. Although virtually all cancer patients can be expected, in varying degrees, to be anxious, depressed, or frightened because of their disease, the majority are still responsible, mentally sound adults. The *parens patriae* rationale would not seem to be applicable to such patients, as it would be in cases of juveniles or the developmentally disabled. Accordingly, the balance weighs heavily in favor of allowing cancer patients to obtain the treatment of their choice. The state's interest in protecting the health of its citizens can be adequately protected in this context by requiring an informed consent by the patient following disclosure of the nature of the proposed treatment, the fact that it has not been proved to be effective by well-controlled scientific studies, and the availability of conventional treatment.

END NOTES

1. *Bardessano v. Michels,* 3 Cal. 3d 780, 788, 18A.L.R. 4th 132 (1970).
2. *Cobbs v. Grant,* 8 Cal. 3d 229, 245 (1972).
3. See Alaska Stat. 09.556; De. Code Ann. tit. 18, 6852; Idaho Code 39-4304; Iowa Code Ann. 147.137 (West); Me. Rev. Stat. Ann. tit. 24; N.Y. Pub. Health 2805-D (McKinney); N.C. Gen. Stat. 90-21.13; Ohio Rev. Code Ann. 2317.54 (Anderson); Or. Rev. Stat. 677.097; Pa. Stat. Ann. tit. 40 (Pivodon); R.I. Gen. Laws 9-19-32; Tenn. Code Ann. 78-14-5; Vt. Stat. Ann. tit. 12, 1908; Wash. Rev. Code 7.70.050.
4. Office of the General Counsel, Texas Department of Health, 1100 West 49th Street, Austin, Texas 78756.
5. 12 Pac. L.J. 915, 928-35 (1980).
6. *Long v. Patterson,* No. 82-3947, Hillsborough Sup. Ct. (Fla. 1982). In 1 Med. Mal. Verdicts, Settlements and Experts 14 (1985).

7. *Sygman v. Kahn,* No. 18778/82, Kings County Sup. Ct. (N.Y. Oct. 4, 1982). In 1 Med. Mal. Verdicts, Settlements and Experts 5 (1985).

8. *Davis v. United States,* No. LR-C-83-978 (E.D. Ark. 1983). In 1 Med. Mal. Verdicts, Settlements and Experts 5 (1985).

9. NORCAL Claims RX, Vol. 4, No. 4 (Oct.-Nov. 1983).

10. *Kremer v. Kaiser Foundation Hosp.,* No. 184,819, San Bernardino County Ct. (Cal. Dec. 14, 1982).

11. *Brown v. Nash,* No. 63471, Suffolk Super. Ct. (Mass. June 19, 1985). In 2 Med. Mal. Verdicts, Settlements and Experts 13 (1986).

12. *Nathanson v. Yarvis,* No. 195/79, Nassau County Sup. Ct. (N.Y. 1979). In 1 Med. Mal. Verdicts, Settlements and Experts 19 (1985).

13. *Ippolito v. LaGuardia Hospital,* No. 8704/82, Queens County Sup. Ct. (N.Y. June 21, 1985). In 2 Med. Mal. Verdicts, Settlements and Experts 8 (1986).

14. *Morrison v. Stallworth,* 326 S.E. 2d 387 (N.C. Ct. App. 1985). In 1 Med. Mal. Verdicts, Settlements and Experts 9 (1985).

15. *Robbins v. Geller,* No. EAC28269, Pomona County Ct. (Cal. Jan. 7, 1982).

16. *Moore v. Preventive Medicine Group,* No. 59642, Santa Monica Sup. Ct. (Cal. 1982). In 1 Med. Mal. Verdicts, Settlements and Experts, 5 (1985).

17. *Huff v. Tracy,* 57 Cal. App. 3d 439, 129 Cal. Rptr. 551 (1976); *Thompson v. National RR Passenger Corp.,* 621 F2d 814 (6th Cir. 1980).

18. 15 A.L.R. 3d 511-13 (1967).

19. 15 A.L.R. 3d 513-14 (1967).

20. 15 A.L.R. 3d 514-16 (1967).

21. C. R. Cramer, *Loss of Enjoyment of Life as a Separate Element of Damages,* 12 Pac. Law J. 972 (1981).

22. *Ferguson v. Vest,* No. 87-L-207 (IL). In 6 Med. Mal. Verdicts, Settlements and Experts 44-45 (1990).

23. *Nussbaum v. Gibstein,* 138 A.D.2d 193, 531 N.Y.S.2d 276 (A.D. 2 Dept. 1988).

24. *Savelle v. Heilbrunn,* 552 So. 2d 52 (La. Ct. App. 1989).

25. Anderson, *Counseling Women on Familial Breast Cancer,* 37 Cancer Bull. 130-31 (1985).

26. Mills, *Prenatal Diethylstilbestrol and Vaginal Cancer in Offspring,* 229 JAMA 471-72 (1974).

27. *Burke v. United States,* No. M-84-425 (Md. 1984). In 1 Med. Mal. Verdicts, Settlements and Experts 9 (1985).

28. *Gorman v. LaSasso,* No. 83-CV-6311, Denver Dist. Ct. (Colo. 1983). In 1 Med. Mal. Verdicts, Settlements and Experts 17 (1985).

29. *Ok-Jae Song v. Smatko,* 208 Cal. Rptr. 300 (Cal. Ct. App. Nov. 16, 1984, as corrected, Dec. 11, 1984).

30. *Barenbrugge v. Rich,* No. 81L8949, Cook County Cir. Ct. (Ill. Oct. 25, 1984). In 2 Med. Mal. Verdicts, Settlements and Experts 17 (1986).

31. *O'Dell v. Chesney,* No. 118-496, Riverside County Ct. (Cal. Jan. 15, 1982).

32. *Mehalik v. Morvant,* No. 45173, Lafourche Parish Ct. (La. 1981) (Note: This case was settled on Dec. 9, 1985).

33. *Brown, supra* note 11.

34. *Glicklich v. Spievack,* No. 80-2150, Middlesex Ct. App. (Mass. Dec. 8, 1983).

35. *Burke v. United States,* No. 83-CV-6311, Denver Dist. Ct. (Colo. 1983). In 1 Med. Mal. Verdicts, Settlements and Experts 9 (1985).

36. *Lauro v. Travelers Insurance Co.,* 261 So. 2d 261 (La. 1972), *writ denied,* 262 So. 2d 787 (La. 1972).

37. American Cancer Society, *Survey of Physicians' Attitudes and Practices in Early Cancer Detection,* 35 CA 197-213 (1985).

38. Woo, *Screening Procedures in the Asymptomatic Adult,* 254 JAMA 1480-84 (1985).

39. *Guidelines for the Cancer-Related Checkup: Five Years Later,* 35 CA–A Cancer J. for Clinicians 194-213 (1985).

40. C. M. Haskell, *Cancer Treatment,* 19-27 (W.B. Saunders Co., Philadelphia 1980).

41. G. Fletcher, *Textbook of Radiotherapy,* 284 (Lea & Febiger, Philadelphia 1980).

42. *Duke v. Morphis,* Superior Court, Tarrant County. (Tex.) No. 352-62434-80. In 4 Med. Mal. Verdicts, Settlements and Experts 43 (1988).

43. *Rudman v. Beth Israel Medical Center,* Supreme Court of the State of New York, County of New York (N.Y.) No. 4764/86. In 4 Med. Mal. Verdicts, Settlements and Experts 46 (1988).

44. *Barnes & Powers v. Hahnemann Medical College and Hosp.,* Common Pleas Court of Philadelphia (Pa.) No. 4031, 1982. In 3 Med. Mal. Verdicts, Settlements and Experts 35 (1987).

45. International Agency for Research on Cancer (WHO), 26 IARC Monographs on the Evaluation of the Carcinogenic Risk of Chemicals to Humans 37-384. (International Agency for Research on Cancer, Lyon, France 1981).

46. K. Falck, et al., *Mutagenicity in Urine of Nurses Handling Cytostatic Drugs,* 1 Lancet 1250-51 (1979); T. V. Nguyen, et al., *Exposure of Pharmacy Personnel to Mutagenic Antineoplastic Drugs,* 42 Cancer Res 4792-96 (1982).

47. D. E. Bergsagel, et al., *The Chemotherapy of Plasma-Cell Myeloma and the Incidence of Acute Leukemia,* 301 New Eng. J. Med. 743-48 (1979); R. R. Reimer, et al., *Acute Leukemia after Alkylating-Agent Therapy of Ovarian Cancer,* 297 New Eng. J. Med. 177-81 (1977).

48. P. H. Plotz, et al., *Bladder Complications in Patients Receiving Cyclophosphamide for Systemic Lupus Erythematosus or Rheumatoid Arthritis,* 91 Annals Intern. Med. 221-23 (1979).

49. H. O. Nicholson, *Cytotoxic Drugs in Pregnancy. Review of Reported Cases,* 75 J. Obstet. Gynaecol. Br. Commonw. 307-12 (1968).

50. M. J. Garrett, *Letter: Teratogenic Effects of Combination Chemotherapy,* 80 Annals Intern. Med. 667 (1974).

51. R. B. Jones, et al., *Safe Handling of Chemotherapeutic Agents: A Report from the Mount Sinai Medical Center,* 33 CA–A Cancer J. for Clinicians 258-63 (1983).

52. R. B. Weiss and S. Bruno. *Hypersensitivity Reactions to Cancer Chemotherapy Agents,* 94 Annals Int. Med. 66, 71 (1981).

53. *Lefler v. Yardumian,* Superior Court, Pinellas County (IL) No. 83-14700. In 3 Med. Mal. Verdicts, Settlements and Experts 35 (1987).

54. *Newman v. Geschke,* Superior Court, Multnomah County (Ore.) No. A8609-05800. In 4 Med. Mal. Verdicts, Settlements and Experts 46 (1988).

55. Cassileth, *Contemporary Unorthodox Treatments in Cancer Medicine,* 101 Annals Int. Med. 105-12, 107 (1984).

56. *Id.*

57. Alaska Stat. 08.64.367; Ariz. Rev. Stat. Ann. 26-2452; Del. Code Ann. 16-4901-05; Fla. Stat. Ann. 500.1515 (West); Idaho Code 18-7301A; Ind. Code Ann. 16-8-8-1-7 (Burns); Kan. Stat. Ann. 65-6b; Ky. Rev. Stat. Ann. 311.950 (Baldwin); La. Rev. Stat. Ann. 40:676; Md. Code Ann. 18-301; Mont. Code Ann. 50-41-102; Nev. Rev. Stat. 585.495; N.J. Stat. Ann. 24:6F-1 (West); N.D. Cent. Code 23-23.1; Okla. Stat. Ann. 63-2-313; Or. Rev. Stat. 689.535; Tex. Rev. Civ. Stat. Ann. 71, article 4476-5a; Wash. Rev. Code Ann. 70.54.1310; W. Va. Code 30-5-16a.

58. Fla. Stat. Ann. 499.035 (West); Kan. Stat. Ann. 65-679a; La. Rev. Stat. Ann. 40-1060 (West); Mont. Code Ann. 42-102; Okla. Stat. Ann. 363-2-313.12; Tex. Rev. Civ. Stat. Ann. 71, article 4476.5b.

59. Nev. Rev. Stat. 585.495.

60. Okla. Stat. Ann. 63-2-313.7 (West).

61. Colo. Rev. Stat. 12-30-113(2).

62. Alaska, Delaware, Florida, Indiana, Maryland, Montana, Nevada, New Jersey, North Dakota, Oklahoma, Texas, and Washington.

63. Idaho, Indiana, and Oklahoma.

64. Arizona, Indiana, Louisiana, New Jersey, Oklahoma, Texas, and Washington.
65. Alaska, Colorado, Delaware, Louisiana, and Maryland.
66. California Health and Safety Code 1701.1 (West 1979).
67. *People v. Privitera,* 23 Cal. 3d 697, 153 Cal. Rptr. 4431, 591 P.2d 919 (1979).
68. Marco, *Laetrile: The Statement and the Struggle, in Legal Medicine* 121-36 (C. H. Wecht ed. 1980).
69. *Rutherford v. United States,* 399 F. Supp. 1208 (W.D. Okla. 1975); *Rutherford v. United States,* 542 F. 2d 1137 (10th Cir. 1976); *Rutherford v. United States,* 424 F. Supp. 105 (W.D. Okla. 1977); *Rutherford v. United States,* 429 F. Supp. 506 (W.D. Okla. 1977); *Rutherford v. United States,* 438 F. Supp. 1287 (W.D. Okla. 1977); *Rutherford v. United States,* 582 F. 2d 1234 (190th Cir. 1978); *Rutherford v. United States,* 616 F. 2d 455 (10th Cir. 1980).
70. *Rutherford,* 442 U.S. 544.
71. *Rutherford,* 399 F. Supp. 1208, 1215.
72. 21 U.S.C. 321 (P) (1) (1980).
73. *Rutherford,* 542 F. 2d 1137.
74. 42 Fed. Reg. 39775-39787 (1977).
75. *Id.* at 39787-39795.
76. *Rutherford,* 438 F. Supp. 1287, at 1294-1300.
77. *Rutherford,* 582 F. 2d 1234.
78. *Rutherford,* 442 U.S. 544.
79. *Id.* at 559.
80. *Rutherford,* 616 F. 2d 455, 457.
81. *Id.*
82. *People v. Privitera,* 23 Cal. 3d 697, 153 Cal. Rptr. 431, 591 P. 2d 919 (1979). For a judicial decision that reached a different conclusion, see *Suenram v. Society of the Valley Hospital,* 155 N.J. Super. 593, 383 A. 2d 143 (1977). The Suenram court was not considering a statute, however, and, in fact, the New Jersey legislature authorized the use of Laetrile shortly after the court's opinion was rendered.
83. California Health and Safety Code 1707.1, which provides as follows: "The sale, offering of sale, holding for sale, delivering, giving away, prescribing or administering of any drug, medicine, compound or device to be used in the diagnosis, treatment, alleviation or cure of cancer is unlawful and prohibited unless (1) an application with respect thereto has been approved under 505 of the Federal Food, Drug and Cosmetic Act, or (2) there has been approved an application filed with the board setting forth: (a) Full reports of investigations have been made to show whether or not such a drug, medicine, compound or device is safe for such use, and whether such drug, medicine, compound or device is effective in such use; (b) A full list of the articles used as components of such drug, medicine, compound or device; (c) A full statement of the composition of such drug, medicine, compound or device; (d) A full description of the methods used in, and the facilities and controls used for, the manufacture, processing and packaging of such drug, medicine, or compound or in the case of a device, a full statement of its composition, properties and construction and the principle or principles of its operation; (e) Such samples of such drug, medicine, compound or device and of the articles used as components of the drug, medicine, compound or device as the board may require; and (f) Specimens of the labelling to be used for such drug, medicine, compound or device and advertising proposed to be used for such drug, medicine, compound or device."
84. *People v. Privitera,* 153 Cal. Rptr. 431, 433.
85. *Id.* at 437.
86. *Id.* at 434.
87. *Id.* at 444.
88. *Id.*
89. For an example of a well-controlled study of the effect of an "unorthodox" cancer treatment, *see* Johnston, *Clinical Effect of Coley's Toxin: I. A Controlled Study,* Cancer Chemotherapy Reports, Number 21 (Aug. 1962).
90. Cassileth, *supra* note 42.

CHAPTER 35 Brain-injured patients

CLARK WATTS, M.D., J.D.

PRIMARY CAUSES OF BRAIN IMPAIRMENT
THE PROCESS
THE DIFFERENTIAL DIAGNOSIS
TRAUMATIC BRAIN IMPAIRMENT
BRAIN RECOVERY
LEGAL CONSIDERATIONS

When referencing the brain, the general term *injured* should be considered in its broadest context. The brain is considered injured when it sustains pathology from whatever cause. Although this is the context in which the term will be used in this chapter, we will focus on the traumatically brain-injured patient because most of the medicolegal implications of brain injury apply to this group of patients.

It is very important for the legal practitioner to understand how the physician will arrive at a diagnosis in these patients, through the process of creating a differential diagnosis. Equally important for the legal practitioner representing brain-injured patients is an understanding of how the brain recovers, and how the injury and the recovery are quantitated. Of additional importance to the legal practitioner is an awareness of obstacles to coverage of brain injuries by insurance interpretations.

PRIMARY CAUSES OF BRAIN IMPAIRMENT

Prior to any discussion of the differential diagnosis of primary causes of brain impairment, it is helpful to understand how one arrives at a differential diagnosis.[1] A differential diagnosis is simply a listing, usually by probabilities, but often without stating the mathematical probabilities, of diseases that it is reasonable to consider in a person suffering from brain impairment. The process of arriving at the differential diagnosis is a relatively simple one, but often poorly understood. It begins, as with all contacts between physicians and patients, with a history and a physical examination to elicit signs and symptoms from the patient. This is followed by correlating the signs and symptoms with the anatomy and physiology of the portion of the brain that

seems to relate to those signs and symptoms. The process of time over which the signs and symptoms have been present is factored in, and the most likely disease categories, based on general pathology, are then extracted from the process. Confirmation of the conclusions at this point is obtained by laboratory tests and, finally, a differential diagnosis of specific pathology is created.

THE PROCESS
Signs and symptoms

Symptoms are those complaints the patient presents to the physician. *Signs* are those findings the physician elicits by physical examination. In eliciting the signs and symptoms of a patient with suspected brain disease, it is important to keep in mind that the brain can express itself in response to disease in only a few ways. The brain may respond to disease by an alteration of the *mental status* of the patient. Usually, an alteration of mental status is an alteration in the level of consciousness. The patient may appear conscious and be awake and alert, lethargic, or obtunded. Or the patient may present in or deteriorate into an unconscious state. An important subset of the mental status examination is a search for any derangements of intellect, orientation, self-awareness, or memory.

The patient with impaired brain function may present with *motor* symptomatology. Most patients with this group of signs and symptoms will be noted to have certain patterns of paresis, or weakness of muscle function. Some will present, however, without significant weakness, but instead will have abnormal movements created by disorders of the nervous system such as spasticity or seizure disorders. The muscles may be unusually rigid or uncoordinated in action. The abnormal movements may be noted during voluntary or involuntary activity.

Pain, such as headaches, is the most common form of *sensory* complaint. The patient may also complain of abnormal sensation, as with paresthesias, or electric-like painful phenomena, or numbness, the presence of dulled sensation. The complaint may be present spontaneously, or only when the physician, in examining the patient, obtains an admission of the symptom. Other sensory complaints may involve visual or hearing difficulties.

Disturbances of *language* are a common complaint of patients with brain impairment. Language disorders can be categorized in several ways, but generally they can be placed into three separate groups, called *aphasias*. In expressive aphasia the person has, as the name implies, trouble expressing himself, that is, trouble making coherent, understandable sentences. The person suffering from receptive aphasia has difficulty receiving communication input and processing it into meaningful language. The verbal expressions of these individuals may appear normal, even quite articulate, but they have no relationship to input received. The person with global aphasia has elements of both and, in the worst cases, may be mute.

Finally, afflictions of the brain may reflect themselves as *disorders of the mind.* This group of presenting signs and symptoms is mainly concerned with emotions, disturbances of reality, and alterations of self-image.

It is rare that the patient will present with a single group of symptoms; more often there will be a constellation of symptoms. For example, a patient presenting with a tumor involving the left side of the brain may complain of lethargy, headaches, numbness and weakness of the right arm and leg, blindness in certain portions of the field of vision, expressive aphasia, and depression.

Consideration of anatomy/physiology

Groups of symptoms and signs may, with some accuracy, be related to anatomy and physiology in the process of localizing the disorder within the brain. The brain consists of four anatomical elements, which are connected anatomically and physiologically. The largest mass of the brain is the *cerebrum,* composed of the two lateral cerebral hemispheres. Each has a frontal lobe anteriorly, a parietal and a temporal lobe laterally, and an occipital lobe posteriorly. The two frontal lobes in association with structures connecting the two cerebral hemispheres in the midline (portions of the limbic "lobe") are functionally related to personality, emotion, and self-image. The posterior aspects of each frontal lobe provide voluntary motor function for the opposite side of the body, whereas the anterior aspects of both

parietal lobes provide conscious sensory function to the opposite side of the body. Brain auditory function is served by temporal lobes as is memory when the temporal lobes are interacting with the frontal lobes. In most individuals, voluntary and conscious speech function is located in the left frontotemporoparietal area of the left cerebral hemisphere, whereas, visual-spatial orientation function is lateralized to the right cerebral hemisphere, particularly the right parietal lobe.

The second element of the brain is the *cerebellum,* located posterior, beneath the cerebrum. This paired structure is responsible, primarily, for involuntary actions of coordination.

Descending down from the middle of the base of the paired cerebral hemispheres, passing anterior to the cerebellum on its way into the spinal canal where it continues as the spinal cord, is the *brain stem,* the third element. It serves as a major pathway for nervous impulses to leave the brain and enter the spinal cord, and to pass from the spinal cord to the brain.

The final element of the brain is the collection of *cranial nerves,* which passes from the various other elements of the brain to structures peripheral to the skull. They conduct impulses to the brain that provide the senses of vision, smell, taste, and hearing; the voluntary functions of the face, such as mastication and sensation; and certain automatic functions of the body such as rhythmicity of the heart and autonomic bowel function.

An example of the importance of considerations regarding localization can be seen in the patient who complains of visual disturbances. If that patient were also complaining of weakness in the left hand, one would consider a lesion in the right cerebral hemisphere that is affecting the nerve fibers of vision as they pass from the eye in front to the occipital lobe in the posterior aspects of the cerebral hemisphere where vision is recognized. On the other hand, if the patient with visual disturbances were also complaining of problems with smell or taste, one might look more anterior, to the region of the eyes, where the eyes are more closely associated with nasal and oral mucosa from which taste emanates.

Considerations of time

In arriving at a differential diagnosis, one must not only consider the patient's signs and symptoms and anatomical/physiological correlations, but one must also factor in the time course over which the symptoms and the signs are present. For example, the patient may very well have a headache precipitated by a minor episode of head trauma. The headache would come on suddenly coincident with the trauma and persist appropriately. A headache similar in intensity and location, however, may have gradually developed over several weeks or months in a patient with a brain tumor. Likewise, a brain tumor may cause hand weakness progressively and slowly over several months, whereas, a stroke, secondary to cerebral vascular embolization, may cause a sudden onset of hand weakness.

General pathology

The general pathology of the underlying condition causing brain impairment may be more accurately suspected once signs and symptoms, potential location, and the dimension of time are considered. Consider an example where the pathology is expected to be present in the brain stem. A collection of signs and symptoms gradually developing over a period of time may suggest the development of a mass lesion such as a neoplasm or an abscess. Such a situation would rarely include the sudden onset of coma. On the other hand, consider a patient who had previously experienced over a period of time intermittent transient numbness and weakness on one side or the other of the face and, occasionally, on both sides. If the patient then develops sudden onset of coma, she or he is more likely to be suffering from a cerebral vascular accident involving the brain stem than to be suffering from a tumor.

THE DIFFERENTIAL DIAGNOSIS

After the physician works through the process of analysis in considering the patient's presenting signs and symptoms, the anatomical and physiological localization of the suspected lesion, the time course for the development and presentation of the suspected lesion, and the general pathologic nature of the suspected lesion, the etiology of the brain impairment may preliminarily be placed into one or more categories of diseases from which a more specific differential diagnosis may be extracted. After providing definitions and examples of the major categories of neurological diseases, we will categorize the traumatic diseases to illustrate the process of developing a specific differential diagnosis.

Disease categories

Brain impairment may occur as a result of disease categorized as follows: genetic, congenital/developmental, degenerative/metabolic, infectious, traumatic, neoplastic, vascular, immunologic, psychogenic, and idiopathic.

Most of the primary diseases of the brain associated with *genetic* disorders are characterized by an underlying error of metabolism. To understand this concept, it is helpful to look at one of the earliest recognized and best understood primary brain disorders produced by a genetic abnormality, phenylketonuria. This disorder, untreated, is seen primarily in children and is highlighted by mental retardation, seizures, and imperfect hair

pigmentation, and is transmitted as an autosome recessive condition. Due to a well-defined genetic disorder, the gene necessary for the activation of an enzyme, phenylalanine hydroxylase, is disturbed and the enzyme is almost completely lacking. As a result, the normal conversion of phenylalanine to tyrosine does not occur. Instead, phenylalanine is converted to phenylpyruvic acid, phenylacetic acid, and phenylacetylglutamine. With the accumulation of these metabolites in the brain, there is interference with normal maturation of the brain, neurofibers within the brain are not properly myelinated (a process of normal insulation), and other widespread and diffuse anomalies develop. Fortunately, in children born with this disorder, urine and blood levels of phenylalanine rise in the first few days and weeks of life and can be detected by a simple screening test.

In general, *congenital/developmental* disorders are those created by a deleterious effect of the environment, either *in utero* or following birth, upon the developing brain. Some years ago a number of the genetic disorders were placed in this category. However, as specific abnormalities in the genome have been identified, the corresponding disorders have been removed from this category. The term *cerebral palsy* refers to a general condition caused by a number of different environmental insults to the developing brain. While its most common presentation is a spastic weakness of all four extremities, some children may experience mental retardation and seizure disorders. The characteristic of this type of congenital disorder is that it is not progressive, although it may appear to be so as the child grows and becomes progressively more disabled in comparison with his or her peers. The etiologic insult may occur before birth, in the perinatal period, or in the first few years of life. Cerebral palsy is believed to be caused by any number of insults including abnormal implantation of the ovum, maternal diseases, threatened but aborted miscarriages, external toxins, or metabolic insults such as maternal alcohol ingestion.

The category of diseases termed *degenerative/metabolic* disorders is usually reserved for those conditions that develop in individuals with previously normal brain development. It is appropriate today to exclude conditions with known genetic bases, even though they express themselves later in life, such as Huntington's chorea, or conditions that are congenital or developmental and, as noted previously, appear to progress as the affected individual is compared with developing peers. Alzheimer's disease was at one time believed to be a classic condition in this category. Individuals in the prime of their senior years develop a rapid dementia associated with specific neuropathologic changes in the brain of unknown etiology. The dementia is rapid and occurs much earlier than would be expected based simply on senility. With recent suggestions that this condition may have an underlying genetic predisposition, it may be more appropriate now to consider it as one of the genetic disorders, noting the appropriateness of genetic counseling. Aside from Alzheimer's disease, the most studied degenerative/metabolic disease of the nervous system is probably parkinsonism. This condition is characterized by a progressive uncontrollable tremor with an associated dementia. The motor disability created by the tremor often progresses much more rapidly than the dementia, so that patients, well aware of their limitations, suffer substantial depression. For some reason certain cells within the brain are unable to manufacture an appropriate amount of an agent, dopamine, which is metabolically necessary for the function of the cells. A large number of patients infected during the influenza epidemic of 1918 developed this condition later in life. However, it is not believed that the majority of the patients today have this problem secondary to viral infection. In fact, the etiology of the condition in most patients today is not at all clear, although because the dementia is similar to that of Alzheimer's, there may be an association. A syndrome identical to parkinsonism has been described in a group of drug abusers who have used n-methyl-4-phenyl-1236-tetrahydropyridine, both intravenously and by inhalation.

Most known *infectious* agents have been reported to cause infections of the brain. Meningitis is a term used to refer to infections of the coverings of the brain, whereas encephalitis is used to refer to an infection within the brain. In addition to the generalized widespread infectious processes these terms suggest, localized brain infections, or abscesses, can also occur. Management is to provide the appropriate treatment based on proper identification of the underlying etiologic agent, whether it is bacterial, viral, fungal, or parasitic. This category of disease lends itself to a simplified discussion of how the physician might use the earlier presented scheme of analysis. A patient who has the fairly rapid development of brain impairment associated with a fever might be considered to have a disease within this category. If widespread impairment ensues that is characterized by nonfocal deficits and suppression of the mental status of the patient, one might consider meningitis or encephalitis. If, however, the disease process appears to be focal in nature resulting in a partial paralysis (e.g., hemiparesis or weakness on one side of the body) one might consider the presence of a more focal infectious process such as a brain abscess.

The *traumatic* category of diseases encompasses everything associated with acute brain trauma. This includes not only diseases caused by disruption of brain tissue, but also diseases caused by systemic illnesses secondary to the traumatic episode, whether or not this trauma directly involves the head. For example, not uncommonly, following trauma to the head, the patient experiences a period of apnea or diminished respiratory effort. If this is not corrected quickly, the patient may suffer hypoxia, or a lack of oxygen, which can damage brain cells. A more comprehensive discussion of traumatic brain disease appears later in this chapter to provide more details of the application of principles for defining a specific differential diagnosis of primary brain impairment.

The category of *neoplastic* diseases contains all tumors that are progressive in development, whether benign or malignant. It includes those tumors that arise primarily within the brain and those that metastasize to the brain from extracranial sites. As suggested by the foregoing comments, it is traditional to describe tumors as benign or malignant. A benign tumor is one that grows more slowly, does not extend beyond the confines of the tumor mass itself, and does not metastasize or spread through the vascular system. The malignant tumor is a more aggressive tumor. It has a shorter time course and may very well spread to other parts of the brain or the body by way of the vascular stream. The malignant tumor characteristically results in death in a shorter period of time than the benign tumor. However, this concept may be deceiving in that a histologically benign tumor placed in a critical location within the brain may cause death quicker than a malignant tumor placed within the brain in a location that is not as critical. All tumors cause impairment by one of two mechanisms. They may produce direct pressure on the surrounding brain. Additionally, they develop a volume that cannot be accommodated safely within the fixed cranial vault. Consequently generalized increased intracranial pressure occurs, which adversely affects the flow of blood in sensitive areas of the brain not directly contiguous with the mass itself.

Most diseases in the *vascular* category affect the blood vessels directly or indirectly. Primarily congenital or developmental conditions, such as aneurysms and arteriovenous malformations, can produce sudden brain impairment by hemorrhage. Arteriosclerosis of the vessels, a degenerative/metabolic condition, may cause sudden impairment by creating an occlusion of the vessels, causing death of tissue from lack of circulating oxygen and nutrients. Occlusions may also occur with embolization of cerebral vessels by arteriosclerotic debris from other sites such as diseased heart valves.

Immunologic diseases are caused by disturbances of the immune system. Multiple sclerosis is such a condition. It is characterized by repeated and progressive bouts of demyleinization of nerve cells and their axons, which are extensions of cells to connect with other cells. These extensions ordinarily contain an insulating material called myelin. As a result of disturbances in the immune system not completely understood, the myelin is recognized by the body as a foreign substance and is placed under lymphocytic attack and destruction. Presentation of the patient will depend on the area of the brain affected, with any combination of signs and symptoms possible.

The category of *psychogenic* diseases refers to those recognized and characterized as diseases of the mind associated with personality disorders, disturbances of emotion, and problems of self-image not placed in one of the preceding categories. Certainly, patients may be depressed as a result of head trauma or disabling conditions such as parkinsonism.

Iatrogenic diseases are those produced as a result of treatment by the physician of other conditions. A patient who develops a blood clot following surgery for a brain tumor due to inadequate hemostasis by the surgeon has developed an iatrogenic hemorrhage.

Idiopathic diseases are those for which there is no known, or reasonably suspected, etiology. As a result of dramatic recent advances in the neurosciences, especially in neuroimaging, these are so few in number that this category is presented only for completeness.

TRAUMATIC BRAIN IMPAIRMENT

The process of establishing a differential neurological diagnosis has changed in the last several years. This change has been brought about by the significant technological advances that have been made in neuroradiology, especially in neuroimaging. Prior to these advances, most differential diagnoses of brain impairment were expressed in terms of the category of diseases with confirmation often left to surgery or autopsy. However, as the result of today's imaging technology, including computerized tomographic (CT) scanning, magnetic resonance imaging (MRI), and other relatively noninvasive high-resolution imaging devices, it is routine to develop a specific list of potential diseases within an individual category. This is the case involving trauma.

The diagnosis of traumatic brain disease usually begins with the identification of a traumatic episode resulting in either blunt or penetrating head injury. Penetrating head injuries generally produce less of a problem in the differential diagnosis because the penetrating offender, usually a bullet, will produce primary brain disruption and some hemorrhage. More challenging is the establishment of a differential diagnosis of traumatic brain disease following blunt trauma.

During blunt trauma, the brain is subjected to forces secondary to acute acceleration and deceleration of the brain within the skull, which is itself undergoing acute acceleration and deceleration. As the result of these forces, a number of pathologic processes ensue. The

brain may be "stunned" by relatively minor head injury without any anatomical or pathologic changes, producing the so-called "concussion." Renewed interest in this condition has occurred because of the exquisite detail of neuroimaging created by MRI. Some believe that through this modality previously unrecognized changes in the limbic lobe, the medial temporal lobe, and the upper brain stem may occur in "concussion" accounting for the characteristic findings of transient loss of consciousness, some degree of retrograde amnesia, and difficulty with mental energy (e.g., lack of motivation), which may exist for weeks or months following the injury. Blood vessels, including both arteries and veins, may be torn, resulting in hemorrhage. This hemorrhage may occur exterior to the brain or within the brain substance. Some portions of the brain may move through greater distances than other portions of the brain, creating shearing injuries at the interface of these moving areas—not to dissimilar from the activity at the fault line during an earthquake. Brain tissue may be disrupted. Mentioned earlier is the fact that, following some severe head injuries, apnea, or loss of normal respiration, may ensue, resulting in hypoxia and other metabolic changes that cause direct injury to nerve cells.

With both CT scanning and MRI scanning, intracranial hemorrhages following head trauma are easily identified. Epidural hemorrhages are arterial in nature and are located beneath the skull but external to the most outer membrane lining the brain, the dura mater. These hemorrhages are usually associated with a skull fracture that lacerates an artery lying between the dura mater and the skull. The hemorrhage may develop rapidly over a period of two to three hours creating increased intracranial pressure and focal pressure on the brain. Recovery is excellent in patients who are operated on with evacuation of the hematoma prior to developing coma, whereas the prognosis is extremely poor in someone who develops coma prior to surgery.

The subdural hematoma forms beneath the dura mater but external to the arachnoid membrane, which is the inner covering of the brain. The blood usually comes from torn veins, and develops more slowly than an epidural hematoma. It is less well localized and is often associated with other injuries to the brain because the force required to tear veins is actually greater than the force required to cut an artery following a skull fracture leading to an epidural hematoma. As the result of the more widespread brain injury that occurs with an acute subdural hematoma, the mortality rate for subdural hematomas is higher than that for acute epidural hematomas in that more patients with acute subdural hematomas are comatose at the time of surgery. Often associated with acute subdural hematomas are intracerebral hematomas, blood clots within the substance of the brain. Although rarely an indication for surgery, their presence does adversely affect prognosis.

Subarachnoid hemorrhage (SAH) occurs between the arachnoid membrane and the surface of the brain. It is rarely focal in presentation and may occur with minor head injuries. While SAH, in and of itself, rarely produces primary brain impairment, it may be associated with the development, days or weeks later, of hydrocephalus, which is caused by the excessive accumulation of cerebral spinal fluid that has been normally produced within the brain but is unable to be normally absorbed because of the presence of blood in the subarachnoid space.

Injuries produced by shearing forces within the brain are rarely, individually, very severe. However, because they may be widespread throughout the brain, collectively they can produce significant brain impairment, which is not treatable other than through the provision of primary support to the patient during the recovery and rehabilitation process. Prognosis of the patient with this condition is extremely varied depending on how widespread the problem is. Patients may remain in coma or they may improve to various stages of function, including to states indistinguishable from the preinjury condition of the patient.

Hypoxia and other adverse metabolic stresses suffered by the brain in the posttraumatic period are a major cause of death or residual disability. For example, most of the patients in the persistent vegetative state probably suffered from these afflictions. When brain cells are subject to these conditions, one of three states may ensue. The brain cell continues to function relatively normally, or is one of a group of cells whose lack of functioning cannot be detected clinically. The second state the cell may move into is that of cell death. Because dead cells do not regenerate, that cell and its colleagues are removed from brain physiology and, depending on the location of the group of cells, the patient will suffer permanent deficit. The third state the cell may find itself in is one of "idling." In this state the cell is alive but is not functioning normally. It will require time for the cell to rejuvenate itself, to recover from the insult, and to begin functioning again.

A discussion of the differential diagnosis of head injuries is not complete without some mention of post-traumatic epilepsy. Seizure activity following trauma may be indistinguishable from nontraumatic epilepsy. The condition is due to the creation of hyper-excitable areas in the brain by the underlying disorder, or the removal of the inhibition of normally excitable brain by the disorder. It is such a generalized nonspecific response to trauma that it has little value in distinguishing for the physician the underlying brain pathology.

Putting it all together, the differential diagnosis of brain impairment begins with a history of head trauma and its attendant metabolic sequelae. The neurological status of the patient is observed over time and correlated with brain anatomy and physiology. Changes in the patient's condition are studied by neuroimaging and other laboratory technologies. Neuropsychological evaluation and response to medical and surgical treatment and rehabilitation are quantified. Through rational and objective analysis of this experience, a specific diagnosis may be made in virtually every instance.

BRAIN RECOVERY

At one time it was believed that cells either functioned or did not function—an all or none phenomenon.[2] Increasingly, it is becoming obvious that cells may function at various levels of activity, depending on influences from surrounding cells. This is an explanation for one phenomenon seen in recovery as the result of rehabilitation. During the time period of rehabilitation, more and more brain cells move from the idling state to the active state. As they do, they exert their influence on surrounding cells, increasing the activity of the cell pool and thus improving the neurological status of the patient. A second phenomenon of rehabilitation is that of relearning. A patient's "weakness" may improve because of the increase in activity of the cell pool as mentioned earlier or as the result of more efficient utilization of the existing cell pool through repetitive behavior during rehabilitation. It is believed, with regard to the first phenomenon, that 90% of the ultimate recovery will be seen within the first six months following injury and the remaining 10% will be seen in the next 1.5 years. The time frame for the second phenomenon is less well understood and may proceed for years. Currently, it is difficult to quantify these two phenomena individually.

Although some believe that through careful neuropsychological testing it is possible to quantitate neuropsychological abnormalities in patients with no deficits on neurological examination and neuroimage evaluation, others believe that adequate research has not been conducted to establish standards for such distinctions.[3] In evaluating these matters, it is important to keep in mind the principle that the greater the lack of correlation between neuropsychological testing and neuroimaging confirmation of underlying residual brain impairment, the more important it is to search for preinjury evidence of neuropsychological abnormalities in order to understand fully the problem presented by the patient in the post-traumatic period.

LEGAL CONSIDERATIONS

In general, the legal considerations for the brain-injured patient vary little from those generally present in common and statutory law related to personal injury torts and contracts. Issues of informed consent generally concern the incompetent. Increasingly patients, particularly the elderly, have created advanced directives, either a durable power of attorney or a living will. The laws related to these matters are generally state specific.[4] The exception is the Patient Self-Determination Act of 1990, a federal law mandating that hospitals that receive federal funds must inform patients of their right to create advanced directives and to have them followed.[5]

The question often arises as to how to handle a matter of termination of treatment to include termination of life support in patients who do not have advanced directives. Once again, the law regarding these matters is generally state specific, ranging from the permitting of a surrogate judgment maker through the use of a standard of the "best interest" of the patient to the requirement of a court-appointed guardian ad litem. The trend across the nation is to permit knowledgeable individuals, usually close relatives and/or friends, to provide evidence of what the patient would have decided. This is of particular note in situations where the patient is in the persistent vegetative state with no hope of recovery and, potentially, years of survival. The U.S. Supreme Court in *Cruzan v. Director*[6] held that although a competent adult has a right to terminate treatment, the state may establish the standard of proof in matters involving the incompetent patient such as one in the persistent vegetative state. In *Cruzan* the Supreme Court upheld the state of Missouri's requirement that the proof be "clear and convincing."

Of major concern to head-injured patients and their families is denial of coverage under health insurance policies.[7] Often the portion of the policy that relates to chronic care or rehabilitation is ambiguously worded. As noted earlier, there are no bright lines between acute care, rehabilitation, and custodial care. These terms and phrases are often self-defined after the fact by adjusters to provide denial. It is important that legal practitioners help medical practitioners understand the legal implications of conclusions such as "no further medical required" or "medically stabilized."

END NOTES

1. A number of excellent treatises are available to which the reader may refer to expand the knowledge base of this section. Especially recommended are D.P. Becker and S.K. Gudeman, *Textbook of Head Injury* (W.B. Saunders, Philadelphia 1989); A.L. Pearlman, and R.C. Collins, eds.; *Neurological Pathophysiology* (3rd ed., Oxford University Press, New York (1984); L.P. Roland, ed., *Merritt's Textbook of Neurology* (Lea & Febiger, Philadelphia 1989); C. Watts et al., *Problems Associated with Multiple Trauma, in Neurological Surgery* (6 volumes), ch. 86 2543-2602 (J. R. Youmans, ed. W. B. Saunders, Philadelphia 1990).
2. P. Bach-y-Rita, *Recovery From Brain Damage,* 6 J. Neuro. Rehab. 191-199 (1992).
3. As evidenced by the conflicting positions contained in the following references, it behooves any lawyer representing clients with brain injuries to become familiar with the subject matter of neuropsychologic testing: H.S. Levin et al., eds., *Neurobehavioral Recovery from Head Injury.* Oxford University Press, New York 1987); G. P. Prigatona, *Personality Disturbances Associated with Traumatic Brain Injury,* G.P. Prigatona, 60 J. Consulting and Clin. Psy. 360-308 (1992); G. P. Prigatano and J. E. Redner, *Uses and Abuses of Neuropsychological Testing in Behavioral Neurology,* II Neurol. Clin. 219-231 (1993).
4. *See* A. D. Lieberson, *Advance Medical Directives* (Clark, Boardman, Callaghan, New York 1992).
5. Omnibus Budget Reconciliation Act of 1990, Pub. L. 101-508, §4206, 4751.
6. *Cruzan v. Director, Missouri Dept. of Health,* 110 S.Ct. 2841 (1990).
7. *See, e.g.,* S. McMath, *Insurance Denial for Head and Spinal Cord Injuries: Stacked Deck Requires Health Care Reform,* 10 Heath Span 7-11 (July/Aug. 1993).

CHAPTER 36

Patients with human immunodeficiency virus (HIV) infection and acquired immunodeficiency syndrome (AIDS)

MIKE A. ROYAL, M.D., J.D., F.C.L.M.*

PATHOGENESIS
TESTING AND TREATMENT
LEGAL RESPONSES

Human immunodeficiency virus (HIV) infection and the subsequent development of the full-blown acquired immunodeficiency syndrome (AIDS) have stimulated more controversy and had more written about them than any other disease process in history. This chapter provides a brief overview of the pathogenesis, testing, and treatment of HIV infection, the legal framework built to deal with the problems that HIV infection and AIDS have created, and the continuing legal and ethical challenges. Those readers desiring greater detail relating to a particular subject area are directed to the *AIDS Bibliography* (published monthly by the National Library of Medicine),[1] the *AIDS Law & Litigation Reporter* (published monthly by the University Publishing Group),[2] and the *AIDS Litigation Reporter* (published twice monthly by Andrews Publications)[3] for up-to-date compilations of the literature, statutes, regulations, and case law. For those interested in the historical case law background, the *AIDS Litigation Project I and II*[4] summarizes the 817 federal, state, municipal, and military cases involving HIV or AIDS through January 1991. Appendix 36-1 lists telephone numbers that individuals may call for additional information related to HIV.

Despite all that has been written and all the attention—legal, political, and otherwise—we seem to be further behind than when we started. According to the World Health Organization, 30 to 40 million people will be infected with HIV by the year 2000. As of January 1, 1994, there were 346,730 cases of AIDS reported in the United States.[5] Of these, 208,897 individuals have died of AIDS. The current estimate of the number of HIV-infected individuals in the United States is 1.5 million. During the past decade, the Centers for Disease Control (CDC) has identified HIV/AIDS as a leading cause of death in the United States.[6] In more than 60 of our largest cities, AIDS has become the leading cause of death among men between the ages of 25 and 44 years.[7] In 1992, it had become the eighth leading cause of death overall (up from ninth in 1991), accounting for 1.5% of all deaths, and the second leading cause of death among persons ages 25 to 44 years (up from third in 1991) accounting for 16.3% of deaths in this age group.[8] While other leading causes of death have remained stable or declined, deaths from AIDS have continued to increase. By the turn of the century, it is expected that AIDS will be the third most common cause of death in the United States.

Though these numbers are quite impressive, they are surely significant undercounts. Studies have shown significant levels of failure to list HIV/AIDS on death certificates.[9] In addition, the CDC recently has expanded the federal AIDS case definition so that it now includes HIV-infected individuals who died from conditions, such as recurrent pneumonia, that would not have been included in the earlier definition (see Appendix 36-2). For example, in 1993 alone, an additional nearly 24,000 cases of AIDS were reported due to the expanded criteria, with the vast majority due to severe HIV-related immunosuppression (CD4 + T-lymphocyte counts 200/cc.)[5]

As the National Commission on Acquired Immune

*The author gratefully acknowledges work from previous contributors: H. William Goebert, Jr., M.D., J.D., F.C.L.M.; Frank T. Flannery, M.D., J.D., F.C.L.M.; Janet B. Seifert, J.D.; and James G. Zimmerly, MD., J.D., F.C.L.M.

Deficiency Syndrome stated in its final report, "the human immunodeficiency virus (HIV) has profoundly changed life on our planet" and if we are to deal with this "expanding tragedy . . . we need a new mind set, a new, less selfish national resolve, a new way of thinking about the epidemic that says this toll of human suffering and death is unacceptable to us."[10]

PATHOGENESIS

AIDS is a disease in which the infected host's immune system is slowly destroyed, thus subjecting the host to a variety of opportunistic infections and malignant conditions that are usually not pathogenic or present in individuals with normal immune systems. Once AIDS is established, it appears to be inevitably fatal. Chang and colleagues studied a cohort of 3699 individuals with AIDS in New York State and noted that the median length of survival was 11.5 months, and that survival had increased over time from 5.3 months pre-1984 to 9.3 months in 1984-1986 and to 13.2 months in 1987-1989.[11] This increased survival time certainly is due to antiretroviral therapy and better treatments directed toward coexistent opportunistic infections.

Studies of long-term survivors with HIV infection (those living more than eight years) have provided a wealth of information about the various features that appear to be important in HIV pathogenesis.[12,13] HIV is now known to be not a single virus, but a heterogenous group of retroviruses [HIV-1, HIV-2, and human T-lymphotropic virus type I (HTLV-1) and type II (HTLV-2) have been identified to date].[14] Although retroviruses have been identified as animal pathogens for nearly a century, their role as the cause of significant human morbidity and mortality has not been recognized until recently. Retroviruses, as opposed to other viruses, cause infection by using the host cell's own machinery (directed by viral reverse transcriptase) to produce viral DNA, which is then incorporated into the host cell chromosome.[15]

HIV is transmitted to human hosts either by infectious viral particles or by cells infected by the virus.[16] The recognition of cell-to-cell transfer of HIV is important because up to 50 to 100 times more virus-infected cells than free viral particles are typically found in body fluids.[17,18] Thus, future efforts directed toward treatment and vaccine development must also consider viral transfer through this route.

Which host cells are infected first after HIV transmission is still not known. Eventually, with acute viral infection, lymphoid tissues (and peripheral blood cells) primarily are involved.[19] It is known that at least four receptors are involved in viral attachment to host cells: the CD4 molecule,[20,21] galactosyl ceramide (Gal-C) on brain and bowel cells,[22,23] and the Fc and complement receptors.[24,25] No doubt others soon may be identified. Once HIV is complexed with antibody, Fc and complement, which are cell surface molecules, can permit infection of host cells through an antibody-dependent enhancement process.[26-28] However, viral interaction with cell surface components is only the first step toward viral entry. It appears that conformational changes in the viral envelope, cleavage of gp120, and other currently undefined steps are necessary for fusion and nucleocapsid entry once attachment has occurred.[29] To make the problem more complicated, each of these steps—attachment, fusion and nucleocapsid entry—appears to be dependent on the viral type and the host cell being attacked.

Once the viral nucleocapsid enters the host cell, the following steps must occur to produce complete HIV particles (virions): uncoating of viral genomic RNA; reverse transcription and host cell synthesis of unintegrated, proviral double-stranded DNA; integration of proviral DNA into the host cell chromosome; host cell synthesis of viral mRNA (transcription); host cell synthesis of viral nucleocapsid and other components (translation); assembly; and finally release of the viral particle. All of these steps, from viral attachment to final assembly and release, provide potential targets for directed therapy.[30]

Over time, possibly due to relatively noncytopathic HIV strains replicating in macrophages, CD4+ T-lymphocyte numbers decrease (by an average of 60 million/L cells per year, as shown by the San Francisco Men's Health Study)[31] and, with the associated breakdown in inhibition of viral replication, more virulent cytopathic HIV strains emerge causing further damage to the immune system and its inevitable consequences.[32] Levy has proposed that it is the increased production of cytokines, such as tumor necrosis factor (TNF)-, or loss of interleukin (IL)-1 production by HIV-infected macrophages that is responsible for the reduced levels of CD4+ cells through apoptosis or programmed cell death.[33]

TESTING AND TREATMENT

The initial HIV screening tests, all ELISA (enzyme-linked immunoabsorbent assay) based, were not very useful for detecting antibodies to HIV in the general populace. Due to sensitivity and specificity problems, a small percentage of erroneous test results were possible, which had profound consequences to the noninfected individual who was found to be falsely positive or the infected individual found to be falsely negative. Fortunately, other more accurate techniques for HIV antibody detection were developed. At the present time, more than 130 commercial tests are available from more than 40 companies.[34]

The problem with the original ELISA tests (and many that are still used today) is that they are based on viral lysate antigens, which may contain components of the host cells in which they are grown.[35] These host antigen contaminants, most commonly the human leukocyte antigen (HLA), create the potential for false-positive results. Non HIV-infected individuals who have HLA antibodies (which may occur from exposure to fetal white blood cells during pregnancy or from blood transfusion) may test positive on such tests.[36] Newer tests, such as the Western blot, indirect fluorescent antibody assay (IFA), and the radioimmunoprecipitation assay (RIPA), avoid these contamination problems by using recombinant or synthetic peptide antigens.[37] Once the amino acid sequence of a particular antigen is determined, it can be constructed from free amino acids with a peptide synthesizer. This relatively pure form of antigen can then be used to create these more specific tests, which if performed and interpreted correctly, *usually* do not produce biologic false-positive results, but even a single erroneous result can have a devastating impact. Unfortunately, with the increased specificity, some sensitivity is lost, because these tests may be too specific to detect all strains of retroviruses. Thus, they remain most useful as confirmatory rather than screening assays, and as might be expected from their complexity, they are also quite expensive. For a more thorough discussion, the interested reader is referred to the review article by Constantine.[38]

Although we have learned a great deal about the pathogenesis of HIV infection, we have not had similar success with the development of therapies for treatment. Only three drugs, zidovudine (AZT), didanosine (dideoxyinosine or ddI), and zalcitabine, are currently approved for use by the Food and Drug Administration (FDA).[39] Promising newer agents and combination therapy are currently under study in clinical trials, which, as a result of public outcry and the nature of the disease, have become significantly streamlined or occasionally cut short when compared to the typical clinical trial for new drugs.[90] In addition, FDA approval for drugs showing efficacy has also been faster. For example, ddI was approved even before definitive evidence of its clinical efficacy was determined.[41]

AZT was first found to have retroviral activity against HIV-1 in 1985.[42] Since that time, several clinical trials have documented its efficacy in delaying the onset of AIDS and its side effects (primarily bone marrow suppression and myopathy); however, it is still not clear when such therapy should be instituted and at what dose.[43] Current recommendations suggest that a daily dose of 500 to 600 mg (typically 200 mg every eight hours) be used.[44] Didanosine was the second drug approved by the FDA for use in treating individuals with

HIV-1 infections who were intolerant or resistant to AZT. Peripheral neuropathy is the main side effect, occurring in up to one-third of patients. Pancreatitis, headaches, and diarrhea are also common. The currently recommended dose is 300 mg twice daily for those weighing more than 75 kg (with appropriate dosage adjustments for those weighing less than 75 kg).[45] Zalcitabine is currently approved only for combination therapy with AZT in those individuals with CD4+ T-lymphocyte counts of less than 300/cc. Doses of 0.375 to 0.75 mg every 8 hours have been shown to be effective with less pancreatitis than earlier studies using higher doses.[46]

On January 20, 1994, the Public Health Service's Agency for Health Care Policy and Research (a private sector panel of physicians, dentists, nurses, social workers, physician assistants, and HIV-infected individuals) released new guidelines to improve the ability of "front line" primary care practitioners to provide early care for newly HIV-infected individuals (see Appendix 36-3). Dr. Philip R. Lee, the assistant secretary for health, Department of Health and Human Services, and head of the Public Health Service has stated that "A key recommendation is that some patients who have not yet developed symptoms be given daily preventive doses of a sulfa drug shown to prevent the onset of *Pneumocystis carinii* pneumonia, a principal killer of HIV-infected persons."[47] In addition, Dr. Lee stated that instituting treatment for those asymptomatic HIV-infected individuals whose CD4+ T-lymphocyte counts fall below 200 cells/cc could help "perhaps thousands of people, extending their lives and preventing debilitating bouts of illness." According to Dr. Lee, the guidelines will help primary care practitioners, who may have had only limited contact with HIV-infected patients, deal with these issues. For those readers wanting more detail about the treatment of HIV infection, the article by Hirsch and D'Acquila is an excellent discussion of the pharmacology of the FDA-approved treatments and promising new agents.[48]

LEGAL RESPONSES

As more individuals live for a longer time with HIV infection, the number of AIDS-related cases in the courts has grown exponentially. Whereas most of these cases continue to involve protection of the rights of HIV-infected individuals, the number of AIDS-phobia cases is increasing.[49] A patchwork of statutory and regulatory efforts, at the federal, state, and local levels, has tried, somewhat successfully, to chart a clear course through the turbulent seas created by the competing needs and rights of society and the HIV-infected individual. Each state and the District of Columbia have enacted a variety of HIV-related statutes, from efforts directed toward public health initiatives to those directed toward protection of individual rights (informed consent in testing, antidiscrimination provisions, and confidentiality protection) (see Appendix 36-4). Complicating this murky picture is ignorance and fear, which have caused some legislatures to waste valuable time considering bills having no sound basis. Those readers desiring a more in-depth coverage of this complex area are directed to an ever-growing body of reviews.[50]

Societal concerns

More than any other aspect of the disease, the fear of transmission, even from casual contact (which has not yet been shown to have occurred), generates strong emotional responses, which have hampered rational attempts to deal with the issue. However, one certainly can understand these emotions. While the chances of acquiring HIV in most circumstances is very low, acquisition in an individual case is an all-or-none phenomenon.

HIV is primarily transmitted through exposure to infected blood or body fluids and perinatally from mother to child. Aside from the health care environment, exposure to infected blood or other body fluids usually occurs in the setting of sexual or other intimate contact, intravenous drug use in which contaminated needles are shared, and blood product transfusion. Of the body fluids, sweat is the only one in which HIV has been searched for and not found, whereas it has been isolated in blood, semen, saliva, tears, breast milk, urine, feces, and other body fluids (*e.g.,* joint fluid, cerebrospinal fluid, ascitic fluid, pleural fluid) to which only health care workers typically would be exposed.

Although nearly 6000 cases of HIV transmission through blood product transfusion were identified through 1993, William T. Teague, president and chief executive officer of The Blood Center in Houston, Texas, stated that "with rare exception, these exposures occurred prior to the spring of 1985, when the nation's blood supply began being tested for anti-HIV."[51] He noted that only about 20 cases of transfusion-associated HIV infection have occurred since the blood supply began to be tested. As a caveat to physicians, many of the recent court cases dealing with this issue turn on questions of proper informed consent with respect to blood transfusions, especially whether autologous and directed donations were discussed preoperatively. A full discussion of the growing number of AIDS transfusion cases is beyond the scope of this chapter; however, interested readers are referred to the sections on blood transfusion cases in the *AIDS Law & Litigation Reporter* and *AIDS Bibliography* or one of the many excellent reviews on the subject.[52]

Health care workers consistently have comprised approximately 5% of the AIDS cases reported to the CDC each year. A similar percentage—about 6%—of the labor force in the United States is employed in the health care industry. Although the majority of those health care workers who have become HIV-infected report engaging in high-risk behaviors (nonoccupational risk factors), a significant number are still at risk from occupational exposure.[53] Because HIV so closely parallels hepatitis B virus (HBV), another blood-borne pathogen, with respect to reduction of transmission risk for health care workers, the CDC has issued "universal precaution" guidelines for prevention of HIV, HBV, and other blood-borne pathogen transmission in health care settings.[54] In addition to focusing on sound hygiene practices to avoid contact with contaminated fluids, a major effort was made to decrease inadvertent needlestick injuries, the major vehicle for HIV transmission to health care workers.[55] With needlestick exposures, the risk of transmission is estimated to be in the range of 1/250 to 1/50, but clearly is dependent on the volume and type of fluid, the number of viral particles in the fluid, and the site of exposure or injection.

Since the reports that six patients contracted HIV from a Florida dentist, the issue of whether to test all health care workers has become quite controversial.[56] In 1991, in an attempt to find a middle ground, the CDC recommended that "exposure prone" invasive procedures be identified and that HIV-infected health care workers potentially should avoid such procedures or inform their patients of their HIV status, but made no recommendations regarding mass testing of health care workers.[57] Congress mandated that the states adopt "equivalent" guidelines to those put forth by the CDC,[58] and the ambiguity in the CDC guidelines has prompted a spectrum of state responses.[59] No doubt as a response to growing concerns of HIV transmission in the dental surgery environment, the CDC did come forward with new recommendations for infection control practices in dentistry.[60] However, with respect to mandatory testing of health care workers, the debate continues.

One part of the debate that has not received as much attention is the issue of cost. Given the extraordinarily low risk of HIV transmission when proper precautions are taken, is the cost of mandatory testing worth the invasion of privacy and potential discrimination? Phillips and colleagues estimate that mandatory testing of all surgeons might avert 25 HIV infections at a total cost of $27.9 million or about $1.1 million per infection with a range of $81,000 (high-risk scenario) to nearly $30 million (low-risk scenario).[61] The cost is sure to be even higher when one factors in the need for periodic testing to identify subsequent conversion after the initial mass screening. However, what is the value of 25 lives devastated by becoming HIV infected? These are questions without easy answers.

Since the first report of HIV in saliva by Groopman and colleagues[62] in 1984, this potential mode of transmission has become the most difficult and troublesome aspect of HIV infection. Although avoidance of passionate kissing substantially decreases any potential likelihood of transmission, the risk of saliva-mediated HIV transmission from less intimate contact theoretically still exists. It may simply be so low as to have escaped detection to this point, especially when other more likely modes of transmission coexist. This theoretical risk is especially bothersome to parents of children in day care centers where fingers and toys may carry saliva from one child to another.

With publicity surrounding HIV infection in athletes,[63] possible transmission of HIV through contact with bloody body fluids has become a recent concern in competitive sports, especially those sports, such as boxing, basketball, and football, where it is not unusual to have blood or body fluids in contact with cuts and scrapes.[64] Even though such transmission has yet to be documented, the risk is certainly there. To address these issues, several organizations have published guidelines in an attempt to balance risks and concerns.[65]

Protection of individual rights

Societal concerns of preventing the spread of communicable diseases and ensuring the safety of the blood supply run squarely into the competing concerns of the HIV-infected individual. Informed consent for testing and confidentiality with respect to test results have become critical issues when one considers the significant potential for discrimination against HIV-infected persons. Physicians often find themselves in the midst of this ethical and legal dilemma when they balance the duty to warn a third party of the potential risk of infection against patient confidentiality concerns. Although most courts have upheld the privacy right of HIV-infected individuals and the majority of states have provided statutory protection for HIV status, there are still no easy answers.[66] An exception to this general rule is often created where the HIV-infected individual is a health care professional and potential exposure to patients occurred, although Arnow and colleagues argue that, even in such circumstances, "look-back" investigations may still be conducted in a manner that protects the identity of the health care professional.[67]

Another area of major concern of HIV-infected individuals, as it is with all individuals with medical problems or disabilities, is ensuring access to medical treatment. Discrimination in medical care has perhaps the most cruel and devastating effects, because it leaves helpless those who are most in need of care. Traditionally, health care professionals had no legal duty to treat any person absent an actual or implied provider-patient relationship. However, the American Medical Association clearly has delineated an ethical duty to treat HIV-infected patients in a specific statement made by the Council on Ethical and Judicial Affairs.[68] With the passage of the Americans with Disabilities Act (ADA) of 1990,[69] Congress imposed a statutory duty on health care providers to provide care to those persons with disabilities, including HIV-infected individuals who qualify under the statute.[70] Hopefully, as knowledge about HIV becomes more widely disseminated, fear can be replaced by understanding and access will become less an issue.

END NOTES

1. *AIDS Bibliography,* U.S. Department of Health and Human Services, Public Health Service, National Institutes of Health, National Library of Medicine, Reference Section, 8600 Rockville Pike, Bethesda, MD 20894 (phone: 301-496-6097; fax: 301-402-1384). Those having access to Internet through FTP (file transfer protocol) can FTP to nlmpubs.nlm.nih.gov and login as "nlm-pubs". The index file in the "aids" directory provides information on the bibliographies available.
2. *AIDS Law & Litigation Reporter,* University Publishing Group, 107 East Church Street, Frederick, MD 21701 (phone: 800-654-8188).
3. *AIDS Litigation Reporter,* National Journal of Record of AIDS-Related Litigation, Andrews Publications, P.O. Box 1000, Westtown, PA 19395 (phone: 610-399-6600).
4. L. O. Gostin et al., *AIDS Litigation Project I and II* University Publishing Group, 107 East Church Street, Frederick, MD 21701 (phone: 800-654-8188).
5. Centers for Disease Control, 43 MMWR 1 (1994).
6. Centers for Disease Control, 42 MMWR 421-22 (1993).
7. Centers for Disease Control, 269 JAMA 2991-94 (1993).
8. Centers for Disease Control, 42 MMWR 869-72 (1993). The death rate from HIV infection in 1992 for persons aged 25 to 44 years was three times as high for black men (136.0/100,000) as for white men (42.1/100,000) and 12 times as high for black women (38.0/100,000) as for white women (3.3/100,000). HIV infection was the leading cause of death for black men aged 25 to 44 years.
9. H. H. Chang et al., *Survival and Mortality Patterns of an Acquired Immunodeficiency Syndrome (AIDS) Cohort in New York State,* 138 Am. J. Epidemiol. 341-49 (1993).
10. National Commission on Acquired Immunodeficiency Syndrome, 270 JAMA 298 (1993).
11. Chang, *supra* note 9.
12. J. A. Levy, HIV Pathogenesis and Long-Term Survival, 7 AIDS 1401-10 (1993). *See also* AIDS: The Unanswered Questions, 260 Science 1254-88 (May 28, 1993), in which are presented a number of articles on AIDS pathogenesis and treatment.
13. J. A. Levy, *Pathogenesis of Human Immunodeficiency Virus Infection,* 57 Microbiol. Rev. 183-289 (1993).
14. N. T. Constantine, *Serologic Tests for the Retroviruses: Approaching a Decade of Evolution,* 7 AIDS 1-13 (1993). *See also* H. M. Barton, *HIV and Hepatitis Testing Raise Complex Questions for Physicians,* 89 Tex. Med. 55-58 (1993).
15. Laurence, *The Immune System in AIDS,* Sci. Am., Dec. 1985, at 85.
16. B. A. Castro et al., *HIV Heterogeneity and Viral Pathogenesis,* 2 AIDS (Suppl. 1) S17-S28 (1988).
17. *Supra* note 12.
18. J. A. Levy, *The Transmission of AIDS: The Case of the Infected Cell,* 259 JAMA 3037-38 (1988).
19. *Supra* note 12.
20. A. G. Dalgleish et al., *The CD4 (T4) Antigen Is an Essential*

Component of the Receptor for the AIDS Retrovirus, 312 Nature 763-67 (1984).

21. D. Klatzmann et al., *Selective Tropism of Lymphadenopathy-associated Virus (LAV) for Helper-Inducer T Lymphocytes,* 225 Science 59-62 (1984).

22. J. M. Harouse et al., *Inhibition of Entry of HIV-1 in Neural Cell Lines by Antibodies Against Galactosyl Ceramide,* 253 Science 320-23 (1991).

23. N. Yahi et al., *Galactosyl Ceramide (of a Closely Related Molecule) Is the Receptor for Human Immunodeficiency Virus Type 1 on Human Colon Epithelial HT29 Cells,* 66 J. Virol. 4848-54 (1992).

24. J. Homsy et al., *The Fc and Not the CD4 Receptor Mediates Antibody Enhancement of HIV Infection in Human Cells,* 244 Science 1357-60 (1989).

25. W. E. Robinson, Jr., et al., *Complement-mediated Antibody-dependent Enhancement of HIV-1 Infection Requires CD4 and Complement Receptors,* 175 Virology 600-04 (1990).

26. *Supra* note 18.

27. Homsy, *supra* note 24.

28. Robinson, *supra* note 25.

29. *Supra* note 12.

30. M. S. Hirsch and R. T. D'Aquila, *Therapy for Human Immunodeficiency Virus Infection,* 328 New Eng. J. Med. 1686-95 (1993). Additionally, the most recent releases of the journals *AIDS, Journal of Acquired Immune Deficiency Syndromes,* and *AIDS Research and Human Retroviruses* provide up-to-date information on current literature. *See also* W. Anderson et al., *Patient Use and Assessment of Conventional and Alternative Therapies for HIV Infection and AIDS,* 7 AIDS 561-66 (1993); S. Burris, *HIV Education and the Law: A Critical Review,* 20 Law, Med. & Health Care 377-91 (1992).

31. W. Lang et al., *Patterns of T-lymphocyte Changes with Human Immunodeficiency Virus Infection: From Seroconversion to the Development of AIDS,* 2 J. Acquired Immune Defic. Syndr. 63-69 (1989).

32. *Supra* note 12.

33. *Id.*

34. *Supra* note 13.

35. D. S. Burke, *Laboratory Diagnosis of Human Immunodeficiency Virus Infection,* 9 Clin. Lab. Med. 369-92 (1989).

36. *Supra* note 13.

37. X. Zhang et al., *Evaluation of a New Generation Synthetic Peptide Combination Assay Designed to Detect Antibodies to HIV-1, HIV-2, HTLV-I, and HTLV-II Simultaneously,* 38 J. Med. Virol. 49-53 (1992).

38. *Supra* note 14.

39. *Supra* note 30.

40. P. Cotton, *Trial Halted After Drug Cuts Maternal HIV Transmission Rate by Two Thirds,* 271 JAMA 807 (1993). Preliminary results of a randomized controlled trial suggesting that the rate of HIV transmission from mothers to infants was cut from 25.5% in pregnant women and their infants who received placebo to 8.3% in those treated with zidovudine caused the study to be halted with less than 60% of the total number of patients originally scheduled to be enrolled. Although the National Institute of Allergy and Infectious Diseases stopped short of making treatment recommendations based on these results, the Pediatric AIDS Foundation stated that AZT must now be offered to HIV-infected women who are pregnant. The CDC estimates that 7000 HIV-infected women give birth each year with approximately 1750 infants who are born with the infection.

41. Hirsch, *supra* note 30.

42. P. A. Furman et al., *Phosphorylation of 3'-Azido-3'deoxythymidine Kinase by Bromodeoxyuridine in Cell Cultures Transformed by Friend Virus,* 83 Proc. Natl. Acad. Sci. USA 8333-37 (1986).

43. M. F. Goldsmith, *HIV/AIDS Early Treatment Controversy Cues New Advice But Questions Remain,* 270 JAMA 295-96 (1993).

44. *Supra* note 30.

45. *Id.*

46. *Id.*

47. Dr. Philip R. Lee, Asst. Secr. of Health, Dept. of Health and Human Services, and head of the Public Health Service.

48. Hirsch, *supra* note 30.

49. D. E. Lanin, *The Fear of Disease as a Compensable Injury: An Analysis of Claims Based on AIDS Phobia,* 67 St. John's Law Rev 77-103 (1993). *See also* L. H. Feffer, *AIDSphobia, A New Entity,* 65 New York State Bar J. 14-15 (1993).

50. *See, e.g.,* H. L. Hirsch, *Social, Legal Medical & Ethical Challenges of HIV Infection (Part I & II),* 39 Med. Trial Tech. Q. 324-56, 461-93; E. A. Gomez, *AIDS: Legal and Ethical Issues,* 16 Trial Diplomacy J. 117-28 (1993); S. F. Hancock, Jr., *AIDS and the Law,* 65 New York State Bar J. 8-13 (1993); J. M. Taraska and J. L. Solomon, *AIDS, Infectious Diseases and the Healthcare Practitioner, in Legal Guide for Physicians* (Matthew Bender & Co. Inc., Albany, N.Y. 1993).

51. W. T. Teague, *HIV from Transfusion Now Very Rare,* Am. Med. News, March 7, 1994, at 20.

52. *See, e.g.,* R. D. Eckert, *The AIDS Blood-Transfusion Cases: A Legal and Economic Analysis of Liability,* 29 San Diego Law Rev. 203-98 (1992); R. C. Howard, *The Jurisdictional and Discovery Issues in Transfusion-associated AIDS Litigation Involving the American Red Cross,* 39 Wayne Law Rev. 207-29 (1992); D. H. Robbins, *AIDS Cases in Federal Court: A Federal Question?,* 61 George Washington Law Rev. 490-521 (1993).

53. M. E. Chamberland et al., *Health Care Workers with AIDS,* 266 JAMA 3459-62 (1991).

54. Centers for Disease Control, *Universal Precautions for Prevention of Transmission of Human Immunodeficiency Virus, Hepatitis B Virus, and Other Bloodborne Pathogens in Health-Care Settings,* 37 MMWR 377-82, 387-88 (1988); *Guidelines for Prevention of Transmission of Human Immunodeficiency Virus and Hepatitis B Virus to Health-Care and Public-Safety Workers,* 38 MMWR (suppl. S-6), 1-37 (1989). *See also* Occupational Safety and Health Administration, *Occupational Exposure to Bloodborne Pathogens,* 29 C.F.R. §1910.1030, 56 Fed. Reg. 64004, 64175 (1991).

55. *Supra* note 53.

56. P. J. Hilts, *AIDS Patient Urges Congress to Pass Testing Bill,* N.Y. Times, Sep. 27, 1991, at A12 (describing testimony of Kimberly Bergalis).

57. *Supra* note 13.

58. Treasury, Postal Services, and General Government Appropriations Act of 1992, Pub. L. 102-141 &634 (1991).

59. M. D. Johnson, *HIV Testing of Health Care Workers: Conflict Between the Common Law and the Centers for Disease Control,* 42 Am. Univ. Law Rev. 479, 533 (1993). This is an exhaustive review of the legal background to mandatory testing. *See also* W. C. Stanton, *HIV in the Health Care Workplace: Challenges Involving HIV-Infected Employees and Physicians,* 14 Whittier Law Rev. 15-40 (1993).

60. Centers for Disease Control, 40 MMWR 1-8 (1991). Note that in 1993 the CDC published guidelines for infection control practices in dentistry. CDC, 42 MMWR 1-12 (1993).

61. K. A. Phillips et al., *The Cost-Effectiveness of HIV Testing of Physicians and Dentists in the United States,* 271 JAMA 851-58 (1994).

62. J. Groopman et al., 226 Science 447-49 (1984).

63. *See, e.g.,* M. Johnson and R. S. Johnson, *I'll Deal With It, Sports Illus.,* Nov. 18, 1991, at 16-27; C. Gray, *AIDS Becomes a Sports Issue,* 146 Can. Med. Assoc. J. 1437 (1992); W. L. Risser, *HIV Makes Caution Necessary in Sports Settings,* 20 Phys. Sportsmed. 190 (1992); L. H. Calabrese and A. LaPerriere, *Human Immunodefi-*

ciency Virus Infection, Exercise, and Athletes, 15 Sports Med. 6-13 (1993).

64. R. A. Goodman et al., *Infectious Disease in Competitive Sports*, 271 JAMA 862-67 (1994).

65. *See, e.g.,* National Collegiate Athletic Association, *Blood-borne Pathogens and Intercollegiate Athletics, in 1993-1994 NCAA Sports Medicine Handbook* 24-28 (M. T. Benson, ed., Overland Park, Kan. 1993); *Committee on Sports Medicine and Fitness, Human Immunodeficiency Virus (Acquired Immunodeficiency Syndrome [AIDS] Virus) in the Athletic Setting,* 88 Pediatrics 640-41 (1991).

66. E. A. Gomez, *AIDS: Legal and Ethical Issues*, 16 Trial Diplomacy J. 117-28 (1993). Many states have passed statutes mandating confidentiality safeguards. *See e.g.,* Pennsylvania's Confidentiality of HIV-related Information Act, 35 P.S. §§ 7601 *et seq.*, Act No. 1990-148; Cal. Health & Safety Code §199.21 (West 1991).

67. P. M. Arnow et al., *Maintaining Confidentiality in a Look-Back Investigation of Patients Treated by a HIV-Infected Dentist,* 108 Public Health Rep. 273-78 (1993).

68. American Medical Association, Council on Ethical and Judicial Affairs, *Ethical Issues Involved in the Growing AIDS Crisis,* Report A, 41st Interim Meeting (Dec. 1987).

69. Americans with Disabilities Act of 1990, Pub. L. 101-336, 104 Stat. 327 (codified at 42 U.S.C. §§ 12101-12213, 47 U.S.C. §§ 225.611).

70. *See, e.g.,* J. Cohen, *Access to Medical Care for HIV-Infected Individuals Under the Americans with Disabilities Act: A Duty to Treat,* 18 Am. J. Law & Med. 232-50 (1992); T. H. Christopher and C. M. Rice, *The Americans with Disabilities Act: An Overview of the Employment Provisions,* 33 So. Tex. Law Rev. 759-800 (1992).

APPENDIX 36-1   Sources of HIV information

- General information: English; 800-342-2437; Spanish; 800-344-7432; TDD Service for the Deaf: 800-243-7889
- General information for health care providers (HIV Telephone Consultation Service): 800-933-3413
- State hotlines for information about HIV-specific resources and counseling and testing services:

Alabama	800-228-0469
Alaska	800-478-2437
Arizona	800-548-4695
Arkansas	501-661-2133
California (north)	800-367-2437
California (south)	800-922-2437
Colorado	800-252-2437
Connecticut	800-342-2437
Delaware	800-422-0429
District of Columbia	202-332-2437
Florida	800-352-2437
Georgia	800-551-2728
Hawaii	800-922-1313
Idaho	208-345-2277
Illinois	800-243-2437
Indiana	800-848-2437
Iowa	800-445-2437
Kansas	800-232-0040
Kentucky	800-654-2437
Louisiana	800-922-4379
Maine	800-851-2437
Maryland	800-638-6252
Massachusetts	800-235-2331
Michigan	800-827-2437
Minnesota	800-248-2437
Mississippi	800-537-0851
Missouri	800-533-2437
Montana	800-233-6668
Nebraska	800-782-2437
Nevada	800-842-2437
New Hampshire	800-324-2437
New Jersey	800-624-2377
New Mexico	800-545-2437
New York	800-541-2437
North Carolina	800-733-7301
North Dakota	800-472-2180
Ohio	800-332-2437
Oklahoma	800-535-2437
Oregon	800-777-2437
Pennsylvania	800-662-6080
Puerto Rico	800-765-1010
Rhode Island	800-726-3010
South Carolina	800-322-2437
South Dakota	800-592-1861
Tennessee	800-525-2437
Texas	800-299-2437
Utah	800-366-2437
Vermont	800-882-2437
Virginia	800-533-4148
Virgin Islands	809-773-2437
Washington	800-272-2437
West Virginia	800-642-8244
Wisconsin	800-334-2437
Wyoming	800-327-3577

- For HIV/AIDS treatment information:
The American Foundation for AIDS Research: 800-39AMFAR (392-6327)
AIDS Treatment Data Network: 212-268-4196
AIDS Treatment News: 800-TREAT-12 (873-2812)

- For information about AIDS/HIV clinical trials conducted by the National Institutes of Health and Food and Drug Administration-approved efficacy trials: AIDS Clinical Trials Information Service (ACTIS): 800-TRIALS-A (874-2572)

• For more information about HIV infection:
Drug Abuse Hotline: 800-662-HELP (4357)
Pediatric and Pregnancy AIDS Hotline: 212-430-3333
National Hemophilia Foundation: 212-430-3333
Hemophilia and AIDS/HIV Network for Dissemination of Information (HANDI): 800-42HANDI (424-2634)

National Pediatric HIV Resource Center: 800-362-0071
National Association of People with AIDS: 202-898-0414
Teens Teaching AIDS Prevention Program (TTAPP) National Hotline: 800-234-TEEN (8336)

APPENDIX 36-2 **1993 Revised Classification System for HIV infection and expanded surveillance case definition for AIDS among adolescents and adults MMWR1992; 41(No.RR-17): 1-19**

SUMMARY

CDC has revised the classification system for HIV infection to emphasize the clinical importance of the CD4+ T-lymphocyte count in the categorization of HIV-related clinical conditions. This classification system replaces the system published by CDC in 1986 (MMWR 1986; 35:334-9) and is primarily intended for use in public health practice. Consistent with the 1993 revised classification system, CDC has also expanded the AIDS surveillance case definition to include all HIV-infected persons who have 200 CD4+ T-lymphocytes/L, or a CD4+ T-lymphocyte percentage of total lymphocytes of 14. This expansion includes the addition of three clinical conditions—pulmonary tuberculosis, recurrent pneumonia, and invasive cervical cancer—and retains the 23 conditions in the AIDS surveillance case definition published in 1987 (MMWR 1987; 36:1-15S); it is to be used by all states for AIDS case reporting effective January 1, 1993.

REVISED HIV CLASSIFICATION SYSTEM FOR ADOLESCENTS AND ADULTS

The etiologic agent of acquired immunodeficiency syndrome (AIDS) is a retrovirus designated human immunodeficiency virus (HIV). The CD4+ T-lymphocyte is the primary target for HIV infection because of the affinity of the virus for the CD4 surface marker. The CD4+ T-lymphocyte coordinates a number of important immunologic functions, and a loss of these functions results in progressive impairment of the immune response. Studies of the natural history of HIV infection have documented a wide spectrum of disease manifestations, ranging from asymptomatic infection to life-threatening conditions characterized by severe immunodeficiency, serious opportunistic infections, and cancers. Other studies have shown a strong association between the development of life-threatening opportunistic illnesses and the absolute number (per microliter of blood) or percentage of CD4+ T-lymphocytes. As the number of CD4+ T-lymphocytes decreases, the risk and severity of opportunistic illnesses increase.

Measures of CD4+ T-lymphocytes are used to guide clinical and therapeutic management of HIV-infected persons. Antimicrobial prophylaxis and antiretroviral therapies have been shown to be most effective within certain levels of immune dysfunction. As a result, antiretroviral therapy should be considered for all persons with CD4+ T-lymphocyte counts of 500/L, and prophylaxis against *Pneumocystis carinii* pneumonia (PCP), the most common serious opportunistic infection diagnosed in men and women with AIDS, is recommended for all persons with CD4+ T-lymphocyte counts of 200/L and for persons who have had prior episodes of PCP. Because of these recommendations, CD4+ T-lymphocyte determinations are an integral part of medical management of HIV-infected persons in the United States.

The classification system for HIV infection among adolescents and adults has been revised to include the CD4+ T-lymphocyte count as a marker for HIV-related immunosuppression. This revision establishes mutually exclusive subgroups for which the spectrum of clinical conditions is integrated with the CD4+ T-lymphocyte count. The objectives of these changes are to simplify the

TABLE 36-1. 1993 revised classification system for HIV infection and expanded AIDS surveillance case definition for adolescents and adults*

CD4+ T-cell categories	Clinical categories		
	(A) Asymptomatic, acute (primary) HIV or PGL	(B) Symptomatic, not (A) or (C) conditions†	(C) AIDS-indicator conditions‡
(1) 500/L	A1	B1	C1
(2) 200-499/L	A2	B2	C2
(3) <200/L AIDS-indicator T-cell count	A3	B3	C3

*The [A3, B3, C1,2,3] cells illustrate the expanded AIDS surveillance case definition. Persons with AIDS-indicator conditions (Category C) as well as those with CD4+ T-lymphocyte counts <200/L (Categories A3 or B3) will be reportable as AIDS cases in the United States and Territories, effective January 1, 1993.
PGL = persistent generalized lymphadenopathy. Clinical Category A includes acute (primary) HIV infection.
†See text for discussion.
‡See Table 36-2.

classification of HIV infection, to reflect current standards of medical care for HIV-infected persons, and to categorize more accurately HIV-related morbidity.

The revised CDC classification system for HIV-infected adolescents and adults* categorizes persons on the basis of clinical conditions associated with HIV infection and CD4+ T-lymphocyte counts. The system is based on three ranges of CD4+ T-lymphocyte counts and three clinical categories and is represented by a matrix of nine mutually exclusive categories (Table 36-1). This system replaces the classification system published in 1986, which included only clinical disease criteria and which was developed before the widespread use of CD4+ T-cell testing.

CD4+ T-LYMPHOCYTE CATEGORIES

The three CD4+ T-lymphocyte categories are defined as follows:

• **Category 1:** 500 cells/ L
• **Category 2:** 200-499 cells/ L
• **Category 3:** <200 cells/ L

These categories correspond to CD4+ T-lymphocyte counts per microliter of blood and guide clinical and therapeutic actions in the management of HIV-infected adolescents and adults. The revised HIV classification system also allows for the use of the percentage of CD4+ T-cells (see Box 36-1).

HIV-infected persons should be classified based on existing guidelines for the medical management of HIV-infected persons. Thus, the lowest accurate, but not necessarily the most recent, CD4+ T-lymphocyte count should be used for classification purposes.

CLINICAL CATEGORIES

The clinical categories of HIV infection are defined as follows

Category A

Category A consists of one or more of the conditions listed below in an adolescent or adult (13 years) with documented HIV infection. Conditions listed in Categories B and C must not have occurred.
• Asymptomatic HIV infection
• Persistent generalized lymphadenopathy
• Acute (primary) HIV infection with accompanying illness or history of acute HIV infection.

Category B

Category B consists of symptomatic conditions in an HIV-infected adolescent or adult that are not included among the conditions listed in clinical Cat-

*Criteria for HIV infection for persons age 13 years: (a) repeatedly reactive screening tests for HIV antibody (e.g., enzyme immunoassay) with specific antibody identified by the use of supplemented tests (e.g., Western blot, immunofluorescence assay); (b) direct identification of virus in host tissues by virus isolation; (c) HIV antigen detection; or (d) a positive result on any other highly specified licensed test for HIV.

BOX 36-1
EQUIVALENCES FOR CD4+ T-LYMPHOCYTE COUNT AND PERCENTAGE OF TOTAL LYMPHOCYTES

Compared with the absolute CD4+ T-lymphocyte count, the percentage of CD4+ T-cells of total lymphocytes (or CD4+ percentage) is less subject to variation on repeated measurements. However, data correlating natural history of HIV infection with the CD4+ percentage have not been as consistently available as data on absolute CD4+ T-lymphocyte counts. Therefore, the revised classification system emphasizes the use of CD4+ T-lymphocyte counts but allows for the use of CD4+ percentages.

Equivalences, given in the table below, were derived from analyses of more than 15,500 lymphocyte subset determinations from seven different sources: one multistate study of diseases in HIV-infected adolescents and adults and six laboratories (two commercial, one research, and three university-based). The six laboratories are involved in proficiency testing programs for lymphocyte subset determinations. In the analyses, concordance was defined as the proportion of patients classified as having CD4+ T-lymphocyte counts in a particular range among patients with a given CD4+ percentage. A threshold value of the CD4+ percentage was calculated to obtain optimal concordance with each stratifying value of the CD4+ T-lymphocyte counts (i.e., <200/L and 500/L). The thresholds for the CD4+ percentages that best correlated with a CD4+ T-lymphocyte count of <200/L varied minimally among the seven data sources (range, 13% to 14%; median, 13%; mean 13.4%). The average concordance for a CD4+ percentage of <14 and a CD4+ T-lymphocyte count of <200/L was 90.2%. The threshold for the CD4+ percentage most concordant with CD4+ T-lymphocyte counts of 500/L varied more widely among the seven data sources (range, 22.5% to 35%; median, 29%; mean 29.1%). This wide range of percentages optimally concordant with 500/L CD4+ T-lymphocytes makes the concordance at this stratifying value less certain. The average concordance for a CD4+ percentage of 29 and a CD4+ T-lymphocyte count of 500/L was 85% (CDC, unpublished data). Clinicians and other practitioners must recognize that these suggested equivalences may not always correspond with values observed in individual patients.

Equivalences for absolute numbers of CD4+ T = lymphocytes and CD4+ percentage*

CD4+ T-cell category	CD4+ T-cells/L	CD4+ percentage (%)
(1)	500	29
(2)	200-499	14-28
(3)	200	<14

*The percentage of lymphocytes that are CD4+ T-cells.

---

egory C and that meet at least one of the following criteria: (a) the conditions are attributed to HIV infection or are indicative of a defect in cell-mediated immunity; or (b) the conditions are considered by physicians to have a clinical course or to require management that is complicated by HIV infection. Examples of conditions in clinical Category B include, *but are not limited to:*
- Bacillary angiomatosis
- Candidiasis, oropharyngeal (thrush)
- Candidiasis, vulvovaginal; persistent, frequent, or poorly responsive to therapy
- Cervical dysplasia (moderate or severe)/cervical carcinoma *in situ*
- Constitutional symptoms, such as fever (38.5°C) or diarrhea lasting more than one month
- Hairy leukoplakia, oral
- Herpes zoster (shingles), involving at least two distinct episodes or more than one dermatome
- Idiopathic thrombocytopenic purpura
- Listeriosis
- Pelvic inflammatory disease, particularly if complicated by tubo-ovarian abscess
- Peripheral neuropathy

For classification purposes, Category B conditions take precedence over those in Category A. For example, someone previously treated for oral or persistent vaginal candidiasis (and who has not developed a Category C disease) but who is now asymptomatic should be classified in clinical Category B.

TABLE 36-2. Conditions included in the 1993 AIDS surveillance case definition

- Candidiasis of bronchi, trachea, or lungs
- Candidiasis, esophageal
- Cervical cancer, invasive*
- Coccidiodomycosis, disseminated or extrapulmonary
- Cryptococcosis, extrapulmonary
- Cryptosporidiosis, chronic intestinal (>1 month's duration)
- Cytomegalovirus disease (other than liver, spleen, or nodes)
- Cytomegalovirus retinitis (with loss of vision)
- Encephalopathy, HIV-related
- Herpes simplex: chronic ulcer(s) (>1 month's duration); or bronchitis, pneumonitis, or esophagitis
- Histoplasmosis, disseminated or extrapulmonary
- Isosporiasis, chronic intestinal (>1 month's duration)
- Kaposi's sarcoma
- Lymphoma, Burkitt's (or equivalent term)
- Lymphoma, immunoblastic (or equivalent term)
- Lymphoma, primary, of brain
- *Mycobactenum avium* complex or *M. Kansasii*, disseminated or extrapulmonary
- *Mycobacterium tuberculosis*, any site (pulmonary* or extrapulmonary)
- *Mycobacterium*, other species or unidentified species, disseminated or extrapulmonary
- *Pneumocystis carinii* pneumonia
- Pneumonia, recurrent*
- Progressive multifocal leukoencephalopathy
- *Salmonella* septicemia, recurrent
- Toxoplasmosis of brain
- Wasting syndrome due to HIV

*Added in the 1993 expansion of the AIDS surveillance case definition.

Category C

Category C includes the clinical conditions listed in the AIDS surveillance case definition (see Table 36-2).

For classification purposes, once a Category C condition has occurred, the person will remain in Category C.

EXPANSION OF THE CDC SURVEILLANCE CASE DEFINITION FOR AIDS

In 1991, CDC, in collaboration with the Council of State and Territorial Epidemiologists (CSTE), proposed an expansion of the AIDS surveillance case definition. This proposal was made available for public comment in November 1991 and was discussed at an open meeting on September 2, 1992. Based on information presented and reviewed during the public comment period and at the open meeting, CDC, in collaboration with CSTE, has expanded the AIDS surveillance case definition to include all HIV-infected persons with CD4+ T-lymphocyte counts of <200 cells/L or a CD4+ percentage of <14. In addition to retaining the 23 clinical conditions in the previous AIDS surveillance definition, the expanded definition includes pulmonary tuberculosis (TB), recurrent pneumonia, and invasive cervical cancer.* This expanded definition requires laboratory confirmation of HIV infection in persons with a CD4+ T-lymphocyte coount of <200 cells/L or with one of the added clinical conditions. This expanded definition for reporting cases to CDC becomes effective January 1, 1993.

In the revised HIV classification system, persons in Subcategories A3, B3, and C3 meet the immunologic criteria of the surveillance case definition, and those persons with conditions in subcategories C1, C2, and C3 meet the clinical criteria or surveillance purposes (see Table 36-1).

*Diagnostic criteria for AIDS-defining conditions included in the expanded surveillance case definition are presented in Tables 36-3 and 36-4.

TABLE 36-3. Definitive diagnostic methods for diseases indicative of AIDS

Diseases	Diagnostic methods
Cryptosporidiosis Isosporiasis Kaposi's sarcoma Lymphoma *Pneumocystis carinii* pneumonia Progressive multifocal leukoencephalopathy Toxoplasmosis Cervical cancer	Microscopy (histology or cytology)
Candidiasis	Gross inspection by endoscopy or autopsy or by microscopy (histology or cytology), culture, on a specimen obtained directly from the tissues affected (including scrapings from the mucosal surface), not from a culture
Coccidioidomycosis	Microscopy (histology or cytology), culture, or detection of antigen in a specimen obtained directly from the tissues affected or a fluid from those tissues
Cryptococcosis Cytomegalovirus Herpes simplex virus Histoplasmosis Tuberculosis Other mycobacteriosis Salmonellosis	Culture
HIV encephalopathy (dementia)	Clinical findings of disabling cognitive or motor dysfunction interfering with occupation or activities of daily living, progressing over weeks to months, in the absence of concurrent illness or condition other than HIV infection that could explain the findings. Methods to rule out such concurrent illness and conditions must include cerebrospinal fluid examination and either brain imaging (computed tomography or magnetic resonance) or autopsy.
HIV wasting syndrome	Findings of profound involuntary weight loss of >10% of baseline body weight plus either chronic diarrhea (at least two loose stools per day for 30 days), or chronic weakness and documented fever (for 30 days, intermittent or constant) in the absence of a concurrent illness or condition other than HIV infection that could explain the findings (e.g., cancer, tuberculosis, cryptosporidiosis, or other specific enteritis).
Pneumonia, recurrent	Recurrent (more than one episode in a one-year period), acute (new X-ray evidence not present earlier) pneumonia diagnosed by both (a) culture (or other organism-specific diagnostic method) obtained from a clinically reliable specimen of a pathogen that typically causes pneumonia (other than *Pneumocystis carinii* or *Mycobacterium tuberculosis*), and (b) radiologic evidence of pneumonia; cases that do not have laboratory confirmation of a causative organism for one of the episodes of pneumonia will be considered to be presumptively diagnosed.

TABLE 36-4. Suggested guidelines for presumptive diagnosis of diseases indicative of AIDS

Diseases	Presumptive criteria
Candidiasis of esophagus	Recent onset of retrosternal pain on swallowing; AND Oral candidiasis diagnosed by the gross appearance of white patches or plaques on an erythematous base or by the microscopic appearance of fungal mycelial filaments from a noncultured specimen scraped from the oral mucosa.
Cytomegalovirus retinitis	A characteristic appearance on serial ophthalmoscopic examinations (e.g., discrete patches of retinal whitening with distinct borders, spreading in a centrifugal manner along the paths of blood vessels, progressing over several months, and frequently associated with retinal vasculitis, hemorrhage, and necrosis). Resolution of active disease leaves retinal scarring and atrophy with retinal pigment epithelial mottling.
Mycobacteriosis	Microscopy of a specimen from stool or normally sterile body fluids or tissue from a site other than lungs, skin, or cervical or hilar lymph nodes that shows acid-fast bacilli of a species not identified by culture.
Kaposi's sarcoma	A characteristic gross appearance of an erythematous or violaceous plaque-like lesion on skin or mucous membrane. (*Note:* Presumptive diagnosis of Kaposi's sarcoma should not be made by clinicians who have seen few cases of it.)
Pneumocystis carinii pneumonia	A history of dyspnea on exertion or nonproductive cough of recent onset (within the past three months); AND Chest X-ray evidence of diffuse bilateral interstitial infiltrates or evidence by gallium scan of diffuse bilateral pulmonary disease; AND Arterial blood gas analysis showing an arterial po_2 of 70 mm Hg or a low respiratory diffusing capacity (80% of predicted values) or an increase in the alveolar-arterial oxygen tension gradient; AND No evidence of a bacterial pneumonia.
Pneumonia, recurrent	Recurrent (more than one episode in a one-year period), acute (new X-ray evidence not present earlier) pneumonia diagnosed on clinical or radiologic grounds by the patient's physician.
Toxoplasmosis of brain	Recent onset of a focal neurologic abnormality consistent with intracranial disease or a reduced level of consciousness; AND Evidence by brain imaging (computed tomography or magnetic resonance) of a lesion having a mass effect or the radiographic appearance of which is enhanced by injection of contrast medium; AND Serum antibody to toxoplasmosis or successful response to therapy for toxoplasmosis.
Tuberculosis, pulmonary	When bacteriologic confirmation is not available, other reports may be considered to be verified cases of pulmonary tuberculosis if the criteria of the Division of Tuberculosis Elimination, National Center from Prevention Services, CDC, are used. The criteria in use as of January 1, 1993, are available in MMWR 1990; 39 (No. RR-13):39-40.

APPENDIX 36-3 Guidelines on evaluation and management of early HIV infection*

AGENCY FOR HEALTH CARE POLICY AND RESEARCH PUBLIC HEALTH SERVICE, DEPARTMENT OF HEALTH AND HUMAN SERVICES, PRESS RELEASE, JANUARY 20, 1994

Disclosure of HIV status

- The practitioner should disclose the presence of HIV to a patient or in the case of children, to the parents or caretakers, in person. Counseling should include discussion of the psychological and medical effects of the illness, available therapies and support services.
- Patients should also be told about federal, state and local reporting requirements and of potential advantages and disadvantages of voluntary disclosure to family, friends and others.

Medical Evaluation and Management

- Detailed medical history-taking, including sexual and substance use history, is crucial and should emphasize review of HIV test results and previous infections.
- Practitioners closely monitor patients' count of CD4 cells beginning with the initial medical evaluation, and every six months thereafter for those with counts above 600 and at least every three months for patients whose counts are between 600 and 200. Monitoring of CD4 count below 200 is dependent on the availability of other interventions.
- Preventive therapy for *Pneumocystis carinii* pneumonia (PCP) begin when a patient's CD4 count drops below 200 or he or she has an episode of disease or other specific symptoms.
- Pregnant women's CD4 cell count be measured when they begin a prenatal care program or at delivery if they have not had prenatal care.
- Patients be screened for *Mycobacterium tuberculosis* and preventive therapy or treatment be started, if warranted. Methods to improve adherence with treatment of tuberculosis should be employed.
- All HIV-infected and sexually active adults and adolescents be checked for the presence of syphilis and other sexually transmitted diseases in the initial medical evaluation and regularly thereafter.

- Patients be offered antiretroviral therapy with zidovudine (ZDV, formerly known as AZT) whose CD4 counts are below 500. Patients should be informed about the potential benefits and risks of early therapy with ZDV, and other options for antiretroviral therapy should be discussed. Pregnant women should be told of possible benefits as well as risks to both themselves and their unborn babies.
- Women be given regular pelvic examinations that include Pap smears.
- Adolescents be assessed based on their level of sexual and physical maturity, and that drug dosages should be adjusted accordingly.
- The provider conduct an oral examination at each visit and recommend that a dentist examine the patient at least two times a year.
- The practitioner also conduct an eye examination and recommend the patient see a qualified eye doctor according to a schedule that varies with their age and symptoms.
- Contraceptive, family planning, and prenatal counseling be given to all HIV-infected women, with the focus on the patient, and that her psychological state, medical and social support network be assessed.
- HIV-infected mothers be informed of the need for contingency planning for future care of their children.
- Patients be provided with access to appropriate clinical trials including women, as well as pregnant women and adolescents.
- The provider should obtain information regarding available case management programs and provide patients access to them.

Consumer Information

- Two accompanying booklets—for persons living with HIV and for caregivers of HIV-infected children—urge readers to learn all they can about HIV infection, see their practitioner regularly, and work in partnership with their provider regarding their care.
- The booklets, which are available in English and Spanish, also recommend that women talk with their provider about family planning, pregnancy, breast feeding and related matters.

---

*Copies of *Early Evaluation and Management of HIV Infection,* an accompanying quick reference guide, and the consumer booklets, may be obtained free of charge by calling 800-342-2437. Those with handset-equipped facsimile machines can get many of these materials by calling AHCPR Instant Fax (301-594-2800) 24 hours a day. The document number for the guideline overview is 940570 and for the quick reference guide for clinicians, 945073.

APPENDIX 36-4 Reporting requirements for HIV infection

By name	Anonymous	Not required
Alabama	Georgia	Alaska
Arizona	Iowa	California
Arkansas	Kansas	Connecticut
Colorado	Kentucky	Delaware
Idaho	Maine	Florida
Illinois	Montana	Hawaii
Indiana	New Hampshire	Louisiana
Michigan	Oregon	Maryland†
Minnesota	Rhode Island	Massachusetts
Mississippi	Texas	Nebraska
Missouri		New Mexico
Nevada		New York
New Jersey*		Pennsylvania
North Carolina		Vermont
North Dakota		Washington†
Ohio		District of Columbia
Oklahoma		
South Carolina		
South Dakota		
Tennessee*		
Utah		
Virginia		
West Virginia		
Wisconsin		
Wyoming		

*Implementation date, January 1992.
†Requires reports of symptomatic HIV infection by name.
Note: Current as of 3/1/94. All states require reporting of AIDS cases by name at state/local level.

CHAPTER 37 Impaired and disabled patients

ALLAN GIBOFSKY, M.D., J.D., F.A.C.P., F.C.L.M.*
HAROLD L. HIRSH, M.D., J.D., F.C.L.M.

Disability is defined as "the inability to engage in any substantial gainful activity by reason of any medically determinable physical or mental impairment which can be expected to result in death or which has lasted or can be expected to last for a continuous period of not less than 12 months." Inherent in this definition are three requirements that must be met in order for disability to be present: duration, absence of substantial gainful activity, and the presence of a medically determinable impairment. Individuals may not be considered disabled if they have earned income greater than a statutory-defined threshold even though they may only be able to work part-time at their previous occupation and are earning substantially less than their previous income.

In establishing disability, several subjective and, as such, somewhat inaccurate measures must be considered. Among these are such nonmedical factors as gender, prior training, expertise, experience, education, social involvement, local or national availability of suitable employment, problems of transportation to and from available employment, and ability to work with others. Disability is also affected by economic, social, and environmental factors—employability, geography, and type of job. The decision includes a consideration of the background of the particular statutory or contractual disability eligibility requirements, as well as calculation of the loss of earning capacity, limitations in everyday living, and socioeconomic status of the disability.

Total disability has been defined as an individual's absence from the usual place of employment or business, or an inability to engage in his or her regular occupation, that is, an inability to do regular work.[1] This specifies no class or category of occupational endeavors or particular occupation. It entails that the individual cannot reasonably be expected to engage in an occupation with due

regard to his or her training, background, experience, and prior income status. Another consideration may be that the individual cannot engage in any or every occupation or have the ability to perform any or all work for compensation or profit.

Permanent and total disability means that the individual is reasonably expected to have a prolonged, persisting incapacity without any reasonable chance of regaining capacity to work at all.

Partial disability connotes an inability to perform one or more work functions. It may mean simply an inability to do all regular duties.

For most individuals, the duration requirement referred to in the preceding definitions is straightforward, because their disability is chronic and will tend to increase with time. In some cases, however, there may be alterations in the individual's ability to work. Musculoskeletal and neurologic conditions in which patients experience frequent exacerbations and remissions (e.g., rheumatoid arthritis, multiple sclerosis) may result in shorter periods of disability, often making it more difficult for certain individuals to meet the duration requirement.

If disability is the result of trauma, in addition to ascertaining the symptoms and signs or physical manifestations, the physician is particularly concerned with pain. Although this is primarily a subjective report of the patient, there may also be objective signs such as dilation of pupils, nervousness, and abnormal blood pressure, pulse, and/or respirations. Pain that is not reported until 24 or more hours following the injury is usually emotional in origin. For disability evaluation purposes, pain can be classified as:

- Severe (precludes the activity precipitating the pain)
- Moderate (tolerated with marked handicap in performance of activity producing pain)
- Slight (tolerated with some handicap in performance of activity producing pain)

*The authors gratefully acknowledge work from the previous contributor: Gary M. Townsend, M.D., J.D., F.C.L.M.

• Minimal (annoying but no handicap in performance of activities).

In evaluating the impact of an injury, the physician determines the following: whether the injury was the direct or primary cause of the disease process (e.g., a compound fracture with an incidental infection or a chest injury with a pleural effusion or pneumonia); whether the injury aggravated or accelerated the activity of a systemic condition (e.g., diabetes, gout, or hypertension); whether a systemic disease process (e.g., bone tumor or osteoporosis) predisposed to a fracture; and, finally, whether the injury and the systemic disease are purely incidental.

In evaluation of disability due to a mental disorder, several factors must be considered, including those which are physiological, psychological, and personal to that individual. Factors considered may include mental deficiency or retardation, personality disorders, sociopathic personalities, psychoneuroses, psychoses, and organic brain syndromes.[2]

The most important requirement of the disability definition is that the individual has a medically determinable impairment. In contrast to the definition of disability, *impairment* has been defined as the presence of a specific disease that is of sufficient severity to justify the conclusion that a substantial reduction in functional ability has resulted.

Impairments must be demonstrable "by medically acceptable clinical and laboratory diagnostic techniques." Objective evidence of a physical or mental impairment is required, and symptoms alone are never sufficient for a determination of disability. Physical or laboratory findings must confirm an underlying condition that could reasonably be expected to produce the symptoms.

The determination of impairment is dependent on the extent of any anatomical abnormality and psychological or physiological (functional) loss.[3] In making the appraisal, the physician considers the nature and extent of the injury or illness, and whether the condition is stable or nonprogressive after maximum rehabilitation. The physician may also take into account the patient's efficiency as to activities of daily living, both in his or her home life and employment.

Impairment is determined by objective measurements and translated into numerical values. Among the factors measured are loss of structural integrity, pathology, pain, and clinical findings, denoting the diagnosis that, in turn, includes anatomical tissue changes, pathology, and physiological disturbances.[4] Among the clinical symptoms are pain, swelling, deformity, and a variety of movements such as jumping, throwing, and bending. Also included in the impairment evaluation is physical capacity—pushing, pulling, grasping, stepping, reaching,

---

BOX 37-1
PHYSICAL REQUIREMENTS OF WORK

Sedentary work
  Sitting
  Lifting ≤ 10 lbs
  Occasional lifting or carrying of small objects
  Occasional walking and standing
  Fine dexterity
Light work
  Lifting of ≤ 20 lbs
  Frequent lifting or carrying of ≤ 10 lbs
  Frequent walking or standing
  Sitting with push/pull arm or leg controls
Medium work
  Lifting ≤ 50 lbs
  Frequent lifting or carrying of ≤ 25 lbs
Heavy work
  Lifting ≤ 100 lbs
  Frequent lifting or carrying of ≤ 50 lbs
Very heavy work
  Lifting of > 100 lbs
  Frequent lifting or carrying of > 50 lbs

---

walking, and stair climbing (see Box 37-1). The questions to be answered are these: Are the limitations due to the disorder, can further problems be prevented, and to what extent are they developed? The examinee's mental capacity and functional ability must be evaluated, and finally the physician must assess whether the impairment is temporary or permanent.

The bases for determining impairment as to activities of daily living include the amount of self-care needed, the ability to communicate, ambulate, and travel, and other nonspecific activities.

When evaluating impairment, the physician utilizes all currently available practical means of diagnosing disease (i.e., laboratory and radiographic studies). Whenever possible, functional capacity is measured and expressed quantitatively, avoiding solely subjective complaints and imprecise terms whenever possible. Impairment is an appraisal of all clinical findings contributing to the determination of a temporary or permanent physical limitation of the body or any of its organ systems.

A severe impairment is one that "significantly limits physical or mental ability to do basic work activities." Basic work activities are defined as those necessary to do most jobs. These include physical functions such as walking, standing, lifting, or handling; the ability to see, hear, and speak; adequate mental capacity; ability for social interaction with coworkers; and the skills to adapt to changes in routine work settings.

The requirement for objective evidence also means

BOX 37-2
DECISION LEVELS IN THE DISABILITY DETERMINATION AND APPEALS PROCESS

1. Eligibility determination by the Social Security District Office
2. Initial disability decision by State Disability Determination Services (DDS)
3. DDS reconsideration of disability denial
4. Administrative law judge (ALJ) hearing
5. Social Security Appeals Council review
6. Federal courts

BOX 37-3
STEPS IN THE DISABILITY DETERMINATION PROCESS

1. Is the applicant involved in substantial gainful activity?
2. Is there a severe impairment present?
3. Does the impairment meet or exceed listed criteria? (for Social Security claims)
4. Can the applicant perform his or her previous work?
5. Can the applicant do any other available work?

---

that a conclusion by the individual's personal physician that he or she is unable to work does not determine the presence of disability. This is the common misunderstanding that physicians and patients have about the definition of disability whether under individual policies or under Social Security (see Box 37-2).

The Social Security regulations contain an extensive listing of impairments for each major body system. Within each category, specific diseases are listed, followed by the findings that must be present in order to confirm the diagnosis and by the measures of disease severity that allow the presumption of a disabling impairment to be reached (see Box 37-3). Because it is not possible to list all diseases, the regulations include the concept of medical equivalency. Under this concept, nonlisted disorders can be considered as medically equivalent to listed ones.

In these instances, the diagnostic evidence required differs, the clinical evidence required for a determina-

tion of impairment is similar. The use of a list of impairments with specific criteria tends to make disability determination more objective and uniform, but this may create problems for applicants who do not meet the criteria.

In conclusion, in determining the degree of extent of disability, a number of conditions are factors, including whether[5]:
- The individual is continuously confined indoors
- The individual is under regular (continuous, weekly, or monthly) treatment by a registered physician
- Bodily injury resulted from accidental means (body injury through an accident)
- The disability began within a certain, specified number of days after the accident
- The injury or sickness will wholly and continuously disable the examinee or be a recurrent problem.

Ultimately, the following must be established[6]:
- Did accidental injury occur?
- Is physical impairment causally related to claimed injury?
- What is the nature and extent of injury?
- How was the injury treated?
- Has all been accomplished that can be expected of treatment?
- Is improvement stationary, and has it reached its maximum potential?
- Will further rehabilitation be beneficial in lessening the extent of disability?
- What are the chances of readjustment to employment?
- What is the extent of permanent physical impairment?
- Was there loss of fundamental ability to use impaired parts?
- Is there permanent disability?

END NOTES
1. McBride, *Disability Evaluation and Ratings,* 1 Lawyers Med. J. 18 (1965).
2. *Meter v. Continental Insurance Co.,* 40 N.Y. 2d 675, 38a N.Y.S. 2d 565, 358 N.E. 2d 258 (N.Y. App. 1976).
3. Marcus, *Psychiatric Disability Litigation: Definitions and Problems,* Med. Trial Tech. Q. Annual 137-40 (1984).
4. *Gunn v. Secretary,* 341 F. Supp. 611 (Ind. 1972).
5. *Supra* note 5.
6. McBride, *supra* note 1.

CHAPTER 38   Pain management

WAYNE HODGES, M.D., Psy.D., F.A.A.P.M.

ONTOGENY OF THE SPECIALTY: PAIN MEDICINE
BASIC CONCEPTS
DIAGNOSTIC PROCESSES
TREATMENT PROCESSES
MEDICOLEGAL/POLITICAL ISSUES IN PAIN MANAGEMENT

ONTOGENY OF THE SPECIALTY: PAIN MEDICINE

That the reader is encountering pain management as a new entry in this text serves to signify its novelty as a science and practice within medicine. Notwithstanding its neophyte status, however, the discipline has a strong scientific and research underpinning with many decades of actual clinical application that have led to the establishment of definite standards of practice. The time-tested procedural approach of medicine (history, physical exam, diagnosis, treatment) applies ever so aptly to the pain patient; however, therein lies the pitfall as well. The pain patient represents an amalgam of physical, psychological, social, economic, and political parameters, which must, to the newcomer, make the pain patient appear much as the first slides under Linnaeus's microscope—a paradoxical picture wherein some organization and structure are obviously present, but the interrelation and meaningfulness are an enigma. Because of this complexity, the disease model that has served medicine so well in other areas is inappropriate. Furthermore, it is inadequate. Beyond that, application of the traditional disease model to the pain patient, especially within the realm of chronic pain, has in the past provided and still continues to provide a fertile field of iatrogenically produced patient debilities. Thus, the physician approaching the pain patient would be well served to remember the following points:

- Although pain medicine is new, it has understood standards of practice.
- Competent, comprehensive, erudite evaluation and treatment of the pain patient must prevail.
- The disease model is inappropriate and must be replaced by the biopsychosocial model of diagnosis and treatment.

- Management, not cure, is often the goal of treatment. Management implies pain relief (even if tentative), prevention of deterioration, and optimization of daily life function.

At least four decades ago, Dr. John Bonica[1] recognized pain as a clinical entity worthy of individualized consideration as opposed to being little more than a secondary accompaniment of an acute trauma, or an even worse myth, the miserable complaints of neurotic individuals who refuse to get well. Pain as sensation and perception received empirical attention in the discipline of experimental psychology even prior to the advent of Bonica's observations. Ancient folk and medical history is replete with pain as a universal problem, frequently with colorful solutions offered for its cure.

It is an unfortunate fact that patients (not the medical profession) are frequently the impetus behind a new specialty in medicine; so it was with pain management. Those suffering acute pain from injury (whether sustained from happenstance or whether sustained from iatros) were often accused, either covertly or overtly, of possessing excessive affinity for controlled analgesics should they cry out for more pain relief postoperatively or during convalescence. It is now a well-documented fact that the acute pain patient sustained undue suffering because of inadequate analgesic medications. Due to the tenacity of these patients in their protests, guidelines encompassing more reasonable and thoughtful analgesia for the acute pain patient have evolved as promulgated in *Acute Pain Management: Operative or Medical Procedures in Trauma.*[2]

The chronic pain patient has been loathed, maligned, and slandered for many years by the medical profession, as well as others. Such malevolence continues to this day.

The chronic pain patient who did not respond to his or her physician caretaker's best efforts (e.g., laminectomy with diskectomy), was told that, with time, pain would go away. The pain often did not go away and neither did the patient. As the patient hovered incessantly at the physician's door much like Poe's raven, physicians assumed that it was unreasonable for the patient not to respond optimally to "excellent care" and that, accordingly, malingering, secondary gain, or psychoneurosis must underlie the patient's continued bemoanings. With rapid order, then, the patient was sent straight to the psychologist/psychiatrist's office for remedy. It did not take the pain patient long to let the psychological practitioner know that the pain was in his *back* and not his *head*.

Having been misunderstood, if not outright betrayed by their primary practitioners, insulted that their pain was psychologically fabricated, and having no extant alternative otherwise, such patients have been wont to frequent the houses of charlatans. The latter patient actions only served to further substantiate, in the minds of the "legitimate" health care providers, that the patient had no *real* medical disorder. Thus, the pain patient slipped through the missing rung in the health care ladder. As with the acute pain patient, with time, the discordant rumblings of chronic pain patients ultimately synchronized into a highly audible symphonic protest. Health care finally responded. Pain management became a specialty.

Formal pain management organizations evolved and standards of practice have been established, albeit with ample latitude between the boundaries governing such practice. The ancient literature reflects numerous considerations of pain, the universal bond of all mankind, but a formal, scientifically oriented treatise was not available until 1953 when Dr. John Bonica published *The Management of Pain,* earning him the venerated title of the "father of pain medicine." Board certification is now granted by two institutions independent of the American Board of Medical Specialties. The American Academy of Pain Management is the oldest accrediting body; the American College of Pain Medicine was established in 1992, and has held two certification examinations as of this date. The American Academy of Pain Medicine is fully represented in the American Medical Association House of Delegates; in this capacity it concomitantly holds membership in the specialty and service society. As of 1994, pain medicine has been recognized by the American Medical Association as a self-designated specialty.[3]

Another multidisciplinary organization, The International Association for the Study of Pain (IASP), established a task force on the guidelines for desirable characteristics for pain management facilities in 1990,[4]

and in 1991, recommendations for a core curriculum of professional education in pain management.[5] Certification standards for pain centers, comprehensive programs wherein pain medicine is practiced, have been established by the American Academy of Pain Management, the Commission on Accreditation of Rehabilitation Facilities, and the Joint Commission on Accreditation of Hospitals. A discussion of the relative merits regarding certification from these various sources has been made by the author elsewhere.[6]

The present epoch is an era of health care expenditure parsimony, and general asceticism is an ever-progressing attitude in patient care. With this in mind, note that outpatient pain treatment programs are likely to be more cost-effective than large, multidisciplinary in-patient programs. Nevertheless, it should be cautioned that a comprehensive pain treatment facility must encompass multidisciplinary elements of management that address the overall complexity of the patient as opposed to a single modality-oriented treatment approach that fails to do so.

BASIC CONCEPTS
The pain medicine specialist

Pain medicine as a new specialty has arisen in the midst of a formidable environment of cost containment, uncontrollable explosions of medical technology, and societal/professional attitude changes with regard to the American physician, adding to the complications facing the birth of any new specialty. Pain practitioners come from a multitude of previously existing specialties in medicine to include representatives from most of the 23 specialties holding membership in the American Board of Medical Specialties. Therefore, the diversity of backgrounds from which pain practitioners arise leads to a lack of a common, uniform base of training and experience. As denoted previously, the IASP established a task force on guidelines for pain treatment facilities that contained recommendations for physician training; likewise, as previously referenced, IASP has also published a *Core Curriculum for Professional Education in Pain Management.*[7] The Accreditation Counsel on Graduate Medical Education (ACGME) has also addressed pain medicine training,[8,9] but as of this date no formal residency in pain medicine exists. Therefore, it is especially pertinent that the pain practitioner be certified by one of the independently certifying institutions mentioned earlier.

By way of desirable characteristics, the specialist in pain medicine will have appropriate licensure to practice medicine and, preferably, a broad spectrum of training to include documented significant exposure to clinical psychology, physiotherapy, and vocational evaluation/rehabilitation; one must have a special appreciation for the musculoskeletal and neural systems. It would, by way of perfection, be requisite for the pain medicine specialist to be a physician, clinical psychologist, physical therapist, and vocational evaluator, with independent boards in anesthesiology, psychiatry, neurology, and orthopedics. One lifetime does not allow the development of such an individual and, accordingly, one must assume the most cogent characteristics of each of these disciplines and integrate them into a polished, well-established physician applying currently available standards of pain management.

Above all, the physician must be capable of a holistic entertainment of the pain patient's unique qualities, or in the words of Sir William Osler, "It is not nearly as important what illness a patient has, as what patient has the illness."

So often medical training forces a dull, plodding adherence to variously accepted standard routines of perception, decision-making, and treatment actions. Although this may serve to have medical practitioners trod a daily path that is safely within medicolegal guidelines, the role of the specialist in pain medicine requires an individual capable of abstraction, ingenuity, and conceptual freedom to identify with and integrate homeopathy and allopathy, the physical and spiritual, and the known with the unknown. No more cogent reminder of these facts exists than within the ancient writings of Plato:

So, neither ought you to attempt to cure the body without the soul, and this . . . is the reason why the cure of many diseases is unknown to the physicians of Hellas, because they are ignorant of the whole which ought to be studied also, for part can never be well unless the whole is well.

Pain: epidemiology and definitions

Incidence. Pain is everywhere present, pandemic, literally affecting masses of people and costing many millions of dollars. An excellent overview of pain's impact, socially and economically, is provided by Turk et al.[10] In this overview, the author notes that there are 20 to 50 million patients plagued with arthritic pain (with 600,000 new victims each year), 25 million migraineurs, 7 million Americans disabled from low back pain, and more than $900 million spent on over-the-counter analgesics—$100 million of this on aspirin alone. This amounts to 20 tons of aspirin per year and prompts the author to recall a statement of levity in characterizing a patient who complained of headache because he or she was experiencing a systemic deficiency in aspirin!

Pain defined. Dr. John Bonica defined pain as "an unpleasant sensory and emotional experience associated with actual or potential tissue damage or described in terms of such damage,"[11] and this definition was ultimately adapted by the IASP. Although a variety of definitions of pain actually exists, all such definitions, irrespective of their idiosyncratic points of emphasis, embody these important facts:

- Pain is subjective and recalcitrant to measurement by laboratory means.
- Pain is an unpleasant perceptual experience with resulting adverse changes psychologically, socially, politically, and economically.

Pain can be categorized as acute, chronic, or chronic benign.

Acute pain. This entity is well recognized by its precipitating cause, usually documentable illness and injury. There are accompanying acute reactions to include both behavioral displays, autonomic changes such as increased blood pressure and pulse, as well as objective documentation of the etiology by standard laboratory procedures (e.g., serology, radiology, and findings on physical exam). Acute pain is usually proportional to the extent of injury or illness and subsides in proportion to the resolution of the lesion. This latter consideration is of major import: When a patient's complaint of pain does not resolve accordingly, the physician should suspect the emergence of chronic pain.

Chronic pain. Time, per se, is not the single criterion by which one makes the diagnosis of chronic pain, but when complaints continue beyond the normal allotted time for appropriate tissue healing or when a patient's complaints greatly exceed known tissue damage, chronic pain is suspicioned. Chronic pain is a disease state that transcends any precipitating cause and becomes an autonomous, independent clinical syndrome. It is not a psychiatric disorder. It is not malingering. Typical autonomic reactions to pain may be absent. It is important to keep in mind, however, that the response of pain complaint can be affected by exogenous variables such as familial rewards for pain, anger at an abusive employer, and disincentives for recovery. The phrase *chronic pain syndrome* is used to describe the overall debility and compromised functioning of the chronic pain patient who has decompensation in all major life-space areas. *Guides to the Evaluation of Permanent Impairment*[12] overviews the eight "D's" of chronic pain, with the presence of at least four of these criteria being adequate to establish a presumptive diagnosis of the chronic pain syndrome:

1. *Duration:* Pain exists beyond the noted occurrence of tissue healing and the chronic pain syndrome can emerge as early as 2 to 4 weeks subsequent to an injury. Obviously, prompt assessment and appropriate treatment/rehabilitation are required.
2. *Dramatization:* Pain patients display marked, verbal, and nonverbal pain behaviors.
3. *Diagnostic dilemma:* Patients will usually have seen a large number of physicians with replete, poorly

coordinated diagnostic studies, many of which have failed to yield anything other than nebulous conclusions.

4. *Drugs:* Patients who evidence a chronic pain syndrome frequently present with a plethora of medications and a history of polypharmacy.

5. *Dependence:* Patients become introverted, passively dependent on not only the health care system but their families and the economic-political system to which they may seem an appendage (i.e., third-party carriers).

6. *Depression:* The chronic pain patient frequently decompensates to a low-grade, ongoing depression that may exacerbate to suicidal ideation and attempts. Depression becomes a way of life. In this author's experience, over an approximately 20-year span of practice, at least 90% of pain patients are clinically depressed.

7. *Disuse:* The patient fears movement, becomes sedentary, and guards against pain tenaciously, usually leading to musculoskeletal deconditioning and ultimate perpetuation of the pain syndrome.

8. *Dysfunction:* The patient becomes essentially an inadequate personality, unable to negotiate normal stresses and strains and decision-making of day-to-day existence. They resort to mere subsistence on the bare necessities and are usually, reciprocally, ostracized by most of the world, oftentimes by the family itself. It has aptly been stated that the chronic pain patient must learn how to live, whereas the terminal patient must learn how to die.

DIAGNOSTIC PROCESSES

The physician practicing as a pain medicine specialist must be an excellent diagnostician. It is to be kept in mind that a *sine qua non* of pain management is early diagnosis and treatment. Delaying appropriate studies constitutes one of the chief factors known to promote debility from underlying but treatable lesions simply due to failure of diagnosis and appropriate therapy. Usually such patients have been exposed to a random, poorly coordinated barrage of physicians and diagnostic procedures. Thus, it becomes the woeful lot of the pain medicine specialist to fuse a seemingly vast array of heretofore inconclusive findings into a meaningful diagnosis with appropriate treatment plans. This is a burden more than a privilege. But it is a burden that, if appropriately shouldered and carried, results in the honor that comes from personal actualization of the principles inherent in the Hippocratic oath and the heartfelt appreciation of one's patients (who in all likelihood were previously misunderstood, discriminated against, and made to feel as an illegitimate, worrisome intrusion on the health care system).

The pain patient may have been exposed to many individual physicians, none of whom specialize in pain management and, accordingly, have had varying idiosyncratic approaches to the solution, usually unsuccessful. An admonishment is due such practitioners who would wade into the deep water of pain management without appropriate preparation: A physician who provides care that would normally be extended by a given specialist will be held to the standards of the particular specialty he or she is attempting to mimic.[13] Because certain specialties frequently encounter the chronic pain patient (e.g., orthopedics, neurology, anesthesiology, psychiatry), there is the temptation to manage the patient's overall pain complaints even when they are well into an obvious chronic pain syndrome. In times past there was no alternative; such specialties, in fact, were called on to deal with these individuals over the long haul. The establishment of pain medicine as a recognized specialty no longer allows the liberty of those who do not so specialize to maintain such patients without the accompanying risk of legal recompense.

The pain medicine specialist, as diagnostician, must be closely attuned to a full differential diagnosis for each patient's complaints. This can be exhausting to the doctor. Exhaustion has never been an excuse in medicine to slack one's duty, as a brief recollection of one's training may, indeed, bring to mind. Yet, in 20 years of managing pain in the private setting, this author has yet to see aortic aneurysm included in the diagnostic work-up of a patient with low back pain syndrome. Likewise, routine screening for prostatic cancer has seldom, if ever, been witnessed by the chapter author. For example, a case is recalled in which an excellent neurosurgeon, known personally to this writer, treated a patient with a previous history of diskectomy/laminectomy whose low back pain complaints continued to grow the older he became. The attending neurosurgeon felt, as many physicians routinely would, that the etiology of the patient's complaints was plain: low back pain syndrome. In this particular case, however, the patient died with metastasized prostatic cancer, which is well known to extend itself early on into the venous cavities of the lumbar vertebrae.

Thus, the examining pain medicine specialist must perform a comprehensive examination concentrating on the musculoskeletal and neurologic systems minimally and on other body systems to include an entire physical when indicated by the nature of the given complaint. With myalgia/arthralgia, comprehensive laboratory studies may be conducted to include, though not be limited to, the following:

1. SMA-24
2. Urinalysis
3. Myopathy profile
4. Rheumatologic profile

5. Serum protein electrophoresis
6. Antibodies to acetylcholine
7. Tuberculin screen.

Certainly, serology and the entire diagnostic process must be individualized so that the studies routinely done have a basis in the differential diagnosis prompted by the given patient's presentation.

Comprehensive roentgenographic studies must be carried out where indicated and at no point should the doctor hesitate to add to plain-film X-rays as needed. The following studies are to be considered in addition:

1. Computerized tomography (CT) scans
2. Magnetic resonance imaging (MRI)
3. Bone scan (triple phase where reflex sympathetic dystrophy is suspicioned)
4. Single photon emission computerized tomography (SPECT) scans (brain and skeleton)
5. Electromyography (EMG)
6. Medical infrared imagery (thermography)
7. Myelography.

Keep in mind that the statistical existence of significant margins of false-positives and false-negatives exists in all studies. There are varying reports to be referenced, but one can estimate a 15% to 20% false-negative rate in EMG studies where there is a need to rule out neuropathy/radiculopathy. Accordingly, it would be a gross error, diagnostically and morally, to conclusively base decision-making simply on the existence of a negative EMG study. One should never assume the patient to be neurotic and then, based on those assumptions, perform hasty, poor physical examinations and diagnostic studies.

Another case in point is that of an approximately 63-year-old white female who was assisted in ambulation to this author's exam table by two of the nursing staff. The patient was wincing and crying out during this entire process, and only with great difficulty could she be placed in the various anatomic positions required for appropriate examination. The patient complained of polyarthralgia and polymyalgia, but particularly the low back. The paperwork that accompanied the patient came from an outpatient urgent medicine center; it indicated that staff had observed the patient leaving their office ambulating and getting into her car in such a manner as if to imply that her pain complaints were inappropriate or feigned; no physical findings were reportedly remarkable. Early in this author's examination sentinel nodes were grossly palpable in the bilateral supraclavicular areas. Bone scan subsequently revealed untreatable, grossly disseminated, metastatic cancer.

At the time of this writing, there is major societal concern over health care costs. Parsimony, as it relates to diagnosis and treatment, is not, in this examiner's opinion, a physician liberty. By training and by the very

inherent nature of the profession, a medical practitioner is to be unbiased in the diagnosis and treatment of the patient to the furthest extent of his or her ability, and *limited only by currently extant diagnostic and treatment methodologies.* Political/societal opinions and forces will vacillate. The physician who is more attuned to political winds then to the patient's actual diagnostic and treatment needs will find the process of dealing with the patient more positively correlated with the vacillations in societal/political events than with the diagnostic and treatment requirements of the patient's disorder. Thus, the question of whether a patient should be allotted all appropriate studies required to diagnose a complaint definitively is not a physician decision factor. If a patient has severe headaches, even in the absence of neurologic deficit, that patient should be recommended for an MRI or CT scan of the brain. Certainly, this would have been preceded by appropriate skull X-ray series. If society and its legislative/political dictates deny the patient this study, then so be it. It is not, to be sure, the decision of the physician to deny it.

This principle becomes of paramount relevance within certain medicolegal arenas such as workers' compensation claims. As an example, this author provides the case of an approximately 40-year-old male who presented with a history of on-the-job injury at a major steel supply. The patient had been struck on the head and neck by a large metal hook swung by a tall crane, knocking the patient unconscious onto other metal debris littering the grounds. Six months after injury, on presentation to this author's office, the patient complained of intractable headache, bilateral upper extremity dysesthesia/paresthesia (left greater than right), and severe cervicalgia with marked decreased range of motion. As part of the differential diagnosis, this author requested an MRI of the cervical spine, which was denied by third-party workers' compensation sources. Moreover, as an apparent political resentment of an effort to fully diagnose the patient's complaints, third-party sources removed the patient to a so-called "work-hardening" program, wherein he was placed on stringent exercises throughout the day. With prolonged, adamant complaints for approximately 2 or 3 additional months, the subsequently attending physician finally conceded that an MRI scan of the cervical spine should be obtained, and upon so obtaining, it reflected herniated nucleus pulposus (HNP) at C5-6. The patient then underwent a diskectomy and was, believe it or not, returned to the "work-hardening" program for several months ensuing. During this time, the patient was again exposed to stringent exercises, especially of the cervical spine, whereupon 1 day he noted marked increase of his neck pain. Ultimately, the patient (fortunately!) exited this program. Approximately a year passed postinjury and this author once again saw the patient for care: He displayed much the appearance of a badly beaten and mistreated dog. He was immediately hospitalized psychiatrically for suicidal depression; subsequent repeat MRI scanning of the neck reflected recurrent HNP at C5-6 central and left of midline with anterolateral mass effect on the thecal sac with cord indentation; disk material protruded into the left C5-6 neural foramen. So as to prevent one having to read between the lines, it can be stated that within this particular example there was more concern granted the third-party workers' compensation carrier and the employer than the patient's diagnostic and treatment needs. The patient suffered many months, underwent failed surgery, sustained another ruptured disk (allegedly during so-called work-hardening exercises), and is now totally debilitated both physically and psychologically. To comply with anything other than the demands of the patient's actual needs is immoral, unethical, and of high legal risk.

When third-party sources (i.e., anyone other than the patient) are requesting patient diagnosis and treatment, the ethical principle promulgated by the American Psychological Association should be adhered to strictly[14]; the physician should be keenly aware of situations wherein there arises a conflict of interest between the patient and the physician's employing source. The physician must clarify the nature and direction of their loyalties and responsibilities and keep all parties well informed of their commitments. The physician must inform the patient as to the purpose and nature of an evaluation, recommended treatments, or training procedure. The physician should avoid exploiting the trust and dependency of such patients as those in chronic pain. Every effort should be made to avoid a dual relationship that could preclude good professional judgment or increase the risk of patient exploitation. When a physician agrees to provide services to a patient at the request of a third party, the physician thereby assumes the responsibility of clarifying the nature of the relationships to all parties concerned. Unfortunately, it is rare or totally nonexistent for these basic ethical and moral principles to guide physician approach to the patient, which becomes of paramount importance within the political-economic context often existing with pain patients.

This author can prompt the reader to attend to the business of patient care no better than an excerpt from an attorney's letter regarding prominent medicolegal issues pertaining to the pain patient:

Pain clinics need to listen to the patient. We are all aware of the practitioner who has already made their mind up as to cause and treatment from the records without talking to the patient. We find many times the patient has a condition that has been overlooked, because *no one will listen to the complaints.*

In addition to the basic history and physical, the chronic pain patient should undergo a comprehensive, multidisciplinary work-up to include a *functional capacity assessment;* the latter optimally should be conducted both prior to and after a comprehensive pain treatment program. A psychological evaluation is, of necessity, a major part of the diagnostic process.

A word of caution is due, however, as it relates to use of the Minnesota Multi-phasic Personality Inventory (MMPI) and the traditional search for elevations in the hypochondriasis and hystriosis scales, pictorially referred to as a "hysterical conversion valley." Documentation reveals that a chronic pain patient complains to such an extent that the hypochondriasis scale will be elevated, and they are very attuned to the affective nature of their painful existence (often elevating the histrionic scale), while denying psychological problems; the latter, because they are so sensitive about being accused of having a neurosis. It is inappropriate and scientifically inaccurate to use the MMPI in this manner without taking into account a global, comprehensive evaluation of the patient.[15] A patient's work-up may also require vocational evaluation and planning when a residual functional capacity is not compatible with the demands of the patient's previous work functions or activities of daily living.

TREATMENT PROCESSES
Multidisciplinary treatment

Treatment of the pain patient is multidisciplinary, meaning that it encompasses appropriately indicated elements of medical, physical, psychological, and vocational modalities of therapy. One is cautioned regarding the false confidence that exists from repletely staffing a center with all manner of disciplines (e.g., psychologist, physical therapist, occupational therapist, kinesiologist, dietician, vocational evaluator, etc.) with the assumption that the magnitude of a center's staff inherently bespeaks of its competence in treating the pain patient. In fact, as alluded to earlier, large multidisciplinary programs are likely not to be cost-effective and the shuffling of a patient from one department to another, simply to document a patient's exposure to a multitude of disciplines, hardly substitutes for a well-physician-supervised, carefully thought through program of attention to medical issues, psychological issues, musculoskeletal reconditioning, and vocational issues.

Musculoskeletal conditioning is a function of cogently thought through physical exercises focused on the individual patient's requirements; these should be carried out under the physician's supervision and orders; musculoskeletal conditioning can often be carried out in a far more cost-effective manner without the patient being needlessly exposed to numerous service departments; the value and technique of physical exercise are no great mystery and can be effectively carried out by any staff member appropriately instructed. Likewise, chronic pain programs are likely to be more cost-effective when delivered on an outpatient basis.

Medication. The medical management of pain consists of thoughtful evolution of a pharmacologic regimen that balances the need to effect maximal pain relief while at the same time obviating the untoward effects of chronic drug regimens. Always, as with any medical practice, the disadvantages of treatment must be weighed against the advantages. A change in thinking that is long overdue is occurring in both acute and chronic pain as it relates to appropriate pharmacologic management. In both of these areas, but especially so in acute pain, patients have been denied adequate dosages and frequency in dosages of analgesics. For many years a somewhat sour, disbelieving attitude of bias pervaded much of the health care system's approach to the patient who requested analgesia. For some reason, the myth developed that patients do not really hurt as much as they say they do, accompanied by another very unrealistic and unfounded belief that various medical procedures do not really cause pain (when in fact they do). Augmenting this unfortunate set of beliefs was the advent of drug crime in America, with resulting stringent restrictions placed by the Federal Drug Enforcement Agency on all avenues of drug use, including that legitimately applied within the medical profession. Thus, to avoid critical scrutiny by another colleague, or just as likely from the Federal Drug Enforcement Agency, a doctor simply forgoes the possible risk of dealing with controlled analgesics, thus leaving the patient alone in the grip of disabling pain.

In actuality, acute pain management has proffered more from the renovation in thinking than has chronic pain. That is to say, it is not thought as illegitimate and disdainful to adequately treat postoperative pain with sufficient analgesics, since, indeed, the patient will be allotted this medication for an objectively limited period of time.

The *Quick Reference Guide for Clinicians*[16] lists the following approaches for use in acute/postoperative pain management:

- Cognitive behavioral interventions (e.g., relaxation, distraction, and imagery)
- Systemic opioids or nonsteroidals to include acetaminophen
- Patient-controlled analgesia, giving the patient a sense of self-management of their pain, often preferable to intermittent injections
- Spinal anesthesia; epidural opioid or local anesthetic intermittently infused versus continuously infused
- Intermittent versus continuous local neural block-

ade (e.g., intercostal nerve block or local anesthetic via intrapleural catheter)
- Physiotherapy (e.g., massage, heat, cold)
- Transcutaneous electrical nerve stimulation

The reader is again referred to the *Quick Reference Guide*, which presents a helpful algorithm for the physician managing acute pain.

Although an increasing number of papers is now appearing in the professional literature advocating the use of long-term opioid analgesics in appropriately selected chronic pain patients, the reality of the matter is that the medicolegal environment has not changed significantly, and the heavy scrutiny of the Federal Drug Enforcement Agency and state medical licensing boards make it a reality that further restrictiveness must exist. This author is not advocating mass application of controlled analgesics for the chronic pain patient; however, the state of affairs is simply being brought to the fore that, for selected groups of patients, more can be done pharmacologically than is currently the case.

It is with some compunction and self-scorn that this author recalls a patient whose care should have been managed appropriately by Class II opioid narcotics *but was not* simply due to the fear of being viewed askance by the Federal Drug Enforcement Agency or the state licensing board. The patient suffered from causalgia of the left lower extremity with a history of numerous past surgical procedures. He suffered bitter pain, at times decompensating into ETOH intake for relief. Over time he changed into an individual of short temperament and impatience, as well as displaying marked agitated depression. Cyclic exacerbations had lead to several attempts at suicide. He had undergone morphine infusion pump and dorsal column stimulator surgical implants with complications and ultimate removal of the devices. He had been on numerous noncontrolled analgesics, as well as numerous Class IV and Class III analgesics. Under the care of this author, he was administered all major treatment modalities typical of a chronic pain center and was none the better. He was sent for consult to the Department of Neurosurgery of a major teaching university, where he was administered a comprehensive intake work-up (as should be done). The conclusion reached was that the patient would not be a viable candidate for a brain implant stimulator due to an undue affinity for controlled analgesics. Undue affinity for analgesics, indeed! The patient ultimately left the care of this author after *rightfully* cursing him out. The patient, in this author's opinion, should have been placed on transdermal long-acting morphine.

One can easily lose sleep pondering the horrible path of existence such patients must trod from day to day. The patient had been told about and had undergone all the current roster of treatments standard for pain centers such as deep muscle relaxation, biofeedback, didactics with pain-coping groups, various forms of physiotherapy, nerve blocks, tricyclic and other related (noncontrolled) medications, and the various philosophies wherein a patient supposedly will feel better by not talking about their pain and not displaying pain behaviors (and with professional staff ignoring pain complaints). The reader is asked to consider placing a torch to one's foot and leaving it there (a probable semblance of causalgia), and at the same time attempting to keep a straight countenance, while someone advises you to think positively, do not emit pain gestures, breath deeply and relax, and go on about your activities! Pain medicine has taken a leap forward from its early origins, but it has tremendous bounds yet to make.

Within the realm of chronic pain, much excitement is astir as more and more so-called "adjuvant" drugs are "discovered" that assist in the management of the pain patient without actually having them on analgesics per se. This thrust to use anything in the pharmacopoeia offering some management advantage stems in part from the reluctance discussed earlier of the prescribing physician to administer medications other than those smiled on by the swing of the pendulum of current fads. Thus, the following classes of medications can be considered without significant medicolegal risk, given appropriate patient assessment and selection as per the *Principles of Analgesic Use in the Treatment of Acute Pain and Chronic Cancer Pain*[17]:

1. Tricyclic antidepressants
2. Antihistamines
3. Caffeine
4. Nonsteroidals
5. Steroids, usually short-term
6. Phenothiazines
7. Anticonvulsants.

The following medications are to be avoided according to the *Principles of Analgesic Use*[18]: benzodiazepines, sedative hypnotic drugs, canabanoids, and cocaine. However, others have found benzodiazepines beneficial.[19] More recently, various empirical usages are receiving wider spread applications in chronic pain management such as serotonergic specific antidepressants, calcium channel blockers, and mexilitine. Certainly, all these adjunctive medications can be of benefit, but it is merely an arbitrary quirk of current societal thinking to assume that we can substitute these medications for analgesics and then hope that all adversity has been precluded—this type of thinking is inaccurate and unacceptable. All the alternative medications denoted have numerous adverse side effects (e.g., phenothiazines and tardive dyskinesia, which is irreversible). The probable reason that any of these medications is beneficial is the fact that there is an alteration of

autonomic and central nervous system modulation of pain, per se, with concomitant alteration of the attentional process—little more, little less.

The Agency for Health Care Policy and Research, which evolved the acute pain management clinical practice guidelines, is pending a similar publication on chronic, malignant pain guidelines.

Various nerve blocks continue to be a major part of the medical regimen in pain management to include central and peripheral blockade, regional intravenous blocks, lumbar epidural steroid blocks, sympathetic blocks, etc. Note that such procedures, however, are to be coadministered within an overall matrix of multimodal therapies so that the effectiveness of any one particular block can be augmented by the complimenting effects of other therapies. Perhaps timeliness of application of certain of the blocks is not of major import, e.g., as per lumbar epidural steroid blocks and low back pain; yet, with other disorders, early administration of appropriate blocks is crucial, e.g., reflex sympathetic dystrophy and stellate ganglion and lumbar sympathetic blocks.

It is the appropriate duty of the physician to order and supervise all elements of the patient's treatment program, remembering that from a medicolegal perspective the physician is "where the buck stops." Thus, a physician cannot easily discharge the responsibility by simply setting initial orders and expecting all departments to follow those orders unless there is adequate medical monitoring as to the continued appropriateness of the orders, staff/patient compliance with the orders, and the assurance that staff members given the assignments are competent.

It is also the physician's responsibility, when indicated, to conduct formal medical impairment examinations using American Medical Association guidelines. In this respect, it was previously standard for the physician not to comment on disability, but rather to limit his or her assessment and opinion to *medical impairment* only. This has changed with the advent of the fourth addition of the *Guides to the Evaluation of Permanent Impairment*.[20] It is now formally recognized that an appropriately trained physician who has knowledge and insight into the patient's disorder, work setting, and familial environment can pass judgment on *disability* in addition to *impairment*.

Behavioral medicine. The impact of clinical psychology on the pain management scene has been major. The very foundation of assessing the pain patient and subsequently prescribing an apt program of treatment closely follows the model of behavioral analysis. As crucial as any neural blockade or medical procedure, the patient who is in chronic pain may be exposed to biofeedback, pain-coping groups, individual and family therapy, bariatric/nutritional management, and stress management.

Physiotherapy. Musculoskeletal conditioning with palliative modalities of physiotherapy is crucial to the treatment of the pain patient. Administration of myofascial stretching/relaxation and anti-inflammatory procedures are greatly beneficial. The patient should receive formal didactics, musculoskeletal conditioning with follow-up homework assignments, and supportive medical appliances to assist along these lines (i.e., home hot and cold packs, mechanical massagers, etc.). It has been noted that many patients who undergo appropriate musculoskeletal reconditioning prior to the advent of scheduled back surgery, in fact, ultimately may not require it. Appropriate before and after treatment functional capacity assessment should be effected in order to determine objectively the abilities of a patient's musculoskeletal system to sustain various activities of daily living and expected work functions.

Vocational assessment/rehabilitation. When a patient's residual functional capacities and documented medical impairment are such that return to previous normal activity levels is not possible, the physician should consult the *Dictionary of Occupational Titles* (U.S. Department of Labor) to accurately recommend job placement if, in fact, return to viable employment is feasible. At times, patients may require job readiness training in order to assist them in their reentry to the employment scene, whereas on other occasions the patient may require total retraining in another work area altogether.

MEDICOLEGAL/POLITICAL ISSUES IN PAIN MANAGEMENT

The chronic pain patient is constantly plagued by pain such that he or she will eventually be controlled by it. The legal, medical, governmental, and economic vectors, which overlap, seem at times to constitute the major sources of attention and activity of involved professional agencies—to the detriment of the actual patient whose condition initially stimulated such activity. A patient comes to the state of chronic pain usually from illness or injury. In many cases of illness, and in most cases of injury, it is a fact of current society that, unless the patient receives appropriate legal counsel, there is open question as to whether or not legitimate attention would be given their problems. Thus, the patient may well have a plaintive attorney and the third-party carrier will have a defense attorney. A rehabilitation supplier and the state board of workers' compensation may also be involved. The industrial setting itself will also maintain personal interest in the outcome. Considered in the following discussion are the recommended principles, philosophies, and concepts necessary for societal, legal,

and governmental sources to adopt in order to assure any semblance of just outcome in the management and disposition of the chronic pain patient.

Sociolegal, economic principles

Chronic pain and chronic pain syndrome must be accepted as legitimate medical disorders and, thereby, legitimate concerns of society. Chronic pain is a disorder marked by subjective complaints, many without objective findings. Alleged disability is more times than not based on the patient's opinion of his or her inability to function. Industry, the employer, and workers' compensation agencies who have the job of administering payment and maintaining a workers' compensation fund stand to lose when a patient claims debility from chronic pain. Accordingly, from a political and economic perspective, there is likely to be much resistance in attributing legitimacy to the patient's claim by such agencies and societal institutions.

Traditional medicine teaches that without "objective findings" the patient is malingering, desires secondary gain, or has a psychologic illness underlying the complaint. A modest survey was conducted by the author to assess major medicolegal issues of concern as viewed by attorneys practicing within the area of impairment/disability from chronic pain. A stated recurrent concern was the difficulty inherent in getting legitimate recognition of a patient's problems due to absence of "objective findings." It seems that medicine, societal agencies, and the attorneys dealing with chronic pain are all obsessed with the perception that unless some "magical tests" can be brought to bear, the legitimacy of the pain patient will not be recognized. On a pragmatic plane, this is certainly the case. It should not be. No test will measure pain. The tenacious search for the proverbial "pinched nerve," or some other anatomic/physiologic abnormality, has lead more than one patient into numerous unneeded independent medical evaluations and repetitive studies. The defending attorney or the workers' compensation/third-party carrier will ask for one independent medical evaluation after the other, knowing that in the chronic pain patient there is unlikely to be clear-cut, hard core tests that will document the patient's underlying etiology.

Having thus obtained the expected ambiguity in findings, the hope is to use the absence of "objective" results to win in subsequent litigation, claiming that indeed the patient has no identified medical disorder to substantiate their complaints. There is no better setting than to tout the old adage: "the absence of evidence is no evidence of absence." Keep in mind that medical technology and testing, though more advanced than ever in civilization, remain inadequate to explain the painful percepts and sensations in the human animal. Malingering is relatively infrequent.[21,22] It is, therefore, because of the inadequacy of our technology and the lack of understanding of medicine in general that a patient's complaints cannot be delineated.

Thus, simply because tests do not exist to explain a patient's woes, no bases exist thereby to conclude that no such woes exist. This author recalls a white male, approximately 28 years old, who presented well-dressed, animated, and in obvious good physical condition. He had been in an automobile accident four months earlier. His left shoulder and left superior dorsal thorax continued to hurt, to evidence crepitus, and to "feel funny." Plain films failed to show any lesion. Examination showed mild compromise in range of motion of the left pectoral girdle and some tenderness to firm palpation of the left scapula and dorsal pectoral girdle musculature. Auscultation, in fact, revealed peculiar sounds of crepitus in the area of the left scapula in general. Bone scan showed four fractured ribs lying hidden underneath the left scapula. On so learning of his findings, the patient was thankful, desired no treatment, and had no litigation. He was merely interested in knowing why he continued to hurt, why he had peculiar noises in his shoulder, and desired definitive medical explanation so as not to have an unforeseen lesion that might later result in undue difficulty. It should never have been necessary for this young man to visit a pain center. Such a diagnosis would have been easier to make by more primary care practitioners. It is this author's conviction, moreover, that he was not properly examined and that proper studies were not obtained due to the fact that he looked young, successful, and in no acute distress, and thereby could be seeking little more than a "green poultice" due to his actual disorder of "compensationitis." One attorney responding to the previously referenced survey summed it up quite well in regards to appropriate management of the pain patient and the inherent difficulties thereof:

In dealing with my clients who have been patients of pain management specialists, I have noted that, for whatever reason, they often improve with their complaints or their symptoms after having been treated by a pain management specialist. Although this is not a criticism of doctors at all, I think sometimes the primary care providers are mostly focused on getting a physiologic injury "healed" by helping a fracture to heal or healing open wounds or other injuries. When the fracture or the wound, or the injury is clinically healed, they have really discharged their primary function in regards to the patient. Sometimes, the pain or disruption of the injury continues, and I believe this is where the pain management practice helps greatly with continuing to care for the patient and taking them to the next level of healing or recovery—getting over continuing physiological or psychological pain.

An added comment would seemingly be in order with regard to objective tests and the absence of yet-to-be developed tests that may ultimately reveal pathology thus far not recognized. A few years back the bone scan was not available. The young patient just described would never have had the fractured ribs diagnosed had it not been for the bone scan. Imagine the number of patients now suffering disorders for which we have no tests; unfortunately, because of the absence of tests to document their complaints, they are dismissed as malingerers or neurotics or as having "compensationitis." To be sure, this author is not advocating the gullible, uninsightful acceptance of any and all complaints and the blithe overlooking of possible untoward intentions of certain patients whose motivations are related more to secondary gain and manipulation than to benefit any real sickness.

What, then, is the crux of this discussion? The facts are simple. The chronic pain patient possesses many ambiguities and intangible complaints that nevertheless forcefully exert real-life, tangible demands from society, i.e., settlements and disability benefits. There is the question of legitimacy, veracity, and patient motivation inherent in this process. Who will ferret out the truths and untruths and thereby establish justice for the patient? *Not the doctor.* The physician is to render a thorough and thoughtful examination with an appropriate roster of medical studies, then act on these with standard, accepted modalities of treatment. In this role, the physician provides a unique and needed element to the overall picture of the pain patient-societal quandary. The physician should go no further. It is the duty and burden of society and its agents to determine through standard channels (i.e., the legal system), whether or not an individual is a malingerer versus legitimate. It is a societal issue of ethics and morality. Only society and its agents can pass judgment on whether a patient who suffers pain should be excused from work. Should a patient who suffers blinding, nauseating migraine headaches be excused from a day's work, or if persistent enough, be termed disabled? Can a patient who says he or she cannot bend over due to back pain be told that he or she can, in fact, bend, should bend, and will bend or be punished socioeconomically? Who is to make the arbitrary decision that reflex sympathetic dystrophy will not qualify as a legitimate source of disability, whereas a ruptured disk in one's back with nerve compression will qualify? Again, it is this author's contention that only society and its agents need reply. It is not that society is *correct;* rather, it is simply the burden of society to make these decisions and not the burden of the individual physician. Indeed, many societal decisions are wrong. But within an ordered society, it is the medicolegal guidelines within which one must operate that prevent the individual from running amok of the system. In avoiding dogmatism as it relates to physician decision making, it is always better to "err on the side of the angels than on the side of the devil."

The physician cannot discriminate against a patient simply because there is the presence of litigation. The physician, ethically, is admonished to keep in mind that any patient in current society may well have legitimate reasons for legal representation. The mere fact that an attorney may be involved constitutes an ill-conceived motivation for the doctor to avoid the patient, whether it be through a deposition or a courtroom appearance.

Legal counsel's duty is to assure that an accurate, comprehensive assessment is presented on the chronic pain patient, fully utilizing the biopsychosocial model. There must be comprehensive medical and psychological assessment and a portrayal of economic factors, with adequate attention to the marked deleterious effects on the patient and family of the chronic pain syndrome. It is furthermore the ethical duty of the attorney to assure that the patient's best interest is kept in mind. A rapid settlement of a patient's claim in order for an attorney to collect "quick money" is a sell-out to the patient and constitutes a major moral infraction no less appalling than a physician who will electively operate on a patient without good indication. There is no sadder sight than to see a chronic pain patient 2 years after settling a claim who is depressed, penniless, and markedly debilitated due to pain but with no recourse because he signed away all of his rights on the recommendation of an attorney who needed a quick $5000.

It is the unfortunate truth as things currently stand that justice can rarely be done the chronic pain patient outside the legal setting. The dynamics and motivations of the various parties involved are such that little justice and resolution can otherwise evolve. Although one might philosophically say that such legal processes are appropriate and the ends worth the means, such a Machiavellian process is seldom worth it to the patient. By the time a courtroom setting is reached, the chronic pain syndrome has grossly evolved and entrenched itself, and all parties are violently inflamed against each other. All have suffered unduly, especially the patient.

END NOTES

1. J. J. Bonica, *The Management of Pain* (Lea & Febinger, New York 1953).
2. *Acute Pain Management: Operative or Medical Procedures in Trauma* (U.S. Department of Health and Human Services Feb. 1992).
3. 8 Am. Acad. of Pain Med. Newsl. (Winter 1993).
4. *Desirable Characteristics for Pain Treatment Facilities and Standards for Physician Fellowships in Pain Management* (International Association for the Study of Pain, 1990).
5. *Core Curriculum for Professional Education in Pain Management* (International Association for the Study of Pain 1991).
6. W. Hodges, *Pain Center Certification: Controversies and Issues,* paper presented at the Annual Conference of the American Academy of Pain Medicine, Scottsdale, Arizona, 1991.
7. *Supra* note 5.
8. 6 Am. Acad. of Pain Med. Newsl. (Dec. 1991).
9. J. C. Gienapp, Executive Secretary, Accreditation Council for Graduate Medicine Education, Personal Communication, Sep. 30, 1991.
10. D. C. Turk et al., *Pain and Behavioral Medicine* 73-74 (The Guilford Press 1983).
11. J. J. Bonica, ed., I *The Management of Pain* 18 (Lea and Febinger, Philadelphia 1990).
12. *Guides to the Evaluation of Permanent Impairment* (4th ed., American Medical Association, 1993).
13. *Medicolegal Primer* 108 (1st ed., American College of Legal Medicine Foundation 1991).
14. *Case Book on Ethical Principles of Psychologists* 77-92 (American Psychological Association 1987).
15. 1 Am. Pain Soc. Bull. (Jan./Feb. 1994).
16. *Quick Reference Guide for Clinicians. Acute Pain Management In Adults: Operative Procedures* (U.S. Department of Health and Human Services Feb. 1992).
17. *Principles of Analgesic Use in the Treatment of Acute Pain and Chronic Cancer Pain* (American Pain Society 1992).
18. *Id.*
19. Fibromyalgia Network Newsl. 7 (Oct. 1993).
20. *Supra* note 12.
21. F. Levitt and J. J. Sweet, *Characteristics and Frequency of Malingering Among Patients with Low Back Pain,* 25 Pain 357 (1986).
22. Social Security Administration 1986 Report of The Commission on the Evaluation of Pain (U.S. Government Printing Office, Washington, D.C. 1986).

GENERAL REFERENCES

Bonica, J. J., et al., I, II *The Management of Pain* (2nd ed., Lea and Febiger, Philadelphia 1990).

Institute of Medicine, *Pain and Disability* (National Academy Press, 1987).

Turk, D. C., et al., *Pain and Behavioral Medicine* (The Guilford Press 1983).

Turk, D. C., and Melzack, R., *Handbook of Pain Assessment* (The Guilford Press 1992).

U.S. Department of Health, Education and Welfare, *Report of the Panel on Pain* (National Institute of Health, Publication 79-1912, 1979).

CHAPTER 39

Occupational health law

CAROLYN S. LANGER, M.D., J.D., M.P.H.

THE OCCUPATIONAL SAFETY AND HEALTH ACT
KEEPING THE WORKER INFORMED
DISCRIMINATION IN THE WORKPLACE
TORT LIABILITY
LEGAL LIABILITY OF THE OCCUPATIONAL HEALTH CARE PROVIDER: MEDICAL MALPRACTICE
CONCLUSION

Occupational medicine is a branch of preventive medicine that "focuses on the relationship among" workers' health, "the ability to perform work, the arrangements of work, and the physical, [biological], and chemical environments of the workplace."[1]

From a medicolegal standpoint, occupational medicine is unique among the medical specialties. In no other specialty do regulatory and legislative mechanisms shape and drive the practice of medicine to the extent found in occupational health. Indeed, an entire federal agency, the Occupational Safety and Health Administration (OSHA), has been established within the Department of Labor to safeguard the rights of this particular class of patients (the worker) and to specifically prevent or minimize the incidence of work-related disorders.

Providers of occupational health services also face unique challenges arising out of their dual loyalty to patients and employers. Can (or should) the occupational physician strive to uphold traditional notions of patient confidentiality, informed consent, and personal autonomy while simultaneously advancing the employer's goals of increased productivity; public goodwill; decreased workers' compensation costs; and promotion of worker, coworker, and customer health and safety? Although dual loyalties to employer and employee create the potential for conflict and impairment of medical judgment, in reality, incidents of conflict occur far less frequently than might be anticipated.[2] Occupational health care providers—whether company employees, independent contractors, or private physicians—can most effectively limit their own liability, promote the health and safety of their patients, and preserve the legal and moral rights of workers through familiarization with occupational health laws and regulations, and by adherence to good medical and risk management principles.

THE OCCUPATIONAL SAFETY AND HEALTH ACT

In 1970 Congress passed the Occupational Safety and Health Act (OSH Act) "to assure so far as possible every working man and woman in the Nation safe and healthful working conditions and to preserve our human resources."[3] This legislation created OSHA, the primary function of which is to (1) encourage employers and employees to reduce workplace hazards, (2) to promulgate and enforce standards that lessen or prevent job-related injuries and illnesses, (3) to establish separate but dependent responsibilities and rights for employers and employees with respect to achieving safe and healthful working conditions, (4) to maintain a reporting and record-keeping system of occupational injuries and illnesses, (5) to establish research and training programs in occupational safety and health, and (6) to encourage development of state occupational safety and health programs.

Coverage

The OSH Act covers all employees and all employers (defined as any person engaged in a business affecting commerce who has employees) with the following exceptions:

1. Self-employed individuals
2. Farms on which only immediate family members of the employer work
3. Working conditions or workplaces regulated by other federal agencies under other federal statutes (e.g., Mine Safety and Health Act of 1969, Atomic

Energy Act of 1954, Department of Transportation regulations, etc.).

4. Government employees.

Federal employees receive protection by an executive order that mandates federal compliance with OSHA regulations. State and municipal government employees may be protected if their states have OSHA approved state plans that explicitly grant them coverage.

Standard setting

OSHA standards encompass four major categories: general industry, construction, maritime, and agriculture. In the absence of a specific OSHA standard for a particular working condition or workplace, employers must adhere to Section 5(b)(1) of the OSH Act—the general duty clause. The general duty clause directs each employer to furnish "to each of his employees employment and a place of employment which are free from recognized hazards that are causing or are likely to cause death or serious physical harm. . . ."[4] Where OSHA has promulgated specific standards, the specific duty clause, Section 5(a)(2) of the OSH Act, mandates that employers "shall comply with occupational safety and health standards . . . promulgated under this chapter."[5]

Section 6(b) of the OSH Act authorizes the Secretary of Labor (hereinafter the Secretary) to promulgate, modify, or revoke any occupational safety and health standard. In adopting standards the Secretary must first publish a Notice of Proposed Rulemaking in the *Federal Register* and allow for a period of public response and written comments (at least 30 days, although usually 60 days or more). At the request of any interested party, OSHA will also schedule a public hearing. After the close of the comment period and public hearing, the Secretary must publish the final standard in the *Federal Register*.

Enforcement

The OSH Act authorizes OSHA (the agency) to conduct workplace inspections. As a result of a 1978 U.S. Supreme Court decision, however, OSHA compliance officers may no longer conduct warrantless inspections without the employer's consent.[6] Because OSHA only employs about 2000 compliance officers to police more than 76.5 million workplaces,[7] the agency has established a priority system for inspections. From highest to lowest, these priorities are (1) imminent danger situations, (2) catastrophes and fatal accidents, (3) employee complaints, (4) programmed high hazard inspections, and (5) follow-up inspections.

Following an inspection, the area OSHA director may issue the employer a citation indicating the standards

TABLE 39-1. OSHA violations and penalties

Violation	Penalty*
Other than serious violation Directly related to job safety and health, but unlikely to cause death or serious harm.	Penalty of up to $7000 per violation is discretionary
Serious violation Substantial probability of death or serious harm. Employer knew or should have known of hazard.	Mandatory penalty of up to $7000 per violation
Willful violation Employer intentionally or knowingly committed a violation or was aware of a hazardous condition and failed to take steps to eliminate it.	Minimum penalty of $5000 per violation up to $70,000 per violation (Willful violations resulting in a worker death may lead to criminal conviction with fines up to $250,000 for an individual, $500,000 for a corporation, and/or imprisonment)
Repeat violation Violation of a previously cited violation.	Fine of up to $70,000 per violation
Failure to correct prior violation Failure to correct a violation before the abatement date.	Penalty of up to $7000 for each day beyond the abatement date

*Note: OSHA may also issue citations and proposed penalties following conviction for falsification of records, reports, or applications; for violations of posting requirements; or for interference with a compliance officer's performance of duties.

that have been violated and the length of time proposed for abatement of those violations. The area director also proposes penalties for these violations. The employer must post a copy of the citation in or near the cited work area for 3 days or until the violation is abated, whichever is longer. Table 39-1 summarizes the types of violations that OSHA may cite and the concommittant penalties that it may propose.

Employers may contest a citation, proposed penalty, or abatement period by filing a Notice of Contest within 15 working days of receipt of the citation and proposed penalty. The area OSHA director will forward the case to the Occupational Safety and Health Review Commission (OSHRC), an agency independent of the Department of Labor. An administrative law judge will rule on the case following a hearing. Any party may seek further review by the entire three-member OSHRC. Commission rulings may, in turn, be appealed by any party to the U.S. Court of Appeals.

KEEPING THE WORKER INFORMED

More than 60,000 chemicals are in commercial use today.[8] Yet, the health effects of many of these substances remain unknown. In fact, it is estimated that more than 32 million workers may be exposed to toxic agents in the workplace.[9] Following passage of the OSH Act, OSHA promulgated a series of regulations to provide workers with more information about the agents in their workplace and to enhance the detection, treatment, and prevention of occupational disorders. Three of these important provisions are

1. The Hazard Communication Standard[10]
2. The Recording and Reporting Occupational Injuries and Illnesses Standard[11]
3. The Access to Employee Exposure and Medical Records Standard[12]

Although employers are ultimately responsible for safeguarding the health and safety of their workers, these regulations have given employees, unions, health care providers, and governmental and nongovernmental agencies a more decisive role in the management of workplace health and safety.

The hazard communication standard

OSHA promulgated the Hazard Communication Standard (HCS) in order to provide workers with the "right to know" the hazards of chemicals in their workplace and to enable workers to take appropriate protective measures. Under the HCS, employers must (1) ensure the labeling of each container of hazardous chemicals in the workplace with appropriate identity and hazard warnings, (2) maintain and ensure employee access to Material Safety Data Sheets (MSDSs), and (3) provide employees with information and training on hazardous chemicals in their work areas. MSDSs list the chemical and physical properties of chemical substances, their health hazards, routes of exposure, emergency and first-aid procedures, and protective measures for their handling and use. The HCS only applies to chemical agents. Furthermore, MSDSs are not subject to methodical review by regulatory agencies. Thus, their quality and adequacy of information vary widely, and they may be of limited use to the clinician in the treatment of exposed workers.

The HCS also contains important provisions for health care provider access to the identities of trade secret chemicals. When a medical emergency exists, the chemical manufacturer, distributor, or employer must immediately divulge the identity of trade secret chemicals to the treating physician or nurse if this information is requested for purposes of emergency or first-aid treatment. As soon as circumstances permit, the chemical manufacturer, importer, or employer may subsequently require the physician or nurse to sign a written statement of need and a confidentiality agreement.

In nonemergency situations, the chemical manufacturer, distributor, or employer must likewise disclose the identity of trade secret chemicals upon the request of a health professional (defined by the regulation as a physician, occupational health nurse, industrial hygienist, toxicologist, or epidemiologist). Prior to disclosure, however, the health professional shall (1) submit a request in writing, (2) demonstrate an occupational health need for the information, (3) explain why disclosure of the chemical identity is essential (in lieu of other information, such as chemical properties, methods of exposure monitoring, methods of diagnosing and treating harmful exposures to the chemical, etc.), (4) enter into a written confidentiality agreement, and (5) describe procedures to maintain confidentiality of the disclosed information. The HCS is a valuable instrument for providing health professionals with information about patient exposures.

Recording and reporting requirements

Soon after passage of the OSH Act, OSHA promulgated standards to fulfill the Act's mandate for the provision of recordkeeping and reporting by employers and for the development of information and a system of analysis of occupational accidents and illnesses. Under 29 C.F.R. 1904, employers with more than 10 workers must maintain a log and summary of all recordable occupational injuries and illnesses. Recordable occupational injuries and illnesses include any occupational (1) fatality (regardless of the span between injury and death, or the duration of illness), (2) lost workday cases (other than fatalities), or (3) nonfatal cases without lost workdays that involve transfer to another job, termination of employment, medical treatment (other than first aid), loss of consciousness, or restriction of work or motion.

Employers must make entries in the log within 6 working days after notification of a recordable injury or illness. Generally, employers use the form OSHA No. 200 ("the OSHA 200 log") to record this information, and must retain the OSHA 200 log for 5 years beyond the year of entry. Employers also often use form OSHA No. 101 or workers' compensation or insurance reports to record supplementary information.

In addition to these record-keeping requirements, the standard further imposes a reporting requirement on working establishments. Employers must report all incidents to the nearest area OSHA office within 8 hours when such accidents result in (1) a fatality or (2) a hospitalization of three or more employees. This requirement applies to all employers, irrespective of the size of their workforce.

Importantly, this standard also grants OSHA, as well as other federal and state agencies, the authority to inspect and copy these logs of recordable injuries and illnesses—although some U.S. circuit courts have upheld the need for a search warrant prior to such inspections. The regulations also ensure employee access to all such logs in their working establishment. These provisions have proved to be a useful source of epidemiologic data to employees, unions, researchers, the Bureau of Labor Statistics, and other agencies.

Access to employee exposure and medical records

Employers have no general duty to collect medical or exposure data on workers. Nonetheless, some specific OSHA standards, such as the lead standard, may require medical surveillance of workers exposed to specific agents. In other cases, employers may voluntarily institute biological and environmental monitoring programs even when not mandated by OSHA. Regardless, to the extent that employers do compile medical and exposure records on workers, they must ensure employee access to these data.

Employers shall make medical records available for examination and copying within 15 days of a request by employees or their designated representatives. The employer is only obligated to provide a worker with access to medical records relevant to that particular employee. Access to medical records of other employees requires their formal written consent. Employers must also provide employees or their designated representatives access to employee exposure records. When an employer lacks exposure records on a particular worker, the employer must provide that worker with exposure data of other employees who have similar job duties and working conditions. Under these circumstances, access to coworkers' exposure records does not require written consent. OSHA has the authority to examine and copy any medical or exposure record without formal written consent.

When medical records do exist on an employee, the employer is required to preserve and maintain these records for the duration of employment plus 30 years. Exposure records must be preserved and maintained for 30 years. Although these record retention requirements are the legal responsibility of the employer, it is recommended that independent contractor physicians who provide occupational health services to companies clarify the ownership and disposition of medical records,

specifying in advance the party to be charged with maintaining the medical records for the required duration.

The three standards discussed in this section—the Hazard Communication Standard, the Recording and Reporting Occupational Injuries and Illnesses Standard, and the Access to Employee Exposure and Medical Records Standard—collectively keep employees informed of the nature and risks of hazardous materials in their workplace, and of any resulting exposure or health effects. By communicating these risks to workers, OSHA seeks to (1) encourage employers to select safer materials and engineering controls, (2) enable workers to use better protective measures and handling procedures, (3) familiarize workers and health care providers with valuable emergency and first-aid information, and (4) minimize health hazards through earlier detection, treatment, and prevention of occupational disorders.

DISCRIMINATION IN THE WORKPLACE

Americans "with disabilities are a discrete and insular minority who have been faced with restrictions and limitations [in the workplace] . . . resulting from stereotypic assumptions not truly indicative of the individual ability . . . to participate in, and contribute to, society."[13] The clinician functions as an important interface between disabled persons and the workplace in a variety of settings: primary care, preplacement physicals, workers' compensation and disability evaluations, etc. It is incumbent on health care providers to make a fair and accurate assessment of workers' functional capabilities in relation to job tasks so as not to reinforce deep-rooted stereotypes about the disabled. Moreover, health care providers can play a key role in safeguarding the rights of workers and in educating employers through familiarization with recent legislative and judicial developments in the areas of employment and discrimination law.

The Americans with Disabilities Act

Congress enacted the Americans with Disabilities Act (ADA) in 1990 in order to eliminate discrimination against the disabled. Although the ADA addresses five separate areas,[14] this chapter focuses exclusively on Title I, employment discrimination.

Title I of the ADA prohibits discrimination against qualified individuals with disabilities in virtually all employment contexts: job application, hiring, discharge, promotion, compensation, job training, and other terms, conditions, and privileges of employment. The act defines disability as:

1. a physical or mental impairment that substantially limits one or more of the major life activities;
2. a record of such an impairment; or

3. being regarded as having such an impairment. "Physical or mental impairment" is further defined as "any physiological disorder, or condition, cosmetic disfigurement, or anatomical loss affecting one or more . . . body systems."[15]

Under the ADA, qualification standards, tests, or selection criteria that employers administer to job applicants must be uniformly applied, job related, and consistent with business necessity. To be consistent with business necessity, a standard must concern an essential function of the job. An employer who denies an amputee a desk job on the basis of strength testing would be in violation of the ADA if, for example, lifting were not an essential job task. Moreover, even when the qualification standards are job related, the employer must first attempt to make reasonable accommodations before excluding disabled workers on the basis of those tests. Examples of reasonable accommodations include modified work schedules, job restructuring, equipment modification, design of wheelchair-accessible workstations, provision of readers or interpreters, etc.

The ADA provides three major defenses to employers charged with discrimination:

1. Selection criteria are job-related and consistent with business necessity, and a disabled individual cannot perform essential job tasks even with reasonable accommodation.
2. Reasonable accommodation would impose an undue hardship on the employer.
3. A disabled individual poses a direct threat to him- or herself or to the health and safety of others in the workplace.

The ADA has several important implications for health professionals—whether they are company salaried or private physicians—who are often called on to perform preplacement physicals of job applicants or return-to-work assessments of injured workers. First, physicians and employers need to recognize that the ADA bars all preemployment (pre-offer) physicals. Employers may continue to administer pre-offer, nonmedical tests (e.g., language proficiency or strength and agility testing) that are job related, but they may only require a medical examination after extending an offer of employment. This offer may be conditioned on the results of the *post-offer, preplacement* physical examination provided that all applicants are subjected to such an examination regardless of disability.

Second, physicians are prohibited from disclosing specific diagnoses to employers. They must treat information from medical examinations as confidential, and must maintain these records in separate medical files apart from personnel records. Once physicians have determined if workers meet the employer's health and safety requirements, they may only inform the employer

about necessary job restrictions and limitations. For example, the ADA would bar disclosure of a diagnosis of epilepsy to the employer, but would permit a report that recommends restricting the employee or job applicant from working at heights or from driving certain types of vehicles.* To make such determinations of functional capabilities and limitations, the physician must insist that the employer provide a written job description that accurately details specific and essential job tasks. Physicians may offer input on ways to achieve reasonable accommodation. However, the employer has the responsibility to make all employment decisions and to determine the feasibility of reasonable accommodation. The physician's obligation is primarily to determine if employees have the ability to perform the essential functions of the job with or without reasonable accommodations, and to ensure that such individuals will not pose a health or safety threat to themselves or to others.

Discrimination denies the disabled the many advantages of employment: prestige, power, self-esteem, economic well-being, social outlets, and access to health insurance and other job benefits. The ADA will have far-reaching consequences in protecting the rights of the disabled and more fully integrating them into the workplace. Health professionals can play a critical role in fostering patient autonomy and educating employers while simultaneously promoting a safe and healthful workplace.

Gender discrimination, pregnancy, and fetal protection policies

As with the disabled, pregnant workers have often represented a disenfranchised group within the workplace. Although the ADA is broad sweeping, it does not shield these women from employment discrimination because "pregnancy" is not considered a physiological disorder under the act's definition of disability. Nonetheless, pregnant workers receive ample protection under both legislative and judicial avenues.[16] The Civil Rights Act of 1964 (Title VII) prohibits discrimination on the basis of sex, and as amended through the Pregnancy Discrimination Act of 1978, further prohibits discrimination against "women affected by pregnancy, childbirth, or related medical conditions . . . for all employment related purposes."[17]

Despite the intent of these laws, a number of industries instituted fetal protection policies (FPPs) throughout the 1980s to exclude fertile or pregnant women from the workplace in order to avert toxic

---

*Workers will often voluntarily disclose their diagnoses to supervisors or first-aid responders on their shift in order to familiarize them with the signs and symptoms of their disease in the event of a medical emergency.

exposures to the fetus. In some instances, companies went so far as to exclude all females—including post-menopausal women—from jobs or job tracks involving potential exposure to toxic substances unless these workers could provide documentation of surgical sterilization. These FPPs were unsound for several reasons: (1) They disregarded reproductive risks to male workers, (2) they assumed that all females in the workplace could or would become pregnant, (3) they essentially required female workers to proclaim their reproductive status to supervisors and coworkers (i.e., females remaining in the workplace were implicitly sterile), (4) they discouraged some women from applying for higher paying jobs, (5) they encouraged other women to undergo unnecessary surgical sterilization solely to retain their jobs, and (6) they overlooked the adverse health effects to the unemployed mother and child from foregone income and health benefits.

In 1991 the U.S. Supreme Court declared these FPPs to be unconstitutional in a case called *International Union, UAW v. Johnson Controls, Inc.*[18] The court held these policies to be discriminatory because they did not apply equally to the reproductive capacity of male employees. Furthermore, the court held that "decisions about the welfare of future children must be left to the parents . . . rather than to the employers who hire those parents."[19]

There are principally only two instances in which employers may discriminate on the basis of gender or pregnancy: (1) Employers may deny employment when sex is a bonafide occupational qualification (BFOQ) reasonably necessary to the normal operation of that particular business or enterprise. Analogously to the ADA, the qualification standards must relate to the essence of the employer's business. For example, a movie producer would be justified in claiming that male gender is a BFOQ when hiring actors for male roles. (2) Under the safety exception, employers may discriminate on the basis of sex in those instances in which sex or pregnancy interferes with the employee's ability to perform the job. For example, airlines are permitted to lay off pregnant flight attendants at various stages of pregnancy to ensure the safety of passengers. In all other instances, women should be treated equally as men in the employment setting as long as they possess the necessary job-related skills and aptitudes.

In light of this legislative and judicial history, the following practices that screen out individual females or the entire class of females might be construed as discriminatory:

1. Implementing FPPs or other policies that exlcude females from the workplace based on gender or reproductive status
2. Applying coercion by providing female—but not

male—workers or job applicants with information on reproductive risks, or by requiring only female workers to sign waivers absolving the employer of liability in the event of an adverse reproductive outcome
3. Administering special tests or medical examinations exclusively to women
4. Using physiological parameters, such as muscle strength, as selection criteria when not a requirement for the job (For this reason, as with the ADA, job descriptions that accurately reflect job tasks are vital.)
5. Using gender as a proxy for physiological parameters even when specific physiological traits (e.g., anthropometrics, muscle strength) are a requirement for the job and a high correlation exists between gender and ability to perform the job. Employers must give each individual the opportunity to demonstrate that she meets the job parameters.

Workers' compensation

Physicians who evaluate and treat workers with job-related injuries or illnesses must acquire a broad understanding of the workers' compensation (WC) system and an appreciation of their role in the legal disposition of WC claims.

WC systems currently exist in all 50 states and in three federal jurisdictions.[20] WC is a no-fault system that evolved in the earlier part of this century to promote expeditious resolution of work-related claims. Injured workers relinquished their rights to bring an action in torts in exchange for a rapid, fixed, and automatic payment. The quid pro quo for the employer was a limited and predictable award. WC pays for medical and rehabilitation expenses and for up to two-thirds of wage replacement.

Unlike tort actions, WC claims do not require a showing of employer negligence. Therefore, even injuries or illnesses due to the employee's own negligence are compensable. Regardless of etiology, the worker, nonetheless, carries the burden of proving by a preponderance of the evidence that a causal relationship exists between an occupational exposure and the resulting injury or illness; i.e., the injury or illness must "arise out of or in the course of employment." Employees are also generally entitled to compensation for work-related aggravation of preexisting disorders. Second, to qualify for WC payments, the worker must prove damages, typically by demonstrating a disability or loss in earning capacity. Even when the occupational exposure results in an injury or illness that produces no disability, the employee may still be eligible for an award if the WC laws in that jurisdiction explicitly provide for such coverage, such as payment for scarring, disfigurement, or damage or loss of function of specific organs or body systems.

Physicians who evaluate and treat injured workers must strive to be objective when documenting physical findings and impairments. Although physicians are not discouraged from making assertions about causality, they must be prepared to support their conclusions in a deposition or courtroom should the claim lead to litigation. It is also incumbent on physicians to familiarize themselves with alternative work and light-duty programs in order to minimize the length of disability.

Confidentiality and WC claims. Patients will often present treating physicians with authorization forms requesting release of medical records to the patient's employer, the employer's attorney, or the employer's insurance company in support of a WC claim. By signing these release forms, patients do *not* waive all rights of confidentiality. It is critical that physicians only disclose information related to the disorder that forms the basis of the WC claim. Several physicians have been sued for releasing confidential information about HIV status that was unrelated to the WC claim, such as ear and sinus problems[21] or head injury with back pain.[22] Patients sued these doctors under various theories: negligence, breach of confidentiality, breach of contract, and invasion of privacy.

TORT LIABILITY

Many WC statutes contain "exclusive remedy" provisions that hold that WC shall provide the exclusive remedy for injuries and illnesses arising out of or in the course of employment. The goals of these provisions are to foreclose remedies in torts and to limit the employer's liability to WC. During the last two decades, however, workers have been attempting to circumvent the exclusive remedy provisions of WC laws in order to pursue a cause of action in torts. As in WC cases, plaintiffs in tort suits may recover for medical expenses and lost earnings—although tort actions are more likely to take into account future promotions and job advancements, thereby yielding a higher award for wage replacement. Moreover, tort suits offer the additional advantage of recovery for certain types of damages unavailable under WC: pain and suffering, punitive damages, loss of consortium, etc.

Despite the greater financial incentive to bring a tort suit, the courts have been reluctant to carve out exceptions to the WC exclusive remedy provisions. The most common doctrines under which employees file tort suits are[23]:

1. Third-party and product liability suits
2. Intentional harm committed by an employer
3. Injury by a co-employee (injuries by co-employee

health care providers are discussed in the following section on medical malpractice)
4. Dual capacity doctrine—the employer assumes a second role or capacity sufficiently distinct from its role as employer such that workers injured by the employer while acting in this second capacity may recover outside of the WC system.

Theoretically, both WC and tort liability should provide employers with the incentive to promote a safe and healthful workplace. However, given the employer's ability to insure and to pass on some of these costs to consumers, the extent to which these goals are accomplished remains unclear.

LEGAL LIABILITY OF THE OCCUPATIONAL HEALTH CARE PROVIDER: MEDICAL MALPRACTICE

What is the legal liability of a physician or nurse who commits medical malpractice while under contract to provide occupational health services to a company's employees? Management hires physicians and nurses—whether they are company salaried or independent contractors—for the benefit of the company, i.e., to assure the fitness for duty of workers.

Historically, physicians and nurses salaried by a company were considered co-employees of other workers. Consequently, their negligent acts and the resulting injuries were regarded as arising out of and in the course of employment. Injured workers were therefore limited by the exclusive remedy provisions of WC laws to recovery under the WC system. However, if the workers could establish that the health care providers were not under the control of the company, but rather were functioning as independent contractors, they could avail themselves of a remedy in torts.

The distinctions between "co-employee" and "independent contractor" have been problematic for the courts. Physicians and nurses often have greater latitude than other employees in their exercise of judgment. At what point do their actions transcend the control of their employers and exceed the scope of employment? Some companies authorize and encourage occupational health care providers to furnish primary care services to employees and even to their families. At what point does the occupational health professional establish a doctor-patient relationship, no longer acting solely for the benefit of the employer, but also for the benefit of the employee?

The courts have developed two tests to determine if an occupational health care provider is the co-employee of an injured worker (in which case the negligent act is covered by the employer's WC policy) or if the occupational health care professional is an independent contractor (and therefore subject to tort liability). Under the *control test,* health care providers are more likely to be presumed company employees when management exerts greater control over their function, operation, and judgment. For example, physicians and nurses act under the control of the company when they must follow predetermined guidelines and protocols in conducting physical examinations (e.g., which forms to use, which lab tests to conduct).

Under the *indicia test,* the court analyzes various indices of control that normally signify employee status. For example, physicians and nurses are more likely to be categorized as company employees rather than independent contractors if they receive a salary, health insurance, and other company benefits; fall under the company's WC and pension programs; work out of company offices; have regularly scheduled work hours; and report to the company's chain of command.[24]

Despite these two tests, the immunity of occupational health care providers continues to erode. Although the control and indicia tests provide useful guidelines concerning the potential liability of the occupational health care provider, their application results in some uncertainty because many physicians and nurses only partially meet these criteria. For example, some physicians may have a part-time private practice and request workers to follow up after duty hours in their private offices. Other physicians may work out of their own offices, but see exclusively company employees. Furthermore, courts appreciate that workers often rely on the results of employment physicals to their detriment; and that physicians have a high degree of skill and training and are in a better position to warn patients of harm and to insure against losses. Thus, although courts were traditionally reluctant—even in the independent contractor setting—to hold that a doctor-patient relationship existed between a prospective or actual employee and the physician conducting the examination at the employer's request and for the employer's benefit, more courts are willing to recognize that the "examination creates a relationship between the examining physician and the examinee, at least to the extent of the tests conducted."[25]

Therefore, the wisest approach for occupational health care providers, whether company employees or independent contractors, is to conduct examinations and treatment with due care and to ensure patient disclosure of results from any tests or exams performed. Physicians must be cautious in following up with patients because attempts to offer advice or to treat may establish a doctor-patient relationship and place their actions beyond the scope of employment. Physicians who want to ensure that employees receive adequate follow-up without risking tort liability should consider sending certified letters to patients advising them of the results

---

BOX 39-1
RISK MANAGEMENT PRINCIPLES FOR OCCUPATIONAL HEALTH CARE PROVIDERS

1. Request job descriptions that reflect essential job functions.
2. For company-employed physicians, provide medical services *only:*
   - to employees (to employees' dependents only if company authorizes in contract and provides malpractice coverage)
   - during normal business or duty hours
   - on company premises (if available)
   - to extent delineated in employment contract
3. Adhere to company policies.
4. Evaluate necessity and purpose of components of physical exams and medical surveillance programs.
5. Do not order unnecessary tests.
6. Ensure that all tests are interpreted by qualified individuals.
7. Inform patients of results of all tests.
8. Ensure adequate/reasonable follow-up (appropriate to circumstances).
9. Good record-keeping—document, document, document!

---

and of the need for follow-up with their own private family doctors or other specialists as appropriate. See Box 39-1 for more detailed risk management principles. Physicians would be prudent to delineate these responsibilities in their contracts with employers. Furthermore, occupational health care providers employed by companies should not rely solely on employers' WC policies, but should also be covered by malpractice insurance.

CONCLUSION

Occupational health care providers are in a unique position to assure worker health and safety. Because they interact with injured workers at every phase of employment—preplacement, preinjury, and postinjury—they have a profound impact on the disposition of job applicants and employees in the workplace. Occupational health professionals place a strong emphasis on prevention. Familiarization with judicial, legislative, and regulatory mandates will enable them to preserve the health and uphold the rights of workers, to educate employers, and to minimize their own liability.

END NOTES

1. From the ACGME Special Requirements for Residency Education in Occupational Medicine, effective Jan. 1, 1993.
2. J. A. Gold, *The Physician and the Corporation,* 3 Bioethics Bull. 1 (Fall 1989).
3. 29 U.S.C. § 651(b) (1988).
4. 29 U.S.C. § 654(a)(1) (1988).

5. 29 U.S.C. § 654 (a)(2).
6. *Marshall v. Barlow's, Inc.,* 436 U.S. 307 (1978).
7. John Miles, Jr., Regional Administrator, OSHA Regional Office (Region I), Boston, Private Communication, Mar. 14, 1994.
8. Office of Technology Assessment, *Reproductive Hazards in the Workplace* 37 (Lippincott Co., Philadelphia 1988).
9. OSHA 3110, *Access to Medical and Exposure Records* 1 (1989).
10. 29 C.F.R. 1910.1200.
11. 29 C.F.R. 1904.
12. 29 C.F.R. 1910.20.
13. 42 U.S.C. § 12101 (a)(7) (Supp. IV 1992).
14. *Americans with Disabilities Act of 1990:* Title I, Employment; Title II, Public Service/Public Transportation; Title III, Public Accommodation & Services Operated by Private Entities; Title IV, Telecommunications; Title V, Miscellaneous Provisions.
15. Note that current drug abusers receive no protection under the ADA because illegal drug use is not considered a disability under the act. However, alcoholics and fully rehabilitated drug abusers may be protected under the ADA (unless they fail to meet productivity and other performance standards that cannot be corrected by reasonable accommodation).
16. 42 U.S.C. § 2000e-2(a) (1988).
17. 42 U.S.C. § 2000e(k) (1988).
18. *International Union, UAW v. Johnson Controls, Inc.,* 111 S.Ct. 1196 (1991).
19. *Id.* at 1207.
20. L. I. Boden, *Workers' Compensation,* in *Occupational Health: Recognizing and Preventing Work-Related Disease* 202 (B. S. Levy, D. H. Wegeman, eds., Little, Brown & Company, Boston 1995).
21. *Doe v. Roe,* 190 A.D.2d 463 (1993).
22. *Urbaniak v. Newton,* 277 Cal. Rptr. 354 (Cal. App. 1 Dist. 1991).
23. Adapted from S. L. Birnbaum and B. Wrubel, *Workers' Compensation and the Employer's Immunity Shield: Recent Exceptions to Exclusivity,* 50 J. of Products Liability 119 (1982).
24. *See, e.g., Garcia v. Iserson,* 33 N.Y.2d 421, 309 N.E.2d 420 (1970), holding that worker's exclusive remedy fell under WC law. The plaintiff could not maintain a malpractice action against a company physician because the injuries arose out of and in the course of employment since the company employed the physician at a weekly salary and took the usual payroll deductions, required the physician to work on company premises during certain scheduled hours, and included the physician in the company's medical plan and WC policy. *See also Golini v. Nachtifall,* 38 N.Y.2d 745, 343 N.E.2d 762 (1975), holding that WC provided the exclusive remedy to the plaintiff injured by a physician who received company salary and benefits and worked in company facilities.
25. *Green v. Walker,* 910 f.2d 291 (5th Cir. 1990), holding that physician who was under contract to perform annual employment physicals was liable for malpractice in failing to diagnose and report cancer to examinee.

GENERAL REFERENCES

Ashford, N.A., and Caldart, C.C., *Technology, Law, and the Working Environment* (Van Nostrand Reinhold, New York, 1991).

Billauer, B.P., *The Legal Liability of the Occupational Health Professional,* 27 J. of Occupational Med. 185-188 (1985).

J. Ladou, ed., *Occupational Medicine,* (Appleton & Lange, Norwalk, Conn., 1990).

CHAPTER 40

Sports medicine

RICHARD S. GOODMAN, M.D., J.D., F.A.A.O.S., F.C.L.M.

SPORTS MEDICINE IN LEGAL TERMS
SPORTS MEDICINE IN MEDICAL TERMS
SPORTS MEDICINE IN SPORTS TERMS

Despite the fact that "sports medicine" has emerged as an independent and widely acknowledged discipline, it still has yet to be categorically defined by the medical and legal professions. Although it is convenient that this detail has not hampered the field's economic growth, it will become critical to the future credibility of athletics health care providers. An update on the legal aspects of sports medicine is the study of the search by the legal profession to define "sports medicine" and the role and responsibilities of the practitioners so that there is a clear delineation of the rights, responsibilities, and liabilities of the participants and other parties involved.

SPORTS MEDICINE IN LEGAL TERMS

The mere conception of the term *legal aspects of sports medicine* would have been foreign to Judge Cordozo, who in the "Amusement Ride" case,"[1] also known as the "Flopper" case, stated: "One who takes part in such a sport accepts the dangers that so far that they are obvious and necessary just as a fencer accepts the risks of a thrust by his antagonist or a spectator at a ball game the chance of contact with the ball." This was also restated in the case where the court ruled: "As an integral part of athletic competitions persons are generally held by their actual and implied consent to the risks of 'injury-causing events which are known, apparent or reasonably foreseeable consequences.'"[2] This assumption of risk by the participant was reiterated in the case of *Benitez v. New York City Board of Education.*[3]

Until recently the only distinction or break in the ultimate and total assumption of risk by the participant in an athletic activity was the potential liability of the team physician in an action for medical malpractice. The liability of the team physician and only the physician was carefully reviewed in a 1981 article in the *Houston Law Review.*[4]

An article by LaCava[5] defined the role for the team physician, and also incidentally gave a clue as to the definition of sports medicine. *Sports medicine* was defined as:

1. Sport biotypology, aiming to establish the athlete's biotype in a sport discipline. 2. Sports physiopathology, i.e., the study of human adaption to physical effort during athletic training. 3. Sport-medical evaluations, i.e., to establish the athlete's conditioning to the effort required. 4. Sports traumatology, aiming to individuate the typical sports injury (athlopathies), treat and possibly prevent them though the study of the biomechanics of each sport discipline. 5. Hygiene and sport, i.e., to fix the hygienic behavior of the athlete and the ambience in which a sport is preformed. 6. Therapeutic sport, i.e., use of a sport for the prevention and treatment of diseases.

SPORTS MEDICINE IN MEDICAL TERMS

The concept of the legal aspects of sports medicine being almost exclusively limited to the duties of the team physician to the members of the "team," with the term *physician* being defined as a licensed medical school graduate, is now undergoing a rapid transition. At present, team trainers, chiropractors, and orthopedists with or without any knowledge of athletics injuries may all legally claim to be practicing "sports medicine"—a "benefit" of the absence of sanctioned guidelines. Many of the aforementioned professionals may be providing excellent care within the limits of their capacities, but the fact still remains that society must take a positive action to protect the public from charlatans by delineating the qualifications required to practice "sports medicine," through the government or the legal community.

SPORTS MEDICINE IN SPORTS TERMS

The concept that sports medicine can include anyone who provides some type of health care to anyone who participates in a physically demanding leisure time activity or physically demanding competitive activity becomes apparent when one reviews *The Year Book of Sports Medicine* published by Mosby.[6] A review of the membership of the publications editorial board reveals that it includes a professor of applied physiology, a director of physical education, a professor of medicine, a head athletic trainer, a professor of medicine, and a professor of orthopedic surgery. Not only are these various professions represented on the editorial board of the *Year Book of Sports Medicine,* but the journals reviewed cover a range of medical specialties, medical subspecialities, related health care fields, and para medical fields including psychiatry, family medicine, cardiology, nutrition, pediatrics, obstetrics and gynecology, physical medicine, physiology, preventive medicine, roentgenology, sports medicine, respiratory diseases, anesthesia, emergency medicine, arthroscopy, chiropractic sports medicine, clinical biomechanics, orthopedics, applied physiology and occupational physiology, athletic training, biomechanical engineering, trauma, and geriatrics.

Therefore, one aspect of this update on the legal aspects of sports medicine is to expand the definition of a practitioner of sports health from that which is limited to a team physician to any of the health care providers involved in the care of participants in a sport and not limited to team physicians or those orthopedists who would limit the definition to "a surgeon who does knee arthroscopy."

Definition of sports

A definition of who practices sports medicine or provides health care to an athlete is of no help to the legal mind without a definition of what is a sport, so we need first to satisfactorily address what properties we will consider to constitute a sport. To avoid the potential disagreements that would result in an effort to formulate our own definition, we recommend the following as a comprehensive standard: an activity involving physical exertion and skill that is governed by a set of rules or customs and is often undertaken competitively.[7] On examination, this denotation may be applied to athletic pursuits as diverse as rock climbing and in-line skating, without being so vague as to logically include everyday heavy lifting or walking. The matter may seem trifling, but it actually carries some import in the deliberation of the issues at hand. Without defining the relevant scope of activities, and subsequent related demands of care, we cannot confine the region of knowledge necessary to adequately address those demands. Specification of the behaviors that are germane to our interests allows us to isolate those skills.

One dictionary defines a sport as "an activity involving physical exertion and skill that is governed by a set of rules or customs and is often undertaken competitively." The United Nations Educational Scientific and Cultural Organization defines a sport as "all forms of physical activity except required programs of physical educa-

tion"[8] and includes activities of personal challenge, such as downhill skiing, sailing, white water paddling, rock climbing, physical contests, and exercise programs in the whole spectrum of such facilities. This definition, therefore, not only includes the team physician, per se, but also the physician who signs a note certifying physical fitness to participate, the trainer, the supervisor, the physical therapist, the coach, the exercise physiologist and the manufacturer, supplier, installer, and maintainer of related equipment.

A discussion of the liability of the equipment industry, however, raises the issue of instructions and warnings. Reviews have revealed that although no squash or racquetball players wearing approved eye guards sustained significant eye injuries[9] it is similarly been found that instructions to wear equipment and use it properly are seldom heeded by the athlete. The legal implications of the use and abuse of labels raise the quote: "As might be expected, warning labels are worthless. In reality, the only preventive measure they provide is to prevent the helmet manufacturer from the assault of innovative plaintiff attorneys."[10] This finding of warning labels is similar to that note regarding the use of bicycle helmets.

Leaving aside at this point the related legal aspects of sports equipment, we return to the discussion of sports medicine and look for the legal definitions. The American Osteopathic Academy of Sports Medicine defines it as follows: "Sports medicine is that branch of the healing profession that utilizes a holistic, comprehensive team approach to the prevention, diagnosis and adequate management (including medical, surgical and rehabilitative techniques) of sports and exercise related injuries, disorders, dysfunctions and exercise related disease."[11]

Another definition is that of David Herbert, in his book *Legal Aspects of Sports Medicine* where he defines it as

the provision, primarily, of medical or allied health care to athletes, exercise, recreations enthusiasts and others and the delivery of preventative primary and rehabilitative care related to the prevention, treatment and rehabilitation of injuries and conditions related to sports and exercise or recreational activity, as well as the rendition of service and advice for fitness and training purposes to individuals who desire to engage in the aforementioned activities and secondarily, the provision of non-medically related services of products of those who are interested in sports, exercise, or recreation, even though in its latter sense the use of the term "medicine" may be inherently inappropriate.[12]

Having thus offered definitions of sports and sports medicine, the legal aspects of sports medicine should therefore be defined as the legal aspects of the "sports medicine staff." This definition of sports medicine may be more practical as it is not practiced exclusively by members of the medical profession, but in reality it includes, as Mr. Herbert said, "The physician, the physician assistant, nurse, therapist, trainer, assistant trainer, student trainers, sport psychologist, chiropractors, podiatrists, dentists, nutritionists, dieticians, fitness training personal, weight training personal, strength training personal and behavioral type motivator."[13] Some or all of these specialties have legal definitions in some or all states. Some have no legal or statutory definitions, and some like medicine are statutorily defined in each and every state in the union, although differently in each state.

Nonlicensed providers of sports medicine have been narrowly averting disaster for years. Jacqueline White's article "Risky Drug Distribution in Training Rooms" described a 1992 study commissioned by the National Collegiate Athletic Association that investigated the drug dispensing practices at 30 U.S. colleges.[14] The report concluded that not only were coaches, trainers and other unqualified athletic department staff furnishing athletes with prescription medication, the drugs were frequently improperly labeled and stored. This case alone should provide fertile ground for more stringent sports medicine standards. As another example, however, former Loyola Marymount University coach Paul Westhead avoided charges in the death of collegiate basketball star Hank Gathers after Gathers, who had idiopathic cardiomyopathy, collapsed on the court.[15]

Concurrent with sports medicine's growth, we've witnessed a proliferation of definitions offering denotative "absolution." A short survey leads us through "The Duty and Standard of Care for Team Physicians,"[16] which engages landmark decisions in topically related cases (e.g., negligence, duty), and eloquently unifies them as a guide for physicians engaged in athletic care. It is a highly pragmatic and useful document, but it fails to address the limits to be placed on nonphysicians who may pose as practitioners of sports medicine. Handicapped by similar weaknesses, the following definition was provided in *Sports Medicine and Physical Fitness:*

Sports medicine: 1. Sport biotypology: aiming to establish the athlete's biotype in a sport discipline. 2. Sports physiopathology: i.e., the study of human adaptation to physical effort during athletic training. 3. Sports-medical evaluations: i.e., to establish the athlete's conditioning to the effort required. 4. Sports traumatology: aiming to individuate the typical sports injury (athlopathies), treat and possibly prevent them through the study of biomechanics of each sport discipline. 5. Hygiene and sport: i.e., to fix the hygienic behavior of the athlete and the ambience in which sport is performed. 6. Therapeutic sport: i.e., use of a sport for the prevention and treatment of diseases.[17]

The American Osteopathic Academy of Sports Medicine has defined it as follows:

Sports medicine is that branch of the healing arts profession that utilizes an holistic, comprehensive team approach to the prevention, diagnosis, and adequate management (including medical, surgical, and rehabilitative techniques) of sports and exercise related injuries, disorders, dysfunctions and exercise related disease processes.[18]

Accredited programs offering residents instruction in athletic medicine are available at a growing number of schools. The University of California at Davis introduces medical students to on-field education,[19] and at Michigan State University, residents participate at training room sessions, practices, and games.[20] In addition, professional organizations such as the American Osteopathic Academy of Sports Medicine, the American Academy of Podiatric Sports Medicine, and the American Academy of Sports Physicians offer certification to health care providers in order to recognize and endorse medical specialists' proficiency in athletics-related disciplines.

Considering the field's increasing prominence, and the public's growing need, the American Medical Association and/or the American Board of Medical Specialties should move to define the field and specify the requirements for its practice. It seems evident and unfortunate that, without guidance from American physicians' leading representatives, sports medicine will find itself at odds with regulatory bodies in the future.

Recognizing, therefore, that the legal aspect of sports medicine in an update raises many more issues than can be answered by reference to court decisions, rules, or regulations, a total overview of the questions raised is addressed next. What risk does the participant in a sport assume? What liability rests on the individual who provided a clearance to participate in a sport, whether it was a physician, a cardiologist, a sports physiologist, a physical therapist, a coach, or a team physician?[21] Does a license to practice that profession decrease or increase the liability, and does the license have to be from the state where the participant lives, or from the state where the event occurred? How much reliability can the participant in any sport, from jogging to professional football, wrestling, and skiing, expect from the manufacturers, fitters, suppliers, resalers, and salespeople of sports-related equipment, including everything from eye protectors, football helmets, motorcycle helmets, ski releases, ski bindings, etc.? How much protection does the manufacturer of such equipment receive from attaching warning labels and instructions on proper use to the equipment? Potential legal liabilities arise out of the use of protective equipment, mats, playground architecture, playground equipment architecture, and positioning of various equipment at sports arenas including photography, video, cameras, benches, and the playing surface itself. Are the other practitioners of sports medicine, i.e., trainers, nutritionists, coaches, held to their legal liability as per statute or the liability of a physician in a similar situation?

In summary, sports medicine implies medical care to athletes. In reality it is health care to active people and is practiced by practitioners who may or may not be licensed in any state and if licensed may or may not be licensed in the state where they are active due to the travel arrangements of the athlete or the team. In addition, because of the plethora of professions and professional licenses covering these activities and the various state licensing procedures and codes regulating the interstate mobility of these practitioners, the need for judicial and legislative action as well as professional standards is apparent.

END NOTES

1. *Murphy v. Steeplechase Amusement Co.,* 250 N.Y. 479, 482 (1929).
2. *Turcotte v. Fell,* 68 N.Y.2d 432, 439 (1984).
3. *Benitez v. New York City Board of Education,* 73 N.Y.2d, 650, 541 N.E.2d 29, 543 N.Y.S.2d 29 (1989).
4. J.H. King, Jr., *The Duty and Standard of Care for Team Physicians,* 18 Houst. L. Rev. 657-703 (1981).
5. La Cana, *What Is Sports Medicine: Definition and Tasks,* 17 J. Sports Med. and Physical Fitness (1977).
6. *The Year Book of Sports Medicine* (Mosby, St. Louis, Mo. 1993).
7. Anne H. Soukhanov et al., eds., *The American Heritage Dictionary of the English Language* 1089 (3rd ed., Houghton Mifflin Co., New York 1992).
8. Ray J. Shepard, *Is Population Involvement in Exercise Programs Increasing, in The Yearbook of Sports Medicine, Supra* note 6, at XV.
9. National Specialty Committee on Standard for Athletic Equipment (NOCSAE), Warning Label (Courtesy of R.E. Smith, Smoll Floriday, Everett JJ > 7 App. Congn. Psychol 43-52 (1993).
10. J.P. DiFiori, *Sports Related Traumatic Hyphema,* 46 Am. Fam. Phys. 807-813 (1992).
11. D. L. Herbert, *Legal Aspects of Sports Medicine,* 7 (Professional Reports Corporation, Canton, Ohio 1990). Cited from The American Osteopathic Academy of Sports Medicine.
12. D.L. Herbert, *Legal Aspects of Sports Medicine* 9 (Professional Reports Corporation, Canton, Ohio 1990).
13. *Id.*
14. Jacqueline White, *Risky Drug Distribution in Training Rooms,* 20 Phys. and Sports Med. 33-34 (Sep. 1992).
15. Dave Berns, *Gathers' Case Leaves Questions,* 20 Phys. and Sports Med. 34-37 (Sep. 1992).
16. King, *supra* note 4.
17. La Cava, *supra* note 5.
18. Herbert, *supra* note 12.
19. J. Tanji, *Hands-on Sports Medicine for Residents,* 17 Physical Sports Med. 83-90 (1989).
20. D. Hough, *Primary Care Sports Medicine in the University Setting,* 12 Physical Sports Med. 69-74 (1989).
21. R.S. Goodman, *The Legal Liabilities of Sports Medicine,* 4 Orthopedic and Sports Med. News 15-19 (McMahon Group, 148 W. 24th Street, New York 1984).

CHAPTER 41 # Forensic use of medical information

CYRIL H. WECHT, M.D., J.D., F.C.L.M.*

BRIEF HISTORY OF FORENSIC MEDICINE
THE ADVERSARIAL PROCESS
EXPERT WITNESSES
THE CORONER'S CASE
FORENSIC PSYCHIATRY AND PSYCHOLOGISTS

Forensic medicine is the area of medicine that concerns itself with the testimony and information to be presented in judicial or quasijudicial settings. For example, medical information and testimony to be presented before hearings and trials as well as formal legal investigations would be considered forensic.

Forensic pathology concentrates on autopsies to be reported in legal settings. There are other areas of forensic medicine, such as forensic toxicology, forensic surgery, forensic pediatrics, and other forensic areas of the health sciences that involve presenting information in a legal forum.

BRIEF HISTORY OF FORENSIC MEDICINE

Medicine as a curiosity, superstition, science, and ultimately a form of self-preservation appears to have originated long before human beings organized into communities capable of governing conduct by a legal system consisting of commonly accepted norms. Unfortunately, our historical knowledge of the interaction between law and medicine is limited by the slow development of an effective recording system. Thus the origin of forensic medicine can be traced back only 5000 or 6000 years. At that time, Imhotep, the Grand Vizier, Chief Justice, Chief Magician, and Chief Physician to King Zozer, was regarded as God of the Egyptians. He was also the first man known to apply both medicine and law to his surroundings.[1]

In ancient Egypt, legal restrictions concerning the practice of medicine were codified and recorded on papyri. Because medicine was shrouded with mysticism, its practice was regarded as a privilege of class.[2] Despite the strong influence of superstition, definite surgical procedures and substantial information regarding the interaction of drugs indicate an awareness that human beings, as opposed to God or demons, could regulate various bodily responses.

Apparently, the Code of Hammurabi (2200 B.C.) was the first formal code of medical law, setting forth the organization, control, duties, and liabilities of the medical profession.[3] Malpractice sanctions included monetary compensation for the victim, as well as the forcible removal of a surgeon's hand.[4] Medicolegal principles can also be found in early Jewish laws, which distinguished mortal from nonmortal wounds and investigated questions of virginity.

Later, in the midst of substantial jurisprudential evolution, Hippocrates and his followers studied the average duration of pregnancy, the viability of children born before full-term, malingering, the possibility of superfetation, and the relative fatality of wounds in different parts of the body. Particularly noteworthy is the continuation of an interest in poisons. The Hippocratic oath includes a promise not to use or advise the use of poisons.[5]

As in Egypt, India restricted the practice of medicine to members of select castes. Medical education was also regulated. Physicians formally concluded that the duration of pregnancy should be between 9 and 12 lunar months. And, again, the study of poisons and their antidotes was given high priority.[6]

Although little medicolegal development occurred during the Roman era, investigations were conducted regarding the cause of suspicious deaths. This process

*The author gratefully acknowledges work from previous contributors: John Dale Dunn, M.D., J.D., F.C.L.M., and Thomas J. Hardy, M.D.

was sufficiently sophisticated to lead one physician to report that only 1 of the 23 wounds sustained by Julius Caesar was fatal.[7] In addition, between 529 and 564 A.D., the Justinian code was enacted, regulating the practice of medicine, surgery, and midwifery. Malpractice standards, medical expert responsibilities, and the number of physicians limited to each town were clearly established. Interestingly enough, although it was recognized that a fair determination of the truth often necessitated the submission of expert medical testimony, such testimony was restricted to the impartial specialized knowledge of the expert.[8] Obviously, this evidence was intended to aid the fact-finder, not to replace the fact-finder's independent conclusion.

Throughout the Middle Ages, issues of impotence, sterility, pregnancy, abortion, sexual deviation, poisoning, and divorce provided the backdrop for much medicolegal development. Investigatory procedures advanced as more homicide and personal injury judgments were rendered. In 925, the English established the Office of Coroner. This office much later assumed the responsibility of the investigation of suspicious deaths.

China's contribution to forensic medicine did not surface until the first half of the thirteenth century. Apparently, medicolegal knowledge had quietly passed from one generation to another, for the *Hsi Yuan Lu* ("the washing away of wrongs") was so comprehensive that its influence can be noted until fairly recently. It was a treatise detailing procedures for cause-of-death determinations and emphasized the importance of performing each step in the investigation with precision. In addition, the book noted the difficulties posed by decomposition, counterfeit wounds, and antemortem and postmortem wounds, and by distinguishing bodies of drowned persons from those thrown into the water after death. Examination of bodies in all cases was mandatory, regardless of the unpleasantness of the condition of the body.[9]

By the end of the fifteenth century, the Justinian code was a lost relic. A new era of European forensic medicine began with the adoption of two codes of German law: in 1507, the Bamberger code *(Coda Bambergensis),* and in 1553, the Caroline code *(Constitutio Criminalis Carolina).*[10] The Caroline code, based on the Bamberger code, required that expert medical testimony be obtained for the guidance of judges in cases of murder, poisoning, wounding, hanging, drowning, infanticides, abortion, and other circumstances involving injury to the person.[11]

Owing to these works, surrounding countries began to question earlier superstitious systems of legal judgment, such as trial by ordeal.[12] Legislative changes followed, particularly in France, and medicolegal volumes began to be published throughout Europe. Most noteworthy

among them was Ambroise Pare's book (1575) discussing monstrous births, simulated diseases, and methods to be adopted in preparing medicolegal reports.[13] In 1602, the extent of medical information had grown such that Fortunato Fidele published four extensive volumes. Even more important, between 1621 and 1635, Paul Zacchia, physician to the Pope, contributed his extensive collection, *Questiones Medico Legales,* discussing such issues as death during delivery, feigned diseases, poisoning, resemblance of children to their parents, miracles, virginity, rape, age, impotence, superfetation, and moles.[14] Limited in accuracy by ignorance of physiology and anatomy, the book nevertheless served as an influential authority of medicolegal decisions of that time.

In 1650, Michaelis delivered the first lectures on legal medicine at Leipzig.[15] The teacher who replaced him compiled *De Officio Medici Duplici, Clinici Mimirum ac Forensis,* published in 1704.[16] This was followed by the extraordinary *Corpus Juris Medico-Legale* by Valenti in 1722.[17] Not only did Germany significantly stimulate the spread of forensic medicine, but particularly after the French Revolution, France's system of medical education and appointment of medical experts further defined the parameters of the field.[18]

So that we are not blinded by the remarkable accomplishments just mentioned, we must remember that "witch-mania," which originated in 1484 by papal edict, was still widely accepted throughout much of the eighteenth century. Thus, with the blessing of the medicolegal community, thousands branded as witches were burned at the stake. Despite the repeal of British witch laws in 1736, alleged witches were murdered by mobs as late as 1760, and "witch doctors" practiced as late as 1838. France is known to have held a witch trial in 1818.[19] As Chaillé so accurately stated,

... with the impotence of science to aid the law, it adopted miracles as explanations, suspicion as proof, confession as evidence of guilt, and torture as the chief witness, summoning the medical expert to sustain the accused until the rack forced confession.[20]

Nevertheless, in England, medical jurisprudence pushed forward, laying the foundation for the depth of information we share today. In 1788, the first known book on legal medicine was published in English.[21] The following year, Professor Andrew Duncan of Edinburgh gave the first systematic instruction in medical jurisprudence in any English-speaking university. Recognition by the Crown was evidenced in 1807 when the first Regius Chair in forensic medicine was established at the University of Edinburgh.[22] Eighty years later, the Coroner's Act defined the duties and jurisdiction of the coroner. As amended in 1926, these obligations included

(1) investigation of all sudden, violent, or unnatural deaths and (2) investigation of all prisoners' deaths by inquest.[23] The 1926 amendment also set forth minimum qualifications for the position of coroner and carefully outlined its jurisdiction in criminal matters.[24] It was not until 1953 that the coroner's jurisdiction in civil matters was defined.[25]

Early American colonists brought the coroner's system, intact, to the United States in 1607.[26] Because the position was held by political appointees, most of whom lacked medical training, their cause-of-death determinations could be based on little more than personal opinion. It is not surprising that controversy concerning the validity of death investigations led Massachusetts, in 1877, to replace the coroner with a medical examiner whose jurisdiction was limited to "dead bodies of such persons only as are supposed to have come to their death by violence."[27] Eventually, New York City and other jurisdictions followed suit, in an attempt to establish a profession of trained experts, qualified to unravel the mystery behind the violent deaths that increased each year as the population expanded. To this end, the medical examiner was given the authority to order autopsies.[28]

During the last half of the twentieth century, considerable advances have been made in the area of forensic medicine. Scientific and technological improvements have provided new fabric and groundwork for jurisprudential development. The question at this point, however, is whether such development will proceed. Medicolegal teaching programs have increased at many universities, medical schools, and law schools. Yet, these programs simply provide a theoretical foundation. The forum of discussion must now proceed from the world of academia to the practitioner's realm.

THE ADVERSARIAL PROCESS

The legal system in the United States is based on the concept that there is a value in the presentation of opposing points of view. The legal process is designed to provide for presentation of opposing points of view and a contest of persuasion. In a nutshell, forensic medicine is the study of all the medically related sciences in a way that concentrates on the persuasiveness of information to be presented in the adversarial process that the law applies to the determination of truth. Legal scholars and practitioners believe in the value of the process and support the concept that one can find the truth best in a legal setting by setting the parties to present conflicts on the facts and the law.

The *reasonable medical certainty* is a legal concept that is difficult for physicians to understand, but it is a purely legal concept. Reasonable medical certainty is a catch phrase meaning "more likely than not" in a medical sense. In other words, if the likelihood of an event is more probable than not, given the facts, the physician can testify with a "reasonable medical certainty." Most physicians feel that the word "certainty" is misleading, but the legal system has no problem with the word. If a physician understands that the legal system weighs and balances the probity and veracity in terms of "more likely than not," then the use of the word "certainty" is more easily understood.

Methods and practice in law and medicine are widely divergent. Practitioners in law attempt to apply general principles to specific fact situations, whereas medicine is a highly individualistic and very flexible application of general scientific information. Most physicians would not consider themselves to be empiric scientists operating within a very structured environment. Medicine requires a great deal of flexibility and artistry.

In the case of law the persuasiveness of an argument always returns to the generally accepted principles; therefore, there is always an attempt to eliminate the uncertain and to mold the arguments to fall foursquare on the previously accepted legal principles. As a result, when lawyers and physicians attempt to resolve conflicts, they invariably start from a different place and sometimes collide before they cooperate.[29]

EXPERT WITNESSES

The layperson, judge, or jury member needs help in order to establish the truth. As a result, experts are allowed to provide testimony to help the fact-finder. The expert is a person who by reason of training, education, skill, experience, or observation is able to enlighten and assist the fact-finder in resolving factual issues. Experts are allowed to provide the specialized information to laypersons, if the court accepts them as experts in the first place. To be accepted properly as an expert, the court must establish that an individual fits the qualifications as stated. One can be qualified by education or experience, but one must ultimately have enough knowledge to enlighten a layperson. A judge usually makes the determination of whether an individual is an expert and that determination sometimes is balanced against the potential for prejudice in the presentation of testimony. For example, even if a general practitioner qualifies as an expert on a neurosurgical procedure, his or her expertise must be recognizably less than the expertise of a neurosurgeon. If the judge feels that the jury will not be able to make that distinction, then the court may exclude the testimony and not qualify the expert.[30,31]

The believability and credibility of a forensic scientist are tested in the courtroom and other legal proceedings. It is no coincidence that the word *examination* is used to describe the process of presenting testimony in a trial or hearing. Direct and cross-examination are, ultimately, a true test of an individual's knowledge of the materials presented. A good cross-examination attempts to test and disprove the assertions that are brought out in the direct examination. The effective and well-prepared attorney is more than qualified to adduce the information that will be relevant and material to the factual issues at hand. The forensic scientist must prepare adequately to clearly present the information in the most persuasive manner possible. Ultimately, a forensic scientist in a legal setting is an advocate. The individual is tested for professional expertise, thoroughness, accuracy, and honesty.[32,33]

Opinion testimony and hypotheticals

After experts are qualified by the court and accepted to give expert testimony, they can give opinion testimony and can also answer hypothetical questions. Experts are allowed to give opinion testimony based on facts that are normally used by experts in forming their opinions. This would include text and journal information as well as the evaluation of the facts and the gathering of evidence that are a part of the information used by experts in the field. For example, frequently experts can use hearsay evidence in the formation of their opinion.

In a court an attorney might present a hypothetical question in order to establish an expert's opinion given certain assumed facts. (Hypothetical questions are questions based on stated assumptions.) If an expert is allowed to give an answer to a hypothetical question, it can be used as persuasive testimony by the opposing parties, given that many times factual disputes cannot be completely resolved. For example, an attorney will ask the expert to assume certain facts that are in dispute and then draw a conclusion. This kind of opinion testimony allows attorneys to advance the version of the facts that their clients offer.

Admission of evidence requires a foundation. Through the use of the testimony of the witness, the validity of the physical evidence can be established. For example, a photograph must be a true and accurate representation of the situation of which the witness has knowledge. Retouched photographs and photographs that misrepresent a scene must be tested by laying the foundation in order that the information can be accepted into evidence. The typical process involves the labeling of an item as an exhibit and then the foundation being laid by a witness, often the expert witness, or through a process of verification so that the exhibit can be accepted as evidence. Photographs, diagrams, demonstrations, models, slides, films, and tapes can be accepted into evidence, provided that the court finds that there is no attempt to misrepresent or deceive.[34]

Courts generally have a problem with accepting books, texts, journals, and treatises as evidence. The problem is that written material can be so easily abused that the courts generally recognize that in-court testimony by a witness is more easily tested and verified. On the other hand, an effective argument can be made that a journal or book, if considered authoritative, can be used because it is written in a nonadversarial context that makes it more likely to be more believable. There are arguments to be made on both sides because, taken out of context, a book can be misleading. In most trial courts, written materials can be used if the expert witness accepts them as authoritative. Textbooks can be used both to contradict the testimony of the expert as well as to support that testimony.[35]

Court-appointed experts

Trial courts have the authority and, in some cases, have exercised the authority to appoint their own experts. Court-appointed psychiatrists, social workers, and other experts are frequently used in complex cases. That does not rule out the use of experts by opposing parties, but it does allow the court to place more weight on the testimony and evidence presented by the court-appointed expert. The credibility question ultimately still lies in the areas of persuasiveness. For example, an ineffective court-appointed expert can be overcome by an effective, believable expert for the plaintiff or defendant or for the prosecution or the defense. In any event, the forensic scientist who is appointed by the court must ultimately stand the test of the courtroom and the direct and cross-examination process.[36]

THE CORONER'S CASE

All unexpected deaths or those that occur under suspicious circumstances should be evaluated by the coroner or medical examiner. The coroner may or may not be a forensic pathologist. Many times the coroner is an official who certifies the cause of death in what are called coroner's cases. The phrase "coroner's case" is the same as the medical examiner's case and is defined as a death under suspicious or violent circumstances or a death that is unexpected, sudden, or without the benefit of an attending physician who can certify the cause of death. In many states patients who die within 24 hours of admission to a hospital or in surgery are automatically considered medical examiner's cases.

A number of economic, political, and social factors influence the activities of a medical examiner's office. Inevitably this results in an inaccurate application of the forensic sciences. For example, in many states there are many deputy medical examiners and only a few forensic pathologists. The forensic sciences are helpful in reducing the error rate on cause of death and in discovering unsuspected causes of death, but expense, time, effort, and social as well as cultural influences affect the rate of autopsies in all circumstances, so the forensic sciences are applied in relatively narrow criminal or suicide circumstances most of the time.[37]

Unfortunately many deaths occur in which legal or economic consequences can be seriously affected by a lack of application of forensic pathology. Insurance and liability considerations should not be ignored. All clinicians should encourage the proper application of forensic pathology and toxicology to assist in an accurate determination of the cause of death. In any event, those cases that qualify, under appropriate state law, should be referred to the medical examiner or the coroner, and only the attending physician who is reasonably convinced of the cause of death should be so confident as to sign the death certificate without consultation with an appropriate forensic pathologist and without encouraging postmortem examination. The autopsy can reveal many things if properly performed.

Forensic pathology involves the use of medical and scientific principles in determining the cause of death. In the case of all deaths that are unexpected, unexplained, violent, suspicious, or not attended by a physician, this area of specialization is applied in the interest of society and the state, both for public health as well as for potential criminal and civil implications. The determination of the cause of death is important in accidental deaths, criminal violence, and public health threats. Appropriate investigation of the cause of death can have serious implications both for the individual involved as well as for the society as a whole.[38,39]

Various aspects of the functions of the coroner/medical examiner are discussed in the chapter on forensic pathology (Chapter 42).

Investigation of the scene of death

Unfortunately, too little evidence is gathered at the scene of a death. More than 50% of death scenes have information and evidence available that will help in the determination of cause of death, but in many cases, information and evidence is not obtained. The scene should be investigated if there is any suspicion of foul play or suspicious circumstances. It has been said that almost 20% of deaths require appropriate medicolegal investigation. Death by violence, in some age groups and ethnic groups, is the most common cause of death. Investigation is required for death that occurs under the following circumstances[40]:

1. Death in a healthy individual
2. Violent, unnatural, suspicious, or unusual death
3. Death of an individual who is not under the continuing care of a physician
4. Death within 24 hours of admission to a hospital or in the operating room
5. Death in other special circumstances, such as those that occur while in legal custody or incarceration.

Scene investigation. An investigation of a scene may be most appropriately handled by the police or a legal investigator. The medical investigator may or may not be the most qualified to examine evidence at a scene or gather the information and physical materials that might assist in the determination of the cause of death. In many states the coroner is a legal investigator and uses the forensic pathologist as medical investigator.

Determination of death. The first duty of a medical examiner or a physician at the scene is to determine death. Lack of respirations, unreactive pupils, lack of response to painful stimulus, and lack of heartbeat as auscultated over the heart are reasonable determinants of death. In special circumstances such as shock, exposure, and hypothermia, the actual determination of death may be difficult.

The scene of death. The adequate medical investigation of the cause of death includes an observation of the scene with the appropriate gathering of physical evidence. The experienced, suspicious, and thorough investigator will gather a number of types of information including (1) a history of the events prior to death; (2) medical history, if available; (3) medications and appropriate medical documents; and (4) physical evidence from the scene. This is particularly important in possible suicides, since there are a number of reasons, civil as well as cultural, to conceal information about suicide. It is appropriate to gather body secretions, excretions, vomitus, and other physical evidence at the scene, and to include clothing and other objects. At that point, all the physical evidence should be labeled and properly packaged so that the chain of custody can be protected.

The chain of custody or the chain of evidence is the unbroken documentation of the possession and protection of physical evidence. The chain of custody or chain of evidence concept is designed to avoid possible tampering with evidence. Essentially, if the actual possession of the physical evidence is properly traced, then that physical evidence is less likely to have been tampered with. That does not rule out the possibility of tampering, but it does allow legal means for assuring the fact-finder that the evidence was collected properly, preserved properly, and presented accurately at the time of trial.[41]

Additional sources of information

Since age and sexual characteristics are frequently determined by examination of the bones, X-rays can make a significant contribution to the identification and the determination of the age and sex of the dead.

Forensic hematology and serology. Numerous markers are available from blood specimens and can assist in the matching and identification process. Basic blood types are obviously well known to the reader, but other markers and characteristics of blood will help in the identification of an individual. As in all cases, blood examination for type and genetic markers can be definite only in an exclusionary process. The finding of certain characteristics can only suggest but not prove the identity, since there are many individuals who carry the same markers.

The development of sophisticated tissue typing and genetic marker techniques has created a tremendous growth in the ability of the forensic specialist. The use of hematology blood types and genetic markers to rule out paternity is well established. Unfortunately, there is no clear test-match to establish paternity, but exclusion of paternity is possible through the tests available at this time. Standard blood typing as well as genetic markers with other kinds of characteristics can be used in combination to rule out the majority of individuals in a paternity-testing situation, but there is a certain, albeit small, percentage of individuals who cannot be excluded by currently available testing. In addition to the use of forensic hematology and serology to deal with paternity cases, tissue and fluid typing tests are available that can be used in rape cases and other criminal situations to implicate a suspect. In addition to blood typing, tissue type testing and secreter tests also can match an individual for certain characteristics. When combined with hair and other external evidence, these tissue and fluid analyses can produce corroborative information to assist the forensic specialist. Forensic hematologists and histologists are capable of examining bloodstains, hair specimens, and other physical evidence to properly match the perpetrator with the crime.[42,43]

Polygraphs. The polygraph continues to be a source of great dispute in courts of law throughout the country. At this time the polygraph is not acceptable on a routine basis in courts of law because it is not considered to be reliable. Because of this unreliability, the courts at this time consider the use of polygraph testing an area of potential abuse, misinformation, and misrepresentation. The ability of individuals to pass polygraphs in spite of the fact that they are telling lies is an area of significant difficulty for trial courts that allows abuse on either side. Although there are strong advocates for the use of polygraph testing, at this point the majority of courts do not accept its use as evidence.

Forensic evidence of cause of death

Blunt force. Blunt force is one of the most common causes of violent death and there are a number of characteristics of blunt force injuries that assist the examiner in the determination of the time and the mechanism of death[44]:

1. Abrasions and lacerations may assist in the evaluation of the mechanism.
2. Bruises and the development of ecchymosis are important indicators, and can be aged.

3. Initial changes create a reddish bruise that becomes purple and begins to develop a yellowish color after a number of days. The body does not bruise after death unless there has been a tremendous injury after death. Characteristics of abrasions, lacerations, and bruises are not necessarily the same shape of the object that causes them, so care must be taken as to the cause of certain kinds of injuries.

Wounds from cuts or stabs. Some common characteristics of deaths and injuries related to sharp instruments and weapons have been noted:

1. Homicide usually involves stabbing through clothes, whereas suicides are usually done to the skin.
2. The amount of bleeding at the scene may indicate the time of survival of the patient.
3. Look for defense wounds, which are small cuts on the hands and arms of the victim.
4. The direction of the attacker and also the dominant hand of the attacker can sometimes be detected by the direction of the pattern of wounds.
5. It may be worthwhile to attempt to determine which wound was the fatal one.
6. Look for other wounds and the possibility of sexual assault.
7. Usually attempts at suicide by knife involve multiple superficial wounds because of the hesitation of the victim. One deep single wound is suspicious for homicide. The homicidal cut throat is usually horizontally positioned rather than diagonally, as in suicide.
8. Homicidal stabbing is more frequent than suicidal stabbing. The position of the stab wounds frequently assist in determining whether it is homicide or suicide.

Asphyxiation. The characteristics of this kind of death depend on the nature of the cause of the asphyxiation and the effort made to resist the asphyxiation. Hemorrhages from severe respiration effort can be found in the conjunctiva and evidence of strangulation or other physical forces might also be found.

Drowning. Drowning deaths can have certain characteristics that require analysis, including the following:

1. Sometimes severe trauma may be associated with drowning. A broken neck is a common predecessor to drowning.
2. There are no definite classic physical findings, but associated injuries may help to determine the cause of death.
3. Persistent foam at the mouth and nostrils may indicate that the patient may have developed pulmonary edema, which is a sign that the patient is a drowning victim.
4. There are characteristic differences in saltwater and freshwater drowning, particularly in the con-

dition of the lungs, which are much lighter in freshwater drowning than in saltwater.

5. Occasionally laryngeal spasm can be the cause of drowning death, which would result in no significant changes in the lungs. Generally this is a diagnosis of exclusion. Some forms of blood and tissue tests can be helpful in the diagnosis of drowning.

Electrocution and fire. Electrocution kills either by direct destruction of vital organs or by causing a cardiac or respiratory arrest. Direct as well as indirect damage can result from fires. The most common cause of death in fires is the inhalation of toxic or asphyxiating gases.

Sudden infant death syndrome (SIDS). Respiratory failure or compromise is the most common cause of infant death from known causes, but SIDS is a peculiar phenomenon that is probably related to abnormal respiratory center development. Characteristics of SIDS include the following:

1. Preponderance of males
2. Generally in the first 6 months of life, with the peak usually in the first 3 months
3. More frequent in cold weather
4. Usually associated with a mild respiratory problem
5. Prematurity and previous respiratory problems frequently present.

In a diagnosis of SIDS, physicians are alert to the possibility of the battered child syndrome.

FORENSIC PSYCHIATRY AND PSYCHOLOGISTS

Psychiatric problems are frequently fraught with legal implications. Forensic psychiatry is critical to determine competence in contract actions, responsibility for torts and crimes, competence to testify, ability to give informed consent to treatment, and particularly competence to stand trial. A related area is testamentary capacity, that is, the ability of the testator to comprehend that he or she is writing a will, is aware of the property involved as well as the objects of bounty, and understands to whom the property will descend at death.

The defense to a criminal charge is predicated at times on insanity. Whether the state recognizes the M'Naughton rule, the ALI rule, the Durham or New Hampshire rule, and whether the defense is diminished responsibility or irresistible impulse, the fundamental questions to be answered are whether a mental disease or illness is present and whether it affected the accused's behavior.

At times, the granting of a divorce or annulment and the award of custody, placement, or adoption are based on the presence or absence of a psychiatric problem.

Similarly, in reproduction situations, the performance of an abortion or a sterilization procedure is conditioned on the psychiatric status of the patient. Artificial insemination mandates an absence of psychiatric problems in the donor or perhaps in his family.

Personal injury and malpractice claims may turn on the presence of traumatic psychoneurosis. In recent years, psychiatric problems related to employment have been the basis for workers' compensation. Strict product liability has also been imposed for psychiatric injury.

Inherent in the etiology and effects of alcoholism and drug habituation and abuse are psychiatric factors; physicians have been held liable for addicting patients to drugs.

Psychiatric problems are often treated along with mental retardation, juvenile delinquency, autism, and hyperactive children. The use of psychosurgery, that is, prefrontal lobotomy, brain ablation and electrode implantation, and electrical convulsive therapy may be used only in indicated circumstances with proper consent.

Forensic psychiatry is critical in determining malingering, sociopathy, sexual psychopathy (rape), and other sex-related problems such as homosexuality, transvestitism, transsexual surgery, pedophilism, and fetishism.

Suicide contemplated because of depression, if recognized, can be prevented. Actually depression, which can be prevented if anticipated and recognized, is seen postoperatively particularly after cardiac surgery, postpartum, in intensive unit care, after transplantation, and incident to dialysis.

Psychiatric malpractice claims frequently involve treatment with medications, usually undertreatment or overtreatment, and toxic reactions — recently, for example, tardive dyskinesia. Infrequently, misdiagnosis and delayed or erroneous treatment are alleged. Intimate therapy has only recently become a cause célèbre and cause of action.

Psychiatric implications occur even in patients with psychoneurosis and personality trait or character disorders, but particularly in schizophrenia, manic-depressive psychosis, the various depressions, and paranoia. Organic brain disease can include epilepsy, cerebral arteriosclerosis, space-occupying lesions, Alzheimer's disease, and a variety of other disorders. These must be distinguished from trauma, infectious metabolic chemical or electrolyte disorders, cortisone intoxication, dehydration and cerebral edema, liver and kidney failure, and other etiologies.

The credibility and qualifications of a psychiatric or psychological expert are subject to the same legal requirements as other expert testimony. The opinions of psychiatric experts are, based on an adequate and intense investigation and examination of the witness, admissible for consideration by the fact-finder. There are frequently conflicting opinions about the psychological state of individuals.

The tests of admissibility for psychiatric and psychological evidence in testimony is the same as that applied to all forms of evidence. The credibility of the expert involved is one factor that complicates the matter of admission of forensic psychiatric and psychological information. The opinions of the mental health expert about criminal and civil matters are subject to cross-examination and rebuttal by other experts.[45]

On the last day of the U.S. Supreme Court's 1992-1993 term, the justices' ruling in *Daubert v. Merrell Dow Pharmaceuticals*[46] changed the rules for the admission in federal courts of testimony by scientific experts.

For nearly 70 years, most federal courts judged the admissibility of scientific expert testimony by the 1923 standard of *Frye v. United States,*[47] i.e., are the principles underlying the testimony "sufficiently established to have general acceptance in the field to which it belongs"?

In *Daubert,* the Supreme Court unanimously agreed that the *Frye* test was supplanted in 1975 when Congress adopted the Federal Rules of Evidence, which included provisions on expert testimony.

In evaluating evidence of DNA identification, medical causation, voiceprints, lie detectors, eyewitness identification, and a host of other scientific issues, litigants and courts must now reconsider admissibility questions under *Daubert.*

The Supreme Court did not reject the *Frye* test on grounds that it was a wrong or poor judicial policy. Rather, the court simply concluded that *Frye* "was superseded by the adoption of the Federal Rules of Evidence."

Rule 702 allows opinion testimony by a qualified person concerning "scientific, technical or other specialized knowledge that will assist the trier of fact to understand the evidence or to determine a fact in issue."

To satisfy that requirement, a court will have to undertake "a preliminary assessment of whether the reasoning or methodology underlying the testimony is scientifically valid and of whether that reasoning or methodology properly can be applied to the facts in issue," according to Justice Blackmun, who wrote the majority opinion.

Blackmun identified four factors that a court should consider in determining whether the scientific methodology underlying an expert's opinion is valid under Rule 702:

1. Whether the expert's theory or technique "can be (and has been) tested"
2. Whether the theory or technique has been "subjected to peer review and publication"
3. What the known or potential "rate of error" is for any test or scientific technique that has been employed

4. The *Frye* standard of whether the technique is generally accepted in the scientific community

Blackmun emphasized that the inquiry under Rule 702 "is a flexible one" that focuses on whether an expert's testimony "rests on a reliable foundation."

The full impact of *Daubert* may not be clear for many years, as courts apply its four-factor test to a broad range of expert evidence.

Blackmun criticized *Frye* as being "at odds with the 'liberal thrust' of the Federal Rules and their 'general approach of relaxing the traditional barriers to "opinion testimony."'" However, he also wrote that an expert's testimony must be "scientifically valid," which requires an independent judgment of validity by the court.

The potential impact of *Daubert* is vast, and courts will have to reconsider the admissibility of many types of scientific evidence.

The *Daubert* decision will eventually affect court rulings pertaining to such areas as polygraph testing, voiceprint analysis, questioned documents examinations, and so-called expert psychological testimony on such subjects as rape trauma syndrome and post-traumatic stress disorder.

END NOTES

1. Polsky, 1 Temple Law Rptr. 15, 15 (1954).
2. Smith, *The Development of Forensic Medicine and Law-Science Relations,* 3 J. Pub. L. 304, 305 (1954).
3. Harper, *The Code of Hammurabi, King of Babylon,* 77-71 (2d ed. 1904).
4. Oppenheimer, *Liability for Malpraxis in Ancient Law,* 7 Trans. of the Medical-Legal Soc. 98, 103-104 (1910).
5. Polsky, *supra* note 1, at 15.
6. Smith, *supra* note 2, at 306.
7. *Id.* at 306-07.
8. Polsky, *supra* note 1, at 15.
9. Wecht, *Legal Medicine: An Historical Review and Future Perspective,* 22 N.Y. Law School L. Rev. 4, 876 (1977).
10. Smith, *supra* note 2, at 308.
11. Polsky, *supra* note 1, at 16.
12. Smith, *supra* note 2, at 309.
13. *Id.* at 309.
14. *Id.* at 310.
15. *Id.* at 310.
16. Chaillé, *Origin and Progress of Medical Jurisprudence,* 46 J. Crim. L. and Criminal 397, 399 (1949).
17. Polsky, *supra* note 1, at 16.
18. Polsky, *supra* note 1 at 17.
19. Chaillé, *supra* note 16 at 400.
20. *Id.* at 400, note 24.
21. *Id.* at 402.
22. Farr, *Elements of Medical Jurisprudence* (1788). [Translated and abridged from the "Elementa Medicinne Forensis" of Johannes Fridericus Faselius.]
23. Polsky, 3 Medico-Legal Reader 7 (1956).
24. *An Act to Amend the Law Relating to Coroners,* 16 & 17 Geo. C. 59 (1926).
25. *Id.* at §1.
26. Thurston, *The Coroner's Limitations,* 30 Med-Legal J. 110, 112-113 (1962).

27. Taylor, *The Evolution of Legal Medicine,* 252 Medico-Legal Bull. 5 (1974).
28. Fisher, *History of Forensic Pathology and Related Laboratory Science in Medicolegal Investigation of Death* in 4 *Guidelines of the Application of Pathology to Crime Investigation* 7 (W. Spitz, ed. 1973).
29. Wecht, *Forensic Sciences* (1984).
30. Lempert, *A Modern Approach to Evidence* (1977).
31. Curran, *Law, Medicine, and Forensic Science* (3rd ed. 1982).
32. Wecht, *supra* note 29.
33. Curran, *supra* note 33.
34. Wecht, *supra* note 29.
35. Lempert, *supra* note 30.
36. Hirsch, *Handbook of Legal Medicine* (5th ed. 1979).
37. Fatteh, *Handbook of Forensic Pathology* (1973).
38. Wecht, *supra* note 29.
39. Fatteh, *supra* note 37.
40. *Id.*
41. Hirsch, *supra* note 36.
42. Wecht, *supra* note 29.
43. Curran, *supra* note 33.
44. Fatteh, *supra* note 37.
45. Curran, *supra* note 33.
46. *Daubert v. Merrell Dow Pharmaceuticals.*
47. *Frye v. United States,*

CHAPTER 42 Forensic pathology

CYRIL H. WECHT, M.D., J.D., F.C.L.M.

AUTOPSIES
FORENSIC PATHOLOGY/HOSPITAL PATHOLOGY: THE DIFFERENCE
RAPE
PATERNITY
CHILD ABUSE
DRUG ABUSE
DNA
CONCLUSION

Forensic pathology is a truly unique and fascinating medical specialty. The training to become a forensic pathologist, as with any medical specialty, is highly specific and comprehensive, including one year of formal instruction in medicolegal investigation after completion of four years of residency training in anatomical and clinical pathology. Although scientifically specialized, the actual practice of forensic pathology cuts across a wide spectrum of everyday life, from the investigation of sudden, violent, unexplained, or medically unattended deaths (the basic jurisdiction of the forensic pathologist) to sex crimes, paternity lawsuits, child abuse, drug abuse, and a variety of public health problems. These are areas in which forensic pathologists regularly find themselves involved; the range and diversity of such a practice provide constant intellectual stimulation and challenge.

AUTOPSIES

There are many important reasons why autopsies should be undertaken to the greatest extent possible. These include a variety of benefits to the family of the deceased, such as identifying familial disorders and assisting in genetic counseling, providing information for insurance and other death benefits, and indirectly helping to assuage grief. There are benefits for the public welfare, such as discovering contagious diseases and environmental hazards, providing a source of organs and tissues for transplantation and scientific research, and furnishing essential data for quality control and risk assessment programs in hospitals and other health care facilities. Autopsies benefit the overall field of medicine, such as the teaching of medical students and residents,

the discovery and elucidation of new diseases (Legionnaire's disease and AIDS), and the ongoing education of surgeons and other physicians regarding the efficacy of particular operations, medications, and so on. There are additional benefits to the legal and judicial systems, such as determining when an unnatural death (accident, suicide, or homicide) has occurred, and enabling trial attorneys and judges to make valid decisions pertaining to the disposition of civil and criminal cases.

In light of all the significant medical contributions and substantial scientific data that have been derived directly and indirectly from postmortem examinations over the past three centuries, it is incredible that in the United States, the Joint Commission on Accreditation of Healthcare Organizations (JCAHO), in 1970, dropped its long-standing requirement that hospitals perform autopsies in a certain percentage of patient deaths in order to maintain JCAHO certification (teaching hospitals, 25 percent; other, 20 percent). Moreover, this is disturbing, considering the increasing number of wrongful death cases involving medical malpractice and other personal injury and products liability claims, as well as thousands of homicides, suicides, and drug deaths each year, all of which require definitive and complete autopsy findings in order to enable individuals to pursue legitimate objectives within the civil and criminal justice systems.

Areas of concern

A surprisingly high percentage of clinicians, hospital administrators, and even pathologists have expressed a general reticence toward any new, concerted effort to increase the number of hospital autopsies. The reasons usually given are economic, educational, and legal. Hospital executives and other nonmedical administrative personnel are constantly seeking ways to cut costs and increase income. Postmortem examinations cost money for the autopsy technician, for the toxicology, chemistry, and bacteriology tests on tissues and fluids, and for various supplies. Pathologists are busy with their other responsibilities and do not get paid extra for autopsies. Attending physicians and house staff rarely attend autopsies and usually do not even seek information later concerning the autopsy.

Attending physicians and hospital administrators are concerned that in certain instances, autopsies may reveal evidence of malpractice and generally may provide additional data for plaintiff's attorneys in medical malpractice lawsuits. Their reasoning is that in the absence of pathological evidence, the plaintiff will have a difficult, even impossible, task proving that the death was directly and causally related to any alleged errors of omission or commission in the diagnosis and treatment of the patient, that is, that there was any deviation from acceptable and expected standards of care on the part of the attending physicians or nurses that led to the patient's demise. In fact, it is the experience of most forensic pathologists that in the majority of cases, autopsy findings help to demonstrate that there was no medical negligence in the patient's treatment. The objective, scientific documentation of the cause and mechanism of death can be the single most important factor in dissuading a patient's family and their attorney from initiating a malpractice action; or, if a lawsuit has been filed, in providing the defendant-doctors and/or hospital with tangible evidence of an advantageous nature. Speculation and conjecture generally help plaintiffs more often than defendant-doctors in medical malpractice cases in which the cause and mechanism of death are relevant issues.

The idea that new technology and improved diagnostic skills have made autopsies obsolete is incorrect and naive at best and intellectually arrogant and scientifically dangerous at worst. Although it is true that certain death cases are so well understood and unequivocally documented that it is not necessary to perform an autopsy, many clinical questions still need to be asked and answered in a majority of deaths. No matter how competent and experienced the treating physician may be and despite highly sophisticated equipment like CT scans and magnetic resonance imaging, there can be no substitute for actually examining organs and tissues at autopsy, insofar as documentation of definitive and accurate diagnoses is concerned.

Recommendations

It would be in the best interests of society, physicians, and the advancement of medical science if more postmortem examinations were to be performed in appropriate cases. Economic considerations and legal trepidations should be outweighed by the need to determine accurate diagnoses and the cause and mechanism of death.

Several professional organizations have suggested that the JCAHO should assist in halting the national decline in the frequency with which autopsies are performed on patients who die in hospitals. Undoubtedly this would be a stimulus to the performance of postmortem examinations, which would enhance teaching programs and assist physicians and hospitals in peer review and risk management programs. For many years, the standards have not prescribed a specific autopsy rate because the appropriate rate varies from hospital to hospital.

However, concerns have arisen that the decrease in use of autopsies may have had adverse effects on medical education, research, and quality assurance programs. The JCAHO has therefore proposed standards that would require hospitals to include the results of autopsies in their quality assurance programs and to develop in-house policies and guidelines that would lead to a higher rate of autopsies.

FORENSIC PATHOLOGY/HOSPITAL PATHOLOGY: THE DIFFERENCE
Hospital versus forensic pathology

Pathology as a discipline tends to conjure up certain thoughts and conceptions in medically trained personnel that fall far short of an adequate explanation of the subspecialty of forensic pathology, although they would adequately apply to hospital pathology. Hospital pathology and forensic pathology, although obviously sharing many common factors in training and scientific procedure, are substantially and significantly different in their approach to death investigation.

Hospital pathologists are charged with ascertaining pathological findings and correlating them with the existing clinical data; in other words, finding morphological changes to explain particular clinical signs and symptoms. A hospital autopsy, therefore, seeks to verify the diagnosis made prior to death and evaluate the treatment rendered pursuant to that diagnosis. The purpose of this exercise is to increase the storehouse of medical knowledge as well as provide a certain degree of quality control. Philosophically, then, hospital pathologists tend to approach their examinations with verification and academic discovery as their objectives. This predisposition can and often does lead to missing subtleties that contraindicate clinical background, diagnosis, and treatment rendered.

Forensic pathology, on the other hand, approaches a death in an entirely different manner. Frequently, the clinical history of the deceased does not exist or is not available so that even if forensic pathologists were intellectually disposed to do so, it would often be impossible to match their findings with clinical observations, diagnosis, or treatment. Perhaps more important to the distinction between hospital and forensic pathology is their jurisdictional spheres. Forensic pathology goes well beyond the hospital setting and investigates any sudden, unexpected, unexplained, violent, suspicious, or medically unattended death. In fact, the word "investigation" tends to distinguish these two disciplines because, for the most part, hospital pathologists limit themselves to an autopsy and review of available clinical data. Forensic pathologists, however, truly engage in an "investigation" that will routinely address the following:

1. *Who* is the deceased? This information, particularly in a criminal situation, is often unknown. Factors such as sex, race, age, and unique characteristics are evaluated.
2. *Where* did the injuries and ensuing death occur?
3. *When* did the death and injuries occur?
4. *What* injuries are present (type, distribution, pattern, cause, and direction)?
5. *Which* injuries are significant (major versus minor injuries, true versus artifactual or postmortem injuries)?
6. *Why* and *how* were the injuries produced? What were the mechanisms causing the injuries and the actual manner of causation?
7. *What* actually caused the death?

The scope of such a medicolegal investigation is obviously broad and comprehensive—as it must be. The information generated may determine whether or not a person is charged with a crime, is sued civilly for negligence, or receives insurance benefits. The information may also determine a myriad of other critical and vitally important issues. Each of these uses pivots on a general determination other than the cause of death that is alien to hospital pathology, namely, the manner of death.

The word "alien" is used because manner of death is a purely legal question and one that only forensic pathologists, armed with the results of their medicolegal investigation, are prepared to address. Hospital pathologists have little opportunity to develop a fair understanding, satisfactory appraisal, and high index of awareness

of the medical, philosophical, and legal problems related to the determination of the manner of death. For them, essentially every death is natural and even medical negligence may go undetected or may be labeled as a natural complication of disease. The fact that drafting and signing hospital death certificates is primarily the responsibility of the attending physician accentuates this trend. Quite often the hospital physician is not inclined to include in the autopsy report a specific cause of death or the full causal chain of events, especially in those instances that might suggest a possible cause for litigation or when several potential causes of death are believed to be present.

None of these comparisons should be construed as an assertion that hospital pathologists are somehow incompetent. Their approach is simply different from that of a forensic pathologist. In addition, hospital pathologists are not charged with the duty of determining the answers to many of the questions that a forensic pathologist must routinely address.

Another problem in which hospital pathologists are usually not interested, are not asked to answer, or deem to be of vague academic interest, is the determination of the time of death and the timing of the tissue injuries. For forensic pathologists, however, the issues of the time of death and time of injuries are crucial to many civil and criminal cases in which they will inevitably become involved, so they must be specifically addressed.

Forensic pathologists are also aware of the crucial importance of the scene and the circumstances of death in the scientific reconstruction and understanding of the autopsy findings. Unlike hospital pathologists, scene visits are frequently undertaken by forensic pathologists to alert themselves to any possible inconsistencies between the death scene and their actual scientific findings.

The approach to the forensic autopsy itself is also different. Forensic pathologists, frequently exposed to the pathology of trauma, fully recognize the importance of a careful external examination, including the clothing, to determine the pattern of injuries and their relationship to the identification of the injurious agent. Hospital pathologists, because their subjects usually die in the hospital, generally have no need to be curious about these factors and are satisfied with a cursory and superficial external examination. Hospital pathologists are, however, more inclined to detect and diagnose microscopic changes of rare natural diseases because of the direction of their work and the academic environment in which they function. On the other hand, forensic pathologists are more alert and familiar with subtle microscopic changes due to poisons, noxious substances, and environmental diseases—in other words, with the microscopic profile of unnatural death.

It is when the issue of determining the manner of death (natural versus unnatural) arises that the two disciplines dramatically diverge in application. Such a determination is really a legal one that is totally foreign to hospital pathologists. As noted, for them every death is natural and they are, therefore, rarely called on to make a differentiation between natural and unnatural. In fact, due to lack of experience and training, most hospital pathologists simply are not qualified to render an opinion on this issue.

Forensic pathologists are intimately familiar with problems of causality and manner of death. Determining the manner of death is a basic responsibility they assume in every investigation, and their background and training reflect this requirement.

The differences between hospital and forensic pathology are obviously multiple and significant. It is important, therefore, to explore some of the more interesting and unique aspects of a forensic pathologist's medicolegal investigation.

Identifying the deceased

One of the first, and often most difficult, problems with which a medicolegal investigation is confronted is simply a determination of the identity of the deceased. Two relatively unknown and helpful forensic scientific disciplines employed in the identification process are odontology and anthropology.

Forensic dentistry. Although the application of medical and other scientific investigative techniques to the field of forensic pathology is not a new idea, most forensic pathologists do not routinely utilize sophisticated dental expertise in their scientific investigations. The possibilities for applying useful techniques for investigation and identification in the area of odontology are multiple in nature. While its total future application in identification will never become as extensive and universal as fingerprinting, the similarities are striking. Dental structures themselves, as well as various dental appliances such as fillings, crowns, and so forth, in a person's mouth tend to be unique to that individual. Odontology is especially helpful in identification because dental structures do not deteriorate rapidly following death and, when the deceased dies of violence that might mutilate the body either by thermal or mechanical means, the teeth frequently survive intact.

Forensic anthropology. Another relatively recent subdivision of the forensic sciences that assists the medicolegal investigation is forensic anthropology. Although anthropology as a science is certainly not new, its accepted and recognized application to legal processes is of fairly recent vintage. To a significant extent, physical

anthropologists may work closely with forensic pathologists and odontologists in such cases as human identification, evaluation of injuries, determination of sex, race, age, and so forth. However, because of their special experience and background, physical anthropologists who are well trained and experienced in their field are able to make unique contributions to these vitally needed areas that other specialists are simply unable to do. Using rather amazing techniques and investigative studies, physical anthropologists can arrive at remarkable and important conclusions. This is not a field of pseudoscientific guesswork. It is a complex, sophisticated, objective accumulation of hard, physical data that should properly occupy a position of top evidentiary priority in a court of law. Physical anthropologists are able to deal with purely skeletal remains, whether they are complete or fragmented, burned bodies, or semiskeletal remains that are decomposed beyond recognition, and ascertain race, sex, age, information helpful in determining the time of death, the cause of death, and more.

Time of death

As mentioned earlier, forensic pathologists must also deal with time of death, a determination that is largely unique to their investigation. Determining when a death occurred can be critical in civil and especially criminal litigation. For instance, placing the moment of death in a time frame in which an accused murderer has indisputable proof of his or her whereabouts obviously militates strongly against conviction. Pinpointing the time of death with unequivocal accuracy cannot be done; but, estimates within certain parameters are possible when based on a number of factors.

Early postmortem changes occurring hours to days after the demise including cooling of the body (algor), pooling of blood in dependent areas (livor), skin discoloration, stiffening (rigor), drying of the ocular bulbs, and fluctuations of the blood glucose levels and other body chemicals such as the potassium concentration of the eye fluids. Our discussion will be limited to the evaluation of those postmortem changes that are most frequently used and accepted in the process of determining the time interval from death to discovery of the body.

Immediately following the death, the body temperature gradually starts to fall until it reaches the ambient temperature (see Table 42-1). The rate of cooling, which varies from 1 to 2° F per hour, is affected by many factors such as the interval since the demise, the temperature of the deceased at the time of death, body mass, the gradient between the temperature of the corpse and the surrounding temperature, the extent of body insulation (clothing and body fat), and environmental conditions

TABLE 42-1. Early postmortem changes*

Change	Onset time from death	Kinetics	Comments
Cooling of body	At death	Average drop in temperature: 2° F per hour in 6 hours, 1 to 1.5° F for each hour thereafter	Measured intrarectally (4 inches deep) with a long 70 to 110° F thermometer (axillary or hepatic temperatures are acceptable)
Postmortem lividity	1 to 2 hours (30 minutes to 6 hours)	†Maximal, 6 to 10 hours; partly fixed, 10 to 12 hours; moveable, 24 to 48 hours; permanently staining, 3 to 5 days	Note color and hue
Postmortem rigidity	1 to 4 hours (30 minutes to 6 hours)	†Complete in 12 to 16 hours, starts to disappear after 24 to 48 hours; may last in lower extremities for 3 to 5 days; may, at higher temperature, disappear in 24 hours	First in small joints, then spreads to larger joints

*In temperate weather. High or freezing temperatures may significantly alter the rate of postmortem changes, that is, accelerating or decelerating them, respectively.
†Minimal to maximal range.

such as humidity and ventilation. Each of these factors affects the configuration of the cooling curve.

After death, the color of the skin turns much paler than in life. Half-an-hour to two hours later, a particular bluish-violet discoloration appears in the dependent parts of the body. This discoloration has been labeled liver mortis or postmortem lividity—the discoloration of death. The lividity is produced by gravitational movement of the blood and its settling in small blood vessels of the dependent skin and tissues.

Initially, the postmortem lividity can be totally or partially blanched by the application of pressure. Later on, however, the blood permeates through the blood vessels into the adjacent tissues, staining them permanently. Occasionally under the pressure of the collecting blood, some of the small blood vessels in the areas of livor may burst and produce small, pinpoint areas of "bleeding" that, to the uninitiated, may appear to be bona fide antemortem hemorrhages and can pose problems in determining the cause and manner of death. The presence of postmortem lividity in nondependent parts of the body undoubtedly indicates movement of the dead body prior to the examination and often is a significant finding, particularly in criminal cases.

It is of paramount importance to note the color and hue of lividity because it may well indicate the primary or secondary cause of death. A pink or cherry red livor, imparting to the body a lifelike appearance, suggests poisoning by carbon monoxide. A similar discoloration may be seen in cyanide poisoning or following prolonged freezing of a body. Dark blue discoloration of the skin may be seen following asphyxia or poor oxygenation of tissues such as that present in individuals with chronic heart or lung disease.

Soon after death (see Table 42-1), the body and

extremities are very flaccid and can be easily moved to any desired position. However, within a relatively short time (1 to 4 hours), the body and extremities exhibit progressive stiffness and resistance to manipulation. This stiffness, which results from chemical changes of the muscular tissues (depletion of high energy compounds and increased acidity), is known as rigor mortis or postmortem rigidity—the stiffness of death. Once the fully established rigor is broken by manipulation of a particular joint, it does not reappear in the same area. When fully developed, the rigor remains unchanged for about 12 hours and then disappears gradually over the next 12 to 24 hours. The presence or absence of rigor is a factor in determining time of death.

Most postmortem changes, including green discoloration of the skin, foul smell, and the like, are due to decomposition of the body (see Table 42-2). Decomposition changes result from two types of processes: (a) autolysis—a decomposition change produced by the release of cell-destructive compounds from the dead human tissues (endogenous digestive enzymes), and (b) putrefaction—decomposition by external or internal bacteria, by fly larvae (maggots), and by insects. In the final stages of decomposition, the internal organs become mushy or liquefied, thereby impairing or destroying the value of their gross and microscopic examination by the pathologist. However, it must be kept in mind that in most cases, even in the presence of marked tissue deterioration, evidence of trauma, such as hemorrhages and fractures, can be recognized and evaluated by the expert.

The determination of the time of death is important in practically every criminal investigation and, in many instances, the fate of the whole case may well depend on it. Unfortunately, the many factors affecting postmortem

TABLE 42-2. Late postmortem changes*

Decomposition changes	Time of appearance	Observation
a. Green discoloration of skin, abdomen, trunk, etc.	1 to 2 days	
Visible purplish-brown subcutaneous veins	5 to 7 days (24 hours in septic infection)	
Skin blisters	5 to 7 days	
Formation of gas (in gastrointestinal tract and tissues)	7 to 9 days	Greatest in areas of loose tissue (scrotum, breast, etc.)
Wet, peeling skin	7 to 9 days	
Greenish-purple swollen face and body	1 to 4 weeks	
Easily detached hair and nails	3 to 4 weeks	Extensive deformation of body
b. Presence of scavengers in body	Generally 2 to 3 days following death	Size of maggots, knowledge of incubation time, and rate of growth help in estimating time since death
c. Mummification	3½ to 6 months	Drying of the body with excellent preservation of physical features. Occurs in warm, dry, and ventilated conditions.
d. Adipocere (changes in fatty components of skin and other tissue, leading to fair preservation of facial and body features)	3 to 6 months	Decomposition (hydrolysis and hydrogenation) of body fats and release of fatty acids occurring under extreme humidity conditions

*The rate of change generally observed in temperate climates. High or freezing temperatures may significantly alter the rate of postmortem changes, that is, accelerating or decelerating them, respectively.

changes make exact determination of time of death precarious. Often, the conditions extant at the scene at the time of death are unknown or unclear. For example, the temperature of the individual at the time of death is usually unknown and presumed to be normal. However, physical activity, brain hemorrhage, or asphyxia may considerably elevate the body temperature prior to death. In individuals who die of sepsis, the temperature of the body may paradoxically increase after death instead of declining. As a result of the metabolic bacteria such as *Clostridia*, the author has witnessed postmortem ballooning by gases and very rapid decomposition of body tissues occurring in just 6 to 8 hours rather than in the usual 5 to 7 days. At the other extreme, bodies buried in snow or at freezing temperatures may be well preserved for extended periods of time and the usual decomposition "clock" does not apply. Even when the estimates of body temperature, rigor, and livor are integrated, the accuracy of the timing of death remains limited to an estimate within reasonable parameters.

The opinion, therefore, of the forensic pathologist as to this most crucial determination when relying on the postmortem changes alone as an index is a carefully calculated estimate based on the evaluation and integration of numerous general and individual variables. This estimate must be expressed as an elastic time interval and not as a definitive pinpoint occurrence in time.

Time of injury

The aging of injuries is defined as the determination of the time interval from the infliction of the injuries to

the death. This evaluation is based on several criteria: (1) changes in the color and consistency of the injured areas as revealed by macroscopic examination and (2) alteration in the microscopic structure of the injured tissue, including inflammatory changes and evidence of repair.

The gradual, grossly observable phases of an injury explained in the time-related kaleidoscopic changes of a periorbital contusion are representative of the gross observations and information thus supplied. From an early bluish-red color, the bruise changes gradually to dark violet. After a day or two, it turns yellow to yellow-green, and on the fourth to fifth day it becomes slightly brown in color before its final absorption and disappearance. These changes are, of course, a result of the chemical alteration in the blood pigment following its dispersion in the tissues as a result of hemorrhage and, when combined with microscopic information, can be helpful in aging an injury.

Naked eye observation must be supported by more refined microscopic examination; otherwise, the age of small injuries may be easily misjudged, while larger injuries with significant hemorrhaging components may appear grossly fresher than in reality due to the masking effect of the bleeding on the tissue reactions. For this reason, the pathologist must specifically examine microscopic sections from each one of the significant areas of injury as well as from the tissues adjacent to the lesion. The latter requirement is considered essential to adequate sampling because the early tissue reaction occurs at the border between the injured and noninjured tissue.

Acute inflammatory changes with the presence of

acute inflammatory cells in small numbers may be seen as early as ½ hour to 2 hours after injury. Evidence of necrosis and increased numbers of acute inflammatory cells indicate a 6- to 8-hour reaction time. Disintegration of red blood cells and acute inflammatory cells indicates an age of about 2 days, whereas the presence of hemosiderin indicates an age in excess of 4 to 5 days. More sophisticated methods of aging of wounds in the early post-traumatic interval rely on special histochemical microscopic methods that are able to clock the time of wounding by determining variations in the enzymatic activity in the area of injury. Note that the aging of an injury is not based on mathematical formulas or calculations, but on the recognition of elastic patterns of tissue reaction within the knowledge, experience, and training of the pathologist. Therefore, if aging of injuries represents a central issue in a particular case, additional examination by an experienced forensic pathologist may be very rewarding.

Manner of death

Several references have been made to the manner of death as opposed to the cause of death; in fact, the concepts are quite different. The cause of death obviously refers to the mechanisms that ultimately result in a demise. Manner of death, on the other hand, pertains to a mechanism of death that was natural or unnatural (suicidal, accidental, or homicidal). As noted earlier, this is a purely legal conclusion by a forensic pathologist, derived from an integration and analysis of the medicolegal investigation, including the history, the autopsy findings, and the cause of death. It can be a complicated and difficult conclusion to reach because natural and unnatural factors often intermingle and combine to cloud the ultimate cause and, hence, the manner of death.

Unnatural deaths can be categorized using the following general rules of thumb:

- The unnatural factor was the major precipitating factor causing death (that is, bleeding due to a tear of the aorta pursuant to chest impact; self-inflicted gunshot wound; stab wound inflicted by another).
- The unnatural factor exacerbated a preexisting natural disease process (that is, minor bleeding precipitating a fatal heart attack).
- The unnatural factor precipitated or caused a natural disease process leading to death (that is, pneumonia secondary to chest trauma).
- The unnatural factor contributed secondarily to the cause of death, preceding or following a natural condition the deceased may have otherwise survived (that is, a driver of an automobile experiences a heart attack and sustains severe blunt force injuries in a crash).

As noted, in those instances in which natural and unnatural causes of death intermingle, the determination of the manner of death becomes complex. Hard questions such as those that follow must be addressed:

- Was the unnatural factor of a sufficiently significant magnitude to contribute to the death?
- Was an unusual cause an inevitable result of natural conditions, or a complication triggered by an unnatural (human) factor?
- What was the time element between the alleged cause and ultimate demise? The longer the lapse, the greater the possibility of an intervening and supervening cause.
- Was there a chain of clinical signs and symptoms between the perceived cause and death?

Traditional autopsy findings generally do not provide the information required to reach a manner-of-death conclusion. A comprehensive medicolegal investigation, however, usually reveals information that, when integrated with autopsy findings, allows the pathologist to draw a reliable conclusion.

Investigations of death due to gunshot wounds will be used here as a medium to show some of the nontraditional means, processes, and findings employed to determine the probable manner of death in gunshot cases. Although quite specific, the techniques discussed offer insight into the scope any comprehensive medicolegal investigation must have with respect to determining the manner of death as well as the nonmedical information that must be gleaned from and entered into a comprehensive investigation.

Firearms account for a large proportion of unnatural deaths in the United States—most notably in homicides, but in suicides and accidents as well. Vital questions such as the following must be answered in such cases:

1. How is the wound size or pattern related to range, direction of fire, and type of bullet?
2. Can the range of the shooting be estimated from the characteristics of the gunshot wound?
3. Can the relative positions of the victim and the source of fire be determined from the pattern and path of the wounds?
4. When several wounds are present, which was inflicted first?

Gunshot wounds are inflicted by rifled firearms, including revolvers, pistols, and rifles, that have the inside of the barrel grooved spirally to give a screwing, stabilizing motion to the ejected bullet. The pattern of the gunshot wound is produced on the target area by the elements ejected from the gunbarrel. Besides the bullet, these elements are other components of various weights and velocities, all falling behind the bullet and dissipating in the air with the increase in range. The elements ejected are the bullet, gases of combustion, primer components, soot, and burnt and unburnt powder.

Contact gunshot wounds (in which the firearm is

actually in contact with the victim at the time of firing) are usually round or oval with abraded or contused borders and surrounded by a rim of soot. The abraded borders are produced by the sides of the bullet passing through the skin. Inside the wound track, powder and soot are present. When the muzzle of the gun is pressed hard against clothing, the hot barrel will "iron" the fabric when forcefully recoiling and thus leave on the clothing a double ring imprint. A similar burned, brandlike mark may be left on the skin. When the contact gunshot wound is located on the skull or face, the blowback of combustion gases rips the skin at the site of entrance producing a stellate, irregular-shaped wound. Such a wound is invariably surrounded by a rim of soot. It should be noted that distant gunshot wounds of entrance produced by ricocheting, tumbling, or deformed bullets may tear the skin and closely mimic the appearance of a contact gunshot wound. Such misleading, distant gunshot wounds, however, lack the soot and powder seen in contact gunshot wounds.

Contact gunshot wounds are most likely to be found in a suicide situation and, when present, alert the forensic pathologist to that possibility. Other factors must, of course, be evaluated such as the location of the wound of entrance (that is, a wound in the back tends to rule out suicide), and whether or not there is a multiplicity of wounds in vital or debilitating locations (which, again, tend to eliminate suicide as well as accident).

In a near-contact gunshot wound, that is, up to ½ inch distance from the muzzle of the gun, the usually round gunshot wound of entrance shows similar features to the contact gunshot wound except for the absence of the gun imprint and a larger rim of soot.

Near-contact wounds are not usually indicative of suicide because persons committing suicide with a gun almost always press the firearm to their body. Near contact wounds are frequently found in accidental situations in which the victim was in close contact with his or her own weapon when it misfired and in homicides.

At medium ranges, that is, from ½ inch to 6 inches, the wound is surrounded by or contains both soot and gunpowder marks. Soot is not seen around the wound when the range exceeds 6 inches, while powder marks may be seen up to 2 feet. The gunpowder marks consist of peppered, dotted bruises and/or abrasions called satellites or stippling, which are produced by grains of burnt and unburnt powder striking the skin. Some of the grains of powder actually become embedded and may be observed under the microscope. The maximum range at which stippling is produced by handguns is 2 feet. The intensity of the stippling varies not only with the range, but also with the kind of handgun, the ammunition, and the type of gunpowder.

Medium-range wounds usually rule out suicide for the reason mentioned earlier and are common in both accidental and homicidal situations. Making the differentiation requires evaluating other factors since range alone is not determinative.

In ranges in excess of 2 feet, the satellite wounds disappear, because gunpowder will not be carried out beyond this range by the explosive blast. The wound is usually round, and surrounded by a rim of abrasion or contusion (the abrasion collar). It is interesting to note that in some instances the edges of the wound may show a black discoloration of dirt or grime. This discoloration should not be confused with soot; it results from bullet contaminants being wiped against the skin upon entry. The grime ring is composed either of dirt clinging to the surface of the bullet and/or of a very thin layer of rubbed lead.

Naturally, a distant gunshot wound almost always allows the forensic pathologist to discount suicide. Self-inflicted accidental situations are likewise improbable. We are left with an accidental wound inflicted by another or homicide, of which this kind of wound is most characteristic.

Once inside the body, the bullet's path throughout the tissues is obviously indicative of the direction of fire. In perforation-type wounds (those entering and leaving the body), however, this determination may be more difficult and often requires correctly identifying the wounds of entrance and exit.

Entrance wounds on the clothing often leave soot and/or gunpowder residue and can be identified with the naked eye or by special techniques such as infrared photography or microscopic examination. On the skin, gunshot wounds of entrance can usually be easily recognized by their round or oval shape, with contused or abraded margins, or stellate-shaped configuration if overlying bone. The shape of the abrasion or contusion rim should be carefully noted. As mentioned before, this rim indicates the area in which the bullet brushed against the skin and, therefore, may be very helpful in determining the direction of fire. A circular rim of equal width indicates a gunfire directed perpendicular to the skin surface, while in any other situation, the rim is wider in the area facing the incoming direction of the bullet.

Exit wounds tend to be more atypical, irregular, or slit-shaped, mimicking a stab wound or blunt trauma tears. Gunshot wounds of exit usually lack external bordering bruises because the bullet emerges from the inside. Interestingly, however, if the bullet exiting the body encounters a material tightly attached or compressed against the skin, such as a belt, the exit wound may show bruising.

The identification of the wound of entrance, the track, and the wound of exit are critical in determining the manner of death. As should be obvious, simply knowing

TABLE 42-3. Gunshot wounds—pattern by manner of death

Manner of death		Potentially fatal wounds	Number of wounds	Range	Body site	Clothing	Neutron activation test‡
Suicide		Single	Usually single*	Contact† or near	Accessible predilection areas (midforehead, temples, left cheek, roof of mouth, left chest)	May be displaced to expose target area (that is, displacement of bra to expose left chest)	Positive on hands
Homicide		Single or multiple	Single or multiple	Any range	Any site	Usually undisplaced	Usually negative on hands of the victim§
Accident	Self-inflicted	Single	Single	Close or medium range (up to 12 inches)	Accessible site	Usually undisplaced	Positive on hands of the victim
	Not self-inflicted	Single	Single	Mostly medium or distant	Any site	Usually undisplaced	Negative on hands of victim

*Very rarely, minor or hesitation wounds may also be present.
†When rigging devices are present, distant range gunshot wounds may be self-inflicted.
‡Gunshot fire residue test (see text).
§Unless the victim has used a firearm prior to death.

the range of fire is often insufficient to rule out one or another manner of death. The direction of fire, however, can be most helpful, especially in potential suicide and self-inflicted accident situations. Angles and entry wounds that would be most difficult to attain by oneself can eliminate these possibilities and direct the pathologist's investigation in the direction of homicide or accidental infliction by another.

The location, pattern, and multiplicity of gunshot wounds are in many cases excellent indications of the manner of death (Table 42-3). One should, however, refrain from being dogmatic and remember that in a small number of cases the typical location and the multiplicity of wounds can be misleading in determining the manner of death. There are cases reported, for instance, in which a suicide victim has had several gunshot wounds. In one case the victim shot himself in the head four times, twice in the right temple and twice in the midforehead. The revolver and the ammunition were old and malfunctioning, and three of the bullets did not perforate the skull, but shaved it and were found embedded beneath the scalp.

Conclusion

Hospital and forensic pathology are very different in their scope and approach to investigating death. Virtually any scientific discipline can come into play during a comprehensive medicolegal investigation. The forensic pathologist's responsibility is to identify the discipline required, understand the information generated, and arrive at logical, scientifically sound conclusions regarding the cause and manner of death.

RAPE

Forensic pathologists often deal with victims of violent crimes and are called on to assist the state in investigating and prosecuting such cases. Comprehension of the legal requirements of a successful legal prosecution makes the forensic pathologist a uniquely qualified medical expert; and, as will be shown, a medical expert is often essential to identify and successfully prosecute a rape case.

In the most basic medicolegal terms, rape is the penetration of female genitalia by the penis of a male without the female's consent. Ejaculation is not a necessary component, nor is force. This repugnant and heinous act ranks as one of the most difficult of all crimes to prosecute because it pivots on the female's consent and usually only the victim and the assailant are present during the commission of the crime so that the only witness as to consent is the "prejudiced" female herself. A thorough scientific examination of the victim and the accused by a forensic pathologist can, however, generate substantive evidence for trial that can greatly assist in an accurate determination as to whether or not a crime has occurred.

Penetration

The first and most obvious element with which the forensic pathologist must deal is the question of penetration. The usual circumstances of rape include the use of force by the assailant to gain access to the female genitalia and to effect penetration. Such violence often leaves injuries in varying degrees depending on the struggle involved and the previous coital experience of the female. In an average-sized adult female, life-threatening and/or severe injuries usually do not result from insertion of the male's penis into the vagina. A young girl who has had no previous coital experience, on the other hand, may show severe stretching or tearing of the labia and vagina from penile entry. A female who engages in coitus frequently may show no damage at all, even in a violent situation. When injuries are found to the musculature or epithelium of the labia or vagina, it strongly indicates penile penetration; however, lack of such injuries does not, by any means, rule out such penetration.

Another indicator that receives considerable attention as evidence of penetration is the condition of the hymen. Fresh injury to the hymen is usually evidenced by blood clots or hemorrhaging, but the inflammatory process generally seen as a result of injury to other tissues is absent. Hymenal injury may, however, occur without penetration by way of masturbation and heterosexual sex play. Fresh rupture and hemorrhaging of the hymen, especially when combined with testimony of rape, is, however, probative evidence of rape.

The presence of seminal fluid in the vagina of the female is usually considered conclusive evidence that penetration has occurred. This neglects, however, the case in which ejaculation occurs while the male is in the mounting position, and the only penetration of the vagina is by the seminal fluid itself. On the other hand, the absence of ejaculatory material at the time of examination is not unusual even in cases in which the crime of rape has actually occurred. Interruption of the act after penetration but before ejaculation can occur, and the rapist is often incapable of achieving ejaculation. Fear of impregnation and disease on the part of the female frequently results in rapid washing with strong antiseptic solutions after the act. These solutions may produce complete removal of seminal material or introduce factors that interfere with the detection of the constituents of seminal material.

An examination of the vaginal lining sometimes generates findings indicative of penetration such as abrasions, bruises, erosions, or vaginal vault tears. Such an examination must, as noted, be tempered by the knowledge that sexually active females often do not exhibit any evidence of this nature. This can even be true of virgin females except that the virgin vagina tends to be demonstrably rugose, and the folds are quickly eliminated by even limited sexual intercourse so that a smooth vaginal mucosa in a purported virgin indicates penetration. Redness and swelling of the vaginal area as well as the swelling and engorgement of the mucosa at the introitus, the clitoris, and the labia minora, like the evidence mentioned earlier, strongly indicate penetration; but, again, these conditions can be the result of digital manipulation and is not, by itself, determinative of penile penetration.

In investigating an alleged penetration, prudent pathologists must factor in all the evidence of which they are aware before reaching a conclusion of penile penetration. The emotion-charged circumstance of an allegation of rape and the resultant pressure to prosecute the actor demand the utmost restraint and care in investigation by the pathologist in order to prevent a miscarriage of justice. As noted at each of the points of evidence of penile penetration, there are physiologically plausible and noncriminal explanations for each finding.

Consent

The next, and infinitely more difficult component of rape to prove, is whether or not the victim consented to the penetration. As already implied, in those instances in which the female offered little or no resistance, the forensic pathologist will be unable to offer much assistance since the investigation focuses on physical findings as opposed to mental intent. Rape is, however, usually accompanied by violence, the evidence of which tends to indicate that penile penetration was nonconsensual.

If force has been used, there is usually evidence of this on the person or clothing of the victim. There may be lacerations from fingernails or other objects, particularly on surface areas of the body from which clothing was forcibly removed. There may be contusions from blows by fists or other objects about the face, neck, and forearms in particular. Contusions on the throat of the female from throttling attempts are also quite common. Bite marks on the breasts, neck, and face occur frequently and areas on the thighs of the female may show contusions or lacerations caused by forcible spreading of the legs to achieve penile entry. Signs may also be present which indicate that the female actively resisted. The fingernails may be broken or bent from use as defensive weapons and debris may be present under the nails such as clothing fibers, hair, and skin fragments from the assailant. Beard hairs and facial epithelium are most common, but any part of the assailant's body surface may be represented.

Again, the presence of wounds does not necessarily mean that valid consent to coitus was not given. Bites, contusions, and lacerations with the fingernails often accompany orgasm, and sadistic or masochistic sexual responses commonly produce minor injuries and may produce severe injuries, even though valid consent to sexual intercourse has been given. Precoital sex play can generate lacerations on the thighs and tearing of the clothing and postcoital fighting may occur, particularly in cases in which remuneration was expected but not forthcoming. Self-inflicted injury has also occurred for the purpose of adding evidence to a spurious claim of rape.

Identification

In the prosecution of a rape case, a critical component always is the identification of the alleged assailant. The forensic pathologist accomplishes this by employing a number of scientific analyses and common sense observations. It is surprising that a suspect frequently is presented for examination literally teeming with evidence of committing the crime even though more than enough time was available to rid himself of much of the evidence.

If penetration of the vagina by the penis was complete, there may be evidence of vaginal epithelial cells on the penis. This examination is based on the idiophilic nature of vaginal epithelium. If ejaculation occurred, seminal material may be present on the male's pubic hair, penis, or clothing. The clothing of the suspect may have physiological fluids or hairs from the female on its surface. The suspect may have skin fragments or hair under his nails and his hands or genital areas may exhibit blood from the victim and/or vaginal secretions.

The general body surface of the male may show signs of injuries such as lacerations and contusions on any part of the body from being struck with fists or other objects. Bites and scratches on the hands and arms of the assailant are common in rape since it is often necessary to silence the female and the arms of the assailant are placed in a vulnerable position. The face is often the first point of defensive attack by a female, so scratches on the assailant's face and neck are also common.

Unfortunately, it is more likely that no signs are present or that explanations other than rape may have produced the evidence found. After visual examination of the alleged assailant, more scientific and definitive analyses are performed on seminal fluid, hair, and clothing to ascertain the identity of the assailant. Each of the constituents of seminal fluid is identifiable, and tests have been designed to relate results to a given male. The finding of spermatazoa is the only single examination that identifies a stain or secretion as seminal in origin. Spermatozoa can be recovered from the vaginal vault by swabbing or washing. In cases in which the deposition of sperm is very recent, swabbing, with direct preparation of a slide for study, is usually sufficient. When more completeness is necessary, however, vaginal washing is carried out. The diluted vaginal contents then must be concentrated, usually by centrifugation, before slides are prepared. The slides are examined microscopically for the presence of motile or nonmotile spermatozoa.

Dried stains require special procedures to free the spermatozoa. The proteinaceous material present in the seminal fluid prevents good wetting by water alone. Dilute acids, bases, and detergents seldom cause spermatozoal damage and are used to free spermatozoa from dried seminal stains.

Spermatozoa adhere tenaciously to various fibers, particularly cotton, so agitation is often necessary to free them. Examination of a contaminated slide generally requires some means of visualizing the spermatozoa. There are many histological stains that are used, but the simplest and most rapid is optical staining using phase-contrast microscopy. The slides are examined not only for the presence of motile and nonmotile spermatozoa, but also for malformed types. The presence of the same percentages of spermatozoa in two different samples is strong evidence of common origin.

The determination of acid phosphatase activity is widely used for identification purposes. This enzyme is present in the prostatic secretion and is especially helpful when spermatozoa cannot be found due to azospermia. Similar phosphatase activity level in samples taken from the victim and the accused tend to strongly indicate that they are the same.

Unfortunately, various chemicals may lead to incorrect results, either in a positive or negative direction. Ethanol and fluoride inhibit prostatic acid phosphatase, and certain physiological conditions, particularly fever, reduce the activity to levels that may not be detectable. By the methods ordinarily used, phenols and acid phosphatases other than prostatic are the most important sources of positive error. Many antiseptic solutions contain free phenols, may easily contaminate the vagina, and are often found because the victims, as earlier noted, try to wash away the crime.

Naturally, hair is very often transferred between the parties by the contact necessary in the crime of rape. The species of hair, and the part of human body from which the hair came, can usually be determined by microscopic examination. Individual hairs may be differentiated somewhat, but a large group of hairs is more readily subject to identification. Until recently, hair was at best eliminative unless other factors were also present. The advent of neutron activation analysis, however, has led to many claims of individuality of hair samples, but as yet is not accepted as a method of positive identification.

The value of clothing fibers may be limited, but when combined with other information, it can generate corroborative evidence. Frequently, the assailant's clothing is stained by the blood of his victim and, in this circumstance, the evidence is most helpful. More often, however, fibers alone are the only available sample and can only show that fibers similar to those of the accused's clothing were found somewhere on the person of the victim. Similarity in fibers is the strongest correlation that can be made because, unlike human hairs, fibers tend to lack strong distinctions, especially man-made material.

Conclusion

There are many specific ways in which the forensic pathologist can be helpful in the prosecution and investigation of a case of alleged rape. Following is a step-by-step review of the investigative process.

1. Examination of the scene. The position of the victim and the state of the victim's clothing at the scene should be carefully noted. Efforts should be made to prevent contamination of the anus or vagina by their discharge during subsequent transportation of the body.
2. Photographs of the body at the scene
3. Identification photographs of the body in the autopsy room
4. Large and close-up photographs of the injuries, especially of the sexual areas
5. Gentle glove examination of the sexual areas: mouth, vagina, and anus. Gloves should be changed or washed when moving from area to area in order to prevent contamination. The physical condition of the hymen should be noted and recorded.
6. Cotton swabbing and aspirates should be taken from the mouth, vagina, and anus for preparation of microscopic slides, acid phosphatase testing, and the detection of seminal fluid. Immediate examination of a "hanging drop" slide preparation should be carried out in order to check for the presence of motile spermatozoa.
7. Speculum examination of the vagina under adequate light to detect the presence of blood, contusions, lacerations, or presence of foreign bodies (fragments of wood sticks, glass, metal, etc.). In fatalities, microscopic sections should be taken from the areas of injury in order to determine their age, according to the patterns of tissue reactions.
8. Careful examination of the anus to check for presence of injuries. The presence or absence of a patulous or scarred anus indicative of chronic anal intercourse should also be noted.
9. At least 20 hairs plucked in their entirety (and not cut) from the head, axillary areas, and pubic area
10. Fingernails should be cut or scraped and marked

accordingly, left and right. Examination of the fingernail scrapings may reveal the presence of skin, cloth fibers, or blood that may be matched to that of the assailant.

11. Very thorough external examination. Suspected bite marks should be swabbed for saliva typing and imprints lifted if possible.
12. In fatalities, a full internal autopsy should be performed that should pay special attention to the pelvic area, to the presence of perforation or other injuries, evidence of pregnancy, and so forth.
13. A full toxicological examination, including analyses for alcohol, barbiturates, sedatives, and narcotics

PATERNITY

An area peripherally related to rape in which the practicing forensic pathologist will become involved is the identification of the father of a child. Paternity actions were, at one time, extremely messy legal actions with charges and countercharges flying as the most intimate and private areas of the parties' lives were explored. The only mode of proof was the testimony of the parties and their witnesses. Naturally, the high emotion occasioned by paternity actions has not changed, but the forensic pathologist's ability to contribute to positive identification has increased enormously. Today's ability to paternity scientifically determine tends to limit or eliminate the heretofore common practice of the accused of producing a number of males (true or false) who had sexual intercourse at or near the time of conception. Paternity, and not promiscuity, is the issue, and scientific testing can offer virtually positive proof of fatherhood.

We are all endowed with certain genetic characteristics by way of the peculiar combination of our genetic heritage. This combination of genes, peculiar to each person, will be found in all cells of the body (excluding, of course, the egg and sperm), and so an analysis of blood cells will generate the information necessary to establish or exclude paternity. The easiest and first approach to scientific proofs of paternity is exclusion techniques. There are two kinds of exclusions:

1. A man can be excluded when both he and the mother lack a gene that the child has, because a child cannot possess a gene lacking in both of its parents.
2. A man can be excluded when the child does not possess a gene that, according to genetic law, *must* have been inherited from the subject male. (An AB blood type male cannot have a blood type O child because, having no other blood genes to contribute, either an A or B will be present in the child of an AB father.)

Exclusion techniques are reasonably well accepted in the courts throughout the United States because of their virtually absolute finality and their well-accepted and long-standing scientific bases. Unfortunately, newer techniques based on both statistical probability and scientific examination that can prove paternity are not so well accepted.

Genetic science has become so advanced that literally hundreds of genetic characteristics, and proofs of the same, have been identified. By sampling just a few of these characteristics in the child, we are provided with a virtually positive identification index of its father. The subsequent application of mathematical techniques can statistically show whether or not a given male is the child's father with virtually no possible error. For example, if one identifies 20 genes in a child that have a frequency of occurrence in the general population of five and the accused male has those same genes, it is 99.7% likely that the accused is the father. Unfortunately, the possibility of error and the relatively recent development of these identification techniques keep them from being widely accepted by our courts.

The peripheral relationship of these two areas lies in the identification process. As noted in the section concerning rape in this chapter, blood from the parties involved in the crime can often be found on the person of each. The genetic identification index mentioned here can be applied to positively identify the rapist. Thus, important evidence of close contact, if not actual penile penetration, can be generated. Going one step farther, the identification of a suspect in a rape situation as the father of a resultant child would be virtually conclusive evidence of penile penetration so that the issue left to debate would be consent.

CHILD ABUSE

The forensic pathologist enters the child abuse drama as an epilogue, and usually does so with much anxiety. The pathologist must identify the pattern of trauma and differentiate abuse from a true accident. This is a great responsibility because the decision of whether or not to prosecute a suspect will often turn entirely on the pathologist's conclusion. On the one hand, it is difficult to imagine a more traumatic and emotionally and psychologically debilitating experience than to be falsely accused of the despicable conduct of child abuse, but, on the other hand, it is equally distressing to allow an abuser to go free to abuse the defenseless once again. Forensic pathologists must, therefore, satisfy themselves that the injuries they so meticulously document are, in fact, the result of abuse; and, at the same time, they must be able to exclude other less sinister explanations for their findings. Since they do not work in a vacuum, forensic pathologists accumulate a tremendous amount of data

from a variety of sources, evaluate its authenticity, and reach a determination of the mode of death after sifting fact from speculation and fantasy.

When and what

The identification of a puzzling association of chronic subdural hematoma and multiple limb fractures of different ages in young children first began to appear in the mid-1940s. Pathologists were unable to correlate the findings with any known disease and were looking for some undiagnosed exotic new disease. The medical profession was apparently psychologically unprepared to accept the concept that parents could seriously maim their own children, and it was not until the mid-1950s that parental violence was identified as the responsible modality for these observations. Since then, multiple studies the world over have more clearly defined the battered child syndrome so that it is now well known. It is convenient, though somewhat artificial, to classify the child abuser into several categories.

The intermittent abuser periodically batters a child, but administers wholly appropriate care between these episodes. These parents do not intend to hurt their children, but are driven by panic or compulsion and tend to be sincerely remorseful afterward. They are often motivated to reform and can be successful in time. The child-victim of these episodes is usually grabbed by a convenient handle—an arm or a leg—and shaken forcefully, resulting in broken bones and joint dislocations.

It is tempting to separate one-time child abusers from the previous group; it is, however, more likely that one-timers are potential repeaters and were only restrained from killing their child by some particular circumstance.

Constant child abusers actually hate the child, and callously and deliberately beat and mistreat it. Their intent is to hurt the child, usually with the rationalization that they are dispensing appropriate discipline. Such an abuser is indifferent to the child's suffering. These people often have personality disorders, are coolly detached from the destructive nature of their actions, and are not inclined toward reform.

In this age of alternative lifestyles and broken families, more and more young mothers look for and find live-in boyfriends. Often these men are affectionate to their girlfriend's children and contribute to their growth and well-being. Frequently, however, the child becomes the innocent victim of an emotional struggle. When resentment builds, either toward the mother or the children themselves, intermittent habitual abuse can be present, with the woman's children becoming the common target of the man's hostility.

The ignorant abuser is perhaps the most tragic,

because the parent means well, but attempts at rearing the children result in permanent injury or death; and these parents are genuinely devastated by the harm they cause. For example, a young mother hears from another mother how she corrects her children's behavior. If her child cries too much, she simply pours pepper into the child's mouth and the child stops crying immediately. Late one afternoon, the young mother's child is cranky and crying, so she pours about "one-half a dixie cup" of pepper into the child's mouth. The child becomes agitated, runs around the house making grunting noises, starts to convulse, and dies in agony. The frantic mother unsuccessfully tries to resuscitate the child and is shattered by its death.

Law versus medicine

The difficult dilemma that faces the forensic pathologist is differentiating abuse from other causes. As already explained, abuse can be an intermittent or even a single event. In the absence of multiple unexplained or unexplainable injuries of varying ages in the child, reaching an unequivocal conclusion of child abuse can be impossible.

As a result of the inability to reach a conclusion about abuse there is a common and serious conflict between medical and legal causality that hampers communication between the pathologist and the prosecutor. The doctor sees an effect, such as a lacerated liver, that may result from several similar but not identical causes. The doctor may be unable to determine "beyond a reasonable doubt" that abuse, to the exclusion of all other mechanisms, caused the results he or she discovers. Because we are legally, ethically, and morally bound not to experiment on children to determine the mechanisms, patterns, and forces involved in the creation of injuries, we can only infer from animal experiments or from retrospective studies of these tragic victims how and with what force a specific injury is produced. The *certainty* of causality aimed for in the law is far from realized, and the pathologist's certainty much diluted.

In a general sense, it is the very nature of a child's life that inevitably includes multiple bumps, bruises, lacerations, and even fractures and dislocations caused by accidents that makes differentiation so difficult for the pathologist. Child abuse cases do, however, tend to present a number of common findings on autopsy along with equally common and perplexing problems of differentiation.

Common findings

The problem for the pathologist with respect to the hemorrhage produced in the battered child is to determine that the trauma found was the result of more than one application of force. With regard to head trauma, for example, it may be difficult to surmise that a unilateral subdural hemorrhage is not due to a fall. If, however, the hemorrhage is multicentric, associated with several external lesions (particularly contusions or lacerations), or more than one abrasion, the implication is that either the child fell more than once after receiving an initial severe craniocerebral injury, or was hit several times, or bounced several times. It will be the pattern and multiplicity of injury that lend aid to the forensic pathologist in reaching a conclusion.

Typically, thoracic damage results from a combination of blows and squeezes. Multiple ribs may be fractured, either posteriorly or anteriorly, and may be displaced resulting in perforated lungs, heart, or liver. These internal injuries can cause excessive hemorrhage into the chest cavity and, if air is sucked into the chest cavity, can produce respiratory difficulty from pneumothorax. With the exception of a pure squeeze, the chest wall contuses more easily than the abdominal wall because the skin is closer to the semirigid ribs. These contusions are very common injuries found in the ignorant abuser situation because they can result from excessive though seemingly innocent squeezing.

The internal organs can, of course, receive trauma from any direction, and an unmarked epidermis can hide extensive internal bleeding and disruption of internal organs. The areas most vulnerable are the points of attachment of an internal organ, especially at the sources of its blood supply, and at points at which blood vessels change direction. One such area is the middle of the superior half of the abdomen. In this area are found several blood vessels changing direction, particularly the branches of the celiac truck and their branches, the hepatic, splenic, and gastric arteries and their branches, as well as the accompanying veins. The loop of duodenum, the ligament of Treitz, and the pancreas are in the retroperitoneal space, while the stomach and transverse colon are in the triangle located in the peritoneal cavity. Compression, whether prolonged as in a hug or squeeze, or momentary, as from a blow, is the mechanism of trauma, and a stretch-stress of sufficient acceleration-deceleration will detach the jejunum from the ligament of Treitz, lacerate the liver, contuse the intestines or stomach, and/or rupture any one of a number of blood vessels criss-crossing the area. Other direct blows, for example, a "kidney punch," may lacerate the kidney from behind, with bleeding into the space around the kidney that can be extensive. In this case, surface contusion is almost always present.

The result

As noted earlier, it is more important for the pathologist to be able to explain whether one blow or many caused the damage than to be able to explain all the lesions by mechanism. A child dying of multiple internal injuries manifesting bruises over the entire body, especially if the injuries are of different ages, is more likely to have been beaten than a child with one contusion in an exposed portion of the body, with internal injuries in the same area. The big problem comes when the parents allege that the child fell down a flight of steps. In this case, a careful cataloging of *all* lesions and on-site study of the steps may resolve the issue.

DRUG ABUSE
Drug abuse/drug excess

Contrary to what appears to be current popular opinion in the United States, drug abuse and drug-related deaths have not really abated since the advent of the sensationalized drug movement in the 1960s and 1970s; what has abated is the attention paid to this problem. Quite simply, the use and abuse of drugs in our society, although perhaps not accepted, are no longer news. This most unfortunate indifference has led to a serious dearth of information and education related to drug abuse and use. The forensic pathologist continues to be confronted with drug-related death that may often have been averted if the deceased had been more informed.

An interesting outgrowth has occurred in drug abuse during the past decade that frequently makes the forensic pathologist's task of determining the cause and manner of death most difficult. The outgrowth is an increasing problem with drug excess as opposed to drug abuse. That is, the multiplicity of drugs available and used, illegally or legally, has increased so dramatically that a demise is often the result of drug combinations rather than the abuse and overdose of a single entity. This problem has become significant in the medical profession as well as on the street.

Physicians are bombarded on an almost daily basis with new, improved, and modified drugs. The volume of drugs available for use in treatment makes it virtually impossible to remain current with every one and, more significantly, to be aware of and understand the ramifications of drug combinations. By themselves, most drugs are therapeutic; but, when prescribed along with other drugs, potentially lethal combinations and synergisms can result. This is an especially insidious problem when a team of physician/specialists treat a patient. Although the specialists may be completely familiar with the drugs they use within their narrow focus, they may well be totally unfamiliar with commonly prescribed drugs for treatment outside their specialty. The tragic result can be the clashing of drugs prescribed by the specialists or a synergistic effect causing untoward results or death.

What is abused and how to detect

At the interface between the law and medicine, forensic pathologists are charged with the responsibility of ascertaining the existence of drugs in the systems of a deceased, determining whether or not said drugs caused or contributed to the demise, and, finally, rendering an opinion as to whether or not drugs were used or abused. Below is a list of some of the more frequently abused drugs a forensic pathologist will identify in practice:

Opiates	Stimulants	Hallucinogens
Heroin	Cocaine	LSD
Morphine	Methamphetamine	Marijuana
Codeine	D-amphetamine	Mescaline
Methadone	Phenmetrazine	Psilocybin
Pethidine	Methylphenidate	Dimethyltryptamine

Depressants	Tranquilizers	Miscellaneous
Barbiturates	Thorazine	Propoxyphene
Glutethimide	Meprobamate	Pentazocine
Methyprylon	Chlordiazepoxide	Deleriants
Chloral hydrate	Diazepam	Amitriptyline
Ethchlorvynol	Oxazepam	
Paraldehyde		

Common scientific methods for detecting the presence of these drugs are gas-liquid chromatography (GLC), thin-layer chromatography (TLC), and spectrophoto-fluorometry (SPF).

TLC is the most widely employed test used to detect and identify drugs. Small amounts of the substance to be analyzed are touched to the edge of a glass plate coated with a thin layer of absorbent powder such as aluminum oxide. The plate is then partially immersed in a solvent that, by way of capillary action, will migrate up the plate carrying the unknown substance with it. Different drugs migrate at different known rates, which helps to identify them. In addition, the test plates are sprayed with various visualizing reagents that color react and, thus, further identify the subject drug. TLC is a highly sensitive and most accurate technique used by forensic pathologists in drug screening.

The SPF test subjects the unknown to a monochromatic light in the ultraviolet or near ultraviolet spectrum that will cause some unknowns to fluoresce. By recording the wavelengths of the light to which the unknown has been exposed and the specific wavelengths at which maximum fluorescence occurs, a unique identifying pattern may emerge representing a physical property of the unknown by which it can be identified.

In the GLC test, a thin tube is packed with an organosilicone liquid coated on a granular support. The unknown is then gasified and passed through the prepared tube and into a mechanical detector that produces peaks. Using the peaks and time required to pass through the tube at a given temperature, certain properties of the unknown can be determined and help in its identification. These are some of the more common techniques employed to detect and identify drugs in a deceased. Their use, however, requires a more basic determination that drugs may have been involved in a death.

Drug death—or not

The frequently subtle differentiation between natural and drug-induced death, or between the death of a person undergoing legitimate medical drug treatment and drug abuse death, may be impossible to achieve in the absence of some forewarning to the investigating pathologist. Pathological findings that could properly be attributed to natural or nondrug-related etiology may well be natural medical complications arising from drug use or abuse. Being unaware of drug-related possibilities could easily make the forensic pathologist's opinion as to manner of death completely inaccurate. A properly conducted investigation, however, tends to reveal certain factors that will alert the pathologist and usually eliminate inaccuracies in the determination.

The pathologist's first hint may come from the deceased. Unexplained coma followed by death or irrational behavior prior to a bizarre act resulting in death, especially in younger people, raises the possibility of a drug-related death. An investigation of the scene of death often reveals evidence such as needles, tourniquets, spoons for heating or measuring drugs, discarded plastic bags, syringes, burned matches, and other drug-related paraphernalia that may well point to a drug-related demise. Even the location of the body when discovered, such as the bathroom (a common place for intravenous injection), may be helpful when combined with other information. Although the autopsy in a suspected drug-related death follows the usual scientific routine, certain findings and observations peculiar to drug users and abusers are commonly found.

During external examination, special care will be taken to find and identify needle marks indicative of the injection of drugs. These marks are often concealed by the abuser in order to reduce obvious evidence of drug use and may be found interspersed with tattoos, between the toes, in the gums, and in creases and folds of skin almost anywhere on the body. Abscesses, scarring, and sores are common due to scratching of the skin surface with contaminated paraphernalia in order to inject drugs intradermally (skin popping). Stains on fingertips from capsule dyes may indicate drug abuse and the color may actually be helpful in identifying the abused drug. Froth exuding from the nose and mouth is a common indicator of severe pulmonary edema and congestion that may result from death due to the use of depressants.

Internal examination usually generates little specific definitive information. The most common finding is

pulmonary edema and congestion that, though nonspecific, is almost a constant and, thus, helpful in identifying drug-related death. The gastrointestinal contents sometimes reveal traces of pills and capsules and, occasionally, the dye from capsules tinge the mucosa with an unnatural color. Examination of the nasal passages and nasopharynx sometimes reveal irritation or even traces of drugs (usually cocaine) that are commonly inhaled through the nose (snorted).

Microscopic examination tends to be nonspecific in drug deaths; but certain findings are more commonly observed in drug deaths than in other kinds of deaths. These include pulmonary edema, congestion, focal hemorrhage, bronchitis and, peculiarly, granulomas. Granulomas result from the intravenous injection of foreign substances such as starch, textile fibers, or talcum, either because these substances are used to dilute or cut the drug being abused or because the injection was sloppy and picked up clothing fibers. It is also not uncommon to find evidence of thrombosis, thrombophlebitis, and viral hepatitis from the use of needles.

As might be expected, the most significant finding will be made during toxicological analysis. Using the earlier mentioned gas-liquid chromatography, thin-layer chromatography, and spectrophotofluorometry, as well as other sophisticated techniques, the forensic toxicologist can identify the presence and concentration of drugs. The samples of choice in these analyses are blood and urine, although nasal secretions, gastric contents, bile, and tissue from the liver, kidneys, or lungs may be necessary to make a definitive determination of drug type and concentration.

DNA

Scientists have successfully analyzed traces of deoxyribonucleic acid (DNA) from single human hairs in research expected to have important applications in crime detection and many other areas. Hair is one of the most frequently found forms of biological evidence at crime scenes, so identification of hair can be of considerable forensic importance.

Analysis of DNA, the substance of the genes, has emerged in recent years as an important aid in solving crimes in addition to its other uses. But there is far too little DNA in a single hair for analysis by conventional means. Less than 10 billionths of a gram of DNA can usually be recovered from a fallen hair. Yet, the most common method of analysis requires several millionths of a gram. Furthermore, the DNA from such a hair is usually degraded, so that only small fragments are available for study.

To cope with these problems, researchers use a relatively new method, called the polymerase chain reaction, to make millions of copies of a DNA fragment. The copy making is known as gene amplification, and it makes enough DNA available from the fragment being studied to permit analysis. The same method can be applied to blood or semen when the sample is too small or too poorly preserved to be studied by conventional means.

As used today, the chain reaction method does not permit absolute identification of the source of a piece of DNA, but if analyzed thoroughly, the material can be used to determine which of several suspects it might have come from and which suspects can be ruled out. This is essentially how blood types are used in deciding whether a sample of blood may have come from a suspect.

However, DNA typing with the new method can discriminate with far greater precision than blood typing. Potentially, the typing can approach the precision of a fingerprint, a degree of accuracy already possible with conventional DNA analysis, provided that a sufficiently large sample is available.

The typing involved in cases for evidence at a crime scene means determining which of several chemical variants of a single gene an individual has. In the research on disease susceptibility, scientists have analyzed HLA genes, a group of genes that are important in human tissue typing to match recipients and organ donors. The techniques used in the analyses of hairs would also be useful in choosing donor organs for transplants, in determining susceptibility, or lack of it, to some diseases, and in research in other fields.

New developments and criticisms

Recently, several molecular biologists have questioned the validity of the technique used in identifying suspects in criminal trials through the analysis of genetic material. Some scientists say that for both theoretical and practical reasons, DNA fingerprinting cannot be counted on to decide with virtual certainty whether a person is guilty of a crime. The problem is that the DNA fingerprints can stretch and shift, like a design printed on rubber, making them difficult, if not impossible, to interpret. Even without these shifts, DNA patterns can be almost impossible to compare, and scientific underpinnings have not been established for determining just how unlikely it would be for DNA fingerprints from two people to match by accident.

DNA evidence, described to proponents as capable of precisely identifying or ruling out suspects based on analyses of the genetic material in a drop of blood or in a semen stain found at the scene of a crime, has been introduced in hundreds of criminal cases. In several instances, the cases were thrown out because of criticisms of the way particular laboratories did the testing.

The National Academy of Sciences has established an expert committee to study the scientific basis of the technique. The Federal Office of Technology Assessment is also studying the method and preparing a report for Congress.

In theory, molecular biologists believe that the use of DNA evidence should work because it relies on the generally accepted fact that individuals have distinctive patterns of sequences of DNA. But, critics say, it is a long way from theory to having a practical test.

CONCLUSION

Virtually any situation involving an interface between law and medicine may call for the specialized expertise of a forensic pathologist. It is their background in both law and medicine that uniquely qualifies forensic pathologists to stand at the nexus and serve as the necessary bridge between these two fields. Presented here was only a small sampling of situations encountered in the daily practice of forensic pathology. Hopefully, the examples have provided a feel for the practical and actual application of this discipline to everyday life as well as the methods and techniques employed in doing so. Most important, it is hoped that the nontechnical nature of forensic pathology has been shown in this chapter; that is, the critical and necessary application of common sense grounded in expertise that is frequently required to reach the conclusions of the manner and cause of death.

Several recent court decisions in various jurisdictions have conferred the benefit of governmental immunity on coroners and medical examiners in lawsuits alleging administrative or professional negligence relating to the determination of cause and manner of death. These judicial rulings are based on the premise that both elected coroners and appointed medical examiners are public officers. Hence, even if their decisions are subsequently proven to have been incorrect, as long as they were made in "good faith" with no evidence of "malice," the pathologist, acting in an official capacity as coroner or medical examiner or their agent, will be entitled to governmental immunity. These decisions are consistent with long-standing concepts set forth in administrative law and common law.

The "Rosario" rule (named after a 1961 case in which it was first enunciated) states that prosecutors must give the defendant's attorney any relevant written or recorded statement made by a witness who is expected to testify in a criminal proceeding. The rule, which has been upheld by the New York Court of Appeals as recently as December 1992, was developed to preserve constitutional guarantees of due process and the right to cross-examine an accuser.

Several cases are now pending in New York and

elsewhere in which defense attorneys in homicide cases have appealed their clients' convictions, stating that the district attorney prior to or during the trial never turned over the medical examiner's original tape recording of the autopsy to the defense. Even if it is argued that such items are the "duplicative equivalent" of material previously given to the defense, a strict application of the Rosario rule could result in a new trial being ordered by the appellate court. Defense attorneys argue that inasmuch as a medical examiner's report is an essential component of every homicide case, that official governmental medicolegal investigative facility (coroner or medical examiner) performs a law enforcement function and has an active relationship with the prosecutor's office.

If the appellate courts in pending cases find that medical examiners have that kind of connection to prosecutors, then the district attorney's office may eventually be responsible not only for turning over the original autopsy tape recording, but also for searching the medical examiner's entire case file for any items (e.g., notes, diagrams, sketches, memos, research material, etc.) to which defense lawyers would be entitled.

GENERAL REFERENCES

Davis and Mistry, *The Pathology Curriculum in US Medical Schools,* III Arch. Pathol. Lab. Med. 1088-1092 (1987).

DiMaio and DiMaio, *Forensic Pathology* (Elsevier Science Publishing Co., New York 1989).

Jachimczyk, *The Postmortem Examination,* 2 Trauma 58 (1961).

Landefeld et al., *Diagnostic Yield of the Autopsy in a University Hospital and a Community Hospital,* 318 New Engl. J. Med 1249-1254 (1988).

Leetsma, *Interpretation of Head Injuries in Infants and Children, in Forensic Neuropathology* (Raven Press, New York 1988).

Sturner, *Sudden Unexpected Infant Death,* in 1971 Legal Medicine Annual (Appleton-Century-Crofts, New York).

Svendsen and Hill, *Autopsy Legislation and Practice in Various Countries,* III Arch. Pathol. Lab. Med. 846-850 (1987).

Wecht, *Relationships of the Medical Examiner,* 14 Cleveland-Marshall Law Rev. 427-441 (Sept. 1965).

Wecht, *The Medicolegal Autopsy Laws of the Fifty States, the District of Columbia, America Samoa, the Canal Zone, Guam, Puerto Rico, and the Virgin Islands* (rev. ed., Armed Forces Institute of Pathology 1977).

Wecht, ed. *Forensic Sciences* (3 vols., Matthew Bender & Co., New York 1982).

Wetli et al., *Practical Forensic Pathology* (Igaku-Shoin Medical Publishers, New York 1988).

CHAPTER 43

Psychiatric patients and forensic psychiatry

MARVIN H. FIRESTONE, M.D., J.D., F.C.L.M.*

MENTAL STATE AND THE LAW
THERAPEUTIC METHODS
CIVIL RIGHTS
PSYCHIATRY AND CRIMINAL LAW
PSYCHIATRIC MALPRACTICE
REFUSAL OF MEDICATION
NEUROPSYCHIATRY AND FORENSIC ISSUES

MENTAL STATE AND THE LAW

Consideration of the role of a person's mental status by the law is by no means a recent development. Writings in the Old Testament, Egyptian, Greek, and Roman laws indicate early attempts by human beings to comprehend and incorporate the role of the mind with the rules of society.[1] As humans developed in sophistication, so did the awareness that human behavior was composed of two parts: muscle activity (*actus rea* in criminal jurisprudence) and mental state (*mens rea* or guilty mind as it is later called). Early recognition of these two components can be traced to the Romans' description of a person's loss of certain mental capacities as *non compos mentis*.

The implementation of psychology and psychiatry in a formal legal forum did not really evolve until the late 1700s. Prior to this time, the pronouncement of insanity or unsoundness of mind was the function of the presiding village or town bishop, pursuant to ecclesiastical law. It was not until around the end of the century that physicians began to be recognized as having special knowledge regarding a person's mental status. For example, in 1788, Doctors John, Willis, and Francis attended King George III for an attack of "phrenzy fever," which in effect was the equivalent of a manic episode.[2] Later, during a subsequent attack, Drs. He-

berden and Baker were consulted for medical advice, as the king's peculiar behavior became more public.

Only a few years later, French physician Philippe Pinel established psychiatry as a cognizable branch of medicine through the writing of his treatise on insanity,[3] while Benjamin Rush of Philadelphia established himself as the founder of American psychiatry by virtue of authoring the text *Medical Inquiries and Observations Upon Disease of the Mind.*[4] Despite these developments, psychiatrists during this time were only infrequently called into court to address the issue of criminal responsibility. In 1828, the medicolegal status of mental illness and true genesis of what is commonly referred to as forensic psychiatry was formally planted by an American, Dr. Isaac Ray, through the writing of his *Treatise of Medical Jurisprudence of Insanity.* The state of legal medicine at that time was aptly illustrated by Ray when he wrote in his introduction: "[T]he English language does not furnish a single work in which the various forms and degrees of mental derangement are treated in reference to their effects on the rights and duties of man."[5]

In the area of criminal law, the evaluation of insanity and competency to stand trial remains a dominant function. However, psychiatrists are also directly involved in a wide number of roles in the criminal justice process as well—from arrest interrogation to sentencing, corrections, and parole review. In many ways, psychiatrists and other mental health professionals have con-

*The author gratefully acknowledges work by previous contributors, Joseph T. Smith, M.D., J.D., F.C.L.M.; Steven B. Bisbing, Psy.D., J.D.; and Harold L. Hirsh, M.D., J.D., F.C.L.M.

585

tributed greatly to the evolution of the modern criminal justice system.

THERAPEUTIC METHODS

The use of various psychotropic medications represents the primary organic therapy used by psychiatrists. Typically grouped into three distinct classes—the antipsychotic drugs, the antidepressants, and antimanic agents—each of these drugs creates a relatively powerful biological action within the body and brain that affects specific symptoms of certain mental disorders. A fourth class comprised of the antianxiety agents, stimulants, and sedative-hypnotic agents, is less symptom-specific, and they produce their chemical effect regardless of the presence of a mental illness.

Electroconvulsive therapy and psychosurgery

Electroconvulsive therapy (ECT) and particularly psychosurgery have experienced a continuous decline in use and popularity since their position of prominence in the 1950s and 1960s. Accordingly, the incidence of litigation involving either of these two treatments is fairly rare.

Psychosurgery procedures, although rarely done today, require in some cases a court order and detailed affidavit demonstrating that a thorough disclosure of all relevant information has been given and an informed and competent consent was obtained.

Psychotherapy

The techniques and therapy procedures employed by psychiatrists differ in many respects from those of other medical doctors. Except for the use of psychotropic medication and the rare application of ECT, the procedures applied by the psychiatrist do not involve the physical contact commonplace in other medical practices. This is because psychiatrists deal with the feelings, emotions, and mental experiences of their patients. In doing so, a primary means of intervention is the use of verbal psychotherapy, a verbal rhetoric wherein the therapist utilizes his or her knowledge, insight, and perceptions of the patient's behavior in an attempt to help the patient to alter maladaptive behaviors or thought patterns.

Psychotropic medications

There now are numerous antianxiety, antipsychotic, and antidepressant medications that have been shown to have therapeutic efficiency. Lithium salts and carbamazepine have also been effective in controlling bipolar (manic-depressive) affective disorders. Several other medications (e.g., thyroxine, propranolol, valproic acid, amantadine, and trihexyphenidyl) have been found to be therapeutic as adjuncts and to control the side effects of other psychotropic medications.

CIVIL RIGHTS
Voluntary hospitalization

There are essentially two ways mentally ill persons can be admitted to a psychiatric hospital or institution. The first is to be involuntarily committed. The other, and more common means, is for the individual to voluntarily sign in, which is similar to a patient entering a general medical facility. In other words, admission is effected through what is legally and clinically presumed to be a free and voluntary action on the part of the patient.

Voluntary or consensual hospitalization of the mentally ill is a relatively new idea. Massachusetts enacted the first voluntary admission statute as far back as 1881, but other states were very slow to follow. In fact, by 1949 only 10% of all mental patients were voluntary admissions. For approximately the next 20 years, states struggled to amend and revise their commitment laws in order to define and establish realistic procedures for voluntary admission. By 1972, most psychiatric admissions were voluntary.

The purpose of voluntary hospitalization for the mentally ill is to dispel the coercion, trauma, and stigma normally associated with involuntary hospitalization, and afford the same opportunity for treatment to mentally ill patients that is available to those suffering from physical illness.

The majority of states now provide for two forms of consensual admission: informal voluntary hospitalization (pure) and formal voluntary hospitalization (conditional). The distinction between these two has to do with the regulations governing discharge. In the case of voluntary informal admission, the patient must be released on request. Some states will limit, by law or policy, the scope of this form of admission due to the potential for patient manipulation. The more formal or conditional form of voluntary admission permits the hospital to detain a patient for a specified period of time following a request for discharge. For example, South Dakota permits "[R]elease within at least five days—excluding Saturday, Sunday and holidays—from request."[6] The conditional release is designed to provide institutions adequate time to evaluate a patient with respect to possibly initiating involuntary commitment proceedings. Initiation of these proceedings thus allows a hospital to detain a patient for either the statutorily mandated time or, in some cases, for as long as it takes to convene a commitment hearing. The rationale behind the allotment of additional time for possible commitment is therapeutic, because it provides patients who may be angry, impulsive, or manipulative an opportunity to reconsider their request for discharge. This extra time also affords the clinical staff a chance to develop outpatient treatment plans if the patient remains undeterred in desiring to leave.

One issue of increasing importance in relation to the idea of voluntary hospitalization of the mentally ill is the question of competency to consent. Presumably, the act of voluntarily entering a psychiatric hospital requires the patient to be legally competent to make such a decision. Many of the first statutes authorizing voluntary commitment made the requirement of competency a specific element. The rationale for such a strict requirement was, at least in part, to prevent clearly incompetent patients from being improperly manipulated by psychiatrists and mental hospitals. This concern is clearly elaborated in the case of *Application for William R.*:

I have previously called to the attention of the organized Bar (see N.U.L.J. Editorial 1/29/58) that the pink form is being increasingly used by the Department of Mental Hygiene for the transfer and admission to state mental institutions, without judicial consideration, of most of the senile aged who do not make positive objection, and that it accounted for more than 1,000 such transfers within a period of nine months in 1957 from Kings County Hospital alone. I pointed out that this is a development of recent date, conceived as a technique for circumventing judicial sanction, due to much criticism by judges and doctors alike of certification procedures of aged seniles to state mental institutions as being morally wrong. This newly used technique effectively shunts seniles into involuntary confinement without awareness by them of their plight and without their actual approval or judicial surveillance. These unwanted seniles may not even hope to escape factually involuntary confinement because the possibility of private care, often provided at a judicial hearing, is denied to them and of course, they cannot thereafter effect their own release.[7]

More recent laws, however, designed to encourage voluntary admission and based on a theory that it ensures needed treatment, omit such requirements in all but a minority of states. The dilemma regarding the issue of a patient's competency to be hospitalized voluntarily remains unresolved. To date, the question of whether a patient by voluntary admission must be competent to exercise an informed consent has not been authoritatively addressed by any court. This lack of judicial scrutiny is largely a consequence of present-day voluntary admission procedures. A person who either has been coerced into voluntarily signing in or lacks the capacity to fully comprehend the consequences of the application for admission is unlikely to have any grounds on which to raise either issue since, at any time, a request for discharge can be made. Such an individual would then be either released pursuant to that request or committed pursuant to state involuntary commitment statutes. In either event, at least in theory, the issue of invalid or improper voluntary admission would have been negated, thereby preventing any court from hearing the significant issues surrounding this aspect of the voluntary admission process.

Rights of the voluntary patient. The rights of the voluntary psychiatric patient are unclear in most cases, and at best, inconsistently applied in courts that have addressed this issue. Primarily, the question of "rights" revolves around three areas: (1) access to in-patient treatment, (2) the legal right to refuse unwanted treatment, and (3) the ability to be discharged when so desired.

To date, there have been no reported cases that have squarely addressed the question of whether there is a "right to in-patient treatment" for the voluntary patient under state or federal law. Individual states have been left to develop their own laws regarding the acceptance and discharge of voluntary patients. For example, a Missouri voluntary discharge statute reads: "He [hospital director] may discharge any voluntary patient if to do so would, in the judgment of the head of the hospital, contribute to the most effective use of the hospital in the care and treatment of the mentally ill."[8]

This seemingly arbitrary basis for discharge is quite similar to statutory language common in admission statutes. The issue of a patient's right to admission is as much a social question as it is clinical, since it undoubtedly encompasses the question of whether individuals unable to afford in-patient psychiatric services may be denied access to such treatment on the basis of economic status. This question remains unresolved.

Similarly, the right to immediate discharge is the subject of much debate. From a practical perspective, most voluntary admissions are accepted on a conditional basis since informal admissions tend to be more costly in terms of staff time and resources (e.g., administrative paperwork must be completed every time a patient chooses to leave). Therefore, the majority of patients are subject to mandatory detention, a provision that greatly limits the patient's freedom to decide when he or she wishes to be released.

The question of whether a voluntary patient has the right to refuse treatment (e.g., psychotropic medication) and remain as a patient has been rejected by at least one appellate court. In *Rogers v. Okin,*[9] the court rejected a lower court's finding of such a right to refuse treatment and instead concluded that applicable state statutes (Massachusetts) provided no such guarantee that voluntary patients had a choice of treatment. Instead, they concluded that state law left decisions regarding the treatment of patients to the judgment and discretion of the hospital doctors and staff.

Despite this holding, the issue of the rights of voluntary patients remains far from settled. For the latest U.S. Supreme Court rulings on this issue, see additional case law material at the end of this chapter.

Involuntary hospitalization

Basis and rationale. Involuntary hospitalization of civil commitment refers to state-imposed involuntary detention or restrictions of personal freedom based on a determination that a person is mentally ill and dangerous to self or others.

The institution of the civil commitment process is based on two fundamental common law principles. The first relates to the right of the government, provided by the U.S. Constitution to the individual states, to take whatever actions are necessary to ensure the safety of its citizens. Commonly referred to as the police power, this authority is limited by the states' constitutions and by the Fourteenth Amendment of the U.S. Constitution.

The other rationale used to justify the involuntary commitment of mentally ill persons is the *parens patriae* doctrine. This concept, which denotes that the state is acting in place of the parent, prescribes that the "sovereign has both the right and the duty to protect the person and the property of those who are unable to care [for] themselves because of minority or mental illness."[10] From a practical perspective, numerous state statutes and case law in an attempt to cut back the broadness of certain state commitment provisions have either abolished the *parens patriae* rationale or made it contingent on a finding of dangerousness (e.g., thereby invoking the salient purpose of the police power).

Commitment standards. The civil commitment process can be viewed in terms of two interrelated elements: (1) the criteria or standards governing whether someone is committable and (2) the procedural rules regulating the process itself.

In nearly every jurisdiction, the basic criteria for involuntary civil commitment are the product of a statute. The wording and interpretation of the various commitment laws differ from state to state but the standards for commitment are generally similar.

Typically, all states require an individual to demonstrate clear and convincing evidence of at least two separate and distinct elements. The first pertains to the individual's mental condition. Nearly every state requires a threshold finding that a person suffers from some mental illness, disorder, or disease.

The second and often more critical requirement is a determination that some "specific adverse consequence" will ensue, as a result of the mental illness, if the person is not confined. Commonly couched in language such as "likely to harm self or others," "poses a real and present threat of substantial harm to self or others," or "dangerous to himself or others," this element is frequently referred to in references as simply the "danger to self or others" requirement. In some states, such as Delaware and Hawaii, this element is extended to harm to property as well as persons.

Closely related to both the mental illness and dangerousness requirements is the standard of "gravely disabled." This standard is somewhat similar to the mental condition requirement, since it typically applies to a person's ability to care for himself or herself. This is not a uniform standard like the other two criteria, but represents an attempt by a minority of states to provide a broader description of the kind of manifest behavior that may prompt commitment. An example of a state statute applying the gravely disabled standard is the following:

Gravely disabled means that a person, as a result of mental or emotional impairment, is in danger of serious harm as a result of an inability or failure to provide for his or her own basic human needs such as essential food, clothing, shelter or safety and that hospital care is necessary and available and that such person is mentally incapable of determining whether or not to accept treatment because his judgment is impaired by his mental illness.[11]

Commitment procedures. Nearly all states provide two basic methods or procedures by which an individual can be taken against his or her will and transferred to a psychiatric facility for detention and examination. The first procedure is referred to as the emergency commitment, which, under appropriate circumstances, permits the commitment of an individual without any prior formal due process hearing. The second procedure is based on a court order that follows a formal hearing, held prior to the confinement of the individual.

The emergency commitment procedure can generally be initiated by any adult who signs a petition under oath, asserting that immediate treatment is needed for the safety of an individual. This petition is typically accompanied by at least one, and sometimes two, certificates of examination by a qualified examiner. These certificates attest that the examiner, commonly a psychiatrist, physician, or clinical psychologist, has concluded that the individual is in need of immediate treatment and is likely to pose a threat of danger to self or others. The executed petition and certificates are then presented to either the police or a mental health facility, in order to effectuate the taking into custody and transportation of the individual to a psychiatric facility. In many states, the police are permitted to take a person they believe requires immediate hospitalization into custody, and to a psychiatric facility without certification by a qualified examiner. However, this form of abbreviated commitment is usually valid for only one day unless a certificate is subsequently executed. In any event, all individuals involuntarily committed under emergency procedures must be provided a judicial-type hearing to ascertain further need for commitment within a statutorily prescribed time, which may vary from one to six weeks.

In the absence of an emergency, most states permit the involuntary commitment of an individual following a more formal admission process. Commonly referred to as commitment by court order, this procedure may also be initiated by any adult who has reason to believe an individual is in need of hospitalization. A petition is filed with the court and in some cases accompanied by at least one certificate executed by a qualified examiner. Pursuant to the submitted petition, regardless of certification, the court is then authorized to order the individual to undergo a psychiatric evaluation. Upon confirmation that the individual indeed needs hospitalization, a formal hearing is scheduled to adjudicate the individual's need for commitment. The hearing serves to determine whether the statutory conditions for commitment are met.

In essence, the basic difference between the two procedures for commitment is the timing of the formal hearing: before court-ordered commitment or after emergency commitment. The procedures described reflect the general form of the two methods used in most jurisdictions, but the precise requirements, procedural safeguard, and time requirements differ greatly from state to state. Therefore, it behooves any clinician, attorney, or advocate involved in this area of law to become thoroughly familiar with the particular state's statutory requirements.

Least restrictive alternative. Up to the late 1960s, a patient civilly committed to a state institution could expect to remain there for a major portion, if not the duration, of his or her life. Commonly criticized as mere human warehousing, the vast majority of mental institutions in America were a miserable failure at achieving anything remotely therapeutic. Usually, the best a civilly committed patient could hope for was bare minimum custodial care. The thought of ever leaving the institution was a fleeting fantasy for many patients, and those who were discharged were rarely any better off than when they were admitted.

It was not uncommon for patients legitimately committed due to mental illness, and posing risk of danger, to remain hospitalized far beyond the time when one or both of these conditions no longer existed. However, since states rarely required the periodic evaluation of those who have been civilly committed, a patient could literally waste away in the hospital despite no longer qualifying for detention. This situation represented a serious abridgement of the civil liberties of mental patients and spurred considerable concern by libertarians, scholars, and civil rights activists.

In 1966, the case *Lake v. Cameron,*[12] (applying D.C. law) signaled a significant advancement in the recognition of civil rights of the mentally disabled. *Lake* involved the involuntary commitment of a 60-year-old woman diagnosed as senile, but not considered a danger to herself or others. Writing for the majority, Chief Judge Bazelon held that a person could not be involuntarily committed to a psychiatric hospital if alternative placements could be found that were less restrictive on a patient's constitutional right to liberty. From this opinion was developed the doctrine of the "least restrictive alternative" (LRA), which at least in theory recognized and sought to protect the liberty rights of patients that were so routinely ignored in the past.

Following the *Lake* decision, numerous states adopted legislation requiring courts to consider less restrictive alternatives, whenever appropriate. In the absence of statutory authority, several lower federal courts upheld the validity of the LRA doctrine based on implied constitutional grounds. This implied reasoning was addressed in the seminal case, *Lessard v. Schmidt:*

> Even if the standards for an adjudication of mental illness and potential dangerousness are satisfied, a court should order full-time involuntary hospitalization only as a last resort. A basic concept in American justice is the principle that "even though the governmental purpose [might] be legitimate and substantial, that purpose cannot be pursued by means that broadly stifle fundamental personal liberties when the end can be more narrowly achieved. The breadth of legislative abridgment must be viewed in light of less drastic means for achieving the same basic purpose. [citations omitted][13]

The LRA doctrine has been applied to numerous other forms of restraint of a patient's liberty within the hospitalization process (e.g., the use of physical restraints and seclusion rooms). In extending the scope of the doctrine to other treatment procedures, respect for a patient's civil rights is acknowledged, the hospitalization experience becomes less stigmatizing, and positive patient-staff relations are fostered.

Despite the social, therapeutic, and psychological value of the LRA doctrine, its application is subject to severe limitations. As Chief Judge Bazelon held in *Lake,* a less restrictive alternative must actually exist in order for the doctrine to apply.

From a practical standpoint this presents a major setback in most cases since such less restrictive alternatives rarely are available. The practical value of the LRA doctrine is, therefore, limited unless the courts take the initiative to create, or order, alternative placements. In the absence of legislative authority, it is extremely doubtful that this is going to happen.

Rights of the civilly committed patient. The right to treatment/habilitation, to the basic necessities of life, to refuse treatment, and to treatment in the least restrictive environment have all been litigated and afforded varying degrees of protection.

The concept of a right to treatment was first articulated in 1960 when Dr. Morton Birnbaum proposed that:

The courts, under their traditional powers to protect the constitutional rights of our citizens begin to consider the problem of whether or not a person who has been institutionalized solely because he is sufficiently mentally ill to require institutionalization for care and treatment actually does receive adequate medical treatment so that he may regain his health, and therefore his liberty, as soon as possible; that the courts do this by means of *recognizing and enforcing the right to treatment;* and, that the courts do this, independent of any action by any legislature, as a necessary and overdue development of our present concept of due process of law. [emphasis in original][14]

A constitutional right to treatment, or to "habilitation," was held to apply to mentally disabled individuals in the landmark case *Wyatt v. Stickney.*[15] The court held that in the absence of the opportunity to receive treatment, mentally disabled individuals in institutions were not patients, but were residents with indefinite sentences. Further, the court stated that basic custodial care or punishment was not the purpose of involuntary hospitalization. The purpose, they concluded, was treatment. In its subsequent opinions, the court developed an extensive remedial plan that was intended to establish minimum constitutional standards for adequate treatment and habilitation of the mentally disabled.

A second basic constitutional right, the right to liberty, was addressed in the Supreme Court decision *O'Connor v. Donaldson.*[16] Donaldson had been involuntarily confined in a state mental institution for almost 15 years and was suing the state for depriving him of his constitutional right to liberty. In the first award ever granted to a mental patient based on a violation of constitutional rights, Donaldson received $20,000 in damages. The court, in addressing the deprivation of liberty that involuntary confinement imposed, concluded that three conditions had to be met in order to justify release: (1) the institution was not offering proper treatment; (2) the patient did not present a danger to self or others; (3) the person was capable of living in the community with the assistance of family or friends. Although these narrow conditions were illuminated in later litigation, *Donaldson* laid the foundation for future constitutional litigation regarding the rights of the mentally ill.

The issue of the right to refuse treatment has not yet been squarely addressed by the U.S. Supreme Court. The issue of whether an involuntarily committed mental patient has a constitutional right to refuse treatment (antipsychotic medication) was before the high court in 1982 in *Mills v. Rogers,*[17] but was sidestepped and sent back to a lower federal court for reconsideration.

Despite the Supreme Court's refusal to decide *Mills,* several lower federal courts have sought to resolve the right to refuse treatment issue. In one of the most noted cases, *Rennie v. Klein,*[18] the Court of Appeals for the 3rd Circuit affirmed the finding that a constitutional right to refuse treatment existed. However, the appeals court differed from the lower court when it adopted a "least intrusive means" analysis. Under this analysis, antipsychotic drugs could be forcibly administered in a non-emergency situation to patients who had never been adjudicated incompetent, only if such treatment was the least restrictive mode of treatment available.

A year after *Rennie,* the U.S. Supreme Court held in the landmark case of *Youngberg v. Romeo*[19] that mentally retarded residents of state institutions had a constitutional right to the basic necessities of life, reasonably safe living conditions, freedom from undue restraints, and the minimally adequate training needed to enhance or further their abilities to exercise other constitutional rights. Of significant importance to future civil rights cases involving the mentally disabled, was the court's deference to the judgment of qualified professionals to establish minimal adequate training and to safeguard a patient's liberty interests. In seeking to minimize judicial interference in the daily administration of institutions, the court held that "liability may be imposed only when the decision is such a substantial departure from accepted professional judgment, practice or standards as to demonstrate that the person responsible actually did not base the decision on such a judgment."[20]

The full impact of *Youngberg* has yet to be determined but at least one significant civil rights case, *Rennie v. Klein,* has been redefined because of it. In 1983, the 3rd Circuit Court of Appeals rejected the "least intrusive means analysis" and adopted the standard of "whether the patient constitutes a danger to himself or others" in determining whether medication can be forcibly administered.[21]

PSYCHIATRY AND CRIMINAL LAW

The purpose and rationale for the system of criminal justice in the United States are based on four fundamental concepts: isolation, retribution, deterrence, and rehabilitation.

As far back as biblical times, the issue of crime and punishment was premised on the notion of intent. The idea of wrongful or criminal guilt inherently required two elements: (1) that the wrongdoer commit an act or misdeed and, more important, (2) that the act was the product of a willing and rational intent. In other words, a crime is made up of two essential components: (1) voluntary conduct *(actus rea)* and (2) intent or guilty mind *(mens rea).*

An exception to a finding of criminal guilt has historically been reserved for minors and the mentally disabled. For example, in Babylonian times Jewish law held that "it is an ill thing to knock against a deaf mute, an imbecile or a minor: he that wounds them is culpable, but if they wound others they are not culpable."[22] Centuries later, a secular pronouncement was contained in the Justinian Digest:

[T]here are those who are not to be held accountable, such is not a madman and a child who is not capable of malicious intention: these persons are able to suffer a wrong but not to produce one. Since a wrong is only able to exist by the intention of those who have committed it, it follows that these persons, whether they have assaulted by blows or insulted by words, are not considered to have committed a wrong.[23]

In 1265, Bracton, Chief Justice of England, wrote the first systematic treatise on English law and in it stated that neither child nor madman could be liable since both lacked the felonious intent necessary for an act to be considered criminal. He likened the acts of an insane person, lacking in mind and reason, to be not far removed from that of a brutish animal.[24] Other notable jurists, including Lord Hale, Chief Justice Mansfield, and Chief Justice Holmes in this country have all recognized the need to excuse from criminal responsibility any person incapable of forming the requisite criminal intent.[25]

Competency to stand trial. Our society's sense of morality dictates that an individual who is unable to comprehend the nature and the object of the proceedings against him or her, to confer with counsel, and assist in the preparation of his or her own defense may not be subjected to a criminal trial. The oft-quoted legal theorist, Blackstone, in defining this common law rule said:

If a man in his sound memory commits a capital offense, and before arraignment for it, he becomes mad, he ought not be arraigned for it; because he is not able to plead to it with that advice and caution that he ought. And if, after he has pleaded, the prisoner becomes mad, he shall not be tried; for how can he make his defense?[26]

Borrowing from this common law principle, one of the fundamental tenets of American jurisprudence is the entitlement of every defendant to be afforded a fair and adequate hearing. In order for this requirement of fairness to be effectuated, it is necessary that the individual litigant be capable of meaningful participation in the ongoing events of the legal process. The requirement that a litigant be competent in order to stand trial is of such moral and philosophical importance to our system of justice that it is considered a fundamental element, and recognized as a constitutional right. In *Pate v. Robinson,* the Supreme Court held "that the failure to observe a defendant's right not to be tried or convicted while incompetent to stand trial deprives him of his due process right to a fair trial."[27]

Despite the constitutional recognition that a defen-

dant must be competent at the time of the trial, the determination and parameters of this fundamental principle have been the source of continued ambiguity. For example, such common mental status criteria as orientation to time and place and the capacity to recollect past events have been found to be insufficient in determining trial competency. Various states have established standards by which to measure a defendant's competency to stand trial. At a bare minimum, it is sufficient to say that the fundamental fairness of law requires at least a finding of competency consistent with the test developed in *Dusky v. United States:* "[T]he test must be whether he has sufficient present ability to consult with his lawyer with a reasonable degree of rational as well as factual understanding of the proceedings against him."[28]

From the general nature of this test, it is easy to see that dispute and controversy are not uncommon in a case where a defendant's capacity is at issue. While numerous federal and state decisions have sought to devise a more objective test, none has been totally successful. As a rule, any substantial impairment that interferes with a defendant's capacity to communicate, testify coherently, or follow the proceedings of the trial with a "reasonable degree of rational understanding" will lead to a determination of incompetency.

The determination of competency is essentially a threefold procedural process. The first step can be characterized as the trigger stage. Both prosecution and the defense, as well as the court, may raise or trigger the issue of incompetency whenever there is a suggestion that the defendant may not be competent to stand trial. In fact, the trial court is under constitutional obligation to recognize and respond to any evidence that the defendant may not be mentally fit for trial. Once the issue has been raised, neither the defendant nor counsel can waive the issue and have the case brought to trial. Fundamental fairness of law requires that a defendant be competent throughout a trial.[29]

After raising the issue of a defendant's competency, it is common procedure for the court to appoint one or more independent experts to conduct a psychiatric examination. Two issues, one procedural and one substantive, are important to note. While in most jurisdictions a question of competency automatically triggers an impartial psychiatric examination, a defendant has no constitutional right to one. Also, the function of a competency evaluation, as opposed to an insanity defense evaluation, is that the sole issue to be decided is whether the defendant is sufficiently competent "at that time" to proceed in his or her own defense during the trial. Evidence of incompetency, insanity, or other forms of incapacity during the commission of the crime are not germane to the question of competency to stand trial.

Following the raising of the question of competency, the court then determines whether there is sufficient evidence to justify a formal hearing. It is at this second stage that the role of a psychiatrist is so vital. Oftentimes the results of a psychiatrist's examination will be persuasive in the court's determination of competency. For example, in the federal court system as well as in some states, if a psychiatric examiner concludes that the defendant is likely to be incompetent, then a judicial hearing on the issue is required. While neither the Supreme Court nor any state has clearly articulated how much evidence of incompetency is necessary to compel a hearing, as a rule, evidence sufficient to raise a bona-fide doubt will suffice the constitutional standards.[30]

At a separate and distinct legal proceeding, the third stage, the competency hearing, takes place. The importance of competency to participate in one's own defense is so fundamental to our system of justice, that a competency hearing can be held at *any time* during a trial proceeding. Typically, the psychiatric expert who initially evaluated the defendant is the prime witness at this proceeding. A competency hearing is similar to and different from a normal trial in several respects. It is similar in that it is adversarial in nature. In addition to the findings of the court-ordered psychiatric expert, both the state and the defense may produce their own witnesses, lay and expert, regarding the defendant's competency, along with any other evidence. Also, the defendant has a right to counsel, and is permitted to cross-examine the other side's witnesses. However, unlike a normal trial, the defendant has no options regarding adjudication before a judge or jury. A competency hearing is typically before a judge. Also, in most states the defendant must prove incompetency by at least a preponderance of the evidence, although in the federal courts it is the prosecutor who must carry the burden. One final but important distinction exists that bears particular note. Due to the special circumstances in which a competency hearing is carried out, the defendant's right to invoke the privilege against self-incrimination is narrowed. The U.S. Supreme Court in *Estelle v. Smith*[31] concluded that a defendant may not claim the privilege against self-incrimination to prevent the examining psychiatrist from testifying about the defendant's competency. However, the Court did rule that the privilege against self-incrimination (Fifth Amendment) may bar the disclosure of statements or any resulting psychiatric conclusions from those statements, if they were made during the pretrial competency hearing or a subsequent sentencing proceeding.

While the involvement of the psychiatric expert in this situation might appear to be somewhat curtailed, the contribution that expert findings and testimony make in a competency proceeding is invaluable to our system of fundamental justice.

The disposition of persons found incompetent to stand trial is procedurally uniform in the United States. However, differences in state statutes provide for a variety of rights and limitations. Traditionally, defendants found mentally incompetent to be tried were automatically referred to a state institution until the time they were found to be competent. In effect, a defendant's stay in a mental hospital, often an institution for the criminally insane, could drag on indefinitely, and often did. Release could only be effectuated if either the defendant was found to be competent, at which time trial proceedings would then be initiated, or if the prosecution dropped the charges. Besides the egregious possibility of a confinement lasting many years, the fact that the defendant was neither tried and convicted of a crime or even commitment procedures was a truly unbelievable injustice. However, in 1972, the landmark case *Jackson v. Indiana*[32] addressed this traditional practice of indefinite commitment of defendants found incompetent to stand trial. In *Jackson* the Court made two significant holdings. First, the Court held that while automatic commitment in and of itself is not prohibited, the length of commitment could not exceed a "reasonable period of time necessary to determine whether there is a substantial probability that he will attain that capacity in the foreseeable future." Also, the Court determined that the state would bear the burden of demonstrating "progress" in the attainment of competency, so that a defendant whose competency does not appear "reasonably foreseeable" must either be formally committed pursuant to standard civil commitment procedures or released.

Insanity defense

Probably no single issue in the annals of criminal law has stirred controversy, debate, and comparison among laypersons, as well as jurists, than the insanity defense. The 1982 jury decision finding John Hinckley not guilty by reason of insanity for the shooting of President Reagan and three other persons stunned the nation, and thrust back into the public consciousness questions regarding the viability and fundamental morality surrounding the defense.

By the mid-eighteenth century, a significant attempt was made to apply some form of cognizable formula for determining insanity. Judge Tracy in the case of *Rex v. Arnold* suggested that one of the essential requisites for determining criminal responsibility was whether the accused was able to distinguish "good from evil" at the time of the offense.[33]

Later in the century, Hawkins wrote an important treatise on the subject, which revised this moralistic standard to the more cognitively based question of "right and wrong."[34] Despite what appeared to be an improvement in providing some form of rule for evaluating insanity, the right-wrong test was short lived.

In 1800, there was a significant broadening of the interpretation of legal insanity by the inclusion of insane delusions as an acceptable ground for the defense. It was in *Hadfield's Case*[35] that the addition of delusions, or false beliefs that are firmly held despite incontrovertible evidence to the contrary, was first accepted by the common law court. Hadfield, a soldier who had suffered severe head traumas during the French wars, attempted to shoot King George III in order to attain martyrdom, which he was convinced was his destiny. Despite the lack of a "frenzy or raving madness" his counsel contended that the delusion was the true character of insanity:

These are the cases which frequently mock the wisdom of the wisest in judicial trials: because such persons often reason with a subtlety which puts in the shade the ordinary conceptions of mankind; their conclusions are just and frequently profound; but the premises from which they reason, when within the range of the malady, are uniformly false—not false from any defect of knowledge or judgment; but, because a delusive image, the inseparable companion of real insanity, is thrust upon the subjugated understanding, incapable of resistance, because unconscious of the attack.[36]

Following counsel's argument, the court practically preempted the proceeding by ordering an acquittal. Some 40 years later, a similar attempt was made on the lives of Queen Victoria and Prince Albert by Edward Oxford. Oxford, like Hadfield, suffered from the delusion of martyrdom and was also acquitted.[37] Despite the notoriety of these two cases, the application of the insanity defense based on delusional beliefs was not widely successful.

In 1843, a very significant change in the legal rule used to determine insanity was created. In the trial of *Daniel M'Naughton*[38] the defendant expressed feelings of great persecution by the Pope and Tories, the political party in power at that time. To rid himself of this torment, M'Naughton decided to kill Sir Robert Peel, the prime minister. Not knowing Peel by sight, M'Naughton lay in wait at his residence and mistakenly shot his secretary, Henry Drummond, who was leaving the prime minister's home. In addition to the numerous medical experts who all testified to M'Naughton's insanity, the court also summoned two physicians who were simply observing the trial. Since neither physician was partisan to the proceedings both were afforded a special degree of credence. Upon their unanimous conclusion that the defendant was indeed insane, Chief Justice Tindal halted the proceedings and the jury promptly found M'Naughton "not guilty by reason of insanity." Several

days following the verdict, Queen Victoria, herself the target of assassination by the insanity acquitee Edward Oxford, summoned the House of Lords to a special session. At this meeting, the Lords were instructed to clarify and more strictly define the standards by which a defendant could be acquitted by reason of insanity. It was out of this session that the so-called M'Naughton rule was developed.[39] The gist of this rule provides that:

The jurors ought to be told in all cases that every man is presumed to be sane and to possess a sufficient degree of reason to be responsible for his crimes, until the contrary can be proved to their satisfaction; and that, to establish a defense on the ground of insanity, it must be clearly proved, that, at the time of the committing of the act, the party accused was labouring under such a defect of reason, from disease of the mind, as not to know the nature and quality of the act he was doing or, if he did know it, that he did not know he was doing what was wrong.[40]

In essence, the M'Naughton rule, often referred to as the "right-wrong" test, has three elements that must be proven in order to establish insanity. The accused, at the time of the crime, must be suffering from some mental illness that caused a defect of reason such that he lacked the ability to understand the nature and quality of his actions or their wrongfulness.

Thus passed the eighteenth-century "good-evil" standard into the "right and wrong" test of the nineteenth century. Moreover, the M'Naughton decision marked the advent of the psychiatric expert witness as the key figure in defenses based on insanity. Henceforth, psychiatrists would be afforded special latitude in offering retrospective opinions regarding the defendant's state of mind at the time of the offense, whether his or her conduct emanated from some form of mental disease, and whether the defendant was cognizant of the wrongfulness of his or her conduct.

For more than a century the M'Naughton test served as the basic standard by which the insanity defense was judged in the United States and Great Britain. Even today, a significant minority of states still apply it in its original form. Despite its extensive utility it was not without later criticism. Notwithstanding its fairly broad language, the M'Naughton test was often narrowly construed as an evaluation of a defendant's cognitive capacity to distinguish right from wrong. Furthermore, its scope of application was greatly influenced by the perception of many psychiatrists that the concept of disease of the mind encompassed only psychosis, to the exclusion of other pathologies.

As advances in psychiatric theory were made, the M'Naughton rule came under increasing attack as being antiquated. The major basis of this criticism was the argument that some forms of mental illness affect a person's volition or power to act without impairing his cognitive functioning. In other words, although many mentally ill individuals might be able to distinguish between right and wrong, they could not control their wrongful actions. To rectify this perceived deficiency, a number of states broadened the M'Naughton rule to include an additional element known as the "irresistible impulse" test.[41] The irresistible impulse test stated in essence, that even though an individual might understand the nature and quality of his act and the fact that it is wrong or unlawful, he is nonetheless compelled to commit the act because of his mental illness. This test basically rests on four assumptions:

[F]irst . . . there are mental diseases which impair volition or self control, even while cognition remains relatively unimpaired; second . . . the use of M'Naughton alone results in findings that persons suffering from such diseases are not insane; third . . . the law should make the insanity defense available to persons who are unable to control their action, just as it does to those who fit M'Naughton; fourth, no matter how broadly M'Naughton is construed there will remain areas of serious disorders which it will not reach.[42]

It is important to note that regardless of whether the irresistible impulse test was developed by state statute or case law it was never used as a sole standard, but as a modification of M'Naughton.

Despite the addition of the irresistible impulse concept to the determination of insanity, this too was believed to be too narrow in light of contemporary psychiatry. In 1954, Judge Bazelon, writing for the U.S. Court of Appeals for the District of Columbia in the decision *Durham v. United States* rejected the M'Naughton rule as too limited and held:

We find as an exclusion criterion the right-wrong test is inadequate in that (a) it does not take sufficient account of psychic realities and scientific knowledge, and (b) it is based upon one symptom and so cannot validly be applied in all circumstances. We find that the "irresistible impulse" test is also inadequate in that it gives no recognition to mental illness characterized by brooding and reflection and so delegated acts caused by such illness to the application of the inadequate right-wrong test. We conclude that a broader test should be adopted.[43]

Accordingly, the court articulated a broader standard that provided that "[a]n accused is not criminally responsible if his unlawful act was the product of a mental disease or defect." Apparently, the purpose of the Durham rule, with the description of mental disease or defect deliberately vague, was to afford greater flexibility to psychiatric testimony in order to circumvent narrow or psychiatrically inapposite legal inquiries.[45,46] As one can imagine, the Durham, or New Hampshire rule as it was sometimes called, created considerable controversy due to its ambiguity and semantically indefinite meaning. However, despite the conflict and dubious import, it was never widely accepted in the legal system. In fact, it was only adopted in three jurisdictions—New Hampshire, Maine, and the District of Columbia. Ultimately, the same Court of Appeals for the District of Columbia that created it abolished the Durham rule in 1972.

In the early 1960s the American Law Institute (ALI) drafted a model provision intended to reasonably bridge the narrowness of the M'Naughton rule and the expansiveness of the Durham test. Incorporated in its Model Penal Code, the ALI standard stated:

A person is not responsible for criminal conduct if at the time of such conduct as a result of mental disease or defect he lacks substantial capacity either to appreciate the criminality of his conduct or to conform his conduct to the requirements of the law.[47]

The ALI test differs from the M'Naughton standard in three ways. First, it incorporates a volitional element to insanity, thereby providing an independent criterion— the ability (or inability) to control one's conduct. Second, the ALI substitutes "lacks substantial capacity to appreciate the wrongfulness of conduct," which, in effect, takes into account a defendant's affective or emotional state instead of simply cognitive comprehension. Finally, the ALI standard does not require a total lack of appreciation of the nature of the defendant's conduct but instead that only "substantial" capacity is lacking. Arguably, the ALI test embraces a broader spectrum of psychiatric disorders sufficient to trigger the insanity defense because it contemplated mental defects as well as diseases.

The ALI test is accepted in a majority of jurisdictions and has been frequently cited as being considerably more applicable than its predecessors. For example, its incorporation of both a cognitive and volitional element of impairment is viewed as more consistent with the contemporary conceptualization of mental illness in general. Its move away from total (e.g., M'Naughton) to substantial incapacity also appears to be realistic in terms of modern psychiatry. It broadens the role of the psychiatric expert by providing additional questions to be addressed, while leaving the responsibility of the ultimate decision up to the jury.

The ALI standard, despite its improvements in incorporating language indicative of advances in modern psychiatry, leaves wide open the interpretation of "mental disease or defect." Most courts, to address this ambiguity, have relied on the definition provided in the case *McDonald v. United States*.[48] In *McDonald,* the court defined mental disease or defect as "any abnormal condition of the mind which substantially affects mental or emotional processes and substantially impairs behavior controls."[49] This definition was created to help add clarity to the *Durham* standard but turned out to provide guidance for courts using the ALI rule. It is important to keep in mind that the insanity defense under the ALI standard is a two-pronged test. In addition to providing the existence of a mental disease or defect, the defendant then had to show that the disease or defect so impaired his or her judgment that he or she was not able to conform his or her conduct to the requirements of the law (volition element).

Diminished capacity. In response to the narrowness and seemingly severe restriction imposed by the M'Naughton standard, the California Supreme Court introduced the concept of diminished capacity in the 1949 case, *People v. Wells*.[50] The defense affords the court the opportunity to take into consideration an individual's mental state as a mitigating factor in certain situations. Typically, the diminished capacity defense is used when a defendant is charged with first-degree murder. In effect, it permits psychiatric testimony regarding a defendant's mental condition at the time of the commission of the crime, in order to address the issue of the defendant's ability to form the requisite intent *(mens rea)* to commit the offense. Thus, in a first-degree murder trial, the defense would attempt to put on psychiatric testimony to demonstrate the accused's lack of capacity to appreciate the nature and quality of his or her conduct. Diminished capacity, unlike the insanity defense, is not a complete bar to criminal responsibility. Its effect, if successfully established, is to mitigate or reduce the criminality of the offense from first-degree murder to second-degree murder, or manslaughter, which would result in a lesser sentence.

At one point, at least 15 states recognized some variation of the concept of diminished capacity. However, due to difficulties in definition, application, and administration, it has often been criticized as producing inconsistent and unfair decisions. Today, the diminished capacity defense is employed by only a small minority of states and has failed to generate the support or fill the gap that its creators had intended it to. In fact, the concept was abandoned in California in 1981,[51] following the successful but highly controversial use of the concept by defense counsel for Dan White, who had a finding of murder for the killing of the mayor and county supervisor of San Francisco mitigated to manslaughter. This case stirred nationwide sentiment because of White's successful use of the "Twinkie defense," in which it was argued that the defendant's heavy consumption of junk food caused an impairment in his mental condition.

Other defenses. The development of the two-pronged ALI test, in addition to broadening the range of behavior that would excuse a defendant from criminal responsibility as compared with M'Naughton, has also opened the door to other forms of "illnesses" that could be considered to form the basis of an insanity defense.

Recently, the courts have begun to address new theories of defense to exculpate criminal behavior. Among these new illnesses is post-traumatic stress disorder, pathological gambling, and most recently, premenstrual syndrome.

Post-traumatic stress disorder (PTSD) is a form of mental condition that develops as a result of some traumatic event such as combat war experience, plane or car crashes, and various natural disasters. The most salient symptoms manifested by an individual suffering from PTSD include recurrent elements and phases of the past trauma in dreams, uncontrollable and emotionally intrusive images, dissociative states of consciousness, and unconscious behavioral reenactments of the traumatic situation.

To date, PTSD has been raised most frequently in criminal cases by Vietnam veterans as a form of insanity defense. Typically, the argument is made that the defendant's criminal behavior resulted from combat in Vietnam. Arguably, situations in which the defendant's criminal actions appeared to suggest some casual connection with a reenactment of a former war experience, in the absence of any other plausible explanation, is the most apropos time to raise a PTSD insanity defense. For example, the two murder trials of Vietnam veteran Charles Heads poignantly illustrate this defense. Following his return from Vietnam, Heads frequently complained of depression, incessant nightmares, and flashbacks. One day in 1977, Heads, reacting to a fog-laden mist that surrounded a field adjacent to his brother-in-law's home in Louisiana, grabbed a rifle from his car and attacked the house. In the ensuing moments, he fatally shot his brother-in-law. Heads claimed that he, for an instant, was reliving combat. However, in his first trial in 1978, the jury rejected this temporary insanity claim.[52]

The Supreme Court suspended his life sentence, due to a serious error by the trial judge, and ordered a new trial. In 1981, a second jury heard his characterization of that fateful day as well as testimony from several veterans regarding their experiences of stress emanating from the war, and found Heads not guilty by reason of temporary insanity stemming from his past combat experiences.[53] This was the first PTSD defense successfully used in a capital case.

However, even under seemingly ideal situations in which the defendant displays fairly clear signs of PTSD, there is no guarantee the defense will be accepted. In addition to demonstrating the existence of the illness, it must also be shown that it so impaired the defendant that it was directly causative of the criminal act. As a note, while a majority of PTSD criminal cases involve war veterans, the defense is certainly not confined to this group.

The second relatively new illness occasionally being asserted as a basis for the insanity defense is pathological gambling. As recognized by the American Psychiatric Association in its mental health diagnostic guide, the *Diagnostic and Statistical Manual of Mental Disorders* (DSM IV), pathological gambling is classified as an extreme impulse control disorder. A person is considered to be a pathological gambler if there is evidence of persistent and recurrent inability to resist the impulse to gamble and when the gambling compromises, disrupts, or damages family, personal, and vocational pursuits.[54] Pathological gambling has had only limited success as a form of insanity defense in light of the conflict between psychiatric experts regarding whether it is a true mental disorder. Also jurisdictions that have dropped the volitional elements from the insanity standard have completely cut out the most salient feature of this disorder. Similarly, courts that apply a somewhat strict view of the "mental disease or defect" part of the ALI rule have tended to conclude that pathological gambling does not meet the cognitive standard. As a result, it is expected that fewer defendants will be able to successfully raise it as a defense.

In the past few years increasing attention has been paid to the subject of premenstrual syndrome (PMS). Researchers, while far from uniform in their description and determination of etiology, appear to have generally accepted the following as requisite criteria for a PMS diagnosis: Symptoms occur cyclically each month; emotional symptoms must be primary symptoms; symptomatic relief coincides with or shortly following full flow of menses; symptoms must be present during every premenstrual phase for at least a year; and symptom severity must be moderate to severe.[55] Recent research indicates that women report a wide variety of symptoms or changes in relation to the premenstrum.[56] Among the most common symptoms cited are hot flashes, changes in libido, acne, changes in energy level (e.g., hypomanic behavior), diminished self-esteem, mood swings, suicidal feelings, irritability, impulsivity, insomnia, and difficulty concentrating. Because of the relative newness of the research surrounding PMS and the corresponding conflict in the medical community regarding its nature, it has generally not proved to be an accepted defense in limiting criminal responsibility. In only a handful of cases in England has PMS been successfully plead to reduce the seriousness of criminal charges. For example, in one case a woman plead that she suffered from a temporary hormonal imbalance during the commission of a murder

and her charge was reduced to manslaughter by reason of diminished responsibility.[57]

In light of the difficulty of establishing PMS as a recognizable mental illness at this time, the likelihood of a successful defense based on it is considered minimal.

Abolition of the insanity defense. Prior to 1930, Washington, Mississippi, and Louisiana had tried without success to do away with the insanity defense. Even before then, as well as after, numerous commentators had sought to abolish the defense.[58,59]

In 1979, Montana became the first state to constructively limit the use of an insanity plea. It amended its Code of Criminal Procedure to delete the section recognizing the insanity defense, which was substantially consistent with the ALI standard. The legislature substituted a new section that limited the relevancy of mental disease to the determination of *mens rea* of criminal intent. The Montana section stated that "Evidence that defendant suffered from a mental disease or defect is admissible whenever it is relevant to prove that the defendant did or did not have a state of mind which is an element of the offense."[60]

Three years later Idaho explicitly abolished the use of insanity as a separate defense to charges of criminal acts. However, like Montana, the Idaho statute recognized that a defendant's mental state may be relevant to the issue of criminal intent.[61] "[N]othing herein is intended to prevent the admission of expert evidence on the issue of mens rea or any state of mind which is an element of the offense, subject to the rules of evidence."[62] Alabama and Utah have followed similar courses in either restricting a plea of insanity to the question of criminal intent or abolishing it altogether.

As alluded earlier, the change in Montana and Utah to a *mens rea* approach is, in effect, a constructive abolition of the use of insanity as a defense. This is because it requires a finding that a person was so impaired that he or she was incapable of forming the intent to commit the act. For example, if a defendant purposefully shoots and kills a person, the defendant will not avoid criminal responsibility by claiming that his conduct was the result of a hallucination, delusion, or some form of thought disorder. A *mens rea* statute would only relieve persons of responsibility if they were unable to form the requisite intent to commit the crime. To establish the lack of intent, it would be necessary to demonstrate that the defendant was completely unaware of what he or she was doing or did not believe the act being committed (shooting a gun at victim) was actually taking place. A common illustration is, if the defendant believed the gun was a banana and that he or she wasn't trying to kill the victim but was, instead, only squirting the victim with banana seeds.

The degree of impairment that this illustration provides should give some indication of just how narrow the *mens rea* approach is. It is highly doubtful that any more than a handful of all insanity acquittees each year would be found nonresponsible under this standard. John Hinckley, Monte Durham, Daniel M'Naughton, Hadfield, and any number of other notable defendants whose insanity trials helped shape the common law in this area would certainly not qualify.

Despite this fact, proponents for abolishing the insanity defense argue that there is no constitutional requirement that a defense of mental illness exist at all.[63] Further, allowances for the lack of *mens rea* comports with the historically held tenet that fundamental morality requires exculpation when a person truly does not know what he or she is doing. It is also argued that the *mens rea* standard is much easier to administer, thereby reducing the likelihood of confusion and complications frequently arising from contradictory expert testimony. Similarly, abolitionists as well as proponents of the *mens rea* test contend that an individual's mental state at the time of the crime would still be considered with regard to treatment, rather than penal, alternatives.

NARROWING THE STANDARD. The American Bar Association's House of Delegates in 1983 passed a resolution to cut back the standard to be used for pleading insanity. This resolution stated: "The ABA approves, in principle, a defense of nonresponsibility for crime(s) which focuses solely on whether the defendant as a result of mental disease or defect was unable to appreciate the wrongfulness of his or her conduct at the time of the offense charged."[64]

In effect the ABA was dropping the volition or irresistible impulse prong from the ALI standard in favor of a strictly cognitive formulation. The reason for this change was basically twofold. Rejecting, but recognizing, certain state efforts to either completely or constructively abolish the defense, the ABA's proposal sought to diminish some of the ambiguity that many had claimed had infected the defense, while still maintaining its moral integrity and foundation. By dropping the volition element and applying the word *appreciate,* the standard would be broad enough to encompass cases of severe reality impairment, and would avoid the often difficult and controversial task of addressing compulsion. Also, commentary supporting this change suggests that this standard is consistent with contemporary psychiatric expertise and avoids the problem of vague or overinclusive interpretations of mental disease.

The American Psychiatric Association, like the ABA, supports a modification of the ALI standard. Carefully considering the evidence that various commentators have advanced regarding the present standards, principally M'Naughton and ALI, as well as other widely circulated alternatives such as the *mens rea* approach, guilty but insane plea, and complete abolition, the APA concluded that a more limited retention of the defense was required. Cognizant of the long history of difficulty jurists and experts have had in defining mental disease and defect, the APA proposed a standard they felt would only encompass individuals with serious disorders and permit relevant psychiatric testimony on the majority of cases where criminal responsibility was at issue. The APA proposed:

A person charged with a criminal offense should be found not guilty by reason of insanity if it is shown that as a result of mental disease or mental retardation he was unable to appreciate the wrongfulness of his conduct at the time of the offense. As used in this standard, the terms mental disease or mental retardation include only those severely abnormal mental conditions that grossly and demonstrably impair a person's perception or understanding of reality and that are not attributable primarily to the voluntary ingestion of alcohol or other psychoactive substances.[65]

Like the ABA, the APA's proposal has dropped the volition element in favor of a solely cognitive standard. The only difference between the two organizations' proposals is the APA's specificity regarding the nature and severity of the mental disease or defect to be considered.

The federal government, as well as the American Medical Association, favors much greater limitations that approximate the *mens rea* alternative. Numerous bills in Congress have urged various legislation ranging from complete abolition, use of a *mens rea* standard, to the creation of a new plea — "not guilty only by reason of insanity." Other proposed legislation included shifting the burden of proof to the defendant to prove he was insane at the time of the offense, (e.g., in the Hinckley trial the government had the difficult task of proving Hinckley sane beyond a reasonable doubt) and to abolish the defense in prosecutions of assassination attempts on the president.

As a sign of changes to come with regard to the federal courts, the Justice Department recommended a comprehensive set of changes affecting a variety of areas in criminal justice. Entitled the Comprehensive Crime Control Act of 1984,[66] several provisions pertaining to the insanity defense were included. In an abbreviated form, those changes included the following: (1) limiting the (insanity) defense to those who are unable to appreciate the nature or wrongfulness of their acts, (2) placing the burden (of proof) on the defendant to establish the defense by clear and convincing evidence, (3) preventing expert testimony on the ultimate issue of whether the defendant had a particular mental state or condition, and (4) establishing procedures for federal civil commitment of a person found not guilty by reason of insanity if no state will commit him.

GUILTY BUT MENTALLY ILL PLEA. In 1975, Michigan became the first state to adopt the alternative plea guilty but mentally ill (GBMI) or guilty but insane (GBI). Presumably dissatisfied with the definitional and procedural problems of the insanity defense and the belief that its abolition was not constitutionally sound, Michigan sought a compromise. Also, Michigan sought to decrease the number of successful insanity pleas in its courts, since a 1974 court held that insanity acquittees must be treated the same as civil committees.[67] In effect, this 1974 ruling permitted a significant number of insanity acquittees to be released from hospitalization fairly quickly. This raised a concern for public safety. To date, 11 other states have enacted similar GBMI legislation, many because of the Hinckley decision.[68]

Because it is at the forefront of this alternative defense plea, Michigan's law has served as a model for other states. Therefore, there is sufficient procedural commonality to permit generalization. When an insanity plea is entered, a psychiatric evaluation is required. Upon the conclusion of the trial, a jury is presented with four possible verdicts: (1) not guilty, (2) guilty, (3) not guilty by reason of insanity, or (4) guilty but mentally ill. The GBMI verdict requires a finding of three factors: (1) the accused was guilty of the crime, (2) mentally ill at the time the offense was committed, and (3) not legally insane at the time of the offense.[69] Most GBMI states require that these factors be proven by a preponderance standard (e.g., 51 out of 100 chances). Following a finding of guilty but mentally ill, the court has the discretion to impose any sentence within the statutorily prescribed limits of the crime committed. Typically, sentencing is geared toward psychiatric care within the confines of a prison. If no treatment is available in prison, probation contingent on outpatient treatment is always an option.

Despite the appearance of a novel alternative incorporating both rehabilitative and retributive aspects, the guilty but mentally ill plea has been hit hard by criticism even in its home state.[70] Opponents of the plea state that it is exceedingly difficult to discriminate between a finding of guilty but mentally ill and not guilty by reason of insanity in light of the similarity in definition. Similarly, there is a concern that juries will misuse the GBMI plea out of ignorance, finding a defendant guilty when a NGRI finding was more appropriate. Also, the title guilty but mentally ill is considered deceptive since it implies some form of mitigation but actually provides no special allowance.

Proponents who tout this alternative on humanitarian grounds because of the treatment element are often confronted by the fact that treatment is not guaranteed, only a criminal sentence.

In effect then, despite a change in name and arguably greater choice of alternatives, a jury's verdict of guilty but mentally ill is basically no different for a defendant than a verdict of guilty.

PSYCHIATRIC MALPRACTICE

The development and emergence of malpractice lawsuits against psychiatrists have been very gradual and seemingly of recent occurrence. Before 1970, civil actions for psychiatric-related injuries were relatively rare. As a medical specialty, psychiatry was considered almost immune from suit because it was generally a difficult area of medicine to build a case against.

An early study of malpractice claims against psychiatrists occurring between the years 1946-1962 cited only 18 cases of negligent or civilly liable conduct.[71] Although this study was restricted to only cases that had been appealed and reported, thus not accounting for cases settled out of court or unreported, the number was still remarkably low. In these early lawsuits, the defendant psychiatrists rarely lost, and when they did, the judgment was generally small. Until the 1970s, the incidence of lawsuits against psychiatrists remained quite low. The reasons for this are likely to be numerous, but certain factors seem inescapable. Due to the intimate nature of the psychiatrist-patient relationship, patients were likely to be reluctant to acknowledge or expose their psychiatric history. Other obstacles included the lack of a commonly accepted method of practice within the profession, which made it difficult to establish a standard of care; the reluctance of other psychiatrists to testify as experts against another colleague; the adeptness of psychiatrists in dealing with a patient's negative experience, thereby avoiding litigation; the difficulty in proving patient injury, in the absence of actual physical harm; and the possible reluctance of the legal profession to delve into an area (of medicine) in which there are few consistent answers.

There has been a steady increase in malpractice actions against psychiatrists since the early 1970s. However, this fact must be seen in context. The incidence of claims against psychiatrists still remains much lower than against other physicians,[72] and the majority of claims do not result in successful verdicts against the psychiatrist.

As the incidence in malpractice actions has increased so has the variety of claims against psychiatrists. Some causes of action reflect acts of negligence or substandard care for which any physician may be found liable. These malpractice areas include negligent diagnosis, abandonment from treatment, various intentional and quasi-intentional torts (assault and battery, fraud, defamation, invasion of privacy), failure to obtain informed consent, and breach of contract. Areas of liability specific to psychiatry include: harm caused by organic therapies (ECT, psychotropic medication, and psychosurgery), breach of confidentiality, sexual exploitation of patients, failure to control or supervise a dangerous patient or negligent release, failure to protect third parties from potentially dangerous patients, false imprisonment, and negligent infliction of mental distress. These claims represent the major causes of action that may be brought against a psychiatrist.

Malpractice actions based on a psychiatrist's use of psychotropic drugs have been fairly infrequent considering the widespread use of this form of treatment during the past 20 years. However, a study of claims filed between 1972 and 1983 against psychiatrists showed that 20% of the actions were related to medication.[73]

A psychiatrist's failure to adequately monitor or provide sufficient warnings and instructions about a drug's side effects provides an opportunity for several different allegations of negligence. For example, in a recent case, *Duvall v. Goldin,*[74] a psychiatrist was sued by a third party who was struck in a car accident by an epileptic patient having a seizure while driving. The plaintiff alleged that the psychiatrist had a duty to inform the patient of the effects of his medication when driving in order to protect other individuals possibly endangered by the patient's conduct. The Michigan Court of Appeals reversed the trial court's dismissal of the case and held that there were reasonable facts raised by the complaint to void summary judgment for the psychiatrist.

Relatives of patients who have committed suicide by taking an overdose of medication frequently file suit, claiming that the psychiatrist was negligent in prescribing the drugs. In the treatment of suicidal patients there always exists the delicate balance between providing clinical treatment, which involves certain risks, and applying protective, less therapeutic, measures. In recognition of this balance, a psychiatrist will not automatically be found liable if a patient commits suicide with medication provided for treatment. Negligence is likely to be found in high-risk situations when either the psychiatrist's choice of intervention (e.g., medication) or manner of supervision was unreasonable under the circumstances.

The last area of consideration, and certainly one of growing concern with regard to liability involving drug treatment, concerns tardive dyskinesia (TD). Despite only a few reported legal cases to date, the frequency and dangerousness of the side effects, coupled with the amounts of damages that have been awarded, have begun to create considerable interest within the psychiatric profession particularly among clinicians who prescribe antipsychotic medication.

Claims of negligence in cases involving tardive dyskinesia are fairly similar to those in other drug treatment suits. Liability can result from the lack of an adequate examination (patient history, physical, or laboratory tests, failure to closely monitor or treat side effects, failure to obtain the patient's informed consent, and failure to project and control drug reactions). The *Clites v. Iowa*[75] case is one of the first decisions specifically dealing with TD and aptly illustrates some of the liability considerations inherent in the issue of drug therapy. The plaintiff was a mentally retarded man, who had been institutionalized since age 11 and treated with major tranquilizers from age 18 to 23. Tardive dyskinesia was diagnosed at age 23 and the plaintiff subsequently sued. He claimed that the defendants had negligently prescribed medication, failed to monitor its effects, and had not obtained his informed consent. A damage award of $760,165 was returned and affirmed on appeal. The court ruled that the defendants were negligent because they deviated from the standards of the "industry." Specifically, the court cited a failure to administer regular physical examinations and tests; failure to intervene at the first sign of tardive dyskinesia; the inappropriate use of drugs in combinations, in light of the patient's particular condition and the drugs used; the use of drugs for the convenience of controlling behavior rather than therapy; and the failure to obtain informed consent.

Informed consent/refusal

A major consideration regarding treatment of the mentally disabled patient is the question of competence to consent to treatment. This class of patients can be divided into two groups—the mentally retarded and the mentally ill. For mentally retarded patients, the degree and ability to understand treatment information is relatively fixed, given the organic nature of their disability. Therefore, if the patient's retardation impairs his or her ability to understand the information to be disclosed, then consent must be obtained from the patient's legal guardian or from the court.

The problems encountered with the mentally ill patient are far less predictable and finite. Questions like "Is the information being understood clearly or is it distorted?" or "Can all of the information be properly assimilated and does the patient have the capacity to express his or her decision?" are important considerations. One commentator aptly illustrated this dilemma by stating:

[H]ow does one obtain consent from a severely ill catatonic schizophrenic who sits and stares at a blank wall all day, refusing to speak to anyone? Certainly if a patient is psychotic or hallucinating and cannot assimilate information about a proposed procedure, he does not have the capacity to reach a decision about the matter in question. Some mental patients are incapable of evaluating information in what most people would call a rational manner. A treatment decision might ordinarily be based on considerations of perceived personal objectives, or long-term versus short-term risks and benefits. But there are patients whose acceptance or rejection of a treatment is not made in relation to any "factual" information. To add to this dilemma, while a mental patient may refuse to give his consent to a procedure, his refusal may only be a manifestation of his illness, having little resemblance to his actual desires.[76]

Another problem confronting the psychiatrist treating the mentally ill patient is the fluctuating periods of lucidity some patients experience. As a rule, for a psychiatrist or any other physician treating a patient of questionable competency, liability will be limited if a reasonable effort was made to determine a patient's competency at the time of consent. If the patient provides consent to treatment, for example, the initiation of psychotropic medication, and then later claims he didn't understand what was disclosed, the question of competency will be evaluated on the reasonableness of the doctor's conclusion of competency. If the patient is not competent, then a psychiatrist or physician will generally be required to seek the consent of the patient's guardian.

Consistent with other common law concepts regarding consent, for example, the forming of a contract or executing of a will, the law will not recognize an agreement that is not the product of a person's free will.

Freedom from coercion, fraud, or duress is the pivotal requisite to ensuring that a patient's consent is voluntary. Any act, subtle or overt, that impinges on a patient's decision-making process may be sufficient to invalidate a patient's consent. For example, a patient who is threatened by the hospital staff, restricted from engaging in favored activities, or forced to do irksome tasks unless consenting to treatment has been subjected to violations of the voluntary requirement. More subtle, but equally coercive, is the physician who emphasizes the consequences of not having a particular treatment and downplaying the risks. The courts are particularly sensitive to the manner, content, and conditions in which information is given and consent is provided when vulnerable patients such as the mentally disabled, elderly, or physically weak are involved.

Exceptions. Under certain circumstances, disclosing risks to the patient and obtaining consent may not be necessary. Psychiatrists and physicians should be wary, however, about relying on an exception, if it can be avoided, because support by the courts is inconsistent.

Four exceptions to obtaining informed consent are commonly recognized, although all four might not necessarily be available in a particular state. In a situation involving a threat of serious injury or loss of life, and when it is impossible to obtain the patient's consent or someone authorized to provide consent on the patient's behalf, the law will imply that a consent "would have been made if the patient were able to." Commonly referred to as the "emergency exception," two considerations must be heeded to avoid liability. First, the patient's condition must be so serious that treatment could not be delayed without risking serious injury. Second, it must be the patient's condition and not the surrounding circumstances that determine the existence of the emergency.

The second exception is when, in certain circumstances, psychiatrists or physicians may have therapeutic privilege to withhold information if they determine that a complete disclosure of possible risks and alternatives might have a significant detrimental effect on a patient's physical or psychological condition. The privilege may apply when disclosure might enhance the risk of the treatment itself or interfere with the patient's ability to make a decision. However, the privilege will not be upheld simply because a doctor believes a patient would refuse the treatment if informed of the risks.

A third exception to the requirement of informed consent is recognized when the patient is incompetent and the procedure contemplated is more of a routine, remedial measure. For example, daily custodial care of incompetent institutionalized psychiatric patients is excepted. However, if informed consent would be required for a specific treatment, for example, the administration of electroconvulsive therapy (ECT), the consent of a guardian or appointed substitute decision-maker is required.

Finally, a patient may waive his or her right to make an informed consent. In other words, a psychiatrist or other physician need not disclose the nature and risks of a treatment when a patient specifically requests that he or she not be told.

Breach of confidentiality

The duty to safeguard closely the confidentiality of any communication that transpires in the course of psychiatric treatment is, in a large measure, the cornerstone of the profession. This obligation of confidentiality is a fundamental concern of all physicians, but none is more keenly sensitive to its paramount importance than mental health professionals. This point is aptly reflected in the ethical codes of the various mental health organizations. For example, Section 4 of the *Principles of Medical Ethics with Annotations Especially Applicable to Psychiatry* reads in part:

> A physician shall respect the rights of patients, of colleagues and of other health professionals, and shall safeguard patient confidences within the constraints of the law. . . . [C]onfidentiality is essential to psychiatric treatment. This is based in part on the special nature of psychiatric therapy as well as on the traditional ethical relationship between physician [psychiatrist] and patient. . . . Because of the sensitive and private nature of the information with which the psychiatrist deals, he/she must be circumspect in the information that he/she chooses to disclose to others about the patient. The welfare of the patient must be a continuing consideration.[77]

In essence, confidentiality refers to the right of a person (e.g., patient) not to have communications given in confidence revealed, without authorization, to outside parties. The issue of confidentiality in a psychiatric perspective embodies two fundamental rationales. First, a patient has a right to privacy that should not be violated except in certain prescribed circumstances. Second, physicians have historically been enjoined (on an ethical basis) to maintain the confidences of their patients. In doing so, the mechanisms of treatment are enhanced and promoted.

Psychiatrists have always been susceptible to ethical sanctions for breaching a patient's confidentiality but liability for monetary damages for such an action is a relatively recent development. Several legal theories exist to provide recovery for breach of confidentiality. Some courts have upheld a course of action involving breach of confidentiality based on an implied contract theory.[78] Accordingly, a psychiatrist is considered to have implicitly agreed to keep any information received from a patient confidential and when he or she has failed to do so the contractual relationship is said to have been broken. In cases based on this theory, damages have typically been restricted to economic losses flowing directly from the breach and excluding compensation based on any residual harm (e.g., emotional distress, marital discord, or loss of employment).[79]

Theories based on the invasion of privacy have frequently supported recovery in numerous cases involving breach of confidentiality. The law defines invasion of privacy as an "unwarranted publication of a person's private affairs with which the public has no legitimate concern, such as to cause outrage, mental suffering, shame, or humiliation to a person of ordinary sensibilities."[80] This theory has limited appeal for some patients since the courts have traditionally held that recovery will be upheld only when there is a public disclosure of personal facts as opposed to disclosure to a single person or a small group.

A minority of courts has upheld claims for breach of confidentiality based on the fiduciary duty of the psychiatrist or patient to safeguard against unauthorized disclosures of information gained during treatment.[81] Similarly, patients have argued that physician licensing statutes and doctor-patient privilege statutes provide a remedy for unconsented disclosures of confidential information.[82] Although this last argument has gained only marginal acceptance, some commentators believe that a trend may soon be initiated to encompass a course of action based on privilege statutes, as well as in contract. Both actions would presumably be based on public policy grounds.

In a number of states, the legal duty to maintain patient confidentiality is governed by mental health confidentiality statutes. These statutes outline the legal requirements covering confidentiality quite comprehensively. For example, in Illinois the Mental Health and Developmental Disabilities Confidentiality Act[83] contains 17 sections covering the duty of confidentiality, exceptions to it, rules and procedures for authorizing disclosures, patient and third-party access rules, penalties or violations, and provisions for civil actions by parties injured by unauthorized disclosures.

Failure to warn or protect

Confidentiality was considered sacrosanct by the psychiatric profession until the Supreme Court of California heard the case *Tarasoff v. Regents of the University of California*[84] in 1976. *Tarasoff* involved a university student from India who became obsessed with a young woman (Tatiana Tarasoff) whom he met at a dance. She clearly indicated she had no interest in the young man. Following this rejection, the young man began individual therapy at the university counseling center. Following several sessions, the treating psychologist concluded that his patient might try to harm Ms. Tarasoff. The psychologist enlisted the aid of the campus police to detain the patient in order to ascertain his eligibility for civil commitment. The police interviewed the patient and concluded that he was rational. Based on his assurances that he had no desire to harm Ms. Tarasoff and would refrain from seeing her, they decided not to detain him. The supervising psychiatrist for the case reviewed the facts to that point and concluded there was no basis for commitment. The patient terminated treatment and two months later killed Tatiana Tarasoff.

Tatiana's parents filed a wrongful death action against the university, the treating psychologist, the supervising psychiatrist, and the campus police. The plaintiffs asserted that the defendants owed a "duty to warn"

Tatiana of the impending danger that the patient posed to her. The California Supreme court agreed. In affirming but modifying their earlier holding (1974) the court held:

> [W]hen a therapist determines, or pursuant to the standards of his profession should determine, that his patient presents a serious danger of violence to another, he incurs an obligation to use reasonable care to protect the intended victim against such danger. . . . Thus [the discharge of this duty] may call for [the therapist] to warn the intended victim or others likely to apprise the victim of the danger, to notify the police, or take whatever other steps are reasonably necessary under the circumstances.

The reaction to both decisions, commonly referred to as *Tarasoff I* and *Tarasoff II,* was immediate, forceful, and frequently vehement. The majority of the early commentary, especially from the psychiatric profession, was critical of the numerous unanswered questions left by the California court. This new theory of liability imposed questions such as the following: Was a duty owed if the threat of danger was not aimed at anyone in particular? What steps did a psychiatrist or therapist have to take to discharge the duty? Was a duty to warn still owed if the potential victim was already aware of the patient's threat or dangerous propensities? How was a therapist's determination of dangerousness to be judged if the profession itself disclaimed the ability to accurately predict future behavior? In some cases these and other questions have been addressed in piecemeal fashion by the numerous "duty to warn/protect" decisions since *Tarasoff.*

The response by the courts following the 1976 California decision has been inconsistent and, at times, confusing. Several courts have followed the holding of *Tarasoff,* concluding that a therapist was liable for not warning an identifiable victim. For example, courts in Kansas and Michigan have ruled that the duty to warn was restricted only to readily identifiable victims.[85] A slightly broader but analogous limitation has been fashioned by decisions in Maryland and Pennsylvania where the courts have recognized a duty to warn only when the victim is "foreseeable."[86]

The second case to apply the *Tarasoff* ruling, *McIntosh v. Milano,*[87] added a slightly broader twist to the duty-to-warn theory. In *McIntosh,* a 17-year-old patient fatally shot a young neighborhood woman. Evidence revealed that the patient had disclosed to the defendant psychiatrist feelings of inadequacy, fantasies of being a hero or important villain, and using a knife (which he brought to therapy one session) to intimidate people. The patient also shared that he had once fired a BB gun at a car in which he thought the victim was riding with her boyfriend. However, the psychiatrist denied that the patient had ever expressed any feelings of violence or made any threats to harm the victim. The parents of the victim claimed that the psychiatrist knew the patient was dangerous and owed a duty to protect the victim. The New Jersey court in denying a motion for summary judgment agreed and held that *Tarasoff* applied, based on the therapist-patient relationship. The court found a more general duty to protect society, analogous to a physician's duty to warn others (in the general public) of persons carrying contagious disease.

Representing the broadest expansion of the *Tarasoff* duty-to-warn theory, was a Nebraska decision on *Lipari v. Sears, Roebuck and Co.*[88] In this case, a patient, who recently had dropped out of the Veterans Administration day treatment program, purchased a shotgun from Sears. Following the purchase he resumed treatment only to drop out against medical advice approximately three weeks later. A month after the second termination he walked into a crowded nightclub and randomly discharged the shotgun, injuring the plaintiff and killing her husband. The plaintiff claimed that the VA should have known the patient was dangerous and that the VA was negligent for not committing him. The court held that Nebraska law recognized a duty to protect society, following the holdings of *Tarasoff II* and *McIntosh.* More significantly, they held that foreseeable violence was not limited to identified, specific victims, but may involve a class of victims (e.g., the general public at large). Two other cases, one in Washington State[89] and another in California have expanded the duty to warn to include victims who were not specified or readily identifiable. Of particular note is the California case, *Hedlund v. Orange County,*[90] in which the victim was a woman in couples therapy with a man with whom she lived. During a session when she wasn't present, the man told the therapist he planned to harm her. While in a car, with her son next to her, the man shot at her. The woman sought damages for herself and her son, who, she claimed, suffered emotional harm. Rejecting the defendant's argument that they owed no duty of care to the young boy, the California court extended the duty to warn to foreseeable persons in close relationship to the specifically threatened victim.

Fifteen days before the *Hedlund* decision, the U.S. District Court in Colorado decided the case *Brady v. Hopper.*[91] The plaintiffs were all men who had been shot by John Hinckley during his attempted assassination of President Reagan. The plaintiffs alleged that the defendant's psychiatrist, John Hopper, knew or should have known that Hinckley was dangerous. Relying heavily on the *Lipari* decision, the plaintiffs claimed that the defendant should have known that the president was Hinckley's intended victim and that they were a class of people reasonably foreseeable to be at risk because of this danger. The court focused its decision on the issue of foreseeability of the risk to the specific plaintiffs involved. While affirming the duty of therapists to protect third parties, the court's conclusion was prefaced with the admission: "[T]he existence of a special relationship does not necessarily mean that the duties created by that relationship are owed to the world at large." In rejecting the plaintiff's claims that the defendant was liable to them, the court concluded: "In my opinion, the specific threats to specific victims rule states a workable, reasonable, and fair boundary upon the sphere of a therapist's liability to third persons for the acts of their patients."

Therefore, under *Brady,* a determination of dangerousness, in general, will not create a duty to protect without a specific threat to a specific victim.

In December 1984, the Court of Appeals for the 10th Circuit, in a three-page opinion, affirmed the district court's opinion in *Brady.*[92] In essence, they deferred to the discretion of the lower court, stating reversal could only be found if there was a gross error in the application of the law.

Cases to date, involving some form of the duty-to-warn theory, can be viewed as falling somewhere on a continuum based on two common factors: (1) a threat (or potential for harm) and (2) a potential victim. At one end is the *Brady* decision with its "specific threat–specific victim" rule and at the other end is *Lipari,* which held that "foreseeable violence" created a duty to protect "others," regardless of whether the victim was identified or specified. In addition, decisions in Maryland, California, Pennsylvania, and Iowa have refused to apply the theory by either rejecting it outright or finding no liability based on the facts of the case.[93]

At present, most courts have held that, in the absence of a foreseeable victim, no duty to warn or protect will be found. Reviewing the cases to date (1986), a few facts stand out. Most notable (at the time of this writing) is the relative absence of litigation that most commentators felt would occur following the *Tarasoff* decision in 1974. Outside of California, the *Tarasoff* theory has been upheld in only four states: New Jersey, Nebraska, Washington, and Michigan. However, it is probably prudent for psychiatrists and other practitioners to conduct their practice as if the duty to protect is law in their state. In spite of the fact that there have been no published affirmations of *Tarasoff*-like cases in more than 40 states, the traditional deference to maintaining confidentiality in a psychotherapeutic relationship is not likely to hold up when balanced against the interests of safeguarding society.

Whatever the extent of the duty imposed by the court, a psychiatrist or therapist will not be held liable for a patient's violent acts unless it is found that (1) the

psychiatrist determined (or by professional standards reasonably should have determined) that the patient posed a danger to a third party (identified or unidentified) and that (2) the psychiatrist failed to take adequate steps to prevent the violence.

The liability considerations that underlie the treatment and care of the dangerous patient generally differ according to the amount of control a psychiatrist, therapist, or institution has over the patient. As a general rule, psychiatrists who treat dangerous or potentially dangerous patients have a duty of care, which includes controlling that individual from harming other persons inside and outside the facility as well as him or herself. On the other hand, the outpatient who presents a possible risk of danger to others creates a duty of care, which may include warning or somehow protecting potential third-party victims. While there may be facts that require an expansion of the duty of care in one or the other setting (in-patient, outpatient), this general distinction is important to more clearly understand the legal issues and preventive considerations that the dangerous patient presents.

The duty of care owed to dangerous or potentially dangerous patients in an in-patient setting is very similar in principle to those duties governing the treatment of suicidal patients. Causes of action alleged by third parties injured by the dangerous or violent acts of an in-patient generally involve one of two situations. In one situation, the in-patient is discharged and shortly thereafter harms a third party. The plaintiff sues whoever made the decision to discharge the patient, claiming that he or she was negligently released. The second general situation is when an in-patient escapes from the hospital and then harms someone. The claim in this scenario is typically that the physician or facility in charge of the patient's care was negligent in either supervision or control of the patient.

In both general scenarios the analysis for determining liability is quite similar. As in cases involving suicide, a treating psychiatrist or other practitioner will not be held liable for harms committed following a patient's discharge (e.g., negligent release) unless the court determines (1) that the psychiatrist knew or should have known that the patient was likely to commit a dangerous or violent act and (2) that in light of this knowledge, the psychiatrist failed to take adequate steps to evaluate the patient when considering discharge. Similarly, in cases involving third parties injured by a dangerous patient who has escaped, the court will evaluate (1) whether the psychiatrist knew or should have known that the patient presented a risk of elopement and (2) in light of that knowledge, whether the psychiatrist took adequate steps to supervise or control the patient. The actions of a psychiatrist in a negligent discharge or negligent control or supervision claim will be scrutinized based on the reasonableness of the actions and the standards of the profession.

Sexual exploitation

From a legal standpoint, the courts have consistently held that a doctor or therapist who engages in sexual activity with a patient is subject to civil liability, and in some cases, criminal sanctions. The reason for this overwhelming condemnation rests in the exploitive, and often deceptive, practice that sex between a health care professional (psychiatrist, physician, therapist, etc.) and patient represents. The fundamental basis of the psychiatrist-patient relationship is the unconditional trust and confidence patients have for the therapist. It is this trust that permits patients to share their most intimate secrets, thoughts, and feelings. As therapy progresses, unconscious feelings of conflict, fears, and desires originating from important relations in the patient's past are said to be "transferred" to the therapist in the present. Known as the "transference" phenomenon, this experience is a common occurrence in psychotherapy and often provides a therapist valuable information to analyze and interpret. Because of the transference phenomenon, a patient becomes vulnerable to the emotions being experienced, for example, love feelings. The therapist, therefore, must conduct the treatment with sensitivity and care. A similar phenomenon, known as "countertransference," also may occur in therapy. This occurs when a therapist experiences unconscious conflicts and feelings toward a patient. As with patient transferences, countertransference feelings should be recognized as important therapeutic information and analyzed in order to gain insight into how to better understand the patient.

When psychiatrists or other practitioners engage in sexual activity with a patient, they have, in effect, exploited the vulnerability created by the therapeutic relationship and breached their legal and ethical duty of exercising due care. From a legal perspective, this breach of duty is probably best described in the landmark case, *Roy v. Hartogs*.[94] The plaintiff alleged that the defendant had engaged in sexual relations with her for approximately 13 months. This eventually caused her extreme emotional and physical deterioration and resulted in two separate hospitalizations. The defendant initially claimed that a New York statute relating to interference with the marital relation prevented sexual activity from being the basis of a malpractice action. The court rejected this claim, stating that not all actions involving sexual activity were barred by the statute. Reinforcing this conclusion the court stated:

[T]here is a public policy to protect a patient from the deliberate and malicious abuse of power and breach of trust by a psychiatrist when that patient entrusts to him her body and mind in the hope that he will use his best efforts to effect a cure. The right is protected by permitting the victim to pursue civil remedies, not only to vindicate a wrong against her but to vindicate the public interest as well.

It is important to note that in addition to sexual activity, other types of behavior that demonstrate a manipulation of the transference phenomenon or therapeutic relation may be subject to civil liability. For example, a Florida court found a psychiatrist guilty of "conduct below acceptable psychiatric and medical standards" when it was discovered that he had told a patient that he loved her and would divorce his wife in order to marry her.[95] In the widely cited case, *Zipkin v. Freeman*[96] the defendant psychiatrist was found guilty of a blatant mishandling of the therapy transference when it was shown that he had manipulated his patient to leave her husband and children, invest in ventures controlled by him, and become his mistress and travel companion.

In addition to civil sanctions, a practitioner may face criminal liability if there is evidence that some form of coercion, usually in the form of tranquilizing medication, was used either to induce compliance or reduce resistance to the initiation of the sexual activity. A psychiatrist or other practitioner may be charged criminally if the sexual activity involves a child or adolescent patient. In a situation involving a minor, no evidence of force or coercion needs to be demonstrated in order to support a finding of criminal liability.

In the landmark case, *Roy v. Hartogs*,[97] expert testimony regarding the status of sexual activity as a practice in the psychiatric profession was provided, which concluded, "there are absolutely no circumstances which permit a psychiatrist to engage in sex with his patient."

However, some therapists do attempt to rationalize their actions. Some of the most common defenses, all of which, to date, have been rejected by the courts, include that the patient consented to have sex, that the sexual relation was not a part of treatment, or that the treatment ended before the sexual relations began.

Abandonment

Once there has been established an agreement (explicit or implicit) to provide medical services, the physician is legally and ethically bound to render those services until the relationship has been appropriately terminated. If a psychiatrist or physician terminates treatment prematurely and the patient is harmed because of the termination, a cause of action based on "abandonment of treatment" may be brought. Generally, in the absence of an emergency or crisis situation, treatment can safely be concluded if a patient is provided reasonable notice of the termination and assisted in transferring the case to a new therapist or physician. Proper transfer of a case typically implies that the original psychiatrist or physician will prepare and make available the patient's records as needed by the new therapist or physician. It is also prudent for the original therapist to provide the patient written, as well as verbal notice, in order to avoid any possible questions regarding the nature, timing, or extent of the announcement of termination. This is particularly important when treating psychiatric patients or persons who are psychologically vulnerable, because there may be a tendency to misconstrue or deny a verbal notice.

The issue of abandonment frequently arises when either no notice of termination has been given or when the extent of this notice has been insufficient in some way. It is this latter situation (i.e., how much notice is necessary) that causes some practitioners problems. While there are no rules or guidelines per se regarding this question, a therapist who decides to terminate treatment for whatever reason is expected to act reasonably when doing so. For example, if there are few therapists in the area in which to transfer the patient's case, the treating therapist should afford the patient a longer notice period in order to locate a replacement. However, if a patient refuses or is unable to locate another therapist, the treating psychiatrist or therapist has no obligation to treat the patient indefinitely. The reasonableness of a psychiatrist's or therapist's notice will therefore be judged on the totality of the circumstances relevant to it.

In that light, patients who are experiencing some sort of crisis or emergency situation require special consideration. For example, a psychiatrist or therapist who is treating a patient who is suicidal or presents a possible danger to some third party is not likely to be considered to be acting clinically or legally reasonable if he or she terminates treatment. From a clinical perspective, such a move may exacerbate a patient's already vulnerable feelings, and prompt the patient to do something that he or she might not have otherwise done. Legally, the courts are not likely to consider a psychiatrist's or therapist's decision to terminate treatment reasonable during a time when continuity of care is most required. Therefore, a psychiatrist or therapist should be wary of ending therapy during a period of emergency and, instead, should hold off termination until a more appropriate time.

Patient control and supervision

The treatment of patients who pose a risk of danger to themselves or others presents a unique clinical and legal challenge to the psychiatric and mental health profession.

A lawsuit for patient suicide or attempted suicide is often brought by a patient's family or relatives, claiming that the attending psychiatrist, therapist, or facility was negligent in some aspect of the treatment process. Specifically, there are three broad categories of claims that encompass actions stemming from patient suicide. The first is when an outpatient commits suicide or is injured in a suicide attempt. Plaintiffs in this situation claim that the psychiatrist or therapist was negligent in failing to diagnose the patient's suicidal condition and provide adequate treatment, typically hospitalization. The second situation is when an in-patient is given inadequate treatment and commits or attempts suicide. Typically, the essence of a negligence claim involving inadequate treatment is that the patient was suicidal and the psychiatrist failed to provide adequate supervision. The last general situation is when a patient is discharged from the hospital and shortly thereafter attempts or commits suicide. Family members, or the injured patient, frequently claim that the decision to release the patient was negligent.

The treatment of suicidal or potentially suicidal patients inherently requires a psychiatrist or other practitioner to make predictions regarding future behavior. Psychiatrists and other mental health providers have frequently disclaimed any ability to predict future behavior with any degree of significant accuracy. In light of this fact, the law has tempered, somewhat, its expectation of clinicians in identifying possible dangerous behavior. In lieu of a strict standard requiring 100% accuracy, the law requires professionals to exercise reasonable care in their diagnosis and treatment of patients at risk.[98] Accordingly, a court will not hold a psychiatrist or other practitioner liable for a patient's death or injury due to suicide if the treatment or discharge decision was reasonably based in light of the information available.

In an attempt to enhance the recovery of patients at risk of suicide, some hospitals use what is known as an open ward policy. This permits a patient considerable freedom of movement within the hospital and minimizes procedures that are constraining, such as seclusion, physical and chemical restraints, and constant observation. In some cases, the courts have recognized the therapeutic value of this procedure and concluded that the professional is in the best position to balance the risks and benefits of increased patient freedom. In doing so, the courts have basically deferred their judgment to the professional, even though the professional's conclusions may later prove to be wrong. This deferment to professional judgment is as much an acknowledgment of the difficulties psychiatrists face in attempting to predict future behavior, as it is an acceptance of certain practices and procedures of modern psychiatry. One 1981 federal district court decision sums up its conclusion this way:

[M]odern psychiatry has recognized the importance of making every effort to return a patient to an active and productive life. Thus the patient is encouraged to develop her self confidence by adjusting to the demands of everyday existence. Particularly because the prediction of danger is difficult, undue reliance on hospitalization might lead to prolonged incarceration of potentially useful members of society.[99]

A few courts have refused to make such a deferment and have, instead, kept to the more traditional evaluation of the reasonableness of the precautions provided.[100]

The issue of reasonableness, whether it involves the diagnosis, supervision, or discharge of a patient, will be measured in terms of the accepted standards of the profession. Expert testimony will be needed to establish or disprove that the defendant psychiatrist failed to exercise the reasonable care other psychiatrists would have used in that or similar circumstances. The risk of liability is greatly enhanced when it can be demonstrated that a practitioner or institution failed to follow its own usual practices and procedures for treating a patient at risk for suicide.

Unusual and experimental therapies. The etiologies of many mental disorders (e.g., schizophrenia and depression) remain among the most perplexing mysteries to social scientists, biological psychiatrists, and researchers today. As a result, psychiatry lacks definitive diagnostic and treatment methodologies. As a result, there is a greater opportunity for variance in treating a particular mental illness or disorder.

Treatments considered unusual or experimental may range from the use of certain lesser known or infrequently administered medication to a method of treatment that is completely unorthodox or unique to the individual applying it. While the majority of practitioners in a particular locale may treat a certain psychopathology in the same manner or with the same type of medication, a treatment is not necessarily negligent simply because it is different. In the few cases that have addressed claims alleging negligence stemming from unusual or experimental treatments, the courts have typically applied the respectable minority standard. This standard states that if a particular treatment or procedure is recognized by a respectable minority in the profession, there will be no finding of a breach of due care.

However, unusual or experimental procedures that involve physical contact that inflict some form of pain on a patient may be malpractice per se, either in terms of negligence or as an intentional tort (e.g., assault and battery). For example, in *Abraham v. Zaslow,*[101] a female patient was subjected to a procedure known as rage reduction of Z-therapy. This experimental procedure involved restraining the patient and tickling and poking her while she was being interviewed by a psychotherapist. There was no evidence to demonstrate any recognition of acceptance of this technique within the psychotherapy profession. The court held that this manner of treatment was an intentional and harmful contact that resulted in the patient suffering severe emotional distress, physical bruising, and internal bodily damage.

REFUSAL OF MEDICATION

In a suit involving constitutional rights, patients at a state mental institution filed suit challenging conditions at their institution. Among the conditions they challenged was the use of psychotropic drugs. The court noted that the drugs cause a number of adverse reactions, the most serious being tardive dyskinesia, which interferes with all motor activity, making speech incomprehensible and breathing and swallowing extremely difficult.

Whatever the constitutional basis for the foregoing decision, a federal district court in Ohio found that the guarantee of due process gives a mental patient the right to refuse psychotropic drugs. The court said that a patient is being deprived of liberty without due process if forced to accept these medications (unless the patient is a danger to himself or herself, or to others). Because the inviolability of one's body is one of the oldest rights recognized in our law, informed consent is essential before treatment, the court related, except in emergencies. Even with mental patients, an unwilling patient lessens the prospects for successful drug therapy. Hospital efficiency is no justification for ignoring constitutional rights, the judge stated. The court suggested that an impartial decision-maker from outside the hospital conduct a hearing before any involuntary treatment with psychotropic drugs.

The court said that mental patients had a constitutional right to refuse treatment, at least in some situations. As a constitutional minimum, the state must have at least probable cause to believe that a patient was in a state of mental health institution could not justify forced drugging, the court said.

The state had no interest that could override the need for patients' consent to treatment unless they were dangerous to themselves or others, the high court said. The state must follow a due process procedure, including some kind of hearing before an impartial decision-maker, before it can involuntarily treat a patient.

The court set out constitutionally required safeguards to be followed in treating mental patients. The use of psychotropic drugs to physically restrain mental patients violated their right to treatment in a humane, therapeutic environment.[102]

A federal appellate court for New Jersey ruled that

involuntarily committed mental patients have a constitutional right to refuse administration of antipsychotic drugs.

A patient in a state mental institution filed suit during his twelfth hospitalization after an involuntary commitment proceeding. A federal trial court recognized a constitutional right to refuse treatment. The appellate court modified the trial court's injunction and incorporated the rules of a state administrative bulletin. The Supreme Court reversed and remanded for reconsideration in light of its decision in a related case.

On remand, the federal appellate court said that the proper standard for determining whether drugs can be administered against the patient's will was one based on accepted professional judgment. The procedures outlined in the state administrative bulletin satisfied the due process requirements for applying the professional judgment standard. The bulletin required a physician to explain the reasons for the medication and to specify risks and benefits, to have procedures for patient consultation with family members, and to provide for a review by other professional staff and meetings with the treatment team.[103]

In *Guardianship of Richard Roe III*,[104] a noninstitutionalized patient was found to be incompetent, and his father was appointed guardian. The father then sought contingent authority to consent to the forcible administration of antipsychotic medication. The Massachusetts Supreme Judicial Court denied this request, holding that, except in an emergency, in cases of forced medication, the "substituted judgment" of an incompetent must be exercised by a judge, not a guardian. If the judge determines that the patient would consent to antipsychotic medication, it should be ordered; if the judge determines that the patient would refuse, then he or she must weigh those state interests that can override the right to refuse. Only an "overwhelming" state interest will suffice. The protection of third parties was seen as a potentially overriding interest in this case, but the court cautioned that a bona fide "likelihood of violence" must be established. The Massachusetts court emphasized that its holding was limited to noninstitutionalized, incompetent individuals and did not apply to patients in state hospitals.

Several involuntarily committed mental patients brought a class action suit in a federal court against officials and staff of a Massachusetts state hospital. They had been forcibly administered antipsychotic drugs during their hospitalization. The drugs administered — Thorazine, Mellaril, Prolixin, and Haldol — had significant adverse reactions, such as tardive dyskinesia, that could be disabling.

The patients claimed that forcible administration of the drugs violated their constitutional rights. A federal trial court agreed and said that patients must consent before the administration of drugs except in an emergency. An appellate court agreed in part but said that a hospital's professional staff should have substantial discretion in deciding where an emergency required involuntary administration of medication.

The U.S. Court of Appeals for the 1st Circuit has delineated the circumstances whereby patients at state mental hospitals may be forcibly administered antipsychotic drugs. The opinion deals with the balancing of the state's police powers and *parens patriae* powers with the rights of the institutionalized patient.[105]

The court first addressed the situation where, in the exercise of its police power, the state may forcibly medicate a mental patient. The district court had said, "A committed mental patient may be forcibly medicated in an emergency situation in which a failure to do so would result in a substantial likelihood of physical harm to that patient, other patients, or to staff members of the institution."

Addressing the difficulty in setting a "clear-cut unitary standard of quantitative likelihood that violence would occur," the court of appeals said. "The professional judgment call required in balancing these varying interests and determining whether a patient should be subjected to forcible administering of antipsychotic drugs demands an individualized estimation of the possibility and type of violence, the likely effects of particular drugs on a particular individual, and an appraisal of the alternative, less restrictive forces of action."

Remanding the case to the district court, the court of appeals summarized its holding on this issue as follows:

The district court should not attempt to fashion a single "more-likely-than-not" standard as a substitute for an individualized balancing of the varying interests of particular patients in refusing antipsychotic medication against the equally varying interests of patients — and the state — in preventing violence . . . [the] court should leave this typical, necessarily ad hoc balancing to state physicians and limit its own role to designing procedures for ensuring that the patients' interests in refusing antipsychotics are taken into consideration and that antipsychotics are not forcibly administered absent a finding by a qualified physician that those interests are outweighed in a particular situation and less restrictive alternatives are unavailable.

As for the use of the *parens patriae* power to justify forcible medication, the court said, "The sine qua non for the state's use of its *parens patriae* power as justification for the forcible administration of mind-affecting drugs is a determination that the individual to whom the drugs are to be administered lacks the capacity to decide for himself whether he should take the drugs." However, "the commitment decision itself is an inadequate predicate to the forcible administration of drugs to an individual where the purported justifications for that action is the state's *parens patriae* power."

The court ruled that "absent an emergency, a judicial determination of incapacity to make treatment decisions must be made before the state may rely on its *parens patriae* powers to forcibly medicate a patient, but as a constitutional matter the state is not required to seek individualized guardian approval for decisions to treat incompetent patients with antipsychotic drugs. What procedural safeguards might be required, short of individualized guardian review, we leave for the present to the district court." The case was remanded to the district court for further proceedings.

The U.S. Supreme Court, nevertheless, believed the case applicable to the patients in *Rogers,* who were citizens of Massachusetts. Because state law had changed, and may in fact provide broader protection to the patient than required under the Constitution, the Court remanded the case for reconsideration.

The Massachusetts Supreme Judicial Court was of the opinion that an involuntarily committed patient is competent to make treatment decisions. Incompetence must be determined by a judge, and only after a patient is judged incompetent can he or she be forcibly administered antipsychotic drugs. There is no state interest great enough to permit involuntary administration of drugs in a nonemergency situation. Forcible treatment is permissible in an emergency and to prevent the immediate, substantial, and irreversible deterioration of a serious mental illness, the court said.[106]

In the case of *Rogers v. Okin* the U.S. Supreme Court ruled that some psychiatric patients have a qualified right to refuse psychotropic, or mind-altering, medication, and that some form of administrative review of this kind of treatment should be instituted. However, the Court did not set definitive guidelines and left it to the states to establish right-to-refuse policies.[107]

A qualified right implies that a patient may exercise the right to refuse medication only if he or she does not present some special condition such as incompetency or dangerousness. If a patient has such a condition and refuses medication, he or she may be forcibly treated. In all the judicial opinions issued so far, the existence of an emergency also serves as justification for overriding patients' refusals.

All the states that recognize the right to refuse medication also have procedures to override the right to emergencies. Only 30 states, however, permit overriding patients' refusals in nonemergencies. The exact procedures that are used to override patients' refusals vary considerably from one hospital to another.

In the 20 states where the right to refuse is qualified by more than the existence of an emergency, competency and commitment standards are used to determine which patients may refuse medication. All but one of these states restrict the right to refuse to competent patients.

Most states that have officially initiated a procedure to implement the right to refuse treatment have provided more than one method—often, more formal methods such as statutes and litigation are followed by the development of more detailed administrative rules and departmental policies.

Despite the existence of these policies, "many people . . . are frustrated about the confused status of this issue." Some are trying to approach the problem in innovative ways, for example, by instituting a multidisciplinary panel to review all medication refusals. Nevertheless, an apparently common approach is to have "written procedures representing official guidelines, but in practice to fail to extend to patients a meaningful right to refuse medication.[108]

NEUROPSYCHIATRY AND FORENSIC ISSUES
Brain damage, dementia, or depression

Mood has been considered man's own best estimate of well-being. It reflects the determinations made consciously or subliminally by the mind. Certain commonly occurring problems, including separation, object loss, illness, and injury have long been known to cause a depressed mood. Interactions of genetic, neurochemical, developmental, and interpersonal factors also influence mood.

The important determination for the neuropsychiatrist, as well as the litigation attorney, is whether the mood of depression is a primary (functional) disorder, a disorder secondary to some loss or injury, or whether it reflects symptoms of some covert underlying illness that it may be masking.

Pseudodementia. *Pseudodementia* has been described as a syndrome that mimics an organic (physical) brain deficit, but is actually a result of primary psychiatric illness. It is usually but not exclusively associated with old age. There is considerable overlap of symptoms in primary depressive disorders and dementing (organic) disorders. The diagnosis of depressive pseudodementia is especially difficult when the depressed mood or affect (emotion) is absent and physical impairments dominate the clinical picture.

Physical illness, pathological changes in the brain, metabolic abnormalities, and some medications affect the individual psychologically, as well as via neurobiological mechanisms. Psychiatrists recognize the necessity of excluding the diagnosis of organic illnesses that present as psychiatric syndromes in assessing patients. *The Diagnostic and Statistical Manual III-R* (DSM III-R) reflects this emphasis.

Metabolic illness can mimic a major depression.

Depressive disorders following head injury and stroke are also common. Because of the overlap of symptoms and differences in prognosis, significant medical and legal implications result from misdiagnosis.

The distinctions between depression and dementia are sometimes difficult for the clinician. The differentiation is only occasionally assisted by laboratory data. The EEG is rarely diagnostic and the CT scan and MRI findings are not reliably correlated with the clinical manifestations. Neuropsychological testing provides a profile of the cognitive deficits and can aid in localizing clinically apparent brain injuries, but in most pseudodementia cases, it simply provides a profile of mixed findings that reflect the clinical picture. Use of more sophisticated tests, such as computerized EEG and PET scans, are likewise unhelpful.

Psychiatric history and mental status examination. It is the clinical psychiatric examination that provides the most important information regarding the cause of the depressive state. A family history of affective or addictive disorders and/or a past history of the patient revealing affective illness or a personality profile that is depression-prone (e.g., compulsive, narcissistic, paranoid types) are significant; in addition, a precipitating event threatening a loss of self-esteem, an acute onset, and/or a rapid progression of depressive symptoms would favor the diagnosis of a primary depressive disorder. In contrast, a more vague presentation, with gradual progression of symptoms and retention of past social skills, or a patient who tends to make adaptive efforts while attempting to conceal, deny, or minimize impairments favors an organic process rather than a primary depressive disorder.

Organic factors that cause depression. For many years clinicians have recognized that depressive disorders, referred to in the DSM III-R as organic mood disorders, accompany brain injury. Depressive disorders may also be caused by toxic or metabolic factors or medications, such as reserpine and methyldopa. Endocrine disorders, cancer of the pancreas, and viral illness are likewise common causes for depression. It is also clear that abused substances cause depression. The most common ones are alcohol and sedatives (barbiturates, antianxiety agents, tranquilizers, and hypnotics).

Prognosis. Character structure (i.e., personality type) is probably the best predictor of recovery from depressive illness. The poorest treatment responses and most chronic courses are in those depressed patients with a primary characterologic diagnosis. Post–brain injury depressive disorders show a natural course similar in length to that associated with functional major depressive disorders. Spontaneous remission of this type of depression generally occurs within one year.

Diagnosis determines the outcome. The diagnosis must be based on data collection from several sources. The history of onset of the illness, related precipitants, development of symptoms and the course of the illness, the background health history of the patient and family, and the developmental history with a focus on personality traits and coping defenses are all important. Findings on physical examination, neuropsychiatric evaluation, laboratory tests, and data from collateral interviews with others who have observed the patient over time must also be obtained for a complete assessment.

The distinction between functional depression and dementia is difficult in the absence of an independent or corroborating history. The developmental course of a primary depression, however, can often be distinguished from post–brain injury depression and dementia by ascertaining which symptoms occurred first: loss of confidence, interest and drive (depression), or impaired memory (especially with respect to new learning), orientation, and ability to think abstractly (dementia). On mental status examination, "near-miss" answers are more likely associated with irreversible organic mental syndromes, whereas "don't know" answers are more characteristic of reversible primary functional depression.

Conclusion. The systematic inquiry of the psychiatric expert witness regarding diagnosis and prognosis parallels the systematic clinical work-up of the patient with depression. The attempt is to identify those patients with reversible disorders. Inquiry regarding the history of the illness, physical and mental status examinations and laboratory data, and organic factors must be considered. Among these factors are the following:

1. *Medication:* adverse responses, toxic effects, effects of withdrawal of medications, reactions to combined medications, drug abuse
2. *Metabolic disorders:* too high or too low levels of blood electrolytes, especially calcium, sodium, and glucose, and disorders of the thyroid gland
3. *Toxic substances:* chronic abuse of alcohol, sedatives, or other addictive agents
4. *Systemic illnesses:* liver, kidney, and/or cardiovascular diseases
5. *Trauma:* birth injuries and head injuries earlier in life, vehicular accidents, or surgical trauma
6. *Tumors:* Either intracranial or extracranial tumors, which have direct or indirect effects on mood and cognition (e.g., pancreatic tumors).

Through inquiry should be made into the patient's history and exposure to the noted organic factors in taking depositions from the patient, the treating physician, and family members. The data collected will aid the psychiatrist retained to do the independent medical examination. A determination must be made of the correct diagnosis, degree of impairment, and prognosis utilizing this information in conjunction with the clinical assessment by the psychiatric expert.

The analysis of head injury claims
Epidemiology

1. More than 500,000 (as many as 7 to 8 million) head injuries occur in the United States per year.
2. Ten percent of victims of head injury die. It is the leading cause of death of individuals under age 35 years.
3. Incidence: 180/100,000; prevalence: 800/100,000. (It is the most common cause for neurologically based anxiety/depression except for migraine.)
4. Five million children/year (200,000) hospitalized; 4000 children die each year.
5. Thirty percent to 50% of head injuries are associated with moderate to severe brain injury and patients are left with permanent residue (or die).
6. Five percent to 10% of those with slight to mild brain injuries have residual neuropsychiatric dysfunction.
7. Five percent of patients with brain injury develop seizures (50% of those with depressed skull fractures), usually appearing one to three months after injury, but can be seen in rare cases after 10 years.

Anatomy and pathology

CONCUSSION. Concussion results from a mechanical impact to the head or an abrupt acceleration-deceleration impact of the brain within the skull, wherein neuron function is immediately impaired. Loss of consciousness is a usual feature, although not always a necessary component. Immediately after the trauma, the patient experiences confused thinking, lethargy, or amnesia. The loss of consciousness is due to neuronal-axonal injuries secondary to rotational forces around the brain stem. The post-traumatic amnesia includes both retrograde and anterograde amnesia. Almost all patients with concussions have a period of amnesia that extends beyond the period of unconsciousness. Persons sustaining simple concussive injuries may have mild resultant neurologic and cognitive/emotional impairments, although most improve and return completely back to normal without any residual brain damage.

The correlation between the length of amnesia and prognosis, especially in patients over the age of 30, is a useful clinical indicator. The following chart is a good rule of thumb for prognosis:

Degree of severity	Duration of amnesia
Slight concussion	0–15 minutes
Mild concussion	15 minutes–1 hour
Moderate concussion	1–24 hours
Severe concussion	1–7 days
Very severe concussion	Longer than 7 days

CEREBRAL CONTUSION. This denotes a patient who has residual neurologic deficit after closed head trauma—a "brain bruise." In this group of patients, diffuse axonal injury in the white matter is the most prominent mechanism of brain damage. The injuries usually occur in the following anatomical regions:

1. The corpus callosum,
2. The brain stem, or
3. Diffuse injury to axons.

These injuries are severe, and usually result in death, although patients may remain in a vegetative state.

TRAUMATIC ENCEPHALOPATHY. This term is used to denote patients with residual clinical evidence of brain damage from trauma. It is not restricted to concussions and contusions, but may be extended to include the sequelae of hematomas, including extradural, subdural and intracerebral hematomas, as well as brain lacerations and open head wounds.

Clinical presentation

INITIAL IMPACT. There is usually a general paralysis characterized by loss of muscle tone (the patient drops to the ground motionless); loss of consciousness, reflexes, and respiration occur for a matter of a few seconds to a few minutes; then the patient goes through a restless phase and regains consciousness. While regaining consciousness, the patient is usually irritable and apathetic. Occasionally the patient is uncontrollable and abusive. It is common for the patient to be nauseated, vomiting, hypothermic, and have alterations in pulse and blood pressure. This unstable confusional period usually lasts less than 24 hours. During this period of time, the patient may appear to be acting in a purposeful manner but frequently will question what has happened and will not recall anything concerning the injury. There will usually be a retrograde amnesia covering hours, days, or even years before the accident. If the patient is not rendered unconscious, he or she will appear dazed, confused, and disoriented. The retrograde amnesia in most cases is less than 30 minutes and usually only a few seconds in duration. The anterograde amnesia is usually much longer, but in most cases of minor injury lasts less than 24 hours. In most cases the retrograde amnesia shortens as the patient recovers. With the passage of time, the patient is able to retrieve details closer and closer to the time of impact to the point where, in the typical case, it is only a few seconds immediately before the accident that are lost forever. Therefore, if initial questioning of the patient soon after the injury does not reveal pertinent information regarding how the injury occurred, these facts may be retrievable at a later time when the amnesic period shrinks. The period of anterograde amnesia is not always predictable. However, it usually exists for the period of time while the patient is in a confused mental state. Since the confusional behavior fluctuates with lucid periods intermingled with periods having more clouding of consciousness, the patient will be left with islands of memory in a sea of amnesia.

During the post-traumatic period, subtle organic behavioral deficits occur that mimic emotional reactions. Although the patient may feel well enough to return to work, there will be subtle difficulties with regards to full comprehension and memory. Performance gradually returns to normal around 35 days after the injury if the patient has suffered an amnesia of less than 1 hour and around 54 days after injury in those with amnesia of 1 to 24 hours. During the recovery period, the patient's difficulties are usually attributed to fatigue, inattention and defects in rapid information processing. Older patients usually have more severe difficulties as do patients who have had previous head trauma, as compared to those patients who are younger and who have had no previous head trauma. The more severe the head injury, the greater the probability of memory problems. In patients with no amnesia, no memory difficulties are found. Emotional reactions include anxiety, fear, insomnia, restlessness, fatigue, and nervousness in as high as 80% of the patients with recent head injury. The emotional reactions are more prominent during the second week after the injury and subside in most patients, as do the other symptoms, during the first month to six weeks after the injury. Headaches and dizziness usually appear during the first 24 hours after injury but may be delayed in their onset for days or even weeks. These symptoms are seen in more than half the patients during the initial post-traumatic period. A "post–concussive syndrome," including concentration difficulties, memory problems, emotional changes, insomnia, headache, and dizziness in the weeks following head injury is a common diagnosis made by physicians. It is expected that half the patients will be symptom free in six weeks. Many patients report persistent subjective complaints that cannot be documented by current available assessment techniques and may represent causes other than the brain injury itself.

Prognosis and speed of recovery. Factors influencing the prognosis and speed of recovery include the following:

1. Preexisting personality or character disorder
2. Previous head injury
3. Alcohol usage
4. Emotional or social pressures
5. Physical exercise.

Clinical findings. Clinical findings usually include a CT scan that is normal, a normal EEG, and the findings discussed in the following paragraphs.

Symptoms lasting longer than a few weeks or a month after injury may have emotional or other reasons for the perpetuation of symptoms, although studies have supported a correlation between preinjury personality or litigation and the development of a post-traumatic syndrome. Other studies have concluded that the syndrome is related to the organic mental changes. Increasingly sophisticated procedures such as brain mapping (CEEG or BEAM), magnetic resonance imaging (MRI), and positron emission computerized tomography (PECT) may well provide important data in the future to clarify whether or not there is a presence of physiological or structural disruption of the brain in such cases.

Pretraumatic neurosis and other personality and social factors (e.g., a history of parental rejection or overprotection, chronic maladjustment, depression, alcohol abuse, and proneness to accidents) have been found to be strong correlating factors with the development of post-traumatic syndrome.

The context in which the injury occurs could be important. Many studies have supported the view of some physicians that those injuries wherein legal awards depend on pain and suffering have a correlative influence on prognosis of the post-traumatic symptoms as well as a combination of job difficulty, marriage difficulty, and declining economic status. Other studies have found no such correlation.

If a person sustains several head injuries over time, the effect of each succeeding injury becomes more significant, recovery is slower, and, eventually, permanent brain damage can result.

Another finding is severe closed head injury, defined by the patient having a post-traumatic amnesic period of at least 24 hours (the average period of amnesia has been greater than seven days). The same syndrome occurs as with minor head injury, although the initial coma (i.e., complete loss of consciousness and nonresponsiveness to pain and other stimuli) is longer (as well as the post-traumatic amnesia) and the confusional behavior during the return to full consciousness is longer.

Permanent neuropsychiatric deficits

PERSONALITY CHANGE. Frontal lobe damage is the most prominent cause of personality change. This is not as readily apparent as motor weakness or language difficulties (aphasias); therefore, these changes must be specifically sought in the neuropsychiatric examination, which should include family members or others who knew the patient prior to the injury. The main features of personality change include apathy, euphoria, irritability, and inappropriate behavior accompanying the personality change. With a carefully done complete mental status examination, features of cognitive disorganization may be found in severely injured patients, including disconnected thought processes, disorientation and conceptual disorganization, emotional withdrawal, and various affective disturbances, including excitement and blunting of affect and motor retardation.

COGNITIVE DISTURBANCES. Early in the recovery period from head trauma, the performance IQ (nonverbal IQ) suffers the greatest drop. The performance IQ improves during recovery, and by six months after injury, both verbal and performance scores have generally stabilized at about equal levels. Lingering cognitive deficits, impaired social judgment, deficient planning ability, and a lack of full insight frequently coexist with normal general intelligence and good physical recovery.

DEPRESSION. Depression with anxiety can be organic or a reactive emotional response to the injury. If the injury is to the left frontal lobe, it is not uncommon to have an organic depression. These depressions are responsive to usual antidepressant medication in therapeutic dosages. Psychotic reactions are known to occur, although they are distinctly uncommon.

Studies relating prognosis to coma and amnesia demonstrate that for patients with coma of more than two months' duration, the full recovery rate is 6%, whereas it is 57% in cases of coma of less than two months. Patients with post-traumatic amnesia of over more than three to four weeks generally have significant mental problems and persistent memory deficits.

Secondary complications

1. Raised intracranial pressure
2. Subdural hematoma
3. Fat embolism
4. Development of post-traumatic epilepsy
5. Progressive dementia; head trauma has been hypothesized to increase the risk of Alzheimer's disease in later life.

Discovery of alternative causes

1. Alcoholism, falls while inebriated
2. Childhood trauma (sports, bicycle riding, skateboard)
3. Physical abuse by family member
4. Drug abuse
5. Preinjury mental disorders
6. Sports and recreation (boxing, football)
7. Occupational hazards
8. Risk-taking recreational activities (motorcycling, car racing, sky diving)
9. Stroke, tumor, genetic, demyelinating disorders, metabolic disorders
10. Dementias (Alzheimers, Pick's, Huntington's)
11. Previous or subsequent head injury

12. Viral encephalopathy (herpes simplex, Japanese B, AIDS)
13. Factitious disorder
14. Malingering
15. Other organic mental disorders.

To assess the preceding alternative causes, depositions of friends, family, employers, and a review of military and school records are critical, along with all medical and hospital records since birth (e.g., birth injuries and childhood illnesses).

Establishment of the facts. Establishment of the facts, especially the course of recovery, includes the following:

1. Documentation of the length of amnesia, unconsciousness, and/or coma.
2. Severity of the above. Are the signs and symptoms consistent with the usual pattern?
3. Are the residua consistent with the usual pattern and with the location of the documented lesions? Residual difficulties that are most common (in decreasing order) are visual-spatial problems, speech problems, memory problems, and problems with executive functioning (frontal lobes).

Testing. Diagnostic and neuropsychiatric testing includes

1. CT scan
2. MRI
3. SPECT/PET scans
4. Neuropsychological testing
5. EEG/computerized EEG (e.g., BEAM)
6. Glasgow Coma Scale and Galveston Orientation Amnesia Test (GOAT).

Dissimulation

1. Conscious
   a. Factitious disorder (motivation to be a patient)
   b. Malingering (motivation for financial or other gain)
2. Unconscious (Conversion Disorder)
3. Neuropsychiatric evaluation
   a. Review of all medical records, past and current
   b. Review of all relevant discovery
   c. Review of past and current school and work performance records
   d. Credit reports (high incidence of credit problems among antisocial persons who malinger)
   e. Military records (for IQ testing as well as disciplinary actions)
   f. Family's depositions and/or interviews with family
   g. Complete mental status examination and psychological testing
4. Criteria evidencing dissimulation
   a. Near misses to simple questions

b. Gross discrepancies from expected norms

c. Inconsistency between present diagnosis and neuropsychiatric findings

d. Inconsistency between reported and observed symptoms

e. Resistance, avoidance, or bizarre responses on standard tests

f. Marked discrepancies on test findings that measure similar cognitive ability

Summary. Brain injuries due to head trauma show some consistent patterns that will aid in assessing the nature and extent of such injuries, as well as in determining the prognosis. The neuropsychiatrist's examination, along with appropriate diagnostic testing, can aid in assessing whether or not the signs and symptoms and pattern of recovery are consistent with the injuries claimed or with a known pattern of head trauma, as well as to provide an indication of prognosis and/or need for additional discovery. Inconsistencies must be explained. Preexisting injuries, factitious disorders and/or malingering should be considered when inconsistencies exist. Appropriate evaluative techniques, and consultations, along with close examination of data collected during discovery, form the bases for such an analysis, along with appropriate neuropsychiatric examination.

END NOTES

1. J. Biggs, *The Guilty Mind: Psychiatry and the Law of Homicide* (Harcourt Brace, New York 1955).
2. M. Guttmacher, *America's Last King: An Interpretation of the Madness of George III* (Scribner's, New York 1941).
3. P. Pinel, *A Treatise on Insanity in Which Are Contained the Principles of a New and Practical Nosology of Maniacal Disorders,* (Sheffield, England, trans. 1806).
4. B. Rush, *Medical Inquiries and Observations Upon Diseases of the Mind,* (Prichard & Hall, Philadelphia 1789).
5. I. Ray, *A Treatise on the Medical Jurisprudence of Insanity,* Little, Brown, Boston 1838).
6. 94 S.D. Codified Laws Ann., §§ 27 A-8-10 & 11 (1984).
7. *Application for William R.,* 9 Misc. 2d 1984, 172 N.Y. S2d 869 (1958).
8. *Goodman v. Parwatikar,* 570 F.2d 801 (8th Cir. 1978).
9. *Rogers v. Okin,* 478 F. Supp. 1342 (D. Mass. 1979), *aff'd in part, revised in part,* 634 F.2d 650 (1st Cir. 1980), *vacated & remanded sub nom Mills v. Rogers,* 457 U.S. 291 (1982), *remanded* 738 F.2d 1 (1st Cir. 1984); *also see Rogers v. Commissioner of Mental Health,* 458 N.E.2d 308 (Mass. 1983), *following the holding of In re Roe III,* 421 N.E.2d 40 (Mass 1981).
10. H. Ross, *Commitment of the Mentally Ill: Problems of Law and Policy,* 57 Mich. L. Rev. 945 (1959).
11. Conn. Gen. Stat. Ann.§ 17-176 (West 1976).
12. *Lake v. Cameron,* 364 F.2d 657 (D.C. Cir. 1966).
13. *Lessard v. Schmidt,* 349 F. Supp. 1078 (E.D. Wisc. 1972).
14. Birnbaum, *The Right to Treatment,* 46 A.B.A.J. 499 (1960).
15. *Wyatt v. Stickney,* 325 F. Supp. 781 (M.D. Ala.), *enforced* 334 F. Supp. 1341 (M.D. Ala. 1971), *orders entered* 344 F. Supp. 373 344 F. Supp. 387 (M.D. Ala. 1972), *aff'd in part, rev'd and remanded in part sub nom.,* Wyatt v. Aderholt, 503 F.2d 1305 (5th Cir. 1974).
16. *O'Connor v. Donaldson,* 422 U.S. 563 (1975).
17. *Mills v. Rogers,* 457 U.S. 1119 (1982).
18. *Rennie v. Klein,* 653 F.2d 836 (3d Cir. 1981).
19. *Youngberg v. Romeo,* 457 U.S. 307 (1982).
20. *Id.*
21. *Rennie v. Klein,* 720 F.2d 266, 269 (3d Cir. 1983).
22. J. Quen, *Anglo-American Criminal Insanity—An Historical Perspective,* 10 J Hist. Behavioral Sci 313 (1974).
23. Justinian Digest 48, 8.2 (Dec. 533).
24. S. Grey, *The Insanity Defense: Historical Development and Contemporary Relevance,* 10 Am. Crim. Law Rev. 555 (1972).
25. *Id.*
26. 4 W Blackstone, *Commentaries* 24 (Clarendon Press, Oxford 1769).
27. *Pate v. Robinson,* 383 U.S. 375, 86 S. Ct. 836, 15 L.Ed.2d 815 (1966).
28. *Dusky v. United States,* 362 U.S. 402, 80 S. Ct. 788, 4 L.Ed.2d 824 (1960).
29. *Drope v. Missouri,* 420 U.S. 162, 95 S. Ct. 896, 43 L.Ed.2d 103 (1975).
30. *Id.*
31. *Estelle v. Smith,* 451 U.S. 454, 101 S. Ct. 1866, 68 L.Ed.2d 359 (1981).
32. *Jackson v. Indiana,* 406 U.S. 715, 32 L.Ed.2d 434, 92 S. Ct. 1845 (1972).
33. *Rex v. Arnold,* 16 How. Sr. Tr. 695 (C.P. 1742).
34. 1 Hawkins, *Pleas of The Crown* 1 (1824).
35. *Hadfield's Case,* 27 State Trial 1281 (1800).
36. *Id.*
37. R. Reisner, *Law and The Mental Health System,* 564 (West 1985).
38. 4 State Tr. N.S. 847, 8 Eng. Rep. 718 (1843).
39. American Psychiatric Association, *Statement on the Insanity Defense* 3 (Dec. 1982).
40. *M'Naughton's Case,* 4 State Tr. N.S. 847, 8 Eng. Rep. 718, 721-22 (H.L. 1843) (per Lord Chief Justice Tindal).
41. A. Goldstein, *The Insanity Defense,* 67 (Yale University Press, New Haven 1967).
42. *Id.*
43. *Durham v. United States,* 214 F.2d 862, 874 (D.C. Cir. 1954).
44. *Id.* at 874-75.
45. D. Weschler, *The Criteria For Criminal Responsibility,* 22 Univ. of Chi. Law Rev. 367 (1955).
46. Goldstein, *supra* note 75.
47. Model Penal Code §4.01 (1962).
48. *McDonald v. United States,* 312 F.2d 847 (D.C. Cir. 1962).
49. *Id.* at 851.
50. *People v. Wells,* 203 P.2d 53 (Cal. 1949).
51. Cal. Penal Code §28(b) (1981): *also see People v. Wh* 117 Cal. App. 3d 270, 172 Cal. Rptr. 612 (1981).
52. *Heads v. Louisiana,* 370 S.2d 564 (La. 1979), *remanded for further consideration* 444 U.S. 1008 (1980).
53. *State v. Head,* No. 106, 126 (1st Jud. Dist. Ct., Caddo Parrish, Oct. 10, 1981).
54. DSM IV 615-18 (4th ed. 1994).
55. R. Haskett and J. Abplanalp, *Premenstrual Tension Syndrome: Diagnostic Criteria and the Selection of Research Subjects,* 9 Psychiatry Res. 125 (1983).
56. R. Haskett and M. Steiner, *Diagnosing Premenstrual Tension Syndrome,* 37 Hosp. and Community Psychiatry 33-34 (1986).
57. *British Legal Debate: Premenstrual Tension and Criminal Behavior,* N.Y. Times, Dec. 29, 1981, at 17.
58. M. Guttmacher, *The Role of Psychiatry in Law* (Thomas, Springfield, Ill., 1965).
59. B. Wooten, *Crime and Criminal Law* (Stevens, London 1963).
60. Mont. Code Ann §46-14-102 (1979).

61. 4 Idaho Code §18-207 Cumm. Supp. (1986).

62. *Id.* at §18-207c.

63. *Supra,* note 92.

64. American Bar Association, *Standing Committee on Association Standards for Criminal Justice — Proposed Criminal Justice Mental Health Standards* (ABA Chicago 1984).

65. 7 Mental Disability L. Rep. 136 (1983).

66. *Comprehensive Crime Control Act of 1984* (Government Printing Office, Washington, D.C. 1984).

67. *See People v. McQuillan,* 221 N.W.2d 569 (Mich. 1974).

68. *See* L. Blunt and H. Harley, *Guilty but Mentally Ill: An Alternative Verdict,* 3 Beh. Sci & Law 49 (1985) [*citing* Alaska, Delaware, Georgia, Illinois, Indiana, Kentucky, New Mexico, Pennsylvania, South Dakota, Michigan & Utah].

69. Mich. Comp. Laws Ann. 768.36(1), enacted in Public Act 1980 of 1975.

70. R. Petrella et al., *Examining the Application of the Guilty but Mentally Ill Verdict in Michigan,* 36 Hosp. and Community Psychiatry 254 (1985).

71. W. Bellamy, *Malpractice in Psychiatry,* 118 Am. J. Psychiatry 769 (1962).

72. P. Slawson, *Psychiatric Malpractice: A California Statewide Survey,* 6 Bull. Am. Acad. of Psychiatry & L. 58 (1978).

73. Clinical Psychiatric News 1 (Oct. 1983).

74. *Duvall v. Goldin,* 362 N.W.2d 275 (Mich. App. 1984).

75. *Clites v. Iowa,* 322 N.W.2d 917 (Iowa Ct. App. 1981).

76. G. Annas, L. Glantz & B. Katz, *Informed Consent to Human Experimentation: The Subject's Dilemma* (Ballinger Cambridge, Mass. 1977).

77. American Psychiatric Association, *Principles of Medical Ethics with Annotations Especially Applicable to Psychiatry* (APA Press Washington, D.C. 1985).

78. *Doe v. Roe,* 93 Misc. 2d 201, 400 N.Y. S.Z. 668 (1977); *Clayman v. Bernstein,* 38 Pa. D&C 543 (1940); *Spring v. Geriatric Authority,* 394 Mass, 274, 475 N.E. 2d 727 (1985).

79. *Spring, supra* note 78.

80. *Doe, supra* note 78.

81. *E.g., MacDonald v. Clinger,* 84 A.D.2d 482, 446 N.Y. S.2d 801 (1982).

82. *E.g., Clark v. Geraci,* 29 Misc. 2d 791, 208 N.Y.S.2d 564 (1960).

83. Illinois Mental Health and Developmental Disabilities Confidentiality Act S.H.A. ch. 91½, §801 (1987).

84. *Tarasoff v. Regents of the University of California,* 17 Cal. 3d 425, 529 P.2d 334 131 Cal. Rptr. 14, 551 P.2d 334 (1976).

85. *Durflinger v. Artiles,* 563 F. Supp. 322 (D. Kan. 1981), *ques. cert.* 234 Kan. 484, 673 P.2d 86 (1983), *aff'd* 727 F.2d 889 (10th Cir. 1984). [Negligent release case applying *Tarasoff* and the duty to warm doctrine to hold that a duty is owed to protect identifiable third parties]; *Davis v. Lhim,* 335 N.W.2d 481 (Mich. App. 1983), *remanded on other grounds* 422 Mich. App. 8, 366 N.W.2d 73 (1985), *on remand* 147 Mich. App. 8, 382 N.W.2d 195 (1985), *on appeal* — N.W.2d — (Mich. July 22, 1986).

86. *Shaw v. Glickman,* 415 A.2d 625 (Md. App. 1985); *Leedy v. Hartnett,* 510 F. Supp. 1125 (N.D. Pa. 1981) (interpreting Pa. law).

87. *McIntosh v. Milano,* 168 N.J. Super. 466, 403 A.2d 500 (1979).

88. *Lipari v. Sears, Roebuck and Co.,* 497 F. Supp. 185 (D. Neb. 1980).

89. *Peterson v. State,* 100 Wash. 2d 421, 671 P.2d 230 (1983).

90. *Hedlund v. Orange County,* 34 Cal. 3d 695, 194 Cal. Rptr. 805 (1983). (Bluebook p. 179).

91. *Brady v. Hopper,* 570 F. Supp. 1333 (D. Colo. 1983).

92. *Brady v. Hopper,* 751 F.2d 329 (10th Cir. 1984).

93. *Shaw v. Glickman,* 45 md. App. 718, 415 A.2d 625 (1980); *Thompson v. County of Alameda,* 27 Cal. 3d 741, 167 Cal. Rptr 70 (1980).

94. *Roy v. Hartogs,* 31 Misc. 2d 350, 366 N.Y. S.2d 297 (Civ. Ct. N.Y. 1975), *aff'd* 85 Misc. 2d 891, 381 N.Y. S2d 587 (App. Term 1976).

95. *Anclote Manor Foundations v. Wilkison,* 263 So. 2d 256 (Fla. Dist. Ct. App. 1972).

96. *Zipkin v. Freeman,* 436 S.W. 2d 753 (Mo. 1968).

97. *Roy, supra* note 94.

98. *See, e.g., Brown v. Kowlizakis,* 331 S.E.2d 440 (Va. 1985).

99. *Johnson v. United States,* 409 F. Supp. 1283 (M.D. Fla. 1981).

100. J. Smith, *Medical Malpractice: Psychiatric Care* 504-05 (1986); *Lange v. United States,* 179 F. Supp. 777 (N.D. N.Y. 1960).

101. *Abraham v. Zaslow,* No. 245862 (Santa Clara City Super. Ct. Cal. Oct. 20, 1970).

102. *Davis v. Hubbard,* 506 F. Supp. 915 (D.C. Ohio 1980).

103. *Rennie v. Klein,* 720 F.2d 266, (N.J. 1983).

104. *Guardianship of Richard Roe III,*

105. *Rogers v. Okin,* 634 F.2d 650 (C.Al 1980).

106. *Rogers v. Commissioner of the Department of Mental Health,* 458 N.E.2d 308 (Mass. Sup. Jud. Ct. 1983).

107. *Rogers, supra* note 105.

108. *Anderson v. Anzoak,* 663 P.2d 570 (Ariz. App. 1982); *Goedecke v. State of Colorado, Department of Institutions,* 603 P.2d 123 (Colo. Sup. Ct. 1979) (*modified on denial of rehearing,* 1979); *In re the Mental Health of K-K-B,* No. 51, 467 (Okla. Sup. Ct. 1980); *A.E. v. Mitchell,* 724 F.2d 864 (Utah 1983); *Rivers v. Katz,* No. 191, N.Y. App. (June 10, 1986).

PART FOUR

Legislative and business aspects of medicine

Practice organizations and joint ventures

ARTHUR J. COHEN, M.D., J.D., F.C.L.M.

PRACTICE ORGANIZATIONS
PRACTICE ORGANIZATIONS AMONG PHYSICIANS
ALTERNATE AND MANAGED HEALTH CARE DELIVERY SYSTEMS
JOINT VENTURES
REASONS FOR JOINT VENTURES
CURRENT NEED FOR JOINT VENTURES
TYPES OF JOINT VENTURES
ORGANIZATIONAL STRUCTURAL MODELS
FINANCING CONSIDERATIONS FOR JOINT VENTURES
LEGAL, REGULATORY, ETHICAL, AND ACCREDITATION CONSIDERATIONS
CONCLUSION

TIONS

...for-service solo practice medicine has been the traditional medical delivery system in the United States. This type of medical practice has begun to diminish in importance in recent years as alternative health care systems have developed. The reasons for this change are many. Technological changes, increasing numbers of physicians, insurance costs including but not limited to medical negligence insurance, and increased educational debt have made it more difficult for the individual practitioner to enter solo practice.

The cost of health care averaged about 11% of the gross national product (GNP) in 1987. In 1985, health care cost about 6% of the GNP. The 1990 projection is that cost expenditures will increase to about 12% of GNP. Approximately $500 billion was spent in 1989, and in 1990 the cost may be as much as $750 billion.[1] Physicians end their education and enter practice with an average debt of $42,000. The Health and Manpower Act of 1965 increased the number of medical schools and medical students.

With health care costs approaching $1 trillion a year, private third-party payers, employers, and the U.S. government are requesting fee-for-service medicine, or asking providers to hold costs down more per day.[2] These demands have led to alterations in the health care delivery system. Both government and private insurance carriers have adopted methods to control costs. The medical marketplace has responded by developing products that deliver equivalent health care at lower cost than in the traditional office and institutional setting. Newer insurance plans also attempt to deal with the changing medical environment.

Physicians have restructured the way in which they practice. Physicians are using partnerships, sharing arrangements, group practices, and multiple-specialty groups to alter their work environment. Groupings of physicians in large practices may lead to economies of scale not achieved by a solo practice. Additionally, physicians have banded together and invested in various types of outpatient services, including radiology services, urgent care centers, surgicenters, insurance companies, medical buildings unions, HMOs, IPAs, and other interlocking business arrangements.

On the purely medical side, technology has permitted the development of outpatient surgicenters, diagnostic radiology and magnetic resonance imaging centers, lithotripter centers, breast-screening centers, and walk-in medical centers.

The insurance industry has responded to consumer demands for manageable health benefit costs by developing new products and introducing methods of controlling costs for services covered under conventional insurance plans. HMOs, PPOs, prospective payments, concurrent review, and second opinions are some of the methods and products being used. Federal and state governments have also acted to limit their financial liability under Medicare, Medicaid, and Social Security disability by limiting fee increases and increasing utilization and quality assurance reviews. The days of open-ended resources are gone. The quest for high-tech quality health care at controllable funding levels has created a realignment of providers in the health delivery system.

Among the topics to be discussed in this chapter are practice arrangements between physicians, physicians' organizations, HMOs, PPOs, IPA, Medicare, and contracts.[3]

PRACTICE ORGANIZATIONS AMONG PHYSICIANS

This section discusses the types of practices within which a physician can function. A physician may be an owner, shareholder, employee, or independent contractor of a practice. The form of the practice or venture is designed to accommodate physician and business needs.

Solo practice, sole proprietor

Advantages. The basic form of business is the solo practitioner, sole proprietor practice. The physician-owner is unincorporated and therefore not subject to the double taxation of a corporation. The employer is not responsible for matching, withholding taxes, thus saving about 7.7% on the payroll expenditures. He or she is free to establish such relationships as necessary to create a practice environment. The practice may be incorporated or unincorporated.

Disadvantages. As with any other proprietorship, the owner is personally responsible for the liabilities of the business on a personal level. This includes IRS regulations (both state and federal), occupancy and use certificates, a medical license, and compliance with all regulations controlling a regular business and a medical practice as well. The theoretical disadvantage of the solo proprietorship is the personal liability of the owner for business losses, debt, and negligence. Until tax reforms, one of the major disadvantages was the limited amount of funds that could be paid into a retirement plan. This differential has diminished because of tax legislation that limited the funding of professional corporation 401-K retirement plans.[4,5]

Sharing arrangements

Sharing arrangements are associations between two or more physicians, wherein they share office space, equipment, and possibly employees. They may also share coverage of hospital and office patients on a rotating basis or when one or the other is not available.

Advantages. Sharing arrangements permit shared overhead expenses, allowing the participants to attain economies not available in a solo practice. Depending on the arrangement, it permits shared capital expenditures, relative savings in rent, salaries, other overhead costs, and assured coverage. The physicians involved may be partners in ventures that provide services to their individual practices, such as real estate, laboratory equipment, X-ray, and computer equipment. The advantages of a solo practice are retained with some lessening of the risks. A sharing arrangement can exist between solo practitioners who are incorporated, unincorporated, or in any other permutation.

Disadvantages. The practices may become so interlocked that to the general public the physicians are regarded as partners and not as solo practitioners. The legal problem is one of expanded liability for what may be deemed a *de facto* partnership. Liability may not only be expanded for day-to-day business dealings but also in the event of medical negligence.[6] The ground rules of the sharing arrangement should be established at the time of its creation. Purchases if jointly made, employee benefits if shared, lease responsibilities, and other aspects of the arrangement should be defined early in the relationship. Once again the danger is that a *de facto* partnership is being created. Maintaining separate employees, records, and billing is evidence of separate medical practices.

A sharing arrangement may be made between solo practitioners, professional service corporation partnerships, other health care providers, and corporations.

Partnerships

As defined in the Uniform Partnership Act that has now been adopted in various forms by 49 states, a partnership is an association for two or more persons to carry on as co-owners, a business for profit.[7] The "partner" may be a legal entity such as a corporation. A partnership is contractual in nature but is regulated and controlled by the partnership act of a given jurisdiction. Being contractual, the parties can structure the relationship to suit their specific needs. The partnership agreement should spell out the relative duties and obligations of the partners. The agreement should cover the right to manage, operate, and share profits and losses.

Partners have several fundamental rights unless specifically otherwise stated in the agreement: (1) equal participation in the management of the partnership business and (2) majority voting rules. Other than in a limited partnership, or by agreement of the parties, profits and losses are shared equally and, theoretically, no partner can draw a salary. Salary is, in reality, profit.

If not created for a specific time, a partnership can be terminated at any time by any partner. The partners can opt to dissolve a partnership at any time. The death of a partner terminates the partnership unless arrangements have been made to carry on the business in the surviving partners' names. Loss of a partner can be chaotic to the business, and the partners should form contingency plans for this eventuality.

Advantages. A partnership has the advantages of shared overhead, formal business arrangements among partners, and the ability to pool capital. Other advantages include equal management, control, and shared profits. The tax consequences, rights and obligations, and liability of a partnership should be assessed prior to its formation.

Disadvantages. Being a partner in a general partnership carries certain rights but also creates obligations and liabilities. A general partner is responsible for the actions of the partners if these acts are made within the scope of partnership business. This extends to negligence as well as commitments for equipment and loans. The partners are also responsible (personally) for business losses. Further, majority rule is generally the case. It is important to determine the relative relationships of the parties and reliability of potential partners before entering this type of business arrangement.[9]

Corporation

A corporation is an artificial entity created by statute as the legal representative of the individuals who contribute to its formation or become shareholders in the entity. It is a creature of statute. Most states have corporate legislation that allows the formation of a personal service corporation. The enabling legislation permits a licensed professional to form this type of corporation. It can be created by one or more individuals who may be professionals. The definition of a professional or description of who can incorporate this type of business is contained within the appropriate state statute.[10,11]

Professionals generally form professional service organizations, which are designated as professional associations (PAs) or professional corporations (PCs). The major difference between a corporation and a partnership is personal liability. A partner has unlimited personal liability for all partnership losses whether he or she individually incurred them or not. In a corporation, losses are limited to the extent of investment; only rarely can personal assets be touched. A personal service corporation presents a unique problem for the physician, because most medical negligence policies are written in the name of the individual physicians with supplemental coverage for the corporation. Thus in the event of a suit for medical negligence, both physician and corporate assets may be at risk if the award or settlement exceeds insurance policy limits.

Professional service corporations can be formed by one or more physicians. The potential liability of a physician in a professional corporation may depend on the quality of the other physicians. Asset management

should be explored by the physicians at the time of corporate inception.[12]

A shareholder is not responsible for the ordinary business losses of a corporation, and there is no problem with dissolution. Taxability is another major difference between a partnership and a corporation. Partners are personally responsible for profits and losses, whereas shareholders are responsible for dividends and salary paid out by the corporation. Until recently, corporations could deposit a greater percentage of salary into a pension plan than could an individual. This dichotomy was rectified by the Tax Reform Act of 1986.

Advantages. Theoretically, limited personal liability, possible pension plan benefits, and continuity in the event of the death of a shareholder are some advantages of incorporation. The practice is often more salable if it possesses a corporate name.

Disadvantages. Among the disadvantages of forming a corporation are double income taxation, matching withholding taxes, and maintaining the corporate entity with regard to records and attorney fees in the cost of doing business.

Independent contractor

A physician may choose to provide services as an independent contractor to an individual physician, health care institution, urgent care center, or any other practice setting available. This is a contractual relationship in which the physician generally has no equity interest. The services may be provided on a continuous or temporary basis.

Advantages. No commitment to office space or overhead, freedom to change positions, retention of mobility, and a fixed work schedule and fixed income on an hourly, daily, or weekly basis are some of the advantages of being an independent contractor. Incentives may be built into the contract, but the issue of providing adequate care without incurring unnecessary costs may be a pitfall.

Disadvantages. The independent contractor may be expendable, may be uninsured, and has no permanency to his or her practice situation. The issue of medical negligence insurance should be examined carefully. The agreement should specify who will provide and pay for the insurance. Generally, if one is employed as an independent contractor by a *locum tenens* agency, malpractice insurance will be provided.

Employee

More and more physicians are starting or remaining in practice as the employee of an institution, another physician, medical group, or other practice setting. The key part of this relationship is the contract between the parties. Among the issues to be considered are salary, incentives, insurance, termination, hospital privileges, and restrictive or noncompetition covenants.

A contract is a written expression of the agreement between two parties and as such rests on parties and the mutuality of the arrangement. Both independent contractors and employee physicians are faced with the same problem. Because they generally lack an equity position in the practice, clinic, office, or other health institution, the provider has to protect his or her position in the community, as well as liability and income. In so doing the contract becomes the gold standard of the working relationship between the parties. The contract should specify responsibility for insurance coverage, tail insurances, and termination. One goal is to protect the individual from termination, just or unjust, without malpractice tail insurance coverage. The written agreement may include a noncompetition clause or restrictive covenant. The validity of these covenants varies with the jurisdiction. If inclusion can be avoided, it should be omitted. If inclusion cannot be avoided, then a cash buyout should be written into the agreement. Before any contract with this type of clause is signed, its force in that jurisdiction should be determined.

Alternate health care facilities

Just as health insurance plans have evolved, facilities providing care have changed. Among the newer types of facilities are urgent care centers (walk-in medical centers), ambulatory surgical centers, diagnostic imaging centers, and free-standing laboratories. These have increased the opportunity for physicians to be employees, independent contractors, or investors. The advantage of being an investor is that the return on equity is related to the investment and thus generates passive income. An employee/owner shares in profits and earns income on a fee for service or salary basis.

The issue of ownership and self-referral is a problem for the health care industry, especially for the provider. The temptations for overutilization and overcharging are great. It has been estimated that a physician-run laboratory is utilized 30% to 40% more than a commercial nonprovider-owned entity. This conflict opens the door to antitrust litigation, Racketeering Influence Corruption Act (RICO), commercial fraud, criminal, and licensure sanctions.

Providers should be wary of the potential for problems with joint ventures of this nature. A joint venture must be able to withstand the scrutiny of state and federal regulators with regard to its actual independence and the bona fide nature of the business. It should be able to show its procompetitive effect upon the market and should not be tied into schemes that, in reality, do nothing more than decrease consumer and insurer access to services and limit fee competitiveness.[14-16]

ALTERNATE AND MANAGED HEALTH CARE DELIVERY SYSTEMS

The first section and this one attempt to artificially divide practice opportunities for physicians. Traditionally, medicine has been practiced solo, as a group, or as a multispecialty practice organized as a proprietorship, partnership, or professional services organization. Within this context provider services have been delivered to the health care consumer on a direct financial basis. Although other physicians have been hospital based or employed, they, too, generally billed the consumer directly. With the advent of Medicare, for the over-65 category, and with the expansion of third-party insurance coverage to employees as part of a negotiated pension and benefit package, the traditional financial relationship of provider to patient changed. Although titled "Alternate and Managed Health Care Delivery Systems" this section might also be called "managed health care."

As insurers began to bear more and more of the burden through direct payments to providers, and as costs soared due to increased benefit packages, the true consumers became the U.S. government and industry in general, and health care insurers in particular. Increased coverage meant increased numbers of health care consumers using more and more health care resources. This led to the creation of alternate facility delivery systems in the form of outpatient surgicenters, diagnostic centers, and urgent care centers. These facilities are, theoretically, able to provide services equivalent to hospitals at a lower cost and more conveniently.

The second area of expansion is in managed health care. Two major concepts were created—health maintenance organizations (HMOs) and preferred provider organizations (PPOs). The principle of these organizations is one of prepayment and negotiated fees for service. The HMO is generally a prepaid plan whereby primary care providers are paid on a monthly capitated basis per enrollee, who pay a relatively nominal coinsurance payment. The PPO is a provider group, assembled by an insurance company, physicians, or entrepreneurs, which provides services on a discounted basis to the consumer.

There are variations of the HMO and PPO; however, for simplicity and for antitrust considerations, they can be described as physician controlled and nonphysician controlled. This difference is important, and its relevance is discussed later in the chapter, together with the concept of physician unions.

Health maintenance organizations

HMOs are available in five main categories: (1) staff model, (2) IPA, (3) group, (4) mixed, and (5) networks. The national membership in HMOs is about 35 million people. The concept of the HMO is not new, but the involvement of the federal government, beginning in 1967, led to the expansion of this type of plan. The term "health maintenance organization" was first coined by Paul Ellwood, in the mid-1960s.[17-19] The Nixon administration pushed federal legislation and financing during the late 1960s and early 1970s, which enabled HMOs to gain a national foothold.[20]

What then is an HMO, and how do the models differ? An HMO is an integrated health care delivery system that combines traditional financial risk with a provider network. The HMO presumes it can contain costs by limiting hospitalizations, specialty referrals, and procedures and shifting some financial risk to the provider. It sells insurance coverage to consumers on a premium basis and attempts to create a provider network that is both competent and cost conscious. The goal in assuming the financial risk is the delivery of quality health care to the enrolled consumer at a controlled and predictable price. To do so the HMO contracts with providers on a per capita basis for primary care and discounted basis for diagnostic and specialty referrals. To enforce the system, many plans use a "gatekeeper" concept wherein the primary care provider determines whether specialty or diagnostic referral is needed. Consumer self-referral is generally excluded from coverage.

HMO models

STAFF MODEL. The staff model HMO consists of HMO-owned clinics staffed by physician employees. Cost savings in this model are achieved by fixed provider costs and HMO ownership of hospitals and ancillary service centers. Control of these cost centers increases profitability for the plan as a whole by decreasing referral, in-patient, emergency room, and diagnostic costs. An example of a staff model HMO is Kaiser-Permanente.

INDEPENDENT PRACTICE ASSOCIATION. This model has two subdivisions. The IPA may consist of providers, primary care and specialist, assembled as a provider group by the plan, and that contracts individually or by group to provide services. The cost of these services is negotiated with the plan and may be on a per capita, fee-for-services, or discounted basis. The IPA in this case consists of physicians who provide a panel that is assembled by the HMO. It is not a provider association created by the physician uniquely to contract services to the HMO.

Provider-created IPAs exist for the purpose of representing and negotiating contracts for the group as a whole with HMOs. It is the physician-controlled HMOs and IPAs that present the highest risk for antitrust litigation. The reason for this is obvious. Within a market, these groups may substantially control the market by either market share or de facto price fixing. The IPA is composed of individual practitioners and group practices.[21]

GROUP MODEL. In this model an HMO contracts for services with independent practice groups; the basis for the contract is discounted or per capita costs in exchange for exclusivity. Hospitals, diagnostic centers, surgicenters, and urgent care centers may be arranged on a similar basis for services not provided by the group.

PRIMARY CARE MODEL. In this form, primary care providers are assembled in a network that serves as the provider panel. The primary care physicians serve as gatekeepers who limit referrals to hospitals, specialists, and diagnostic centers. The HMO usually will contract for specialty services.

MIXED MODELS. The mixed model may be any combination of the preceding systems. This system is more complex to assemble, but it may allow an HMO to tailor services to a specific market need.

All HMOs attempt to control costs by various means. The first method is to limit covered services for enrollees to a specific provider network. The second method is to have a copayment fee, which is usually nominal. The third method is to limit services to the primary care physicians, the so-called gatekeepers who determine whether specialty referral and diagnostic testing are necessary. The HMO contract removes the right of self-referral. Additionally, the contract between the insurance company and providers tends to put the providers at financial risk for overutilization of services. These services may be diagnostic tests, specialty referrals, or hospitalizations. Agreements may vary, but the contract will usually create holdback amounts of about 10% to 20% of the capitation rate, discounted rate, or fee-for-service rate. Frequently, the HMO will also create a pool for diagnostic testing and hospitalizations. If the primary care physician has a low referral or utilization rate at the end of each quarter or year, the HMO will pay a bonus to the provider. The provider is at risk because he or she bears part of the cost of the patient's care and derives no benefit from overutilization of services.

PPOs. Preferred provider organizations evolved as another form of managed health care. An HMO is considered an integrated managed health care system in that it assumes risk for patient care. It integrates the financial aspects of an insurance company, acts as a provider network, and manages the services delivered to control cards. A PPO is a different concept, however. The PPO is an actual managed care plan; it is not an insurance company. This permits the PPO to escape most of the state, federal, and insurance regulations that apply to an HMO. The PPO contracts with physicians who deliver services on a discounted basis. The employer or administrator of the PPO is able to offer financial incentives to enrollees in the form of lower health care costs. The physicians, in turn, agree to abide by the utilization and quality assurance controls implemented by the PPO. The beneficiary is responsible for a deductible and coinsurance fee for services rendered. If the beneficiary sees a physician or obtains a service outside the panel, financial disincentives are imposed in the form of higher deductibles and coinsurance payment.[22]

Corporate structure of HMOs and PPOs. PPOs and HMOs have diverse corporate structures. They range from independent entrepreneurial companies to physician-hospital joint ventures. The ownership and management involvement of physicians presents the greatest antitrust hazard. Physician-owned PPOs and IPAs may appear to be vehicles for price fixing and not bona fide joint ventures.[23]

The corporate structure ranges from large publicly held corporations to small physician/investor-owned companies. It is the ownership and control of these smaller companies that has an impact in antitrust litigation. The key to avoiding FTC investigation is maintaining an arm's-length relationship between the physicians and management of these companies. The day-to-day business of the PPO and HMO should be conducted independently of the physicians. Specifically, fee structures should be negotiated and set by the plan administrators, not by the providers.

Changes in the health care delivery system associated with the advent of managed care in the traditional, HMO, and PPO setting, have involved providers in the area of corporate medicine. The proliferation of joint ventures between physicians, hospitals, insurance companies, IPAs, and physicians' "unions" in multiple business combinations has horizontally and vertically integrated the health care system. Unless these new ventures, which include the providers, create a bona fide business, with self-management, that does not control or fix prices, act in an anticompetitive fashion, or somehow generate efficiencies to offset their inherent anticompetitive nature, they may be illegal per se. If, in fact, the venture is a horizontal merger, it may be treated as a cartel and deemed to be a cartel and per se illegal or tested under the "rule of reason."[24,25]

If the venture is a merger of services that integrates resources, the antitrust standard is the rule of reason, which is due to the realities of the marketplace. The tests in these situations are the preservation of competition in the marketplace, increased market penetration, or increased efficiency, for example. The joint venture—including all aspects of the health delivery system-providers, physician-sponsored IPAs, or physician unions—may face antitrust scrutiny and be able to pass the per se and rule of reason test.[26]

To avoid antitrust problems with cooperative undertakings, it is necessary to create a bona fide business that pools resources, enabling the joint ventures to bring efficiencies and competition to the marketplace, and to avoid the creation of sham ventures whose underlying goal is to introduce price-fixing or anticompetitive changes into the marketplace.

Antitrust issues affecting alternative delivery systems

Alternate health care delivery systems include HMOs, PPOs, clinics, IPAs, and various combinations of these entities. The organizational structure may determine possible antitrust considerations. The danger of a Sherman Antitrust Act violation increases with provider inclusion in ownership and control of the business. The role of the provider is multiple. As the health care provider, the consumer relies on his or her judgment with regard to referrals and the provision of basic health care needs. A participatory role in an HMO, PPO, or other entity may create an inherent conflict of interest.

As an investor, the goal is increased profitability. This can occur through referrals to other physician-owned entities, denial of service, overutilization, control of the market through self-referral, or large numbers of provider enrollments. A second factor is the potential for price fixing. The numbers of providers involved in the business may lead to *de facto* price fixing unless there is proof of fees being structured by administrators or other third parties without physician control. The fixed fee structure should affect only those physicians within the network so that the overall market effect is limited and, in fact, is competitive with other providers within the area.

The Sherman Act defines two basic tests: *per se* and *rule of reason* in determining violations. Per se restraints are those that are so obviously anticompetitive that detailed studies are not required to determine their effect on the economy[28,29]; examples are group boycotts and refusals to deal. The rule of reason test is more complex. It requires a more elaborate analysis of the business involved. Among the elements explored are the type of business, type of restraint, history, and reason for its imposition.[30-32]

The true test may be the bona fide nature of the business. PPOs, HMOs, and IPAs range from physician owned and controlled to entrepreneurial control. The plans may be nonphysician owned, partially provider owned, or some permutation that dilutes physician involvement. The independent company, PPO, or HMO that is run as a separate entity with no provider ownership or control over marketing, participation, or fees is the least likely to encounter antitrust problems. An independent plan marketed to consumers and enlisting providers without their ownership participation is the safest approach. This organization mode contains no elements of vertical or horizontal integration.

A provider-owned and provider-run business contains elements of horizontal and vertical integration. The more integrated it is, the more likely that antitrust questions will be raised. Similarly, in a smaller market, the utilization of one medical group or hospital may create an antitrust problem even though the providers do not own or control the business entity.

PPOs are generally considered procompetitive because they tend to lower consumer fees and generate competition among physicians. They may, in fact, be anticompetitive and a sham designed to set fees in a geographical area.[33] The ownership and contractual arrangements among physicians in a PPO are subject to horizontal and vertical analysis. The *Maricopa* case found that the establishment of minimum prices was price fixing per se and a violation of the Sherman Antitrust Act.

A 1982 case found that a physician-owned and -operated insurance company, associated with a local medical society, was capable of concerted action also in violation of the antitrust law.[34,35] A physician-owned company could avoid these issues if the fee structure were determined by independent management with limited physician control in an environment where the number of providers is limited. In this scenario the physicians do not determine fees nor do they constitute a significant percentage of practitioners.

Refusal of a group of dentists to submit X-rays to insurance claims review has been held to be a group boycott. In order to be a conspiracy in restraint of trade, both the conspiracy and restraint have to be proven by the government.[36]

The classic fee-for-service system in the United States has consisted of many small provider-owned businesses functioning competitively in the marketplace. As managed health care systems evolved, the tendency has been to integrate physicians into the system as owner/providers. This leads to increased market penetration by the HMO, PPO, or IPA. Increased provider participation eases marketing because patients will be more likely to enroll if they can continue treatment with their "regular doctor." The business danger of this integration is that increasing numbers of providers will lead to increasing market control and decreased competitiveness. The degree of market share and provider participation may be illegal at certain threshold levels. The combination of physicians may represent substantial market power and control. Fees set by this group may substantially affect other nonparticipating physicians. Associations of physicians as IPA, HMOs, PPOs, or large clinics may be anticompetitive by their very nature.

Regardless of the bona fide nature of the company initially, the exclusion of providers and the collective impact on fees in a community are in violation of public policy. An inherent contradiction exists in the government's attitude toward alternative delivery systems. Federal legislation guarantees the penetration of HMOs in the health care market. Yet, the creation of these entities as joint ventures by physicians and hospitals invites close governmental scrutiny if they are too large or successful in controlling the market share.[37]

Two recent cases[38,39] contain in-depth discussions of the application of the Sherman Act in the health care market. HMOs as a newer type of insurance product are placed within the context of Sherman and Clayton Acts violations. The application of state statutes and the development of an HMO that requires exclusion of health providers and facilities is by nature antitrust in concept. The impact may be acceptable if the market is not dominated by the HMO or IPA. *Ocean States* places the HMO in the context of competition, pricing, and advertising. It takes a more liberal attitude in allowing competitive pricing and marketing between HMO companies.

The gist of these cases is that there is a fine line between antitrust violations and acceptable patterns of behavior. The legitimacy of the business and physician inclusion is in management and ownership.[40-42]

Exclusion or exemption from the Sherman Act is limited. This rule applies to essential facilities. An HMO, PPO, or IPA will not fall within this exemption. Exclusion is a primary concept of the PPO. The theoretical goal is the assembly of a group of efficient, high-quality providers. The danger is that many will exclude the few. In the essential facility exclusion, all "providers" could theoretically be members without antitrust violations.[43,44] A dichotomy exists between provider- and nonprovider-controlled companies. The provider-controlled and -operated companies are more likely to be scrutinized because of market impact, provider exclusion, possible price fixing, and decreased competitiveness. The degree of physician ownership and control is important in that who participates, who is excluded, how fees are determined, and marketing may all be part of a Sherman Act violation.

The provider mix is important. Exclusion of certain allied health professionals despite market demands can be indicative of antitrust violations. Membership and membership allocations, termination, and allocation of resources are potential areas of contention.[45,46] Termination of membership or noninclusion may raise questions of due process as well as antitrust issues. Refusal to provide a membership application or unfairness in the consideration of an application raises issues analogous to medical staff issues. Due process issues do not determine the validity of an antitrust suit but raise other potential issues for the PPO, HMO, or IPA.[47]

Health delivery systems that integrate groups of physicians should be prepared to undergo scrutiny for possible horizontal price fixing or vertical market control. Avoiding Sherman Act violations requires that the joint venture between physicians, institutions, and insurance companies be bona fide joint. The fact that a group of physicians forms an IPA, HMO, or PPO is not illegal. The key is that the group is competitive, is at risk, and does not control a disproportionate percentage of the health care market. *Maricopa* indicated that a PPO operating as a joint physician venture will be viewed as a "single firm competing with other sellers in the market."[48]

It is the nature of a PPO to offer fixed prices to consumers. The consumer has no financial incentive to choose a provider within the network. Price competition does not exist among the providers but between groups of providers within the market area. If the rule of reason test is applied to this scenario, it is likely that the loss of price competition will be found to be internal to the PPO, HMO, or that the loss of price competition will be internal to the PPO, HMO, or IPA and not to the marketplace as a whole. The overall effect on the marketplace is minimal.

A 1988 FTC consent order, in the matter of Preferred Physicians, Inc., was brought pursuant to Title 15 U.S.C. Section 41 of the Federal Trade Commission Act. The fact scenario was relatively simple. In response to market pressures from third-party payors to reduce fees or discount services, a group of physicians formed a PPO and agreed not to compete with each other. The noncompetition agreement dealt with all the third-party payors. The majority of the members had staff privileges at the largest hospital in Tulsa. The net effect was to limit access to the hospital and to fix prices with tremendous market impact. The order of the consent decrees provided that these business practices would stop, but also gave PPO the right to continue to do business if the providers were free to contract with any other HMO or PPO. The PPO itself could also enter joint ventures provided the physician remained free to participate in other plans and joint ventures.[49]

The FTC has taken a strong position with regard to the health care industry. Its inquiries run the gamut of contracts, advertising, boycotts, and discrimination against allied health professionals. As the size of the health care delivery grows, any threats to competition and attempts to control markets will be vigorously pursued. Physicians who seek to enter joint ventures should be cognizant of the fact that these ventures will be closely scrutinized to determine if antitrust violations are occurring, or if they adversely affect the marketplace or other health professionals.

JOINT VENTURES

Changing patterns of health care utilization have led to creative associations of health care providers, institutions, and others to either capture or maintain control of their market share. New forms of technology and newer applications of old technology have led to the evolution of alternative mechanisms of health care delivery systems.

Changes in reimbursement and increasing competitive pressures have led to declining market share for both physician and institutions alike. In an attempt to compensate for these declines in both patient and cash flow, physicians, hospitals, and other types of health care providers have joined forces to restore and prevent losses. One of the more popular concepts is the joint venture. In recent years the joint venture has become a frequently used method to capitalize on new opportunities in the health care market. Physicians are the partners most often chosen by hospitals, and other entities, to participate in this investment vehicle. The most common arrangements involve ambulatory care centers, free-standing diagnostic centers, and managed health care delivery systems. As mentioned, alternative health care delivery systems include HMOs, PPOs, and preferred physician associations. Ambulatory care ventures include outpatient diagnostic facilities, urgent care centers, free-standing surgicenters, and free-standing rehabilitation centers, for example. Diagnostic centers include magnetic resonance imaging centers, mammography centers, radiology services and laboratories, to name a few. Other concepts include what are, in effect, real estate syndications, or equipment purchase and lease-back arrangements.

Little guidance has been forthcoming on the legality of joint ventures. Only a few cases have been prosecuted and these have dealt with fraudulent billing. Although the Inspector General Office of the Department of Health and Human Services has issued intermediary letters of interpretation, these are not legally binding. Joint ventures between physicians, health care providers, institutions, and businesspersons are a new and rapidly proliferating phenomenon. The legality of these ventures turns upon federal and state laws and regulatory policy. Each venture requires that both federal and state law be researched as to the venture's legality. Unfortunately, there may be no clear-cut law that can be simply found and applied. Rather, extrapolations and analogies may have to be drawn from vague or loosely related laws and situations. A further problem is the pyramiding of governmental regulations. When such regulations are involved, it is almost impossible to ascertain the various regulatory agencies' positions without asking them directly. Ultimately, the joint venture may be forced to proceed on the basis of a series of educated guesses. A syndicated real estate venture might be legitimate, whereas a physician-owned lithotripter may not be. Variations in state law make it extremely difficult to apply one type of experience to another state without adequate research into that jurisdiction's laws and regulations.

The proliferation of joint ventures has led to increasing federal and state scrutiny requiring the utmost care in the creation and management of these entities, so that questions of fraud and Medicare, Medicaid, and insurance violations can be avoided. The combination of increasing health care costs ($600 billion in 1989) and the opportunity to overutilize these services has led to increasing government scrutiny on both a state and federal level.

The remainder of this chapter is an attempt to provide various legal, ethical, and financial frameworks through which the venture participants must pass. It will also attempt to discuss some of the possible pitfalls. This chapter is not intended to give specific legal advice; instead, it provides a primer for the creation of a joint venture.

What are joint ventures?

A joint venture is an association of two or more persons or entities to carry out a business enterprise for profit for which purpose they combine their resources. This suggests creation of a new entity having managerial, financial, and productive capacity to enter or serve a new market. The agreement between the parties may establish a completely new entity or utilize preexisting entities to serve new markets or provide a new product. It would seem that the creation of a completely new venture having independent management, facilities, and autonomy is advisable to avoid legal, medical, and tax problems. The independence of the joint venture should be stressed to prevent questions as to whether or not this is a bona fide business. This may be an important issue if questions of fraud, individual liability, corporate liability, or other matters arise.

REASONS FOR JOINT VENTURES

Joint ventures are created to meet hospital, physician, and business goals. Their raison d'être may not be solely for capital formation.

Hospital goals

In addition to raising capital, hospitals may develop relationships with physicians, insurance companies, and others to develop "new profit centers" within the hospital or in an outpatient setting; to create alternative delivery systems to satisfy third-party payors; to increase and enhance market penetration of the physicians and hospital; to alter hospital-patient mix, limit debt financing, and increase community support for the hospital; and to cement the relationship with physicians and other

providers who support the institution. This list could be extended ad infinitum, but the goal is increased profitability by controlling costs, penetrating the patient care market on both an "in-" and "out-" patient basis, and securing the support of the local community and health providers.

Physician goals

Physician goals for entering joint venture agreements with one another or with hospitals are multiple: entering new service areas; creating outpatient facilities; increasing or maintaining market share; controlling costs; sharing financial risk; and participating in investment opportunities and acquiring capital management, and marketing skills that might otherwise be more expensive to acquire. Joint ventures also allow physicians to invest and profit in areas that might otherwise be closed to them. An example is the participation in radiology or laboratory service either as an investor in a corporation or as a limited partner.

CURRENT NEED FOR JOINT VENTURES

Health care costs are spiraling in excess of the inflation rate. When Medicare, Medicaid, and health care benefits were first created, health care resources appeared to be unlimited. Physicians and hospitals were not concerned about cost, patient mix, testing, and lengths of stay. Admission patterns were not closely monitored, and reimbursement appeared unlimited. However, as more and more individuals gained access to the health care system, and as diagnosis and treatment became more complex and expensive, third-party payors, including the U.S. government, began to institute controls to limit the rise in health costs. Physicians, hospitals, and outpatient facilities all face increasingly close scrutiny with regard to how the health care dollar is spent.

The introduction of prospective payment systems (PPSs) based on diagnostic related groups (DRGs) changed the physician-hospital relationship radically. Since the DRG has a certain dollar amount of reimbursement, the patient mix and length of stay of patients became vital to hospital survivability. Insurers are also placing increasing pressures on the hospital and physician. The proliferation of HMOs, preadmission criteria and approval, and prospective monitoring have also become factors in viability. Increasing numbers of physicians and other health care providers are also under pressure to maintain profitability and quality care.[50]

TYPES OF JOINT VENTURES

Joint venture permutations are innumerable. They include physician-physician, physician-hospital, realtor-physician, and almost any other combination imaginable.

They run the gamut of life retirement centers to physician-owned laboratories and surgicenters. Because these ventures have increased in such numbers, the federal government, through proposed legislation and Medicare regulations, is attempting to limit access to certain investment vehicles.[51] Increased capital requirements created by new equipment and treatment modalities have forced providers and institutions to reassess their relationship.

A joint venture may arise between physicians, hospitals, investment capital firms, insurance companies, and businesses—in many different types of arrangements. The types of joint arrangements created may involve real estate, equipment, leases, sales and lease-backs, and so on. The tax advantages and benefits of each venture determine the type of arrangement.

ORGANIZATIONAL STRUCTURAL MODELS

Five basic organizational structures exist for joint ventures with various combinations applied. The models are: (1) contractual, (2) corporate, (3) partnership (limited and general), (4) franchises, and (5) venture capital.

Contractual model[52]

The contractual model has the simplest structure, because the entire joint venture is contained in a contract between the parties. This could involve a service agreement lease, for example. Physicians could lease land from a hospital for the construction of a building that is then leased back to the hospital. The ultimate legal question may be whether or not this is a bona fide entity if the issue were to arise with regard to liability. The advantages are obvious. The hospital does not have to contribute capital and the builders have a leased building with a guaranteed rate of return.

Features. No separate legal entity is formed. The relationship is defined by the contract itself and is based on the relative strengths and weaknesses of the contractees.

Advantages. Simple to organize and understand, it requires no new corporations or infrastructure. The contractual relationship is one of preexisting entities.

Disadvantages. The contractual relationship creates new liabilities for the parties with little in the way of new tax advantages.

Corporate model

The corporate model creates a new entity owned by the shareholders. The joint ventures may be a combination of physicians, hospitals, or other investors. Shares may be owned by individuals, corporations, or partnerships. Ownership need not be limited to physicians or hospitals.

Features. The corporation is a legal entity acting through its board of directors. Joint ventures enter into preincorporation agreements establishing terms of participation. The board has the day-to-day authority to run the business and set policy. The preincorporation agreement might describe the business plan, but this would not be incorporated into the bylaws of the corporation.

Advantages. The corporation is a distinct legal entity. It possesses the power to expand on its own without further joint venturer participation or increased risk. In effect, the corporation creates an arm's-length situation, which may protect the investors from legal responsibility if a bona fide business exists. This may be particularly important with regard to Medicare and Medicaid participation. Being incorporated may also facilitate obtaining a certificate of need.

Disadvantages. The corporation is generally subject to double taxation. Compliance with state and federal blue-sky laws may be necessary. The corporation requires the creation of a new infrastructure with regard to bank accounts, payrolls, liability insurance, and management.

The "MeSh" model

The MeSh model is a joint venture created between hospitals and physicians with equal ownership and equal participation in management. The joint corporation could be created for one venture or to undertake a series of developments in the area of ambulatory care. The advantage of this mode is the bringing together of the hospital and staff to develop outpatient care and potentially increase hospital admissions.

General partnership model

A general partnership is the association of two or more persons who act as co-owners of a for-profit business. Profits and losses are equally shared. The partnership agreement states the rights and duties of the partners. Each is equally responsible for both losses and debt, and share equally in profits generally. The partnership agreement may specify any arrangement the partners may wish to institute. The partnership is subject to the specific statutes of the jurisdiction in which it is created.

The advantages of the partnership are single taxation and joint ownership and management. The major disadvantage is that each general partner is obligated for the losses, debts, and liability of the business. It also may be subject to scrutiny by third-party payors with regard to fraud. Certificates of need, accreditation, and licensure may be more difficult to obtain.

Limited partnership model

A limited partnership consists of at least one general partner who is responsible for the management of the business. There can be one or more limited partner investors who have equity ownership to the amount of their investment but are not involved in the management.

Advantages. The advantages are similar to a general partnership; however, limited partners are not responsible for losses in excess of their contributions. General partners in a limited partnership may be incorporated, thus preserving limited liability for themselves.

Disadvantages. The limited partners gain security and limit their losses but are barred from exerting day-to-day control over the business. Management participation of a limited partner may expose them to the liability of the general partner.

Franchise model

This model may be more popular in the area of primary care. It enables the hospital or institution to capitalize on its reputation. The concept is no different from any other franchise. In exchange for its name and support services the hospital is able to enlist the support of physicians in the community. The franchiser may exert control over site planning, services, and management. The actual practice of medicine is at the discretion of the practitioner. The franchiser may or may not be a hospital. The goal is to present a standardized service and to increase market penetration. The participation of the practicing physician may be that of partner, employee, or shareholder.

Venture capital model

The venture capital corporate model may become prevalent in the future. With the advent of increasingly restrictive legislation, the physician-owners may be forced out of small investments. The corporate model, by involving many investors (both physician and nonphysician) may evolve into the best vehicle for obtaining equity interests in medical facilities and services while avoiding government restrictions.

The venture capital corporation may serve as a general partner or may be the developer of patient services. The venture corporation may allow individuals, including physicians, to participate with limited financial risk and a relatively secure return on capital.

FINANCING CONSIDERATIONS FOR JOINT VENTURES[53,54]

State and federal interest in the nature of joint ventures and referral patterns may affect the type of venture and finance arrangements selected by the joint ventures. The Stark amendments,[55] RICO,[56] and changes in tax legislation[57] have opened physician joint venture to increasing governmental review.

Basic types of financial arrangements will be discussed; however, these should be assessed with a view to setting up an arm's-length transaction between the investors and newly created venture. The goal is to design a deal that is legal and will withstand attacks on the basis of antitrust, fraud, RICO, tax, and possible criminal and civil sanctions. Arrangements where physicians "self-refer" to a service or facility where they have a financial interest are suspect.[58]

Conventional financing

A loan may be for a term, a revolving line of credit, or a demand line of credit. In general, a loan involves a set amount, for a certain term with a specified rate of interest. It may be for interest only with a balloon payment or amortized over a set length of time. The interest may be specified or vary according to a specified formula such as prime rate.

Tax-exempt bonds

Tax-exempt bonds issued by a state or the political subdivision of a state may be exempted from federal taxation. They generally are not tax free in the state issued unless the state waives the right to tax the bonds. At least 75% of the bonds issued by the state or a political subdivision must be used in a tax-exempt trade or business as specified in section 501-c-3 of the IRS code.

Industrial development bonds are bonds issued to create nonexempt businesses, which are defined as entities with more than 25% of the proceeds used to finance nonexempt businesses. Tax-exempt status is determined on a case-by-case basis.

Public and private equity and debt offering

Securities registration statements for public offering must be filed, and the requirements are time consuming and costly. Exemptions to the filing and disclosure requirements exist; these include insurers of securities, incorporators of businesses, and all offers of sales in which 80% of the sales, proceeds, revenues, and assets remain in one state for the first six months. Resales must be made within the same state nine months after the sale. The aggregate offering price must be less than $1.5 million, and the SEC must clear the offering 10 days before the offer of sale.

Private equity offerings are exempted from requirements to file a security statement under Section 4(2). The requirements to qualify for the exemption are precise and statutorily mandated. The dollar amount must be less than $500,000, regardless of the number of investors. Alternatively, the offering can be for less than $5 million and 35 or fewer unaccredited investors and an unlimited number of accredited investors. An accredited investor must have a net worth exceeding $2 million or a net income in excess of $200,000 for the last two years. In some states an offering limited to less than 50 or 35 investors, depending on the state, may be exempt under state blue-sky laws.[59]

Debt offerings are subject to the same general requirements.

Venture capital

Venture capitalists are risk takers who gamble that a gain will be achieved by private or public sale of a newly established business. Venture capitalists have not entered the health care industry until recently. With the advent of ambulatory care and the opportunity to reap large profits, venture capitalists have assisted in starting up ambulatory health care companies. In return for their capital, they assume a large degree of control and a large percentage of profits.

Limited partnership syndications

Limited partnership syndications are subject to full and adequate disclosure requirements. Benefits to the limited partners are passed through the business, and losses are limited to the amount of each partner's contribution. The partnership and limited partners' tax consequences should be assessed at the inception of the venture. The effect of interest payments, depreciation, and property valuation must be made according to IRS regulations. Federal, local, and state regulations applicable to the limited and general partners should be researched. The partnership should register with both the IRS and state.

Equipment lease financing

Equipment may be acquired for the purpose of leasing to a health care facility or medical practice. The facility may be a hospital, ambulatory care center, or physician's office or clinic. The advantages may be accelerated depreciation, guaranteed rent, and capital conservation for the lessee.

The terms of the lease financial arrangements, maintenance agreements, sublease, replacement, or acquisition by the lessee are all subject to negotiation as part of the contract.

Management contracts

Management contracts may be used to conserve capital or to direct cash flow out of a nonprofit to a profit center.

Franchising

The medical franchise works in much the same way as any other franchise operation. The franchisee may be a physician working for a walk-in medical center who is given the right to "buy-in" or assume the ownership and control of a particular service. The franchiser recaptures the developmental costs through the sale of a device with exclusive rights to an area. There is a trade-off in that the franchisee may not be as autonomous as an independent owner/manager.

Nonprofit corporate financing—subventions

This financing vehicle is a form of investing in a nonprofit corporation similar to purchasing stock in a for-profit corporation. Holders of subvention certificates have subordinate rights to those of creditors of the nonprofit corporation. Redemptions may not exceed the original value of the subvention certificate, plus any periodic payments or accruals.[60]

LEGAL, REGULATORY, ETHICAL, AND ACCREDITATION CONSIDERATIONS

The ramifications of joint ventures are multiple and interlocking. Not only are security regulations at a state and federal level brought to bear, but the structure of the venture leaves both the participants and entity open to litigation. Increased costs and growing provider networking and referrals to physician-owned facilities create potential antitrust issues, Medicare and Medicaid violations, fraud, and possible RICO violations.

Ethical considerations

The medical literature, legislative subcommittees, insurance carriers, and the public all question the entrepreneurial aspects of joint ventures between physicians, hospitals, diagnostic facilities, and treatment centers. The suspicion is that a system of self-referral will lead to overutilization with concomitant increases in health care costs.

The issue of "silent rationing" by insurers is becoming apparent.[63] This affects the ventures that investors are building. Since the investment strategy can be (1) to create a service, (2) to capture market share by creating an HMO or PPO, or (3) to control delivery systems, insurers are more likely to do prospective and retrospective studies of diagnostic testing and treatment within a geographical area. Florida requires that physician-investors reveal the potential conflicts of interest in referring a patient to a laboratory facility where the physician holds an interest. The Omnibus Budget Reconciliation Act of 1989 is designed to end this type of self-referral pattern.[64]

Examples of federal intent are P.L. 99-272, which allowed the secretary to establish a system of tracking each physician providing Medicare services with a unique identifier.[65]

Mark-ups were eliminated with the Deficit Reduction Act of 1984. A "direct billing" requirement was instituted to prevent a physician from ordering a laboratory test on a Medicare beneficiary and "marking up" the prices charged.

In a real sense, the ethical and legal issue of fee-for-service medicine for patients at facilities owned by the referring physicians alone or in conjunction with another institution has been raised by increasing health care costs.[66-68]

Reimbursement

The goal of hospitals, physicians, and other providers is to tap both part B payments and increase services to non-Medicare, private-pay patients, thus avoiding the prospective of fixed payment reimbursement systems. As such, outpatient facilities such as surgicenters, walk-in medical centers, laboratory, and X-ray diagnostic centers permit the parties to tap into new markets and avoid limitations.[69]

Taxation

Qualifying a joint venture corporation for tax-exempt status, Section 501 of the Internal Revenue Code elucidates those organizations that may qualify for tax-exempt status. Among the relevant sections are 501-c3-4. These sections specify that the venture must be set up exclusively for charitable, educational, scientific, or religious purposes. The caveat is that the venture may not have income from the operation of a business not related to the exempt business. Income from these sources may be taxable, and the charity runs the risk of losing its tax-exempt status.

Unrelated business: taxable income

Tax-exempt organizations may generate taxable income by diversifying their services. The issue of taxability will depend on the service rendered. Direct provider joint enterprises such as urgent care centers or surgicenters will be taxable. Management services offered to physicians or other providers may not be taxable. The problem can be obviated by creating a totally separate profit-making joint venture. Profits passed through the parent tax-exempt entity would be taxable.[70-72]

Taxation: general comments

The joint venturers should determine the tax consequences of the business at its inception. It may be advantageous to make estate and equipment purchases as partners and lease these items to the joint venture. Subchapter S corporations are another consideration. The net effect of these transactions should be calculated before the inception of the venture.

The merits of hospital-physician joint ventures versus physician-physician joint venture are another area to address.

Licensure and accreditation

Licensure. Joint ventures may be organized between physicians or hospitals, or by physicians alone. The free-standing urgent care or surgicenter may be organized and run solely by and for the benefit of the physicians who provide services, or they may be open to physician and nonphysician investors. These permutations may be determined by state licensing requirements.

A hospital-run facility may fall under the general licensing and certificate-of-need regulations (if any) of the particular state; each state's statutes must be reviewed. In most states free-standing surgicenters, HMOs, and diagnostic facilities are highly regulated, whereas an urgent care center may be treated as a physician's office, with little or no regulation imposed.[73]

Regardless of the specific state regulations that regulate these centers, generally accepted legal precepts will apply. Each facility must be able to deliver the type and quality of services it advertises. The appropriate staff, equipment, and ancillary support services must be provided to maintain acceptable standards of care. As will be discussed, failure to maintain these standards opens the door to litigation not only with the physicians and entity but also to the investors.[74]

Voluntary accreditation

The Joint Commission on Accreditation of Healthcare Organizations (JCAHO) has approved standards applicable to free-standing urgent care centers. The 1990 *Accreditation Manual for Hospitals* contains these standards. The Accreditation Association for Ambulatory Care has been established by the National Association for of Freestanding Emergency Centers. This voluntary association provides an *Accreditation Handbook* that should be used as a guide to the establishment and management of free-standing urgent care centers. Standards are suggested concerning medical records, patient rights, and services provided by the facility.

Utilization review

Utilization review (UR) is a function of the services in an office or institutional setting. UR may be voluntary or involuntary. Hospital UR is performed under state and JCAHO sanction. UR is an attempt to define the type and frequency of services rendered at a particular institution. Unlike quality assurance and risk management, it does not, of itself, provide a methodology to correct deficiencies.

UR may be imposed by third-party insurers, HMOs, PPOs, and is imposed by Medicare and Medicaid. The goal is to determine through preadmission certification, Medicare DRG, validation concurrent review, and transfer and discharge planning, the scope and projected costs of services delivered.[75]

Securities regulation

Securities regulation depends on the type of financing, numbers of investors, dollar amounts, and jurisdiction. It is also affected by the nature of the venture. Creation of general or limited partnerships, corporations, real estate syndicates, lease-purchase agreements, and combinations of the above all influence the type of offering. The physician-hospital agreement may differ from the physician-physician agreement, which may differ from the entrepreneur who puts together a turnkey operation and enlists physician support by selling shares in the endeavor.

The key is to obtain legal opinions with regard to state and federal legislation before the venture is created. Additionally, if an HMO, PPO, or insurance company is created, state and federal laws will have to be reviewed. State and federal security regulations must be assessed and the necessary documentation provided for investors.

Corporate practice of medicine

Corporations are generally prohibited from practicing medicine.[76] The standards established by a facility or other type of venture must reflect standards promulgated by health care providers and not by the partnership, corporation, or any other type of entity. The goal is to provide quality care while avoiding interference with the provider-physician relationship. The JCAHO, state, federal, and voluntary accrediting agencies strive to maintain provider control over standards of care.

Joint ventures may create managed health care entities, diagnostic facilities, treatment centers, or other types of health care delivery mechanisms. In each of these cases the role of the nonprovider manager and investor should be kept separate from the care delivered.[77] To avoid pitfalls the organization should structure the relationship of the providers, specify the type of facility, and delineate the responsibilities of the nonprovider managers and owners.[78-80]

Fraud, abuse, and ethical considerations

Medicare and Medicaid fraud and abuse. Medicare has prohibited the solicitation, receipt, or payment of any fee directly, indirectly, overtly, or covertly for the referral of a Medicare or Medicaid beneficiary for a covered item of service, whether it be for goods, services, facilities, or other benefits. The advent of physician-owned ventures has opened an area of potential abuse. For example, one of the earliest types of a physician joint venture was the small commercial "pass-through" laboratory. In this scenario a group of physicians forms a commercial laboratory that performs "stat" lab work only and refers other tests to a larger commercial laboratory. Profits are generated on the price differential between the cost of the services and the actual cost of the test, plus the administrative costs of the laboratory. The physician-investor receives a dividend based on his or her financial interest. In and of itself this arrangement has not been illegal until recently.

The inspector general for Health and Human Services has estimated that a physician-controlled laboratory performs about 30% more tests on an equivalent Medicare population than a comparable nonphysician-owned laboratory. Current Medicare regulations provide up to $25,000 in fines and up to five years imprisonment for violators of Medicare regulations.[81]

State statutes may also apply. Florida has a statute that penalizes a provider for unnecessary laboratory testing.[82] Joint ventures have to be attuned to the difference between kickbacks and returns on investments and equity. In 1983, the inspector general published a booklet entitled "Kickbacks Are Illegal," which recommended the creation of arm's-length transactions, where provider patterns are not controlled and monies are distributed in the form of dividends, which are not tied to referrals.

The Judicial Council of the AMA has ruled that physicians can engage in commercial ventures, but they should be aware of potential conflicts of interest. If the physician's commercial interest conflicts with patient care, alternative arrangements should be made.[83]

The Stark bill is designed to deal with the issue of physician-owned laboratories and self-referral. The bill is an extension of federal fines and imprisonment. The subsequent legislation is designed to create a method that tracks physician referrals by assignment of an identifier number.[84]

Legislation enacted in 1987 allows the inspector general of the DHHS to exclude a person from Medicare participation if he or she engages in a prohibited remuneration scheme. The act also requires that the secretary of DHHS promulgate regulations known as "Safe Harbor" as of October 1989, but these are still pending. Although the Stark bill pertains to clinical laboratory services, the issue is much broader. Physicians' referrals may also create violations.[85]

Fraud in general. The Racketeering Influence Corruption Act of 1970 (RICO) was written to deal with the entry of organized crime into legitimate businesses. It has been utilized to prosecute health care providers and organizations that engage in certain activities prescribed in the statute. The statute has a broad and, seemingly, simplistic application. The courts have defined the limitations broadly. In effect it prevents a person from investing or acquiring an enterprise through a pattern of racketeering activity; conviction of a criminal act is not necessary. The "pattern" of activity is two or more acts within a 10-year time frame.[86]

With physicians' increasing participation in arrangements that depend on patient referral in order to generate revenues, the situation becomes more confusing. In effect, the physician enters a fiduciary relationship with regard to the patient, and the statutes are extensions of this obligation. Abrogation of this obligation leads to penalties that are being extended by legislative imposition, judicial interpretation and criminal enforcement.[87] The problems involve laboratories, diagnostic studies, denial of care or limitations of care, and self-referral. State commercial bribery laws should also be investigated. The RICO statute allows the recovering party to obtain legal fees and treble damages. Federal and state criminal sanctions may also be imposed.[88-91]

Antitrust restrictions

The antitrust laws affecting health care providers are the (1) Sherman Antitrust Act, sections 1 and 2; (2) Clayton Act, section 7; and (3) Hart-Scott-Rodino Antitrust Improvements Act of 1976. Physician activity is not excluded from antitrust litigation. In fact, there is a greater need for governmental action to impose criminal and civil penalties with the advent of interlocking relationships of providers, third-party payors, and diagnostic and treatment centers.

Section 1 of the Sherman Act has four predicates to establish a violation of the act. The parties must engage in a conspiracy that engages in or promotes anticompetitive practices within an identifiable service area and that adversely affects interstate commerce. Violation of this section is a felony with fines of up to $1 million for a corporation and $100,000 for an individual. An individual can be imprisoned for up to three years. The federal government is presently attempting to formulate sentencing guidelines for the employees of a corporation.

Section 2 can be asserted against an individual or entity without evidence of conspiracy or collusion. The goal of this section is to prevent the monopolization of a single market. Section 2 prohibitions may be asserted against a single entity, such as a hospital, medical staff, group of investors, or any combination thereof.[92]

Arizona v. Maricopa Medical Society dealt with the issue of fee schedules. In this case "violation of section 1 occurred even though the providers acted in order to limit health care costs."[93] The agreement between two health care facilities violated the law by creating a per se price-fixing conspiracy. The court found objectionable the fact that all practitioners were treated the same without regard to skill or training. If the limitations were not equally binding on all practitioners, the problem might have been avoided.[94]

For example, if competing groups of physicians and their managers competed for health care dollars and the managers alone established the fee schedule independent of provider and other bidders, the statute would not be violated.

Legitimate joint ventures create the possibility for in-

tegrated services at reduced costs without violation of antitrust laws. Joint ventures can be created to integrate health delivery services on a horizontal, vertical, or independent basis.[95] Joint ventures must not be a subterfuge for an illegal scheme. "Even if a joint undertaking meets certain economic criteria designed . . . to identify the creating of new productive capacity, it will not be characterized as a joint venture for antitrust purposes if it is merely a subterfuge."[96] Therefore, even if the venture is a "legitimate integrated operation," it still must meet the test of Section 1, the "rule of reason" test. In addition, Section 7 of the Clayton Act must be satisfied as part of the rule of reason analysis.

Two questions must be answered to hold a joint venture illegal: (1) Is it likely that one of the parent groups would enter the market without the joint venture? (2) Is it likely that if one entered the market the other would remain a competitor or enter the market as a competitor? The Clayton Act renders a joint venture unlawful if it lessens competition or creates a monopoly. If, on the other hand, the venture expands consumer services and increases consumer options, it is probably lawful.[97]

In determining the impact of a joint venture, the type of service or organization relevant to market demand and impact on a particular area must be assessed. A PPO, HMO, or other type of provider network might be acceptable in an area of intense competition, whereas the same concept would be a violation of the antitrust statute in a smaller or less competitive market. The issues of antitrust arise with hospitals, physician provider organizations, group competition, exclusion from hospital staffs, exclusion from provider groups, and the horizontal or vertical integration of combined services. Tying arrangements between physicians, group boycotts, and other strategies that tend to exclude a specific group are subject to scrutiny.[98]

In *Hyde v. Jefferson Parrish Hosp.*, the court upheld the precept that limitations are acceptable and do not violate antitrust laws if restraints (in this case PPO membership) are a reasonable by-product of improving quality, cost-effectiveness, or competitiveness in the marketplace. Exclusion of a specific provider group may lead to a statutory violation. See *Weiss v. York Hosp.* for the reverse fact pattern.[99]

Parker v. Brown, a 1943 case, established an exclusionary principle for state-related activity. The state exemption would apply if the acts in question concern a state-controlled activity. Conceivably this could apply to the creation of HMO or PPO joint ventures between hospitals and providers, which integrate the market both horizontally and vertically to exclude other competition.[100]

Further extensions of exclusionary acts were defined

in *UMW v. J. Pennington* and *Presidents RR Conference v. Noerr Motor Freight, Inc.* HMOs are creatures of legislation.[101] They are highly regulated both on the state and federal level. The federal statute, 42 U.S.C. Section 300, and federal regulations, 42 C.F.R. Part 110, provide these entities with the right to enter state markets. In effect, although the state may regulate these entities, they cannot exclude them from state markets. They are subject to state regulation, but, in effect, are given a slight market advantage in developing their products. In certain cases this may, in fact, be anticompetitive, but as a public policy it is an acceptable breach.[102,103]

A venture may be horizontally and vertically integrated in certain situations. An HMO has an advantage in accepting or refusing providers, developing hospitals, and utilizing certain laboratory services.[104] Venture partners should be aware that a horizontally integrated delivery system may be more anticompetitive than a vertically integrated system.

Group negotiation with nongovernmental entities may also be exempted from federal and state antitrust statutes. Insurance companies may not be treated in the same manner as other businesses and remain a regulated business where the state may control premiums.[105]

Antitrust, RICO, and the joint venture

Increasing pressures in the marketplace are beginning to create financial and professional burdens for physicians and hospitals. The "learned" professions are no longer immune from antitrust litigation.[106] Recently, there has been a trend to utilize both the RICO and the Sherman Act legislation on behalf of physicians who were excluded or removed from hospital staffs. The use of the combined forces of these two statutes represents a potentially powerful plaintiff's weapon in the event a joint venture unlawfully affects the market environment to the exclusion of a provider.[107,108] Even the peer review process, although statutorily protected, may fall within the purview of these statutes if certain conditions[109,110] are met.

Insurance regulations

Joint ventures may create insurance companies. Since the advent of HMOs, physicians, hospitals, and other joint venturers have joined forces, in many combinations, to provide health insurance plans to consumers. The HMO was the first and probably the most popular method of uniting physicians. By accepting the economic burden of the patients, the HMO falls under the jurisdiction of both HMO and state insurance regulation. Where there is a conflict, federal laws will control. PPOs may also fall under the purview of the state insurance statutes. Legislation with regard to the PPOs

may be much less onerous than that applicable to HMOs and other types of insurance companies.[111]

Qualifying as an insurance company, HMO, PPO, or combination of these will obligate the joint ventures to comply with federal HMO legislation if they intend to become "federally qualified." State law controls HMOs and PPOs, under state insurance regulations. These imply reserve requirements, approval of policies, re-insurance, and reporting requirements. The joint ventures may be unable to sell the product even if the business is in compliance with all regulations. As investors, the physicians and other providers have to maintain an arm's-length relationship to avoid any questions of price fixing. The plan itself, whatever the product mix, may be compelled to offer certain types of benefit packages and may not be allowed to exclude or rate insureds.[112]

In a nutshell, prepaid plans or insurance company joint ventures are subject not only to state and federal insurance regulation but may also subject the investor to RICO, antitrust, and tort litigation.

Liability issues

There is a growing trend in the United States to hold organizations independently responsible for their acts. The concept of corporate negligence has begun to permeate the medical arena. As a result, PPOs, HMOs, hospitals, and other entities such as laboratory services, urgent care centers, and diagnostic centers are potentially liable for negligence, regardless of provider affiliation.[113-116]

Additionally, there is the potential for employers and the insurance network to be liable, because patients in prepaid plans are forced to select physicians from the panel chosen by the plan and indirectly by the purchaser of the insurance. This expanded liability imposes on the joint ventures an obligation to follow through with credentialing, peer review, quality assurance, and risk management where required.

A further component of the problem is the limitation of care provided. The HMO and PPO tend to try to limit referrals and laboratory testing. Under the guidelines established by the joint venture, this may indicate a breach in the standard of care. As physicians, hospitals, health care providers, and venture capitalists enter the health care arena, their liability exposure mushrooms. In considering a joint venture with diversified services, it behooves the investor to explore the potential for personal liability.

One way to limit loss exposure is to institute risk management programs. Florida was one of the first states to initiate mandatory risk management as a component of health delivery systems.[117]

The integration of utilization review, quality assurance, and risk management may decrease potential loss exposure. The Health Care Quality Insurance Act of 1976 created a national data bank for reporting physicians and providing data to certain organizations to credential physicians. Failure to properly credential an individual could open the way for civil litigation against a hospital if its linkage to a joint venture is too close.

Contractual alternative dispute resolution

Joint ventures are complex business arrangements that bring together diverse institutions and individuals. Frequently investors are not as sophisticated as the joint-venture formers might believe. Other than the full-disclosure agreements, the initial contracts between the joint venturers, providers, and others might include an arbitration or mediation clause.

Issues may arise with regard to control, contracts, capital contribution, and debt assumption. Investors should attempt to ascertain the duties and obligations of each investor when first confronted with a proposed venture.

CONCLUSION

Increasing market competition and capital requirements have brought together different combinations of providers, hospitals, and businesspersons; frequently their interests are not the same.

The formation of a joint venture can subject investors to antitrust litigation, RICO litigation, and increased exposure to negligence, both medical and corporate. In addition, investors may have conflicts within their investor groups.

Increasing governmental intrusion affects the methods used to create a joint venture, both with regard to legal requirements and capital contributions. Nevertheless the area of integrated service, new markets, and providing a valuable service for the health care consumer offers an exciting challenge for physicians and hospitals.

END NOTES

1. Lawrence K, Altman with Elisabeth Rosenthal 2/18/90, Lisa Belkin, Feb. 19, 1990, N.Y. Times series; Feb. 18, 19, 20, 1990.
2. *Health Care in the 1990's,* Hospitals (July 1990).
3. Paul Starr, *The Social Transformation of American Medicine* (Basic Books 1982).
4. Tax Reform Act of 1986, sections relating to 401-K pension plans.
5. *1989 United States Master Tax Guide* (Prentice Hall 1989).
6. *Insiga v. LaBella,* 14 Fla. L. Weekly 214 Apr. 21, 1989.
7. Uniform Partnership Act, *see* Am. Jur. 2D.
8. Florida Statutes 1988 §§ 620 *et seq.*
9. Uniform Partnership Act § 18.
10. Am. Jur. 2D *Corporations generally.*
11. Fla. Stat. § 607, Professional Service Corporations 766.101 1988.
12. Fla. Stat. 607.
13. *Physicians' Responses to Financial Incentives,* 322 New Eng. J. Med. 1059-63.
14. "Stark Amendment," Omnibus Reconciliation Act of 1989. Pub. L. 101-386.
15. Entin and Persky, *Emergicenters: The New Kid on the Block,* Legal Aspects Med. Pract. 10-12 (Dec. 1985).
16. Hirsh, *Alternative Health Care Delivery Systems,* Pract. Mgmt. Anesthes. 10-12 (Sep. 1985).
17. *Preferred Provider Organizations,* InterQual, 1983 and more recent editions.
18. Marion Laboratories, HMO and PPO Digests, 1988 obtainable from Marion Laboratory.
19. *The Flowering of Managed Care,* Med. Econ. (Mar. 5, 1990).
20. Starr, *supra* note 3.
21. In the *Matter of Preferred Physicians, Inc.,* Docket C-3222, dealt with a PPO, but the general principles could be applied to physician-run IPAs.
22. *Preferred Provider Organizations* (American Association of Preferred Provider Organizations, 11 E. Wacker Drive, Suite 600, Chicago, Ill.).
23. *FTC Investigating Price Fixing among "Sham" PPOs.* Managed Health Care (Apr. 9, 1990) [hereinafter cited as *FTC Investigating*].
24. *National Society of Professional Engineers v. United States,* 435 U.S. 679 (1979) [hereinafter cited as *Professional Engineers*].
25. *Arizona v. Maricopa County Medical Society,* 456 U.S. 332 (1982) [hereinafter cited as *Maricopa*].
26. Hyman and Williamson, *Fraud and Abuse: Setting the Limits of Physician Entrepreneurship,* 320 New Eng. J. Med. 1275-78 (May 11, 1989).
27. Marc Rodwin, *Physicians and Conflicts of Interest: The Limitations of Disclosure,* 321 New Eng. J. Med. 1405-08 (Nov. 16, 1990).
28. *Wilk v. AMA,* 895 F.2nd 352 1990.
29. *FTC v. Indiana Federation of Dentists,* 476 U.S. 447 1986.
30. *NCAA v. Board of Regents of the University of Oklahoma,* 468 U.S. 85 1984.
31. *Jefferson Parrish Hospital District No. 2 v. Hyde,* 466 U.S. 2, 1984.
32. *Professional Engineers, supra* note 24.
33. *FTC Investigating, supra* note 23.
34. *Maricopa, supra* note 25.
35. *Nurse Midwife Associates v. Hibbett,* 549 F. Supp. 1185 (M.D. Tenn. 1982).
36. See Indiana Dental Case #29.
37. Brodley, *Joint Ventures and Antitrust Policy,* 95 Harv. L. Rev. (1978).
38. *Capital Imaging Associates v. Mohawk Valley Medical Associates, Inc. and Mohawk Valley Physicians Health Plan, Inc.* (Nov. 24, 1989).
39. *Ocean State Physicians Health Plan, Inc. v. Blue Cross and Blue Shield of Rhode Island,* 883 F.2 1101 (Aug. 21, 1989).
40. *Id.*
41. *Capital Imaging, supra* note 38.
42. *Maricopa, supra* note 25; *FTC Investigating, supra* note 23.
43. *Maricopa, supra* note 25; *Wilk v. AMA, supra* note 28.
44. *United States v. St. Louis Terminal,* 224 U.S. 383 (1912).
45. *Wilk, supra* note 28.
46. *Weiss v. York Hosp.,* 745 F.2nd 786 (1984).
47. *Northwest Wholesale Stationers, Inc. v. Pacific Stationery and Printing Co.,* 105 S.Ct. 2613 (1985).
48. *Wilk, supra* note 28; *Maricopa, supra* note 25.
49. PPI, Inc. Consent Decree.
50. Steinwachs, *A Comparison of the Requirements for Primary Care Physicians in Health Maintenance Organizations with Projections Made by GMENAC,* 314 New Eng. J. Med. 217-22 (1986).
51. Stark Bill P.L. 101-239 § 6204.
52. Rosenfeld, *Joint Venture Organizational Models,* 12 Topics in Health Care Financing 38-44 (Winter 1985).

53. G. J. Rahn, ed., *Hospital Sponsored Health Maintenance Organizations Issues for Decision Makers* (American Hospital Association).
54. *See generally* Kepner, *Primer Series for Health Care Professionals: Capital Formation and Debt Financing Process* (1985).
55. Stark Bill Pub. L. 101-239.
56. RICO Bill 1970 add # 18 U.S.C. 1961.
57. See 1986 Tax Reform Act.
58. *Physicians' Responses to Financial Incentives,* 322 New Eng. J. Med. 1059-63 (Mar. 1990).
59. 70 Pa Statute § 1-2 or 3(d)e Supp. 1984-1985 Fla. Stat. ch. 517 § 517.051 (1988).
60. RICO.
61. 64 Pa. Code § 202.091 (Supp. 1984-1985) Fla. Stat. § 621 (1988).
62. Pa. Cons. Stat. § 412.3 (Supp. 1984-1985).
63. "Health Rationing," *Wall Street J.,* Mar. 27, 1990.
64. Omnibus Budget Reconciliation Act of 1989, see conference report.
65. Pub. L. 99-272 Consolidated Budget Reconciliation Act of 1985.
66. Radovsky, *United States Medical Practice Before Medicare and Now—Differences and Consequences,* 332 New Eng. J. Med 263-67 (Jan. 25, 1990).
67. Hyman and Williamson, *Fraud and Abuse: Setting the Limits on Physician Entrepreneurship,* 320 New Eng. J. Med. 1275-78 (May 11, 1989).
68. Rodwin, *Physicians and Conflicts of Interest, the Limitations of Disclosure,* 321 New Eng. J. Med. 1405-08 (Nov. 16, 1989).
69. *Preferred Provider Organizations,* 9-1 (InterQual, Chicago 1983).
70. CCH, 1989 US Master Tax Guide Tax Exemptions discussion.
71. IRC § 5(b) (13) (1954).
72. O'Donnell and Taylor, *The Current Status of the Hospital Property Tax Exemption,* 322 New Eng. J. Med. 65-68 (Jan. 4, 1990).
73. Fla. Stat. 395.002 (1988) as an example of surgicenter regulation.
74. Racketeering Influenced Fraud and Corruptions Act enacted as part of the Organized Crime Control Act (1970) 18 U.S.C. 1961 *et seq.*
75. Grimaldi and Micheletti, *Diagnosis Related Groups, A Practitioner's Guide* (Pluribus Press 1983).
76. Pa. Cons. Stat. § 421.3 Supp. 1984-1985.
77. McNair, *Structural Issues in Creating and Operating Alternative Health Care Delivery Systems, in Preferred Provider Organizations and Alternative Health Care Delivery Systems* (Pa. Bar Assn. Oct. 1984).
78. Fla. Stat. 766.01-Medical Review Committees.
79. *A Physician's Guide to PPOs* (Health Services Policy Group, AMA, Chicago 1983).
80. Marion Laboratories, Inc., 1988 Marion Managed Care Digest, HMO and PPO edition.
81. 42 U.S.C. § 1395, *cf.,* 42 U.S.C. 1396b Federal Medicare Fraud; *see also* 62 Pa. Cons. Stat. § 1401 and Fla. Stat. 766.11 (1988) (ch 766).
82. *Id.*
83. *Report of the Judicial Council of the American Medical Association, December 1984,* JAMA 2425 (1984).
84. "Stark" Pub. L. 101-239-§ 6204.
85. *See* RICO Stat. pl 91-452 U.S.C. 1961-1968 (1970).
86. *Id.*
87. *Id.,* 28, 30, 31.
88. *See* Pub. L. 98-369, The Deficit Reduction Act of 1984; Pub. L. 00-272, The Consolidated Omnibus Budget Reconciliation Act of 1985; Pub. L. 100-93, The Medicare and Medicaid Patient and Program Protection Act of 1987.
89. For a review article on RICO, *see* The National Law Journal, Health Law Column (Aug. 28, 1989).
90. Fla. Stat. 766.111-Unnecessary Laboratory Testing; 409.226-Medicare/Medicaid Fraud, 1988.
91. Sedima, *SPRL v. Imrex Co.,* 473 U.S. 479 (1985), conviction of crime not necessary to bringing of RICO case.
92. *Arizona v. Maricopa County Medical Society,* 457 U.S. 332 (1982).
93. *Id.*
94. *Id.*
95. *Cf. generally,* Brodley, *Joint Ventures and Antitrust Policy,* 95 Harvard L. Rev. 1521-26 (1982).
96. Report of the Adjunct Task Force on Antitrust Aspects of Third Party Payment Negotiations, Legal Development Report N. 2 at 31 (Sep. 1983).
97. 39 A.L.R. Fed. 774-Antitrust and the Learned Professions.
98. *Jefferson Parrish Hosp. District v. Hyde,* 466 U.S. 2 (1984).
99. *Weiss v. York Hosp.,* 745 F.2nd 786 (1984).
100. *Parker v. Brown,* 317 U.S. 341 (1943).
101. *United Mine Workers v. J. Pennington,* 381 U.S. 657 (1965); *Eastern RR Presidents Conference v. Noerr Motor Freight, Inc.,* 365 U.S. 127 (1961).
102. *Cal. Motor Transportation v. Trucking Unlimited,* 404 U.S. 508, 513 (1972).
103. *Sandcrest Outpatient Services v. Cumberland County Hosp. Systems,* 853 F.2nd 1139 (4th Cir. 1988).
104. *Fla. Stat. Health Maintenance Organizations Act Fla. Stat. § 641 (1988).*
105. *Cf. Union Labor Life Insurance Co. v. Pireno,* 458 U.S. 119; *Group Health and Life v. Health Ins. Co. v. Royal Drug Co.,* 440 U.S. 205; *National Gerimedical v. Blue Cross,* 452 U.S. 378 (1981).
106. 39 A.L.R. 774-Learned Profession Exemption in Federal Antitrust Litigation.
107. *Patrick v. Burget,* 108 S.Ct. 1658 (1988) (antitrust aspect of medical review committees).
108. *U.S. v. Hughes,* 895 F.2nd 1135 (Criminal Sanctions).
109. *Northwest Womens Center v. et al.,* 889 F.2nd 2294 (1989).
110. *Boczar v. Manatee Hospital and Health Systems, Inc.* no.8-1867-CIV-T-17T US District Court for the Middle District, Tampa, Fla. 2/21/90.
111. Fla. Stat. 407.13 & ch. 627.
112. Federal statute controls basic regulations for HMOs unless they choose to be "nonqualified"; also need to review specific state legislation with regard to PPO legislation.
113. *Darling v. Charleston Memorial Hospital,* 32 Ill. 2nd 326, (1966), 211 N.E.2nd 253.
114. *Pedrosa v. Bryant,* 101 Wash. 2nd 226 677 P.2nd 166 (1984).
115. *Insinga v. Labella,* 14 F.L.W. 214 (Apr. 21, 1989).
116. Seventeen states have adopted corporate liability in some form: Arizona, California, Colorado, Georgia, Illinois, Michigan, Missouri, Nebraska, Nevada, New Jersey, New York, North Carolina, North Dakota, Texas, West Virginia, Wisconsin.
117. Fla. Stat. 766.110, 395.041, 641.55, 624.501.

CHAPTER 45

Coproviders and institutional practice

EDWARD E. HOLLOWELL, J.D., F.C.L.M.*

BARRY H. BLOCH, J.D.

STATE LICENSURE
PRACTICE IN A HEALTH CARE INSTITUTION
PEER REVIEW
SUPERVISORY LIABILITY
RADIO CONTROL AND PREHOSPITAL CARE
INDEPENDENT CONTRACTORS
OSTENSIBLE AGENCY
CONSULTANTS AND REFERRING PHYSICIANS
NURSING AND OTHER TECHNICAL PRACTICES IN THE HOSPITAL
CONCLUSION
INSTITUTIONAL PRACTICE: HISTORICAL ORIGINS
LIABILITY OF HOSPITALS AND MEDICAL STAFF PHYSICIANS
MEDICAL STAFF CREDENTIALING
NATURE AND TYPE OF STAFF MEMBERSHIP
STAFF APPLICATION AND RENEWAL
CONSIDERATIONS FOR ACCEPTANCE OR REJECTION
LEGAL PROTECTIONS AVAILABLE TO THE PHYSICIAN
AVAILABLE REMEDIES TO AGGRIEVED PHYSICIANS
GUIDELINES FOR HOSPITAL AND MEDICAL STAFF CREDENTIALING
MEDICAL STAFF PEER REVIEW
RISK MANAGEMENT PRINCIPLES
HOSPITAL PRIVILEGES AND DUE PROCESS
HOSPITAL-REQUIRED MALPRACTICE INSURANCE

Physicians do not practice alone. That fact is unalterable in our complex medical care system. Physicians depend upon the expertise and competence of technicians, nurses, paramedics, administrators, nurse's aides, orderlies, medical records personnel, and even maintenance and repair staff, just to name a few coproviders. In addition, it is important to recognize that the relationships of coproviders are necessarily bilateral. The competence of the individuals working together are additive rather than independent. It is obvious that the observations and efforts of all those who provide care for a patient affect the outcome, and as a result the legal interdependence of coproviders is unavoidable. The more complex that health care becomes and the more technical the capabilities of health care providers, the greater the interdependence of coproviders. Further, when coproviders work together smoothly and professionally, the professionalism and teamwork is evident to the patient; this tends to minimize malpractice and malpractice claims. It is often the feeling or perception that something was wrong that influences a patient to seek an attorney and file a claim. Good teamwork

*The authors gratefully acknowledge the contributions of the previous authors to this chapter: John Dale Dunn, M.D., J.D., F.C.L.M.; James B. Couch, M.D., J.D., F.C.L.M.; Marvin Firestone, M.D., J.D., F.C.L.M.; Gary N. Hagerman, LL.B., F.C.L.M.; and H. William Goebert, Jr., M.D., J.D., F.C.L.M.

635

catches errors before untoward results occur by preventing substandard care from being given. It also creates the perception in the patient that he or she is receiving competent, efficient, and high-quality health care.

The definition of coproviders in the context of the health care system can be expanded beyond the imagination. For example, the competence of the line worker involved in the manufacturing process of a piece of medical equipment could, in the most extreme assessment of the nature of "coproviders," affect the performance of nurses and physicians who use a particular piece of equipment.

This chapter's first part focuses on the health care providers who are directly involved with the patient and who have some form of professional licensure or responsibility for patient care. These persons are physicians, nurses, dentists, podiatrists, licensed psychologists, vocational nurses, registered technicians, and other personnel who work in the health care system and directly affect the provision of care to the patient. In addition, the nature of relationships that create coexisting responsibilities and duties will be discussed.

This chapter's second part explores legal aspects concerning the hospital, the institution in which these people work together. It focuses primarily on the hospital's legal relationship to the patients it serves and to the physicians who serve on its staff and committees.

STATE LICENSURE

Licensed professionals are obligated not only to act within the authority and parameters set out by their own licensure act, but are, in most states, required to report other professionals if they know or should have known that those professionals were acting in violation of their own licensure acts. For example, state laws require that physicians report the incompetence of another physician if it has the potential to harm a patient. Physicians are also required to report the incompetence or impairment of a nurse or any other health care provider, since licensure creates a public duty that, at times, can override the natural instinct not to be a "tattletale."

Once the physician has been reported to his or her licensing board, the board will meet with the physician if the board believes the problem can be remedied informally. The licensing board may even ask the physician to voluntarily surrender his or her license if it is necessary to protect the public. Whether the license is surrendered or not, the physician can be diverted to a supportive program if he or she acknowledges the existence of a problem. If the physician refuses to acknowledge the problem, the board can formally charge the physician with violating the state's licensing act and order the physician's appearance before it at a formal hearing. At hearing, the board usually receives evidence

and testimony and then makes findings of fact and forms conclusions of law as to the alleged violation and appropriate sanction. Most states permit a sanctioned physician to request a stay of the sanction and to bring an appeal of the board's decision before a court of law.

PRACTICE IN A HEALTH CARE INSTITUTION

Apart from the responsibility created by state licensure laws to report professional impairment or incompetence or other acts in violation of licensing law, institutional environments may create an additional burden and duty for professionals to be aware of and to monitor the competence of coproviders in the same institution. The interdependence of professionals within a particular institutional environment is best exemplified by the hospital, but it exists in other health care settings such as nursing homes, mental health institutions, and outpatient settings. Obvious examples would be the responsibilities of the medical staff to the institution to monitor the quality of health care in the hospital as outlined by state licensure laws, voluntary accreditation standards, and common sense, as well as the common law.

In many cases institutions, which normally have to depend on the quality of peer review processes that are delegated to the medical staff, have been found liable for failure to discover the incompetence of an individual practicing within that institution.[1] This well-established common law is based on a reasonable interpretation of the Standards of Accreditation of the Joint Commission on Accreditation of Healthcare Organizations (JCAHO), which are voluntary. In addition, the common law is based on interpretation of state licensure laws that require quality assurance programs to be effective in the hospital setting, medical association and society standards, and are well articulated to protect the interests of the public, and the institutional duty to provide quality care, which ultimately resides at the level of the governing body.

In addition to the responsibility for the competence and quality of performance of peers, coproviders are responsible for preventing the incompetence or impairment of a professional at another level—either above or below their own level—from harming the public in general or an individual patient. For example, nurses would be obligated to report an impaired, incompetent, or otherwise deficient physician, but they would also be required to report a technician who fails to function at an acceptable level.

PEER REVIEW

Quality assurance programs in hospitals depend on the process of peer review, because coproviders with the same professional training are the best judges of the competence and capability of their peers and colleagues.

The process of quality assurance is described best in terms of problem solving and the promotion of desired levels of patient care. Although it is easy to talk in generalities about the importance of quality, the actual process of quality assurance is very difficult in the health care setting, but the duty to provide good and effective peer review is clear.

Quality assurance programs

All health care institutions, health care provider groups, HMOs and managed care programs, and others directly or indirectly responsible for patient care necessarily deal with the developing field of quality assurance in health care. Small area analysis and comparison of health care practices as well as widespread inconsistencies in approaches to various disease processes and surgical problems have created great concern and even governmental intervention in attempts to standardize approaches to health care problems. The unfortunate by-product of this concern and standardization is that it is difficult to be certain of the relative benefits of the various approaches to problems. It is clear that many management approaches are effective, and diversity in health care should not be discarded for a theoretical and unproven cost or quality benefit. In medicine as well as in other "arts," there are many ways to skin a cat. Recently the *Journal of the American Medical Association* inaugurated a regular column on clinical decision making, which specifically states as its goal and objective the ongoing study of the problem of variation in clinical approaches to medical problems.[2]

In this setting, it is still important to eliminate deviations below and outside of acceptable medical practice, particularly those deviations that put patients at risk. Therefore, the JCAHO, medical societies, medical professional organizations, and others are actively involved in attempting to establish standards for practice. The American Medical Association has recently undertaken a study of standards in cooperation with Rand Corporation, and some 20 medical specialty societies have published some form of "standards."

Standards of care

Quality assurance peer review and coprovider relationships are dependent on perceptions of what are considered to be appropriate standards of care. Unfortunately, the legal system and the professional liability litigation in particular have confused the concept of standards in a way not easily explained.

This does not mean that it is impossible to reconcile institutional practice with understanding these standards. What is necessary is the acknowledgment that quality assurance and risk management must work in tandem, with each complimenting the other to assure that medical care is provided that meets the patient's needs and interests. An understanding of those needs is the first step because the legal system defines them in terms of the duties the health care provider owes to his or her patients:

1. To use his or her best judgment in care and treatment
2. To exercise reasonable care and diligence in the application of his or her knowledge and skills
3. To act in compliance with the standard of health care required by law.[3]

Thus, risk management and quality assurance programs must be used to constantly educate the institution's staff regarding how to fulfill these duties during the day-to-day provision of health care.

Normative versus actual standards of care

Elsewhere in this text the issues regarding standards of care are defined more completely, but it is important to recognize that generally courts define standard of care in terms of that degree of skill and expertise normally possessed and exercised by a reasonable and prudent practitioner with the same level of training in the same or similar circumstances.

What this means in a courtroom becomes quite a different thing. Too often, medical testimony presented in a courtroom deals with issues as they relate to "normative" standards rather than "actual" standards. In actual fact, physicians hope to perform at one level but actually perform at another level. For example, the work of John Holbrook, M.D. (personal communication), an emergency physician interested in risk management in Massachusetts, shows that after a review of more than 100,000 emergency department records, fewer than 5% of patients presenting to the emergency department with a headache actually received a fundoscopic examination. Whether this would be an actual standard that is acceptable is subject to debate, but it cannot be ignored as a reality. In a courtroom, the normative standard is described for the benefit of the judge or jury as expected performance recited by a "medical expert" adequately and sometimes superlatively qualified to discuss a particular area of professional expertise. It may not be an actual standard but rather a "normative" standard defined as the degree of skill and expertise that we strive to achieve rather than actually achieve as average prudent practitioners.

In the quality assurance setting, it is important for those involved in the definitions of standards and practices to recognize the difficulties of defining appropriate standards of care and evaluating coproviders. Within those parameters it is still possible to define unacceptable deviance and deal with it appropriately as part of the peer review mechanism.

Normally quality assurance programs are described in terms of the "controlled loop" process of identification of a problem, discussion and evaluation resulting in proposed action, real action, and then reevaluation to determine whether the problem has been properly managed. If a hospital medical staff or health care organization, such as a managed care program, a medical group, a prehospital care service, or other professional organizations responsible for patient care, does not establish a quality assurance program, it is difficult to imagine how they will carry out the duties of professionals to monitor health care provided, the quality of performance of coproviders, and the satisfactory outcome of professional health care activities.

Disciplinary activities in peer review

Practicing with coproviders necessarily results in disciplinary peer review actions when unacceptable and incurable deviance is identified. It is important for those involved in peer review and quality assurance matters that have a direct impact on an individual practitioner to be aware of the concept of due process and the laws of the state and nation that govern disciplinary and peer review activities in the health care setting. The Health Care Quality Improvement Act of 1986[4] is a federal bill that provides for the following: (1) subject physician must be notified of an organization's intent to bring disciplinary action; (2) that subject physician must have an opportunity to respond, request a hearing if he or she desires, and prepare a defense; (3) adequate notice of the nature of the charges must be given; (4) an opportunity for advice and counsel of the subject physician's choice, including an attorney, must be provided; (5) a fair hearing with an impartial panel of noncompeting peers must be available to perform the hearing; (6) the physician must be given an opportunity to examine the evidence against him or her, prepare a defense, cross-examine witnesses, and present arguments in his or her favor; and (7) a written opinion must be provided by the hearing panel if disciplinary action is recommended along with the written decision of the health care governing body or final arbitrator.

If a subject physician decides to sue members of the panel or the institution for engaging in the disciplinary activity and if the defendant institution or peer review panel members can show that the disciplinary action was undertaken in the "reasonable belief" that it was for the furtherance of good health care and with no malice or inappropriate motivations, then after the defendants prove that the suit was brought inappropriately, they can collect damages for expense of defense and court costs. The federal law provides for this remedy in order to encourage physicians to participate in peer review. On the other hand, a failure on the part of an institution or a professional to participate in peer review creates potential liability under the common law theories described earlier.

SUPERVISORY LIABILITY

Physicians supervise nurses, technicians, assistants, paramedics, and at times other physicians. This supervision is done by phone, by radio, or in person. The physician's responsibility and liability for such supervision are directly proportional to control over the actions of the other and knowledge of the other's actions.

Special responsibilities exist in the case of physicians who are supervising their own employees because direct vicarious liability exists for any actions of employees. The special status of nurse practitioners and physician's assistants, who carry out delegated duties, requires that physicians formally report to the state the existence of their relationship to a physician's assistant or a nurse practitioner and formally create delegated standard orders and other protocols to provide for proper guidelines. In addition, in many states definite limits are placed on the nature of the supervision that might be provided. In most states, the physician must be physically available to the nurse practitioner or physician's assistant, but in many states the ability of these employees to act within their standing orders is relatively liberal, including the use of signed prescription pads. State medical practice acts provide that a physician can delegate any responsibility to a properly trained person; this reverts to the basic issue of the physician's judgment of that person's qualifications. There are obviously extremes, such as a physician delegating neurosurgery to a physician's assistant, but other apparent extremes are common practice in the United States, such as nurses harvesting veins for cardiovascular surgeons.

Vicarious liability is that liability normally associated with an employer/employee, master/servant relationship. Employee physicians, nurses, technicians, and others create automatic liability for the employer. *Borrowed servants* are employees of another used for carrying out the activities of the "borrower." The liability of one who borrows another's servant is proportional to the amount of control exercised by the borrowing person. For example, in the health care setting, the "captain of the ship" theory at one time was used in order to deal with the problem of liability for nurses and others in the operating room. Common sense eventually demanded that courts recognize that surgeons do not directly control the administrative duties of others in the operating room. Scrub technicians, circulating nurses, anesthesiologists, and others working in the operating room setting, although they must defer to the judgment and authority of the surgeon on the case, obviously have separate and independent duties and responsibilities proportional to their professional competence. It is therefore unreasonable to make the surgeon liable for an improper sponge, needle, or instrument count, just as it would be inappropriate for a surgeon to be responsible for the conduct of an anesthesiologist who does an improper intubation. If the problem comes to the attention of the surgeon and he or she fails to act in the patient's interest, then liability increases proportionately, but the primary responsibility still lies with that person who acts independently regardless of the level of professional expertise and who has separate and independent ministerial duties and authority.

RADIO CONTROL AND PREHOSPITAL CARE

An interesting and important area of medical care that involves the delegation of medical practice to a remote person is the use of radio control for prehospital care. Separate and independent duties and responsibilities are created for licensed prehospital care personnel [paramedics or emergency medical technicians (EMTs)]. In addition, it is important to recognize that prehospital care services are required by law to have a medical director who establishes proper medical care/prehospital care protocols and monitors the competence of the prehospital care personnel through a functioning quality assurance program.

The physician who either directs or controls the paramedic at the scene has the same liability as a physician who would direct or control a nurse and has ultimate responsibility for the patient. In the case of radio control, the physician has a responsibility proportional to his or her knowledge of the situation, recognizing that the physician is dependent on the eyes, ears, and observational skills of the paramedic or EMT.

Appropriate prehospital care protocols are still widely variable in the United States. Variations easily result from the diverse qualifications of persons working in prehospital care settings, from personal opinions of medical directors, and from different state laws. State law specifically designates levels of skill in terms of basic care providers, special skill care providers, and full paramedic level providers. National and state registry and licensure all are a part of the definition of these various levels of skill. The control of prehospital care personnel is very similar to the type of remote control that exists when patients are in the hospital and nurses are used as observers reporting to physicians the condition of a patient and then carrying out appropriate therapeutic and diagnostic orders.

In the end, the health care professional who delegates responsibilities to others or controls others by providing care directly and in person or remotely by phone or radio is still responsible to act in a professional manner and within acceptable standards of care. A professional duty

to monitor the professional competence and ability of coproviders at, above, or below one's level of licensure or professional skill is a controlling factor and a legal principle that must be accepted by all professionals. In the institutional setting, coproviders are codependent and coresponsible. Even though direct responsibility may not exist, indirect responsibility for general considerations of quality assurance requires vigilance and appropriate action when problems and an incompetent coprovider are identified.

INDEPENDENT CONTRACTORS

The status of an individual as an independent contractor is a labor, employment, and tax consideration as well as a consideration that affects professional liability. If a person works as an employee, the vicarious liability is direct, but if that person is an independent contractor, the liability would be in proportion to the amount of control exercised. For example, many physicians function as independent contractors in various settings, but they exercise independent judgment with regard to their professional practice. The independent contractor concept is one that properly suits a professional role, because professionals are licensed as individuals and are responsible for making personal professional decisions with regard to care of patients. However, hospitals, health care facilities, and professional individuals are still responsible for monitoring the competence of the independent practitioner.

OSTENSIBLE AGENCY

In most states, certain independent contractor relationships have been found to be ineffective to deflect liability from the other contracting party. For example, in a hospital-based physician situation, an independent physician contractor may be the only one available to the patient, and therefore the hospital may be automatically considered to be vicariously liable through ostensible agency, by using the agent physician for carrying out some of its institutional responsibilities.[5] When the patient has no way of knowing that the physician is not an employee or when the hospital uses the physician just as the hospital would use an employee, then many states accept the concept that the hospital would therefore be vicariously liable for the physician's actions. This area has not been as well defined outside the hospital-based physician situation, because other members of the medical staff are more independent. The concept generally has widespread support in the case of hospital-based physicians when patients present to a hospital and have no choice as to which physician to pick.[6]

Independent contractors working within a hospital setting or in a medical group are still subject to the same basic peer review and quality assurance controls, and therefore the institution or the professional organization could be considered liable if it fails to properly conduct the following: (1) proper credentialing and application; (2) adequate peer review and quality assurance review; (3) monitoring of physicians for ongoing appropriateness of care, continued education if indicated, and proper recertification, relicensure, and other matters related to ongoing practice requirements; and (4) proper corrective and disciplinary action taken when a physician performs inappropriately or below the standard of care.

Under some state common law decisions, the medical staff may be considered liable for poor peer review. This liability of a health care institution as outlined in the common law has been extended to the medical staff when the medical staff knows that a physician has become incompetent and fails to take corrective action.[7]

CONSULTANTS AND REFERRING PHYSICIANS

The basic rule that applies here is that a consultant and the referring physician share responsibility for the patient's care based on the proportion of knowledge and control and the foreseeability for potential harm. For example, if the general practitioner refers the patient to a neurosurgeon for a neurosurgical problem, his or her responsibility for the case decreases in proportion to his or her knowledge of the problem, control over the care given the patient, and actions taken in response to any problems identified.

Failure to choose an appropriate consultant can occasionally create liability for the referring physician, particularly if the choice of consultant is based not on the competence of the consultant, but on other financial or personal relationships. If the consultant is known to be incompetent and it can be proven that the referring physician used that consultant anyway, then the liability would revert to the referring physician.

Substitutes and sharing on-call time can create some liability if one shares call or chooses a substitute who is incompetent. This would generally depend on the fact circumstances. For example, if a physician going on vacation is not careful in his or her choice of a competent substitute, the patient could easily consider that failure to take proper care in choosing a substitute as potential liability for the departing physician. In the case of sharing call with another physician, the responsibility is less because the other physician is independent. However, if a physician using shared call knows that another physician sharing call is incompetent or impaired, then he or she exposes the patients in his or her practice to that physician and would be considered liable in proportion to his or her knowledge of the incompetence or impairment of the call-sharing physician.

NURSING AND OTHER TECHNICAL PRACTICES IN THE HOSPITAL

State nurse practice acts and hospital protocol and procedure are controlling with regard to the appropriateness of nurses' professional activities. The physician is not responsible for designing protocols and policies, although the medical staff is generally responsible for the quality of care in the hospital.[8] In the case of a hospital setting or other health care institutional setting, administration generally includes nursing administration and therefore sets policy for the nursing practices within that institution. The medical staff provides overall oversight for the governing body on the quality of care provided in the institution, but depends on the nursing administration to develop policies and protocols for nursing care. The physician would be responsible for incompetence or impairment of a nurse or an inappropriate nursing action.

The physician should either intervene to prevent patient problems or a deterioration in patient condition or report the events so that actions can be taken by the health care institution. Failure to take those actions to ensure that the professional staff of the hospital is functioning in a way that provides quality patient care could result in liability for the physician. The same responsibilities exist for nurses toward other nurses or technicians and for technicians with regard to other professional personnel in the hospital.

Professionals within a hospital or health care institutional setting assume liability in proportion to their knowledge of the problem and their ability to effect change. Within the institution, following protocol and procedure for registering complaints and attempting to provide for corrective action satisfy the responsibilities of the individual. The failure of the institution to act after being informed would create a separate institutional liability.

The state medical practice acts, state nurse practice acts, and federal law[9] provide immunity for people who report in good faith the incompetence, impairment, or inappropriate practice of another professional.

CONCLUSION

The health care environment requires cooperation and teamwork. Physicians are dependent on many other health care professionals in a health care institution to ensure good patient care. These interdependencies are unavoidable and are increasing in magnitude and complexity; therefore, it is important to understand that, generally, the liability and the legal responsibility of those working on a team are easy to analyze. The degree of duty and responsibility is in proportion to the amount of control and knowledge of potential for foreseeable harm. The health care professional is obligated to take actions to protect the interest of patients, who are innocent parties in the health care environment. A failure to act in the interest of good patient care or in the protection of the public welfare creates liability. Apart from concern about becoming a codefendant because of a failure to discipline or supervise, health care professionals should consider the fact that there are many different ways to fail the patient, including allowing another to harm the patient. The public responsibility of licensed health care professionals is the "brother's keeper" responsibility. Health care institutions, on the other hand, have a separate and independent corporate responsibility to ensure quality of care within their organizations. Failure to require proper credentials, inappropriate hiring practices, and failure to develop proper quality assurance and peer review within the institution places the governing body and the institution at great risk if patient harm results from that failure.

INSTITUTIONAL PRACTICE: HISTORICAL ORIGINS

Hospitals evolved in this country during the eighteenth, nineteenth, and early twentieth centuries along the lines of the European (particularly the British) model as charitable institutions and, in some cases, as almshouses for the poor. Because of this focus, many hospitals were affiliated with or originated from various religious orders. Arising from this development was the doctrine of charitable immunity of hospitals from legal liability.[10] This case finding represented a natural outgrowth of their origins and services primarily to the downtrodden in society.

It was not until the 1870s, when university teaching hospitals and municipal hospitals began to appear, that secular institutions began to flourish. Despite this shift away from religious institutions, hospitals continued to enjoy insulation from legal liability, retaining charitable immunity, primarily because of their origins.

Evolution of functional hospital organization and management (1914-1984)

Early in this century the organization of hospitals began to evolve into bipartite and tripartite institutions. The leading case to perpetuate this separation was *Schloendorff v. New York Hosp.,* a New York appellate court decision in 1914.[11] The administrative staff was regarded as the governing body responsible for the overall administration of the hospital, while the medical staff was in charge of rendering patient care. The artificial separation was promulgated in the courts by their erecting a distinction between the "purely ministerial" acts performed by the hospital administration contrasted to medical acts performed by members of the hospital medical staff:

It is true, I think, of nurses, as of physicians, that in treating a patient, they are not acting as servants of the hospital. But nurses are employed to carry out the orders of the physicians, to whose authority they are subject.... If there are duties performed by nurses foreign to their duties in carrying out the physician's orders, and having relationship to the administrative conduct of the hospital, the fact is not established by the record.[12]

This medical/ministerial act dichotomy continued after *Schloendorff,* although the functional distinction between hospital administration and medical staffs became increasingly blurred: For example, it got to the point at which administering the right blood by transfusion to the wrong patient was a "ministerial act" in *Necolauff v. Genesee Hosp.,*[13] while administering the wrong blood to the right patient was a "medical act" in *Berg v. N.Y. Society for the Relief of the Ruptured and Crippled.*[14]

This distinction was finally abrogated in 1957, in *Bing v. Thunig*[15] in which a New York appellate court overturned *Schloendorff.* Since *Bing,* both regulatory and common law in the health care field have evolved to reflect the interrelationships and interdependencies of the hospital and its medical staff. The JCAHO guidelines also reinforce the essence of this corporate relationship.[16] This view of the medical staff as an integral component of the hospital corporation has been confirmed in the decision of *Johnson v. Misericordia County Hosp.*[17] The antitrust case of *Weiss v. York Hosp.*[18] may have muddied the water somewhat by referring to the medical staff as being independent to the extent that it may be the "sole decision maker." Nevertheless, in terms of more practical economic realities, it seems clear that for both hospitals and their medical staffs to survive and, perhaps, thrive in the increasingly competitive health care marketplace, each must emphasize its common directives and capitalize on them in forming new partnerships. To paraphrase Benjamin Franklin, we must hang together or, surely, we shall hang separately.

Evolution of the legal responsibilities for quality assurance in the hospital

The movement away from captain of the ship doctrine. The evolution of the legal responsibilities for quality assurance within the hospital paralleled to a great extent the organizational changes throughout this period. A major development in establishing the legal view that the hospital is more than just a physician's workshop, but with independent responsibilities of its own, arose from the decision of *Tonsic v. Wagner.*[19] In that decision, the Supreme Court of Pennsylvania overturned their "captain of the ship" holding in *McConnell v. Williams* in which a hospital might escape liability for the negligent acts of employees temporarily under the direction of independently contracting physicians: "But such an employee can be temporarily detached, in whole or in part, from the hospital's general control."[20] Thus, the *Tonsic* decision firmly established the principle that a hospital should be held liable for the negligent act of any of its employees even if under the supervision of a nonemployee at the time.

The extension of hospital liability to the acts of independent contractors—apparent agency. The doctrine of apparent agency has substantially contributed to the demise of the independent contractor defense for the hospital. One of the most important judicial pronouncements concerning this came again from the Superior Court of Pennsylvania in the case of *Capan v. Divine Providence Hosp.* First, the changing role of the hospital creates a likelihood that patients will look to the institution rather than the individual physician for care. Thus, a patient frequently enters the hospital seeking a wide range of hospital services rather than personal treatment by a particular physician. It would be absurd to require such a patient to be familiar with the law of *respondeat superior*, so to inquire of each person who treated (plaintiff) whether he or she is an employee of the hospital or an independent contractor. . . . Similarly, it would be unfair to allow this secret limitation on liability contained in a doctor's contract with the hospital to bind the unknowing patient.[21]

LIABILITY OF HOSPITALS AND MEDICAL STAFF PHYSICIANS
Hospital admissions

Nonemergency. In general, a hospital has no duty to admit a patient. However, it must not discriminate by race, color, or creed. Under limited circumstances, based on statutory (governmental hospitals), contractual (subscribes to an HMO or other similar arrangement), or common law (injury caused by the hospital), the hospital may have a duty to admit.

In hospitals wherein clinical research is mandated by the government, the institution is usually allowed discretion to refuse admission, even if the patient may meet criteria for admission. A teaching hospital, however, may not admit a patient contingent on the patient's participation in the teaching program. Otherwise, the patient's constitutional right of privacy would be invaded.

Even if a patient otherwise has a right to be admitted, if there is no medical necessity or if the hospital does not possess the services needed, the hospital need not admit the nonemergency patient.[22] The principle of *no duty to admit* reflects judicial restraint in dictating how a hospital should allocate scarce medical resources. Although many of the cases supporting this common law principle date back to the turn of the century, the majority of the courts continue to apply this doctrine today.[23]

Special circumstances may exist that obligate a hospital under common law doctrines to admit a patient if a prior relationship existed between the hospital and patient or where the hospital was the cause of patient injury, i.e., has placed the person in a position of peril. Such circumstances exist if the original injury or complication of treatment occurred as the result of the hospital's acts or omissions or the hospital begins to provide care to the patient. The hospital may be liable for abandonment if admission is denied under such circumstances.

Emergency. The national trend of the law is to impose liability on hospitals for refusal to treat emergencies or if negligent care is provided in their emergency departments. Theories on which courts have based such liability include the following: (1) reliance, (2) agency *(respondeat superior)*, (3) apparent authority ("holding self out"), (4) corporate negligence, and (5) nondelegable duty. These theories are discussed next.

RELIANCE THEORY. If the patient relies on a well-established custom of the hospital to render aid in an emergency situation, the hospital may be found liable in refusing to provide the necessary care or for providing negligent care.

In *Wilmington General Hosp. v. Manlove,*[24] the hospital was found liable under this theory when a child needing emergency care was not admitted to the hospital after the child's private pediatrician could not be reached to approve the admission. In *Stanturf v. Sipes,*[25] the hospital was held liable when the administrator refused to approve the admission because of the patient's inability to pay. The court stated:

> The members of the public . . . had reason to rely on the [hospital], and . . . that plaintiff's condition was caused to be worsened by the delay resulting from the futile efforts to obtain treatment from the . . . [hospital].[26]

AGENCY THEORY. If the emergency department personnel who deviate from the applicable standard of care and cause harm to the plaintiff are considered "servants" of the hospital, there is little problem in holding the hospital vicariously liable under the doctrine of *respondeat superior*. A servant is defined as "a person employed to perform services in the affairs of another and who with respect to the physical conduct in the performance of the service is subject to the other's control or right to control."[27] Other than house staff, staff physicians are usually considered "independent contractors" rather than "servants." Courts must determine that an agency relationship exists based on an analysis of the facts of the case before holding a hospital liable under this theory.[28]

In *Thomas v. Corso,*[29] the hospital was found liable

when the emergency room nurse failed to contact the on-call physician. In *Citizens Hosp. Ass'n. v. Schoulin,*[30] a similar case, based on nursing negligence in failing to report all the patient's symptoms to the on-call physician, failing to conduct a proper examination, and failing to follow the physician's directions, the court found the hospital liable under *respondeat superior.*

APPARENT AUTHORITY. A hospital may be found vicariously liable for an emergency room physician's negligence, even if the physician is considered an independent contractor, where the facts establish apparent authority (also referred to as "ostensible agency" or "agency by estoppel"). This is the theory of "holding itself out" by the hospital. The hospital will be found liable when it permits or encourages patients to believe that independent contractor/physicians are the hospital's authorized agents. The "holding out" must come from the hospital—not the physician.

The landmark case on which this theory is based is *Gizzi v. Texaco, Inc.*[31] In *Gizzi,* Texaco was held liable for its representations to the public, "You can trust your car to the man who wears the star." This advertisement was sufficient to support the jury's finding against Texaco for the apparent authority it vested in an independent contractor/dealer who sold a used car in which the brakes failed, injuring the purchaser. Texaco did not profit from the sale but was aware that the dealer was engaged in this collateral activity.

CORPORATE NEGLIGENCE. The doctrine of corporate negligence is based on an independent duty of the hospital for the medical care rendered in its institution. Like the apparent agency theory, it holds the hospital liable for an independent contractor/physician's negligence. However, it is based on the hospital's independent negligence in allowing an incompetent physician to practice on its premise.

NONDELEGABLE DUTY. The main reason for employers to utilize independent contractors is to "farm out" services that may be of benefit to the employers but that they may not be willing or able to provide themselves. They also may wish to avoid legal liability for such services. The immunity from liability may be misused or abused. The independent contractor immunity is therefore riddled with exceptions.[32]

For public policy reasons, certain duties delegated to an independent contractor have been determined not to confer immunity on the employer. These exceptions have been termed "nondelegable duties." They usually represent situations wherein the employer's duty is important, urgent, or very imperative. Employers possessing such responsibilities cannot avoid liability by delegating those responsibilities to an independent contractor.

In *Marek v. Professional Health Services, Inc.,*[33] the health service was held liable even though it entrusted the reading of a patient's chest X-ray film to a competent independent contractor/radiologist. The theory on which liability rested was nondelegable duty. The Alaska Supreme Court held in a landmark case of first impression that the hospital is vicariously liable as a matter of law for negligence in its emergency department.[34] Such a duty "may be imposed by statute, by contract, by franchise or by charter, or by common law."[35] As discussed in this landmark case, the hospital had a nondelegable duty to provide nonnegligent care in its emergency department, based on its state license as a general acute care hospital, JCAHO standards, and its own bylaws.

Statutory bases for hospital liability for emergency room care

In *Guerro v. Copper Queen Hosp.,*[36] a privately owned hospital operated only for employees of one company was held liable for refusing treatment to an illegal alien who sought care. The Arizona Supreme Court reasoned that the state licensing statute precluded the hospital from denying emergency care to a patient.

A federal law, the Emergency Medical Treatment and Active Labor Act, commonly referred to as the "anti-dumping" statute, is contained in the miscellaneous provisions of the Budget Reconciliation Act (COBRA) of the Ninety-ninth Congress.[37] This statute is a codification of common law regarding theories of liability and duties of the emergency department. It applies to all hospitals that participate in Medicare and other government medical assistance programs created by the Social Security Act.

The law has had a significant impact on emergency medical care in hospitals. It has improved the chances of plaintiffs and their counsel to recover damages from hospitals because it eliminates the requirement to prove some of the elements of medical negligence. It governs hospitals with an emergency department wherein a patient with an emergency medical condition or a woman in active labor seeks medical care. If such a patient is "transferred" from the health care facility to another facility or is discharged, the patient may recover damages for "personal harm" if the condition worsens during or after such transfer or discharge. The patient must prove only that the condition was not "stabilized" at the time of transfer and that the condition deteriorated because of the transfer. To avoid liability, the attending physician or other medical personnel at the hospital must sign "a certification that, based upon the information available at the time, the medical benefits reasonably expected from the provision of appropriate medical treatment at another facility outweigh the increased risks" of transfer.

In addition to the certification requirement, the transfer must also be an "appropriate transfer." Although the signed certification is a simple enough procedure for the hospital to incorporate within its medical record forms, the requirements that will satisfy the transfer include all the following: (1) "the receiving facility . . . has available space and qualified personnel . . . has agreed to accept transfer . . . and to provide appropriate medical treatment"; (2) "the transferring hospital provides . . . appropriate medical records of examination and treatment"; (3) "transfer is effected through qualified personnel and transportation equipment"; and (4) "such other requirements as the Secretary [of Health and Human Services] may find necessary. . . ." Presumably, the physician or other medical personnel who transfers the patient has the requisite knowledge of the staffing and competence of the receiving facility and has sought agreement for acceptance by the receiving facility before transfer. These requirements seem applicable whether the receiving facility is an outpatient clinic, nursing home, day care program, or a more intensive treatment center.

Although the physician must be acting as an employee or under contract with the hospital and the hospital must be a participating Medicare provider for the penalty provisions of this law to apply, such employment status is not required for recovery of damages that are allowed under state law. In addition, the hospital will be liable for damages under this statute or state law whether or not the involved physician is considered an independent contractor under state law.

This federal law seems to preempt state law that "directly conflicts with any of its requirements." It further provides for federal jurisdiction and allows the injured individual to obtain "such equitable relief as is appropriate," giving the federal court discretion to award damages it considers to be warranted. Legal action may be brought up to two years after the violation.

A patient who suffers "personal harm" resulting from violation of provisions of this law will be entitled to those damages allowed under the state's substantive law of personal injury and wrongful death statutes. In addition to these damages, penalties of up to $25,999 per violation against the hospital and involved physician alike are applicable to provider hospitals and their employed or contracted physicians.

Finally, the hospital receiving the transferred patient is also indemnified against any financial losses by the transferring hospital if the transferring hospital has violated the statute. Hospitals are no longer to be considered the "doctor's workshop." The modern hospital represents an integrated center for delivery of health care services, possessing in-house staff and independent contractor/physicians with an array of staff privileges. The hospital can farm out professional services; however, based on public policy and other legal considerations, the trend of the law is to hold the hospital liable for harm resulting from negligence in handling admissions and transfers of patients in its emergency department. As hospitals have become more profitable and business oriented, the adversarial relationship and the law governing hospitals, patients, and physicians have changed. Although there is no duty for nonemergency admissions by hospitals, under emergency circumstances, the trend of the law is for hospital liability if the patient is harmed as a result of denial of admission or improper care.

Corporate liability of hospitals

No doctrine exemplifies the notion of a hospital as a corporate entity with subsidiary components functioning interdependently to deliver a health care product better than the judicially pronounced theory holding hospitals corporately liable for the quality of care delivered by members of its medical staff, whether they are employees or purely independent contractors. Under the doctrine of corporate liability, it is the hospital itself that may be held directly liable for its own negligence in assuring the quality of health care delivered within its walls.

This doctrine of the direct corporate liability of hospitals is traceable to the famous case of *Darling v. Charleston Memorial Hosp.*[38] In the *Darling* case, a patient was admitted through the emergency room of a private, nonprofit hospital for treatment of a broken leg, and was attended by a hospital staff physician who was rotating on emergency duty. The attending physician was not skilled in orthopedic work, and a cast was improperly applied so that circulation to the leg was blocked. Although the patient subsequently complained about the leg, and the nurses involved in his care observed the discoloration of his toes, nothing was done. When he was finally examined by another physician, the leg required amputation. The court's decision against the hospital could have been based on a finding of apparent agency on the grounds that the plaintiff had no reason to think that the hospital's attending physician was not employed by the hospital. However, the court went further in holding the hospital itself directly liable for breaching its own duty of care to the patient, in failing to "require consultation with a member of the hospital surgical staff skilled in such treatment, or to review the treatment rendered to the plaintiff; and to require consultants to be called in as needed."

The court recognized the hospital's own central role in the overall treatment of the patient, thereby requiring the hospital itself to become directly involved in the health care delivery process. Hospitals could be held directly liable for their own corporate negligence in providing health care services. Prior to this case, the corporate duties of hospitals were limited to three areas, unrelated to direct patient care:

1. The duty of reasonable care in the maintenance and use of equipment
2. The availability of equipment and services
3. The duty of reasonable care in the selection and retention of employees.

Now after *Darling* and its progeny, hospitals must be much more mindful of their selection and retention of staff physicians.[39-43]

MEDICAL STAFF CREDENTIALING
Evolution of the basic hospital-physician relationship

The rights, duties, and protections afforded to the hospital and its medical staff have traditionally been analyzed by reference to the quality and quantity of the delivery of patient care. The law recognizes that the governing body of the hospital must establish the qualifications of physicians who are admitted to the hospital staff and monitor the quality of medical care delivered to hospital patients.

The hospital is generally protected under the law when its decision whether to appoint or reappoint is based on considerations related to the quality of medical care rendered within the hospital. Such considerations may involve an assessment not only of the physician's technical and clinical competence, but of other relevant factors such as his or her ability to cooperate with coworkers and support staff.

The hospital governing body, while it has the duty to ensure the quality of patient care in the hospital, has neither the expertise nor the proximity to specific situations to monitor adequately the actual delivery of medical services. Accordingly, the hospital governing body delegates much of its quality assurance responsibilities to the medical staff, while the governing body retains the ultimate monitoring or oversight responsibility. The medical staff organization through committee structure provides the actual quality assurance mechanism by which the institution's quality of care may be maintained through following the hospital's and medical staff's bylaws, rules and regulations, standards of performance, and procedures for peer review.

The professional and economic significance of hospital staff privileges

The hospital, with its special care facilities and interaction of experts and trained professionals, became the major centralized provider of medical services in the country many years ago. Modern methods for practicing medicine are such that a physician who is denied access to a hospital facility may be severely hampered in his or her practice. Gaining and retaining clinical privileges in at least one hospital has become practically essential for most physicians to practice medicine.

Still, staff privileges are just that: privileges. There is no fundamental or constitutional right to practice at a particular hospital.[44] In some jurisdictions, however, the profession of a valid license may create a right to appointment in the absence of actual incompetence.[45] The current revolution in health care financing and competition is adding yet another layer of complexity to this decision-making process. As physicians seek to attain or retain clinical privileges on the one hand, hospitals and medical staffs are becoming more selective with respect to whom they grant clinical privileges. In some cases, as part of long-term strategic planning, whole departments of clinical services may be eliminated or curtailed substantially due to the changing economics and reimbursement climate and patient population needs. All of these developments have brought the dilemma of hospital corporate liability versus physician staff privileges disputes into bold relief. These issues are discussed in more detail later in this chapter. The remainder of this part deals with the various types of staff privileges available, the process involved in obtaining and retaining them, and the protections, theories of liability, and remedies available in the denial, deferral, limitation, or withdrawal of these staff privileges.

NATURE AND TYPE OF STAFF MEMBERSHIP
Active medical staff

The active staff consists of practitioners who meet certain basic educational, training, and background experience requirements; who regularly admit patients to the hospital, or are otherwise involved in the care of hospital patients, or participate in a teaching or research program of the hospital; and who actively participate in the staff's patient care audit and quality assurance activities.

Each active medical staff member retains responsibility within his or her area of professional competence (as prescribed by clinical privilege delineation determinations) for the daily care and supervision of each patient in the hospital for whom he or she provides services.

Consulting staff

The consulting staff consists of practitioners who are members of the active staff of another hospital where he or she actively participates in the patient care audit and other quality assurance activities, and who is of recognized professional ability in a specialized field and is not a member of another category of the medical staff. Consulting staff members cannot admit patients and their clinical privileges are limited to their particular area of expertise.

Courtesy staff

The courtesy staff consists of practitioners who admit a limited number of patients per year, and is the member of another hospital's active medical staff, where he or she actively participates in patient care audit and other quality assurance activities.

Affiliate staff

This group shall consist of practitioners, who are not active, but have a long-standing relationship with the hospital. These practitioners may not admit patients or be eligible to hold office or vote in general staff and special meetings.

Outpatient staff

This staff consists of practitioners who are regularly engaged in the care of outpatients on behalf of the hospital or in a program sponsored by or associated with the hospital, who do not wish to assume all the responsibilities incumbent on active staff membership. Each outpatient staff member retains responsibility within his or her area of professional competence for the daily care and supervision of patients under his or her care, while actively participating in the patient care audit or other quality assurance activities required of the staff.

Honorary/emeritus staff

Members of this staff are practitioners who are not active in the hospital, but are being honored for their outstanding accomplishments or reputation. These members may also be former members of the active staff who have retained and may retain admitting and clinical privileges to the extent recommended by the medical board and board of directors.

House staff

Members of this group are either fully licensed physicians or physicians who have received appropriate certification from the state medical board authorizing them to enter postgraduate study in a particular hospital. They may admit patients within the specialty department to which they are assigned with the approval of an active staff member in that department who is responsible for the care of that patient, and exercise clinical privileges as established within the residency training program.

Allied health professional staff

This represents a group of nonphysician health care providers, such as podiatrists, nurses, or psychologists, who may provide specified patient care services under the supervision or direction of a physician member of the medical staff. They may write orders to the extent established in the rules of the staff and department to which they are assigned, but not beyond the scope of their licenses, certificates, or other legal credentials. The 1990 JCAHO *Accreditation Manual for Hospitals* accommodates the entry of these nonphysician providers into the hospital's health care delivery system.

STAFF APPLICATION AND RENEWAL
The public/private hospital distinction

Constitutional and statutory protections typically have imposed more restrictions on public hospitals in the area of staff privileges decisions. Increasingly, however, acts of formerly private hospitals have come under an increasing level of scrutiny similar to that for public hospitals.

The two most common theories of medical staff guarantees advanced by physicians have been (1) that the hospital has a fiduciary relationship with the public because of its tax-exempt status, as well as its health and charitable activities, and (2) that by virtue of the hospital's receipt of certain public monies (e.g., Hill-Burton funds), its acts amount to "state action." Such hospital acts were therefore claimed to be subject to the Fifth and Fourteenth Amendments to the Constitution, requiring due process of law for the benefit of persons otherwise being deprived of life, liberty, or property rights. This justification finds its specific application to the physician appointment and reappointment process through the analysis of staff privileges as a necessary means of guaranteeing the liberty right of practicing one's profession.

Delegation of credentialing decisions to the medical staff

The governing body of the hospital (while ultimately responsible for the quality of care delivered) delegates to the medical staff the decision-making process for physician credentialing. The medical staff ordinarily then delegates these specific functions to a select credentials or peer review committee to make these determinations. Initial appellate decision-making authority for these determinations is usually passed to a medical executive committee. The composition of this committee is variable but is usually comprised of clinical department and division chiefs, or service and section heads as well as medical and hospital administrative personnel.

The process

A current or aspiring member to a medical staff submits a completed application including proof of medical education, licensure, board eligibility or certification, supporting materials including recommendations concerning current clinical competence and ethical practice, recent (five years) ongoing as well as adverse claim experience, and a completed privileges delineation request form to the secretary of the medical staff or the hospital administrator. Following this, the physician may be interviewed by the department chair who prepares a written report and recommendation concerning staff appointment and clinical privileges, which is then transmitted to the credentials committee.

Following initial processing, the application for past record is reviewed by the credentials committee. The credentials committee then transmits to the medical executive committee (sometimes known as the medical board) a written report and recommendation as to staff appointment, category, department, and clinical privileges delineation, including special conditions.

The medical executive committee then forwards to the executive director for transmittal to the board of directors a written report and recommendation for clinical privileges to be granted with any special conditions to be attached to the appointment. Physicians receiving adverse determinations may follow an appellate procedure roughly paralleling the foregoing process.

CONSIDERATIONS FOR ACCEPTANCE OR REJECTION

The following represent general criteria considered in the staff privileges decision-making process:

1. Education, training, background, and experience
2. Need in the department
3. Ability to work with others
4. Ability to meet eligibility or other requirements specified in bylaws
5. Freedom from conflict of interest
6. Utilization of hospital experience facilities
7. Maintenance of professional, liability insurance
8. Willingness to make a full-time commitment to the institution
9. Whether the hospital is the physician's primary in-patient facility
10. Status of medical record-keeping and risk management experience
11. Freedom from false or misleading information
12. Current clinical competence, ethical practice, and health status
13. A willingness to comply with bylaws and regulations
14. Continuing medical education as required
15. Evidence of previous or current action taken in licensure or privilege matters.

Several of the preceding criteria might carry potential antitrust implications if applied to deny or limit clinical privileges in some contexts. Curtailment, based on these criteria, should specify with considerable particularity why privileges were denied, deferred, or limited.

LEGAL PROTECTIONS AVAILABLE TO THE PHYSICIAN
Hospital and medical staff bylaws

It is well settled under the law that hospitals acting through their medical staffs must comply with their own internal procedural rules (i.e., bylaws). Failure to do so, at the very least, will invite judicial review. Upon finding a significant failure, a court could nullify the whole process and require the hospital to review the physician's qualifications again in accordance with all internal policies, procedures, and bylaws. Examples of particular procedural rules that should appear in bylaws include (but are not limited to):

1. Adequate notice to the physician of the adverse decision
2. Making available a fair hearing process for aggrieved physicians
3. Communicating adequately to physicians the factors governing the credentialing decision
4. Allocating properly the burden of proof during the hearings.

Contract theory of medical staff bylaw

In Pennsylvania and some other states, the medical staff bylaws may be viewed as part of a contractual relationship between the hospital and members of its medical staff, so that modifications may only be made pursuant to amendment procedures established in the bylaws themselves. At least in Pennsylvania, as well as other states adopting this approach, it may be considered a breach of contract for a hospital to violate procedural protections afforded under its medical staff bylaws in the physician credentialing process.

There may have been an inadequate number of court decisions to make it clear whether any such breach would make available to aggrieved physicians the whole panoply of common law contractual remedies. It is also unclear whether this contractual analogy may apply to the situation of an applicant who is not yet a member of the medical staff.

Protection from economic harm

There may be some protection from tortious interference with a physician's ability to practice his profession. In many jurisdictions (e.g., New Jersey), this has been recognized as a valid claim under tort law. In general, the presence of an intent to deny privileges without legal justification is sufficient to permit this type of claim to go forward in litigation. In addition, interference with trade or business may be alleged as a violation of the federal or state constitution, if the hospital is considered to be a public institution as discussed earlier. If two or more individual staff members or other persons conspire to deny privileges wrongfully, a "restraint of trade" claim may also be possible (i.e., a Sherman Act Section 1 violation as discussed later in the antitrust subsection). In addition to possible claims under federal antitrust laws, some state courts (notably New Jersey) also permit these suits.

Protection from defamation

Physicians involved in the credentialing process are usually seen to be protected from defamation, or "the holding of a person up to ridicule, in a respectable and considerable part of the community." Typically, the hospital and medical staff may have available several defenses to the claim by physicians that they have been defamed during the credentialing process.

First, no liability from defamation will attach to the hospital or its staff if the allegedly defamatory statements are true. Second, the physician applicant consents to the making of these statements by voluntarily going through the credentialing process. Third, public policy requires that persons who are asked to give statements to assist in the credentialing process should be protected by the law for such statements, to ensure that they are given without fear of reprisal and to ensure that the best possible decisions are made to assure patient safety and welfare. In most contexts, this is a qualified privilege. In the absence of malice, this privilege applies to physicians and others involved in credentialing decision—physicians, in making comments, must make them in a proper setting for statements to be protected.

Due process protection

In the case of hospitals owned or controlled by public agencies or private hospitals acting under the color of state law by having a fiduciary relationship with the public, substantive and due process safeguards may become available to physicians seeking to attain or retain staff privileges.

Substantive due process requires that the reasons behind the denial of a physician's staff privileges must be rational and not arbitrary or capricious. Claims based on an alleged violation of substantive due process may involve, for example, challenges to per se rules imposed by the hospital, such as minimum educational requirements (beyond those required for licensure) or board certification in a clinical specialty.

Procedural due process requires that the physician receive adequate safeguards concerning the process itself in determining whether he or she should be granted staff privileges at a particular hospital. A significant number of federal court decisions have held that denial

of privileges by a private health care provider is not sufficiently regulated or controlled by the state to invoke federal jurisdiction.[46,47] However, it is now becoming clear that regardless of whether the hospital concerned is public or private, a physician has a federally protected right to due process.[48,49] These procedural safeguards may include (but not be limited to):

1. Notification of the adverse determination[50]
2. If the physician requests a hearing, written notice of the charges with sufficient specificity to give the physician adequate notice with sufficient specificity of the reason for an adverse ruling[51]
3. Adequate time to prepare a defense[52]
4. Opportunity for prehearing discovery[53]
5. A hearing panel composed of impartial fair-minded physicians[54]
6. Appearance before the decision-making panel
7. Assistance of legal counsel during the hearing
8. Cross-examination of witnesses
9. Presentation of witnesses and evidence in defense[55]
10. Transcript of panel hearing available for review prior to appellate hearing[56]
11. Written decision from the panel for judicial review.

Employment practices discrimination

A newer possible theory that physicians might be able to assert comes under the umbrella of employment practices discrimination. Although this cause of action historically arose in occupations other than medicine, it may be available, at least, to employed physicians. Another type of action might become available to physicians who have lost or failed to obtain staff privileges as a result of their having made prior written or oral statements critical of peers or of the policies of the hospital at which he or she has lost privileges. A relevant court decision in this connection is *Novosel v. Nationwide Insurance Co.*[57] There the federal appeals court in Philadelphia upheld an employee's right to sue his employer, where he may have been wrongfully discharged for having asserted a right protected by an important public policy, namely, freedom of speech and political association.

Antitrust safeguards

Approximately 26% of this country's physicians are involved in exclusive contracts with hospitals. These contracts with radiologists, pathologists, anesthesiologists, and, sometimes cardiologists or emergency physicians have become the subject of Sherman Act antitrust challenges in recent years. To invoke a violation of Section 1 of this act, a plaintiff must assert the following:

1. That the parties against whom the antitrust action

is brought have agreed among or between themselves (i.e., conspired) to engage in activities that restrain trade

2. That the effect of this conspiracy is to restrain trade and is anticompetitive in nature
3. That these anticompetitive practices affect consumer choice of services in a relevant market population covered by the agreement or conspiracy
4. That these anticompetitive practices have a substantial and adverse impact on interstate commerce.

Aggrieved parties have also alleged violation of Section 2 of the Sherman Antitrust Act. Section 2 prohibits the willful acquisition or maintenance of monopoly power in a relevant geographic market within which the provider of services operates, and as a practical matter to which the purchaser of those services may turn for these services. Acquiring or maintaining the power to control market prices and exclude competition in such an area could amount to a Section 2 violation involving monopolistic practice. Section 2 violations do not require a conspiratorial agreement. Assuming that federal jurisdiction may be established by showing that anticompetitive practices have a substantial adverse impact on interstate commerce, an analysis of the merits of an antitrust claim in a credentialing case may proceed.[58] In the most famous recent case analyzing the merits of an antitrust claim concerning the staff privileges of an unsuccessful applicant to a closed medical staff of anesthesiologists, the U.S. Supreme Court, speaking through Mr. Justice Stevens, held that this type of exclusive contract did not violate Section 1 of the Sherman Antitrust Act.[59]

The theory of liability was that through the vehicle of this exclusive contract, consumer choice was limited because the anesthetic services of the hospital were illegally "tied to" its surgical services (i.e., if you went to a hospital to undergo surgery, you had to accept the exclusive panel of anesthesiologists). The Supreme Court, however, held that there was no shortage of other hospitals with comparable services in the New Orleans area from which patient/consumers could choose other surgeons and anesthesiologists for their operations.

Justice O'Connor and three other justices concurred in the result, but stated that this type of practice should have been sustained because it was justified by matters of medical and administrative efficiency (i.e., it satisfied rules of reason while not constituting an illegal practice according to federal antitrust laws). This decision (though not finding an antitrust violation) may be most significant to the health care industry by confirming that relationships among hospitals, physicians, and their patients are subject to the same antitrust principles that apply to others involved in commercial activities. This

decision may be just as notable for what it does not say. For example, exclusive contracts in the areas with only one hospital near state borders, which involve services with independent markets, may well violate Section 1 of the Sherman Act. Clearly, now that health care is regarded by the courts as a commercial activity, the range of antitrust violations may well increase depending on the specific facts and circumstances in each case.

In 1984, the 3rd Circuit Court of Appeals reconfirmed the applicability of traditional commercial analysis to the activities of hospitals and their medical staffs in excluding certain groups from staff membership.

In *Weiss v. York Hosp.,* Dr. Malcom Weiss had filed a Sherman Act antitrust action as a member of a group (osteopathic physicians) who had been excluded from membership on the hospital's medical staff.[60] The lower court had found that this group boycott by York Hospital and its medical staff violated Sections 1 and 2 of the Sherman Act. The 3rd Circuit Court of Appeals in Philadelphia, while reversing the Section 2 violation finding, concurred with the lower court that this practice violated Section 1 of the Sherman Act. The appellate court found that regardless of whether or not the medical staff was acting as an agent or independently of the hospital in this practice, there was a conspiracy among individual staff physicians to exclude osteopathic physicians.

This case confirmed that regardless of whether or not the medical staff is an entity separate from the hospital, individual physicians compete with each other and, thus, may conspire to limit competition in violation of Section 1 of the Sherman Act. With the dramatically increasing numbers of M.D.'s, D.O.'s, D.D.S.'s, D.P.M.'s, D.C.'s, M.S.N.'s, P.A.'s and other health care professionals, the impact that this case should have on future efforts by M.D.'s to boycott certain non-M.D. groups cannot be overstated.

AVAILABLE REMEDIES TO AGGRIEVED PHYSICIANS

A physician denied clinical privileges may be entitled to a variety of remedies if he or she prevails in litigation against the hospital. The remedy usually depends on the infraction. An injunction may be available. The court may prevent the hospital from denying or curtailing staff privileges (permanently or at least until a full hearing and final decision is made by the hospital concerning appointment or reappointment).

To obtain injunctive relief, a physician must show that he or she could be harmed irreparably if the injunction is not granted. However, even if a physician can show this and gets an injunction, this finding will not act to prevent the hospital from denying staff privileges based on subsequent events. Furthermore, injunctive relief is inappropriate if internal hospital administrative remedies have not been exhausted or are still available as prescribed by hospital and medical staff bylaws. In appropriate circumstances (usually limited to federal cases involving public institutions), a court may order a hospital to appoint or reappoint a physician or at least to grant a hearing or other procedural safeguards during the credentialing process.

Another remedy is monetary damages—compensatory or punitive. Compensatory (or civil) damages may be justified if the court finds that the hospital or its medical staff interfered with the physician's right to practice his or her profession, or that the denial of privileges was part of a conspiracy to violate the applicant's civil rights. Such damages must be proven by the physician, based on (1) his or her inability to admit patients to the hospital, (2) the denial of privileges at other hospitals due to the bad publicity generated by this adverse decision, (3) the physician's loss of patients and/or income because of the denial, or (4) the loss of the physician's professional standing or reputation in the community.

Punitive damages are unlikely to be imposed except when the denial of privileges was the result of legally willful, wanton conduct that the court seeks to prevent in the future by making an example of the defendants.

Any of these remedies may be sought by a group or even an entire class of physicians or nonphysician medical personnel. A class action may be brought in which the allegation concerns discriminatory exclusion of minorities, osteopathic physicians, dentists, nurse practitioners, physician assistants, chiropractors, podiatrists, or others.

GUIDELINES FOR HOSPITAL AND MEDICAL STAFF CREDENTIALING
Hospital and medical staff bylaws

There are many key people primarily responsible for staff privileges decisions. These department chairs and members of the medical executive and credentials committees must be well versed in the procedural and substantive safeguards provided to physicians by law and by the hospital and medical staff bylaws, rules, and regulations.

In determining whether to appoint or reappoint a physician, the decision-makers should identify the specific reason or reasons for restricting staff privileges. The medical executive and credentialing committee should specify as many reasonable grounds for denial as possible and, whenever appropriate or relevant, should reference these grounds to medical staff bylaw provisions.

Grounds for denial or limitation of privileges should be adequately documented. They must be reasonably related to a legitimate purpose or purposes, preferably in furtherance of the hospital's overall mission. Moreover, the hospital, through its medical staff and executive committee, should be sure that its actions demonstrate that it applies these grounds in a nondiscriminatory fashion, using principles of fair play and due process as established in its hospital and medical staff bylaws.

Specific measures to minimize liability

There are other more specific measures a hospital can and should take to minimize its potential liability exposure in credentialing matters.

First, the hospital must ensure that it complies with the various statutes, regulations, and informal requirements governing the conduct of the hospital and its medical staff. This crucial goal should be achieved by drafting the hospital and medical staff bylaws carefully and clearly in accordance with the guidelines of the state department of health, the JCAHO, and the Department of Health and Human Services. Further, if the hospital accepts Medicaid patients, its bylaws should comply with the guidelines of the state department of public welfare. Of particular importance, the medical staff bylaws must comply with state department of health regulations and JCAHO guidelines regarding the classification and delineation of privileges. They should provide mechanisms for review of decisions affecting clinical privileges including guarantees that physicians may be heard at each step of the process. Even when the medical staff sets out to adopt bylaws that are as straightforward as possible, it should ensure that credentialing and hearing procedures are fully and clearly set forth and followed.

Second, the hospital should implement measures during the application and reapplication process that will reduce the likelihood that a rejected physician will have a basis for subsequent legal action. For example, during the initial evaluation or reevaluation of a physician, an interview between the physician and the chairman of the department of service is advisable. This interview should be more than cursory; it should be designed to determine the extent of the physician's commitment to the hospital and to identify any problems that might arise during the credentialing process.

The hospital should verify the applicant's credentials and solicit written recommendations. Effective September 1, 1990, the facility must also query the National Practitioner Data Bank to check for reports of privilege actions or malpractice settlements on the applicant. For physicians just out of training, professors and program directors should be asked to submit evaluations. The hospital should specify that it will use the comments to assist in evaluating the physician's suitability for clinical privileges in the hospital, and may communicate the substance of the comments to the physician. After it has cleared this with the commentators, it should scrutinize all solicited and unsolicited information for bias.

Third, the hospital should notify in writing all physicians whose requested privileges are denied or restricted. The notice should sufficiently detail the reasons, supported by adequate documentation. The decision should be communicated as being irrevocable and mandated by an interrelated combination of factors, rather than because of one or another specific reasons. This reduces the likelihood that the applicant will attempt to challenge the decision by challenging one of its bases. The hospital must scrupulously avoid irrelevant or potentially prejudicial considerations (such as "the hospital already has enough female obstetricians"). Physicians involved in the decision-making process for a potential competitor may be advised to recuse themselves or to abstain in the voting process. It should base its decision primarily on its need to maintain high-quality medical care. The hospital must communicate the reasons to the physician with appropriately chosen language. Hospital counsel may assist in this drafting.

Fourth, the hospital should maintain thorough documentation throughout the evaluation period. This provides protection to the hospital, medical staff, and individual members of the credentials and executive committee in the event of subsequent litigation by rejected physicians. The hospital, through its medical staff and various committees, should also take steps to enable applicants to withdraw gracefully prior to a formal denial of privileges, if that would be the likely outcome of a full review.

Minimizing due process claims

Procedural due process. Hospitals should satisfy procedural safeguards during the credentialing process to avoid claims by rejected physicians that they were not treated fairly or had an inadequate opportunity to be heard. At a minimum, the hospital should provide timely notice to physicians concerning the restriction of privileges, or of adverse decisions by the credentialing or executive committee or the governing body. Additional safeguards may include:

1. Independent legal counsel for the physician during the formal hearing process (although this may not extend to representation during the hearing itself)
2. Liberal discovery by the physician and his or her attorney before formal hearing
3. The right to cross-examine evaluators
4. Right of appeal to the governing board
5. Notification in writing of all adverse decisions and the reasons for them.

Substantive due process. Courts have recognized that there are many permissible justifications for denying or restricting clinical privileges. One such justification is the

physician's inability to meet the legitimate eligibility requirements specified in the bylaws. These eligibility requirements may relate to the physician's education, the length or nature of the physician's residency, the amount or nature of the physician's professional liability insurance coverage, or other specifics regarding the physician's training, experience or competence, ethical practice, or adherence to professional standards practiced. Another legitimate reason for denying or restricting privileges is the perceived inability of the physician to make a full-time or otherwise adequate commitment to the responsibilities expected of staff members. This inability may be due to the physician's conflicting commitments at other hospitals, or simply because the physician does not choose to commit to the hospital's operational and administrative needs. If the physician would be a particular asset to the staff, however, the hospital may wish to extend to him or her courtesy or consulting privileges. It is similarly appropriate to deny clinical privileges to a physician who fails to meet any other requirements imposed by the hospital or medical staff bylaws, such as the failure to submit the necessary references or to attend a sufficient number of meetings or pay dues.

As a final example, the hospital may base its denial on "interaction considerations." These may include the physician's poor patient relations, his or her uncooperative or disruptive behavior, or any similar perceived inability to contribute to the supportive atmosphere of trust and cooperation essential to the successful administration of the hospital and the delivery of high-quality health care.

Many other substantive criteria have been legitimately used by hospitals to justify restrictions or denials of clinical privileges. Some criteria, however, may have anticompetitive overtones. In the current procompetitive health care climate, these criteria should be evaluated carefully before being used as a basis for justifying the restrictions of a physician's clinical privileges, regardless of their legitimacy. Some of these suspect criteria may include, under appropriate circumstances, the services in the department, the lack of need for the physician's specific services, or any other alleged overburdening of the hospital's facilities.

MEDICAL STAFF PEER REVIEW

On May 17, 1988, the U.S. Supreme Court decided one of the most important cases affecting the medical staff peer review process in this century. In *Patrick v. Burget*,[61] the Court held that where medical staff peer review was not actively administered or supervised by the state, physicians sitting on peer review committees were not entitled to absolute immunity from federal antitrust actions, if their actions to exclude other physicians from staff membership were for anticompetitive or other reasons not directly related to improving the overall quality of care.

The *Patrick* decision established constraints on physician peer review, the reasons for excluding physicians from medical staffs, and the procedures employed in achieving this. Following *Patrick,* physicians may not be excluded primarily for economic, as opposed to quality of care, considerations. Moreover, to escape federal antitrust liability, the peer review must allow physicians undergoing evaluation full fair hearing protection to ensure adequate procedural due process. A number of approaches can be employed by medical staff physicians and their hospitals to limit their federal antitrust liability. Specifically, some of these include (but are not limited to) the following:

- Rewrite medical staff bylaws to ensure that all requisite procedural due process safeguards protecting the evaluated physician are in place and are enforced fairly.
- Have each medical staff peer review member establish his or her freedom from economic conflicts of interest before making recommendations that could adversely affect the staff privileges of another potentially competing physician.
- Have physician peer reviewers subject their own requests for continuing staff membership and clinical privileges to review bodies constituted by professionals not sitting on the same committees or departments that are chaired by the physician being evaluated to avoid possible claims of undue influence.
- Have as chairs of credentialing committees and other sensitive medical care review committees, salaried physician executives who are not dependent on referrals from physicians being evaluated.

As instructed by the U.S. Supreme Court, if physician peer reviewers are still not satisfied with the protections afforded by the *Patrick* decision, they may look to the Congress—specifically to the protections from federal antitrust immunity following from compliance with the Health Care Quality Improvement Act of 1986.[62]

The Health Care Quality Improvement Act of 1986

In an attempt to minimize the problem of unqualified physicians hopping from state to state and to improve the process of physician credentialing in general, the Congress, on November 14, 1986, passed the Health Care Quality Improvement Act. This act, in conjunction with the Medicare and Medicaid Patient Protection Act of 1987 and the Social Security Amendments of 1987, created a National Practitioner Data Bank, which will collect, store, and release information on the nation's 6 million health care practitioners, including:

- The details of any professional liability actions filed against them following the implementation of the bank
- The circumstances behind any licensure restrictions
- Whether or not they have had their staff or clinical privileges restricted for a period of more than 30 days at any hospital or other health care entity
- The facts behind any professional society membership loss or restriction.

Hospitals and other health care entities must access this information concerning all physicians and nonphysician health care practitioners whenever these persons are subject to credentialing or recredentialing. Failure to do so will result in the hospital or health care entity losing the act's limited federal antitrust immunity provisions. In any corporate liability or similar action it will be presumed that the hospital or other health care entity has knowledge of these practitioners' credentials (or relative lack thereof).

- The hospital must also request information from the clearinghouse routinely, every 2 years, concerning all licensed health care practitioners with medical staff membership or clinical privileges at the hospital.
- The act allows the Secretary by regulation to provide for disclosure of clearinghouse information affecting a particular physician or health care practitioner, to that person.
- Procedures would also be established for disputing the accuracy of such information.
- The act enables parties involved in medical malpractice actions, including plaintiffs' lawyers, to obtain access to information held by the clearinghouse.

RISK MANAGEMENT PRINCIPLES

One area in which risk management is particularly necessary involves exclusive contracts between hospitals and physicians. They are usually permissible, however, they must have rational reasons to support their existence. Legitimate reasons for exclusive contracts include (but are not limited to):

1. Controlling the efficient administration of a specific type of medical service
2. Limiting the department's size to cope with bed limitations and the hospital's overall mission
3. Maintaining the economics of hospital operations
4. Optimizing the effective use of personnel and technologies by having such controlled by only one physician group
5. Promoting uniform teaching and research methodologies
6. Limiting the utilization of certain technological equipment to those most qualified.

When negotiating exclusive contracts, it is usually unwise to specify too narrowly in the contract language the reasons for entering into the exclusive arrangement. Overspecification might restrict the hospital's maneuverability in the event that the exclusive contract is challenged on specific antitrust grounds. The exclusive contract should delineate reasons for its existence, but it is better to frame these reasons in general terms, such as those specified in the previous paragraph. Similarly, it is better to specify several reasons for the exclusive arrangement rather than merely one reason. Some lawyers feel it may be best simply to use broad language supporting the hospital's goal of optimal medical care within the limitations of the facilities and resources available.

Hospitals and their staff physicians have become more economically interdependent than ever. Both must be continually conscious of how their present health care practice styles may economically affect their ability to continue to provide good quality care in the future. A hospital's ability to compete effectively will soon be related directly to its ability to influence the economic aspects of its physician's medical practice styles. Similarly, a physician's ability to compete effectively will soon depend on his or her ability to gain ready access to the extensive resources of at least one economically viable hospital with state-of-the-art technology and high-quality personnel.

Hospitals have a legal right and duty to maximize the quality of care provided on the one hand, but they also must afford certain safeguards to physicians in the appointment and reappointment process. The key to minimizing litigation is to strike a delicate balance between the private rights of physicians to practice medicine and the public rights of patients to reasonable medical care.

Hospitals (and physicians) face unprecedented economic pressures to compete effectively in a buyer's market. Exclusive arrangements between hospitals and physicians in an attempt to insulate themselves from this free market competition may subject them to the risk of treble damages arising from Sherman Act Section 1 or 2 violations. These arrangements must be reasonable in light of the practices of comparable institutions, local market conditions, and the medical as opposed to the economic motivations behind such agreements.

The practice of medicine in America is in the midst of an unprecedented economic transformation. This metamorphosis will carry into the next century. The traditional providers, including in-patient hospitals and fee-for-service private practitioners, must take the lead to respond to this changing environment. These providers have the unique skills and resources that permit them to compete effectively with virtually any new alternative health care delivery system, without compromising the quality of care or the integrity of the medical profession.

HOSPITAL PRIVILEGES AND DUE PROCESS*

Due to the increasing number of practicing physicians[63] and expanding theories of liability against hospitals based upon the granting of privileges[64] or the failure to restrict or revoke privileges,[65] there are now a significant number of judicial decisions dealing with the entire privileging process. This article will discuss the legal issues involved with special emphasis on the due process rights that must be accorded to a physician when his or her[66] privileges are denied, reduced, or revoked.

The nature of a physician's interest in hospital privileges

For the great majority of physicians the use of hospital facilities is necessary for the pursuit of their profession.[67] Although a physician does not have a constitutional right to practice medicine in a hospital,[68] the obtaining of a medical degree and a license to practice medicine does give him a property interest which is given certain constitutional protection. In *Anton v. San Antonio Community Hospital,*[69] the court described this interest as follows: "...the essential nature of a qualified physician's right to use the facilities of the hospital is a property interest which directly relates to the pursuit of his livelihood."[70] The court in *Unterhiner v. Desert Hospital District of Palm Springs*[71] stated: "A doctor who has been licensed by the state to practice medicine has a vested right to practice his profession and it cannot be said that there are no elements of a right to be admitted to a hospital."[72] Since the states and their subdivisions are prohibited by the United States Constitution from depriving any person of property without due process of law,[73] a hospital must afford a physician substantive and procedural due process when it acts with regard to his hospital privileges.[74]

Private versus public hospitals. Numerous decisions have dealt with the distinction between private and public hospitals.[75] When a public hospital is involved there is no question that the hospital is acting as an agency of the state.[76] In cases involving a private hospital there usually must be a finding that the hospital's actions constituted state action or were done under color of state law.[77] This requirement of state action has been found where the hospital receives substantial federal or state funds,[78] licensing by the state,[79] or even contributions from the public during the hospital's annual fund drive.[80] Some courts have chosen to focus on the responsibilities of the hospital rather than the rights of the physicians and have held that a private hospital occupies a fiduciary trust relationship between itself, the medical staff and the public and the actions of the hospital are,

---

*From Hagerman, 13 *LAMP* 51 (July 1985).

therefore, subject to judicial review.[81] In cases involving judicial review of hospital decisions regarding privileges, California has done away with the distinction between private and public hospitals altogether.[82]

Although there are a significant number of federal court decisions which hold that denial of privileges by a private health care provider is not sufficiently regulated or controlled by the state to invoke federal jurisdiction,[83] it is now becoming clear that no matter whether the hospital concerned is public or private, a physician has a federally protected right to due process[84] and the right to be free from arbitrary action on the part of a hospital.[85]

Initial privileges versus existing privileges. The majority of decided cases dealing with hospital privileges involve a physician whose previously granted privileges are revoked or reduced.[86] Some cases, however, deal with the physician's rights upon his initial application for privileges.[87] It has been pointed out that a physician who has had privileges has more of a "vested" interest than one who is newly applying.[88] In California the extent and nature of judicial review depends upon whether the decision of the hospital involved an initial application or existing privileges. In cases involving existing privileges the court is to make an independent judgment review in order to determine whether the decision of the hospital is supported by the weight of the evidence. In cases involving new applications the court is to make a substantial evidence review in order to determine whether the decision of the hospital is supported by substantial evidence in light of the whole record.[89]

Even though a doctor applying for new privileges may have less of a vested interest than one who has already been granted privileges, he must be afforded due process which is adequate to safeguard his interest in pursuing his profession and the hospital cannot act arbitrarily or discriminatorily with regard to his application.[90]

The physician's due process rights in hospital proceedings

Hospital proceedings which affect a physician's privileges usually occur on four different levels. At the first level there may be a complaint brought against a physician who already has privileges by a patient, another physician, the administrator of the hospital or even the board of directors.[91] At the second level a committee of the hospital, usually the credentials committee when a new application for privileges is involved, or the executive committee of the medical staff where existing privileges are involved, conducts an inquiry into whether the subject physician's privileges should be granted, denied, restricted, or revoked. No reported cases have been found which give the physician any due process rights at these two levels. Once a decision has been made by a committee or other authority within the hospital which may adversely affect the physician's present or requested privileges, the physician should be given the following due process rights.

Notification of the adverse recommendation. Once an adverse recommendation has been made which, if approved by higher authority, will result in denial, revocation or restriction of a physician's privileges, the physician must be notified and informed of his right to request a hearing before a panel established to review his privileges or application for privileges.[92]

Written notice of the charges. If the physician requests a hearing he must be given written notice of the charges that will be presented against him at the hearing.[93] The charges must be sufficiently specific to give the physician adequate notice of the nature of the charges.[94] A few courts have noted with apparent approval the practice of providing the physician with the hospital chart numbers of those cases which substantiate the charges against him.[95] While this may be sufficient in view of the reasonable assumption that the physician can read his own charts, one court has said that the charges must state "in reasonable fullness the nature of the criticism in each case."[96]

Adequate time to prepare a defense. After the physician has been advised of the charges against him, he must be given adequate time to prepare his defense.[97] The time interval between notification and the hearing date will necessarily vary somewhat according to the circumstances and the extent and complexity of the charges that the physician must defend against.

Pre-hearing discovery. The physician or his attorney sometimes wishes to conduct discovery prior to the hearing before the panel. Courts have reached different decisions on this issue depending on the nature of the discovery sought. In *Garrow v. Elizabeth General Hospital*,[98] the court held that the information that was relied upon in making the adverse recommendation should be made available to the subject physician prior to the hearing so as to enable him to make adequate preparations for his defense. Similarly, in *Suckle v. Madison General Hospital*,[99] the court held that the physician had a right to access all relevant hospital and medical records during the period in which he was preparing a response to the charges. In cases where the discovery sought is more formal in nature, however, it has not been allowed.[100] This is in keeping with the often made statement that in hospital due process proceedings the doctor is "not entitled to a full blown judicial trial."[101] In *Woodbury v. McKinnon*,[102] the physician involved was not allowed to conduct discovery by means of depositions and interrogatories to obtain evidence to support his contention that other members of the medical staff were not as good as he was.

A hearing panel composed of impartial, fair-minded doctors. The panel charged with the responsibility of giving the physician his due process hearing must be composed of physicians who are impartial and fair minded.[103] If any physician on the panel actively participated in the investigation of the subject physician or made the original adverse recommendation he will be subject to challenge on the grounds of bias or lack of impartiality.[104] In other words, if the functions of investigator, prosecutor and judge are being carried out by the same person a fair hearing will be presumed to be unavailable and actual bias need not be shown.[105] Courts have recognized, however, that prior involvement by a hearing panel member on some other level will not disqualify that person from sitting on the panel if the involvement was not substantial and did not bring about the adverse recommendation under review.[106] The following additional factors have been identified as having a high probability of destroying impartiality: (1) the panel member has a direct pecuniary interest in the outcome; (2) the member has been personally involved in a dispute with the subject doctor or has been the target of his criticism; or (3) the panel member is embroiled in other matters involving the physician whose rights he is determining.[107] As stated in *Applebaum v. Board of Directors*[108]: "Biased decision makers are constitutionally impermissible and even the probability of unfairness is to be avoided." If the hospital is a small one and the matter has been particularly vitriolic and disruptive, consideration should be given to having physicians from outside the immediate hospital area sit on the hearing panel. It has been said, however, that the physician under review is "not entitled to a panel made up of outsiders or of doctors who had never heard of the case and who knew nothing about the facts of it or what they supposed the facts to be."[109]

In some instances the physician or his attorney has sought to *voir dire* the panel members in order to discover any bias or lack of impartiality. In *Duffield v. Charleston Area Medical Center, Inc.,*[110] the subject physician asked for and received permission to examine all members of the panel before the hearing began. The trial court in *Hackethal v. California Medical Association and San Bernadino County Medical Society,*[111] concluded that the subject physician's *voir dire* of the panel members was unduly restricted and this was found to be a denial of procedural due process. Because a physician has a vital interest in having a fair and impartial panel it appears that he should have a reasonable opportunity to question the panel regarding any matters that may bear upon their objectivity or lack thereof.

Appearance before the panel. The right to personally appear before the decision-making panel and be heard has been held to be essential.[112] As stated in *Grannis v.*

Ordean[113]: "The fundamental requisite of due process of law is the opportunity to be heard." The opportunity to speak on one's behalf must also be given at a time when it will be effective. As the Court said in *Lew v. Kona Hospital,*[114] "The fundamental requirement of due process is the opportunity to be heard at a meaningful time and in a meaningful manner." Thus, in a case where all the proceedings leading up to a letter of termination of privileges were done in secret and without any opportunity to be heard it was found that the doctor had not received due process and his privileges were reinstated.[115]

Assistance of legal counsel during hearing. To date only one jurisdiction has recognized the right of a physician to have his legal counsel assist him in a hospital due process hearing. In *Garrow v. Elizabeth General Hospital,*[116] the Supreme Court of New Jersey examined the issue and found that in view of the physician's substantial interest in such proceedings, the ability of an attorney to marshall the evidence, counter adverse testimony and present argument on the doctor's behalf tipped the balance in favor of allowing the physician the right to an attorney at mandated hospital hearings.[117] The court also pointed out that the attorney would be subject to the control of the person in charge of the hearings.[118] A few courts have held that it should be within the discretion of the hearing panel as to whether legal counsel may attend the hearing and actively participate.[119] Other courts have noted the participation of counsel for the physician without indicating whether the allowance of counsel in such proceedings is required in order to satisfy due process.[120]

Cross-examination of witnesses. Although some courts have held that a physician is not constitutionally entitled to cross-examine witnesses who testify against him at the hearing,[121] the better rule clearly appears to be that a physician does have the right to confront and cross-examine any witnesses who appear and testify against him.[122] Due process means fair procedure[123] and to allow a witness to testify against the physician without being subject to cross-examination would certainly seem to violate the rules of fair play.

Presentation of witnesses and evidence in defense. The right of a physician to present witnesses and evidence in his own behalf has been clearly recognized.[124] This is an integral part of fundamental fairness which has been equated with procedural due process.[125]

Transcript of panel hearing. It is advisable to have an accurate record made of the due process hearing so that any objections raised by the subject physician can be reviewed in a hospital appellate review of the panel's decision.[126] In addition, without an accurate record it may be difficult for a court to determine whether the physician was accorded due process at the hearing.

Written decision from panel. The decision of the panel should be written so that it can provide a record for hospital and judicial review.[127] A copy should be given to the physician.[128] In reaching its decision the panel must not rely on *ex parte* communications which were not made known to the doctor in question and the decision must be based upon evidence that was presented at the hearing and to which the physician had an opportunity to respond.[129] The decision of the panel should be based on substantial evidence.[130]

The fourth level of hospital proceedings concerning a physician's privileges is appellate review of the decision of the hearing panel and a final decision by the governing authority. Hospital bylaws normally provide a mechanism whereby the physician can obtain review of the panel decision by an appellate review committee.[131] The physician is usually allowed to submit a written statement of his position to the committee, but the right to make an oral statement is within the discretion of the appellate review body.[132] New or additional evidence not raised during the due process hearing nor otherwise reflected in the record will be allowed to be introduced at the appellate review level only under unusual circumstances.[133] After the appellate review committee issues its decision the final decision must be made by the highest governing authority of the hospital. The final hospital decision is transmitted to the physician concerned and the hospital proceedings are then complete.[134]

The scope of judicial review of hospital decisions

It is now well established that courts have jurisdiction to review hospital decisions which adversely affect a physician's privileges.[135] In addition to jurisdiction based upon alleged violations of rights guaranteed by the Fifth and Fourteenth Amendments, federal courts often find jurisdiction under 42 U.S.C. § 1983[136] in conjunction with 28 U.S.C. § 1343(3).[137] However, the extent of judicial review in such cases is limited.[138] If the Court finds that the physician was afforded due process in the hospital proceedings[139] and the hospital neither violated its bylaws[140] nor acted in an arbitrary or capricious manner,[141] the decision of the hospital will be upheld. This limited review is necessitated by the court's lack of medical expertise as was pointed out in *Laje v. R.E. Thomason General Hospital*:

Judicial intervention must be limited to an assessment of those factors which are within the court's expertise to review. For this reason, our cases have gone no further than to require that the procedures employed by the hospital are fair, that the standards set by the hospital are reasonable, and that they have been applied without arbitrariness and capriciousness.[142]

It has also been said that "The decision of a hospital's governing body concerning the granting of hospital privileges is to be accorded great deference."[143] Therefore, once the court has determined that the decision of the hospital is "supported by substantial evidence and was made using proper criteria, after a satisfactory hearing, on a rational basis, and without irrelevant, discriminatory and arbitrary influences, the work of the court [comes] to an end."[144]

Conclusion

In light of current judicial concepts of due process it appears that the distinction between public and private hospitals will continue to lose viability where physicians' hospital privileges are concerned. It is also expected that more jurisdictions will follow New Jersey in allowing the physician to be represented by counsel at the due process hearing. Because the panel hearing is by far the most important proceeding for the physician, this seems both sensible and fair.

Although a physician applying for privileges may be seen as having less of a vested interest than one who has previously enjoyed them, it is apparent that both are equally entitled to due process. In every case the hospital must be guided by fundamental fairness; keep in mind the words of the U.S. Supreme Court in *Hannah v. Larche*[145]: "Due process is an elusive concept. Its exact boundaries are undefinable, and its content varies according to specific factual contexts."

HOSPITAL-REQUIRED MALPRACTICE INSURANCE*

The increased number of suits against health care providers, the increased number of health care providers in each suit, and the increased amount of awards and settlements has created unrest, tension, and distrust between hospitals and their medical staff. Physicians have a decerebrate posturing response to being named in a malpractice suit. They have a lesser "knee jerk" response when having to pay malpractice insurance premiums. Hospitals are developing the same responses due to escalating malpractice premiums and claims. Their corporate assets are being threatened. Their costs continue to escalate. The inevitable government regulation that results has added to their problems. When the hospital requires insurance for staff privileges, the effect is similar to adding sodium to water. The resulting explosion not only damages the hospital and its medical staff, but also involves the legal community, the state and federal legislature, and ultimately, as always, the public.

The National Association of Insurance Companies' 1975-1978 study showed over 70% of paid claims

*From Goebert, 13 *LAMP* 1 (Nov. 1985).

are a result of physician activity occurring in the hospital.[146]

Hospitals have increasing legal "corporate responsibility" for physician activities. The trustees of hospitals have "fiduciary responsibility" to maintain corporate assets. Joint and several liability makes hospitals the "deep pocket" for uninsured or poorly insured physician staff members.

Physicians have not only patient care requirements, but also hospital functions such as teaching, emergency care, emergency coverage, and committee functioning, especially in credentialing and policy making. The line between physician patient care activity and hospital patient care activity becomes more and more indistinct. Hospitals and their physician staff look to each other for support but once sued, look to each other for money. There is a major problem which is legally frequently solved by hospitals paying more than their fare share to the injured patient.

Is mandatory fiscal responsibility as a requirement for staff privileges a viable answer? In some states, hospitals require this and in some states the requirement is linked with licensure. We shall discuss what happens with the two approaches. In the mid-1970s in response to the "malpractice crisis," Alaska, Hawaii, Idaho, Kansas, Kentucky, North Dakota, and Pennsylvania all required physicians to carry professional liability insurance as a condition of obtaining and maintaining licensure. In Hawaii, the Hawaii Medical Association sought to enjoin the state from enforcing the malpractice insurance requirement against them by a preliminary injunction.[147] This suit was dismissed but the licensing board did not enforce the requirement so the next year Hawaii legislatively deleted it. Also, Alaska repealed the requirement in 1978.[148] Now individual hospitals are reacting by requiring financial responsibility as a condition for staff privileges.

Kentucky and North Dakota ruled the requirement unconstitutional. Kentucky found the statute a violation of due process.[149] The legislature had arbitrarily imposed and restricted the practice of medicine, mainly because all health care providers were being considered inherently negligent or financially irresponsible. There had not been a legislative finding that such was the case. North Dakota, on the other hand, found their entire statutory malpractice changes to be unconstitutional.[150] When addressing the mandatory insurance provision, the court specifically withheld a final decision but did have serious doubts as to the constitutionality of requiring malpractice insurance for all physicians without regard to their ability to pay when the law was silent on the effect of some physicians' inability to pay the premiums.

On the other hand, Pennsylvania, Idaho, and Kansas

ruled in favor of the law. Pennsylvania stated there existed a rational relationship with the requiring of insurance and public interest in assuring compensability.[151] There is no unconstitutional denial of equal protection or a denial to pursue one's occupation. Idaho remanded the malpractice statutes back to the lower courts for further investigation, but they had no problem stating that protection to patients who may be injured as a result of medical malpractice is in the public welfare and compulsory insurance is constitutional.[152] The Kansas Supreme Court also found their statute constitutional.

These cases are important because they give the legal arguments both pro and con for allowing a state to specifically regulate the medical profession by requiring insurance. They address the right to engage in a lawful occupation, the police power of the state, and substantive due process of individuals guaranteed by the constitution. Some courts only required a rational reason for the legislature to require insurance. Other states require a more serious constitutional scrutiny than the rational basis analysis, since the regulation is not truly related to competence and does put some burden on the individual's right to engage in a lawful profession. Close scrutiny will balance the respective interest of both the physician and the public.[153]

Can hospitals require malpractice insurance as a condition of privileges? Yes, but in the absence of a statute, state hospitals would have the same type of scrutiny placed on them as state statutes had in the paragraphs above. In an earlier case, a California hospital which required malpractice insurance as a condition of admission was challenged successfully. The rule was arbitrary and not related to the state's regulation of physicians.[154] Following this case, the California legislature passed a law allowing hospitals to require malpractice insurance and this was found constitutional.[155] In 1977 a survey of U.S. community hospitals showed that out of 4478 hospitals, 26.4% require physicians to have a minimum amount of malpractice insurance.[156]

When private hospitals require malpractice insurance for staff privileges, physicians present a number of arguments.[157] First is "state action" because the private hospital is receiving either state and/or federal funds and therefore the court has jurisdiction to determine if an impermissible imposition infringed on constitutional rights of the physicians' civil rights.[158] The physicians will allege a breach of contract action since hospital privileges were given for a longer length of time. The hospital is taking away privileges without a showing that the physician is unqualified or unskilled. Many of the physicians have been members of the hospital committees and have been on the teaching staffs of universities, and all have state licensure. Some arguments show a violation of the antitrust provisions of the Sherman Act if any of the deciding physicians involved with denying privileges are in competition with the doctor being restricted.[159] A number of cases have addressed the question of a hospital acting under the color of state law. These have found that the specific activity complained of by the physician being denied privileges must be related to the way that the state is acting on the private hospital. There must be a nexus between state action and denial of privileges. These cases show that the granting of funds from Hill-Burton monies, Medicaid, Medicare payments, training of residents from state institutional programs, use of tax-free bonds, hospital licensure and inspection by the state, and reporting of privileges revocations to a state board all are state actions or federal actions but none have a required nexus. The restricted physician must show that those state actions have something to do with a denial of privileges when the physician does not have insurance.[160-162] The due process hearings required in civil right actions under U.S.C. §§ 1983 have not been upheld, but state courts have said that hospitals need to show or need to give due process to physicians prior to a revocation of privileges.[163] The test in these cases is whether or not a hospital acts arbitrarily and capriciously or denies the physician due process. Physicians have also argued that they are unable to afford the insurance, that they do not have a big enough practice, they have an indigent patient population in their practice, and therefore the public will suffer.[164-166]

Hospitals argue, on the other hand, that this is not arbitrary and capricious. It is rational policy supported by good fiscal management and preservation of the hospital resources.[167] The requirement is not excessively burdensome and can be met by providing insurance or fiscal responsibility. The hospital must be able to show that it has done everything necessary to obtain facts supporting the above. Meetings with concerned individuals should have been held; a review by the medical staff executive committee; surveys of the doctors, letters to other hospitals, letters to insurance people finding out the costs and alternatives, and attempts at legislative tort reform, are all things that would be helpful to a hospital initiating these actions.

The courts have supported and allowed the hospitals to initiate such action. Florida,[168] Arizona,[169] Louisiana,[170] and Indiana[171] have all heard arguments both pro and con and ruled in favor of the hospital and against the restricted doctor as long as procedural due process and prior notice was afforded to the doctor. Doctors scream but the courts have not listened.[172,173]

Courts have addressed the California legislative policy of allowing a hospital to require malpractice insurance, and stated that the interests of society that are served by such insurance requirement is not so arbitrary that it would be considered unreasonable. The amount of insurance established by the hospital and the requirement that the insurance company must be admitted to do business in California were reasonable.[174]

The final argument in favor of this policy is that the real reason for such a policy is the requirement that the hospital pay its fair share of liability and the physician pay his/her fair share of liability. In *Holmes,* the situation is summarized as follows:

We cannot ignore the realities of modern procedural practice. If a patient is injured while in the hospital regardless of who is at fault, the hospital will almost always be joined as a codefendant. Despite the outcome of such an action, the hospital must expend valuable financial resources in its own defense, and will, if innocent of wrongdoing, be more likely to recover its expenses from the tortfeasor physician if that physician is insured. If, indeed, some conscientious lawyer decides not to include the hospital in an action where the finger of negligence points directly and solely to the doctor, we can be certain it will only be because the physician does indeed have malpractice insurance.[175]

The hospital has the right to take reasonable measures to protect itself and the patient it serves. We cannot say, as a matter of law, that the hospital board's attention to its medical staff's malpractice insurance is unlawful, arbitrary, or capricious. As a practical matter, we cannot say it is irrational or unreasonable. In *Pollak,* the court states:

We find the plaintiff (physician) has no liberty or property interest sufficient to invoke the due process requirements of the Fourteenth Amendment. While the right to practice an occupation is a liberty interest protected by the Fourteenth Amendment, . . . plaintiff is not precluded from exercising that right by the insurance requirements in order to continue his membership on the hospital staff. . . . Requiring its staff physicians to carry insurance and to submit proof to the hospital of that fact is surely a reasonable exercise of financial responsibility on the part of the hospital.[176]

Basically, the hospital has three alternatives regarding malpractice insurance:

1. To utilize the information regarding the physician's malpractice as one of the criteria used to decide upon appointment or reappointment
2. To require malpractice coverage as a condition of appointment or reappointment
3. To take no policy position

The first two of these are legally permitted. The last does not solve the problem. The hospital can avoid much internal stress by recognizing that this problem is a shared or joint problem with the medical staff. The hospital should involve the staff in trying to solve the problem. Alternatives can be searched for and harmony fostered.

END NOTES

1. *Darling v. Charleston Community Hosp.,* 200 N.E. 2d 149 (Ill. Sup. Ct. 1965); *Elam v. College Park Hosp.,* 183 Cal. Rptr. 156 (1982); *Corletto v. Shore Memorial Hosp.,* 350 A. 2d 534 (N.J. Sup. Ct. 1975).
2. D. M. Eddy, *Clinical Decision Making: From Theory to Practice — The Challenge,* 1 JAMA 287-90 (1990).
3. *E.g., Wall v. Stout,* 310 N.C. 184, 192, 311 S.E. 2d 571 (1984); *see also Physicians, Surgeons, Etc.,* 61 Am. Jur. 2d §167, 298-99 (1981).
4. 42 U.S.C. § 11111 *et seq.*
5. *Brownsville Medical Center v. Garcia,* 704 S.W.2d 68 (Tex. App. Corpus Christi 1985).
6. *Smith v. Baptist Memorial Hosp. System,* 720 S.W.2d 618 (Tex. App. San Antonio 1986, *writ ref. n.r.e.*).
7. *Corletto, supra* note 1.
8. *Accreditation Manual for Hospitals,* Standard M.S. 6 *et seq* (JCAHO, Chicago, Ill. 1990).
9. *Supra* note 4.
10. *McDonald v. Massachusetts General Hosp.,* 120 Mass. 432, 21 A. 529 (1876).
11. *Schloendorff v. New York Hosp.,* 211 N.Y. 125, 105 N.E. 92 (1914).
12. *Id.* at 132 and 94.
13. Necolauff v. Genessee Hosp., 296 N.Y.S. 936, 73 N.E.2d 117 (1947).
14. *Berg v. N.Y. Society for the Relief of the Ruptured and Crippled,* 154 N.Y.S. 455, 456 (1956).
15. *Bing v. Thunig,* 2 N.Y.2d 656, 143 N.E.2d 3 (1957).
16. *Cf. generally,* Joint Commission on Accreditation of Healthcare Organizations, *Accreditation Manual for Hospitals,* Medical Staff Section.
17. *Johnson v. Misericordia County Hosp.,* 99 Wis. 2d 708, 301 N.W.2d 156 (1981), *aff'd,* 99 Wis. 2d 78, 301 N.W.2d 156 (1981).
18. *Weiss v. York Hosp.,* 745 F.2d 786 (1984).
19. *Tonsic v. Wagner,* 329 A.2d 497 (1974).
20. *McConnell v. Williams,* 361 Pa. 355, 65 A.2d 243 (1949).
21. *Capan v. Divine Providence Hosp.,* 410 A.2d 1282 (Pa. Super. Ct. 1979).
22. *People v. Flushing Hosp. and Medical Center,* 471 N.Y.S.2d 745, (N.Y. Cir. Ct. 1983), where the hospital was charged with a misdemeanor when it refused emergency care because the hospital was full; *People ex rel. M.B.,* 312 N.W.2d 714 (S.D. 1981), where the South Dakota Supreme Court ruled that a lower court exceeded its jurisdiction by ordering an admission when no space was available; *contra, see Pierce County Office of Involuntary Commitment v. Western State Hosp.,* 97 Wash. 2d 264, 644 P.2d 131 (1982), where the Washington Supreme Court interpreted a state mental health statute to require admission of all patients who presented to the hospital, despite a lack of space.
23. *See, e.g., Fabian v. Matzko,* 236 Pa. Super. 267, 344 A.2d 569 (1975).
24. *Wilmington General Hosp. v. Manlove,* 54 Del. 15, 174 A.2d 135 (1961).
25. *Stanturf v. Sipes,* 447 S.W.2d 558 (Mo. 1969).
26. *Stanturf, supra* note 25, at 562.
27. Restatement (Second) of Agency §220 (1958).
28. *See, e.g., Smith v. St. Francis Hosp.,* 676 P.2d 279 (Okla. App. 1983).
29. *Thomas v. Corso,* 265 Md. 84, 288 A.2d 379 (1972).
30. *Citizens Hosp. Ass'n. v. Schoulin,* 48 Ala. 101, 262 So.2d 303 (1972).
31. *Gizzi v. Texaco, Inc.,* 437 F.2d 308 (3d Cir. 1971).
32. *See* F. Harper, F. James, Jr., and O. Gray, *Law of Torts,* 26.11, 60-94 (2d ed. 1986) for a discussion of the immunity rule and its exception.
33. *Marek v. Professional Health Services, Inc.,* 179 N.J. Super. 433, 437 A.2d 538 (1981).
34. *Jackson v. Power,* 743 P.2d 1346 (Alaska 1987). In a comparison case, *Harding v. Sisters of Providence,* no. 371 (Alaska Oct. 16, 1987), liability was extended to an independent contractor/ radiologist's negligence on the basis of a nondelegable duty owed by the hospital to its patients.
35. W. Prosser and W. Keeton, *Law of Torts* §71 at 511-2 (5th ed. 1984).
36. *Guerro v. Copper Queen Hosp.,* 112 Ariz. 104, 537 P.2d 1329 (1975).
37. 42 U.S.C. §1395dd (Apr. 7, 1986).
38. *Darling v. Charleston Memorial Hosp.,* 33 Ill.2d 326, 211 N.E.2d 253 (1965); *cert. denied* 383 U.S. 946 (1966).
39. *Fiorentino v. Wagner,* 227 N.E.2d. 296 (1967).
40. *Moore v. Board of Trustees of Carson City Hosp.,* 495 P.2d 605 (Nev. 1972).
41. *Mitchell City Hosp. Authority v. Joiner,* 229 Ga. 140, 109 S.E.2d 413 (1972).
42. *Purcell v. Zimbleman,* 18 Ariz. App. 75, 500 P.2d 335 (1972).
43. *Corletto v. Shore Memorial Hospital,* 138 N.J. Super. 302, 350 A.2d 534 (1975).
44. *Hayman v. Galveston,* 273 U.S. 414, 47 S.Ct. 363 (1927).
45. *Porter Memorial Hosp. v. Harvy,* 279 N.E.2d 583 (1972).
46. *Lubin v. Crittenden Hosp. Ass'n.,* 713 F.2d 414 (8th Cir. 1983).
47. *Cardiomedical Assoc. v. Crozier-Chester Med. Ctr.,* 536 F. Supp. 1065 (E.D. Pa. 1982).
48. *Northeast Georgia Radiological Assoc. v. Tidwell,* 670 F.2d 507 (5th Cir. 1982).
49. *Klinge v. Lutheran Charities Ass'n. of St. Louis,* 523 F.2d 56 (8th Cir. 1975).
50. *Silver v. Castle Memorial Hosp.,* 497 P.2d 564, *cert. denied* 409 U.S. 1048, 93 S. Ct. 517 (1972).
51. *Cristhilf v. Annapolis Emergency Hosp. Ass'n., Inc.,* 496 F. 2d 174 (4th Cir. 1974).
52. *Id.*
53. *Garrow v. Elizabeth General Hosp.,* 79 N.J. 549, 401 A.2d 533 (1979).
54. *Klinge, supra* note 49, at 60.
55. *Branch v. Hempstead County Memorial Hosp.,* 539 F. Suppl 908 (W.D. Ark. 1982).
56. California Medical Association-California Hospital Association, *Uniform Code of Hearing and Appeal Procedures* §3(e).
57. *Novosel v. Nationwide Insurance Co.,* 721 F.2d 894 (1983).
58. *Cardiomedical Association, Ltd., v. Crozier-Chester Med. Ctr.,* 721 F.2d 68 (1983).
59. *Jefferson Parish Hosp. District No. 2 v. Hyde, M.D.,* 466 U.S. 2.104 S.Ct. Rptr. 1551 (1984).
60. *Weiss v. York Hosp.,* 745 F.2d 786 (1984).
61. *Patrick v. Burget,* 486 U.S. 94, 900 F.2d 1498 (1988).
62. Health Care Quality Improvement Act of 1986 (Pub. L. 99-660, as amended by Pub. L. 100-93 and 100-177).
63. Tarlov, *Special Report, Shattuck Lecture — The Increasing Supply of Physicians. The Changing Structure of The Health-Services System and The Future Practice of Medicine.* 308 New Eng. J. Med. 1235 (1983).
64. *Johnson v. Misericordia Community Memorial Hosp.,* 99 Wis. 2d 708, 301 N.W.2d 156 (1981); *Annot.* 51 A.L.R.3d 981 (1973).
65. *Purcell, supra* note 42; *Elam v. College Park Hosp.,* 132 Cal. App. 3d 332, 183 Cal. Rptr. 156, *modified,* 133 Cal. App. 3d 94a (1982).
66. Hereinafter "his" will refer to both sexes.

67. *See Falcone v. Middlesex County Medical Society,* 34 N.J. 582, 170 A.2d 791 (1961).

68. *Hayman v. Galveston,* 273 U.S. 414, 47 S.Ct. 363, 71 L.Ed. 714 (1927); *Sosa v. Bd. of Managers of Val Verde Memorial Hosp.,* 437 F.2d 173 (5th Cir. 1971).

69. *Anton v. San Antonio Comm. Hosp.,* 19 Cal. 3d 802, 140 Cal. Rptr. 442, 567 P.2d 1162 (1977).

70. *Id.* at 814, 140 Cal. Rptr. at 454, 567 P.2d at 1174.

71. *Unterthiner v. Desert Hosp. Dist. of Palm Springs,* 33 Cal.3d 285. 188 Cal. Rptr. 590, 656 P.2d 554 (1983).

72. *Id.* at 297, 188 Cal. Rptr. at 598, 656 P.2d at 562.

73. U.S. Constitution amend. V, XIV.

74. *Klinge, supra* note 49; *Christhilf, supra* note 51. *Woodbury v. McKinnon,* 447 F.2d 839 (5th Cir. 1971).

75. *See, e.g., Silver v. Castle Memorial Hosp.,* 53 Haw. 475, 497 P.2d 564, *cert. denied,* 409 U.S. 1048, 93 S.Ct. 517 (1972) and cases cited therein; note, *The Physician's Right to Hospital Staff Membership: The Public-Private Dichotomy,* 485 Wash. U.L.Q. (1966).

76. *Foster v. Mobile County Hosp. Bd.,* 398 F.2d 227 (5th Cir. 1938).

77. *See, e.g., Suckle v. Madison Gen. Hosp.,* 362 F.Supp. 1196 (W.D. Wis 1973), *aff'd,* 499 F.2d 1364 (7th Cir. 1974).

78. *Christhilf, supra* note 51.

79. *Schlein v. Milford Hosp.,* 423 F. Supp. 541 (D. Conn. 1976).

80. *Sussman v. Overlook Hosp. Ass'n.,* 231 A.2d 389, 95 N.J. Super. 418 (1967).

81. *Silver, supra* note 75; *Garrow, supra* note 53; *Greisman v. Newcomb Hosp.,* 40 N.J. 389, 192 A.2d 817 (1963).

82. *Anton, supra* note 69; *Ascherman v. St. Francis Memorial Hosp.,* 45 Cal. App. 3d 507, 119 Cal. Rptr. 507 (1975).

83. *Lubin, supra* note 46; *Cardio Medical Assoc. supra* note 47, and cases cited therein.

84. *Northeast Georgia Radiological Associates v. Tidwell,* 670 F.2d 507 (5th Cir. 1982); *Klinge, supra* note 49.

85. *Citta v. Delaware Valley Hosp.,* 313 F.Supp. 301 (E.D. Pa. 1970); *Avol v. Hawthrone Comm. Hosp. Inc.,* 135 Cal. App. 3d 101, 184 Cal. Rptr. 914 (1982); *Kelly v. St. Vincent Hosp.,* 102 N.M. 201, 692 P.2d 1350 (1984).

86. *See generally* Comment, *Hospital Medical Staff Privileges: Recent Developments in Procedural Due Process Requirements,* 12 Willamette L.J. 137 (1975).

87. *Sosa v. Bd. of Managers of Val Verde Memorial Hosp.,* 437 F.2d 173 (5th Cir. 1971); *Foster v. Mobile County Hosp. Bd.,* 398 F.2d 227 (5th Cir. 1968); *Schlein, supra* note 79; *Sussman v. Overlook Hosp. Ass'n., supra* note 80; *Unterthiner, supra* note 71.

88. *Unterthiner, supra* note 71.

89. *Unterthiner, supra* note 71; *Anton, supra* note 69.

90. *Foster, supra* note 76; *Schlein, supra* note 79; *Sussman, supra* note 80; *Unterthiner, supra* note 71.

91. *Avol, supra* note 85.

92. *Silver, supra* note 75; *see Accreditation Manual for Hospitals,* Standards for Medical Staff, standard Ill, 104 (JCAHO 1983); California Medical Association-California Hospital Association, *Uniform Code of Hearing and Appeal Procedures,* 32 (1972).

93. *Cristhilf, supra* note 51; *Garrow, supra* note 53.

94. *Suckle v. Madison Gen. Hosp.,* 362 F.Supp. 1196 (W.D. Wis. 1973), *aff'd,* 499 F.2d 1364 (7th Cir. 1974); *Silver, supra* note 50. However, specificity that amounts to pleading of evidence is not constitutionally required. *Truly v. Madison Gen. Hosp.,* 673 F.2d 763 (5th Cir. 1982).

95. *Woodbury, supra* note 74; *Branch v. Hempstead County Memorial Hosp.,* 539 F.Supp. 908 (W.D. Ark. 1982); *Anton, supra* note 69.

96. *Suckle, supra* note 94, at 1211.

97. *Crishilf, supra* note 51; *Miller v. Eisenhower Med. Ctr.,* 27 Cal. 3d 614, 166 Cal. Rptr. 826, 614 P.2d 258 (1980); *Silver, supra* note 50.

98. *Garrow, supra* note 53.

99. *Suckle, supra* note 94.

100. *Woodbury, supra* note 74; *Hackethal v. California Med. Ass'n. and San Bernardino County Medical Society,* 138 Cal. App. 3d 435, 187 Cal. Rptr. 811 (1982).

101. *Klinge, supra* note 49, at 60.

102. *Woodbury, supra* note 74.

103. *Klinge, supra* note 49; *Citta, supra* note 85; *Hackethal, supra* note 100; *Applebaum v. Board of Directors,* 104 Cal. App.3d 648, 163 Cal. Rptr. 831 (1980).

104. *E.g., Applebaum, supra* note 103.

105. *Citta, supra* note 85.

106. *Duffield v. Charleston Area Med. Ctr., Inc.* 503 F.2d 512 (4th Cir. 1974); *Hoberman v. Lock Haven Hosp.,* 377 F.Supp. 1178 (M.D. Pa. 1974).

107. *Hackethal, supra* note 100; *Applebaum, supra* note 103.

108. *Applebaum, supra* note 103, at 657, 163 Cal. Rptr., at 840.

109. *Klinge, supra* note 49, at 63.

110. *Duffield, supra* note 106.

111. *Hackethal, supra* note 100.

112. *Christhilf, supra* note 51; *Poe v. Charlotte Memorial Hosp., Inc.,* 374 F. Supp. 1302 (W.D. N.C. 1974).

113. *Grannis v. Ordean,* 234 U.S. 385 at 394, 34 S.Ct. 779 at 783, 58 L.Ed. 1363 at 1369 (1914).

114. *Lew v. Kona Hosp.,* 754 F.2d 1420 at 1424 (9th cir. 1985).

115. *Poe, supra* note 112.

116. *Garrow, supra* note 53.

117. *Id.*

118. *Id.* at 558, A.2d, at 542.

119. *Anton, supra* note 69; *Silver v. Castle Memorial Hosp.,* 53 Haw. 475, 497 P.2d 564, *cert. denied,* 409 U.S. 1048, 93 S. Ct. 517, 34 L.Ed.2d 500 (1972).

120. *Laje v. R.E. Thomason Gen. Hosp.,* 564 F.2d 1159 (5th Cir. 1977); *Citta, supra* note 85; *Miller v. Eisenhower Med. Ctr.,* 27 Cal. 3d 614, 166 Cal. Rptr. 826, 614 P.2d 258 (1980).

121. *Woodbury, supra* note 74; *Kaplan v. Carney,* 404 F.Supp. 161 (E.D. Mo. 1975); *Sussman v. Overlook Hosp. Ass'n,* 95 N.J. Super. 418, 231 A.2d 389 (1967); in *Woodbury* and *Kaplan* no witnesses testified at the hearing.

122. *Cristhilf, supra* note 51; *Branch, supra* note 55; *Poe, supra* note 112; *Hackethal, supra* note 100; *Silver, supra* note 50.

123. *Poe, supra* note 112.

124. *Branch, supra* note 55; *Hackethal, supra* note 100; *Silver, supra* note 50.

125. *Garrow, supra* note 53.

126. Section 3(e) of the California Medical Association-California Hospital Association *Uniform Code of Hearing and Appeal Procedures* provides: "Record of Hearing. The judicial review committe may maintain a record of the hearing by one of the following metehods: a shorthand reporter present to make a record of the hearing, a recording, or minutes of the proceedings. The cost of such shorthand reporter shall be borne by the party requesting same."

127. *Silver, supra* note 50.

128. *See Klinge, supra* note 49, at 60.

129. *Duffield, supra* note 106; *Suckle, supra* note 94; *Silver, supra* note 50.

130. *Storrs v. Lutheran Hosp. & Homes Society of America,* 661 P.2d 632 (Alaska 1983); *see Laje, supra* note 120; *Sosa, supra* note 87; *Kaplan, supra* note 121.

131. *See* Hershey and Purtell, *Medical Staff Bylaws.* Art. XVI (1985).

132. *Id.* at §16.6-2.

133. *Id.* at §16.6-5.

134. *See generally Klinge, supra* note 49.

135. *E.g., Christhilf, supra* note 51; *Garrow, supra* note 53; *Silver v.*

Castle Memorial Hosp., 53 Haw. 475, 497 P.2d 564, *cert. denied,* 409 U.S. 1048 93 S. Ct. 517, 34 L.Ed.2d 500 (1972).

136. "Every person who, under color of any statute, ordinance, regulation, custom, or usage, of any state or territory, subjects, or causes to be subjected, any citizen of the United States or other person within the jurisdiction thereof to the deprivation of any rights, privileges, or immunities secured by the Constitution and laws, shall be liable to the party injured in an action at law, suit in equity, or other proper proceeding for redress.

137. *E.g., Daly v. Sprague,* 675 F.2d 716 (5th Cir. 1982).

138. *Lew v. Kona Hosp.,* 754 F.2d 1420 (9th Cir. 1985); *Klinge, supra* note 49; *Silver, supra* note 50.

139. *E.g., Woodbury, supra* note 74.

140. *E.G., Northeast Georgia Radiological Assoc. v. Tidwell,* 670 F.2d 507 (5th Cir. 1982); *In re Murphy v. St. Agnes Hosp.,* App. Div. 2d, 484 N.Y.S.2d 40 (1985); However, failure to strictly comply with the bylaws will not be fatal if due process if given. *Kaplan v. Carney,* 404 F.Supp. 161 (E.D. Mo. 1975); *Avol, supra* note 85.

141. *E.g., Foster, supra* note 87.

142. *Laje, supra* note 120, at 1162.

143. *Id.; see* Hollowell, *Decisions About Hospital Staff Privileges: A Case for Judicial Deference,* 11 Law Med. and Health Care 118 (1983).

144. *Woodbury, supra* note 74, at 846.

145. *Hannah v. Larche,* 363 U.S. 420 at 442, 80 S. Ct. 1502 at 1514, 4 L. Ed.2d 1307 at 1321 (1960).

146. Bulletin of the American College of Surgeons (Mar. 1982).

147. *Hawaii Medical Ass'n. v. State of Hawaii,* No. 49777 (Hawaii, 1st Cir. Feb. 4, 1977); Haw. Rev. Stat. §§4538, 67136 (1976); Haw. Rev. Stat. §§4538, (1977).

148. Alaska Stat. §§08.64.215a (1976); *repealed* 1978 Alaska Sess. Laws §§40 ch. 177.

149. *McGuffy v. Hall,* 557 S.W.2d 401 (Ky. 1977).

150. *Arenson v. Olson,* 270 N.W.2d 125 (N.D. 1977).

151. *McCoy v. Commonwealth Board of Medical Education and Licensure,* 37 Pa. Comwlth. 530, 391 A.2d 723.

152. *Jones v. State Board of Medicine,* 97 Idaho 859, *cert. denied* (1976).

153. These constitutional issues are thoroughly discussed in Muranaka, *Compulsory Medical Malpractice Insurance Statutes: An Approach in Determining Constitutionally,* 12 U.S.F.L. Rev. 599 (Summer 1978).

154. *Rosner v. Peninsula Hospital District,* 224 Cal. App. 2d115, (1964).

155. *Wilklerson v. Madera Community Hosp.,* 192 Cal. Rptr. 593 (Cal. App. 1983).

156. Unpublished results prepared by D.L. Matthews, Projects Director, American Hospital Association Hospital Data Center, in Association with Andrew J. Korsak and Ross Mullner.

157. *Propriety of Hospitals' Conditioning Physicians' Staff Privileges on His Carrying Professional Liability or Malpractice Insurance,* 7 A.L.R. 4th 1238 (1981).

158. *Action of Private Hospital as State Action Under 42 U.S.C.S. §§1983 or Fourteenth Amendment,* 42 A.L.R. Fed. 463.

159. *Watkins v. Mercy Hosp. Medical Center,* 520 F.2d 894 (9th Ctr. 1975).

160. *Pollack v. Methodist Hosp.,* 392 F.Supp. 393 (E.D. La. 1975).

161. *Kavka v. Edgewater Hosp., Inc.,* 586 F.2d 59, *cert. denied* (7th Cir. 1978. reported *sub nom., Musso v. Suriano*).

162. *Asherman v. Presbyterian Hosp. of Pacific Medical Center, Inc.,* 507 F.2d 1103 (9th Cir. 1974).

163. *Silver v. Castle Memorial Hosp.,* 53 Haw. 475, 497 P.2d 564 (1972); *Silver v. Queen's Hosp.,* 63 Haw. 430, 629 P.2d 1116 (1981).

164. Laird, *Requiring Liability Insurance Is Unfair,* Am. Med. News 20 (Apr. 24, 1981).

165. Lufton, *Hospital Privileges Revoked: Malpractice Insurance Ruling Awaited,* Am. Med. News (Sep. 4, 1981).

166. *Hospital Privileges, Restraint of Trade, and Professional Liability,* 10 Neurosurgery 285 (1982).

167. *Sosa, supra* note 87.

168. *Maxie v. Martin Memorial Hosp. Ass'n., Inc.,* No. 82330Ca (Fla. Cir. Ct. May 24, 1983).

169. *Holmes v. Maricopa,* 473 P.2d 477 (Ariz. 1977).

170. *Pollack, supra* note 160.

171. *Renforth v. Fayette Memorial Hosp. Ass'n., Inc.,* 383 N.E.2d 368 (Ind. Ct. App. 1978).

172. Doudera, *Can or Should a Hospital Require Its Medical Staff to Obtain Malpractice Insurance,* 6 Med. Legal News 16 (Summer 1978).

173. *Professional Liability Insurance As a Requirement for Medical Staff Privileges,* 10 Neurosurgery 788 (1982); *Professional Liability Insurance as a Condition for Staff Membership,* 80 J. Med. Soc. N.J. 334 (May 1983).

174. *Wilklerson, supra* note 155.

175. *Holmes v. Hoemaku Hosp.,* 473 P.2d 477 (Ariz. 1977).

176. *Pollack, supra* note 160.

GENERAL REFERENCES

Couch, J., and Caesar, N., *Physician Staff Privileges Disputes—A Risk Management Guide for Hospitals and Medical Staffs,* 81 Philadelphia Med. (Sep. 1985).

Couch, J., and Caesar, N., *Cooperation between Hospitals and Physicians for Better Cost Effective Medical Care Delivery—The Health Care Joint Venture,* 81 Philadelphia Med. (Oct. 1985).

Couch J., Caesar N., and Steigman W., *The Legal and Economic Significance of Hospital Medical Staff Appointments and Exclusions,* 81 Philadelphia Med. (Feb. 1984).

Couch, J., Caesar, N., and Steigman, W., *The Effect of Some Recent Antitrust Decisions Regarding Hospital Medical Staff Privileges,* 81 Philadelphia Med. (June 1985).

Creech, *The Medical Review Committee Privilege: A Jurisdictional Survey,* 67 N.C.L. Rev. 179 (Nov. 1988).

Furrow, *The Changing Role of the Law in Promoting Quality in Health Care: From Sanctioning Outlaws to Managing Outcomes,* 26 Hous. L. Rev. 147 (Jan. 1989).

Gnessin, *Liability in the Managed Care Setting,* 471 PLI/Comm 405 (Sep. 1, 1988). *Practising Law Institute Handbook Series, Managed Health Care in 1988: Legal and Operational Issues.*

Hall, *Institutional Control of Physician Behavior; Legal Barriers to Health Care Cost Containment,* 137 Pa. L. Rev. 431 (Dec. 1988).

Harvard Law Review Association, *Antitrust-State Action-Private Parties Immune from Liability When Acting in an Official Capacity: Sandcrest Outpatient Services v. Cumberland County Hospital System,* 853 F.2d 1139 (4th Cir. 1988), 102 Harv. L. Rev. 1080 (Mar. 1989).

Hollowell, E., *The Medical Staff: An Integral Part of the Hospital or a Legal Entity Separate from the Hospital?* (May 1985) (presented at the Twenty-fifth Annual International Conference on Legal Medicine, New Orleans, La.).

Joy, *The Health Care Quality Improvement Act of 1986: A Proposal for Interpretation of Its Protection,* 20 St. Mary's L.J. 955 (Oct. 1, 1989).

Rosenberg, *Independent Practice Associations: Moving Toward an Integrated Medical Group Model,* 471 PLI/Comm 197.

Southwick, A., *Hospital Liability, Two Theories Have Been Merged,* 4 J. Legal Med. 1-50 (1983).

CHAPTER 46   Cost containment and reimbursement

HAROLD L. HIRSH, M.D., J.D., F.C.L.M.*

COST CONTAINMENT
MEDICARE PROGRAM OPERATIONS
MEDICAID
FRAUD AND ABUSE IN PROVIDER CONDUCT
DIAGNOSIS-RELATED GROUPS (DRGs)
PEER REVIEW ORGANIZATIONS

COST CONTAINMENT

Vigorously cutting reimbursements for medical services has become a social policy, enforced by governmental regulation and incorporated into private insurance plans. Another particularly vigorous enforcement of this cost containment policy, by regulating licensure and relicensure, has been considered or adopted by state legislatures. Thus, as a condition of licensure or relicensure, Massachusetts, for instance, has mandated that all physicians caring for a Medicare patient must accept the fractional fee of Medicare assignment as the full fee.

The prospects are that there will be erosion in the quality of care when downscales of ±50% reimbursement are to purchase same-scale 100% service. In an effort to stem that tide, licensure boards have formed medical quality assurance boards armed with sanctioning power and licensure control. The courts have been very clear that such measures are the legitimate exercise of sovereign power to protect the health and welfare of its citizenry.

In the midst of these relatively abrupt changes, there has also emerged an additional risk of increased malpractice exposure when courts believe that there has been an insufficient vigor in physician resistance to medically inappropriate decisions even if resulting from design defects or other inappropriate policies of cost containment. With that coupled to governmental sanctions and the even more ominous threat of licensure sanctions, physicians will be besieged by a rapidly enlarging body of case law defining just how they are to realistically maintain quality standards and expectations within accepted standards of practice and cost containment requirements.

Within the last few years cost control has become much more important for health care organizations as the competitive environment within which they operate has undergone significant changes. Four key changes are (1) a change in the reimbursement basis for Medicare from a cost-based reimbursement to a prospective payment system based on diagnosis-related groups (DRGs); (2) private industry directly negotiating with health care organizations for volume discounts; (3) the entry of entrepreneurs into the health care market who frequently target the more profitable activities for their ventures; and (4) the disappearance of certificate of need (CON) laws or their significant modification, which will remove the franchise protection that an organization received when granted permission to add a service.

Most hospitals attempt to promote cost-effective practices by physicians. Federal law forbids the use of financial incentives to control services to Medicare or Medicaid patients.[1] Some hospitals use cost-effectiveness criteria in clinical privilege decisions. Courts have generally upheld these criteria if they are properly developed and fairly applied.[2]

Two fundamentally different mechanisms operate to contain health care costs: competition and regulation.

Health maintenance organizations

In an effort to contain the inflationary costs of health care, several different approaches have been taken to shunt the cost away from the individual. Health maintenance organizations (HMOs) have become prevalent throughout the country. These organizations pay one premium, which covers all medical care. In return, a participant must be willing to receive care from a

---

*The author gratefully acknowledges work from the previous contributor: James B. Couch, M.D., J.D., F.C.L.M.

specified group of providers. Medicare recipients are encouraged to join HMOs that participate in the Medicare program. With this type of coverage, any deductible required under Medicare is usually eliminated.

Preferred provider organizations

Preferred provider organizations (PPOs), also developed relatively recently, are similar to HMOs in the sense that they refer their members to a designated group of providers (i.e., physicians). Under a private PPO contract, a company would agree to provide medical coverage for its employees limited to the providers within the PPO. In return, the PPO would offer medical care at lower rates.

Prospective payment system (PPS)

The Social Security Amendments of 1983 [hereinafter referred to as Prospective Payment System (PPS)] that pertains only to Part A was enacted specifically to control costs. It represented a dramatic change in the way in which hospitals are reimbursed. It was a revolutionary change; not only did it totally restructure the way in which Medicare reimbursed hospitals, but the federal government also became involved in the setting of specific prices for hospitals for the first time. Unlike other governmental rate setting, however, it applies only to one payer, the federal government, and to Medicare patients. To ease the rigidity of the legislation, additional payments are allowed for cases that are determined to be "outliers."

Managed care and competition

One of the many reform proposals currently in vogue is something called *managed competition,* in order to achieve the desired cost containment which would impose the necessary fiscal discipline.

Managed competition is a theory that seeks to combine market forces and government regulation into a system of universal access and cost control. In contrast, managed care, in broad terms, is a system of controlling the costs of health care through a separate entity, such as an HMO. This entity establishes certain guidelines and procedures to prevent unnecessary expenditures. It screens physicians and compiles lists of approved physicians from which patients covered by the plan choose. Similarly, it enters into contracts with particular hospitals, and patients covered by the plan have to go to an approved hospital for in-patient or outpatient care.

The managed care entity also implements controls to assure that the care provided is necessary and appropriate and provided in a cost-effective manner. These controls include, for example, preadmission certification,

concurrent review, discharge planning, case management, and expanded quality assurance and utilization review.

Managed competition's aim is to set about restructuring the market for health care so that those paying for it have more power and more incentive to negotiate better services at more reasonable prices, and so that those delivering care focus more on efficiency and the quality of the care being rendered.

Managed competition would organize employers, individuals, and health plans into large purchasing groups, or cooperatives. The buzz word for these groups is HIPC, for health insurance purchasing cooperative.

Each purchasing group, or HIPC, would then negotiate with provider networks and agree on a package of health services for the HIPC's subscribers, the price for those services, and how those services would be delivered. Individuals would enroll in the HIPC either through their employer or directly with the HIPC, and would then be able to choose their coverage from among the provider networks with which the HIPC has contracts. Ultimately, Medicare and Medicaid beneficiaries and the uninsured would be enrolled in HIPC's as well.

Essentially, managed competition seeks to harness the enormous group purchasing power of employers and large numbers of individuals to purchase health services at, for want of a better analogy, wholesale or discounted prices. Managed competition would force provider networks to compete for business on the basis of price and quality, for a standard package of benefits. It would also implement numerous controls and safeguards to assure the quality and cost efficiency of the health services being provided.

On the other side, health insurance companies, hospitals, and physicians (the providers) would also be organized into networks. These provider networks would have to provide a minimum package of basic benefits.

On the provider side, the networks could be organized in different ways such as standard HMOs, PPOs, independent practice associations (IPAs), traditional fee-for-service networks similar to Blue Cross/Blue Shield, or even a hybrid such as a large multiple-employer plan that develops its own network of hospitals and physicians.

MEDICARE PROGRAM OPERATIONS

The 1965 amendments to the Social Security Act[3] added Title XVIII to the Act. Title XVIII established a two-part program of health insurance for the aged known as Medicare. Persons are eligible to participate in Part A, the hospital insurance program, if they (1) are 65 or older and are receiving retirement benefits under Title II of the Social Security Act or the Railroad

Retirement Act, (2) qualify under a special program for persons with end-stage renal (kidney) disease, or (3) qualify under the special transitional program. Persons not qualifying otherwise who are 65 or older may still participate in Part A by paying premiums. Anyone age 65 or older who is a U.S. citizen or has been a permanent resident alien for five years may elect to enroll in Part B, a program of supplementary medical insurance. Medicare applies to all qualified people without regard to financial need. It is administered federally, so it has nationally uniform benefits. Provider relations and payments are federally administered on a regional basis, so some regional variations exist. Although Medicare is otherwise free for qualified recipients, there is a deductible that must be met. As soon as a person signs up for Social Security, he or she is automatically enrolled in Parts A and B of Medicare.

Claims must be presented to trigger reimbursement. Until 1983 reimbursement under Part A was based on the allowable costs of the facility providing the care, but was subject to several reimbursement limits. This was changed by the Social Security Amendments of 1983,[4] so that payment to hospitals for in-patient care is based on a prospectively determined amount per discharge according to the patient's diagnosis and the facility's location.

Beneficiaries have to pay certain deductible and coinsurance payments. Some hospitals and physicians routinely waive deductibles and copayments. However, at least one state has forbidden this practice.[5] There is some concern that waivers may be viewed as violations of Medicare antifraud and abuse laws. Federal courts and agencies have refused to rule on this issue.[6]

The coverage of Part A includes a specified number of days of care in hospitals and extended care facilities for each benefit period plus posthospital home care. Provider payment under Part B is based on "reasonable charges," which are subject to numerous arbitrary limits.[7]

The secretary of the Department of Health and Human Services (DHHS) has the overall responsibility for Medicare. The operation of the program has been assigned to the Health Care Financing Administration (HCFA). Congress authorized the delegation of much of the day-to-day administration to state agencies and public and private organizations operating under agreements with the secretary of DHHS. Most payment claims are processed by private agencies that have entered agreements to serve as "intermediaries" for Part A or "carriers" for Part B. They make initial determinations about whether services provided to beneficiaries are payable by the program and how much payment is due. Hospitals must be cautious in acting on information provided by intermediaries and carriers. The Supreme Court ruled in 1984 that HCFA could recover Medicare overpayments from a provider despite the fact that the overpayments were due to erroneous information from the intermediary.[8] The Court stated that providers are expected to know the law and cannot rely on information provided by government agents.

Participating providers

Providers may opt to be participating, i.e., paid directly by Medicare, or nonparticipating, where Medicare pays the patient directly. Nonparticipating physicians who bill more than the maximum allowable actual charge (MAAC) can be assessed substantial civil money penalties and barred from Medicare payments for up to five years.[9]

To be a participating provider of services and receive payments from Medicare, a hospital must sign an agreement with HHS and meet the conditions of participation.[10] The only exception is that Medicare will pay for some emergency services in nonparticipating hospitals.

The participating provider agreement specifies that the hospital will not bill Medicare patients for services except for (1) deductible and coinsurance payments required by law and (2) charges for services that Medicare does not cover. Charges can be made for noncovered services only if the patient has been given adequate notice that they are to covered.

A hospital is deemed to meet the conditions of participation if it is accredited by the Joint Commission on the Accreditation of Healthcare Organizations (JCAHO) or the American Osteopathic Association (AOA) unless a Medicare inspection indicates noncompliance.[11]

Conditions of participation

Medicare also has standards for hospital operations, called *conditions of participation.*[12] They are not licensing standards, but hospitals must comply to qualify for Medicare payments for most services to Medicare beneficiaries. The Medicare law provides that hospitals accredited by the JCAHO or AOA are deemed to meet most conditions of participation unless a special Medicare inspection finds noncompliance.[13]

Physician's orders

In September 1985, the Medicare system introduced a new form to obtain written physician's orders. These forms, titled 485, 486, and 487, were mandated as a requirement for participation in that program. The 485 form is the primary physician form and the other forms are addendums to it. All providers of services must complete the information using these forms and combine this into one order per patient. In addition, this physician–signed form must accompany monthly invoices for service.

Regulated fees

Regulation is the primary consideration in this part of the chapter.

State statute and judicial interpretation. Although *Kartell v. Blue Shield of Mass.*[14] applies to Massachusetts, it may be used as precedent in other jurisdictions. In Massachusetts, Blue Cross-Blue Shield controls approximately 70% of the market share as a third-party payor. Blue Shield of Massachusetts patient-subscribers by agreement must go to doctors who participate in Blue Shield if there is to be reimbursement for health care services.

Blue Shield also has an agreement with the participating physicians that says, in effect, that they assign to Blue Shield the right to reimburse them for services rendered at a rate or sum that Blue Shield determines the services are worth. This results in an effective "lock-in of the pars" and a confiscatory relationship, wherein doctors must accept discounted fees. Furthermore, the doctors are prohibited from balance-billing the patient.

Some physicians in Massachusetts sought legal redress against these confiscatory payment practices, alleging monopolistic restraint of trade in violation of the Sherman antitrust laws. The U.S. Supreme Court has declined without comment to hear an appeal from the federal 1st Circuit Court of Appeals. Thus the highest court overturned the federal district court's finding of monopoly, and substituted an affirmation of the legality of Blue Shields's practices of discounting fees and prohibiting balance billing.

Before the appeals court decision, the Massachusetts state legislature passed a law prohibiting balance billing.[15] Now it would appear that both the statute and the court's ruling have etched in stone the constitutionality of the provision. The second fee regulation is recent legislation that will make mandatory, as a condition of continued licensure, the obligatory care and treatment of all Medicare and Medicaid recipients.[16]

Limits on physician fees

In the case of *Massachusetts Medical Society v. Dukakis,*[17] the AMA and the Massachusetts Medical Society challenged a state law that prohibited physicians, as a condition of licensure, from charging Medicare patients more than the "reasonable charge" as determined by the Medicare carrier. The federal court of appeals upheld the Massachusetts law. The Supreme Court declined to review the case. Massachusetts has passed a law making it illegal to refuse to treat a patient because his or her name appears on a listing of personal injury plaintiffs. The patient may recover actual damages or $1000, whichever is greater, plus attorney fees for violation of the statute.

Waiver of deductibles

The Colorado Supreme Court has upheld the constitutionality of a state statute (876-5A-52) that prohibits providers from routinely waiving health benefit plan deductibles and coinsurance requirements.

The Colorado statute makes such waivers a misdemeanor and subjects violating providers to disciplinary action.

Diagnostic test billing

The HCFA has revised rules on physician billing for diagnostic tests under the Omnibus Budget Reconciliation Act (OBRA) of 1985.[18] Under that provision, a physician who purchases diagnostic tests, such as X-rays, EKGs, and EEGs, from an outside supplier may not "mark up" the cost of the tests in billing the Medicare program. The new provision states that, effective with services rendered on or after April 1, 1988, "global billings" (i.e., billings covering a single fee for both the technical service of taking a diagnostic test and the professional service of interpreting the test) are allowed only where the billing physician personally performed or supervised the test. Global billings are no longer accepted where the physician purchased the test from an outside supplier.

Medical records

To participate in the Medicare reimbursement program, a hospital must have a medical records department that meets the specifications set forth in applicable federal regulations and must maintain medical records that "contain sufficient information to justify the diagnosis and warrant the treatment and end results."[19]

Medicare proposes, disposes, and imposes

In response to the rapidly rising health care costs of the 1980s, Congress enacted Section 2306 of the Deficit Reduction Act of 1984, which revised the then-existing Medicare reimbursement program. Section 12076(a) modifies 42 U.S.C. 1395(u)(b), freezing both Medicare's prevailing and customary charge levels for the 15-month period beginning July 1, 1984, at levels no higher than those set in the preceding 12 months, beginning July 1, 1983.

Second, Section 2306(c) requires physicians to decide before October 1 of each year whether they will be participating or nonparticipating physicians.

Under Section 2306, a two-tiered system is created because physicians can charge their private patients their current fee, but are limited to billing their Medicare patients at the frozen 1982 or 1983 level. Section 2306 particularly infringes on the rights of those doctors who decide not to participate. In essence, the nonparticipating physician has no contract with DHHS, but is bound by DHHS's decision to freeze physician fees.

Part B claims processing

Medicare carriers, which are private insurance companies operating under contract to the HCFA, are responsible for processing and paying Part B claims. Claims for Part B services may be submitted to the carrier by the beneficiary, or by the physician or supplier furnishing the services under an assignment from the beneficiary.[20]

Before payment can be made on claims for Part B services, it must be determined that the beneficiary is covered for Part B benefits, that the charge made was reasonable, that the beneficiary's Part B deductible or applicable coinsurance amounts have been satisfied, and that the services were medically reasonable and necessary. A carrier's initial determination regarding these matters is issued in an Explanation of Medicare Benefits (EOMB). The carrier is required to act on claims within 60 days of their receipt.[21]

Claims denials

Some claims are denied because the services or supplies are specifically excluded from coverage by the Medicare statutes (e.g., personal comfort items and routine check-ups) or by previously issued HCFA coverage determinations with nationwide applicability.[21] Some are denied on purely technical bases, and others for not being medically "reasonable and necessary" under 42 U.S.C. Section 1395y(a)(1)(A).

Carriers are required to disclose the interpretative materials, guidelines, and clarifications used with respect to coverage determinations made in the areas of extended care, home health agency, and durable medical equipment benefits.[22]

Basis of denial

The basis on which a claim is denied is critical to the right of a physician or supplier, acting as the assignee of the beneficiary, to appeal. The EOMB is required to contain sufficient information to enable the recipient to determine the basis of the denial.[23]

A supplier of services has appeal rights only with respect to claims denied on certain grounds, namely, as not medically reasonable and necessary, as constituting custodial care, or, in the case of home health agency services, because the patient is determined not to have been home-bound or not to have needed skilled nursing care on an intermittent basis.[24] Denials on other bases may be appealed only by a beneficiary. The physician or supplier may, however, participate in the appeal indirectly by representing the beneficiary in such an appeal, but it may not make any charge to the beneficiary for doing so, and in some cases it must waive its right to seek payment from the beneficiary for the claim being appealed.[25]

Medicare waiver of liability provisions

The ability of an assignee to appeal also depends on the applicability of the Medicare "waiver of liability provisions" to the denial in question.[26]

Under the Medicare waiver of liability provisions, when a claim is denied as not medically reasonable and necessary, as constituting custodial care, or with respect to home health services because it is determined that the patient was not confined to home or did not require skilled nursing services on an intermittent basis, the claim is still paid notwithstanding this determination, if the services were (1) provided under an assignment[27] and (2) neither the beneficiary nor the assignee knew or could reasonably have been expected to know that payment would not be made for such services under the program.[28]

The statute specifically provides, however, that a person will be deemed to have knowledge that payment is not available for particular Part B services if the person has received notice that claims of such types would not be covered in all or in certain circumstances. Such notice may take the form of either a general notice to the medical community or a notice to a particular supplier of Part B services.[29]

When an assignee is denied waiver of liability by virtue of his or her knowledge, but the beneficiary neither knew nor could reasonably have been expected to know that the services were not covered, the program will apply that amount as an overpayment against the assignee, and the assignee will not be allowed to collect from the beneficiary.[30]

The waiver of liability determination is a two-stage process. First, it is determined whether the claim was denied as not medically reasonable and necessary.[31] This determination is critical because the waiver of liability provisions do not apply at all to Part B services that have been denied on certain grounds, such as constituting a personal comfort item, a routine physical, or elective cosmetic surgery.[32] Next, it must be determined whether the beneficiary and/or the assignee knew or had reason to know that the claim would not be covered.

It is important to recognize that a waiver of liability puts the beneficiary and the assignee on notice that the Part B services in question are not covered, at least under the circumstances of the claim in question. Thus, in the future, such claims would not qualify for waiver of liability and might even constitute false claims under fraud and abuse laws.[33]

As to a particular Part B service, waiver of liability

would continue to be available for claims in process and claims for services rendered prior to notification that the services were not covered.[34] A Part B supplier may not pursue the underlying coverage dispute in its own right if its liability has been waived as to a particular Part B service. But because an adverse coverage determination can have so great an effect on future claims, a Part B supplier whose liability with respect to a particular service has been waived should consider pursuing an appeal on behalf of the beneficiary in an effort to reverse the underlying coverage determination.

In a bid to drive physicians into Medicare participation (accepting assignment 100% of the time), Congress has created a regulatory obstacle course for nonparticipating physicians. The recently passed OBRA promises fee updates to participating physicians, but usually takes them away from nonparticipating physicians. In an attempt to entice physicians into signing Medicare participation agreements, Congress added some additional benefits. In addition to the full 3.2% increase in the Medicare prevailing charges effective January 1, 1987, participating physicians:

- Are listed in Medicare directories available to the public
- Receive faster payment
- Benefit from a new hospital referral rule that states that beginning in October, hospital personnel who refer a Medicare patient for outpatient care must identify the referral physician as either participating or nonparticipating. If the physician is nonparticipating, the hospital must also identify (if practicable and qualified) a participating physician.

Procedural fairness for supplier or beneficiary

The case of *Bowen v. Michigan Academy of Family Physicians*[35] involved the availability of judicial review of Medicare regulations governing physicians. A unanimous Supreme Court held that DHHS regulations affecting physician services under Medicare can be challenged in federal court.

OBRA[36] significantly expanded the statutory appeal mechanisms for Medicare Part B claims for Part B services and supplies furnished on or after January 1, 1987. The decision to appeal depends on the physician's or supplier's waiver of liability status, the nature of the original denial, and the types of services or supplies furnished.

Court of appeals

Appeals from Part B claims denials may involve the following levels of review: a request for reconsideration of the carrier's initial determination, a carrier fair hearing, a hearing before an administrative law judge, or a judicial review. Each appeal level involves slightly different procedures.

A review of and denial of a claim may be requested either by the beneficiary or by the physician or supplier that furnished the service under assignment. A request for review must be filed within six months with the carrier, the Social Security Administration (SSA), or the HCFA. Review is limited to the submission of written evidence. No hearing is held, and the carrier will either reaffirm or reverse its original determination.

Carrier reconsideration

As mentioned previously, the initial determination with respect to a claim by a Part B carrier is issued as an EOMB.[37] A request for review must be filed within six months with the carrier, the SSA, or the HCFA. At this level, review is limited to the submission of written evidence. No hearing is held, and the carrier will either reaffirm or reverse its original determination. The reconsideration determination is issued as a new EOMB.[38]

An expedited appeals process is also available if requested within 60 days of the initial determination and will provide redetermination within three days. Unfortunately, if the redetermination is unfavorable, the hospital will not be reimbursed for the pending redetermination if the DRG has already expired. In this case the patient is responsible for incurred hospital costs.

Carrier fair hearing

A beneficiary, or the physician or supplier who has furnished services under assignment, is entitled to a "fair hearing" before the carrier when the amount in controversy is at least $100 within six months and the carrier's determination after reconsideration is unsatisfactory, or a claim has not been acted on by the carrier within 60 calendar days after receipt by the carrier.[39] A physician who has not taken assignment also has this right as to a claim denied on the grounds of not being medically reasonable and necessary.[40] Part B claims may generally be aggregated to meet the $100 requirement if they relate to similar or related services to the same beneficiary or the same assignee, and involve common issues of law or fact.[41]

This written request must be filed within six months, however, with provision for extending this time limit for "good cause." At the fair hearing, claimant or a representative (an attorney or other individual, including the physician or supplier who furnished the services) may appear.[42] A claimant may also elect to present written evidence only or have the hearing conducted by telephone. The carrier, however, may not require that a hearing be held by telephone.[43]

The fair-hearing officer may consider questions such as the reasonableness of charges, whether the services were medically reasonable and necessary, whether the services were "covered services," whether deductibles and copayments have been met, and whether payment may be made under the waiver of liability provisions. The decision is final and binding on all parties to the hearing, unless it is reported and revised, or further appealed.[44] A claimant may request reopening, but the decision to reopen is within the hearing officer's discretion. These decisions may be reopened only by the carrier for any reason within one year, for good cause between one year and four years, or at anytime if fraud is involved or if an error on the face of the evidence prejudiced the claimant.

When the appeal involves services for which payment has been denied as not medically reasonable or necessary, however, the physician or supplier wishing to represent the beneficiary must waive, in writing, any right to payment from the beneficiary for the services or supplies at issue, and may not charge the beneficiary in connection with such representation.[45]

Administrative hearings

If the amount in controversy is $500 or more, a hearing may be requested before an administrative law judge (ALJ) by the beneficiary, the physician, or supplier who accepted assignment, or a nonassignee physician regarding a claim denied as not medically reasonable and necessary.[46] Part B claims may be aggregated if they involve the delivery of similar or related services to the same individual, or common issue of law and fact arising from services furnished to more than one individual.[47]

The Medicare statute specifically limits the authority of ALJs to overturn national coverage determinations issued by HCFA[48]; and in other cases involving only a question of law (e.g., a challenge to the validity of a regulation), ALJs are required to make expedited determinations when there are no material issues of fact in order to permit a claimant immediate judicial review.[49]

Judicial review

If the amount in controversy is $1000 or greater, for a single claim or under the same aggregation rules that apply for ALJ hearings, judicial review of an unfavorable ALJ hearing decision can be pursued in the U.S. district court for the district in which the beneficiary, a physician or supplier who accepted assignment, or a nonassignee physician — as to a claim denied as not medically reasonable and necessary — resides or has its principal place of business. Such review must be instituted within 60 days of the mailing of the ALJ's decision, by filing a complaint against the secretary of DHSS. An unfavorable district court decision may be further appealed in the usual manner for federal court decisions.

The Medicare statute limits the authority of the courts by denying the power to overturn a national coverage determination on the sole ground that it was not issued in accordance with notice and comment requirements of the Administrative Procedure Act. Further, prior to invalidating a national coverage determination on substantive grounds, the court must remand the issue to the secretary for a reasonable opportunity to supplement the record and substantiate or revise his or her determination.

The statute also prohibits judicial review of regulations and policy instructions, addressing methods for determining the amount of payment under Part B that were issued prior to January 1, 1981. The statute does not, however, appear to prohibit a court from reviewing the interpretation or application of such rules in particular situations.

The U.S. Supreme Court has recently issued a decision that will have a significant favorable impact on hospitals,[50] skilled nursing facilities, home health agencies, and other providers participating in the Medicare program.

In *Bethesda Hosp. Ass'n. v. Bowen,*[50] the Court ruled that the Provider Reimbursement Review Board *must* exercise jurisdiction over appeals by providers that "self-disallowed" costs in their cost reports. "Self-disallowance" is the deliberate omission from cost reports of claims the provider otherwise believes allowable but that the HCFA holds to be nonallowable under its regulations.

The Medicare statute states that a carrier fair hearing is a prerequisite to an ALJ hearing, even when the amount in controversy is $500 or greater.[51] Section 1395ff of the statute provides for an ALJ hearing with respect to amounts in controversy of $500 or greater. Section 1395u(b)(3)(C) of the statute authorizes fair hearings with respect to amounts in controversy of "at least $100, but less than $500." When read together these sections indicate that, when the amount of controversy is greater than $500, a claimant need not submit to a carrier fair hearing before requesting an ALJ hearing.

A written request for an ALJ hearing must be filed with the carrier, an SSA office, or HCFA within 60 days of the notice of the fair hearing decision.[52] These ALJ hearings may be conducted either in person or by the submission of written evidence and argument. In the Omnibus Budget Reconciliation Act of 1987 (OBRA 1987), Congress directed a study of the feasibility of conducting such hearings only by telephone.[53] There is concern, however, that such hearings may not produce the required full and fair evidentiary hearing with respect to all types of claims, and that the cost-effectiveness of telephone hearings has not been established.

Provider Reimbursement Review Board

Hospitals can appeal payment decision to the Provider Reimbursement Review Board (PPRB) in the case of larger amounts or to their Medicare intermediary in the case of smaller amounts. When the issues being appealed apply to several hospitals, group appeals are frequently pursued to reduce the cost to individual hospitals. The secretary of DHHS has the authority to modify the decisions of the PRRB or the intermediary. The final decision of DHHS concerning a payment issue can sometimes be appealed to the federal courts. However, the number of issues that can be appealed has been substantially limited.

In their present form, the regulations bar Medicare from making payment with respect to any item or service to the extent that "payment has been made or can reasonably be expected to be made promptly . . . under a workmen's compensation law or plan . . . automobile or liability insurance policy or plan (including a self-insurance plan) or under no fault insurance."[54] In addition, Medicare is generally secondary to employer group health plan coverage.[55]

To assure that Medicare does not pay for services for which another party may be liable, Medicare provider agreements require Part A providers to maintain a system to identify primary payors other than Medicare during the admission process.[56] To facilitate this screening, the *Medicare Hospital Manual*[57] includes a checklist for hospital admission clerks to use in order to identify circumstances under which Medicare is not the primary payor. This checklist includes specific questions regarding the beneficiary's illness or injury, and the availability of other health insurance sources. There is no parallel requirement for Part B providers to screen Medicare beneficiaries about other insurance coverage.

If, as a result of preadmission screening, the provider discovers that third-party insurance coverage is available, the provider must seek reimbursement from the third-party payor before submitting a claim to the Medicare program.[58] According to the HCFA, "[i]f a provider learns that an automobile, medical or no fault insurance company may pay for covered services, it must bill the insurance company as a primary insurer."[59] However, if the claim is contested by an automobile, medical, or no-fault insurer, or if for any other reason there is a substantial delay in resolving the claim (i.e., 120 days or more), the Medicare program may make payments to the provider on the condition that it will be reimbursed out of any claim proceeds received by the beneficiary in the future.[60]

Under the Medicare Supplemental Program (MSP) provisions, Medicare providers are free to bill third-party payors their full charge rates for services rendered. Since full "retail" charges almost always exceed the amount payable by Medicare, payment of the provider's charges by a third party routinely eliminates Medicare's secondary liability entirely. However, if the amount received from the third-party payor is for any reason less than the total Medicare payment, Medicare will pay any additional reimbursement up to the amount normally payable by the mm program.

Because hospitals may collect up to their full charges from third-party payors and because provider agreements specifically require preadmission screening, it is important that hospitals correctly utilize the screening process to identify third-party payment sources.

In some circumstances, a provider may also be the potential third-party payor. For example, a Medicare beneficiary may initiate a medical malpractice action against provider that self-insures for malpractice liability. In such cases, the provider takes on additional obligations and liabilities toward the Medicare program.

Because the Medicare program is not obligated to pay for services when another payor is primarily liable, even if the payor is the provider itself, all payments made by the Medicare program for services necessitated by the tortious actions of a third party are conditional payments that may be recovered by the Medicare program.[61] Once a third-party payor is identified, the Medicare program may attempt to recoup any Medicare payments it has already made.[62] Recoupment may be accomplished either through direct collection or be offset against any monies owed by the Medicare program to the provider.[63]

If the liable third party, in this case the self-insured provider, enters into a malpractice settlement agreement and makes payment to the Medicare beneficiary without reimbursing the Medicare program, the beneficiary will have 60 days after receipt of the settlement to reimburse the Medicare program.[64] If the beneficiary fails to pay that amount within 60 days, the Medicare program will be entitled to demand payment from the provider's self-insurance fund even though the fund has already reimbursed the beneficiary.[65] Therefore, if the beneficiary does not reimburse Medicare, the provider may be required to pay for the same services twice — once in the form of the settlement, and a second time in the form of a repayment to the Medicare program.

Given the Medicare program's ability to collect payments from a third-party payor without regard to whether the third-party payor has already paid for medical expenses in its settlement with a beneficiary, a provider should structure any malpractice litigation settlement so that a portion of the settlement goes directly to the Medicare program. Alternatively, the provider should reduce the amount of the settlement and reimburse Medicare directly for any conditional payments that may have been made.

Finally, the obligation to repay the Medicare program may not be avoided by refusing to characterize the settlement as a payment for medical expenses. According to the *Medicare Intermediary Manual*, the Medicare program's ability to recoup payments from liability settlements is not contingent on the way the settlement is characterized by the parties:

[A]ny payment by a liability insurer, except payment under a no fault clause in a non-automobile policy, constitutes a liability insurance payment whether or not there has been a determination of liability. Regardless of how amounts may be designated in a liability award or settlement, e.g., loss of consortium, special damages or pain and suffering, Medicare is entitled to be reimbursed for its payments.[66]

Therefore, even if the settlement agreement designates that the payment is for something other than medical care, the Medicare program will nevertheless seek reimbursement.

Secondary payer

In the case of *American Hosp. Ass'n. v. Sullivan,*[67] a U.S. district court permanently enjoined the HCFA from enforcing Medicare regulations that required providers to bill the Medicare program and accept Medicare rates for services rendered to Medicare beneficiaries, notwithstanding that a third party was legally liable for the beneficiary's injury or illness, and the third party's liability insurance carrier would have paid the provider at a higher reimbursement rate. As a result, hospitals are now free to bill the liability carrier directly, or to take other appropriate collection action, such as filing a lien against liability insurance proceeds, as long as the liability carrier is expected to pay promptly.

MEDICAID

Medicaid is a joint federal-state program designed to provide medical assistance to individuals unable to afford health care. Although the Medicaid program is authorized by federal law (Title XIX of the Social Security Act), states are not required to have Medicaid programs. Each state must pass its own law to participate. Under Medicaid the federal government makes grants to states to enable them to furnish (1) medical assistance to families with dependent children and to aged, blind, or disabled individuals whose income and resources are insufficient to pay for necessary health services, and (2) rehabilitation and other services to help such families and individuals obtain or retain the capability for independence or self-care. The secretary of DHHS is responsible for administration of federal grants-in-aid to states under Medicaid.

Medicaid is different from Medicare in that it provides medical assistance for categories of persons in financial need, whereas Medicare provides medical assistance primarily to people 65 years of age or older without regard to financial need. Medicaid varies widely among the states; Medicare is uniform. Medicaid is financed by general federal and state revenues; Medicare is financed by a special tax on employers and employees for hospital insurance and by contributions by beneficiaries and the federal government for supplementary medical services. Medicaid is basically a welfare program; Medicare is considered a form of social insurance.

Beneficiaries and scope of benefits

Any state adopting a Medicaid plan must provide certain minimum health benefits to the categorically needy. The categorically needy include individuals receiving financial assistance under the state's approved plan for Supplemental Security Income (Title XVI of the Social Security Act)[68] or for Aid to Families with Dependent Children (Title IV-A of the Social Security Act).[69]

Under the "spend-down" option, the individual eligible under Medicaid can qualify for financial assistance under the state plans except for certain characteristics that Medicaid requires to be ignored. States have the option of including other persons within their Medicaid plan as medically needy if (1) they would qualify for assistance under one of the preceding programs if their incomes were lower and (2) their incomes would be low enough to qualify for assistance under that program if they were permitted to subtract the health care expenses they have already incurred.

Eligible recipients must apply to the designated state agency before Medicaid will pay for the services they receive. State Medicaid plans must meet many conditions before they can be approved, but states are permitted substantial flexibility in the administration of their own programs.

States are required to provide only five basic services to the categorically needy, but are free to provide additional optional services. As a result of this flexibility, all states have developed Medicaid programs. States may decide, within federal guidelines, who in addition to the categorically needy will be eligible for medical assistance.

Although the states are given wide latitude in the administration of their programs, they are sensitive to federal direction because 50% or more of the financial support for Medicaid comes from the federal government.

Fee control

The Wisconsin Medicaid program distinguishes between individuals who require care at "skilled nursing facilities" and those requiring care at "intermediate care facilities." Generally, an in-patient certified as requiring a level of care different from the existing level is transferred to an appropriate facility. However, if the patient's attending physician concludes that transfer is likely to do more harm than good, the patient is permitted to remain in the existing facility, provided that the physician also concludes that the patient will be able to receive the appropriate care.

The DHHS interpreted its regulations to require automatic and immediate transfer of a patient without taking into account the attending physician's assessment of any "transfer trauma." Accordingly, it objected to the Wisconsin law and withheld $300,000 of Medicaid payment from the state. The case finally reached the U.S. Supreme Court in *Wisconsin Dept. of Health and Social Services v. Bowen*.[70] Subsequently, the DHHS negotiated a settlement of the case with the state of Wisconsin. The settlement was favorable to the procedures desired by the state. Thus this case helped to establish the point that the federal government should not override the reasonable medical judgments of attending physicians.

Institutional providers of services generally become participants in the Medicaid program by contracting with the state to provide services to Medicaid recipients in exchange for the payment permitted by the state. Payment cannot be collected from the patient except to the extent permitted by federal law. Noninstitutional providers generally are not required to enter into any contract with the state, but participate merely by treating Medicaid recipients and then billing the state. States may directly reimburse physicians who provide covered services to the medically needy, or they may pay the individual beneficiaries, leaving them with the obligation to pay the physician. Payment for physician services can be made only if the physician agrees to accept charges determined by the state as the full charges.

The 1981 amendments to the Medicaid law increased the latitude of the states to determine the services to be covered and the amount of payments. States are generally free to establish their own methods of payment for in-patient hospital services as long as the costs do not exceed the Medicare payment for the same services. However, in 1989 a federal appellate court ruled that the Colorado Medicaid payment system violated federal law because it did not meet the costs incurred by efficiently and economically operated hospitals in treating Medicaid patients.[71] Many states have reduced services. When Tennessee reduced the covered days of in-patient care from 20 to 14, the reduction was challenged as a violation of the federal laws prohibiting discrimination against the handicapped because they generally need longer stays. The Supreme Court rejected this challenge in 1985, ruling that the handicapped nondiscrimination law does not guarantee equal results from Medicaid services.[72] The Court did not rule on whether the limit

was consistent with the Medicaid law. Lower courts have ruled that limits on the number of in-patient days, such as South Carolina's 12-day limit, are consistent with the Medicaid law.[73]

Other states placed new limits on payment to providers. Some states have adopted prospective payment systems for Medicaid similar to the Medicare payment system.[74] Minnesota went one step further in its nursing home payment system. Minnesota will pay nursing homes through its Medicaid system only when the nursing home agrees not to charge non-Medicaid patients more than Medicaid pays for comparable care. This system has been upheld by both the federal and the state courts.[75] In 1985 a Minnesota court ruled that neither the state nor Medicaid patients could stop a nursing home from phasing out participation in Medicaid.[76]

Some states using cost-based payment systems calculate reimbursable costs assuming facility occupancy is at least a certain percentage, such as 85% or 90%. These formulas have generally been upheld by the courts.[77]

California and Illinois have implemented programs of selective contracting with hospitals to provide services to Medicaid patients. These programs use a combination of competitive bidding and negotiations to select the contracting hospitals. These states obtained federal waivers of the Medicaid requirement that patients have freedom-of-choice of providers.[78]

Medicare and Medicaid exclusion regulations

On January 29, 1992, the DHSS Office of Inspector General (OIG) issued final regulations derived from the Medicare and Medicaid Patient and Program Protection Act of 1987 (MMPPPA), which became effective on September 1, 1987.[79]

Implementing the OIG's statutory expanded authority to punish violations of the Medicare or Medicaid program is now authorized under MMPPPA of 1987.[80] The OIG is now fully empowered to exclude providers and suppliers that violate program rules.

The MMPPPA gave the secretary of DHSS new grounds for excluding violators from the program and also consolidated many of the secretary's preexisting rights of exclusion. The secretary's new authority under the MMPPPA was subsequently delegated to the OIG.[81]

The final regulations provide for both mandatory and permissive exclusions from program participation. Mandatory exclusion will be imposed on any individual or entity convicted of a crime related to the delivery of any program-covered item or service, as well as any patient abuse or neglect, whether or not the patient involved was a program beneficiary.[82] The mandatory exclusion period will be not less than five years and can be even longer if certain "aggravating factors" are present. Aggravating factors include, for example, a violation that causes a program loss of $1500 or more; a violation that is committed over a period of one year or more; criminal punishment imposed by a court that includes incarceration; or a convicted individual or entity who has a prior criminal, civil, or administrative sanction record.[83] Mitigating factors may be considered only as an offset against aggravating factors to keep the mandatory exclusion at not more than 5 years; mitigating factors may not be considered to reduce the mandatory exclusion period below the 5-year minimum.

Permissive exclusion may be imposed for numerous acts or omissions, some relating to the program and some not.[84] This may be imposed on an individual or entity convicted under federal or state law of fraud, theft, embezzlement, breach of fiduciary duty, or other "financial misconduct" (1) in the delivery of health care items or services (even if not relating to the program) or (2) with respect to any act or omission in a program operated by, or financed in whole or in part by, any federal, state, or local government agency.[85] Permissive exclusion may also be imposed for conviction under federal or state law of (1) obstruction of an investigation of certain criminal misconduct or (2) a criminal offense relating to controlled substances.

Permissive exclusion may be imposed for a variety of other acts and omissions as well, including (1) loss, suspension, or revocation of licensure, or suspension or exclusion from any state or federal health care program; (2) submission of Program claims "substantially in excess of ... usual charges or costs"; (3) furnishing of items or services "substantially in excess" of a patient's needs, or of a quality that fails to meet professionally recognized standards of health care, whether or not the patient is covered by the program; (4) failure by an HMO that is a party to a Medicare risk contract, or that provides items or services under a state Medicaid plan, to substantially provide the medically necessary items or services that are required under the contract or plan; (5) failure to disclose information or grant immediate access to the secretary, state survey agencies, or other authorized entities when required by the program to do so; (6) failure to comply with a corrective action plan required by HCFA; (7) an individual's default on the repayment of scholarship obligations or loans made or secured in whole or in part by the secretary in connection with the health professions; and (8) certain billing violations by physicians in making program claims.[86]

Permissive exclusion may also be imposed for any action that the OIG determines would serve as a basis for imposition of a civil monetary penalty or criminal penalty for violation of Section 1128A of the Social Security Act[87] (submission of false claims) or Section 1128B of the Social Security Act[88] (the antikickback statute, prohibiting the payment of remuneration in exchange for or to induce the referral of program business). Exclusions in such circumstances may be imposed whether or not such civil or criminal penalties are actually imposed, and, in the case of the antikickback statute, regardless of whether the individual or entity may be able to prove that the remuneration was also intended for some legitimate purpose.[89]

When an exclusion is imposed, whether mandatory or permissive, it will apply to Medicare, Medicaid, all other state health care programs, and all other federal nonprocurement programs. An excluded individual or entity that submits or causes the submission of a program claim during the exclusion period will also be liable for civil monetary penalties and criminal sanctions.

FRAUD AND ABUSE IN PROVIDER CONDUCT

A number of recent developments in the area of Medicare/Medicaid fraud and abuse law have shed new light on government efforts to define the scope of prohibited patient referral and physician compensation arrangements.

Medicare fraud: civil monetary penalties

Physicians should keep in mind that the secretary of DHHS has been authorized[90] to impose civil monetary penalties and program suspensions against health care providers for submitting false or improper Medicare and Medicaid claims. Some of the penalties have been Draconian.

The 1977 amendments to the 1972 Medicare-Medicaid fraud and abuse provisions of the Social Security Act make receiving or offering any "remuneration" a felony, subject to prosecution by the Department of Justice. The purpose of these amendments was to reduce the potential for defrauding the Medicare and Medicaid programs.

In April 1985, the U.S. Court of Appeals for the 3rd Circuit sharply expanded the definition of a violation by affirming a conviction in the case of *United States v. Greber.*[91] The appeals court ruled that, even if a medically necessary service were performed, payments made to a physician in connection with tests performed by a laboratory can be the basis for Medicare fraud if any portion of the payment is intended to induce future referrals.

This case says that receiving monies from such endeavors (including joint ventures) will be considered illegal payments—bribes or kickbacks—for referring patients to such organizations as laboratories, hospitals, nursing homes, and manufacturers of durable medical equipment.

This decision has been upheld in *Government of the Virgin Islands v. Lee,*[92] *U.S. v. Ryan,*[93] *U.S. v. Quaisi,*[94] and *U.S. v. Brantley.*[95]

Medicare and Medicaid fraud and abuse

Abuse is a broader term than fraud. While fraud requires deliberate deceit, the government considers it abuse to operate a hospital in a manner that is inconsistent with accepted principles of medical practice and business and that results in excessive and unreasonable expenditures by Medicare and Medicaid. In general, abuse is subject to civil sanctions, such as suspension of payments, suspension from the program, and repayment of overpayments, rather than to criminal sanctions.[96]

Those who are involved in providing services and supplies for Medicare and Medicaid patients are subject to strict antifraud abuse acquirements. Misrepresentations in claims and reports are felonies, subject to a maximum penalty of $25,000 and/or five years in prison. For example, in 1987 a federal appellate court upheld a Medicaid fraud conviction of a physician for using improper billing codes on claims.[97]

Kickbacks, bribes, rebates, and other inducements for referrals of Medicare and Medicaid patients are all felonies. Both payment and receiving inducements are also offenses. In 1989 a federal appellate court ruled that any payment to induce future referrals can be a violation even if the payment is for actual services.[98] The court decided that a payment for professional services is permitted only if it is wholly and not incidentally attributable to the delivery of goods and services. Also in 1989 another federal appellate court upheld the convictions of an ambulance company and a hospital training director who was paid by the ambulance services for serving as its part-time training consultant.[99] The director served on the hospital committee that wrote specifications, reviewed bids, and recommended contracting with the ambulance company. The court ruled that he did not have to be in a position to make a referral, but could violate the statute by being in a position to recommend or arrange a referral.[100]

Congress has prohibited directly some referrals by a physician to a facility of which the physician has an ownership interest.[101] Stricter restrictions have been proposed, so the status of these proposals should be checked before checking physician investment in ventures. Some state laws also regulate such referrals.[102]

Hospitals must be careful when structuring business relationships with physicians and other providers to assure that any payments are not considered forbidden kickbacks.[103] However, there is no governmental or judicial authoritative guidance as to what conduct is permitted.[104-106] Regulations have been proposed to define "safe harbors," conduct that will not be considered a violation.[107]

Limitations

Patient records can be relevant to fraud and abuse investigations. The general federal criminal statute of limitations is five years.[108] The specific civil statute of limitations for civil money penalties is six years.[109]

In 1981 the Social Security Act was amended to permit DHHS to impose civil money penalties and assessments for filing false claims. Penalties of $2000 per item or service and assessments of twice the amount claimed may be imposed. Civil money penalties can be imposed for false or fraudulent claims for payment or for services that were not provided as claimed, and for an improper billing, e.g., a claim made in violation of a payment assignment agreement, a participating agreement with the Medicare or Medicaid programs, or a limitation on charges imposed at the state level. Providers can be held liable even if they did not personally submit a bill, if the provider should have known or had reason to know that inappropriate billing practices were occurring.[110] Thus, a physician might ultimately be held liable for the improper actions of his or her office manager or billing clerk.

Several other practices may also create civil monetary penalty liability.[111] For hospital providers, the submission of false or misleading information that could affect the decision as to when a hospital in-patient should be discharged may result in such liability. Illegal inducements to physicians to limit Medicare- or Medicaid-covered services can also result in civil money sanction.[112]

Preliminary investigation and negotiations

Investigations of improper billing matters are similar to those for alleged antireferral fee violations. As with other OIG matters, if the OIG determines through its investigation that a civil money penalty is appropriate, it will often make an informal settlement offer early in the process. Such offers should be considered carefully by the provider, but only after its counsel has analyzed the validity of the case against it.

The OIG has a great deal of discretion in determining the amount or severity of any penalty, and it can depend, in part, on the wealth and liquidity of the provider. In many cases, the preferable approach is to negotiate the best deal possible informally with OIG, to avoid the time, expense, and a potentially unfavorable result, such as a large fine, impossible payment terms, or program exclusion, of an administrative hearing.

Administrative hearing

If an acceptable settlement cannot be reached, a formal sanctioning process begins. The first step is a notice to the provider that outlines in detail the nature and basis for the penalty and explains the available appeal procedures.[113] The appeal procedures include a right to a hearing and submission of a written argument before an ALJ before any sanction is imposed.[114,115] However, at the hearing, there can be substantial discovery, evidentiary, and cross-examination rights. The provider is entitled to be represented by counsel.

The evidentiary burden rests on the OIG to show that the provider committed an offense for which civil money penalties can be imposed.[115] It is very important, however, that the provider present as full and complete a defense as possible. Any legal defenses not presented at the administrative level may generally not be asserted on appeal.[116]

If the ALJ renders an adverse decision, it may be appealed to the secretary of DHSS, then to the U.S. Court of Appeals, and possibly the Supreme Court.[116] Although a monetary penalty can be stayed while the matter is being considered by the secretary, it cannot be delayed while the matter is pending before the U.S. Court of Appeals.

The amount of the penalty is initially determined by the OIG; however, it may be increased or decreased by either the OIG or the secretary.[117] The maximum penalty for inappropriate billings is a fine of $2000 for each false claim, as well as a damage assessment for twice the amount improperly billed.[118] Because a "claim" can mean each separate line item on a bill, the final amount of the penalty can be many times the amount of the bill itself.[119]

In determining the amount of the penalty, the OIG may not always impose the maximum penalty and is required by regulation to take into consideration (1) the nature of the false claim, (2) the degree of the provider's culpability, (3) the existence of any prior offenses, and (4) the financial condition of the provider. Other aggravating or mitigating circumstances, including the presence or absence of a deliberate scheme to defraud the government, may also be considered.[120]

In 1989 the Supreme Court ruled that the constitutional prohibition against double jeopardy limits the amount that can be claimed in a governmental civil penalties suit after a criminal prosecution for the same conduct.[121] This may have little practical significance because (1) the government can avoid this limit by pursuing the civil suit simultaneously with the criminal prosecution and (2) the limit does not apply to civil penalty suits by private persons.

Other federal criminal and civil penalty statutes can be applied to wrongful acts related to Medicare and Medicaid.[122] In one case, the grounds for the lack of medical necessity was the improper way in which the procedures were performed.[123]

The False Claims Act

The False Claims Act (FCA) imposes liability on any person who "knowingly" presents a false or fraudulent claim for payment to the U.S. government. The statute defines "knowingly" to mean that the person presenting the claim (1) has actual knowledge of the falsity of the claim, (2) acts in deliberate ignorance of the truth or falsity of the information in the claim, or (3) recklessly disregards the truth or falsity of the information presented in the claim.[124] The statute, as amended in 1986, expressly provides that "no proof of specific intent to defraud is required." Under the 1986 amendments to the FCA, the damages that may be awarded for a violation of the act are three times the amount of the actual damages sustained by the government, plus a penalty of not less than $5000 or more than $10,000 for each false claim submitted.

In *United States v. Lorenzo*,[125] Dr. Lorenzo, a dentist, was found to have received $130,719.10 for claims submitted to Medicare that were determined to be improper. Statutory penalties on this amount resulted in a judgment against Dr. Lorenzo in the amount of $18,806,157.30. This is believed to be the largest judgment to date under the FCA.[126] The court pierced the veil of Dr. Lorenzo's various corporations to hold several of them, as well as Dr. Lorenzo himself, liable for the judgment.

The doctrine of "piercing the corporate vein," used in *Lorenzo*, has been invoked in many cases, typically by creditors seeking to recover from shareholders of corporations made insolvent by shareholder activities, e.g., *DeWitt Truck Brokers, Inc. v. W. Ray Flemming Fruit Co.*,[127] but also in government actions against individual defendants, e.g., *United States v. Pisani*,[128] an action to recover Medicare overpayments to a physician's wholly owned professional corporation.

In *United States v. Diamond*,[129] a physician who received a total of $549.04 from 39 false claims was found liable to the government for $78,000. A penalty of $1,791,000 has been assessed against one provider.[130]

Prospective payment system

As noted earlier, the Social Security Amendments of 1983[131] established a Medicare and Medicaid PPS based on DRGs to pay hospitals for in-patient care. The system has been modified by numerous amendments.[132,133] All Medicare in-patients are divided into 477 DRGs based on their principal diagnoses. The principal diagnosis is the one chiefly responsible for the admission. Medicare will pay for 475 of the groups. Groups 469 and 470 involve unacceptable diagnoses and invalid data.

With a few exceptions, the hospital receives one payment for the entire admission based on the DRG and facility location, unless the patient becomes an outlier, requiring an extraordinarily long stay or a high total cost for the case. Medicare makes an extra payment for outliers. Another exception is that capital costs, direct educations costs, and kidney acquisition costs are not included in the prospective payment; they are paid on a cost basis.[134]

An adjustment for indirect medical education costs increases payments to hospitals with medical residency programs.[135] Children's hospitals, long-term hospitals, psychiatric hospitals, and rehabilitation hospitals are exempt from the PPS so they can continue to receive cost-based payment from Medicare.[136] Psychiatric and rehabilitation units of general hospitals can apply for an exemption.

There is an adjustment for some hospitals that serve a disproportionate share of low-income or Medicaid patients, are sole community providers, or experience other extraordinary circumstances.[137]

Under the PPS the incentive is to minimize services and shorten stays. Hospitals lose money if services exceed the prospective payment, and they can keep savings when services cost less than the payment.

Interhospital transfers may be affected by the change to prospective payment. Those fashioning the PPS wanted to make one payment to be shared by all hospitals that provided care to the patient, but the act did not authorize shared payment. The hospital from which the patient is finally discharged receives a full prospective payment based on the patient's DRG. The hospital that cares for the patient before transfer is paid a per diem rate equal to the prospective payment for the DRG divided by the average length of stay for that DRG. The transferring hospital can qualify for additional payment if the patient becomes an outlier due to high costs.

Prospective payment based on DRGs may be replaced with other payment mechanisms. One proposal is *capitation,* in which an amount would be paid for each covered person regardless of use of services.[138]

The passage of the Tax Equity and Fiscal Responsibility Act (TEFRA) has significantly influenced the health care payment system by changing the amount and type of reimbursement hospitals receive for in-patient services. This law focuses on prospective reimbursement policies for hospitals based on DRGs. Hospitals are no longer paid separately for various laboratory studies,

previously reimbursed under Part B of Medicare. Now, all costs are paid under Part A of Medicare. The PPS does not regulate and therefore has not affected physician fees, pharmaceuticals, and technology.

Medicare billing to join electronic superhighway

Currently, 79 different companies across the country—many of them giant insurers like Blue Cross-Blue Shield or Prudential—are under contract to process bills for Medicare. The firms use 14 different computer systems to process bills for Medicare's 36 million beneficiaries. The government allows many of the companies to have rules on whom to pay and what is covered that differ from region to region.

By the end of the decade, one giant nationwide computer system will electronically pay nearly all of the one billion bills Medicare handles each year. Beneficiaries will merely hand their Medicare cards to their doctors, hospitals, laboratories, or nursing homes to make sure their bills get paid.

The Medicare Transaction System (MTS), as the new system is to be called, will eliminate many of the current steps and save an estimated $200 million a year while eliminating the requirement to file separate paper claims. Local companies that help in processing will have instant access to all the information in the MTS system.

DIAGNOSIS-RELATED GROUPS

Diagnosis-related groups (DRGs) have ushered in a greater physician awareness of cost containment. Under the DRG system promulgated under TEFRA,[139] Medicare reimbursement to a hospital is a predetermined, fixed payment based primarily on diagnosis rather than on actual services performed or time occupying the hospital. Each patient is assigned to a DRG category on the basis of age, sex, discharge status, procedures, and diagnosis or diagnoses. The same reimbursement, unless for "exceptional" cases, will be made to the facility whether the patient is hospitalized for 7 days or for 15 days for the DRG. In the designation of DRG, only 3% to 4% of cases can be classified as exceptional.

Hospital payment is determined by a formula that includes final diagnosis plus an economic factor and current area labor costs. At the end of the year of operation under DRGs, a reconciliation takes into consideration uncompensated care and changes in the total amount of payment from each source, and other factors. The hospital then receives a final reconciliation payment or the federal government obtains a release.

Effects of TEFRA and DRGs on physician-hospital practice

The only physicians principally mentioned in the legislation and in the regulations promulgated thereunder are those who are "provider-based," designated as PBPs.

Under TEFRA, hospitals are reimbursed by Medicare only for certain services rendered on behalf of the provider, namely, administrative duties. Reimbursement for services rendered to individual patients by a physician is paid only to that physician, and such payments cannot be assigned to the provider. The principal group to which this applies is the full-time salaried employee-physician, including anesthesiologists, pathologists, and radiologists.

Physician role in DRGs

Physicians now must be more discriminating when determining whether a patient should be admitted. The hospital must rely on the medical staff to aid in preventing overutilization. This is definitely to the economic detriment of the many physicians who accept assignment under Medicare.

The physician must cooperate with the hospital to effect an economically favorable picture. Under no circumstances, however, should the physician compromise patient care. If a physician disagrees with the DRG recommendations or the hospital's Utilization Review Committee (URC), those disagreements should be made in writing, documenting the medical rationale. This will support the physician's interests regardless of what forum questions arise in, either as defendant in a medical malpractice action or as party to a suit against the hospital for denial or restriction of staff privileges. The physician should maintain an objective an attitude as possible in dealing with hospital administration. The physician must certify that the discharge diagnosis and other pertinent information used to determine payment are correct. If the physician has any question, he or she should consult with the proper hospital personnel before certifying the discharge diagnosis. Incorrect information could result in administrative and/or criminal sanctions in addition to malpractice vulnerability.

A profile of each physician's practice patterns is made to determine which physicians, if any, are responsible for repeated financial losses. Unless the physician can justify a prolonged hospital stay and the studied performed, the hospital may take adverse action.

Those physicians who overutilize, injudiciously admit, order studies indiscriminately, and discharge in an untimely way will not be reappointed to the staff or will be suspended from the staff. Such a physician does have the right of appeal.

To avoid physician-hospital confrontations, many hospitals are employing "DRG enhancers" or coordinators who are responsible for accommodating physicians' medical decisions. This person reminds the physician when he or she is approaching the reimbursement rate limit.

Legal implications of DRGs

Courts have ruled that it is legal and constitutional for the federal government to impose DRG reimbursement on providers.

In a landmark case, a Medi-Cal patient sought approval for a recommended surgical procedure and attendant acute care hospitalization as a result of an arteriosclerotic condition. Medi-Cal authorized the surgical procedure and 10 days of hospitalization for that treatment. Complications resulted and a question arose as to the medical necessity of a postoperative stay in the hospital. That request was denied. Plaintiff then claimed that the denial was a negligent act that resulted in a premature discharge ultimately necessitating an amputation of the plaintiff's right leg. At the trial level the jury found in favor of the plaintiff, *Wickline,* holding that Medi-Cal was negligent in handling this case and awarded the plaintiff $500,000.[140]

The Court of Appeals found that the Medi-Cal program was "absolved from liability . . . as a matter of law," because the responsibility for allowing a patient to be discharged from the hospital was that of the treating physician, not the health care payor. It is for the treating physician to decide the course of treatment medically necessary, including hospitalization terms. Medi-Cal did not override the medical judgment of the treating physician at the time of the discharge, nor was it given any opportunity to do so. Therefore, there could be no viable cause of action against it for the consequences of that decision.

Physicians have a legal duty to treat to the level of the usual and customary standard. There is also a concomitant duty to provide all the care that is medically necessary or indicated. When patient care is not authorized or otherwise is obstructed, it is imperative for physicians to document the circumstances. Physicians must explain the problem to their patients, describe the care needed, and help patients to resolve the dispute with the carrier or hospitalize the patients. Physicians who blindly accept erroneous restrictions or decisions may be liable for the consequences.

A physician must inform the patient of the consequences of not receiving necessary care and management whether the patient chooses to refuse treatment or whether the treatment will not be reimbursed under current legal rules. The patient may volunteer to pay for care or services that may not be allowed under the DRGs.

The Wilson decision

In *Wilson v. Blue Cross of Southern California,*[141] the estate and heirs of Howard E. Wilson, Jr., sued his insurance carriers and a URC for wrongful death arising from a utilization review decision. The plaintiffs claimed that Wilson had been prematurely discharged from a psychiatric hospital based on the URC's determination that Wilson's continued in-patient hospitalization was not "medically necessary." Wilson committed suicide two weeks after the discharge.

The trial court granted summary judgment for the defendants based on the *Wickline* decision, finding that Wilson's attending physician was solely responsible for Wilson's discharge and any resulting harm, because the physician failed to appeal the review decision. The same division of the California court of appeal that had authored the *Wickline* opinion reversed the *Wilson* judgment, finding that, under California tort law, the defendants could be held liable for Wilson's death if their actions were a "substantial factor" in his demise.

Distinguishing the factual underpinnings of the *Wickline* holding, the *Wilson* court held that none of the public policies inherent in the statutory and regulatory law governing utilization review in the Medi-Cal program applied to Wilson's commercial insurance policy, and thus the general rule of California tort liability applied with full force and effect. Principally relying on the deposition testimony of Wilson's attending physician, the court found that there was sufficient evidence to raise triable issues of fact as to whether the defendants' actions were a substantial factor in causing Wilson's death. If so, liability would be found.

The Corcoran decision

In *Corcoran v. United HealthCare, Inc.,*[142] the Corcorans had brought an action against United HealthCare, Inc., a URC, and Alabama Blue Cross, an insurance administrator, seeking damages for the wrongful death of their unborn child and the emotional distress they suffered as a result of the death. Notwithstanding the high-risk nature of Mrs. Corcoran's pregnancy and the recommendation of her physician that she be hospitalized for the remainder of her pregnancy so that the fetus could be monitored around the clock, United determined that hospitalization was unnecessary, authorizing instead 10 hours per day of home nursing. During a period when no nurse was on duty, the fetus went into distress and was lost.

The trial court granted summary judgment on the grounds that plaintiffs' cause of action was preempted in its entirety by the Employee Retirement Security Act (ERISA) and that no remedy for their claims was provided for under ERISA. Given that the insurance program in *Corcoran* was admittedly an ERISA plan, the principal question on appeal was whether plaintiffs' claims "related to" that plan. If they were related, they would be preempted by ERISA under Section 514(a), 29 U.S.C. Section 1144(a). The defendants argued that plaintiffs' claims "related to" the insurance plan because the URC's decision was a benefit determination under the terms of the health benefits plan. In contrast,

plaintiffs argued that the URC's determination constituted medical advice and, therefore, did not "relate to" the plan.

The court of appeals disagreed with both arguments, finding that the URC "gives medical advice . . . in the context of making a determination about the availability of benefits under the plan," and "makes medical decisions as part and parcel of its mandate to decide what benefits are available under the . . . plan." Based on this finding, as well as its determination that plaintiffs' action sought a remedy "for a tort allegedly committed in the course of handling a benefit determination," the court of appeals affirmed the trial court's holding that their claims were preempted by ERISA. Although clearly troubled by the result and also recognizing that Congress could not have anticipated the issue of utilization review liability when it drafted ERISA's broad preemption provisions, the court nevertheless found that plaintiffs' claims were preempted and that no remedy was available for what may have been a serious utilization review error.

In analyzing the scope of liability in the utilization review area, both *Wickline* and *Wilson* focused heavily on the issues of how utilization review decisions affect the delivery of medical treatment, and in particular whether such reviews merely determine the availability of insurance benefits or virtually constitute medical decisions themselves. *Wickline* set the stage for future personal injury lawsuits based on erroneous utilization review decisions and defective cost containment mechanisms.

The holding in *Wilson* expanded utilization review liability overnight. Whereas *Wickline* appeared to provide protection to payors and URCs from utilization review liability by placing legal responsibility in the majority of circumstances squarely on the backs of providers, especially attending physicians, *Wilson* clarified that, for utilization review in the private sector, the legal responsibility for bad outcomes might be shared by providers, payors, and URCs, because each might be found to have been a "substantial factor" in the outcome.

Just as *Wilson* seemingly expanded medical review liability for third-party payors and URCs overnight, the holding in *Corcoran* drastically reduced their exposure to such liability in most instances, because the vast majority of health insurance programs in this country are ERISA plans. If the *Corcoran* decision is followed in other jurisdictions, third-party payors and URCs will be immune from tort liability for personal injuries resulting from most of their utilization review decisions.

Not only does the *Corcoran* holding foreclose any remedy for injuries caused by the withholding of necessary medical care pursuant to utilization review, it also results in placing sole responsibility for such injuries on providers. It is therefore imperative that providers exercise all available appeal rights if they disagree with a utilization decision.

The case law relative to the liability of health care providers and insurers or care by managed care plans and insurance companies is evolving. It is fairly clear that a physician will incur liability if a patient is injured by the delay or denial of necessary care for any reason, including utilization review or cost containment. In addition, the utilization review company or named care plan might also incur liability in certain circumstances, such as where treatment, although questionable, may be available.

A California jury recently awarded $89 million to the family of a cancer patient who died after her HMO refused to pay for a bone marrow transplant.[143] The jury found that Health Net had indeed breached its contract, breached the covenant of good faith and fair dealing, and inflicted emotional distress through its "reckless" denial of coverage. Under California law, reckless acts satisfy the intent element of intentional infliction of emotional distress. The jury ordered Health Net to pay the $212,000 in medical expenses, and awarded the family $12.1 million in compensatory damages and $77 million in punitive damages.

In a similar case, Blue Cross refused to pay for a mastectomy in a patient with breast cancer. A New York Supreme Court[144] characterized Blue Cross conduct as "not only morally reprehensible, but shows an indifference to the human condition." It found that Blue Cross claim review procedures constituted not only a wrong to the plaintiff individually, but was conduct "which could foster a great harm upon the public in general," and therefore the Court allowed the claim for punitive damages for breach of contract.

As the movement toward managed care progresses, the potential legal liabilities are quickly becoming evident. HMOs and other insurers face potentially enormous liabilities if they rely too heavily on economics in deciding whether or not to pay for their insured's treatment. Besides compensatory and punitive damages, new theories of recovery against health insurers are being advanced, including the so-called claim for "tortious interference with the physician-patient relationship."

In another case,[145] the court found both the physician and HMO liable for malpractice based on the physician's compliance with the HMO's utilization decision. The patient, complaining of intermittent chest pains, presented to the primary care physician. The physician who was assigned to this patient by the HMO ordered a Holter monitor tracing. After the tracing was begun, the HMO informed the physician that the test would not be covered, and the tracing was discontinued without being read. Shortly thereafter, the patient suffered a massive myocardial infarction. The Holter tracing was then read and showed T-wave changes predictive of cardiac problems. The court found the physician negligent for not providing necessary care. The HMO, in its capacity as the employer of the physician, not as the insurer, was also found liable for malpractice.

Health insurers should regularly review their claims handling procedures, have qualified professionals who can properly evaluate proposed treatments, and render payment decisions on a timely basis. There should be an adequate appeals mechanism and when the insurer rejects one treatment it should strive to reach an understanding with the insured by seeking possible alternative courses of treatment, if available. Standards should be applied as consistently as possible and the insurer should work with the insured and his or her physician in reaching a compromise.

As a result of a recent decision,[146] hospitals that serve large numbers of low-income patients can challenge a regulation (42 C.F.R. 412.106) that allowed reimbursement for Medicaid patients only for the days allowed by the state Medicaid program rather than for the time the patient was hospitalized. Another court held[147] that these hospitals may obtain adjustment of any unworkable restrictions under the statuatory framework and obtain judicial review if such adjustments are arbitrarily denied.

Consequences/sequela

Under the structure of the prospective payment system, it is financially rewarding for a hospital to discharge Medicare patients as early as possible, regardless of the situation and at times to the patient's detriment and death.[148]

Closely associated with the problem of premature and inappropriate discharges is the problem of hospital discharge planning. This hospital-provided service has been seriously taxed under PPS due to an increased caseload and, consequently, fails sometimes because it is overburdened.

Since Medicare patients are 65 years of age and older, they frequently suffer from several chronic and significant medical problems due to their advanced age. As such, they do not easily fit into the rigid categories of the DRG system; they need individualized consideration and care. Subsequently the DRGs do not accurately predict actual hospital costs.

The fiscal needs of the hospital that encourages underutilization may be completely at odds with medically indicated care. The physician is placed in a difficult position between his or her economic dependence on the hospital and his or her own ethical and professional conscience. It is when concessions are made that problems arise.

PEER REVIEW ORGANIZATIONS

In 1982 the TEFRA[149] created utilization and quality control peer review organizations (PROs) to conduct peer review of care of federally funded patients. The Social Security Amendments of 1983 modified the role of PROs to focus their efforts on the potential problems created by prospective per-case reimbursement based on diagnosis-related groups.[150]

The PROs and similar private third-party payor systems are focused primarily on expenditure reduction, so they do not fulfill the hospital's responsibility to review the quality of physician performance. Some elements of these review programs can assist, but hospitals must have their own systems of review.

PROs randomly review cases on the basis of six areas: (1) admission, (2) transfer to psychiatric units, (3) procedure review, (4) outliers, (5) reimbursements (with seven days) and (6) DRG validation.

The two most significant changes implemented in 1989 as a result of amendments to the act[151] are mandatory physician and hospital profiling and the "quality intervention" program.[152]

Profiling

Under the act PROs must maintain profiles for all providers, physicians, and hospitals who participate in the Medicare program. Profiling is specifically designed to identify providers who fall more than two standard deviations below the statistical norm. Once identified, these providers will be subjected to more focused review, which in turn can lead to the imposition of sanctions.

The physician profiles include an analysis of denial rates for admissions and readmissions, mortality rates, and lengths of stay for premature discharges. Hospital profiles include an analysis of such factors as average length of stay per DRG per quarter, average number of discharges per DRG per quarter, noncompliance with PRO review procedures, mortality rates, frequency of procedures identified for quality objectives, and readmission rates.

Quality intervention plan

Under the quality intervention plan (QIP), PROs must carry out (1) quality problem identification activities; (2) identification of the source of each quality problem (i.e., physician, hospital, or both); (3) assignment of a severity level and a corresponding point total to each quality problem; (4) quarterly profiling and computation of weighted severity scores; and (5) mandatory implementation of intervention and/or sanction.

On review, patient care that does not violate any generic utilization screens or indicators may still be sanctionable if a review of the QIP factors evidences an alleged quality problem.

Under the QIP, each quality problem must be assigned one of three severity levels, with a corresponding point value, as follows: (1) medical mismanagement without the potential for significant adverse effects on the patient (Level I, 1 point); (2) medical mismanagement with the potential for significant adverse effects on the patient (Level II, 5 points); and (3) medical mismanagement with significant adverse effects on the patient (Level III, 25 points). The term "significant adverse effect" is defined as (1) unnecessary prolonged treatment, complications, or readmissions, or (2) patient mismanagement that results in anatomical or physiological impairment, disability, or death.

Once each quality problem is identified, the PRO must determine which health care provider is responsible for the problem—the physician, the hospital or skilled nursing facility, or a combination—and assign severity levels and corresponding point totals to the responsible parties.

After the review and allocation of responsibility is completed, a notice is sent to the offending provider or providers. Each provider has a maximum of 30 days, including mail time, to "discuss" the alleged quality problem with the PRO. This gives the provider an opportunity to offer exculpatory or mitigating information in writing to the PRO. The PRO will make a final determination based on all available information, and the provider may be assigned a point total.

The points accumulated by each provider are compiled by the PRO on a quarterly basis and maintained as a separate "QIP profile" distinct from the utilization profiling statistics. A complicated intervention system then becomes applicable, whereby accumulation of a certain number of points by any particular provider automatically triggers prescribed acts of intervention by the PRO. These acts of intervention and their corresponding triggers include (1) automatic notification to the provider (3 points in any quarter or 5 points per bi-quarter); (2) mandatory provider education, including, in the case of a physician, for example, telephone and/or in-person discussions with the provider, reading of suggested literature, and continuing medical education courses (10 points in any quarter); (3) "intensification" of review, including 100% retrospective review of all cases (15 points in a quarter); (4) other interventions, including, but not limited to, concurrent or predischarge review or prior approval or preadmission review (20 points in a quarter, which could occur from a single Level III violation); and (5) coordination with licensing and accreditation bodies, including federal and state agencies responsible for the professional licensure of the provider (25 points in any quarter, which could also occur from a single Level III violation). Hospitals should be aware that payment to them may be denied as the result of a violation being assessed against them or their physicians.

Sanctions

Sanctions may be imposed at any level if a particular quality problem or series of problems meets the definition of a substantial, gross, or flagrant violation. Sanctions may include suspension from the Medicare program for up to six months.

PROs may exercise a more lenient intervention or a more severe sanction, depending on individual circumstances, thus effectively overriding the intervention triggers. However, it must submit a written explanation to HCFA, which constitutes a disincentive to such action and gives providers all the more reason to submit persuasive responses to all PRO notices.

The HCFA has revised the Medicare PRO "Scope of Work" (SOW), the document that defines the duties of PROs.[153] HCFA characterizes the fourth SOW as a fundamental change in the way PROs carry out their responsibilities, placing less emphasis on dealing with individual concerns, and focusing more attention on improving health care generally. This will be accomplished by analyzing patterns of care and outcomes, and furnishing educational feedback to providers based on the information derived from this analysis.

Health care quality improvement initiative

The primary new component in the HCFA PRO fourth SOW is the Health Care Quality Improvement Initiative (HCQII), which provides for the systematic identification and examination by PROs of significant trends or changes in trends in patterns of care. The PROs will provide feedback and work with hospital administrative and medical staff to improve processes and outcomes for Medicare beneficiaries. The PROs will use baseline data to observe whether provider performance is progressing toward identified benchmarks. The data for HCQII projects will ultimately come from a uniform clinical data set (UCDS).

Case review

PROs will still be required to perform individual case review of care rendered to an HCFA-selected sample of Medicare beneficiaries. This retrospective review will consider quality of care, admission, discharge, invasive procedures, documentation, coverage, DRG coding, and outliers. PROs will continue to make medical necessity decisions and to monitor hospital compliance with Medicare notice and attestation requirements.

Notices of quality problems are now called notices of quality *concerns,* and the PRO is still expected to maintain a profile of quality concerns that contains thresholds to trigger intervention, although the numerical rating system that is used will not be disclosed.

One significant change in individual case review under the fourth SOW is an increased emphasis on documentation. If a reviewer deems a chart to be incomplete, rather than devoting time to seeking out the missing materials, the PRO will issue a "technical denial" of the claim in question, and any prior reimbursement already made on the claim will be recovered unless and until the documentation defect is corrected. Documentation will also be an increasingly important element of quality review.

END NOTES

1. 42 U.S.C.A. §13201a-7a(b) (1989 Supp.).
2. *E.G., Mizell v. North Broward Hosp. Dist.,* 175 So.2d 583 (Fla. 4th DCA 1965); *Edelman v. John F. Kennedy Hosp.,* No. C-2104-80 (N.J. Super. Ct. Jan 25, 1982), *cert. denied,* 475 A.2d 585 (N.J. 1984), as discussed in Medical staff, Hospital Law Manual 49 (Mar. 1987); Miller, *Use of Hospital Data in Medical Staff Discipline,* 1 Topics in Hosp. L. 37 (Dec. 1985).
3. Pub. L. No. 89-97, 79 Stat. 290 (1965).
4. Pub. L. No. 98-21, 97 Stat. 65 (1983), as amended by Pub. L. No. 98-369, 98 Stat. 1073 (1984); 42 C.F.R. §§405.470-405.477 (1988).
5. *Parrish v. Lamm,* 758 P.2d 1356 (Colo. 1988).
6. *West Allis Mem. Hosp., Inc. v. Bowen,* 852 F.2d 251 (7th Cir. 1988).
7. E.g., 42 U.S.C.A. §1395u(b) (1989 Supp.).
8. *Heckler v. Community Health Services,* 467 U.S. 51 (1984).
9. 42 U.S.C.A. §1395u(b) (3) (G), (j) (1989 Supp.).
10. 42 U.S.C.A. §1395x(e) (1983 & 1989 Supp.); 42 C.F.R. pt. 482 (1988); *e.g.,* 42 C.F.R. §§405.1101-405.1137 (1988).
11. 42 U.S.C.A. §§1395aa, 1395bb (1989 Supp.); *Cospito v. Heckler,* 742 F.2d 72 (3d Cir. 1984), *cert. denied,* 471 U.S. 1131 (1985) (not improper delegation to Joint Commission because HHS retains ultimate authority).
12. 42 U.S.C.A. §1395x(e) (1983 & 1989 Supp.); 42 C.F.R. pt. 482 (1988).
13. 42 U.S.C.A. §§1395aa(c), 1395bb (1983 & 1989 Supp.); *see also* Holthaus, *HCFA's Surprise Surveys Can Be Costly,* 63 Hosps. 50 (July 20, 1989).
14. *Kartell v. Blue Shield of Massachusetts,* 542 F.Supp. 782 (D.C. 1982), as amended (1982).
15. Ann. Laws. Mass., Chapter 112, § 2, p. 17, paragraph 7, 1987.
16. Pub. L. 98-21, Title 6, Prospective Payment for Medicaid Hospital Services, Amends Title 42, Social Security Amendments.
17. *Massachusetts Medical Society v. Dukakis,* 815 F.2d 790 (1st Cir. 1987).
18. Omnibus Budget Reconciliation Act of 1985, Pub. L. 99-272, 42 U.S.C. § 1395 et seq., effective Aug. 1, 1986.
19. *Bethesda Hospital Ass'n v. Bowen,* 485 U.S. 399 (1988).
20. 42 C.F.R. §§ 405.1672-405.1686; *see also* Haley, *Important Medicine and Medicaid Changes in OBRA 93,* 8 Health Care Law Newsl. 14-18 (Dec. 1993).
21. 42 C.F.R. § 405.801; *see also* Blanchard, *Appeals from Medicare, Part B. Claims Denials,* 3 Health Care Law Newsl. 15-19 (Sept. 1988); Blanchard, *Strategies for Addressing Increased Denials of Medicare Part B Claims,* 3 Health Care Law Newsl. 12-16 (Aug. 1988).
22. *See* 42 U.S.C. §§ 1395y(a)(6) and (7); *Medicare Coverage Issues Manual,* Medicare & Medicaid Guide (CCH) ¶ 27,200.

23. Omnibus Budget Reconciliation Act of 1987 § 4035(c)(2) (December 21, 1987), effective June 1, 1988.
24. *See David v. Heckler,* 591 F. Supp. 1033, 1042-45 (E.D.N.Y. 1984).
25. 42 U.S.C. §§ 1395pp(d), 1395u(1).
26. 42 U.S.C. § 1395ff; *see Medicare Carrier's Manual* § 12019; *see also* 42 C.F.R. §§ 405.870-405.872.
27. *See* 42 U.S.C. § 1395u(b)(3)(B)(ii)).
28. 42 U.S.C. § 1395pp(a); 42 C.F.R. § 405.330.
29. 42 C.F.R. §§ 405.334-405.336; *Medicare Carrier's Manual* § 7300.5.
30. 42 U.S.C. § 1395pp(b); 42 C.F.R. § 405.332.
31. 42 U.S.C. § 1395y(a)(1).
32. *See Medicare Carrier's Manual* § 7300.2C.
33. 42 U.S.C. §§ 1320a-7a and 1320a-7b.
34. *See* 42 C.F.R. § 1395pp(a)(2).
35. *Bowen v. Michigan Academy of Family Physicians,* 476 U.S. 667 (1986); *see also* 42 U.S.C. § 1395ff; 42 U.S.C.A. §§405(h), 1395ff, 1395ii (1983); *Heckler v. Ringer,* 466 U.S. 602 (1984).
36. *Supra* note 18.
37. 42 C.F.R. §§ 405.807-405.810; *see also* Manning, *Medicare Appeal Rights Update,* 3 Health Care Law Newsl. 3-4 (Oct. 1988).
38. *See Medicare Carrier's Manual* § 12010.2.
39. 42 U.S.C. § 1395u(b)(3)(C); *see* 42 C.F.R. §§ 405.811-405.835; *see also Manual* ch. XII.
40. *See* 42 C.F.R. § 405.820; *Manual* § 12015H.
41. 42 U.S.C. § 1395pp(a)(1).
42. *See* 42 C.F.R. §§ 405.835-405.850.
43. *See Manual* § 12017D.
44. *See Manual* §§ 12100.5-12100.15.
45. 42 U.S.C. § 1395ff(b)(1).
46. 42 U.S.C. § 1395ff(b)(2)(B).
47. 42 U.S.C. § 1395ff(b)(2)(B).
48. OBRA 1987 § 4082(b).
49. 42 U.S.C. § 1395y(a)(1). 42 U.S.C. § 1395ff(b)(3)(A).
50. *Bethesda Hosp. Ass'n v. Bowen,* 485 U.S. 399 (1988).
51. *See Manual* § 12015B.
52. 42 U.S.C. § 405(b).
53. OBRA 1987 § 4037(b).
54. 42 U.S.C. § 5y(b)(2)(A)(ii); *see also* Yood, *The Medicare Secondary Payor Provisions, Possible Rewards and Pitfalls,* 7 Health Care Law Newsl. 5-12 (Oct. 1992).
55. 42 U.S.C. § 1395y(b)(2)(A)(i),(b)(1)(A).
56. 42 C.F.R. § 489.20(f).
57. *Medicare Hospital Manual,* HCFA Pub. 10, § 301.
58. 42 C.F.R. § 489.20(g).
59. *Medicare Intermediary Manual,* HCFA Pub. 15-1, § 3419.4.
60. *See Medicare Carrier's Manual,* HFCA Pub. 14, §§ 3338.3, 3338.8; MIM §§ 3489.3F., 3489.8.
61. 42 C.F.R. § 411.24.
62. 42 C.F.R. § 411.24(b).
63. 42 C.F.R. § 411.24(d).
64. 42 C.F.R. § 411.24(h).
65. MIM § 3419.7.
66. 42 C.F.R. § 411.24(i).
67. 1990 U.S. Dist. LEXIS 10327 (D.D.C. 1990); Rodriguez, *Recent Federal Case Enjoins Enforcement of Medicare Secondary Payer Regulations,* 5 Health Care Law Newsl. 13-17(Nov. 1990).
68. Title XVI of the Social Security Act.
69. Title IV-A of the Social Security Act.
70. *Wisconsin Dept. of Health and Social Services v. Bowen,* 485 U.S. 1017 (1988).
71. *Amisub (PSL), Inc. v. Colorado Dep't of Social Servs.,* 879 F.2d 789 (10th Cir. 1989), *rev'g* 698 F.Supp. 217 (D. Colo. 1988).
72. *Alexander v. Choate,* 469 U.S. 287 (1985).
73. *Charleston Mem. Hosp. v. Conrad,* 693 F.2d 324 (4th Cir. 1982).
74. *E.g.,* Michigan, *Medicare & Medicaid Guide* (CCH) ¶15,600; *see also Presbyterian-Univ. of Pa. Medical Center v. Commonwealth,* 553 A.2d 1027 (Pa. Commw. Ct. 1989).
75. *Minnesota Ass'n of Health Care Facilities, Inc. v. Minnesota Dep't of Pub. Welfare,* 742 F.2d 442 (8th Cir. 1984), *cert. denied,* 469 U.S. 1215 (1985); *Highland Chateau, Inc. v. Minnesota Dep't of Pub. Welfare,* 356 N.W.2d 804 (Minn. Ct. App. 1984).
76. *LaZalla v. Minnesota,* 366 N.W.2d 395 (Minn. Ct. App. 1985); *accord Catir v. Commissioner of Dep't of Human Servs.,* 543 A.2d 356 (Me. 1988).
77. *E.g., Haven Home, Inc. v. Department of Pub. Welfare,* 216 Neb. 731, 346 N.W.2d 225 (1985); *Humphrey v. State, Dep't of Mental Health,* 14 Ohio App. 3d 15, 469 N.E.2d 981 (1984).
78. *Medicare & Medicaid Guide* (CCH) ¶¶14,625.23 [waivers], 15,560(IV)(1) [California], 15,582(III)(1)[Illinois].
79. Pub. L. No. 100-93.
80. *See* 57 Fed Reg 3298 *et seq.* (1992) (amending 42 C.F.R. pts 1000-1004 and adding 42 C.F.R. pts 1005-1007); *see also* Conn, *Final Medicare and Medicaid Exclusion Regulations Published,* 7 Health Care Law Newsl. 3-6 (May 1992).
81. *See* 53 Fed. Reg. 12999 *et seq.* (Apr. 20, 1988).
82. *See* 57 Fed. Reg. at 3331 (to be codified at 42 C.F.R. § 1001.101).
83. *See* 57 Fed. Reg. at 3331 (to be codified at 42 C.F.R. § 1001.102).
84. *See* 57 Fed. Reg. at 3331-40 (to be codified at 42 C.F.R. §§ 1001.201-.1701).
85. *See* 57 Fed. Reg. at 3331 (to be codified at 42 C.F.R. § 1001.201(a)(2)).
86. See 57 *Fed. Reg.* at 3331-32 (to be codified at 42 C.F.R. §§ 1001.301-.401).
87. 42 U.S.C. § 1320a-7a.
88. 42 U.S.C. § 1320a-7b.
89. *See* 57 Fed. Reg. at 3334 (to be codified at 42 C.F.R. §§ 1001.901-.951).
90. Sections 1128A and 1128(c) of the Social Security Act, 42, U.S. 13201-71 and 13201-7(c); *see also* Rodriguez and Blacker, *Recent Developments in Medicare and Medicaid Fraud and Abuse,* 4 Health Care Law Newsl. 12-17 (July 1980); Lee, *Civil Money Penalties: A Costly Action for Medicare Program Violations,* 4 Health Care Law Newsl. 8-11 (Sept. 1989); Lindeke, *Medicare and the False Claims Act Program Violations Result in $18 Million Judgement,* 6 Health Care Law Newsl. 3-6 (May 1991); Manning, *Medicare and Medicaid False Claims Prosecutions: Your Clerks' Mistake Can Subject You to Criminal Prosecutions,* 9 Health Care Law Newsl. 16-20 (July 1994).
91. *United States v. Greber,* 760 S.2d 68 C.A.3 (1985), *cert. denied;* U.S. 988 (1985).
92. *Government of Virgin Islands v. Lee,* 775 F.2d 514, C.A. 3 (1986).
93. *U.S. v. Ryan,* 828 F.2d 1010 C.A. 3 (1987).
94. *U.S. v. Quaisi,* 779 F.2d 346 C.A. 6 (1985).
95. *U.S. v. Brantley,* 786 F.2d 1372, C.A. 7 (1986).
96. *E.g., Haven Homes, Inc. v. Dep't of Pub. Welfare,* 216 Neb. 731, 346 N.W.2d 225 (1985); *Humphrey v. State, Dep't of Mental Health,* 14 Ohio App. 3d 15, 469 N.E.2d 981 (1984).
97. *Medicare & Medicaid Guide* (CCH) ¶¶14,625.25 [waivers], 15,560 (IV)(1) [California], 15,582 (III)(1) [Illinois].
98. 42 U.S.C.A. §1320a-7b (1989 Supp.).
99. *United States v. Larm,* 824 F.2d 780 (9th Cir. 1987), *cert. denied,* 198 S.Ct. 1957 (1988).
100. *United States v. Kats,* 871 F.2d 105 (9th Cir. 1989); *accord United States v. Gerber,* 760 F.2d 68 (2d Cir. 1985), *cert. denied,* 474 U.S. 988 (1985); *see also United States v. Lipkis,* 770 F.2d 1447 (9th Cir. 1985); *but see United States v. Porter,* 591 F.2d 1048 (5th Cir. 1979).
101. *United States v. Bay State Ambulance,* 874 F.2d (1st Cir. 1989).
102. Pub. L. No. 101-239, §6204 (1989); Iglehart, *The Debate Over Physician Ownership of Health Care Facilities,* 321 New Eng. J. Med. 198 (1989); Morse & Popovits, *Stark's Crusade: The Ethics*

in Patient Referrals Act of 1989, 22 J. Health & Hosp. I. 208 (1989).

103. *E.g.,* Fla. Stat. §458.331(1)(gg) (1987); *Respiratory Therapeutics, Inc. v. Foster Medical Corp.,* 542 So. 2d 1010 (Fla. 3d DCA 1989).

104. *West Allis Mem. Hosp. v. Bowen,* 852 F.2d 251 (7th Cir. 1988).

105. Baldwin, *Justice Dept. Firm on Waiver Policy,* 15 Mod. Healthcare 33 (1985).

106. *Bakersfield Community Hosp. v. Sullivan,* No. 89-1056-TPJ (D.D.C. Aug. 8, 1989) *as discussed in* 17 Health L. Dig. 15 (Sep. 1989); Burda, *Judgement Refuses to Rule on Hospital Sale,* 19 Mod. Healthcare 7 (Sep. 1, 1989).

107. 54 Fed. Reg. 3,088 (Jan. 23, 1989).

108. 42 U.S.C. § 3282.

109. 42 U.S.C. § 1320a-7a(c)(1).

110. 42 U.S.C. § 1320a-7a(a)(1); *In the Matter of the Inspector General v. Silver,* CMPL Docket No. C-19.

111. 42 U.S.C. § 1320a-7a(a)(3).

112. 42 U.S.C. § 1320a-7a(b)(1).

113. 42 C.F.R. § 1003.109.

114. 42 U.S.C. § 1320a-7a(c)(2).

115. 42 C.F.R. § 1003.116.

116. 42 C.F.R. § 1003.114. 7a(e).

117. 42 U.S.C. § 1320a-7a(e).

118. 42 U.S.C. § 1320a.

119. 42 U.S.C. § 1320a-7a(a); 42 C.F.R. §§ 1003.103, 1003.104.

120. 42 C.F.R. § 1003.106.

121. *United States v. Halper,* 109 S.Ct. 1892 (U.S. 1989).

122. *E.g.,* 18 U.S.C.A. §286; 18 U.S.C.A. §287; 18 U.S.C.A. §371; 18 U.S.C.A. §494; 18 U.S.C.A. §495; 18 U.S.C.A. §1001; 18 U.S.C.A. §1002.

123. *See United States v. Radetsky,* 5351; 2d 556 (10th Cir. 1976), *cert. denied,* 429 U.S. 820 (1976); 18 U.S.C.A. §§1001, 1002; 18 U.S.C.A. §1341; 18 U.S.C.A. §§ 1961-1963; 18 U.S.C.A. §1018; 18 U.S.C.A. §1505; 31 U.S.C.A. §231.

124. 31 U.S.C. §3729.

125. *United States v. Lorenzo,* 1991 (E.D. Pa. 1991).

126. 31 U.S.C. § 3729 (1988).

127. *DeWitt Truck Brokers, Inc. v. W. Ray Fleming Fruit Co.,* 540 F.2d 681 (4th Cir. 1976).

128. *United States v. Pisani,* 646 F.2d 83 (3d Cir. 1981).

129. *United States v. Diamond,* 657 F. Supp. 1204 (S.D.N.Y. 1987).

130. *Mayers v. United States Dep't of Health & Human Servs.,* 806 F.2d 995 (11th Cir. 1986), *reh'g. denied,* 813 F.2d 411, *cert. denied,* 108 S. Ct. 82 (1987); *see also Chapman v. United States Dep't of Health & Human Servs.,* 821 F.2d 523 (10th Cir. 1987); *Scott v. Bowen,* 845 F.2d 856 (9th Cir. 1988).

131. Pub. L. No. 98-21, 97 Stat. 65 (1983).

132. Pub. L. No. 98-369 (1984); Pub. L. No. 99-272 (1985); Pub. L. No. 99-509 (1986); Pub. L. No. 100-203 (1987); Pub. L. No. 100-360 (1988); Pub. L. No. 100-647 (1988).

133. Pub. L. No. 98-21, 97 Stat. 65 (1983), as amended, which is codified primarily at 42 U.S.C.A. §1395ww (1989 Supp.); 42 C.F.R. pt. 412 (1988).

134. 42 U.S.C.A. §1395ww(g), (h) (1989 Supp.); 42 C.F.R. §§412.90, 412.100 (1988).

135. 42 U.S.C.A. §1395ww(d)(5)(B) (1989 Supp.); 42 C.F.R. §412.118 (1988).

136. 42 U.S.C.A. §1395ww(d)(1)(B) (1989 Supp.); 42 C.F.R. §412.23 (1988).

137. 42 U.S.C.A. §1395ww(d)(5)(C), (F) (1989 Supp.).

138. Baldwin, *Administration Expects to Begin Study to Find "Something Better" than PPS,* 15 Mod. Healthcare 32 (July 19, 1985); Wallace, *Capitation System Tops Agenda—IICFA Official,* 15 Mod. Healthcare 52 (July 5, 1985).

139. Tax Equity and Fiscal Responsibility Act of 1982, Pub. L. No. 97-248, 1982 U.S. Code Cong. & Admin. News (96 STAT.) 324; Social Security Amendments of 1983, Pub. L. No. 98-21 1983 U.S. Code Cong & Admin News (97 STAT.) 65.

140. *Wickline v. California,* 192 Cal. App. 3d 1630, 228 Cal. Rptr. 661 (1986), *review granted,* 231 Cal. Rptr. 560, 727 P.2d 753 (1986), *review dismissed,* 239 Cal. Rptr. 805, 741 P.2d 613 (1987) (originally published at 183 Cal. App. 3d 1175 (1986); *see generally,* Morreim, *Cost Containment and the Standard of Medical Care,* 75 Calif. L. Rev. 1719, 1748 n. 124 (1987) and *Wickline v. State: The Emergency Liability of Third Party Health Care Papers,* 24 San Diego L. Rev. 1023 (1987).

141. *Wilson v. Blue Cross of Southern California,* 222 Cal. App. 3d 660, 271 Cal. Rptr. 876 (1990).

142. *Corcoran v. United Healthcare, Inc.,* 965 F.2d 1321 (5th Cir. 1992), *cert. denied,* 113 S.Ct. 812.

143. *Fox v. Health Net,* ___ Cal.Rptr. ___ (1994).

144. *White v. Blue Cross and Blue Shield of Greater New York,* 146 Misc. 2d 125, 549 N.Y.S.2d 598 (1989).

145. *Elsesser v. Hosp. of the Philadelphia College of Osteopathic Medicine,* 802 F. Supp. 1286 (E.D. Pa. 1992).

146. *Jewish Hospital, Inc. v. Secretary of Health and Human Services,* 19 F.3d 270 (C.A. 6, 1994).

147. Rye, *Psychiatric Hospital Center, Inc. v. Shalala,* 846 F.Supp. 1170 (S.D.N.Y. 1994).

148. Staff Report of The Senate Special Committee on Aging. Impact of Medicare's Prospective Payment System on the Quality of Care Received by Medicare Beneficiaries.

149. *Supra* note 139.

150. Pub. L. No. 98.21 §602.97 Stat. 167 (1984).

151. Peer Review Improvement Act of 1982, Pub. L. No. 97-248, Title I. §§ 141-50, 96 Stat. 381-95 (1982), 42 U.S.C. §§ 1320c *et seq.* (1988).

152. Godes, *Pro Reviews: Understanding the System,* 6 Health Care Law Newsl. 7-11 (Jan. 1991).

153. 58 Fed. Reg. 12042 (Mar. 2, 1993).

CHAPTER 47

Physician as an employer

CHARLES G. HESS, M.S., M.D.

HAZARD COMMUNICATION STANDARD
BLOODBORNE PATHOGENS STANDARD
WORKERS' COMPENSATION
UNEMPLOYMENT COMPENSATION
CLINICAL LABORATORY IMPROVEMENT AMENDMENTS

Most physicians, acting as employers, are well aware of their financial obligations (withholding taxes, FICA, and unemployment insurance) to the government. They are less familiar, however, with "other" governmental obligations overseen by agencies with acronyms like OSHA and HCFA. In addition, many federal laws have been passed in America since 1963 that have profoundly affected the practice of medicine—the Equal Pay Act of 1963, Civil Rights Act of 1964 (title VII), the amended Age Discrimination in Employment Act of 1967, the Equal Opportunity Act of 1972, the Medical Waste Tracking Act of 1988, the amended Americans with Disabilities Act of 1990, and the Family Leave Act of 1993.

This chapter deals with aspects of employee safety (the Hazard Communication Standard and Bloodborne Pathogens Standard), employee benefits (workers' compensation and unemployment compensation) and employee performance (Clinical Laboratory Improvement Amendments).

HAZARD COMMUNICATION STANDARD

Noncompliance with the Hazard Communication Standard by physician employers can result in substantial monetary penalties (per violation). There are almost 600,000 chemical products in existence in the United States, with new ones being introduced each year.[1] Some of these chemicals pose serious problems for exposed employees. The Occupational Safety and Health Administration (OSHA) issued, in 1983, a regulation called "Hazard Communication" that applied to employers in the manufacturing sector. Under the Hazard Communication Standard (HCS), the employee is required to be informed of the contents of the law, the hazardous properties of chemicals encountered in the workplace, and measures (such as safe handling procedures) needed to protect employees from these chemicals. The law was expanded in 1988 to include employers in the nonmanufacturing sector such as the physician-employer; thus, HCS became the first regulation to concern itself especially with the health and safety of medical employees.[2] HCS was revised in February 1994.

Duties

Under the "general duty clause" of this law, the physician-employer "shall furnish a place of employment which is free from recognized hazards that are causing or are likely to cause death or serious physical harm to his or her employees."[3] The physician-employer is required to post the Job Safety and Health Protection Poster (OSHA Form 2203) in his office or clinic. Any fatal accident or accident that results in the hospitalization of three or more employees must be reported to the nearest OSHA office within 8 hours.

Under HCS, each physician-employer who has one or more employees exposed to a hazard is required to develop a written program to protect those individuals. This "Hazard Communication Plan" (HCP) must outline those health and safety policies and procedures placed into effect by the employer to protect his or her workers. The stated purpose of the HCP is to reduce the occurrence of illnesses, injuries, and fatalities in the workplace.

Hazardous chemicals

A complete inventory must be taken once a year of all products in the office or clinic. HCS requires that all chemicals imported, produced, or used in a workplace undergo a "hazard determination." This evaluation, which may be relegated to an employee, should include not only medical supplies (such as isopropyl alcohol and bleach) but also office supplies (such as copier toner and correction fluid).[4] There are essentially two ways to determine whether or not a product is considered hazardous. One way involves writing the product's manufacturer or distributor for a material safety data sheet; the other way involves comparing chemicals in office products with those on one of four lists.[5] For a hazard determination, OSHA recommends use of the following four lists:

Noncarcinogenic chemicals
1. OSHA's "Toxic and Hazardous Substances"[6]
2. ACGIH's "Threshold Limit Values (TLV) for Chemical Substances and Physical Agents in the Work Environment"[7]

Carcinogenic chemicals
3. The National Toxicology Program's "Annual Report on Carcinogens"[8]
4. The International Agency for Research on Cancer's "Monographs."[9]

Most consumer products containing hazardous chemicals that are used in the office are cleansers.[10] Medications that are dispensed by a pharmacist to a health care provider for direct administration to a patient are exempt.[11] Drugs in solid form (pills or tablets) are also considered exempt; until recently, most injectables and other medications used in an office were also considered exempt from HCS.

Material safety data sheets (MSDSs)

An MSDS is an informational sheet furnished by a product's manufacturer to the user in order to identify the hazardous characteristics of the product. Every hazardous product must have an MSDS, provided by the manufacturer or distributor upon written request. In 1986, OSHA developed Form 174 to provide a universal form that would meet the HCS requirements. Use of the form is not mandatory, but all the information on the form is required by OSHA.

Once a year, requests should be made for MSDSs on all hazardous products that have been changed or are new to the office. Such sheets should be kept for five years.[12] Under the revised HCS, MSDSs may be kept on a computer disk or microfiche (rather than paper) as long as there are "no barriers to employee access."[13] Drug package inserts cannot be accepted in lieu of MSDSs under the present rule.[14] Drug samples, if not used in the office, do not require MSDSs. After an MSDS is obtained, it has to be "rated" in order to create a hazard label. This is best done using a modification of the method suggested by Suchocki.[15]

Hazard labels

Under HCS, the employer is required to label, tag, or mark hazardous chemicals in the office or clinic. The purpose of the label is to serve as an "immediate warning" and as a "reminder of more detailed information" in the MSDSs. Instead of labeling specific containers, OSHA also permits the posting of proper information on the front or back sides of cabinet doors where hazardous materials are stored.[16] The label must show the identity of its hazardous chemical or chemicals and any appropriate hazard warnings. There is no single labeling system recommended by OSHA. The most widely used label is that developed by the National Fire Protection Agency (NFPA 704 Standard).[17] The hazard label represents a condensed, "shorthand" version of relevant data on the MSDS.[18]

Training program

Finally, HCS requires employers to provide a training program for all employees exposed to hazards in the routine performance of their duties. The aim of this program is to provide all staff members with a clear understanding of the topics mandated by the standard. Employees must be trained at scheduled staff meetings or special staff meetings. The training can be done by the employer or one or more employees, to which certain topics have been assigned. Each training session must be documented on an employee training log.

BLOODBORNE PATHOGENS STANDARD

The second federal law to concern itself with the safety of medical employees was the Bloodborne Pathogens Standard (BBP) of 1991, by OSHA. The intent of this law is to reduce exposure in the health care workplace to all bloodborne pathogens, particularly the hepatitis B virus (HBV) and the human immunodeficiency virus (HIV). HBV infection is considered the major infectious bloodborne occupational hazard to health care workers; the Centers for Disease Control (CDC) estimate that there are approximately 8700 such infections in health care workers in the United States each year, causing approximately 200 deaths.[19] With regard to HIV, CDC estimates that about 1,000,000 Americans are infected with the virus; as of September 1, 1993, CDC had logged nearly 400,000 AIDS cases, with about 200,000 deaths.[20] There are reports of at least 24 workers who apparently were infected with HIV through occupational exposure to blood or other potentially infectious materials.[21]

Exposure control plan

Any employer having at least one employee with occupational exposure is required to have a written

"Exposure Control Plan" (ECP). The stated purpose of the plan is to eliminate or minimize occupational exposure to blood and other potentially infectious materials. The employer is required to make a copy of this plan available to all employees and any OSHA representative. It must be reviewed and updated at least once a year.

Exposure determination

Each employer who has one or more employees with occupational exposure is required to perform an "exposure determination." The exposure determination list consists of the following[22]:

1. A list of job titles in which *all* employees have occupational exposure
2. A list of job titles in which *some* employees have occupational exposure
3. A list of all tasks (or groups of closely related tasks and procedures) that identify certain employees within a job classification where some but not all employees have occupational exposure.

Exposure incident

The ECP must also explain how the employer will evaluate the circumstances surrounding exposure incidents.

Exposure control

BBP was drafted so that employees will be protected by performance-oriented standards. The specific provisions of the ECP are an effort to make clear "what is necessary" to protect employees. It is the responsibility of the physician-employer to limit worker exposure through implementation of the following categories of control[23]:

1. Universal precautions
2. Workplace controls
3. Personal protective equipment
4. Housekeeping policies
5. Hazard communication policies
6. Hepatitis B program
7. Training program.

Universal precautions. OSHA's method for reducing worker exposure to bloodborne pathogens is based on the adoption of "universal precautions" as the foundation for a plan of infection control. Under BBP, workers are required to exercise universal precautions to prevent contact with blood or other potentially infectious materials.

Workplace controls. Workplace controls are of two types: engineering controls and work practice controls. Engineering controls reduce the risk of occupational exposure by confining or isolating infectious materials.

Examples of engineering controls are sharps containers, biosafety cabinets, and self-sheathing needles.

Work practice controls reduce employee exposure by altering the manner in which a procedure is performed. The employer is required to incorporate the following work practice controls into the ECP:

1. *Washing hands:* Employers are required to provide hand-washing facilities that are readily accessible to employees.
2. *Handling blood:* Mouth pipetting or suctioning of blood or other potentially infectious materials is prohibited.
3. *Handling equipment:* Equipment used for diagnosis or treatment must be examined prior to servicing or shipping and must be decontaminated unless the employer can demonstrate that decontamination of such equipment is not feasible.
4. *Handling personal items:* Employees must not keep food and drink either in refrigerators, freezers, shelves, or cabinets or on countertops or benchtops where blood or other potentially infectious materials are present.
5. *Handling sharps:* Employees must not bend, break, or shear contaminated needles and other contaminated sharps.

Personal protective equipment. When engineering and work practice controls are insufficient to eliminate exposure, then personal protective equipment (PPE) must be used "to prevent or minimize the entry of materials into the worker's body."[24] BBP states that "when there is occupational exposure, the employer shall provide, at no cost to the employee, appropriate personal protective equipment such as, but not limited to, gloves, gowns, lab coats, face shields or masks and eye protection, and mouthpieces, resuscitation bags, pocket masks, or other ventilation devices."[25] OSHA places the responsibility of protecting employees directly on the employer.

Housekeeping policies. BBP requires employers to keep workplaces "in a clean and sanitary condition." Under housekeeping policies, the employer is required to schedule, and then to implement, a written agenda for cleaning and decontaminating the office, including

1. Cleaning of surfaces
2. Cleaning of equipment
3. Cleaning of linens
4. Discarding of regulated waste.

Hazard communication policies. BBP requires the use of hazard communication through labels or signs to ensure that employees receive adequate warning in order to eliminate or minimize their exposure to bloodborne pathogens. Such labels are to be affixed to refrigerators and freezers containing blood or other potentially infectious material, as well as other containers used to store, transport, or ship blood or other potentially infectious materials. Red bags or red containers may be substituted for labels.

Hepatitis B program. The employer is required to make the hepatitis B vaccine available to all employees who have occupational exposure. To those who have had an exposure incident, the employer is also required to obtain a postexposure evaluation and a medical follow-up.

Training program. Training about the hazards associated with blood and other potentially infectious materials must be provided by the employer to all employees with occupational exposure. The only requirement of the person conducting the training is that he or she be knowledgeable in the subject matter. The employer is required to keep training records for all employees with occupational exposure for three years from the date on which the training occurred; the same rules that apply to medical records also apply to training records.

WORKERS' COMPENSATION

Two methods of obtaining compensation open to the temporarily unemployed worker are workers' compensation insurance (WCI) and unemployment insurance. Since 1976, all 50 states offer sick employees some form of compensation for lost wages and medical expenses.[26] WCI gives the employee a legal way to receive benefits for work-related illnesses or injuries. Employers are required to offer WCI to employees injured while performing their assigned tasks in all but three states (New Jersey, South Carolina, and Texas).[27] Any individual working for a noncharitable company or corporation who incurs a job-related injury is eligible under present state laws. Some states exclude employers with fewer than five employees, domestic workers, temporary workers, and casual workers, such as gardeners, newspaper vendors, and charity workers.

Types of WCI

Each state is responsible for administering its own program of WCI. The employer pays premiums for the WCI based on the employee's job and the involved risk in the performance of that job. State legislatures offer four kinds of coverage[28]:

1. State compensation fund
2. Employer self-insured program
3. Commercial insurance program
4. Combination program.

Types of claims

To obtain workers' compensation benefits, an employee must receive an on-the-job injury. He must be physically injured while performing a service in his job

description that is required by the employer. He does not have to be "on company property" at the time of the injury. Claims under WCI are of five types[29]:

1. *Nondisability:* A "nondisability" claim covers medical expenses for a minor injury. In these cases, which are easily adjusted, the employee, after treatment by a doctor, continues to work or returns to work within a few days.
2. *Temporary disability:* A "temporary disability" claim covers medical expenses for a more serious injury, together with payment for lost wages (usually about two-thirds of the employee's regular salary). Each state has a specified waiting period before salary replacement can begin. Because of the uncertain course of an injury, these claims are more difficult to adjust. Temporary disability status ends when the worker is once again employed, although not necessarily in the same capacity as before the injury.
3. *Vocational rehabilitation:* A "vocational rehabilitation" claim covers the cost of retraining for both temporary and permanent cases. It affords the opportunity for employment to those individuals who are unable to return to their former positions.
4. *Permanent disability:* A "permanent disability" claim refers to an employee's lessened ability to compete for job opportunities. In such cases, a doctor has determined the injury to be "permanent and stationary"; the individual is unable to return to his or her former position because of a permanent impairment. Assignments are made on the basis of partial disability (i.e., 20%, 60%, or 90% loss) or full disability (100% loss). Examples of partial disability include the loss of an eye or a leg. Full disability means the individual will not be able to work in any capacity.
5. *Death of employee:* A "death of employee" claim refers to death benefits paid to the dependents or survivors of a fatally injured employee.

Records

In workers' compensation cases, a "contract" exists between the physician and the insurance carrier—not the physician and the patient.[30] In the case of a physician-employer, it is best, to avoid a conflict of interest, to refer the employee to another physician for a work-related injury.[31] The doctor who treats the patient is required to accept the workers' compensation approved fee as full payment for services rendered.

When an employee first seeks treatment for an injury, a First Report of Injury Form should be completed. The time limit for filing varies, depending on the state, from 1 to 10 days.[32] The report should be made in quadruplicate, with copies to the State Compensation Commission or Board, the insurance carrier, the patient's employer, and the compensation case file.

A detailed, narrative progress report should be filed to report any significant change in an employee's medical or disability status.[33] The report should be made in duplicate, with one copy going to the insurance carrier, the second to the compensation case file.

Appeals

Employers are required to post a statement of employees' rights to WCI, together with the name and address of the insurance carrier, in a highly visible area of the workplace. In some instances, claims for workers' compensation are denied because the employee fails to report the injury to his or her supervisor or employer. In other instances, the employer may deny the reported injury is work related because of the rising costs of insurance coverage. Claims that are denied by the employer have to be appealed to the State Compensation Commission or Board. If the appeal is unsuccessful, the patient will have to pay his or her own medical expenses.

UNEMPLOYMENT COMPENSATION

The Federal Unemployment Tax Act offers states an incentive to develop their own programs by agreeing to bear the costs of administering those state programs meeting the federal guidelines. The joint federal-state system of unemployment compensation or unemployment insurance (UI) provides insured employees with partial replacement for lost wages. It is funded primarily by a tax on the employer. More than 85% of this nation's workers are covered by UI.[34] UI covers both full-time and part-time employees; excluded from this coverage are some government workers, some farm workers, some domestic workers, casual workers (such as babysitters and newspaper carriers), children employed by parents, employees of religious organizations, elected officials, and railroad workers.[35]

Federal provisions

The federal law requires an employer to pay a payroll tax on each employee's wages. Under the Federal Unemployment Tax Act, as amended in 1985, the tax rate is 6.2% of the first $7000 paid to each employee of employers with one or more employees in 20 weeks of the year or a quarterly payroll of $1500.[36] Because states also have unemployment taxes, the employer is granted partial credit against the tax for payments made to a state unemployment fund. A credit of up to 5.4% is allowed for taxes paid under state insurance laws meeting all requirements of the federal act (leaving the federal share at 0.8% of taxable wages).[37] Employers are also granted a federal credit for any decrease in the state tax because of favorable employment experience.

State provisions

Each state, as well as the District of Columbia, Puerto Rico, and the Virgin Islands, operates its own program of UI. If a state program complies with the federal law, it qualifies for federal funds to help pay unemployment benefits. To be eligible for those benefits, an employee must have worked a certain number of weeks, or earned a specified minimum amount, or both of these. Payments are made according to benefit schedules or stipulated formulas based on prior wages, employee tenure, number of dependents, and state law. Payments are generally available for up to 26 weeks.

CLINICAL LABORATORY IMPROVEMENT AMENDMENTS

The Clinical Laboratory Improvement Amendments (CLIA) are almost entirely performance oriented. CLIA was passed in 1988 to ensure the accuracy of laboratory tests performed on human specimens. The physician is no longer able to perform tests on patients in his or her office without legal permission from the federal government. Most of the regulations became effective on September 1, 1992.

Certification

All laboratories under this law must obtain one of five certificates: the Health and Human Services (HHS) certificate—or a registration certificate, certificate of waiver, certificate of physician performed microscopy, or a certificate of accreditation. Even if only one test is performed (and even if no charge is made for that test), the Health Care Financing Administration (HCFA) requires the physician-employer to obtain a certificate. Once an application is received, HCFA may issue a registration certificate, together with a CLIA number (for requests for laboratory testing reimbursement made to Medicare or Medicaid third-party payers after January 1, 1994).

A registration certificate permits a laboratory to continue operations for two years or until a determination of compliance can be made, whichever is shorter. The certificate of accreditation can be issued by the Commission on Office Laboratory Assessment (COLA) to those laboratories (including POLs) desiring an alternative to federal inspections under CLIA. Also, a laboratory in a state with a federally approved licensure program may choose to receive a state license in place of a CLIA certificate, provided it complies with the regulations of that state.

Categories of tests

Present laboratory tests, numbering about 10,000, have been classified according to the degree of difficulty in the performance of the test.[38] This ranking initially resulted in a three-tier organization of tests into categories called waived, moderate complexity, and high complexity, to which a fourth category (physician-performed microscopy) was added in February 1993.

A laboratory that limits itself to performing waived tests is essentially exempt (except for manufacturers' instructions) from CLIA requirements. Procedures classified under physician-performed microscopy must be performed personally by the doctor, in conjunction with an examination of the patient in the office. Laboratories performing waived and physician-performed microscopy tests are not subject to routine inspections, but are subject to random compliance and complaint investigations. Those laboratories performing physician-performed microscopy, moderate-complexity, and high-complexity tests must fulfill certain requirements for personnel standards, patient test management, quality control, proficiency testing, and quality assurance.

Personnel standards

Each laboratory performing nonwaived tests must meet certain personnel standards (PS), which are tied to the complexity of the testing process. The rules, which differ for moderate-complexity testing and high-complexity testing, list very detailed personnel responsibilities and qualifications; qualifications are based on formal education, laboratory experience and/or laboratory training.[39] Laboratories performing tests in the moderate-complexity category must employ a laboratory director, technical consultant, clinical consultant, and testing personnel.

Patient test management

Each laboratory performing nonwaived tests is required to have in place a system assuring the correct performance of the entire testing process, beginning with the preparation of the patient and ending with the distribution of test results. Patient test management (PTM) consists of two parts: (1) written policies and (2) documentation (to verify the former).[40] The regulations require written policies for:
1. Preparing patients
2. Processing (collecting, preparing, identifying, storing, transporting, and discarding) specimens
3. Reporting results.

With regard to test results, "normal" or "reference" ranges must be available, but they do not have to be printed on reports. The laboratory is also required to develop a written policy (or protocol) to follow when a life-threatening or "panic" value occurs. The protocol demands that the individual ordering the test or the individual responsible for utilizing the test results be notified immediately when any test result indicates an immediate danger to a person's life.

With the second part of PTM, three documents are required: the test requisition, the test record (patient log), and the test report, all of which must be kept for a minimum of two years. Tests can only be performed on the oral, written, or electronic (computer) order of an "authorized person." That authorized person will usually be the doctor (or another state-authorized individual). Written requests must be signed by the authorized person; oral orders are permitted as long as written orders are obtained within 30 days. The "three R's" of PTM allow a laboratory to track and positively identify patient specimens as they move through the complete testing process. Specific information must be contained in these three documents in order to comply with the law.

Quality control

Manufacturers of instruments, kits, and test systems usually provide guidelines for quality control (QC) of their products. One kind of internal QC procedure involves the use of QC samples; these samples, similar to patient specimens, have known test results. QC samples, when run at the same time as patient specimens, can provide the operator with a "within run" check to confirm test results.[41] Each laboratory performing nonwaived tests is required to develop and follow written QC procedures that monitor the quality of the analytic testing process of each test method. Of the two sections on QC, one contains general requirements, and the other, special requirements for specialties or subspecialties.

Laboratories using uncleared tests must follow the full QC rules. Full QC rules are also required for all tests of moderate complexity that have been cleared but modified or developed in-house and for all tests of high complexity.

Proficiency testing

One way of making sure a particular laboratory's performance is in line with that of other laboratories performing the same analysis involves the testing of unknown samples from an outside source. Just as QC samples provide a type of internal QC, proficiency testing (PT) offers a kind of external QC. Each laboratory performing tests of moderate or high complexity must enroll in an approved PT program for all specialties or subspecialties in which it desires to be certified. The PT provider must be either a private, nonprofit organization or a federal or state entity. PT is being implemented in stages to enable previously unregulated laboratories to comply with the new rules under CLIA. Newly regulated laboratories must enroll by January 1, 1994. To allow time for these laboratories to learn the PT process, they will not be penalized for failures until 1995 (unless those failures constitute a serious threat to patient health).

Once the laboratory has been enrolled, the PT provider will send samples to its subscriber three times a year; each shipment includes five samples for that "event." The samples, whose values are not known, are run along with the laboratory's regular workload of patient specimens. It is unlawful to send portions of PT samples to other laboratories for "comparison" studies. The final results are sent to the PT provider, together with an attestation form signed by both the operator and the laboratory director. For most tests, the minimum passing score is 80%.[42] Any laboratory failing two consecutive or two out of three testing events will be subject to sanctions (including cancellation for that specialty, subspecialty, or test.)

Quality assurance

Every laboratory performing nonwaived tests must implement and follow written policies and procedures for a quality assurance (QA) program designed to monitor and evaluate the quality of the total testing process. CLIA is the first standard to require a QA program as part of the law. It is the responsibility of the employer, as laboratory director, to assure the accuracy of test results and the adequacy of laboratory services. In a POL, laboratory testing may be done by two workers or one worker and the director; in such cases, all members should make up the QA committee. The QA committee is responsible for making sure that "quality" evaluations take place and that corrective actions take place whenever problems are identified. To reach this goal, at least seven key "elements" must be addressed; a QA audit check list should include the following[43]:

1. *Procedure Manual* (written policies and procedures; review every one, three, or six months)
   - All listed procedures are currently performed and have been approved, signed, and dated by the director; if the directorship has changed, these procedures have been reapproved, signed again, and dated again by the current director.
   - All modifications of current procedures have been approved, signed, and dated by the director.
   - All copies of discontinued procedures have been kept for at least two years.
2. *Personnel Standards* (every 12 months for present staff; every 6 months for new staff)
   Annual review of personnel competence has been documented:
   - Testing personnel have been observed processing (collecting, preparing, identifying, storing, transporting, and discarding) specimens.
   - Testing personnel have been observed performing tests after introducing new instruments or new methods.
   - Testing personnel have been observed perform-

ing tests on previously analyzed samples or PT samples.
   - Testing personnel have been observed performing calibration checks as well as instrument maintenance.
   - Testing personnel have been observed regarding problem-solving skills.
   - Testing personnel have been observed recording and reporting test results.
   - New personnel have received appropriate education and training for their testing responsibilities.
3. *Patient Test Management* (review every one, three, or six months)
   - All criteria for referral of specimens to a reference laboratory have been met; the "turnaround" time for receiving results from a reference laboratory has been found acceptable.
   - The information obtained on all test requisitions and test records has been complete and accurate.
   - Test results that appear inconsistent with relevant criteria (such as patient age, sex, diagnosis, distribution of test results, and relationship with other test parameters) have been identified and evaluated; the number of incorrect test reports has been noted.
   - Based on a random review of final test reports compared to the original worksheets or printouts, test results have been checked for completeness and accuracy, and the number of incorrect reports has been found acceptable; any incorrect result has been corrected or replaced with a corrected copy on the patient's chart.
   - All efforts to store and retrieve test results have been successfully performed.
   - For all specimen rejections and inoperable tests, the course of action stated in the manual has been followed.
4. *Quality Control* (review every one, three, or six months)
   - The manufacturer's recommendations or written protocols for all instruments, kits, or test systems have been followed; all test procedures, as well as the reporting of results, have been performed as outlined in the manual.
   - On each day of testing, control procedures using at least two levels of control materials have been performed and documented.
   - QC results have been reviewed for each "run" to determine if they are in the established range; if the results have been out of limits, this has been evaluated and documented.
   - When the QC result has not been appropriate, the handling of the patient's test results has been

recorded; where problems or errors have occurred, corrective actions have been instituted and documented.

□ All expired reagents, materials, and supplies have been discarded.

5. *Proficiency Testing* (review after receipt of PT results)

□ The laboratory has been enrolled in all applicable PT.

□ For tests with no PT, the accuracy and reliability of those test results have been checked (at least twice yearly).

□ PT results have been reviewed and recorded; all PT documents have been retained by the laboratory for at least two years.

□ For all unsatisfactory PT results, an investigation has been conducted as to possible causes of error; any corrective action taken has been documented.

6. *Complaint Investigations* (review every one, three, or six months)

□ All complaints reported to the laboratory have been documented; the number of complaints has been noted.

□ Any trend with regard to the complaints received has been noted.

□ The resolution of all complaints received has been achieved; when appropriate, corrective actions have been implemented and documented.

7. *Quality Assurance Review* (review every month)

□ All of the previous key elements required for quality assurance have been reviewed and evaluated with the specified frequency.

□ All data collected for each element or for other problems have been reviewed and evaluated by the QA committee.

□ For all problems that have been identified, corrective actions have been devised and documented.

□ For all unsolved problems, either progress has been documented or alternative actions have been devised and documented.

□ Any trend with regard to the problems discovered has been noted.

□ All problems, including breakdowns in communication among laboratory personnel, actions, and resolutions have been discussed and documented.

□ All QA reviews have been approved, signed, and dated by the director.

END NOTES

1. A. McLaughlin and J. Pendergrass, *Hazard Communication— a Compliance Kit* A-1 (U.S. Government Printing Office 1988).
2. L. Traverse, *The Generator's Guide to Hazardous Materials/Waste Management* at 119 (Van Nostrand Reinhold, New York 1991).
3. J. Suchocki et al., *The Safety Resource Guide for OSHA Compliance* at 7 (Eagle Associates, Ann Arbor 1990).
4. Program Notes, Eagle Associates, Inc. Seminar, given by Joseph Suchocki (Apr. 1990).
5. Suchocki, *supra* note 3, at 11.
6. 29 CFR 1910, Subpart Z, Toxic and Hazardous Substances, Occupational Safety and Health Administration (OSHA).
7. *Threshold Limit Values (TLV) for Chemical Substances and Physical Agents in the Work Environment,* (American Conference of Governmental Industrial Hygienists (ACGIH), 6500 Glenway Ave., Bldg. D-5, Cincinnati, OH 45211).
8. *Annual Report on Carcinogens,* (National Toxicology Program, 5285 Port Royal Rd., Springfield, VA 22161).
9. *Monographs* (summary), (International Agency for Research on Cancer, 49 Sheridan St., Albany, NY 12210).
10. Suchocki, *supra* note 3, at 12.
11. *Hazard Communication Changes,* Am. Prac. Adv. at 116 (Apr. 1994).
12. *The Illusive Material Safety Data Sheet,* Am. Prac. Adv. at 120 (Mar. 1993).
13. *Supra* note 11, at 117.
14. *Alert for Material Safety Data Sheets!,* Am. Prac. Adv. at 77 (Jan. 1993).
15. Suchocki, *supra* note 3, at 17.
16. *Questions and Answers,* Am. Prac. Adv. at 10 (Aug. 1992).
17. National Fire Protection Agency (NFPA) 704, *Standard System for the Identification of the Fire Hazards of Materials,* (1990).
18. Suchocki, *supra* note 3, at 15.
19. *Occupational Exposure to Bloodborne Pathogens,* (summary), 29 C.F.R. Part 1910.1030 at 64032.
20. *CDC Study Puts Number of HIV-Infected at about 1 Million,* Am. Med. News at 14 (Jan. 24/31, 1994).
21. *Supra* note 19, at 64055.
22. *Bloodborne Pathogens Program,* All-Med News at 2 (Feb. 1992).
23. C. Hess, *All-Med's OSHA Compliance Office Manual* (All-Med Press, Houston 1992).
24. *Supra* note 19, at 64124.
25. *Supra* note 19, at 64177.
26. W. Rom, *Environmental and Occupational Medicine* at 1351(2nd ed. Little, Brown and Company, Boston 1992).
27. M. Fordney, *Insurance Handbook for the Medical Office* at 297 (3rd ed., W. B. Saunders Co., Philadelphia 1989).
28. J. Rowell, *Understanding Medical Insurance* at 202 (Medical Economics Books, Oradell 1990).
29. *Id.* at 202.
30. Fordney, *supra* note 27, at 305.
31. L. Gant, *The Physician New to Practice* 6(All-Med Press, Houston 1994).
32. Rowell, *supra* note 28, at 205.
33. *Id.* at 207.
34. Rom, *supra* note 26, at 1353.
35. D. Lacey, *Your Rights in the Workplace* at 8/5 (Nolo Press, Berkeley 1992).
36. M. Hoffman, ed., *World Almanac and Book of Facts* at 150 (Pharos Books, New York 1992).
37. *Id.*
38. *CLIA '88 Compliance,* at 4 (American Proficiency Institute 1993).
39. P. Fleury and C. Kaczmarek, *Clinical Laboratory Improvement Workshop* at 7-12 (Physician's Viewpoint Services, Houston 1992). Personnel Standards prepared with the assistance of Patricia Fleury.
40. *Patient Test Management System Trilogy,* Am. Prac. Adv. 61 (Dec. 1992).
41. *Supra* note 38, at 9.
42. *Regulations for Implementing Clinical Laboratory Improvement Amendments of 1988: A Summary,* 267 JAMA at 1731 (Apr. 1992).

CHAPTER 48

Medical technology

C. GORDON HECKEL, M.D., J.D., F.C.L.M.*
MAX KARL NEWMAN, A.B., M.D., F.A.C.P.
DONALD L. NEWMAN, M.D.
STEVEN E. NEWMAN, M.D.

DIAGNOSTIC TECHNOLOGY
CARDIAC SYSTEM
NEUROLOGICAL SYSTEM
DERMATOLOGY
BLOOD VESSELS
GASTROINTESTINAL
CYSTOSCOPY AND ARTHROSCOPY
LEARNING TECHNIQUE
LABORATORY TESTS
BIOMEDICAL EQUIPMENT MANAGEMENT

Health care is a particularly dynamic field. The application of modern science and technology has enhanced the ability of practitioners to diagnose ailments earlier and with greater accuracy than ever before. Treatment not previously available may cure, alleviate symptoms, or even postpone disability or death. Some of the new developments may have been overpublicized, leading to unfounded or unrealistic public expectations.

Some of the enhanced risk of malpractice litigation and liability arises from technological gains. Obviously, were it not possible to use new devices and techniques, there would be no suits over failure to do so. Recent court decisions in certain jurisdictions have permitted juries to deliberate over patients' claims of this kind.

There are a number of legal considerations incident to new technology. With extensive experience and advances in technology, computerized tomography (CT) and positron emission tomography (PET) scanning, magnetic resonance imaging (MRI), and other diagnostic modalities have expanded the scope and value of these devices. The recent advances in medical technology have been incredible and are giving physicians a vast armamentarium of diagnostic and therapeutic modalities. That is the good news. The bad news involves the legal requirement to "keep abreast" or "up-to-date."

The physician today not only has a professional obligation but a legal duty to know what is available, what is the test of choice, and when to use it. These requirements will be tempered by what is available to the physician.

DIAGNOSTIC TECHNOLOGY
Thermography

Thermography is a diagnostic modality for measuring surface body heat, or the lack of, in aiding diagnosis and monitoring therapy of the neuromusculoskeletal system from head to toe. Infrared scanners detect the heat differences on the body surface, which can be indicative of underlying pathology. The procedure determines the physiologic and pathologic change of the underlying microcirculation under sympathetic nervous system control. The temperature pattern communicates information regarding the nature, extent, and severity of the soft/support tissue injury when due to trauma. It is an objective, demonstrable picture of the pathologic process. However, it must always be correlated with the clinical examination to indicate why the pain process exists (since pain is always subjective, but is a valid pathologic condition).

Criticism of the thermographic modality has been intense, because it provides medicolegal information when other imaging modalities, such as electromyography and nerve conduction with evoked potentials, myelography, MRI and CT, and regular X-rays, are normal or questionable. Much of the detractive attitude

*The authors gratefully acknowledge work from previous contributors: Harold L. Hirsh, M.D., J.D., F.C.L.M., and Michael J. Schaffer, D.Sc.

is directed toward its misuse rather its scientific accuracy. To credit or discredit thermography, the procedure should be thought of as scientific and not adversarial.

In comparative studies, the following observations have been made. Where normal lumbar spines (asymptomatic) have been imaged in preemployment X-rays, abnormality of 57% was present in 1172 lumbar spines.[1] Where the imaging was done with myelography in asymptomatic back patients, extradural defects and bulging was found in 24% (myelography done for other levels).[2] In studies on asymptomatic backs by electrophysiological studies (EMG and nerve conduction), more than 20% to 25% demonstrated abnormal motor unit action potentials.[3] With the current intensive use of CT and MRI, where back studies demonstrate disk bulges, protrusions, spinal canal abnormalities, more than 20% were in asymptomatic backs.[4,5] Hence, no more criticisms can be made of thermography as to false-positives than of other modalities of diagnosis. Consequently, thermography is never used alone, but is correlated with clinical examination and the other imaging modalities when they are indefinite.[6]

To enhance the effectiveness, computerized equipment and thermal cooling are now available, permitting more uniform visualization. The color scales alter automatically and maximum focusing occurs. This permits consistency for comparison of results in laboratories so equipped (i.e., symmetries, colors, and dermatome distribution). Where disk bulging is described by other imaging procedures, the physiologic effect on the annulus is to stimulate the sympathetic nervous system, producing a vasoconstriction (cold) or vasodilatation (hot) of the peripheral vessels along the dermatome. This permits objective proof of the subjective complaints of pain, burning, and numbness.

From a medicolegal standpoint, the rules of evidence concerning admissibility of thermographic finding during trial may vary from jurisdiction to jurisdiction, and even within the same jurisdiction. In the past, eight states and the District of Columbia have espoused the *Frye* case or general acceptance standards under the same.[7] Many states have now moved away from this standard as a precondition for accepting novel scientific procedures. More recently, the *Williams* standard (relevancy approach) is based on the Second Circuit U.S. Court of Appeals.[8] Similarly, the Federal Rules of Evidence (FRE) have moved away from general acceptance. Some people believe that local renditions have modified the *Frye* standard to permit admissions of novel scientific methods. Specifically, FRE 702 provides "If scientific or technical, or otherwise technical specialized knowledge will assist the trier of fact or (help) determine the fact in issue, a witness qualified as an expert by knowledge, skill or experience, training or education, may testify thereto in the form of an opinion or otherwise." FRE and the *Williams* case reflect a significant trend on admission of thermographic procedure. FRE, at the discretion of the trial court, permits admissibility in more than 42 states. Most recently the *Daubert* decision would influence the acceptance of thermography as a valid objective imaging procedure.

Roentgenography

Xeroradiography. In conventional film radiographs, density and thickness differences are detected by film density difference or film contrast in the image. In addition to similar broad area contrast differences seen in film radiography, xeroradiography accentuates each interface of thickness difference with edge enhancement. Xeroradiographic images, therefore, provide additional information about the radiographed object that is especially useful when the inherent density differences in the radiographed object are small (e.g., body soft tissues). Xeroradiography has been applied in soft tissue imaging, as well as nonmetallic foreign body localization, bone radiography, and angiography.

The advantages of xeroradiography are that with the wide latitude of density portrayal and edge enhancement, one can simultaneously evaluate the bone structures and soft tissues. In trauma, evaluation of airway disease, and joint problems, this can be employed effectively. Airway evaluation is facilitated by the ability to delineate the pharynx, larynx, respiratory tree, and soft tissues at the same time despite their great X-ray attenuation differences. Foreign body localization is aided by the edge enhancement effect that renders many foreign bodies visible that would not otherwise be seen on conventional radiography. Therefore, these examinations may have significant evidentiary value in trauma cases and cases in which there is a question as to the presence of a foreign body. Another potential use would be in forensic radiology, especially to determine death by strangulation.

X-rays. X-rays penetrate through the body tissues and affect a photographic film in varying degrees, depending on the amount of density that the rays must pass through. The bony structure of the body is readily demonstrated by this medium. Similarly, certain abnormalities of the lungs and heart can be demonstrated. It requires, however, special materials and studies to demonstrate anything in the circulation or, in most cases, in the gastrointestinal tract.

X-rays normally refer to the photographic record of such a study. Fluoroscopy reveals the same findings on a fluorescent screen, but without a permanent record in the form of a photographic film. The following is a list defining the usual X-ray views that are taken: AP refers to anterior-posterior and means that the rays pass from the front of the body through to the back before striking the photographic film. A PA view, or posterior-anterior view, is one in which the rays pass in the opposite direction. Lateral view is one in which the rays pass from one side of the body through to the other before striking the photographic film. Oblique views are views in which the rays pass through obliquely between the two planes of the body. Stereo views consist of two views taken from slightly different angles, resulting in a stereoscopic view, or one having depth when placed in a proper viewing box. The result is similar to the old stereopticon slides in which one gains a three-dimensional effect. Planigrams are special views made by moving both the film and X-ray tube, resulting in a blurring in all but a given level within the body. This clear area can be positioned at a predetermined depth in the body tissues, and often brings out findings that are obscured in a normal X-ray by overlying shadows.

A myelogram or pantopaque study is a special study to outline the spinal canal, which is not ordinarily visible by routine X-rays. It is made by withdrawing a small amount of spinal fluid and replacing it with a special material that casts a heavy shadow within the spinal canal. By use of other special material, namely barium, studies can be made of the gastrointestinal tract, and such a study is commonly referred to as a GI or gastrointestinal series.

Proton radiography. Proton radiography is a technique to improve the diagnosing and detecting of abnormalities such as tumors in the brain, breasts, or other organs, as well as hard-to-detect valvular insufficiencies of the heart. It not only produces better images of the abnormalities, but does so with one-twelfth the radiation exposure of X-rays. The procedure uses accelerated protons—elementary particles that form the nuclei of hydrogen atoms—rather than X-rays to penetrate the subjects to produce the internal images.

Photon imaging

Imaging with photons refers to the formation of a replica of an object. What is seen is not the object but the photons reflected from the surface of the object. Photons are generated when the charged particles go from a higher to a lower energy state. The concept originates in the electromagnetic spectrum, and partakes of the physical characteristics of oscillation and frequency (wavelengths). The visible photons are reflected from an opaque surface, like the skin, transformed into electrical impulses with the thermographic unit, form a visible image on a closed-circuit television screen, and photographed. When photons penetrate the body as radio waves (MRI) or X-rays (CT scan, PET, SPECT, DSA),

the ability to visualize the anatomical and physiological structures results.

Recent advances in neuroimaging techniques of the closed head injury permit more accurate and speedy diagnosis, within minutes of trauma, of the extent of anatomic and physiologic damage to the brain tissue. The techniques include the following:

1. *Diffusion-weighted MRI:* It detects the rush of water through the injured brain cells, giving objective information as to size, location, and severity of the damaged ischemic area, as well as the potential of drugs to ameliorate the results of the pathological condition. Repeat testing affords prognostic information "within a few minutes." As always, correlation with the neurological examination is necessary.

2. *Perfusion MRI:* It is faster than PET or SPECT scanning. While taking ultrafast images, a standard contrast agent is intravenously injected to enhance the MRI image. Normal tissue loses the MRI image signal, and traumatized areas that are ischemic do not.

   Usually, both diffusion-weighted and perfusion MRI procedures are advised in tandem, so as to give a complete picture of the traumatized area that is ischemic.

3. *Echoplanar imaging:* This procedure utilizes ultrasound equipment. It details the degree of brain tissue damage. It is much faster than the preceding two MRI procedures. Visualization is achieved in seconds and allows for rapid localization.

4. *Holographic process (Voxel):* It gives a 3D image of the brain. It can also be used for any anatomic area, preceded by MRI and CT scanning, or even ordinary X-rays. It is noninvasive and generates images from digital data of the scans. This permits early treatment, especially surgical procedures, by visualizing the anatomic structures as they appear in the body or cranial vault anatomically. To make the hologram from CT and MRI images, a holographic laser camera takes films that are similar to ordinary X-ray film, but the image appears in 3D. This equipment has been developed by the Vozel Co. of California, and has been adequately tested in many radiographic laboratories in this country and overseas.

Nuclear magnetic resonance imaging (MRI). Nuclear magnetic resonance tomography is capable of producing cross-section images similar to those obtained by CT. Unlike CT, it does not use ionizing radiation, but rather utilizes an apparently safe interaction between magnetic fields, radio waves, and atomic nuclei. In addition, it shows hydrogen density in thin slices rather than depicting tissue electron density as does CT. The pictures obtained by this new imaging technique are potentially more useful than those obtained by CT.

The strength of the MRI signal depends on the hydrogen density and on the magnetic relaxation times (T_1 and T_2) that are dependent on temperature, viscosity, and magnetic interaction. The intrinsic differences in hydrogen density and T_1 and T_2 of fat, muscle, blood, and bone are major determinants of contrast in the MRI image. Since these differences are significantly greater than those of the equivalent determinant of X-ray contrast (electron density), there is much more contrast in an MRI image than in its X-ray equivalent.

It has been reported that in certain instances, MRI tomography has proved superior to CT. While CT distinguishes tissues on the basis of a single window-level control for X-ray attenuation, MRI tomography can provide the equivalent of three window-level controls for hydrogen and T_1 and T_2.

MRI imaging can readily distinguish brain tumors from normal brain tissue, not only on the basis of altered anatomy, but also on the basis of high water content due to hypervascularity or reactive edema. This technique can also detect multiple sclerosis and other demyelinating diseases, and also atherosclerotic plaques in the carotid arteries. Images of the temporal and posterior fossae at the base of the skull are clearly superior to those provided by CT, particularly because of a lack of bone artifacts. MRI tomography can demonstrate structures that have never been visualized by CT scanning, such as the substantia nigra in the brain stem.

A 15-kilogauss MRI scanner has captured the first sodium MRI images of human beings in the world. Such images can yield information that may in the future be used to noninvasively delineate areas of tissue damage caused by stroke, heart attack, kidney disease, and other disorders.

Called a multinuclear scanner, the MRI unit is said to be powerful enough to produce images of the nuclei of several different elements, including sodium, phosphorous, and hydrogen. It is also capable of separately imaging hydrogen compounds, such as fats, carbohydrates, and metabolites.

With MRI, we are able to do chemical analysis of a human body point by point and study the body's various compounds. The stronger the magnetic field, the more compounds we can see. The implications of this for the diagnosis and management of disease are enormous.

Never before have we been able to look inside the human body with such detail and clarity. With these high-resolution scans, we now can distinguish small structures in the gray matter of the brain, for example, that may play a role in diseases such as Alzheimer's, Parkinson's, and Huntington's.

Sodium imaging differs from the more familiar hydrogen (or proton) imaging in that hydrogen pictures describe anatomy, while sodium images detail function. A cell that is damaged, dying, or dead will show an increase in sodium.

The researchers also have obtained phosphorus images from animals and anticipate producing such images from humans in the future. Phosphorus images are expected to involve longer scan times than sodium images because of the lower concentration of phosphorus in human tissue. (At present, it takes 35 minutes to obtain 32 slices for a sodium study.) Techniques to increase imaging speed are under development.

Computerized tomography (CT). The CT image is a cross-sectional radiographic view of the body that can be used for the identification of many disease entities and anatomical anomalies.

Computed tomography works on the same principle of different absorption characteristics of body tissues, but the detectors used are much more sensitive than X-ray film. Unlike a conventional X-ray image of the head that reveals the bone of the skull and the soft tissue of the scalp, a CT scan of the head depicts a slice of the brain with its convolutions and ventricular system. The slice is so-called because the CT image depicts a tomographic plane of the area studied equivalent to a cross-sectional anatomical specimen. Although injection of an intravenous contrast agent may be necessary in some cases to differentiate normal tissues and organs from invasive abnormal lesions, CT is a painless, noninvasive imaging procedure that carries no more radiation than a conventional barium enema exam. Major improvements have occurred in CT scanners since the original machine.

CT has become a diagnostic tool of major importance for all parts of the body. In some cases, it may be the only way to rule in or out a serious disease, especially the presence or absence of a tumor. It can also eliminate the need for other diagnostic procedures or, when necessary, be an effective adjunct to the planning and follow-up of surgery, radiation therapy, and chemotherapy.

Reconstructive or computerized tomography is a new imaging concept that employs mathematical principles that were formerly used in astronomy and electron microscopy to form images of orbital and molecular structures. The difference is that with the present application, pictures of structures in the body are created.

Any summary description of presently and potentially available CT units is necessarily dated. Advances are continually made in this highly competitive area. Augmented imaging and display capabilities of dedicated small computers with regard to flexibility, independence, and convenience are occurring. The computer-based image processing, analysis, and display techniques potentially contribute additional information to the computerized tomographic capabilities.

Computerized axial tomography represents an appropriate use and adaptation of existing technology to the health sciences. The potential of tissue characterization from quantization of X-ray absorption offers the promise of markedly improving diagnostic specificity. Because of public awareness, the great immediate acceptance by the medical profession, and the potential economic impact in health cost and planning, the use of these images as evidence is increasing.

Positron emission tomography (PET scanning). PET is an imaging technique that measures the location and concentration of physiologically active components (i.e., metabolism of the organ), and allows the detection of atrophy, necrosis, and scarring, especially for head injuries and brain disorders. It is superior in these aspects to MRI and CT scanning, and is also used in heart trauma.

Single-photon emission computerized tomography (SPECT). SPECT produces three-dimensional images of the concentrated radiopharmacals with an organ. It does not require a cyclotron, as in PET scanning, to activate the pharmaceutical—technetium 99 or iodine 23—and the image is reconstructed as in CT.

Radionuclide imaging. Radionuclide studies are diagnostically useful in selected situations. Radionuclide bone scans with technetium 99m, methylene diphosphonate (MDP), or a similar radiotracer are helpful in the diagnostic evaluation of musculoskeletal injuries. Gaseous metastases are best detected by radionuclide study. Bone scans have been reported to be 96% accurate in detecting nonvertebral metastases.

Radionuclide techniques can be used to visualize myocardial perfusion, particularly during stress, and are thought to be a somewhat more sensitive test for coronary artery disease than the stress ECG. The addition of CT techniques can give a three-dimensional view of cardiac muscle perfusion.

Another technique, in which radioactive tracers are selectively taken up by irreversibly damaged myocardium, can detect myocardial necrosis as early as 4 hours after an infarction, but it is most sensitive 36 to 48 hours afterward. Nuclear medicine studies have their greatest value several days after a suspected or acute myocardial infarction.

Some persons will prefer radionuclide scanning for detecting pulmonary embolism. Use of the renal scan as a diagnostic test has been advocated because this procedure gives excellent visualization of the renal parenchyma. Radionuclide studies have been useful in the evaluation of functioning adrenocortical tumors and hyperplasia.

One advantage of radionuclide scans is that the entire body can be visualized, and they can be used in the diagnosis of abscesses by indium-treated leukocytes.

However, the isotope concentrates in all inflamed tissues and is therefore less specific in some situations than among other imaging techniques.

Radionuclide scanning is proving valuable in screening for the spread of malignant disease and in studying physiological processes. It will differentiate a pseudo mass from a true mass.

Ultrasound. The use of reflected sound waves from interfaces of different densities in the body to create anatomical images has become another important diagnostic modality. This imaging technique has the capability to portray detailed anatomical structures by a noninvasive method that does not appear to have clinically significant biological effects.

The basic principle of ultrasonic imaging involves the detection of reflected sound waves. The acoustic waves are initially generated by a transducer that, after sending the sound wave into the patient, also acts as a receiver to record the reflections from structures in the body. The transducer crystal is excited by a brief electrical signal that thickens the crystal by several microns. As the signal is released, the crystal returns to its former size. With these periodic changes in thickness, the skin surface (to which the transducer is applied) is moved, setting up periodic waves of compression and decompression within the tissues underlying the patient's skin. The transducer relaxes after the signal is sent, and in this state acts as a receiver for the returning wave pulses (echoes). Returning acoustic waves push and pull at the transducer face, and, because of a property of the crystal substance, generate electrical signals. From a knowledge of the speed of sound waves in tissue and the time lapse between signals, the distance from the transducer to the interface creating the echo is determined.

The echoes, after being converted to an electrical signal whose amplitude is proportional to the strength of the reflected ultrasound energy and whose occurrence in time is proportional to the delay in time of the reflected energy, can be made into an image form by modulating the intensity of an electron beam that sweeps the face of an oscilloscope. When the electron beam strikes the phosphor on the oscilloscope face, light is emitted in proportion to the intensity of the exciting electron beam. In brightness-modulated display (B-scan), the echo information is displayed as intensified points of illumination on a cathode-ray tube, on which the location of the intensified point is proportional to the delay time in the detected signal and the brightness is proportional to its energy content. The multiple data points thus provide a two-dimensional cross-sectional visualization of anatomical structures. This image can be taken from the viewing display by exposing a photographic or X-ray film to the oscilloscope face. This range of reflected ultrasonic energy is then assigned a shade of gray in the copy format in a continuous fashion according to the characteristics of the film.

To better visualize small echoes from anatomical structures, gray-scale capability has been added to B-scan systems. This has been achieved by the use of scan conversion storage tubes. With this type of electronic storage tube, the electrical charge is stored at any given location in direct proportion to the signal imposed on it.

Ultrasound has been utilized most effectively in obstetrics and gynecology, but has gained quite extensive use in cardiac examinations because of its ability to accurately record physiological, time-varying events such as cardiac valve motion. More recently, with improved resolution, abdominal imaging with ultrasound has been extensively employed for many medical abnormalities. It is particularly useful in determining whether a tumor is a fluid-filled cyst or a solid lesion. Liver, kidney, splenic, and pancreatic abnormalities are also readily diagnosed by this imaging technique.

A significant new development in ultrasonography has been multicrystal transducer fabrication that allows real-time imaging. "Real time" refers to the ability to image physiological events through rapid electronic circuitry placed in the reception mode. This cycle is repeated for each element in sequence with a repetition of many complete frames per second.

The video signal of returning echoes for each element is displayed as intensity or brightness spots (B-mode) on the vertical axis of the video monitor that correspond to the relative position of each element in the transducer. All data are stored on magnetic videotape for subsequent examination and photography. A wide field of view diminishes the chance of error due to improper transducer positioning or angulation.

Ultrasound compression technique. An ultrasound test of the lower extremities using a simple compression technique can assume a vital role as a quick screen for deep vein thrombosis. The easy-to-administer test requires no special equipment except a conventional ultrasound scanner and relies on compression to locate the venous thrombi. A normal vein collapses on light pressure from the ultrasound transducer, but the presence of a thrombus prevents compression of the vessel walls, giving a positive scan.

The ultrasound test requires only 10 to 15 minutes and is an easily learned technique. The test has become routine at hospitals, and use of venography has fallen dramatically.

Digital image processing. Digital image processing can be defined as computer manipulation of the original image to produce a new or processed image. Image enhancement is used to make certain features more apparent visually. Deriving a functional image allows the depiction of the spatial distribution of some parameter other than the one that was imaged directly. It can be used in addition to echocardiography, radionuclide imaging, and computed tomography.

CARDIAC SYSTEM
Electrocardiogram and vectorcardiogram

The role and medicolegal status of the electrocardiogram (ECG) is well established. The vectorcardiogram is a recording of the changes in spatial orientation, direction, and magnitude of the electrical activity generated by the heart. Unlike the conventional scalar ECG, which records the voltage developed during the cardiac cycle on a time scale, the vectorcardiogram demonstrates the sequence, direction, magnitude, and distribution of forces generated by the heart. The ECG and the vectorcardiogram present, in different forms, information derived from a single series of electrical events.

Pneumatic antishock garment (MAST)

External counterpressure supplied by inflation of the pneumatic antishock garment (MAST) may help to control massive bleeding, particularly in the presence of shock. When this measure fails to stop pelvic blood loss, arterial injuries should be suspected; arteriography may be lifesaving. The source of bleeding can be defined and transcatheter embolization of the bleeding arteries can then be performed, using either autologous clot or synthetic thrombogenic agents.

Angiography

Subtraction angiography is a technique by which the fluoroscopic X-ray image is digitized, and the computer subtracts the image made before the injection of the contrast medium from that made after the injection of the contrast medium. This subtracts, or eliminates, the bony structures, allowing excellent vascular images to be obtained free of the overlying vertebrae. The contrast material is injected intravenously rather than through arterial puncture and catheterization.

Coronary arteriography is the study of the anatomy of the coronary vessels in living subjects employing roentgenographic contrast material. It is useful in the study of atherosclerosis and other structural abnormalities affecting the coronary circulation. "Arteriography" and "angiography" are not really synonymous, the latter referring to all blood vessels rather than arteries alone, but in general usage and in this discussion the terms are used interchangeably.

Selective coronary arteriography permits the determination of the presence and severity of vascular obstruction and the detection of collateral vessels. An important application of this technique is the postoperative assessment of direct (endarterectomy, vein graft) and indirect (mammary artery implantation) myocardial revascularization procedures. The patency of the implant as well as collateral vessel formation and progression of obstructive disease may be determined.

Selective coronary angiography is often performed as part of each preoperative catheterization in patients beyond middle age. The coronary angiogram may be helpful in deciding whether some of the patient's symptoms are caused by coronary atherosclerosis (i.e., angina pectoris in the presence of aortic stenosis), and which vessels may be used if selective coronary perfusion is required during surgery.

Patients who have proven or suspected coronary artery disease may be considered for surgical treatment if response to medical therapy is inadequate. Selective coronary angiography is essential, since application of direct and indirect myocardial revascularization procedures requires detailed knowledge of the severity and distribution of obstructive lesions, and the extent of "runoff" (qualitative blood flow) and collateralization. Angiography of venous bypass grafts is performed shortly after surgery so that nonpatent grafts may be reconstructed.

Cardiac catheterization

The term *cardiac catheterization* refers to several techniques that permit the intubation of the chambers of the heart and great vessels. Positioning of catheters in these structures makes possible measurement of pressure, sampling of blood, and the injection of certain substances to evaluate function and structure.

Catheterization procedures are performed in laboratories equipped with special roentgen equipment and apparatus to monitor and record pressure curves and detect indicator substances. Blood and respiratory gas analyses and other chemical studies are carried out in the "support" laboratory. Although many aspects of thermodynamic function and cardiovascular structure can be evaluated by cardiac catheterization, the type and amount of data required at each study will vary with the lesion in question.

The use of clinical catheterization techniques to obtain information about basic cardiac functions increases the capacity to evaluate cardiac performance and follow the natural history of disease. Replacement of electrodes (via a catheter) in both the right atrium and right ventricle permits the sequential recording of electrical activity. This record delineates the site of conduction disturbances (His's bundle electrogram).

Pressures in the cardiac chambers and great vessels may be recorded continuously. The physician identifies the site of origin of a particular pressure curve by locating the catheter tip on fluoroscopy and recognizing the curve form.

The information recorded at cardiac catheterization may be used to calculate data that permit more sophisticated cardiac evaluation. By means of appropriate formulas the valve areas, cardiac output, vascular resistance, and shunt flows may be determined. More basic parameters of cardiac function, such as the tension-time index, cardiac work, and the rate of systolic ejection, may be determined and are useful in assessing the performance of the heart.

Abnormal communications between cardiac chambers (atrial or ventricular septal defects), between vessels and chambers (sinus of Valsalva–right atrial fistula), or between vessels (patent ductus arteriosus) permit "shunting" of blood from areas of higher pressure to areas of lower pressure. Duration of systole and diastole can be measured directly from pressure traces.

Natural components of blood, such as lactate and pyruvate, may be detected and measured, as well as substances (dyes, gases, radioactive materials) injected for special studies. In appraising the therapeutic efficacy of antianginal agents, determination of coronary blood flow has an immediate practical value.

Evaluating myocardial metabolism provides an explanation, in chemical terms, for some clinical occurrences. Myocardial ischemia, the condition most frequently evaluated, is the foremost example of the useful application of this technique. This determination has assumed added significance in light of the need to evaluate the effects of coronary artery reconstructive surgical procedures on coronary blood flow.

Most cardiologists agree to catheterizing all patients proposed for surgery. The information thus obtained usually substantiates the clinical diagnosis, sometimes reveals unsuspected cardiac lesions, and is often helpful in determining the type of surgical procedure required. Moreover, the extent of the procedure may be more accurately determined in the presence of multiple lesions.

Left ventriculography performed at the time of cardiac catheterization permits evaluation of the systolic excursion of the chamber wall, which helps determine the site of mammary artery implantation. Moreover, it helps determine the feasibility and possible benefits of surgical removal of an aneurysm or noncontractile area. Left ventriculograms taken in systole and diastole can be used to calculate the amount of blood ejected with each contraction (ejection fraction), an important parameter of ventricular function.

Cardiac catheterization performed at regular intervals following cardiac surgery permits assessment of immediate and long-term results. The rapidity of postoperative hemodynamic changes may be determined, and deterioration that might require reoperation can be detected. Moreover, the data recorded here and in similar cases (operated and nonoperated) give the surgeon a benchmark for deciding when in the course of a specific lesion, surgery offers the greatest promise, if at all. Postoperative evaluation permits assessment of anatomical and physiological changes following surgery, in addition to allowing recognition of remaining defects. Following myocardial revascularization, implanted vessels, bypass grafts, and endarterectomized vessels will be assessed for patency and filling of collateral vessels.

Patients with symptomatic heart disease of undetermined type may be treated more efficiently when a proper anatomical diagnosis is established.

Constrictive pericarditis may be demonstrated and cured surgically, silent valvular lesions may be detected, and the presence of significant coronary disease established, in patients with atypical angina pectoris.

A small percentage of patients have asymptomatic heart disease that cannot be definitely diagnosed clinically but may have pathological manifestations that would require surgery.

Occasionally it becomes necessary to catheterize a patient to obtain information for other than medical reasons. Thus atypical chest discomfort in a patient who should be excluded from some occupations (e.g., airplane pilot) may be evaluated by selective coronary catheterization and angiography to ascertain the presence of coronary artery obstruction.

A hemodynamic evaluation in the presence of functional or organic heart murmurs (e.g., a systolic ejection murmur at the left sternal border that may be functional or represent pulmonic stenosis or idiopathic dilation of the pulmonary artery) may benefit the patient in terms of employability or insurance coverage. In a younger patient, participation in athletics and choice of career, such as military service, may depend on information obtained at cardiac catheterization.

Echocardiography

Echocardiography or ultrasound cardiography is a technique in which echoes from pulsed high-frequency sound waves are used to locate and study the movements and dimensions of cardiac structures, such as valve leaflets and chamber walls. The ultrasound beam *tracks* the motion of the cardiac structures over a period of time. Thus, in its simplest terms, echocardiography is a time-motion study.

Information gleaned from echocardiography can be used to pinpoint certain specific abnormalities and malfunctions and furnish direction for diagnostic study. The advantage of this technique is that it is noninvasive (does not use injected contrast media). Because echocardiography can be performed by mobile equipment at the patient's bedside or in the office, it is both a valuable

screening device for early diagnosis and a useful technique for observing serial changes over an extended period. Even with a low index of suspicion it can be fruitfully employed without any morbidity or inconvenience.

Echocardiography has certain limitations. Although it yields important diagnostic information for many lesions, for others, it is much less definitive. It often furnishes corroborative information, as in mitral insufficiency. In many disorders, it must be used in conjunction with cardiac catheterization to give a complete picture.

Echocardiography can directly visualize intracardiac events. The technique is now useful in establishing diagnosis and evaluating the severity of the following disorders:

- Mitral stenosis and insufficiency
- Tricuspid stenosis
- Pericardial effusion
- Idiopathic hypertrophic subaortic stenosis
- Prolapsed mitral valve leaflet syndrome
- Atrial tumors (myxomas and thrombi)
- Atrial septal defects
- Malfunction of prosthetic valves
- Ebstein's anomaly
- Multiple congenital defects of neonates and infants.

Other than for diagnosis of lesions, echocardiography and ultrasound cardiography are also useful in assessing cardiac function. Clinically relevant measurements, such as cardiac output and ejection fraction, can be made in both the resting and dynamic state to assist in evaluating the heart, both as muscle and pump. Echocardiography can yield direct recordings of the motion of the mitral valve leaflets, the interventricular septum, the left ventricular and atrial walls, and the aortic anulus. In addition, it allows measurement of the size of the cardiac chambers and of the changes in chamber dimensions with cardiac activity. It also permits recognition of abnormal filling defects, such as atrial tumors. The echocardiogram has the advantage of directly displaying these events. In general, echocardiography is used in conjunction with other diagnostic tools and is not the final diagnostic step, especially when surgery is contemplated.

Phonocardiography

Phonocardiography is a graphic recording of external pulse waves (carotid and jugular) or of chest wall movement (apexcardiography). It is an external manifestation of the intracardiac mechanical occurrences that produce them. The technique allows for the recording of heart sounds and correlating them with other extracardiac events, such as the external carotid pulse or apexcardiogram (apical chest wall movements).

It has proven useful in diagnosis and teaching. The limitations of the externally recorded carotid pulse and apexcardiogram for timing heart sounds are inherent in their representing only indirectly intracardiac events.

Respiratory impedance pneumography

Respiratory impedance pneumography measures both rib cage and abdominal movements and computes rate and tidal volume with a microprocessor system. It is the only modality established as accurate. It has proved useful in early detection of pulmonary catastrophes caused by pulmonary embolism, acute pulmonary edema, bronchospasm, and aspiration of gastric contents. It is also useful for weaning patients from mechanical ventilation.

Digital subtraction angiography

Digital subtraction angiography employs subtraction from the initial image by computer, after an injection of a chemical bolus. It is used mainly in injuries and disease of the heart and arteries.

Cardiac pacemaking

Pacing the heart is a form of therapy. This success in the treatment of heart block led to broadened indications for temporary and permanent pacemaker implantation. Managing bradycardias not related to heart block, prophylaxis against heart block in certain cases of acute myocardial infarction, terminating atrial and ventricular tachyarrhythmias inhibiting atrial and ventricular extrasystoles and tachycardias, and assisting cardiac output during recovery after cardiac surgery now lie within the widened therapeutic use of pacemakers. Reliable control of the heartbeat in patients with bradycardia caused by complete heart block is a reality. It has become an established mode of therapy for management of complete heart block.

Automatic implantable cardioverter-defibrillator

The automatic implantable cardioverter-defibrillator (AICD) is an electronic unit intended to prevent sudden cardiac death in high-risk patients. It is designed to sense when ventricular tachycardia or fibrillation occurs and automatically terminate them with high-energy, synchronized electrical shocks. This therapeutic modality has resulted in an impressive decrease in sudden death mortality. The potential risks and dangers associated with the AICD in high-risk patients are moderate and often unavoidable.

Holter recording

A Holter recording is a continuous magnetic tape recording of a patient's ECG, customarily recorded for a period of 10 to 24 hours. Standard electrodes are attached to the patient's chest and leads connected to a compact portable tape recorder. The recorder can be carried over the patient's shoulder like a camera while he or she is active, or placed beside the patient during rest or sleep. The patient follows his or her normal or prescribed routine during the recording period and keeps a diary, noting the time of any symptoms experienced or any unusual activity performed. When the recording is completed, the patient returns the tape and recorder along with the diary.

Special instrumentation operated by skilled personnel is utilized to examine the tape recording for arrythmias, conduction abnormalities, and other morphological changes. Detected abnormalities are printed, with time preference, on standard ECG chart paper for detailed analysis by the physician.

The performance of a Holter recording thus has three distinct and separable phases: obtaining the recording on the patient, analyzing the recording for abnormal phenomena, and interpreting the significance of the detected phenomena within the context of the total clinical picture presented by the patient.

Patients who have had a major myocardial infarction may benefit from continuous ECG monitoring, according to a study that showed a direct link between silent ischemia and sudden death. The monitoring may help physicians identify those patients who might benefit from aggressive therapy, such as bypass surgery or angioplasty.

NEUROLOGICAL SYSTEM
Electrophysiologic testing

Electrophysiologic testing modalities are used in determining neural damage in the central nervous system (CNS) as well as the peripheral nervous system (PNS). The EEG is also used to determine brain damage and abnormal function. The nerve conduction is used for motor and sensory peripheral nerve damage, along with the late reflexes, i.e., F-latency and H-reflex, and occasionally the blink reflex. A further extension of testing partakes of evoked potentials, which monitor the CNS and the sensory PNS.

Electromyography. Electromyography (EMG) demonstrates the MUAP on an oscilloscope screen, accompanied by sound produced in the audioamplifying system (may be computerized). A videotape can be produced for displaying the abnormalities and can demonstrate the same under legal auspices. Thus, the effects of trauma can be objectively demonstrative evidence of the trauma. Information as to the patency of motor nerve roots due to bulging or ruptured disks, when combined with clinical examination, verify the nerve damage. The MUAP is characterized by its duration, amplitude, insertional potentials, interference pattern, and spontaneous motor unit activity frequency, and the morphologic characteristics of the MUAP, as well as recruitment. These objective characteristics demonstrate evaluation as to nerve root irritation or compression, peripheral motor neuropathy, or myopathic changes associated with the traumatic incident. Therefore, this type of modality is useful in determining the presence of ruptured intervertebral disks, severed or severely damaged peripheral motor nerves, and skeletal muscle abnormalities.

Nerve conduction. Nerve conduction is both sensory and motor of the mixed peripheral nerve or the individual sensory or motor nerve. The same apparatus is used. Surface electrodes are usually used; needles are used only in certain circumstances. When the myelin sheaths of the nerve are damaged, sensory nerve conduction is slowed; when the axone is damaged, slowing of the motor component results. However, both pathological states may be present. To further augment these observations, the late reflexes are included: H-reflex for the sensory and F-latency for the motor portions of the peripheral nerve. The blink reflex may be included in the conduction studies. Epidural nerve conduction improves the aptitude for the diagnosis of nerve root entrapment problems in the spinal column. This procedure supplements and aids in the conventional EMG studies done for "ruptured disks" compressing nerve roots.[9]

Evoked potentials of the somatosensory group. This study is conducted by the physician physiatrist or neurologist. It is a test of the sensory pathways of the CNS and PNS. Stimulation of the peripheral nerve with a cephalic recording serves to observe the polarity and latency, amplitude, and dispersion. Recordings may also be made at the spinal cord levels to further localize the pathologic lesions. The limb lengths and the body size are also taken. Testing is done such that side-by-side differences are noted. Uses are that of determining peripheral nerve trauma, radiculopathies, plexopathies, demyelinating disease, and injuries (M.S.). CNS patterns are that of visual evoked potentials, brain AEP, and SSEP abnormalities due to spinal and cerebral trauma.

Surface electromyography. This procedure is carried out with a surface electrode attached. For situations in which the surface electrode is moved, it is termed scanning electrode surface EMG. These procedures measure the quantity of electrical activity of striated (skeletal) muscle.[10] This is of value in psychophysiologic and chronic pain assessment.

Electroencephalography

An electroencephalograph (EEG) is a standardized procedure that is an extension of the clinical study of cerebral disease.

The EEG records amplify brain rhythms typically from 16 simultaneous areas of the scalp, usually with a pen writer on moving paper, resulting in voltage/time graph. The procedure is painless and does not require the input of the patient. Patients keep their eyes closed yet remain awake. Activating procedures to elicit abnormal brain rhythms typically include hyperventilation for a minimum of three minutes, stroboscopic visual stimulation at multiple flash frequencies, and either spontaneous or medication-induced sleep.

The average procedure should include a minimum of 30 minutes of recording time. Special procedures may include recording continuously over 24 hours, all-night sleep studies, sleep deprivation, and, rarely, chemical stimulation. It is not usually necessary to discontinue medications for an EEG (e.g., anticonvulsants in patients suspected of having seizures).

Indications for performance and the type of EEG selected may improve its sensitivity dependent on the suspected diagnosis: epilepsy (seizures, space-occupying cerebral conditions such as tumors, hemorrhage, abscess), strokes and other vascular disease, brain injury from trauma (concussion with, or without loss of consciousness), metabolic disease and coma, brain death, and other diseases, e.g., multiple sclerosis. Frequently, serial records are necessary to demonstrate evolution of suspected abnormalities. The sensitivity of the EEG is dependent on multiple factors, and the absence of abnormality is not considered to indicate absence of the suspected disease. Although most studies will detect abnormal electrical brain activity during a seizure, approximately half the studies will appear normal between seizures. Similarly, the sensitivity of this study is limited in the other indications above. Conversely, there are some EEG abnormalities that might have no clinical significance. As with all laboratory results, they are meaningful only in relation to the clinical findings.

Evoked potentials utilize computer averaging techniques to detect minute brain responses from ongoing brain electrical activity. Detection and quantification of sensory abnormalities not otherwise confirmed electrophysiologically may be clinically helpful when symptoms indicate, e.g., visual evoked potentials, brain stem (auditory) evoked potentials, somatosensory (motor) evoked potentials, and dermatosensory (sensory) evoked potentials. The caveats of recording techniques are even more critical than for a standard EEG and take into account the patient's interference in test performance, stimulus strengths, artifact rejection ratios, and reproducibility of the responses, all of which can affect the quality of interpretation.

Interpretation of EEG recordings requires several years of training and experience. The person reading should have been recognized as meeting or exceeding the standards of the examining board, to enhance accuracy and consistency of reliability of interpretation.

Pain

Pain is a specific disease entity[11] "sometimes relieved by simple suggestion, and other times resistant to destructive neurosurgery." Pain is one of the most common symptoms and one of the most challenging.[12] In simple terms, it is an unpleasant sensory and emotional experience with actual or partial tissue damage, or described in terms of such damage. The specialist is frequently termed an *algologist* (usually a physiatrist or neurologist). The two pain-oriented groups studying the problems are the American Academy of Pain Medicine and the American Academy of Pain Management.

Pain experience has two major components: (1) a localizing component, which produces the somatic sensation (points to pathology and diagnosis); and (2) an alerting and affective component, which is involved in chronic pain. The latter accounts for the extensive medicolegal confrontations (and equally accounts for the extensive employment of multiple and repeated examinations). The anatomy and physiology cannot be detailed here: Nociceptive nerves, present in all tissues and sensory, respond to noxious stimuli of pathologic conditions (injury), transmit the irritation to the spinal cord, and end in the brain, being modified in the entire pathway by endorphins and enkephalins, etc. The brain collates the information and, based on previous experiences, gives the sensation of pain. To validate the pain organically, all recording equipment is used at these anatomic levels. Many of the objectifying procedures have been mentioned in the body of this section (and chronic pain is medically objective by massive thick medical charts).

The following technological procedures are used to validate pain existence.

1. *History and physical examination:* It is described as mild, minor, mediocre, moderate, substantial, severe, quite severe, very severe, extremely severe, profoundly severe, total, etc.[13] Regardless of the test employed, the positive or negative causes for pain must be correlated with the physician history and physical.
2. *Psychological testing:* This must take into account the age, sex, cultural background, educational level, and impending litigation status.
   a. The MMPI test is used most often; the abbreviated form has 399 questions.[14] High scores usually indicate hypochondriasis, depression, hysteria.
   b. The Eysenck Personality Test (EPI) measures stability versus neuroticism, and introversion versus extraversion. Indicates stability of reaction to stress and tendency to break down.[15]
   c. The Beck Depression Inventory has 21 items for measuring depression.[16,17]

There are as many variations of psychological tests as there are psychologists[18]:

1. *Anatomic:* X-rays (plain, myelographic with contrast and CT), CT, ultrasound scan, MRI.
2. *Physiologic:* thermography, electrodiagnostic (EMG, NC, EP).
3. Spinal cord evaluation with Faro-Metrecom.
4. *Mechanical:* Provides an objective and quantitative method to determine the association of pathological conditions and pain production.
   a. *Pressure threshold meter (PTM):* Determines the minimum amount of pressure to produce a pain sensation. Where trigger points, fibrositic nodules, or an inflammatory reaction is present, their anatomic presence can be compared over injured areas, validating the pain complaints.
   b. *Pressure tolerance meter:* Used with the PTM concomitantly. Determines the sensitivity to pain and tenderness, comparing injured and noninjured sites.
   c. *Tissue compliance meter:* Documents the muscle spasm present due to peripheral nerve, nerve root, or muscle injury. Muscle spasm is painful.
   d. *Dynamometer:* Measures skeletal or striated muscle strength in terms of percentage of normal as compared to normal side. This area can be correlated with pain produced on the clinical examination of the injured part.
   e. *Electrical skin resistance recording:* Measures the activity of the sympathetic nerve fibers contained in the peripheral sensory nerve.

These evaluations are dependent on repetitions. Where inconsistent, they indicate no injury or recovery from injury. Where repetition is consistent in findings, they represent actual reasons on an anatomic and physiologic level for the logical complaints of pain. Hence, a mechanical test validates values both for the plaintiff and defense—assuming clinical correlation with the physical examination and other imaging procedures.[19]

DERMATOLOGY
CO_2 laser

Because it is absorbed by the water that is present in tissue, the CO_2 laser has become the most useful system in dermatology and in some other surgical disciplines as well.

Percutaneous laser thermal angioplasty has extended the technique for coronary arteries. Until recently the laser procedure has been used in the treatment of high-grade stenoses in the coronary arteries, but the technique now has been extended to use in peripheral blood vessel obstruction.

BLOOD VESSELS
Argon laser

The argon laser is a new weapon for treating peripheral vascular disease involving a blockage in the leg vessels. This technological tool is used to aid balloon angioplasty, in which a tiny balloon is inflated in a blocked vessel to open up the passageway.

With the laser, physicians are now able to use angioplasty to treat more patients suffering from advanced vascular disease. In the past, the only option these patients had was bypass surgery.

The treatment, formally known as *laser-assisted percutaneous transluminal angioplasty,* is used to treat those patients whose arteries are completely blocked. Because of this obstruction, a balloon catheter cannot penetrate the vessel. With the argon laser, however, the physician can open a channel through the blockage. Then the balloon can be inserted in the artery to clear the remaining obstruction.

The technique will benefit those who suffer from poor circulation in the legs, cramps in their calves, pain in the legs when resting or walking, or sores on their feet that do not heal.

The procedure is performed with the patient under light sedation and local anesthesia, and no surgical incision is necessary. Patients usually spend no more than a day in the hospital. Most return to their normal activities within two to three days after the procedure.

Results thus far indicate that the laser-assisted procedure is successful in keeping vessels open, but only further studies will tell how angioplasty's long-term results stack up against those of bypass surgery.

Because argon laser light tends to scatter, it can cause thermal damage to cells and tissues over a relatively broad area. Therefore, rather than using it as an incisional tool, clinicians use it as a semiselective, somewhat imprecise instrument for treating a variety of vascularized and pigmented lesions, including port-wine stains, Kaposi's sarcoma, and café-au-lait macules.

Study indicates that ALAR has significant potential for increasing salvage of femoral artery graft with late failure, recanalization of segmented occlusions of the artery and, most important, to open segmentally occluded distal popliteal arteries in order to convert a below- to an above-knee bypass.

Penile plethysmography

Penile plethysmography has become an increasingly useful tool to help tell whether sexual impotence is psychological or organic and to diagnose and rehabilitate various types of sex offenders. The technique, which measures the increase in blood flow into the penis during sexual arousal, has also been used in the resolution of litigation revolving around the origin of the plaintiff's impotency. The device is a silicon rubber sleeve that fits around the penis and measures changes in blood volume by its effect on the electrical resistance of a thin layer of mercury contained between the two walls of the sleeve.

For diagnosing the origin of an individual's impotence, penile plethysmography is used to determine the frequency and extent of "sleep erections" that occur during the night. In a normal individual, tumescence occurs from four to six times per night during the deep-sleep stage marked by rapid eye movement (REM). Men who are impotent because of diabetes, spinal cord injury, or other "organic reasons" do not react the same way during REM sleep. In practice, the degree and frequency of penile tumescence are recorded as a fluctuation in a curve or jagged pattern on the readout sheet of a standard physiological polygraph. The sleep erection test has the unique advantage of offering an objective appraisal of the level of male sexual function.

Penile plethysmography has also proved useful in diagnosing and rehabilitating various categories of sex offenders. For example, studies indicate that the technique can differentiate among rapists who assault women frequently, those who add violence to the rape act, and those who choose children for their victims. The distinction is made by playing sexually provocative tape recordings to the subject, who is hooked up to the penile plethysmography, and then recording how he responds to different sexual stimuli. Others use the technique to differentiate homosexuals who prefer physically mature males (androphiles), pubescent males (ebophiles), and younger children (pedophiles) and aid in the rehabilitation of the latter.

As for rehabilitation use, once it has been objectively determined with penile plethysmography that the sex offender no longer responds to the critical sexual stimulus, the prognosis after release is clearly improved. Sex offenders who show continuing erotic interest in deviant stimuli could be retained for treatment after release. Penile plethysmography has been used in conjunction with biofeedback in the attempted rehabilitation of a transvestite exhibitionist. After using penile plethysmography to evaluate the man's sexual arousability and to determine the kind of sexual stimuli that attracted him, a biofeedback system is used by hooking the subject up to an alarm that goes off every time that the man is aroused by the stimuli that feed his deviation. After several months, the man can be rehabilitated.

GASTROINTESTINAL
Endoscopy

Among the techniques that should almost be routine as an extension of the physical examination is endoscopy. With the advent of fiber optic instruments, it has become much easier and less hazardous to perform endoscopic procedures.

Until the advent of fiber optics in 1952 and further modifications over subsequent years, the source of light was a small, incandescent bulb somewhere along the shaft of the scope. The risk from burns due to the heated bulb resulting in fires supported by the nitrous oxide anesthetic, and glass injuries from broken bulbs, far outweighed the advantages of laparoscopy. In the fiber optic instrument, the source of light is outside the body and the illumination itself is carried along a flexible cable and along the scope by minutely thin fibers that are covered with glass fibers with a low index of refraction. This property carries the light forward instead of outward where it would be dissipated.

1. *Gastroscopy* is valuable in helping to determine whether a gastric ulcer is benign or malignant. Endoscopy has become an increasingly routine technique in the approach to selected patients with upper gastrointestinal bleeding.
2. *Sigmoidoscopy* is important in the diagnosis of colonic cancer because approximately 50% of large intestine malignancies are within the reach of the sigmoidoscope; and small rectosigmoid tumors may be missed on examination after a barium enema because of the tortuosity and redundancy of the intestine in this area. Sigmoidoscopy also permits inspection of the mucosa for edema, erythema, friability, or ulceration.
3. *Colonoscopy* with fiber optic equipment permits the direct examination of the mucous membrane beyond the customary 25 centimeters of the rigid sigmoidoscope.
4. The basic principle of *laparoscopy* is relatively simple. A hollow tube is inserted into an artificially gaseous-distended abdomen to give additional observing and working space. A lighted, fiber optic scope, with lenses properly placed to visualize the pelvic field, is inserted in the region of the umbilicus and an assist, or operating instrument, may be inserted between the symphisis tubes and the umbilicus. This method enables one to visualize and evaluate the abdominal cavity and its contents.

Peritoneal lavage

Peritoneal lavage is very safe; serious complications are rare. The liberal use of peritoneal lavage can prevent delay in diagnosing significant injury in patients who have sustained blunt abdominal trauma. However, retroperitoneal injuries such as those involving the duodenum still pose a diagnostic problem because these injuries cannot be reliably detected by peritoneal lavage.

The extreme sensitivity of peritoneal lavage in detect-

ing hemoperitoneum has led to concern about unnecessary laparotomy. In one recent series, significant abdominal injury was not found at surgery in 23 of the patients (32%) with a positive lavage. Postoperative complications occurred in three of these patients (13%); two developed bowel obstruction and one developed pancreatitis.

Recent developments in surgery have changed the definition of what constitutes a significant abdominal injury. Splenic injuries, the most common consequence of blunt abdominal trauma, are treated much more conservatively than in the past, and liver lacerations, the second most common injury, are often treated without drains or other intervention. These developments have precipitated investigation of other diagnostic approaches in blunt abdominal trauma, such as CT, ultrasound, arteriography, and intense observation. Although these measures may be of adjunctive value, the risks of undetected serious abdominal injury far outweigh the risks of unnecessary surgery. Certainly, peritoneal lavage, with its proven safety and sensitivity, is the single most important diagnostic measure that the first-contact physician can initiate in victims of blunt abdominal trauma.

CYSTOSCOPY AND ARTHROSCOPY

Cystoscopy employs a cystoscope, an instrument to examine the interior of the urinary bladder. *Arthroscopy* is available to inspect joints such as the knee, hip, shoulder, and elbow.

LEARNING TECHNIQUE
Biofeedback

Biofeedback can no longer be viewed as an experimental technique since research studies and clinical applications have been conducted in major medical centers for more than 20 years. Biofeedback is basically a learning technique that has been found to be very helpful in the treatment of a number of stress-related and psychophysiological symptoms, as well as for general relaxation and muscle rehabilitation. This technique employs instrumentation to mirror psychophysiological processes of which the individual is not normally aware, and which may be brought under voluntary control. Biofeedback provides a person with immediate information about his or her own biological conditions, such as muscle tension, skin surface temperature, brain wave activity, galvanic skin response, and heart rate. An additional benefit, of course, is that the individual becomes an active participant in the process of health maintenance.

In the biofeedback instrument, the signal transducer receives information from the patient and converts it into a form that is measurable by instruments. The amplifier expands the electrical signal into a manageable quantity. Then, the signal processor extracts the wanted part of the information in the signal and filters out or discards the rest. The display converts the energy of the reduced signal into a particular stimulus or variable sensation that is made available to the patient, that is, light or sound. A patient completes the feedback loop by producing the original signals, perceiving the feedback, and then reacting to it.

There are several different types of biofeedback instruments. The EMG biofeedback instrument is designed to observe the EMG or responsive activity of the muscles of the body. The individual learns not only how to reduce muscle tension, but more important, how to control muscle spasms and activity in various areas of the body. The opportunity for immediate feedback of information from specific muscle areas allows the individual to learn what activities, exercises, positions, postures, and stretches will help, or possibly make the tension or spasm worse.

Since every person is different, the EMG instrument will help to design an individualized program of exercises and to trigger techniques that will help to reduce bodily stress, tension, and resulting pain. This is not a diagnostic EMG as utilized by a neurologist, but a device that feeds back immediate visual and audio information to the individual.

For example, in using EMG biofeedback, the patient's muscular activity is picked up by electrodes placed over the skin surface and small voltage charges are recorded as motor units fire. Of course, it is not surprising that patients can learn to control muscle activity with biofeedback, since the skeletal muscle system is under voluntary control. What is surprising is the degree to which this control can be learned. Numerous studies show biofeedback to be quite useful in treating several disorders, including anxiety disorders, tension headaches, muscle spasms and tics, spasmodic torticollis, blepharospasm, essential hypertension, and muscle reeducation. In managing anxiety and stress-related disorders, some physicians are employing biofeedback training as an adjunctive tool in the overall treatment program for their patients. Other illnesses and disabilities that have been successfully treated are nerve injuries, temporomandibular joint pain, bruxism, subvocalization, stuttering, both fecal and urinary incontinence, asthma, insomnia, phobias, and cerebral palsy.

Brain wave patterns can be observed, analyzed, and controlled with EEG biofeedback. From this description, one would get the impression that it is similar to diagnostic tools employed by neurologists. But EEG biofeedback is not a diagnostic procedure—its main function is to help patients observe and control brain wave or thinking patterns, as a visual guide or indicator of tension states. It is especially helpful in the treatment of insomnia, pain, and obsessive focusing on thoughts of pain, and in training obsessive-compulsive thinkers to relax their minds. This technique can also be applied in treating phobic disorders, anxiety states, gastrointestinal distress, and in helping to uncover unconscious material in psychotherapy.

In thermal biofeedback, peripheral blood flow, or vasodilation and constriction, is measured with temperature biofeedback. Dilation or constriction of the peripheral vessels leads to changes in blood flow that the patient learns to control with the aid of a thermistor placed on the skin surface of the dominant hand and fingers. Minute changes in temperature are fed back to the patient immediately that allow him or her to identify what techniques help facilitate vasodilation and relaxation. This provides for a deep sense of relaxation of the autonomic system and stabilization of the vascular system. It is especially helpful in the treatment of migraine headaches. Raynaud's syndrome, hypertension, and even more important, in identifying how the body reacts to physical and emotional stress. Autogenic training is very often incorporated in the treatment.

Clinical uses of thermal biofeedback involve temperature training that helps the patient learn to regulate blood flow in the periphery, generally the hands and/or feet. But it is much more than that. As we know, the peripheral vascular system has no significant parasympathetic innervation. The sympathetic nervous system causes the contracting of the smooth muscles in blood vessel walls and this results in vasoconstriction. To increase blood flow to the hands, the blood vessels dilate via a decrease in sympathetic activity. This is controlled by the hypothalamus. Therefore, in learning to warm the hands, we can infer that the patient is training his or her hypothalamus and associated machinery. The patient is trying to achieve a normalization of hypothalamic homeostasis.

In galvanic skin response (GSR) biofeedback, minute changes in the skin potential and conductance are measured on the GSR, or dermograph, biofeedback instrument. Changes are affected by emotions, survival responses—for example, injuries (i.e., fight or flight responses)—breathing patterns, thoughts, and overall tension levels. It is a very sensitive and responsive instrument that is helpful in the treatment of GI distress, stress reactions, hypertension, hyperventilation patterns, and in overall arousal levels. This instrument can easily demonstrate how irregular and increased breathing rates can increase internal tension levels. Many patients will deny hyperventilating until they are attached to the GSR biofeedback instrument. They will then immediately become open to learning more appropriate responses and breathing patterns that are conducive to relaxation. The key at this point is to help them incorporate these learned responses into their daily lives.

Skilled listening

Primary care is sought at the level of more than 650 million visits yearly. According to the National Ambulatory Medical Care Survey, the average office visit is 16.1 minutes, although 70% are less than 15 minutes. This results in a deficit doctor-patient relationship. Skilled listening would reduce the reaction of the patient to the hurried professional exposure as well as the decision to litigate. The American Bar Association recently studied the problem in relation to physicians they represented in malpractice. Three-fourths of claims were made by poor doctor-patient relationship. Hence the coding of claims as failure to diagnose or lack of informed consent actually represent communication failures. When patients deliberately withhold information, it is usually due to the physician's behavior, for instance, acting impatient and interrupting the patient. Most patients do not return to their concerns but await the physician's continued interrogation (which may be influenced by a poor night's sleep or physician bias). Hence, it pays to allow the patient to speak freely, and intersperse personal questions as to family, sporting events, and the like. It behooves the physician to use verbal devices such as "good, what do you think?" Allowing the patient adequate time to express himself or herself results in better information, leading to a better clinical diagnosis. In summary, taking the time to listen results in these benefits: time saving, more patient and physician satisfaction, a quicker and more accurate diagnosis, and a reduced incidence of malpractice.[20]

LABORATORY TESTS
Blood

A complete blood count (CBC) is a study of the number of both red and various types of white cells in a given amount of blood, for which normal figures have been established. These will be referred to by their names, and commonly used abbreviations, followed by what is considered a normal quantity.
- RBC (red blood cells): 4½ to 5 million
- WBC (white blood cells): 7000 to 10,000
- Differential count: percentage of various types of white cells
- Polys (leukocytes): 50% to 60%
- Lymphocytes: 35% to 40%
- Monocytes: 4% to 8%
- Eosinophiles: 1% to 2%
- Basophiles: 1% to 3%

The cells are also studied for their shape and any other variations and comment is made if these are abnormal.

A hemoglobin (Hb) (chemical component of red blood cells) determination is given as a percentage and in weight by grams. A lowered RBC count, or hemoglobin loss, indicates anemia.

A sedimentation rate is a study of how fast the red blood cells settle out of a fluid suspension in a period of one hour. The usual normal range for men is 0 to 9 millimeters in one hour, while for women the range is 0 to 20 millimeters in one hour. If the rate exceeds these maximum figures, it indicates the presence of tissue destruction, or is often interpreted to indicate the presence of inflammation somewhere within the body.

Serological tests are laboratory tests made on the blood serum that, when positive, usually indicate the presence of an infectious disease. There are a few diseases that may give a false-positive reading.

Urine

A urinalysis is a study of a urine specimen, by which the specific gravity or density of the solids is determined, as well as the acidity or alkalinity. In addition, a test is made to determine the presence or absence of sugar, which if present, is usually considered as abnormal; and the presence or absence of albumen that if present, is also usually considered abnormal. The specimen is also studied microscopically to determine the presence of any unusual number of blood or pus cells, other cells, or casts, which are simply microscopic groups of cells that are plastered together.

The examination of urine is extremely important in that many pathological conditions or metabolic disturbances can be detected by changes that occur in the nature of the urine. Certain substances may be present that are not normal constituents of urine, or the proportions of the normal constituents may be altered. Another substance not normally present is acetone.

Microbiology—gene testing

The procedures for testing DNA and genes are the newest techniques with high medicolegal value in paternity suits, death causes, and the like. The various procedures are followed through with the polymerase chain reaction (PRC), electrophoresis, and nucleide sequencing.

BIOMEDICAL EQUIPMENT MANAGEMENT

Biomedical equipment is complex equipment with a patient connection that is used for diagnosis, therapy, and monitoring of patients. It also includes housekeeping equipment such as testing, data processing, and record-keeping devices that do not have a direct patient connection, but are complicated enough to warrant special consideration.

In the 1960s this equipment was relatively simple and could be bought, used, and maintained with minor on-the-job training. Between 1970 and 1975, largely as a result of the introduction of integrated circuits, the sales of patient monitoring equipment tripled,[21] complexity increased, and the safety of the patient became a matter of concern. In the 1970s, the medical device industry grew from $3 billion to $12 billion in total shipments in 1980.[22] At the same time, product liability litigation and awards increased, and in 1976 the Food, Drug, and Cosmetic Act was amended to establish the Food and Drug Administration's (FDA) Bureau of Medical Devices to regulate medical device manufacturers.[23] Also, during this period, a substantial number of new professional and institutional standards were generated by such organizations as the Joint Commission on the Accreditation of Healthcare Organizations (JCAHO), the National Fire Protection Association (NFPA), and the Association for the Advancement of Medical Instrumentation, to govern hospitals' arrangement and use of the equipment.

For their part, hospitals reacted by establishing three levels of effort for the handling of their biomedical equipment[24]:

Level 1: Corrective maintenance whereby broken equipment is repaired
Level 2: Preventive maintenance to assure the operational reliability of the equipment
Level 3: Management to assure the quality and cost effectiveness of the equipment.

Corrective maintenance

The amount of corrective maintenance that is done by a hospital varies substantially according to both the information provided by the manufacturer and the skills of the hospital staff. Any of four modes may apply[25]:

1. The manufacturer provides adequate information and diagnostic facilities with which component failures can be identified and repaired by the hospital staff.
2. The manufacturer's documentation and diagnostic facilities are limited, in which case the hospital either:
   a. Has sufficient spare circuit boards to substitute in the equipment until the failed board is found for returning to the manufacturer for repair, relatively inexperienced staff being adequate for this mode;
   b. Employs sophisticated test equipment and trained staff to identify the failure; or
   c. Executes contracts for manufacturer or maintenance contractor support that can be expensive, annual maintenance contracts often cost as much as thirty percent of the capital equipment cost.

Preventive maintenance

Preventive maintenance is done under formal protocol to assure the operability of the equipment. The JCAHO requires that it be done at least semiannually;

this frequency may be decreased, if the Hospital Safety Committee agrees, after actual failure rates have been taken into account.[26]

Typically, the preventive maintenance protocols for equipment are generated by the manufacturer who is inclined to include excessively complex and time-consuming tests as protection against product liability. In this event, the hospital maintenance personnel, pressed by multiple priorities and economic restrictions, can find that they are unable to allocate the time and manpower necessary for compliance with these procedures.[27] Under such circumstances, hospitals tend toward substituting simplified protocols that enable them to meet the only standard actively imposed on them, namely, passing the JCAHO and/or state inspections. This attitude is typified by such claims as "our maintenance program is fine, it got us through our survey without citation."[28]

Of late, this effort has been further complicated both by the widespread proliferation of microprocessors in the equipment and the flexibility they afford. A switch may no longer have a single function but multiple functions that are selected by software programs. In just 15 years, from 1970 to 1985, the number of controls and displays on the anesthesia machine grew by a factor of 5 and the alarm indications by a factor of 20.[29]

Management

Effective equipment management enables the hospital to avoid abuse and to assure proper operation and maintenance of the equipment. This management should be established with five objectives: to select good equipment, to comply with the standards, to assure proper use, to monitor performance, and to support improvements.

Select good equipment. This objective, applied to new equipment, demands that the shortcomings of the old equipment are known, the needs and constraints of the hospital are defined, and the new equipment is properly selected to meet these needs and constraints.

Shortcomings of the old equipment can be indicated by the presence of idle equipment, excessive repair costs, excessive incident reports and malpractice actions, and queues of people waiting to use the equipment. They may be caused by equipment limitations such as excessive gadgetry or early obsolescence. The alternatives, however, are inadequate inventory, status control, inadequate maintenance, or operator instruction.

The selection of equipment needs to be based on logical analysis rather than emotion. Certain features, such as portability, maintainability, operability, reliability, adaptability, safety, and suitability for the environment, are factors for consideration. The effect of the equipment on the facility services such as furniture, water, space, cooling, heating, lighting, power, and drainage also may have to be considered for assessing implementation and operating costs. A balance sheet to determine the cost/benefit of the equipment is appropriate for the selection process. On the one side of the sheet will be the capital amortization and operating costs; on the other will be income and, most important, the intangible assets such as quality, frequency of use, potential for risk, and potential for better procedures, accuracy, communications, availability, and skills mix.

In addition, the opinions of others are applicable. Manufacturer demonstrations of the most suitable equipment should be arranged at the hospital or by site visits to determine the opinions of the technical and clinical users. The FDA's Center for Devices and Radiological Health runs a voluntary reporting system for manufacturer-detected anomalies. These reports are available to the public. The Emergency Care Research Institute, a private organization, also publishes regular hazard bulletins and the results of its literature searches of professional publications. These reports are available to the subscribers of its service.

Comply with the standards. Failure by hospitals to demonstrate compliance with regulations and professional standards can place in question the hospitals' concern for patient care. Under the category of standards, it behooves the hospital to be aware of the mistakes of others and changes in the standard of care created by product liability case law.

From the biomedical equipment aspect, the FDA places some biomedical devices in its Class 1 for which general controls are adequate to assure safety and effectiveness. It places more hazardous devices in Class 2 for which general controls and performance specifications are required. These performance specifications can include maintenance procedures that presumably are to be adopted by the hospital. The hospital licensure authorities, moreover, are expected both to demand that the equipment be type-approved by an acceptable standards testing laboratory and to specify the laboratories acceptable to them. The laboratories normally accepted include the Underwriters Laboratory, ITT Research Institute, Canadian Standards Association, Underwriters Laboratory of Canada, and City of Los Angeles Electrical Testing Laboratory.[30] Accordingly, manufacturers need to get their type-approvals from one of these laboratories. Equipment not tested by acceptable laboratories will probably require additional hospital evaluation in order to convince the licensure authority of their safety and efficacy.

From the hospital construction and equipment aspect, the NFPA has issued National Fire Protection Association Standard NFPA-99 for Health Care Facilities that brings into one document the relevant standards, recommended practices, and manuals developed by the

association.[31] These are professional consensus standards that, as such, are not mandatory for the hospital, but that have some parts adopted as mandatory by hospital licensure and accreditation authorities. The Association for the Advancement of Medical Instrumentation also develops standards for biomedical devices based on the consensus viewpoint of its clinician, engineer, and manufacturer membership.[32]

From the hospital operations aspects, the JCAHO, in its *Accreditation Manual*, includes a chapter on "Plant Technology and Safety Management" governing the administration of biomedical equipment. This chapter covers, in particular, the needs for an inventory, testing at less than six-month intervals unless exempted, and test records, as well as the need for a corrective maintenance procedure, user/operator instructions, and operator training.[33]

Continuous supervision is required in the hospital to assure that the hospital complies with these guidelines and standards, and any changes thereto.

Assure proper use. It is appropriate for assuring proper use that purchased equipment be inspected on delivery to see that it meets the manufacturer's specifications and does the job for which it was ordered. Studies indicate that, on delivery, as much as 40% of some high-technology equipment does not meet manufacturer specifications[34]; acceptance demonstrations are often demanded, therefore, from the manufacturer to validate performance.

Much biomedical equipment operates in an integrated system. In many cases the equipment hardware is controlled by software programs that, in turn, follow the direction of mathematical algorithms. These programs and algorithms are essential to the performance of the hardware, yet may be treated as proprietary information by the manufacturer. Possibly, the hardware will need building services and operating and maintenance staffs who will in turn need equipment-specific organization, procedures, and training. Finally, both the hardware and the staff may have to be configured to act under contingency conditions in which some form of partial operation is continued.

Depending on the magnitude of the system, its implementation should be in accordance with good engineering practice. Such practice includes the provision of facility and equipment interface specifications; layout diagrams; contractor specifications and liaison; on-site installation and checkout support; as-built drawings; operating and maintenance manuals; acceptance test specifications and demonstrations; in-service training; recommended spare parts lists; and warranty, loaner, and corrective maintenance support.

The JCAHO lists many of the regulations, policies, and procedures that should be produced by hospital departments for using the equipment properly, ranging from anesthesia equipment testing before use to special care unit actions in the event of a breakdown in essential equipment.[35] It also requires that there be identification, development, implementation, and review of departmental safety policies; a hazard surveillance program; an incident reporting system including a recall system; provision of safety-related information for operation; an in-service training program; monitoring of the safety program; and a reference library of patient safety documents.

Instruction manuals have grown in size and complexity, and, due to frequent software changes in equipment, are obsolete early. In consequence, manufacturers tend to limit the number of copies of the manuals they supply to one or two copies per machine regardless of the number of users, and the users, not having readily available copies or time to study the mass of information, tend to rely on repetitive practical experience.

As a result, greater emphasis is being placed on the hospital to supplement inadequate manuals and on equipment-oriented seminars and mandatory in-service training to assure the proper use of the equipment. Audience attention is enhanced when it is recognized that, in general, physicians support the use of the equipment, nurses are reluctant to deal with extra complications, and administrators need to be satisfied that the equipment is worthwhile.

Monitor performance. The performance of the biomedical equipment needs to be constantly monitored to assure that the equipment performs properly its assigned function. Part of the operator training will be to observe and detect wrongful results. Preferably, weekly technical inspections are made to solicit operator comments and to observe the technical performance firsthand. Manufacturers should therefore be encouraged to provide adequate simulation and test means in their systems for confirming proper performance with minimum pertubation.

Equipment investigations, especially those in response to incident reports, need to be carefully conducted to resolve equipment shortcomings such as design weaknesses including failure to anticipate usage, incorrect assembly, inadequate testing or labeling, failure to warn and instruct, and user errors. These investigations should be done in the presence of witnesses and the manufacturer's representative as appropriate. Should future litigation be possible, then the equipment needs to be withdrawn from service, its status and the positions of controls and alarms recorded, and any inspection or testing done in such a way that the equipment is not substantially affected.

In the early 1970s, the emphasis was on electrical safety procedures for protecting personnel from the chances of electrical shock. This was broadened by a demand for risk management whereby corrective action was assessed according to the propensity for patient harm. Now the emphasis has been changed again to one of cost-effectiveness to reflect on a monetary basis the value of the systems. Accordingly, widespread use is being made of personal computers throughout hospitals at the departmental level to measure the performance of the hospital services, schedule staff and patients, process medical data, and provide statistical records. Normally, this use of personal computers has the advantage of allowing easier and faster program modification to meet departmental requirements than can be furnished by a central hospital system.

Support improvements. During system implementation and performance evaluations, it may be found appropriate to make equipment modifications, or special units, adaptors, and cables to integrate the systems or improve its operation. Such improvements will apply to the hardware or software, in which case it is appropriate that the changes be properly checked out, documented, and approved for quality. Hospital procedures, drawings, manuals, and warranties may require amendment to assure safety and efficacy, and special in-service training given to reflect the changes.

With respect to hospital-fabricated devices, the FDA recognizes two categories of devices[36]: (1) custom-built devices made for a specified physician for a specified physician for a specified patient and (2) investigational devices that are covered by an investigational device exemption. These devices will be under the control of the hospital's investigational requirements board alone, or in conjunction with the FDA, depending on whether they constitute a nonsignificant or significant risk, respectively. While it is not specifically spelled out, it is recommended that all hospital-originated devices receive the same treatment as that described earlier for improvements if they are to be used by staff or on patients.

Implementation

Biomedical engineering is constituted with three subspecialties, the breakdown being bioengineering to research medical devices, medical engineering to develop and design the devices in the industrial environment, and clinical engineering to maintain and manage the devices in the hospital environment.[37] To implement the five objectives discussed, a larger hospital will set up a clinical engineering department comprising a number of clinical engineers to perform the management function and to support, when needed, the biomedical equipment technicians doing the maintenance function.

Because biomedical equipment in the hospital embraces all engineering specialties including mechanical, electrical, electronic, control, computer, and environment engineering, it is appropriate that the clinical engineering staff be broad-based. Preferably, the engineers will have engineering degrees and be licensed professional engineers, and/or board certified by the International Certification for Clinical Engineering and Biomedical Technology. The department commonly reports to the administration as a core function, or operationally to a clinical department with funding controlled by the administration.

To handle the increase in the amount and complexity of the biomedical equipment, many hospitals have encouraged standardization and pooling of some equipment for common use. For this, a group of critical care technicians is often added as a separate entity reporting to a clinical department to store, prepare, calibrate, and manage the pooled equipment for any of the clinical departments using it. Preferably, these critical care technicians are trained to assume the initial responsibility for identifying, perhaps by substitution, the equipment needing repair. By virtue of their supportive operational relationship with the clinical departments, they are also able to identify educational needs and coordinate engineering in-service training. By so doing, the critical care technician group acts as a valuable integrating medium for the clinical engineering department and its diverse clients.[38]

It is pertinent to note that the U.S. hospital system is in a state of reorientation affecting implementation of maintenance and management. Current reports indicate that multihospital chains run more than 30% of the hospitals, and investor-owned chains are operating 1000 acute care hospitals in addition to home-care services, retirement homes, and health spas. Moreover, nonprofit hospitals are establishing for-profit subsidiaries, while individual entrepreneurs are developing free-standing surgical and emergency centers, "Docs-in-a-Box" offices, and a variety of clinics. These changes require that clinical engineers provide shared services on a multihospital basis, either as a centralized service for the hospital chain, or as an independent service for the fragmented configuration. It is expected that such centralization will create additional management burdens, and fragmentation may cause smaller facilities to be undersupported for economic or geographic reasons. Either way, care is needed to assure that the changes are not allowed to affect the standard of care provided by the service.

Now, with the emphasis on cost-effectiveness, hospitals are being reimbursed under the Medicare program for senior citizens according to the diagnosis and not the treatment. Under this diagnosis–related group (DRG) concept, should the profit margin between reimbursement and treatment cost be inadequate, a hospital may have to curtail capital acquisition, improve or discontinue practicing those procedures with negative profit margins, or reduce the overhead services. Other reim-

bursement programs are expected to adopt this DRG concept and so create a developing need for data processing services to monitor profit margins and reassign priorities.

In the next decade the clinical engineering department will be involved more deeply in three areas: (1) technology assessment, to expand the equipment selection function by assessing such factors as the scope of operation as an extension of an existing service or as a new service requiring new staff resources; the capability for optimum levels of quality, affordability, financial, and liability risks; joint venture on free-standing environment; and life expectancy[39]; (2) training to improve the man-machine relationships, developing audiovisual aids, interactive training techniques, and less material to communicate better on equipment matters; and (3) computer applications in performance evaluation by means of online record-keeping and database management.

It has been said that biomedical equipment takes some of the guesswork from patient care decisions. It improves patient care when it is properly selected and maintained, and when it is used by people who understand it and know what to do if the expected does not happen. If any of these components are missing, the patient's well-being may be in jeopardy.[40]

END NOTES

1. *Pre-Employment Studies by X-Rays in Asymptomatic Patients: 1172 Spines, The Bony Abnormalities Equal 57%,* Med. J. Australia (Jan. 1984).
2. E. M. Hiteselburger et al., *Myelography in Asymptomatic Backs,* 28 J. Neurosurg. 204 (1968).
3. M. K. Newman et al., Unpublished data. Electrophysiologic studies (EMG and nerve conduction). More than 20% to 25% of asymptomatic patients demonstrate abnormal motor unit patterns in back observations.
4. A. Fisher, *Thermography in Differential Diagnosis and Documentation of Painful Conditions, in Current Therapy in Physiatry* (W. B. Saunders, Philadelphia 1984).
5. M. K. Newman et al., *Infrared Imaging, Thermography, Medical and Legal Evidentiary Rule Value,* presented at 24th Annual Meeting. ACLM, Scottsdale, Ariz., May 1984.
6. M. K. Newman et al., Paper presented at the Defense Practice Seminar, Academy of Workers Compensation, Law and Medicine for the Defense, New Orleans, La., 1985.
7. *Frye v. U.S.,* 293 F. 1013 (D.C. Cir. 1923).
8. *William Standard,* 583 F. 1194 (2nd Cir.), *cert. denied,* 439 U.S. 1117 99 S. Ct. 1025, 59L Ed. 2d 77 (1978).
9. R. D. Sine et al., *Epidural Nerve Condition,* 75 Arch PMR 17-24 (Jan. 1994).
10. E. L. Thompson, *Surface Electromyography, Electrical Activity of Muscle,* Mayo Clinic Bull. (Aug. 1989).
11. J. J. Bonica, 1, 2 Management of Pain, (2d ed. Lea & Febiger, Philadelphia 1990).
12. *Pain Discussion,* Sci. Am. Med. 1-17 (1989).
13. E. McBride, *History and Physical Examination* (Lippincott, Philadelphia 1953).
14. I *Handbook of Psychological Tests, An MMPI Handbook,* (University of Minnesota Press, St. Paul 1960).
15. M. R. Bone, *Pain: Its Nature and Analysis and Treatment, in*

Eyesenck Personality Test (EPI) 45-50 (Churchill & Livingstone, London, 1984).

16. *Beck Depression Inventory,* 4 Arch Pysch 561 (1961).

17. N. H. Hendler, *Four Stages of Pain* 1-8 (Wright-Boston, PSG, 1982).

18. R. Cailliet, *Pain Series* (F.A. Davis Co., Philadelphia 1993).

19. S. D. Hodge, Jr., John Wiley Publications, John Wiley & Sons, Inc. 1994, Supplement (current thru Aug. 1, 1993).

20. *Skilled Listening,* Ariz. Med. (Sep. 1992); *also* H. Beckman and R. I. Frankel, *title?,* 5 HMO Pract. 114 (July/Aug. 1991).

21. Stetler, *The Medical Device Amendments of 1976 — Prediction for the Future,* 11 Med. Instrum. 199 (May/June 1977).

22. Schoellhorn, *Industries Achievements and the Task Ahead,* Med. Device & Diagnost. Industry (Mar. 1982).

23. Federal Food, Drug and Cosmetic Act (as amended 1976). Pub. L. 94-295.

24. Shaffer, *Integration of Clinical Engineering into the Hospital Organization,* Hosp. & Health Services Admin. 72-81 (Sep./Oct. 1983).

25. Shaffer, *Medical Equipment Maintenance,* Clin. Eng. News (Mar. 1974).

26. Joint Commission on Accreditation of Healthcare Organizations, *Plant, Technology and Safety Management,* in *Accreditation Manual for Healthcare Organizations* (1985).

27. Ben-Zvi, *An Urgent Plea for Realistic Preventive Maintenance Procedures,* 16 Med. Instrum. 115-16 (1982).

28. American Society for Hospital Engineering, *Medical Equipment Management in Hospitals* (2 ed. 1982).

29. Schreiber, *Safety Guidelines for Anesthesia Machines,* North American Drager (B86-001 MP10M) (1984).

30. Shaffer & Gordon, *Clinical Engineering Standards, Obligations and Accountability,* 13 Med. Instrum. 209-15 (1979).

31. National Fire Protection Association, Standard for Health Care Facilities (1984).

32. Shaffer, *supra* note 30.

33. National Fire Protection Association, *supra* note 31.

34. Ben-Zvi, *The Selection and Evaluation of Medical Instrumentation,* 5 Med. Instrum. 428 (Jan./Feb. 1971).

35. *Supra* note 26.

36. *Supra* note 23.

37. *Medical Engineering Program Expectations,* 61 IEEE Eng. in Med. & Biology Group Newsl. 7-10 (1977).

38. Shaffer et al., *Clinical Engineering Education in the High Technology Hospital,* 18 Med. Instrum. 280-82 (1984).

39. Millenson & Slizewski, *How Do Hospital Executives Spell Technology Assessment?,* Planning, Health Maintenance Q. (1st Quarter 1986).

40. Hargest, *A Clinical Engineer's Viewpoint of Medical Instrumentation,* 14 Med. Instrum. 215-17 (July/Aug. 1980).

CHAPTER 49

Research and experimentation

CYRIL H. WECHT, M.D., J.D., F.C.L.M.*

HISTORICAL BACKGROUND
BENEFIT VERSUS RISK RULE
CRIMINAL AND CIVIL LIABILITY
INNOVATIVE THERAPY
RADIATION EXPERIMENTS
QUESTIONABLE HUMAN RESEARCH AND EXPERIMENTATION PRACTICES
CONCLUSION

HISTORICAL BACKGROUND

Few subjects in the medicolegal field have raised as much widespread controversy since World War II as the question of human experimentation and clinical investigation. Exposés of activities by the CIA, the Department of Defense, and other federal agencies involving the deaths of innocent victims, who were unknowing, involuntary guinea pigs, have raised many moral and ethical questions for the entire country. Ever since the Nuremberg trials following World War II, medical researchers and other professional scientific personnel involved in clinical investigation have been made aware of the medicolegal hazards and pitfalls of improper, illegal human experimentation. The Declaration of Helsinki and Codes and Guidelines adopted by the American Medical Association and other national professional organizations, as well as by the Department of Health and Human Services (DHHS), have served to emphasize the importance and necessity of having well-defined principles for all medical experimenters and researchers using human subjects in their studies.

The World Medical Association (WMA) addressed this controversial subject in 1949 at its meeting in London, at which time a rather strict International Code of Medical Ethics was adopted. It said in part: "Under no circumstances is a doctor permitted to do anything that would weaken the physical or mental resistance of a human being except from strictly therapeutic or prophylactic indications imposed in the interest of the

patient." However, by 1954, the WMA had become uncomfortable with its commitment exclusively to the individual patient. That year, the organization adopted its "Principles for Those in Research and Experimentation," which, while warning that there must be "strict adherence to the general rules of respect of the individual," also explicitly recognized that experiments may be conducted on healthy subjects.

By 1964, the WMA had clearly abandoned the individual patient-centered commitment of 1949 in a new set of recommendations, "because it is essential that the results of laboratory experiments be applied to human beings to further scientific knowledge and to help suffering humanity."

Today, not only the regulations of the WMA, but also those of the Nuremberg Code and the U.S. government justify a human experiment if the risks compare favorably with the foreseeable benefits to the subject or to others. Hence, the Hippocratic tradition regarding human experimentation has been amended to include a concern for suffering humanity—and, of course, for scientific progress.

Yet, this same commitment to benefit society may also have opened the door for the type of experimentation that includes the injection of hepatitis virus into mentally retarded children. That is, a "Willowbrook" becomes possible once experimenters can convince themselves that the risks are outweighed by the possible benefits, including the potential benefits to people who were not included in the experiment.

Some scientific researchers have been irritated by the institution of codes and guidelines and continue to insist that they should be permitted to use their own best moral

---

*The author gratefully acknowledges work by the previous contributor, Harold L. Hirsh, M.D., J.D., F.C.L.M.

and ethical judgment as professional people. While the majority of these persons would, of course, apply a high level of moral and ethical judgment, experience has demonstrated all too frequently that even highly experienced researchers can be carried away with a particular project and engage in activities that not only are in violation of the existing civil common law and criminal codes, but are in opposition to traditional medical morals and ethics. For all these reasons, it is essential that physicians and other scientists who directly or indirectly engage in any kind of experimentation or clinical investigation involving human beings be fully aware of all the legal ramifications and potential problems associated with this area of professional activity.

The late eminent Harvard Medical School anesthesiologist and medical ethicist, Dr. H. K. Beecher, claimed that human experimentation beyond the boundaries of medical ethics was being carried out to an alarming and dangerous degree by clinical investigators in the United States. He claimed that these investigators were more concerned with furthering the interests of science than with the good of the individual patient. He found 12 of 100 consecutively reported studies involving experimentation with human subjects, appearing in a highly respected medical journal in 1964, to be seemingly "unethical." Beecher concluded: "If only one-fourth of them is truly unethical, this still indicates the existence of a serious situation." In the prestigious *New England Journal of Medicine,* he found 50 examples of unethical experimentation described or referred to in various articles.[1]

Government-sponsored experimentation

Medical experimentation on humans has a long history, but public concern over it is a comparatively recent development. One of the more spectacular recent examples of unethical human experimentation was partially revealed in June 1975 by the Commission on CIA Activities Within the United States, the so-called Rockefeller Commission. In its chapter on domestic activities of the CIA's Directorate of Science and Technology, the Commission's report described some of the CIA projects involving drug experimentation on humans, noting that most of the records of such experiments had been destroyed. The report minimized the consequences of the experiments to the subjects involved, many of whom had not even been informed that they were subjects of an experiment.

One of the CIA experiments was described more specifically, although still in casual, almost indifferent terms:

The Commission did learn, however, that on one occasion during the early phases of this program (in 1953), LSD was administered to an employee of the Department of the Army without his knowledge while he was attending a meeting with CIA personnel working on the drug project.

Prior to receiving the LSD, the subject had participated in discussions where the testing of such substances on unsuspecting subjects was agreed to in principle. However, this individual was not made aware that he had been given LSD until about 20 minutes after it had been administered. He developed serious side effects and was sent to New York with a CIA escort for psychiatric treatment. Several days later, he jumped from a tenth floor window of his room and died as a result.

The General Counsel ruled that the death resulted from circumstances arising out of an experiment undertaken in the course of his official duties for the United States Government, thus ensuring his survivors of receiving certain death benefits. Reprimands were issued by the Director of Central Intelligence to two CIA employees responsible for the incident.[2]

As if to suggest that the experiment perhaps had nothing to do with the death, the report added a gratuitous footnote: "There are indications in the few remaining Agency records that this individual may have had a history of emotional instability." The individual was not identified in the Commission's report.

The report went on to conclude that "it was clearly illegal to test potentially dangerous drugs on unsuspecting United States citizens," and recommended that "the CIA should not again engage in the testing of drugs on unsuspecting persons." Not a word about medical ethics, international codes, or anything else to indicate any genuine moral concern—not even a suggestion that the unknowing subjects of the experiments ought to be located and informed. This was how a prestigious governmental commission perceived its obligations and performed its duties.

Fortunately, the news media were not satisfied with this incomplete disclosure. The identity of the victim in the specific incident described by the Commission was soon determined to be Dr. Frank Olson, a civilian Army employee. His "history of emotional instability" consisted of visits to a New York psychiatrist, retained by the CIA, *after* he had been subjected to the CIA's drug experiment. When the detailed circumstances of the experiment and Dr. Olson's death became widely publicized, the president of the United States expressed public apologies to his widow and children. Ultimately, after a suit had been filed, the case was settled privately and quietly by a $2 million payment from the government.

Other examples of governmental drug experimentation on humans also came to public attention. One involved a 42-year-old hospital patient, Harold Blauer, who died in January 1953, approximately 2.5 hours after receiving an injection of a mescaline derivative. (Mescaline is an hallucinogenic drug derived from a type of cactus plant and is similar to LSD in its effects on the mind.)

Mr. Blauer, along with an undetermined number of other patients, had been given injections of mescaline derivatives during the course of a 29-day project conducted by the New York State Psychiatric Institute under an Army contract. At no time was there knowledge on the part of any of the patients or their families as to the nature of the experiment, nor was any informed consent obtained.

Some comments by the acting Mental Hygiene Commissioner of New York State, Dr. Hugh F. Butts, following disclosure of the circumstances of Mr. Blauer's death, are especially relevant:

It was not uncommon practice at that time for medical and psychiatric researchers to use drug treatment without the detailed knowledge and special consent of patients. This was thought necessary to avoid false reactions.

Such practices could not occur today because patients are protected by laws and regulations which have been specifically enacted to prevent such occurrences.[3]

Following the public disclosures of the Olson and Blauer cases, the news media turned up numerous other instances of unethical experimentation with hallucinogenic drugs on unsuspecting human subjects involving several government agencies. At least 7000 persons had been so treated by the U.S. Army alone. The Rockefeller Commission report had also alluded to experiments on "unsuspecting persons in normal social situations," on both the West and East Coasts during the 1950s and 1960s.[4]

Later, it was learned that the U.S. Atomic Energy Commission, predecessor to the Energy Research and Development Administration, sponsored and monitored various experiments from the 1940s through the 1960s on human subjects, including children, in which the subjects were exposed either to radiation or to the highly toxic metal plutonium. In the radiation tests, 79 inmates of the state penitentiary in Oregon, male and female, were exposed to doses of radiation to determine the effects on the reproductive organs. No follow-up studies had been performed in recent years, but as a result of the disclosure, prison officials agreed to conduct medical evaluations to detect adverse aftereffects.

In the plutonium exposure tests, 18 men, women, and children, all thought to be terminally ill, were injected with plutonium in amounts ranging from 2 to 145 times the maximum permissible dose under current standards. The subjects were not told what the substance was. The injections were performed between 1945 and 1947 at various hospitals in four different states. Astonishingly, although all the subjects were thought to be terminally ill at the time, three were still alive 40 years later.[5] Obviously, aside from the ethics of the experiment itself, such long survival of "terminally ill" patients raises serious questions about the ability of researchers to determine such conditions in their choice of subjects.

LSD

The Justice Department recently settled a lawsuit by nine Canadians, who asserted that the CIA, unknowingly to them and their relatives, made them the subjects of mind-control experiments in the 1950s. The plaintiffs were patients of a psychiatrist who received money from the CIA to do research into drugs that could be used to control human behavior. According to government records, the nine plaintiffs were not told they were the subjects of experiments. They were subjected to heavy doses of the hallucinogen, LSD, powerful electric shock treatment two or three times a day, and doses of barbiturates for prolonged periods of drug-induced sleep.

Documents that became public showed that the CIA had used private medical research foundations as a conduit for a 25-year, multimillion dollar research program to learn how to control the human mind.

Through a front organization called the Society for the Investigation of Human Ecology, the agency funneled tens of thousands of dollars to pay for an array of experiments that involved LSD, electroshock therapy, and a procedure known as "psychic driving," in which patients listened to a recorded message repeatedly for up to 16 hours.

The Nuremberg Code

Of course, there is nothing new about medical experiments on humans. Galen founded the experimental science of medicine prior to 200 A.D., and there are references to medical experiments on human subjects in the oldest literature. Nonetheless, public awareness of ethical and legal problems posed by medical research involving human subjects did not coalesce until the post–World War II trials at Nuremberg, where more than 25 "dedicated and honored medical men" were accused of having committed war crimes of a medical nature against involuntary human subjects. According to Telford Taylor, chief prosecutor at the Nuremberg Military Tribunals, the defendants' "advances" in medicine were confined to the field of "thanatology"—the science of death. Of the 25 defendants, only 7 were acquitted; 9 were sentenced to prison; and the remaining 9 were sentenced to death.

After it became known, through these trials, what the Nazis had done under the guise of medical and scientific research, there developed what has been referred to as the Nuremberg Code (see Appendix 49-1). The Nuremberg Code was the forerunner of the subsequent codes and guidelines that were adopted by different agencies and organizations in the ensuing decades. It addressed the question of what constitutes valid, legal, moral, and ethical experimentation. However, it did not explicitly deal with the subject of children. Probably nobody at that time thought it would be necessary. But it did deal with the subjects of consent, the voluntariness of consent, the right of a patient to withdraw if he or she wished, and the basic question of doing things in conformance with proper medical standards and safeguards. The Nuremberg Code prompted more interest and concern in these problems.

Declaration of Helsinki

In 1964, the World Medical Association promulgated a code that came to be known as the Declaration of Helsinki (see Appendix 49-2). The Declaration of Helsinki was, in essence, adopted and given the imprimatur of the American Medical Association in November 1966. It was referred to as "Ethical Guidelines for Clinical Investigation by the AMA." Earlier in 1966, the Public Health Service of the United States had issued some guidelines that were subsequently revised later in the year. Recently, the DHHS has also been attempting to draft some guidelines.

Children as subjects

Apart from international codes, there have also been a number of court decisions in this country bearing on the questions of ethical experimentation and informed consent, particularly in reference to children. Under existing case law, although it is often forgotten, a parent cannot say to a neighbor or friend or a research team of scientists: "Take one of my children and if you wish to do something that is not going to be beneficial or advantageous to him, go ahead and do it anyway because I, the parent, give you permission." A parent cannot legally do that. We are a nation governed by laws, and the law is clear in this regard. Neither parents, legal guardians, administrators of homes and hospitals for retarded children, government officials, or university research teams, individually or collectively, are empowered to ignore or circumvent a basic and important concept of Anglo-American law, namely, that you cannot commit an assault and battery on another human being.

In 1944, the U.S. Supreme Court, in *Prince v. Massachusetts,* stated: "Parents may be free to become martyrs themselves, but it does not follow they are free in identical circumstances to make martyrs of their children before they reach the age of full and legal discretion when they can make that choice for themselves."[6] *Prince v. Massachusetts* has never been overruled by a subsequent U.S. Supreme Court decision.

Some people refer to an earlier case in Mississippi, *Bonner v. Moran,*[7] in which a 15-year-old boy was apparently conned by an aunt into going to a hospital to give skin transplants for his cousin, the aunt's son, who

had been burned. The boy did, but there was some question as to whether the mother of the donor really knew the facts of the treatment and the risks to her own son. She subsequently brought legal action against the hospital, but the court was far less than unequivocal in giving its opinion as to whether or not the mother could recover in damages. That case is sometimes quoted in defense of experimentation without consent, but the circumstances and facts were very peculiar and special for that case. There was good evidence to indicate that while the consent was not originally obtained from the mother, the procedure and risks were subsequently made known to her because the son went back repeatedly for more skin transplants and for treatment.

In any event, until such time as the Supreme Court definitively rules otherwise, or until contrary legislation is enacted by the U.S. Congress, the law prohibits experimentation on humans without informed consent. Furthermore, it is illegal to conduct experiments that are tantamount to assault and battery.

Rather than considering this subject as an academic or legalistic question, one should consider some specific examples. During and following World War II, physicians developed an awareness that excessive oxygen could produce a condition known as retrolental fibroplasia (RLF) in children, which leads to blindness. In most instances, this condition was observed in premature infants who had been placed in an excessive quantity of oxygen. So it was decided to conduct an experiment, with no real informed consent from the parents and obviously not from the babies, in which one group of babies was placed in an excessive quantity of oxygen and another in an atmosphere with a much reduced amount of oxygen. Six of the babies became totally and permanently blind.[8]

Consider another experiment. Red blood cells are broken down in the liver of the human body. In some infants the liver fails to excrete bilirubin, the major degradation product in the breakdown of erythrocytes. Furthermore, in infants, unlike adults, bilirubin has the capacity to pass the blood/brain barrier and to precipitate in the brain a dangerous condition that can lead to permanent brain damage and, in some instances, death. Research had previously established that a chemical found in human breast milk seemed to alter, revise, or impede the biochemical processes within the liver by which bilirubin was normally excreted. But the researchers wanted to see if that was also true *in vivo.* Therefore, they prepared an experiment in which this chemical compound in significant dosages was given to babies. The experiment confirmed that there was a rather fast, quite substantial build-up of the bilirubin level in these children, with the possibility of subtle brain damage as a result. There was permanent brain damage in some of those children.[9]

In another situation, at Children's Hospital in Boston, there was great interest in the natural defense mechanisms of the human host in reaction to an organ transplant. Boston is a leader in the medical field, and Children's Hospital is one of its finest health care facilities. Yet, here is what they did in designing and conducting an experiment. Without obtaining any kind of an informed consent (in most of the cases, it was questionable whether they even obtained a basic consent, that is, the traditional kind that sufficed before the concept of informed consent developed in the medical malpractice field in the early 1960s), they performed a thymectomy on babies and youngsters who were undergoing surgery for various cardiovascular problems. They took out the thymus gland, which is known to play a role in the body's immunological defense mechanisms. They then attached a piece of skin on these children from unrelated individuals, in order to determine what the bodily reaction of the thymectomized child would be to the skin that had been placed on his or her body. This was very interesting and important research. But was there any possible danger to the thymectomized youngster? And did not the parents, at the very least, have the right to have an intelligent, informed discussion from the physicians about what the possibilities of subsequent damage might be?

At Willowbrook State Hospital, Staten Island, New York, some researchers wanted more information about hepatitis in an epidemiological environment. They reasoned that in such an institution, the patients might get hepatitis anyway at some time in the future. So they took retarded youngsters, with no informed consent and most probably without any kind of consent, and gave them orally a fecal extract containing hepatitis virus to see what the medical results would be. They also did a supplemental clinical investigation in which they directly injected hepatitis virus into still other retarded children.[10]

Here is yet another example. Linoleic acid is known to be an essential nutrient, the deprivation of which has been shown to produce serious problems in animals. The effects of its deficiency have also been noted clinically in children. Nevertheless, at the University of Texas at Galveston, from 1956 to 1962, 445 babies, without informed consent, were deprived of linoleic acid. Seven of those children are known to have died of conditions directly related to the deprivation of this essential nutrient. Many others became seriously ill with a variety of dermatological conditions, pneumonia, and other conditions.[11]

In Pennsylvania in 1973 there was an exposé of another deplorable situation at the Hamburg State Home and Hospital in Berks County. It was shown that retarded children, with no consent of any kind obtained from their parents, not even informed consent, were

injected with a meningitis vaccine. The vaccine had not been approved by the FDA and was not on the clinical market, but it was given to these children nevertheless. Said the researchers at a later date, "We thought that the administrator of the hospital was the legal guardian for these children for all purposes, and he told us it was all right to go ahead and do it." Following hearings before the Department of Health, Education, and Welfare and the Department of Justice in Harrisburg, the Commonwealth of Pennsylvania put an end to that experiment and to other similar experiments that had not received approval or that had not been reviewed by appropriate agencies and authorities.

Ethics and fetal research

For years, scientists who wanted to do research involving human embryos and fetuses have found themselves in a Catch-22 situation. They could do their work with impunity and receive federal funds for it, so long as an ethics advisory board approved their proposals. The catch is that the board does not exist, and has not existed for nearly a decade.

The research on fetuses has thrived, although it has remained in the ethical shadows. The testing of new methods for prenatal diagnosis or *in vitro* fertilization, among other things, has been financed with profits from infertility treatments and standard prenatal diagnosis. The research at issue involves either embryos, including those created by *in vitro* fertilization, or intact fetuses obtained from miscarriage or hysterotomy, an early form of cesarean birth.

The ethics board was originally created in 1974, partly in response to fetal research in the 1960s and 1970s, which took place without federal restrictions. Although many experiments were unremarkable, some were profoundly objectionable. In the early 1960s, scientists at one university immersed 15 fetuses obtained from abortions in a salt solution to see whether they could absorb oxygen through the skin. One lived 22 hours. Another experiment at another university examined the fetal brain's metabolism of glucose; the researchers used heads severed from live human fetuses.

At the same time, more researchers were working on *in vitro* fertilization, in which eggs removed from a woman's body are mixed with sperm and one or more resulting embryos are implanted in her uterus. To develop the method, research with human embryos was required. After the U.S. Supreme Court struck down most restrictions on abortion in 1973, Congress appointed a commission for the protection of human subjects and asked it to rule on fetal research.

The commission ruled that fetal research was permissible. But it also ruled that no one could subject a fetus to be aborted to any more risk than one that was to be carried to term. It was an extremely restrictive policy, the commission recognized, but there was an out: An advisory board would decide, on a case-by-case basis, when this "minimal risk" standard could be waived. However, the ethics board was dissolved before it had a chance to rule on any case, and the DHHS has declined to appoint a new one.

Adult experimentation

Of course, there have been similar problems in experiments with adults. Some of these have been widely publicized.

Between February 1945 and July 1956 at the Brooklyn Jewish Chronic Disease Hospital, injections of cancer cells were given to elderly hospital patients, with no actual or meaningful permission having been obtained from them or their families. Malignant tumor cells were injected directly into the veins of elderly people suffering from advanced parkinsonism, multiple sclerosis, and other kinds of severe neurological disorders. The principal researcher in that case was Dr. Chester M. Southam from Sloan-Kettering Institute, who subsequently had his license suspended temporarily by the state of New York. When asked why he had not injected himself in the experiments since he had said that it was quite safe, he replied: "Well, you know there is always a possibility of some harm and let's face it, there simply are not too many cancer researchers around."[12]

The infamous Tuskegee syphilis study, initiated and monitored by the U.S. Public Health Service, was not terminated until 1972. In Macon County, Alabama, some 400 black men with syphilis, of a total of 600 subjects in the study, were deliberately deprived of treatment from 1932 on, purportedly to study the effects of allowing the disease to take its natural course. At least 28 of these men, and possibly as many as 107, are known to have died as a result of the disease. It has been argued that in 1932, the cure for syphilis was ineffective and sometimes worse than the disease, but certainly this was not true in the 1950s, 1960s, and 1970s, during which time the "experiment" was continued and regularly reported.

This incredible experiment was thoroughly evaluated and criticized extensively by a specially appointed committee. In the *Final Report of the Tuskegee Syphilis Study Ad Hoc Advisory Panel*, Department of Health, Education, and Welfare (Washington, D.C., 1973), one of the panelists, Jay Katz, M.D., stated:

> In conclusion, I note sadly that the medical profession, through its national association, its many individual societies, and its journals, has on the whole not reacted to this (Tuskegee Syphilis) study except by ignoring it. One lengthy editorial appeared in the October 1972 issue of the *Southern Medical Journal* which exonerated the study and chastised the "irresponsible press" for bringing it to public attention. When will we take seriously our responsibilities, particularly to the disadvantaged in our midst who so consistently throughout history have been the first to be selected for human research?[13]

Geriatric research

In Philadelphia in 1964 and 1965, 13 elderly nursing home patients died as a direct result of drug experiments conducted on behalf of one of the large pharmaceutical manufacturers. The experiment had two stages. One drug was used to induce nervous system disorders and then another was introduced to control them. Although the Food and Drug Administration (FDA) was aware of the experiment and prepared a report on it in 1967, the report was withheld for many years and not released until the *Philadelphia Bulletin* obtained it under the Freedom of Information Act.[14] There was much doubt as to whether informed consent had been obtained in this experiment.

Reporting on his observations from 50 field inspections by the FDA in 1972, Dr. Alan B. Listook, Medical Officer in the FDA's Bureau of New Drugs, stated the following:

> We have seen consent forms of senile patients signed "X-(her mark)" and have found others executed posthumously. On one occasion, where the obtainment of consent was the major reason for the FDA to conduct an investigation, we visited the subjects of the study, and discussed their understanding of the document they signed. It turned out that the women were not fully aware that they were participating in an experiment of any kind. They were not aware that they had been given a medication which had not been proven to be safe and effective.[15]

More than three years later, exactly the same kind of problem was reported again in a study conducted at a "distinguished university hospital and research center," not otherwise identified.[16] According to this later study, of 51 pregnant women who had signed a consent form in an experiment on the effects of a new labor-inducing drug, 20 did not know they were the subjects of research, even after the drug had been administered, and did not learn of it until they were interviewed by the follow-up investigator. Most of the 51 women had not been aware that any hazards were involved and had been informed only that a "new" drug was being tested, and not that it was an experimental drug. Yet, many of these women were referred to the hospital for study by their own private physicians. Whether the private physicians were aware of the true nature of the experiment is not stated, but in any case, it is clear that having one's own doctor is no safeguard in these matters.

The whole area of new drug investigations is a jungle from the standpoint of research ethics, quite apart from the specific question of informed consent. Again, a quote from the remarks of Dr. Listook is appropriate:

We have had examples of physicians submitting case reports recording the administration to subjects of much more new drug substance than was available to them. We have had police departments report the finding of case lots of investigational drugs by the roadside in trashcans.

On occasion we find records of months of treatment on an index card. We have looked at records of patients reported as having been treated for intractable angina and found no mention of heart disease, no ECG's, and no noted treatment. We frequently find that laboratory results reported to the FDA cannot be substantiated by records in the physician's office or by contact with the clinical laboratory where the work was said to have been done.

In institutions such as mental hospitals or geriatric facilities, we often see therapy prescribed that makes a study impossible to interpret and thus invalid. Major tranquilizers are given during the study of psychoactive compounds: vasodilators are given during the study of drugs being evaluated for the same purpose. Investigational drugs are discontinued without the investigator's knowledge, and adverse reactions go unreported because of lack of communication or lack of awareness on the part of the ward staff.

I could quote horror stories about paroled inmates and discharged mental patients reported as being treated in situ for weeks after their release; of therapy duration and dosage and hospital clinical courses that did not approximate those reported. . . .

We have come across individuals who were able to care for patients in their offices while they were on extended European vacations. Others, while not quite so versatile, have been able to come up with large patient populations for the treatment of widely divergent types of disease. We have the internist who does a study on an antiobesity drug and a few months later is found to be utilizing the same patients in the study of an antihypertensive. In our review of the case reports we find no hypertension reported in the first study.[17]

In view of such findings, it would seem that these researchers were not being meticulous about getting informed consent. Yet, it is from this very area—the development of new drugs—that we most often hear the arguments being advanced that research must not be fettered and that those of us who insist on adhering to the law are obstructing scientific progress.

BENEFIT VERSUS RISK RULE

In situations in which there is no potential therapeutic benefit to the subjects, it is customary to distinguish four levels of human experimentation.[18]

1. Benefit is reasonably believed to exceed the risk to the patient, and the study involves a patient who consents to this low-risk diagnostic or therapeutic procedure by coming to the physician. The patient is given information and shows that it is understood. He or she is not a subject, but rather a patient, and the needs of the patient come before any effort to gain knowledge. There is no legal problem in such a situation, except, of course, the one that physicians must contend with in all therapeutic situations—namely, obtaining an informed consent.

2. Benefit is reasonably considered to at least equal the risk, if not possibly exceed it. The patient is a volunteer. He or she may be a subject also, but if so, the relationship between the volunteer and the physician is made quite clear. At this level, we have a controlled experiment, but everyone knows what's happening, and there is definitely a strong possibility—in fact, a probability—that the project may be of some therapeutic benefit to the patient.

3. The risk exceeds the benefit to the patient, but the risk is balanced by possible benefit to society. Here, the highest possible degree of informed consent is essential. Experiments in this field are still permissible, including those on children, provided the highest degree of informed consent is obtained from the patient or subject.

4. Risk exceeds benefit. The individual is either both the subject and the patient or purely just a subject. Consent from the individual either has not been obtained or has been obtained through deceit, the force of authority, or other improper means.

Usually, the last category is the issue. Because medical research trials frequently require that a convenient, stable subject population be followed over a period of weeks or months rather than days or hours, the medical scientist naturally turns to "captive" groups whose availability can be controlled. These groups include

- Hospitalized or institutionalized patients
- Children
- Mentally abnormal persons
- Prisoners
- Persons under discipline (armed forces and police force)
- Laboratory assistants and medical students.

In all these groups, there are factors present that tend to make the individuals involved susceptible to pressures or influences that induce them to give their consent to experimentation. For example, prisoners hope for probation, soldiers for promotion, and students for higher grades. Use of such groups for medical experimentation is not invariably improper, but experiments conducted on such persons raise the question as to whether the consent obtained, if any, may have been the result of coercion or other influences that would place the project in category 4.

In recent years, medical research in prisons has been prohibited in many states. The National Commission on Protection of Subjects has recently released its recommendations on allowable research on prison inmates. They are very stringent recommendations that would virtually eliminate such research from American prisons.

This problem was particularly relevant in the case of children as experimental subjects. In the Hamburg State Home and Hospital case mentioned earlier, studies were initially undertaken without an informed consent. Indeed, there was *no* consent obtained at all. The physician in charge of the study "thought" that the administrator of the hospital was the legal guardian of these mentally retarded children!

Sometime later, the physicians did send some kind of generalized consent form to the parents, and some of these were signed and returned. However, there is no question at all from a legal standpoint that this kind of consent is not a valid informed consent and would not hold up in the courts of Pennsylvania, even if the parents had been the subjects.

What if the pharmaceutical company involved with that meningitis vaccine felt it was essential to learn what the effects of that vaccine on children would be? Could that company, with its thousands of employees in this country and abroad, including all their research teams and top administrators, have gone to their employees and asked for volunteers?

Inasmuch as the meningitis vaccine that was being tested was of no direct therapeutic benefit to the children who were to receive it, even the parents within the pharmaceutical company could not have given a legal consent for their own children. Such experimentation would be considered assault and battery. And no one—not even a parent—can give legal consent to have assault and battery committed on another human being.

Every one of these experiments on children involved subjects who did not have the necessary intellectual capacity to give a truly informed consent. They may have been legally adjudicated *non compos mentis,* or perhaps they merely had been socially and economically deprived to an extreme degree, but invariably they were incapable of giving an informed consent.

It is imperative that everyone in positions of authority within government, medical institutions, health care facilities, and custodial homes appreciate that no matter what the altruistic and projected humanitarian aspects of medical research may be, human beings cannot be subjected to medical experimentation without a proper informed consent having been obtained from them. In the case of minors (especially retarded children), elderly or senile persons who are suffering from serious diseases and do not have a full grasp of their mental faculties, or people who are imprisoned or otherwise subject to coercion, very serious moral and ethical principles must be carefully considered by the research team before undertaking any experiments that place the subjects at risk.

No legitimate reason or justification exists for further delay or governmental procrastination on this subject.

There is absolutely no question from a legal standpoint that experiments of this nature are in violation of the law and are against basic concepts of medical morality and ethics. Physicians and scientists, as well as governmental officials in charge of hospitals, homes, and institutions of various kinds, should realize that the civil and criminal laws pertain to them, also.

CRIMINAL AND CIVIL LIABILITY

While the *Hyman v. Brooklyn Jewish Chronic Disease Hosp.*[19] case makes mention of the "experimentation" question, it is of little value in ascertaining the legal guidelines for experimentation. The court confined itself to the narrow issue of whether a director of a membership corporation has a right to inspect the corporate "records." In this case, the court held that possible corporate liability gives the director the right to inspection. As to the liability for the experimentation, the court ventures no unnecessary opinion. Assuming that experimentation is carried on under approved scientific techniques, it may be instinctive to consider possible liabilities, viewing a researcher-subject relationship under criminal, tort, and contract law, recognizing that the categories are not always mutually exclusive.

Criminal liability, in the absence of statute, will attach when there is an intended harm constituting homicide or mayhem, or an unintended harm resulting from negligence by commission or omission of such character that it extends beyond ordinary negligence and is considered culpable negligence.

If a volunteer dies during or as a result of "experimentation," the criminal liability, if any, would be for homicide—murder or manslaughter.

The Pennsylvania statute (typical of most states) defines the crime of murder as:

All murder which shall be perpetrated by means of poison, or by lying in wait, or any other kind of willful, deliberate and premeditated killing or which shall be committed in the perpetration of, or attempting to perpetrate any arson, rape, robbery, burglary, or kidnapping shall be murder in the first degree. All other kinds of murder shall be murder in the second degree. The jury before whom any person indicted for murder shall be tried, shall, if they find such person guilty thereof, ascertain in their verdict whether the person is guilty of murder of the first or second degree.

Murder is the unlawful killing of another with malice aforethought, express or implied.[20]

It is highly unlikely that a properly conceived and reliably approved research project undertaken by a competent specialist would qualify as an act of murder. If the research provides a strong possibility of death or severe injury, known in advance to the scientist in charge, malice may perhaps be implied. The statute provides a further definition:

Manslaughter, however, may be found without malice. Where the practice is such as to constitute a gross ignorance or culpable negligence or such a complete disregard of life or health, the courts have found voluntary or involuntary manslaughter.

Although no case involving experimentation that resulted in a conviction for voluntary or involuntary manslaughter can be found, it has been established that where such charges are brought, consent does not usually constitute a defense to criminal liability.

Professor Kidd of the University of California School of Law raises the question with specific reference to experimentation:

How far can one consent to serious injury to himself? The analogies are not close. Abortion, except for therapeutic reasons, is a crime, and the consent of the woman is no defense for the doctor. A person can not legally consent to his own death; it is murder by the person who kills him... A person may not consent to serious injury amounting to a maim.[21]

In general, criminal negligence in a physician (experimenter) exists when the physician exhibits gross lack of competency, inattention, or wanton indifference to the patient's safety, either through gross ignorance or lack of skill. It is assumed that the same standards would be applicable to scientists engaging in human experiments:

In case of permanent injury or disease rather than death, the possible criminal charge would be mayhem. This crime at common law and by statute generally is also founded on malice and as such would be governed by the [same considerations alluded to above].[22]

Basic to the law of torts, a second area of consideration as to the legal consequences of experimentation is the right of the individual to "freedom from bodily harm," so that any unauthorized invasion, or even threat, to the person constitutes grounds for liability. Consent is usually achieved through the use of a release, either written or oral, allowing the patient's person to be physically handled. In the normal doctor-patient relationship, there usually is ample basis for finding informed agreement on the part of the patient for ordinary procedures by virtue of the recognized relationship between the parties. It is assumed that the physician is acting in good faith for the personal benefit of the patient who, by seeking professional assistance, may be assumed to consent to the treatment and diagnoses given. In an experimental situation, the inference of consent is not so easily drawn, and there seems to be more of a need for formal consent:

There is scant legal authority on this problem (but)... abundant expert testimony is usually available to show that subjecting a patient to experimentation without disclosure and consent is contrary to the customs of surgeons and thus

negligent, even though there may be no technical slip in actual performance of the experiment.[23]

Specific to the problem of experimentation, tort liability may arise in cases of nontherapeutic, unnecessary, and legally questionable procedures involving criminal liability and public policy. For instance, in situations such as abortion and euthanasia, cases may be found in which, despite consent, the physician was held to tort liability. In none of these areas has there occurred experimentation by a scientist on humans for nontherapeutic reasons. In some states, a contract action is permitted on the theory breach of an implied agreement to treat with proper care and skill; the essence of the research contract lies in the complete understanding of the parties:

The medical research procedure by definition and by nature is a deviation from normal practice, even though all the specific elements involved may be well established, simply because medical practice ordinarily does not encompass employment of human beings primarily for the advancement of knowledge. There is no implicit understanding that conventional methods will be used and that the patient will be released as soon as his condition warrants. Consequently, the researcher has a more specific responsibility for full disclosure of his purpose, method, and probable consequences. Achieving a meeting of the minds is a far more critical element in the research contract.[24]

Assuming there is a complete understanding, a research contract will probably provide a defense against liability in a reasonable execution of the contract obligation or performance of the experiment. However, such a contract is unlikely to serve as a complete bar to an allegation of negligence. The patient's own performance under the contract will not be the subject of a decree for specific performance by a court of equity as they are for "personal services."

In conclusion, it would seem that medical practice, generally conceived to be diagnosis, treatment, and care, is governed by state statute and supporting administrative licensing and regulatory bodies. Medical research experimentation on human subjects would appear to be outside the scope of these rules:

Case law, insofar as it appears to recognize medically related activity, generally characterizes such research as experimentation and holds it to be outside legitimate medical practice. Reported cases have not yet considered modern controlled medical research as such, and have not yet established limits within which human research may be pursued. Cases which have involved conduct labeled experimentation have been decided basically on issues of disclosure or consent, negligence, lack of qualification, improper activity (quack procedures, medicines or devices) or unlicensed practice of medicine usually arising in cases of departure from accepted diagnosis, therapy or other practice.[25]

Despite the Nuremberg Code, the Declaration of Helsinki, the AMA Ethical Guidelines, and numerous other declarations of similar import, apparently many physicians, scientists, and governmental officials still think that because humane benefits may be derived from these experiments in later years, anything is justified today, particularly if the groups being used as guinea pigs consist of retarded children, senile persons, prisoners, or other unfortunate groups with various physical, psychological, or economic handicaps.

A special national commission has been proposed to review all the various facets of this sensitive, important, and complex matter. This group is to have a dual purpose: first, to establish basic principles and guidelines that would be uniformly applicable in all proposed projects involving human experimentation; and second, to consider, evaluate, and approve each new research proposal involving any kind of experimentation on humans. Legislation would have to be enacted to require that all such proposals be submitted and approved before being implemented. Membership in such a commission should necessarily be broad, extending beyond the medical and scientific professions, and all its decisions and records should be subject to public disclosure.

In 1982, the President's Commission for the Study of Ethical Problems in Medicine and Biomedical and Behavioral Research completed a two-year examination of federal rules and procedures for conducting research with human subjects. The commission concluded that most government supervisory agencies have insufficient data on compliance, and a review of a few well-documented (and widely reported) cases of misconduct on the part of research scientists showed that government oversight can be improved. However, the public must keep a balanced perspective.

Because successful therapies for humans can only be established by tests on human subjects, medical progress depends on the participation of volunteers in research to test new therapies.

The prerequisites for such experimentation include at least the following: a reasonable theoretical base for the belief that therapy may be useful; preliminary tests on nonhuman subjects; a careful weighing of the possible benefits and expected risks of the experimental therapy, as well as an assessment of the available standard therapies; and the genuine voluntary consent of the human subject.

The presidential commission's study demonstrates that federally funded institutions need well-defined procedures for responding to reports of misconduct, ranging from falsified data on patient's/subject's charts to conducting studies with drugs not cleared for tests on humans. Some procedures should protect from reprisal those who report their concern (the so-called "whistle-blowers"). Such procedures also should protect scientists accused of misconduct from publicity and loss of federal funds, at least until a preliminary finding is made that the accusations have some basis in fact. For the sake of all concerned, the institutional response should be prompt, thorough, and fair.

The 23 governmental agencies and institutions involved in research on human subjects (e.g., the DHHS and the National Science Foundation) need clearly defined standards for investigations and sanctions.

INNOVATIVE THERAPY

To understand the concept of innovative therapy, it is useful to consider first the activities referred to as standard medical practice.

Standard practice was defined by the National Commission for the Protection of Human Subjects of Biomedical and Behavioral Research as "interventions that are designed solely to enhance the well-being of an individual patient or client and that have a reasonable expectation of success. The purpose of medical or behavioral practice is to provide diagnosis, preventive treatments or therapy to particular individuals."[26]

The commission was established by Congress.[27] Its purpose was to conduct a comprehensive investigation and study to identify the basic ethical principles that should underlie the conduct of biomedical and behavioral research, evaluate existing guidelines for the protection of human subjects, and make appropriate recommendations to the Secretary of Health, Education, and Welfare concerning further steps, if any, to be taken.

The commission identified innovative therapies as a class of procedures that were "designed solely to enhance the well-being of an individual patient or client," but had not been tested sufficiently to meet the standard of having "a reasonable expectation of success." Innovative therapies have been defined as activities "ordinarily conducted . . . with either pure practice intent or with varying degrees of mixed research and practice intent" that have been sufficiently tested to meet standards for acceptance or approval.

Dale H. Cowan[28] has stated that the difference between innovative and standard practices may be simply the difference between a beginning and an advanced level of the practice of medicine. However, as noted by R. J. Levine, in referring to the Belmont Report,[29] the attribute that defines innovative therapies is the "lack of suitable validation of (their) safety and efficacy," rather than their "novelty." A practice might not be validated because there is (1) a lack of sufficient testing to certify its safety and efficacy for an intended class of patients or (2) evidence that previously held assumptions about its safety and efficacy should be questioned.

The FDA proposed a major change in the rules for reporting side effects from drug trials in 1993. This proposal came on the heels of publicly released information indicating that several people had died after having been given a new drug for hepatitis B in a series of experimental drug trials. Five out of 15 patients who took the drug for four weeks or more died. It was determined in retrospect that five other patients in earlier experiments most probably died as a result of taking that same drug, or its experimental predecessor. The drug involved was fialuridine; in the earlier experiments, it was a closely related drug, filacytosine. None of the deaths was reported to the FDA by the scientists or the drug companies, supposedly because the individuals conducting the experiments "assumed that the deaths had not been caused by the drug."

In late 1993, articles appeared in newspapers throughout the world dealing with the use of cadavers in car crash tests at Heidelberg University in Germany. These experimental studies had been partly financed by the U.S. National Highway Traffic Safety Administration. Similar tests reportedly had been conducted at the University of Virginia and at the Medical College of Wisconsin, and also at Wayne State University in Detroit, the latter at the behest of the Centers for Disease Control and Prevention (CDC). Many questions were raised about whether or not an informed consent had been obtained by the legal next-of-kin before these corpses were used. The tests in Germany included the dead bodies of 200 adults and 8 children. German law permits the use of cadavers for research as long as the relatives' consent is obtained.

In 1976, John Moore, a 33-year-old male, was diagnosed with hairy-cell leukemia at the Medical Center of the University of California at Los Angeles (UCLA). His treating physician was Dr. David W. Golde, a hematologist and researcher at the UCLA Medical Center. A splenectomy was performed as part of the treatment. Dr. Golde recognized the commercial and scientific value of Mr. Moore's spleen and other bodily tissues and materials at the time he recommended the splenectomy. The spleen was taken to a hospital research unit to develop a cell line for commercial use. Golde and another researcher, Quan, then developed and patented a cell line from Moore's cells that produced lymphokines, a genetic product of considerable commercial value. The two researchers, a pharmaceutical company, and UCLA entered into a contract with the Genetics Institute worth more than $330,000 for the products that would be developed from this patented cell line over a three-year period.

Following the splenectomy, Mr. Moore returned to the hospital on several occasions over a seven-year period at the request of Dr. Golde, and had samples taken of his blood, skin, bone marrow aspirate, and sperm. These were done specifically for commercial and not therapeutic purposes. Mr. Moore was never informed at any time by Dr. Golde of these research activities, or of the commercial value of his cells. When Moore ultimately discovered that his cells had been used to develop this cell line, he sued the researchers, various companies, and UCLA. The trial court dismissed all the claims, but an intermediate appellate court reversed and held that Moore had stated a cause of action for conversion. On appeal, the California Supreme Court, two justices dissenting, reversed and held that Moore had no property interest in his cells and, therefore, no cause of action for conversion. However, the court unanimously held that Moore had set forth facts sufficient to state a cause of action for breach of fiduciary relationship and lack of informed consent against Golde for failing to disclose his research and commercial interest prior to the splenectomy, and prior to the removal of Moore's other body tissues and blood in subsequent visits to UCLA. A petition for writ of certiorari to the U.S. Supreme Court was denied.

CONCLUSION

A discussion of the liability of a physician for experimental procedures including human research requires an initial examination of the two competing interests that must be balanced in any experimental situation. There is the obvious interest of the patient to be free from the abuses to which uncontrolled experimentation can lead—from the most grotesque examples of the atrocities of Nazi Germany to the violation of the rights of individuals to be free from becoming unwilling participants in any form of experimentation. The interest of the physician and the interest of society as a whole must be balanced against the interest of the individual. If physicians are limited strictly to previously established procedures, all innovation and progress in the field of medicine would cease. The courts have recognized both of these interests in attempting to deal with the problem of when the physician should bear the burden of the effects of experimental procedures.[32] They have laid down the principle that one who experiments with an innovative treatment is responsible for all the harm that follows. Later cases articulated the need for the advancement of medicine, and in these cases the court stated that it is a recognized fact that, if the general practice of medicine is to progress, a certain amount of experimentation must be carried on.

Complicating the problem of balancing these interests is the difficulty of defining experimentation.[33,34] Courts have confused judgmental decisions and experimentation. In the opinion of one court, a physician is presumed to have the knowledge and skill to use some innovation;

In general, practices or therapies that are standard or accepted have risks and benefits that are known. Additionally, some basis exists for thinking that the benefits outweigh the risks. By contrast, the potential benefits and risks of innovative therapies are less well known and predictable. Consequently, their use exposes patients to a greater likelihood that the balance of benefits and risks may be unfavorable due either to the therapies being ineffective or entailing greater, possibly unknown, risks. Thus standard medical practice can be distinguished from innovative therapies on the basis of the extent of knowledge that exists regarding their likely risks and benefits.

The commission described experimentation or research as

[A]n activity designed to test a hypothesis, permit conclusions to be drawn and thereby to develop or contribute to generalizable knowledge (expressed, for example, in theories, principles, and statements of relationships). Research is usually described in a formal protocol that sets forth an objective and a set of procedures designed to reach that objective.[30]

Levine defined research involving humans as

[A]ny manipulation, observation, or other study of a human being—or of anything related to that human being that might subsequently result in manipulation of that human being—done with the intent of developing new knowledge and which differs in any way from customary medical (or other professional) practice.[31]

The distinction between innovative therapy and experimentation can be drawn by focusing on the four levels of research listed previously. Like research, innovative therapy generally represents a departure from standard medical practice.

Federal regulations require that all research involving human subjects conducted by the DHHS, or funded in whole or in part by a grant, contract, cooperative agreement, or fellowship from DHHS, be reviewed by an Institutional Review Board (IRB) established at each institution in which the research is to be conducted. The regulations define research as "a systematic investigation designed to develop or contribute to generalizable knowledge." The regulations further specify minimum requirements for the composition of IRBs and require that each institution engaged in research covered by the regulations must file a written assurance to the secretary of DHHS that "it will comply with the requirements set forth in (the) regulations."

To approve research by the regulations, IRBs must determine that a number of requirements are satisfied.

1. Risks to the subjects are minimized.
2. Risks to the subjects are reasonable in relation to anticipated benefits, if any, to subjects, and the importance of the knowledge that may reasonably be expected to result.
3. Selection of the subjects is equitable.
4. Informed consent will be sought from each prospective subject or the subject's legally authorized representative.
5. When appropriate, the research plan makes adequate provision for monitoring the data collected to ensure the safety of the subjects.

RADIATION EXPERIMENTS

In December 1993, the U.S. Department of Energy publicly disclosed that for the last six years it had ignored clear evidence of extensive illegal experiments conducted by distinguished medical scientists in the nation's nuclear weapons industry that took place over a period of three decades following World War II, in which various groups of civilians were exposed to radiation in concentrations far above levels that are considered safe at this time. These experiments, conducted at government laboratories and prominent medical research institutions, involved injecting patients with dangerous radioactive substances, such as plutonium, or exposing them to powerful radiation beams. Allegedly, this work was undertaken to determine what the effect of radiation would be on soldiers and civilians if a global atomic war occurred.

The experiments dealing with testing radiation on humans are listed in the table on page 722.

Other experiments of a similar nature took place at a state school in Fernald, Massachusetts, from 1946 to 1956, in which as many as 125 mentally retarded teenage boys were given radioactive iron and calcium in their breakfast cereal. Consent forms sent to the parents indicated that this study was intended to help researchers better understand human metabolism and nutritional needs. No mention was made that radioactive elements would be utilized.

Records from the Massachusetts Institute of Technology indicate that 23 pregnant women at the Boston Lying-In Hospital (now part of Brigham and Women's Hospital) were injected with radioactive iron in the early 1950s in order to allow researchers to study maternal-fetal circulation. In yet another experiment conducted around the same time at Massachusetts General Hospital, patients were given radioactive iodine to study thyroid function and body metabolism, even though the researchers acknowledged they did not know what the long-term effects would be.

Altogether, as of early 1994, U.S. government officials acknowledge that more than 30 experiments involving the use of radioactive materials or radiation, in which the subjects or their parents and guardians were not apprised of the true nature of the studies and, therefore,

Location(s)	Date	People affected	Experiments
Vanderbilt University, Nashville	Late 1940s	About 800 pregnant women	Subjects were studied to determine the effect of radioactive iron on fetal development. A follow-up study of children born to the women found a higher-than-normal cancer rate.
Oak Ridge National Laboratory, Oak Ridge, Tennessee	Mid-1970s	Nearly 200 patients with leukemia and other cancers	They were exposed to high levels of radiation. The experiments ended after a 1974 government memorandum said the study had done little to benefit the patients.
University of Rochester, Oak Ridge Laboratory, University of Chicago, and the University of California Hospital in San Francisco	1945-1947	18 people	Subjects were injected with high concentrations of plutonium, apparently without their informed consent. Many patients were chosen because medical specialists believed they suffered life-threatening illnesses.
Oregon State Prison	1963-1971	67 inmates	Prisoner's testicles were exposed to X-rays to help researchers understand the effects of radiation on production and function of sperm. The inmates signed consent statements indicating that they were aware of some of the risks, but the statements did not mention that radiation could cause cancer.
Washington State Prison	1963-1970	64 inmates	A similar study subjected prisoners to high levels of radiation. The purpose was to determine the minimum dose that would cause healthy men to become temporarily sterile.
Columbia University and Montefiore Hospital in the Bronx	Late 1950s	12 terminally ill cancer patients	Subjects were injected with concentrations of radioactive calcium and strontium-85, another radioactive substance, to measure the rate at which radioactive substances were absorbed into various human tissues.

Sources: The Department of Energy, the Atomic Energy Commission, and Congress.

could not have given legally acceptable informed consent, took place during a three-decade period beginning in 1946. There may well have been several more that are yet to be uncovered.

The government had previously resisted paying compensation to any of these individuals. However, from October 1991 to May 1993, the government spent $47.1 million to reimburse the legal expenses of the private corporations that operated its nuclear weapons plants. Now, the present Energy Secretary, Hazel O'Leary, has proclaimed her definite intention to obtain compensation for all victims of these unethical experiments.

It is important to note that some of these tests were first disclosed in 1986 in a report to Congress by the General Accounting Office. However, when Representative Edward J. Markey of Massachusetts, chairman of the congressional committee that reviewed this report, asked the government for more information and urged full disclosure of all such experiments, he was firmly and repeatedly rebuffed by both the Reagan and Bush administrations.

It should be noted that a senior official of the Atomic Energy Commission, in a 1950 memorandum to one of the prominent physician-scientists involved with some radiation experiments in the Boston area, observed that these medical experiments might have "a little of the Buchenwald touch." Thus, it would appear that both the government officials and medical researchers who planned and conducted these radiation experiments were aware that these studies violated the 1947 Nuremberg Code, which was adopted after the Nazi war crimes trials, and is regarded as the universal standard for experiments involving human beings.

QUESTIONABLE HUMAN RESEARCH AND EXPERIMENTATION PRACTICES

In addition to the large number of alleged illegal experiments involving radiation and radioactive compounds, several other highly controversial situations have been brought to light in the past few years involving research projects and experimentation, in which informed consent, official and academic guidelines, and

other applicable legal and ethical considerations were ignored by the physicians, scientists, and officials in charge of those studies.

The Medical University of South Carolina was accused of testing pregnant women for illicit drug use without their consent, and then transmitting that information to local law enforcement officials. This drug testing program was apparently adopted as a means of forcing drug-addicted women who were pregnant to stop using drugs by threatening them with jail if they refused to cooperate with the hospital's regimen of prenatal visits and also attend an established drug treatment program. Almost all the women in the program were African-Americans, and several of them were actually arrested and prosecuted for illicit drug use as a result of the disclosure of this information by the university hospital to the police. Dr. Charles R. McCarthy, formerly chief of the Office of Protection of Research Risks at the National Institutes of Health, concluded that this project "fits the definition of an experiment." He indicated that federal rules regarding human experimentation require that subjects give informed consent before being made part of an experiment, and that the patient has the right to refuse to participate and still be given appropriate and necessary medical treatment.

The *Boston Globe* recently reported that the infamous Timothy Leary, the 1960s drug guru, gave inmates at the Concord State Prison in Massachusetts doses of psilocybin, a powerful hallucinogenic drug, without their knowledge or consent. This compound can produce hallucinations, perception distortion, and psychosis, and is considered to be psychologically addictive. These tests took place in the 1960s when Leary was a faculty member at Harvard University. He was eventually fired from his position at the prison by state officials, although not until these illegal tests had been under way for many years.

In late 1993, a rash of international articles reported that postmenopausal women were being impregnated with donated eggs fertilized with their husbands' sperm. In England, a 59-year-old woman gave birth to twins, and a 61-year-old Italian woman also gave birth following such a procedure. Numerous cases of a similar nature were also reported in France. Harvested eggs from aborted female fetuses were permitted to mature, and then via artificial insemination, were used to impregnate these elderly women. This experimental process, which had first been utilized in mice by Dr. Roger Gosden, a research scientist in Edinburgh, Scotland, has raised many ethical questions, and has precipitated specific legislation in France and elsewhere that would ban the use of such a technique in postmenopausal women.

In the summer of 1993, two French physicians were charged with manslaughter in connection with the death

of a child, who died after contracting Creutzfeld disease, a rare viral illness that attacks th following a long incubation period. Several oth dren were thought to have been afflicted also, not yet died. This disease, which is incurable a to rapid dementia and death, developed follo administration of pituitary gland extracts children who suffered from dwarfism. The glands had been acquired from 1983 to 1 corpses in Bulgaria and Hungary. Many of the donors had been patients in psychiatric hosp infectious wards.

A current controversy with fascinating ethical overtones is that of human cloning. sponsored research dealing with *in vitro* fe (IVF) has been held in abeyance since 1980, b the Clinton administration attempted to ga support for research on IVF and the result embryos. The "NIH Revitalization Act of 199 the requirement for ethics board scruti research proposals.

A scientific debate has yet to resolve the exactly "What is a clone?" Dr. Robert George Washington University Medical Cen his findings at a meeting in October 1 American Fertilization Society. He claim cloned human embryos, splitting single e identical twins or triplets. Because human s frozen and used at a later date, it could be parents to have a child, and years later, u frozen embryo to give birth to an identical as an organ donor for the older child. A t already been developed for making iden animals (e.g., cattle) by dividing the embry times and letting the new clusters of cells two genetically identical organisms.

In 1993, an internationally known med Dr. Peter Wiernik, publicly admitted his provided illegal injections of an experimer brain tumor patients in 1987, "using th guinea pigs." Dr. Wiernik acknowledg cover-up in an agreement worked ou prosecutors earlier in 1993, whereby h and reprimanded, but not subjected to ecution. The patients, all of whom were t have since died, were told about the expe of the drug, but were not informed approval from the Food and Drug (FDA). Dr. Wiernik had received FDA this drug, interleukin-2 (IL-2), in kidne ments. However, he gave leftover IL-2 geons for treatment of patients with br treatments had never been approved

yet courts have in the past mislabeled that area of permissible judgment as "experimentation." However, any time a physician's procedures do not follow accepted medical practice, he or she is moving in the direction of experimentation and the distinction between innovation and experimentation becomes blurred. On the other hand, the courts have determined that the mere fact of departure from the drug manufacturer's recommended dose does not make the departure an "experiment." A procedure does not rise to the level of an experiment if the physician has previously used the method successfully, the procedure has been described in the literature, and the choice has been reasonably and prudently calculated by the physician to accomplish the intended purpose. However, surely it is not enough that the intentions of the physician be reasonable to find that a previously unapproved procedure is not an experiment.

When drawing the line between experiment and judgment becomes difficult, the courts are likely to be influenced by the fact that no approved therapy is available. The physician then is faced with the choice of no treatment or innovation. And in examining the type of innovation chosen by the physician, the court will look at the rationale of the physician in making that choice and the extent to which that choice was a significant departure from previous standards of care.

Another factor that has been proposed as being important in deciding what is considered "experimentation" is the distinction between the curable and the terminally ill patient. It has been argued that the terminally ill patient with no hope of recovery from accepted medical procedures should be free to choose from any form of treatment and should not be restricted in his or her choice by laws that were designed to protect the patient from the risks of experimentation. A distinction between curable and terminally ill patients is not valid, however, when the protection of the rights of an individual from the use of experimental drugs are concerned. It has been held that a physician treating terminally ill patients with an unapproved drug may be subject to criminal penalties.[35] The U.S. Supreme Court has ruled that the Federal Food, Drug and Cosmetic Act, which restricts the use of experimental drugs, contains no exemptions for the terminally ill patient.[36]

Although a number of courts have recognized a legal right to recover for damages resulting from experimentation by the physician, no cases to date have actually turned on the issue of experimentation alone. The courts have seemed reluctant to base liability squarely on the issue of experimentation, perhaps because the issue of experimentation is composed of a number of elements. Instead, they have employed a number of other legal theories for finding liability.

The first and most important is that of informed consent. One court has stated that without informed consent for an investigational procedure a physician commits a battery.[37] Liability for experimental procedures has been predicated on the lack of informed consent of the patient in a number of cases.[38] In one case involving psychosurgery on a mental patient and that procedure was totally novel and unrelated to any previously accepted procedure, the lack of knowledge on the subject made a knowledgeable consent impossible.[39] However, most courts have accepted the idea that an informed consent is possible even when the knowledge surrounding the procedure is limited. Some believe absolute liability should be imposed on the physician for experimental procedures because they amount to abnormally dangerous activity under 402(a), Restatement (Second) of Torts. However, informed consent before the administration of an investigational drug amounts to voluntarily encountering a dangerous activity that bars recovery under 402(2).

If a physician adopts a method not recognized as sound by the medical community, the physician may be liable if it injures the patient in any way. Any variance from established standards can lead to liability. This "any variance" approach has been modified by most courts. It is generally recognized that where competent medical authorities are divided, a physician will not be held liable if he or she follows a form of treatment advocated by a considerable number in the profession. This represents the "respectable minority" approach.[40]

It is important to consider whether the physician undertook a form of treatment that a reasonable and prudent member of the medical profession would undertake under the same or similar circumstances. This standard is an appropriate one, but in the area of experimentation there is a need for more specific guidelines to be articulated by the courts.[41] For example, the test might include factors such as (1) the qualifications of the physician in question to do the particular procedure involved, (2) the rationality of the procedure based on the extent of departure from accepted procedures and the indication of need for the procedure under the circumstances, and (3) the risk of the procedure versus the benefit to be derived from it.

A third legal theory used in experimentation cases is based on the patient's right of privacy. The right to control one's body is part of the right of privacy inherent in our Constitution. Experimentation has been considered a violation of this right.

The physician may be able to guard against liability for experimental procedures with a covenant not to sue. The patient agrees prior to treatment not to sue if injured as a result of the experimental treatment. When the procedure, though experimental, may have some value and represents a last chance for help, the physician may secure an agreement not to sue if it is not helpful, provided the patient is fully advised.

In addition to the case law that has developed regarding experimentation, there is some federal and state statutory law in this area. Most important within the federal province is the Federal Food, Drug and Cosmetic Act and the regulations promulgated thereunder. These are designed to regulate the influx of "new" drugs in the market. Section 505(i) of the Act[42] exempts from premarketing approval drugs intended solely for investigational use if they satisfy certain criteria. Experimental drugs are available only to authorized investigators. At authorized institutions their use (as well as any experimental procedure) is subject to the IRB under the regulations of the DHHS. The board examines (1) the knowledge to be gained from the study, (2) prior experimental and clinical findings to determine the necessity and timeliness of using human subjects, (3) potential benefits to the subjects, (4) potential risks and procedures to minimize them, (5) confidentiality procedures, (6) the consent process, and (7) the proposed subject population.

The approval of a study does not mean that the investigator is then insulated from personal liability for harm suffered by the subjects in the study, but it substantially decreases the risk, especially with regard to liability based on failure to secure a subject's informed consent. These procedures are not universally mandated by law, but they apply when research is supported by DHHS funds or submitted to the FDA.

State statutes designed to protect subjects from the risks of experimentation tend to focus on specific matters rather than setting general guidelines for review of research.[43] These statutes regulate investigational drugs, fetal research, psychosurgery, confidentiality of information, and privacy. Only the state of New York statutorily requires institutional review committees for human research. Their function is basically the same as that of the IRB.[44] The state of Louisiana is the only state that defines the crime of human experimentation.[45] State statutes regulating human experimentation are a reasonable exercise of the state's police power.

END NOTES

1. Beecher, *Ethics and Clinical Research,* New Eng. J. Med. 37ff (June 8, 1973). [See also Beecher, *Experimentation in Man,* published as a report to the Council on Drugs of the American Medical Association, 169 JAMA 461-78 (1959) (republished by Charles C. Thomas, 1959).]
2. Commission on CIA Activities Within the United States, *Report to the President* (June 1975).
3. Associated Press dispatch, Washington D.C. (Aug. 13, 1975).
4. UPI dispatch, Salem, Oregon (Mar. 4, 1976).
5. UPI dispatch, Washington, D.C. (Feb. 22, 1976) (E. Delong).
6. *Prince v. Massachusetts,* 321 U.S. 158 at 170 (1944).
7. *Bonner v. Moran,* 126 F.2d 121 (D.C. Cir. 1941).
8. Pappworth, *Human Guinea Pigs: Experimentation on Man* (1967).
9. The New Republic, Dec. 3, 1966 at 10.
10. 288 New Engl. J. Med., 755, 791, 1247 (1973).
11. Med. World News, April 13, 1973 at 4.
12. Med. World News, June 5, 1964 at 6; 151 Science 663 (1966).
13. Med. World News, Aug. 18, 1972 at 15; Curran, *Legal Liability in Clinical Investigations,* 289 New Engl. J. Med. 730 (1973).
14. The Philadelphia Bulletin, Nov. 16, 1975 at 1.
15. Hosp. Trib., May 14, 1973 at 1.
16. Barber, *The Ethics of Experimentation with Human Subjects,* 234 Sci. Am. 25 (Feb. 1976).
17. Hosp. Trib., May 14, 1973 at 1.
18. *Human Experimentation,* Med. World News, June 8, 1973 at 37ff.
19. *Hyman v. Jewish Chronic Disease Hosp.,* 206 N.E.2d 3381 N.Y. (1965).
20. 18 Purdon's Statutes §2501 *et seq.;* 18 Pa. C.S.A. §2501 *et seq.*
21. Kidd, *The Problem of Experimentation on Human Beings: Limits of the Right of a Person to Consent to Experimentation on Himself,* 117 Science 211, 212 (1953).
22. *Id.*
23. *Id.*
24. *Id.*
25. *Id.*
26. The commission was established by Congress in Title II, Part A, §201(a) of the National Research Service Award Act of 1974, Pub. L. No. 93-348, 88 Stat. 142. The purpose of the commission was to conduct a comprehensive investigation and study to identify the basic ethical principles that should underlie the conduct of biomedical and behavioral research, evaluate existing guidelines for the protection of human subjects, and make appropriate recommendations to the Secretary of HEW concerning further steps, if any, to be taken. *Id.* at §202(a)(1)(A) (Hereinafter referred to as the Commission.).
27. *Id.*
28. Cowan, *Innovative Therapy Versus Experimentation,* Tort and Insurance L.J. (Summer 1986).
29. National Commission, *The Belmont Report: Ethical Principles and Guidelines for the Protection of Human Subjects of Research* (DHEW Pub. No. (OS) 78-0012 (1978) (hereinafter referred to as the Belmont Report.)
30. *Supra* note 26.
31. Levine, *The Boundaries Between Biomedical or Behavioral Research and the Accepted and Routine Practice of Medicine,* Belmont Report, Appendix I (Paper No. 1, DHEW Pub. N. (OS) 78-0013 (1978).
32. *Carpenter v. Blake,* 60 Barb. (N.Y.) 488, *revised on other grounds,* 50 N.Y. 696 (1872).
33. *Fortner v. Koch,* 272 Mich. 273, 261 N.W. 762 (1935).
34. *Brooks v. St. Johns Hickey Memorial Hosp.,* 269 Ind. 270, 380 N.E.2d 72 (1978).
35. *People v. Privitera,* 23 Cal.3d 697 (1979).
36. *U.S. v. Rutherford,* 582 F.2d 1234, *cert. granted* 99 S.Ct. 1042, 439 U.S. 1127, *cert. denied* 99 S.Ct. 1045, 439 U.S. 1127, *revised,* 99 S.Ct. 2470, 442 U.S. 544, *on remand,* 611 F.2d (1979).
37. *Gatson v. Hunter,* 121 Ariz. 33, 588 P.2d 326 (1978).
38. *Ahern v. Veteran's Administration,* 537 F.2d 1098 (1976).
39. *Kaimowitz v. Michigan Dept. of Mental Health,* (Civil No. 73-19434-AW) Cir.Ct. Wayne Co., Mich. (1973).
40. *Colton v. New York Hosp.,* 414 N.Y.S.2d 866 (1979).
41. *Fiorentino v. Wegner,* 272 N.Y.S.2d 557 (1966).
42. Federal Food, Drug and Cosmetic Act, § 501(i), 21 U.S.C. 335(i).
43. California Health and Safety Code §§24176-24179.5 and 26668.4.
44. New York Public Health Law 2440-2446 (Supp. 1976).
45. La. Stat. Ann. Title 14, 872 (1974).

APPENDIX 49-1   The Nuremberg Code

The Nuremberg Code* provides

1. The voluntary consent of the human subject is absolutely essential. This means that the person involved should have legal capacity to give consent; should be so situated so as to exercise free power of choice, without the intervention of any element of force, fraud, deceit, duress, overreaching, or other ulterior form of constraint or coercion; and should have sufficient knowledge as to enable him to make an understanding and enlightened decision. This latter element requires that before the acceptance of an affirmative decision by the experimental subject, there should be made known to him the nature, duration, and purpose of the experiment; the method and means by which it is to be conducted; all inconveniences and hazards reasonably to be expected; and the effects upon his health or person which may possibly come from his participation in the experiment.

   The duty and responsibility for ascertaining the quality of the consent rests upon each individual who initiates, directs or engages in the experiment. It is a personal duty and responsibility which may not be delegated to another with impunity.

2. The experiment should be such as to yield fruitful results for the good of society, unprocurable by other methods or means of study, and not random and unnecessary in nature.

3. The experiment should be so designed and based on the results of animal experimentation and a knowledge of the natural history of the disease or other problem under study that the anticipated results will justify the performance of the experiment.

4. The experiment should be conducted as to avoid all unnecessary physical and mental suffering and injury.

5. No experiment should be conducted where there is *a priori* reason to believe that death or disabling injury will occur; except, perhaps, in those experiments where the experimental physicians also serve as subjects.

6. The degree of risk to be taken should never exceed that determined by the humanitarian importance of the problem to be solved by the experiment.

7. Proper preparation should be made and adequate facilities provided to protect the experimental subject against even remote possibilities of injury, disability or death.

8. The experiment should be conducted only by scientifically qualified persons. The highest degree of skill and care should be required through all stages of the experiment of those who conduct or engage in the experiment.

9. During the course of the experiment the human subject should be at liberty to bring the experiment to an end if he has reached the physical or mental state where continuation of the experiment seems to him to be impossible.

10. During the course of the experiment the scientist in charge must be prepared to terminate the experiment at any stage if he has probable cause to believe, in the exercise of good faith, superior skill and careful judgment required of him that a continuation of the experiment is likely to result in injury, disability, or death to the experimental subject.

*Source: *Trials of War Criminals Before the Nuremberg Military Tribunals,* Vol. I and II, *The Medical Case* (U.S. Government Printing Office Washington, D.C. 1948).

APPENDIX 49-2   The Declaration of Helsinki

The Declaration of Helsinki* provides

It is the mission of the doctor to safeguard the health of the people. His knowledge and conscience are dedicated to the fulfillment of his mission.

The Declaration of Geneva of The World Medical Association binds the doctor with the words: "The health of my patient will be my first consideration" and the International Code of Medical Ethics which declares that "Any act or advice which could weaken physical or mental resistance of a human being may be used only in his interest."

Because it is essential that the results of laboratory experiments be applied to human beings to further scientific knowledge and to help suffering humanity, The World Medical Association has prepared the following

*Source: 67 Annals Int. Med., Supp. 7 at 74-75 (1967).

recommendations as a guide to each doctor in clinical research. It must be stressed that the standards as drafted are only a guide to physicians all over the world. Doctors are not relieved from criminal, civil, and ethical responsibilities under the laws of their own countries.

In the files of clinical research a fundamental distinction must be recognized between clinical research in which the aim is essentially therapeutic for a patient, and the clinical research, the essential object of which is purely scientific and without therapeutic value to the person subjected to the research.

BASIC PRINCIPLES

1. Clinical research must conform to the moral and scientific principles that justify medical research and should be based on laboratory and animal experiments or other scientifically established facts.
2. Clinical research should be conducted only by scientifically qualified persons and under the supervision of a qualified medical person.
3. Clinical research cannot legitimately be carried out unless the importance of the objective is in proportion to the inherent risk to the subject.
4. Every clinical research project should be preceded by careful assessment of inherent risks in comparison to foreseeable benefits to the subject or to others.
5. Special caution should be exercised by the doctor in performing clinical research in which the personality of the subject is liable to be altered by drugs or experimental procedure.

CLINICAL RESEARCH COMBINED WITH PROFESSIONAL CARE

1. In the treatment of the sick person, the doctor must be free to use a new therapeutic measure, if in his or her judgment it offers hope of saving life, reestablishing health, or alleviating suffering.

   If at all possible, consistent with patient psychol-

ogy, the doctor should obtain the patient's freely given consent after the patient has been given a full explanation. In case of legal incapacity, counsel should also be procured from the legal guardian; in case of physical incapacity the permission of the legal guardian replaces that of the patient.
2. The doctor can combine clinical research with professional care, the objective being the acquisition of new medical knowledge, only to the extent that clinical research is justified by its therapeutic value for the patient.

NONTHERAPEUTIC CLINICAL RESEARCH

1. In the purely scientific application of clinical research carried out on a human being, it is the duty of the doctor to remain the protector of the life and health of that person on whom clinical research is being carried out.
2. The nature, the purpose, and the risk of clinical research must be explained to the subject by the doctor.
3a. Clinical research on a human being cannot be undertaken without his free consent after he has been informed; if he is legally incompetent, the consent of the legal guardian should be procured.
3b. Consent should, as a rule, be obtained in writing. However, the responsibility for clinical research always remains with the research worker; it never falls on the subject even after consent is obtained.
4a. The investigator must respect the right of each individual to safeguard his personal integrity, especially if the subject is in a dependent relationship to the investigator.
4b. At any time during the course of clinical research the subject or his guardian should be free to withdraw permission for research to be continued. The investigator or the investigating team should discontinue the research if in his or their judgment, it may, if continued, be harmful to the individual.

Case index

A

Abbott Laboratories v. Portland Retail Druggists Association, 190
Abraham v. Zaslow, 606
Ackerman v. TriCounty Orthopedic Group, P.O., 41
Albala v. City of New York, 366
Alexander v. Knight, 337
Alexander v. The Superior Court of Los Angeles County, 110
Allaire v. St. Luke's Hospital, 366
Allen v. Mansour, 388
American Hospital Association v. Sullivan, 670
Anderson v. O'Donoghue, 40
Anton v. San Antonio Community Hospital, 114, 653
Apple v. Jewish Hospital and Medical Center, 40
Applebaum v. Board of Directors of Barton Memorial Hospital, 114, 655
Application for William R., 587
Arizona v. Maricopa County Medical Society, 183, 184, 631

B

Baby Boy Doe v. Mother Doe, 452, 468
Baker v. Barber and Talmage, 40
Banks v. Goodfellow, 30
Barbara A. v. John G., 437
Barber v. Superior Court, 419-420
Barenbrugge v. Rich, 502
Barnes & Powers v. Hahnemann Medical College and Hospital, 503
Barry v. St. Paul Fire and Marine, 226
Belmar v. Cipolla, 112
Benitez v. New York City Board of Education, 554
Berg v. N.Y. Society for the Relief of the Ruptured and Crippled, 641
Berry v. Moench, 336
Bethesda Hospital Association v. Bowen, 668
Bhogaonker v. Metropolitan Hospital, 112
Bilonoha v. Zubritzsky, 35
Bing v. Thunig, 34, 641
Blue Cross v. Insurance Department, 225

Board of Curators of the University of Missouri v. Horowitz, 95
Bonbrest v. Katz, 366, 444
Bonner v. Moran, 457, 714
Bost v. Riley, 161
Bouvia v. Superior Court, 427
Bowen v. Kendrick, 434
Bowen v. Michigan Academy of Family Physicians, 667
Boyd v. Albert Einstein Medical Center, 166
Braden v. St. Francis Hospital, 163
Brady v. Hopper, 602
Breithaupt v. Abram, 290-291
Brillo v. Arizona, 388
Broadcast Music, Inc., v. Columbia Broadcasting System, Inc., 183
Brown v. Nash, 500
Buck v. Bell, 437
Burke v. United States, 502

C

California Liquor Dealers v. Midcal Aluminum, Inc., 189
California Savings and Loan Association v. Guerra, 448
Cannon v. University of Chicago, 93
Canterbury v. Spence, 284
Capan v. Divine Providence Hospital, 642
Carey v. Population Services International, 470
Carroll v. Otis Elevator Co., 143
Cechman v. Travis, 479
Chase v. Independent Practice Association, 165
Chicago Board of Trade v. United States, 182, 183
Citizens Hospital Association v. Schoulin, 643
City of Akron v. Akron Center for Reproductive Health, Inc., 445
Clanton v. Vonltaam, 348
C.M. v. C.C., 439
Cobbs v. Grant, 284
Cockrum v. Baumgartner, 449
Colby v. Carney Hospital, 35
Commonwealth v. Cass, 444
Communale v. Traders and General Insurance Company, 223

Cooper v. Sisters of Charity of Cincinnati, 135
Copperweld Corp. v. Independence Tube Corp., 187
Corcoran v. United HealthCare, Inc., 677
Corleto v. Shore Memorial Hospital, 158
Cowe by Cowe v. Forum Group, Inc., 444
Cox v. Haworth, 161
Craig v. Boren, 94
Cramer v. Morrison, 447
Cruzan v. Director, Missouri Dept. of Health, 412, 515
Custodio v. Bauer, 449
Custody of a Minor, 462, 464

D

Darling v. Charleston Memorial Hospital, 158, 644
Daubert v. Merrell Dow Pharmaceuticals, Inc., 120, 142, 148, 565, 692
Davis v. U.S., 499
Davis v. Virginia Railway Co., 148
DeGenova v. Ansel, 166
DeLuca v. Merrell Dow Pharmaceuticals, Inc., 147
Depenbrok v. Kaiser Foundation Health Plan, Inc., 165
DeWill Truck Brokers, Inc., v. W. Ray Flemming Fruit Co., 674
Dexter v. Hall, 28
Dietrich v. Northampton, 366, 444
Doe v. Pickett, 471
Doe v. Puget Sound Blood Center, 328
Doe v. Roe, 336
Dohn v. Lovell, 436
Dos Santos v. Columbus-Cuneo-Cabrini Medical Center, 185-186
Doyle v. Giulicci, 82
Duffield v. Charleston Area Medical Center, Inc., 655
Duke v. Morphis, 503
Durham v. United States, 594
Dusky v. United States, 591

E

Elam v. College Park Hospital, 105, 162
Elizabeth Bouvia v. Riverside General Hospital, 410
Ellis v. Miller Oil Purchasing Co., 143
Enright v. Eli Lilly & Co., 366
Estelle v. Smith, 592

F

Federal Trade Commission v. Ticor Insurance Co., 189
Ferguson v. Vest, 500-501
Fields v. McNamara, 332
Fiorentino v. Wenger, 158
Frazier v. Metropolitan Life Insurance Company, 224
Fridena v. Evans, 162
Frye v. United States, 148, 565

G

Garner v. Ford Motor Company, 332
Garrow v. Elizabeth General Hospital, 654, 655
Gereboff v. Home Indemnity Company, 231
Gideon v. Johns-Manville Sales Corp., 145
Gilbert v. General Electric Company, 448
Gizzi v. Texaco, Inc., 643
Gloria C. v. William C., 367
Gonzales v. Nork, 160
Gooding v. University Hospital Building, Inc., 135
Gorman v. LaSasso, 502
Goss v. Lopez, 95
Government of the Virgin Islands v. Lee, 673
Gowan v. Carpenter, 436
Grann v. Ordean, 655
Grazia v. Sanchez, 81
Griswold v. Connecticut, 445
Grodin v. Grodin, 367, 445
Group Life and Health Insurance Company v. Royal Drug Company, 226
Guardianship of Richard Roe III, 607
Guerro v. Copper Queen Hospital, 643

H

Hackethal v. California Medical Association and San Bernadino County Medical Society, 655
Hadfield's Case, 593
Hagler v. Gilliland, 142
Hamil v. Bashline, 136
Hamilton v. Hardy, 434
Hammonds v. Aetna Casualty & Surety Co., 336
Hannah v. Larche, 656
Harrell v. Total Health Care, Inc., 165
Harris v. McRae, 445
Harron v. United Hospital Center, Inc., 185
Hart v. Brown, 382, 457
Harte v. Sinai Hospital of Detroit, 81
Hartke v. McKelway, 144
H.B. v. Wilkinson, 460
Head v. Colloton, 383
Hedgecorth v. United States, 144
Hedlund v. Orange County, 602
Hickman v. Group Health Plan, Inc., 450
Hicks v. United States, 136
Hizer v. Randolph, 135
H.L. v. Matheson, 473
Hodgson v. Minn., 473
Holland v. Metalious, 373
Hospital Building Co. v. Trustees of Rex Hospital, 182
Howat v. Passaretti, 348
Howell v. Spokane & Inland Empire Blood Bank, 327
Howitt v. Superior Court of Imperial County, 106, 115
Huang v. Board of Directors, 115
Hudson v. Rausa, 41

Humpers v. First Interstate Bank of Oregon, 337
Hyde v. Jefferson Parrish Hospital, 631
Hyman v. Brooklyn Jewish Chronic Disease
　　Hospital, 718

I

In Interest of E.G., 460
In Interest of Karwath, 464
In the Matter of Karen Quinlan, 412
In the Matter of the Marriage of Hodge and Hodge, 448
In the Matter of Spring, 462
In re A.C., 368, 452
In re "Agent Orange" Product Liability Litigation, 146
In re Baby Doe, 438
In re Baby M., 442-443
In re Conroy, 32
In re Estate of Fish, 30
In re Green, 467
In re Guardianship of Hayes, 469
In re Guardianship of Pescinski, 383, 457
In re Hofbauer, 464
In re Jamaica Hospital, 368
In re Moyer's Estate, 373
In re Richardson, 382-383, 457
In re Sampson, 467
In re Seiferth, 467
In re Simpson, 468
In re T.H., 472
In re Wanglie, 414
Inabnit v. Berkson, 331
Ind. Planned Parenthood v. Pearson, 474
Insinga v. LaBella, 159
International Union v. Johnson Controls, 448

J

Jaap v. District Court, 331
Jackson v. Indiana, 592
Jackson v. Waller, 145
Jacobs v. Theimer, 450
Jacobson v. Massachusetts, 465
Janney v. Housekeeper, 277
Jefferson Parrish Hospital District No. 2 v. Hyde, 184-185
Jefferson v. Griffin Spaulding County Hospital, 368
Jenkins v. United States, 145
Johnson v. Matviuw, 39
Johnson v. Misericordia Community Hospital, 105, 161,
　　641
Joiner v. Mitchell County Hospital Authority, 162
Jorgensen v. Meade Johnson Laboratories, 366

K

Karp v. Cooley, 383
Kartell v. Blue Shield of Mass., 665
Killebrew v. Johnson, 435

Kimble v. Los Angeles City Board of Education, 114
Kirk v. M. Reese Hospital and Medical Emergency, 163,
　　324
Kirker v. Orange County, 379
Klaxon Co. v. Stentor Electric Mfg. Co., 22
Klink v. G. D. Searle & Co., 434
Knapp v. Palos Community Hospital, 111
Knier v. Albany Medical Center Hospital, 164
Kremer v. Kaiser Foundation Hospital, 499
Kruegar v. St. Joseph's Hospital, 164

L

Laje v. R.E. Thomason General Hospital, 656
Lake v. Cameron, 589
Landeros v. Flood, 478
Lauro v. Travelers Insurance Co., 502
Lee v. Page, 388
Lefler v. Yardumian, 504
Leno v. St. Joseph Hospital, 374
Lessard v. Schmidt, 589
Lew v. Kona Hospital, 655
Lipari v. Sears, Roebuck and Co., 602-603
Little v. Little, 383, 458
Lochner v. New York, 19
Long v. Patterson, 499
Lowry v. Henry Mayo Newhall Memorial Hospital, 39
Luka v. Lowrie, 459
Lundahl v. Rockford Memorial Hospital, 159

M

MacDonald v. Klinger, 333, 337
Maher v. Roe, 445
Malahoff v. Stiver, 441
Maltz v. New York University Medical Center, 111-112
Marcelletti v. Bathani, 479
Marciniak v. Lundborg, 449
Marek v. Professional Health Services, Inc., 643
Massachusetts Medical Society v. Dukakis, 665
Matchett v. Superior Court, 110
Mathew v. Eldridge, 107
Matoff v. Ward, 151
Matter of Grand Jury Subpoena Duces Tecum, 316
Matter of Westchester County Medical Center, 412
Matthews v. Eldridge, 95
Mayfield v. Gleichert, 36
McClellan v. Health Maintenance Corporation of
　　Pennsylvania, 165
McConnell v. Williams, 641-642
McDermott v. Manhattan Eye, Ear & Throat Hospital,
　　389
McDonald v. Massachusetts General Hospital, 34
McDonald v. United States, 594-595
McFall v. Shrimp, 382
McIntosh v. Milano, 602

McLain v. Real Estate Board of New Orleans, Inc., 187
McMahon v. Young, 150
M.D., P.C. v. Kuriansky, 316
Mduba v. Benedictine Hospital, 158
Mehalik v. Morvant, 502
Menendez v. Superior Court, 323-324
Michael H. and Victoria D. v. Gerald D., 448
Miller v. Eisenhower Medical Center, 114
Mills v. Rogers, 590
Mississippi State Board of Psychological Examiners v. Hosford, 316
Mitts v. HIP of Greater New York, 165
Mohr v. Williams, 290
Monusco v. Postle, 432
Moore v. Preventive Medical Group, 500
Morrison v. Stallworth, 500

N

Nathanson v. Kline, 288
Nathanson v. Yarvis, 500
National Gerimedical Hospital, 190
National Society of Professional Engineers v. United States, 182
Necolauff v. Genesee Hospital, 641
Neil v. Brackett, 30
Newman v. Geschke, 504
Nicoletta v. Rochester Eye and Human Parts Bank, 375
Northern Pacific Railway v. United States, 183
Northern Trust Co. v. Upjohn Co., 144
Northwest Wholesale Stationers, Inc., v. Pacific Stationery and Printing Co., 186
Novosel v. Nationwide Insurance Co., 648
Nussbaum v. Gibstein, 501

O

O'Bannon v. Town Court, 490
O'Connor v. Donaldson, 590
O'Dell v. Chesney, 502
Ohio v. Akron Center for Reproductive Health, 474
Ohligschlager v. Proctor Community Hospital, 160
Owen v. Kerr-McGee Corp., 149
Owens v. Concrete Pipe & Products Co., 145

P

Pamela P. v. Frank S., 437
Parker v. Brown, 188, 631
Pate v. Robinson, 591
Patrick v. Burget, 36-37, 186-187, 651
Pederson v. Dumouchel, 158
Pedroza v. Bryant, 163
People v. Pierson, 467
People v. Privitera, 207, 506
People v. Wells, 595
People v. Wharton, 323-324

Perkins v. Volkswagen of America, Inc., 145
Pickle v. Curns, 162
Pinsker v. Pacific Coast Society of Orthodontists, 108
Planned Parenthood Federation, Inc., v. Heckler, 471
Planned Parenthood of Central Missouri v. Danforth, 472
Planned Parenthood of Southeastern Pennsylvania v. Casey, 472, 474
Planned Parenthood v. Casey, 365, 434, 446
Poelker v. Doe, 445
Pogue v. Hospital Authority of DeKalb County, 159
Polischeck v. United States, 162
Powell v. Florida, 376
Presidents RR Conference v. Noerr Motor Freight, Inc., 631-632
Prince v. Massachusetts, 714
Purcell v. Zimbelman, 163
Purdy v. Public Administration v. County of Westchester, 324

R

Raglin v. HMO Illinois, Inc., 165
Raleigh Fitkin-Paul Morgan Memorial Hospital v. Anderson, 368
Ravenis v. Detroit General Hospital, 162, 375, 384
Redding v. St. Francis Medical Center, 112, 113
Rennie v. Klein, 590
Renslow v. Mennonite Hospital, 366
Rex v. Arnold, 592
Reynolds v. Mennonite Hospital, 163
Rhee, 113, 115
Richardson v. Richardson-Merrell Dow, 147
Rimer v. Rockwell International Corp., 145
Robbins v. Geller, 500
Robbins v. HIP of New Jersey, 165
Rochin v. California, 290
Roe v. Wade, 19, 277, 365, 369, 381, 445, 450, 472
Rogers v. Okin, 587, 608
Rosenblum v. Tallahassee Memorial Regional Medical Center, Inc., 111
Roy v. Hartogs, 208, 604
Ruby v. Massey, 470
Rudman v. Beth Israel Medical Center, 503
Rusk v. Akron General Hospital, 96
Rust v. Sullivan, 445
Rutherford v. United States, 505-506

S

Sanders v. Ajir, 95
Sard v. Hardy, 436, 449
Savelle v. Heilbrunn, 501
Schleier v. Kaiser Foundation Health Plan of Mid-Atlantic States, 165
Schloendorff v. New York Hospital, 34, 275, 641
Schmerber v. California, 291

Scull v. Superior Court, 315
Searcy v. Auerbach, 478
Simonson v. Swenson, 337
Sindell v. Abbott Laboratories, 139
Sirianni v. Anna, 382
Sloan v. Metropolitan Health Council, Inc., 165
Smith v. Hartigan, 440
Smith v. Pearce, 144
Sorrels v. Eli Lilly & Co., 366
South High Dev. Ltd. v. Weiner et al., 166
Southeastern Underwriters Association v. U.S., 224
Sparkman v. McFarlin, 468
Stachan v. John F. Kennedy Memorial Hospital, 379
Standard Oil Co. of New Jersey v. United States, 181, 182
Stanturf v. Sipes, 642
State of Missouri ex rel. Wichita Falls General Hospital v. Adolph, 389
State v. Jaggers, 316
State v. Killory, 207
State v. Koome, 473
State v. McCoy, 149
State v. Wickstrom, 444
Stephen K. v. Roni L., 437
Stokes v. Children's Hospital, Inc., 148
Strunk v. Strunk, 383, 457
Suckle v. Madison General Hospital, 654
Summit Health, 187
Superintendent of Belchertown State School v. Saikewicz, 413, 462
Sygman v. Kahn, 499

T

Taft v. Taft, 368
Tarasoff v. Regents of the University of California, 269, 322, 601
Teital v. Reynolds, 332
Terrell v. Garcia, 449
T.H. v. Jones, 471
Thomas v. Corso, 642-643
Thompson v. Sun City Community Hospital, 135, 136
Thornburgh v. American College of Obstetricians and Gynecologists, 445
Todd v. Sorrell, 389
Tonsic v. Wagner, 641-642
Town of Hallie v. City of Eau Claire, 189
Trans-Missouri Freight Association, 181
Trans-World Investments v. Drobny, 332
Trial of Daniel M'Naughton, 593
Tucker v. Lower, 379
Tucson Medical Center v. Misevch, 160

U

UAW v. Johnson Controls, 369
UMW v. J. Penington, 631-632

United Pacific Insurance Co. v. Buchanan, 28
United States v. Addyston Pipe & Steel Co., 181
United States v. Aluminum Co. of America, 188
United States v. Brantley, 673
United States v. Crosby, 31
United States v. Diamond, 674
United States v. Greber, 672
United States v. Joint Traffic Association, 181
United States v. Lorenzo, 674
United States v. Pisani, 674
United States v. Quaisi, 673
United States v. Trenton Potteries Co., 183
University of California Regents v. Bakke, 93, 94
Unterhiner v. Desert Hospital District of Palm Springs, 653

V

Valtakis v. Putnam, 479
Vanaman v. Milford Memorial Hospital, 160
Verkennes v. Corniea, 367
Villareal v. Chun, 81
Von Goyt v. State of Alabama, 332

W

Wade v. Bethesda Hospital, 468
Wagner v. International Railway Co., 368
Wallace v. Labrenz, 462
Weber v. Stoney Brook Hospital, 463
Webster v. Reproductive Health Services, 445-446, 474
Weiss v. York Hospital, 631, 641, 649
Wells v. Ortho Pharmaceutical Corp., 435
Wenninger v. Muesing, 331
We're Associates Co. v. Cohen et al., 166
Wickline v. State of California, 165
Wilk v. American Medical Association, Inc., 182, 186
William Standard, 692
Williams v. Good Health Plus, Inc., 165
Williams v. Health America, 166
Williams v. Hofmann, 375
Wilmington General Hospital v. Manlove, 642
Wilsman v. Sloniewicz, 436
Wilson v. Blue Cross of Southern California, 165, 676
Wisconsin Dept. of Health and Social Services v. Bowen, 671
Withrow v. Larkin, 110
Woodbury v. McKinnon, 654

Y

Youngberg v. Romeo, 475, 590
Younts v. St. Francis Hospital and School of Nursing, 459

Z

Zipkin v. Freeman, 604

Subject index

A

Abandonment, 121-122, 134
  physician-patient relationship, 270
  psychiatry, 604-605
Abortion, 445-447
  minor, 446-447, 472-474
    bypass procedure, 472-473
    parental consent, 472
    parental notification, 473-474
Abuse, 672-679; *see also* Child abuse
  administrative hearing, 674
  disclosure, 321
  limitations, 673
  Medicaid, 673
  Medicare, 673
  preliminary investigation and negotiations, 673-674
Abuse of process, physician countersuit, 216
Abusive therapy, 207
Acceptance, contract law, 49
Accessibility, arbitration, 81-82
Accessory after the fact, 200-201
Acquired immunodeficiency syndrome (AIDS), 516-530
  duty to warn, 325-326
  legal responses, 518-520
  pathogenesis, 517
  protection of individual rights, 520
  societal concerns, 519-520
  surveillance case definition, 523-528
  testing, 517-518
  treatment, 517-518
Act of God, contract law, 52
Active euthanasia, 425
Acute pain, 536
Administrative law, 21
Advanced health care directive, 411
  statute, by state, 90
Adversarial process, 560
Adverse reaction reporting, pharmaceutical product liability, 169-170
Advertising, pharmaceutical product liability, 172-173
Aesculapius, 6-7

Age Discrimination in Employment Act, medical record, 304
Agency theory, 642-643
AIDS; *see* Acquired immunodeficiency syndrome
Alcoholism
  crime, 203, 329
  treatment records, 304
Aleatory contract, 220
Alternate health care facility, 620
Alternative dispute resolution, 78-84
  Administrative Dispute Resolution Act, 79
  arbitration, 80
  benefits, 79
  checklist, 85-86
  endorsements, 78
  fact-finding, 80
  federal action, 79
  guidelines, 85-86
  mediation, 80
  methods, 79-81
  no-fault compensation option, 80-81
  no-fault plan, 80
  practice tips, 83-84
  statutory malpractice arbitration, 79
Alternative medicine, statute, 89
Alzheimer's disease, 492
Amended Uniform Anatomical Gift Act, 393-397
American College of Legal Medicine, 6
American legal system, 17-23
Americans with Disabilities Act, 94, 548-549
  medical school, 96
Anencephaly, organ donation, 379-382
Angiography, 696-697
Anticipatory repudiation, 54
Antitrust law, 180-191
  alternate health care delivery system, 622-624
  boycott, 186-187
  concerted refusals to deal, 186-187
  conduct violations of, 181-188
  credentialing, 648-649
  defenses, 188-190
  exclusive dealing, 184-186

explicit and implied exemption, 189-190
Federal Trade Commission, 191
guidelines of 1993, 191
health care reform, 191
history, 180-181
insurance contract, 64
joint venture, 631-632
market allocation, 187
merger, 188
monopolization, 187-188
Noerr-Pennington doctrine, 190
per se rule, 181-188
price-fixing, 183-184
state action exemption, 188-189
statute, 87
tying, 184-186
Apparent agency
hospital, 642
independent contractor, 642
Apparent authority, 643
Appeal, 23
licensure, 103
peer review, 110
Arab medical ethics, 7
Arbitration, 81-83
accessibility, 81-82
alternative dispute resolution, 80
contract law, 62
enforcement, 81, 82
evaluation, 82-83
in health care, 80
practicality, 82
system design, 83
Argon laser, 702
Arrest, crime, 209
Arthroscopy, 703
Artificial insemination, 438-439
Asphyxiation, 563
Assisted suicide, 200-201
Assumption of risk
informed consent, 286-287
pharmaceutical product liability, 174
Autoauthentication, medical record, 307-408
regulatory and accrediting issues, 307-408
Automatic implantable cardioverter-defibrillator, 699
Autonomy, 425-426
Autopsy, 567-568

B

Bad faith
insurance contract, 64
liability insurance, 223-224
Battered child syndrome, 476-477
Battery, 120-121, 275

tests requested by police, 289-291
Behavioral medicine, pain, 541-542
Bias, judicial review, 114-115
Bill of Rights, 18
Bioethics, 354-355
Biofeedback, 703-705
Biological death, 404
Biomedical equipment
corrective maintenance, 706
implementation, 708-709
improvements, 708
management, 705-709
performance, 708
preventive maintenance, 706
selection, 706-707
Blood bank, duty to warn, 326
Blood tests, 705
Bloodborne pathogen, 684-687
exposure control plan, 684-685
exposure determination, 685
exposure incident, 685
hepatitis B, 686
housekeeping policies, 685
personal protective equipment, 685
training program, 686
universal precautions, 685
workplace controls, 685
Blunt force, 563
Borrowed servant, 638
Boycott, antitrust law, 186-187
Brain damage, 451-452, 608
Brain death, 404, 405-406
criminal law, 406-407
Brain-injured patient, 509-515
brain recovery, 514
differential diagnosis, 511-513
disease categories, 511-513
legal considerations, 514-515
primary causes, 509
process, 509-511
signs and symptoms, 509-510
Breach of confidentiality, 122, 336
psychiatry, 600-601
Breach of contract, 53, 336
physician-patient relationship, 267
Breach of contract or warranty to cure, 122-123
Breach of duty, 119
Breach of loyalty, 336
Breach of privacy, 336
Bylaws violation, 115

C

Capacity, 27-33
competency, 28-29

Capacity—cont'd
  contract law, 52
  definition, 27
  generally, 27
Cardiac catheterization, 697-698
Cardiac pacemaking, 699
Case, defined, 23
Causation, pharmaceutical product liability, 173
Center for Health Care Studies, 11
Cerebral contusion, 610
Certification, Clinical Laboratory Improvement
      Amendments, 687
Charitable immunity, 34-35
  respondeat superior, 34, 35
Chemotherapy, oncology patient, 503-504
Child; *see* Minor
Child abuse, 475-479
  battered child syndrome, 476-477
  forensic pathology, 579-581
  reporting, 477-479
    immunity, 41-42
    negligent failure to, 478-479
  state liability, 479
Chinese medical ethics, 7
Christian medical ethics, 7
Chronic pain syndrome, 536-537
Civil trial, 70-77
  closing argument, 76
  commencement of action, 70-71
  cross-examination, 75-76
  direct examination, 74-75
  discovery, 72-73
  judgment, 76
  jury instruction, 76
  jury selection, 73-74
  motion, 71-72
  motion in limine, 73
  opening statement, 74
  pleading, 71
  post-trial proceedings, 76-77
  service of process, 70-71
  trial practice, 73
Claims-made coverage, insurance contract, 65
Clinical faculty, physician-patient relationship, 267
Clinical Laboratory Improvement Amendments, 687-
      690
  categories of tests, 687-688
  certification, 687
  patient test management, 688
  personnel standards, 688
  proficiency testing, 688-689
  quality assurance, 689-690
  quality control, 688
Closing argument, civil trial, 76

CO_2 laser, 701-702
Code of ethics, American Medical Association, 7
Code of Hammurabi, 6
Common law, 21-22, 130
Comparative fault, 126-127
  pharmaceutical product liability, 174
Comparative negligence, 126-127
  oncology patient, 500
Compensation for loss of chance, 134-136
Competency, 27-33
  areas, 28-31
  areas of law, 44-45
  capacity to contract, 28-29
  consent to die, 32
  definition, 27
  generally, 27
  informed consent, 31-32
  to stand trial, 591-592
  testamentary capacity, 29-31
    legal requirements, 30
    undue influence, 30-31
  to testify, 31
    general legal test, 31
  tests of, 45
  will, 29-31
    undue influence, 30-31
Competition, cost containment, 663
Computerized medical record, 306-307
Computerized tomography, 694-695
Conception, 437-444
  assisted conception, 437-438
  nontraditional parentage, 437-438
Conceptus, 364
Concussion, 610
Condition diagram, 307
Conditions of participation, Medicare, 664
Confidentiality, 122, 240, 312-313
  court decisions, 336-337
  educational use of patient information, 313-314
  erosion of patients' rights, 313
  health care team responsibility, 313
  medical record, 301
  organ donation, 383
  peer review, 110
  psychiatry, 600-601
  workers' compensation, 551
Conflict of interest, 12
  peer review, 106-107
Conscience clause, fetus, 369
Consent; *see also* Informed consent
  ability to, 282-283
  authority to give consent, 282
  causes of action, 284-285
  consent to die, competency, 32

disclosure, 335
drug research, 292
exceptions to material disclosure, 283
experimental procedure, 292
family, 276-278
human subject research, 291-292
legal dimensions, 278
minor, 276
phantom physician, 289
refusal of, 288
scope, 276
spouse, 276-278
tests requested by police, 289-291
traditional consent, 274-276
Uniform Anatomical Gift Act, 293
Consent form, 281-283
Conservator, 32
Consideration, contract law, 49-50
Consortium, 137-138
Conspiracy, 201
Constitution, 17-20
Consultant, coprovider, 640
Consultation, disclosure, 280
Contagious disease, duty to warn, 325-328
Contraception, 433-435
    minor, 470-472
        parental consent, 471
        parental notification, 471-472
Contraceptive deception, 437
Contract law; *see also* Specific type of contract
    acceptance, 49
    act of God, 52
    arbitration, 62
    background, 46-48
    beginning of modern systems, 47
    capacity, 52
    collection, 57-58
    consideration, 49-50
    contract types, 62-66
    defenses, 50-53
    duress, 51-52
    enforcement, 46
        breach of contract, 53
        contract elements, 48-50
        court review of contract, 53
        equitable estoppel, 53
        parole evidence rule, 53
        performance, 53-54
        procedure of suit in contract, 53
    fraud, 52
    illegal terms, 50-51
    impossibility, 52
    indemnification, 62
    judgment enforcement, 57-58

liquidated damages, 61
measure of damages, 56-57
misrepresentation, 52
mistake, 52
mutuality of obligation, 49-50
negotiation, 58-60
    use of counsel, 60
noncompetition clause, 61-62
offer, 48-49
prenegotiation considerations, 59
process, 58-59
public policy, 50-51
quasi contract, 60
rationale, 46-48
reading a contract, 60-62
reasons for enforcing, 47-48
relief for third parties, 57
remedies, 56-58
Roman law influences, 47
rules of interpreting language, 54-55
standard sections, 60-61
statute, 55-56
undue influence, 51-52
verbal contract, 58
Contract of adhesion, 51-52
Contract theory of medical staff bylaw, 647
Contract warranty
    health maintenance organization, 165-166
    independent practice association, 165-166
    managed care organization, 165-166
    preferred provider organization, 165-166
    professional association, 165-166
    professional corporation, 165-166
Contributory negligence, 126-127
    oncology patient, 500
Controlled substance, statute, by state, 91
Controversy, defined, 23
Coprovider, 636-641
    consultant, 640
    independent contractor, 639
    licensure, 636
    nursing, 640
    ostensible agency, 639-640
    peer review, 636-638
        disciplinary actions, 638
        normative *versus* actual standards of care, 637-638
        quality assurance program, 637
        standards of care, 637
    practice in health care institution, 636
    radio control for prehospital care, 639
    referring physician, 640
    supervisory liability, 638-639
    technical practices in hospital, 640
Coroner, 561

Coroner's case, 561-564
  determination of death, 562
  forensic evidence of cause of death, 563-564
  forensic hematology, 562-563
  polygraph, 563
  scene of death, 562
  scene of death investigation, 562
  serology, 562-563
Corporate liability, hospital, 644-645
Corporate negligence, 156-167, 643
Corporation, 619
Cost containment, 662-680
  competition, 663
  health maintenance organization, 662-663
  managed care, 663
  Medicare, 663-670
  preferred provider organization, 663
  prospective payment system, 663
  Provider Reimbursement Review Board, 669-670
Countersuit, 213-218
Covering physician, physician-patient relationship, 267
Credentialing
  active medical staff, 645
  affiliate staff, 646
  allied health professional staff, 646
  antitrust law, 648-649
  application, 646-647
  available remedies to aggrieved physicians, 649-650
  consulting staff, 645-646
  courtesy staff, 646
  criteria, 647
  defamation, 648
  due process, 648, 651
  employment practices discrimination, 648
  guidelines, 650-651
  honorary/emeritus staff, 646
  hospital and medical staff bylaws, 647, 650
  house staff, 646
  measures to minimize liability, 650-651
  medical staff delegation, 646
  nature of staff membership, 645-646
  outpatient staff, 646
  physical legal protections, 647-649
  procedural due process, 651
  protection from economic harm, 647-648
  public/private hospital distinction, 646
  renewal, 646-647
  substantive due process, 651
  type of staff membership, 645-646
Criminal law, 208-212
  alcoholism, 203
  arrest, 209
  attempted crime, 205
  burden of proof, 208
  causation, 202

  constitutional safeguards, 208
  defenses to, 201-202
  detention, 209
  double jeopardy, 211-212
  duress, 204
  elements, 199-200
  excuses, 202-204
  fetal interests, 367-368
  forensic psychiatry, 590-598
    competency to stand trial, 591-592
    defenses, 592-598
    diminished capacity, 596
    insanity defense, 592-598
  by health care providers, 197-205
  impossible crimes, 205
  inchoate crimes, 204-205
  justified killings, 204
  legal technicalities, 208
  lesser included offenses, 200
  mental illness, 203
  Miranda warning, 209
  mistakes of law, 203-204
  necessity, 204
  against person, 205-208
  plea bargaining, 210
  prevention, 204
  privileged conduct, 204
  protection against self-incrimination, 211
  psychiatric patient, 590-598
    competency to stand trial, 591-592
    defenses, 592-598
    diminished capacity, 596
    insanity defense, 592-598
  right to counsel, 209-210
  right to jury trial, 210-211
  searches, 209
  starting criminal prosecution, 210
  trial, 211
  understanding criminal law, 198-199
  vicarious culpability, 200-201
  warrant, 209
  witnesses, 211
Criminal liability, physician-assisted dying, 416-417
Cross-examination, civil trial, 75-76
Cryopreservation
  embryo, 443-444
  gamete, 443-444
Curbstone consultation, physician-patient relationship, 267
Cystoscopy, 703

D

Damages, 138-139
  pharmaceutical product liability, 174
Data-based performance monitoring, 244-245

Death, 404-422
  authorization of autopsy, 408-409
  cause, 408
  custody of body, 408-409
  defined, 406
  disposal of remains, 408-409
  drug abuse, 582
  impingement of technology, 405
  moment of, 404
  President's Commission for the Study of Ethical
      Problems in Medicine and Biomedical and
      Behavioral Research, 406
  pronouncement, 405-407
  traditional formulation, 405
  unnatural, 573
Death certificate, 206-207, 407-408
Declaration of Geneva, 7
Declaration of Helsinki, 727-728
  experimentation, 714
  research, 714
Defamation, 134
  credentialing, 648
  physician countersuit, 216-217
Defense of property, 204
Dementia, 608
Depression, 608
  diagnosis, 609
  organic factors, 609
  prognosis, 609
Detail person, pharmaceutical product liability, 173
Detention, crime, 209
Diagnosis-related group, 675-679
  consequences, 678-679
  Corcoran decision, 677-678
  legal implications, 676
  physician role, 676
  Wilson decision, 676-677
Diagnostic technology, 691-696
Digital image processing, 696
Digital subtraction angiography, 699
Diminished capacity, 596
Direct examination, civil trial, 74-75
Direct liability
  health maintenance organization, 165
  independent practice association, 165
  managed care organization, 165
  preferred provider organization, 165
  professional association, 165
  professional corporation, 165
Disability, 531-533
  defined, 531
  discrimination, 548-551
  pain, 531-532
  partial, 531
  permanent and total, 531

  total, 531
Disclosure
  about patients, 312-338
  abuse, 321
  alternatives, 280
  approved, 320
  burden of proof, 285
  but for rule, 285-286
  consent, 335
  consultation, 280
  deceased patient, 335
  defenses, 338
  discharged patient, 335
  disclosure, 321
  duty to warn, 322-328
  evidentiary proof, 285-286
  exceptions to material disclosure, 283
  family, 333-334
  Freedom of Information Act, 321-322
  governmental agency access, 321
  hospital role, 281
  incompetent patient, 335
  limitations, 329
  medical record, 332-333
  minor, 334-335
  occupational disease, 322
  oncology patient, 496, 497-498
  prognosis, 280
  public health, 322
  reasonable and legitimate interest, 333-337
  referral, 280
  risks, 279-280
  scope, 279-280
  standards developed by courts, 280-281
  state public records laws, 321
  statutory breaches, 336
  statutory duty, 320
  statutory requirements, 286
  substance abuse, 329
  substances and devices, 321
  surrogates, 334
  test results, 279
  third parties, 334, 335-336
  tort, 336-337
  vital statistics, 320-321
  who is responsible, 281
  workers' compensation, 321
Discovery, 329-333
  civil trial, 72-73
  formal, 330-331
  informal, 331
  licensure, 101
  rules, 329-330
Discrimination
  disability, 548-551

Discrimination—cont'd
    fetal protection policies, 549-550
    gender discrimination, 549-550
    pregnancy, 549-550
District court, 25
DNA, forensic pathology, 582-583
Do-not-resuscitate order, 289, 413-414, 418, 419
    medical futility, 414-415
Doctrine of severability, 54
Documentation, telephone management, 346
Double effect treatment, 425
Double jeopardy, 211-212
Drowning, 563-564
Drug
    duty to warn, 324-325
    liability, 168-175
    pain, 540-541
    strict liability, 123
    telephone management, 347-348
Drug abuse
    death, 582
    forensic pathology, 581-582
Drug research
    consent, 292
    pharmaceutical product liability in testing, 169
Due process
    credentialing, 648, 651
    peer review, 107
        definition, 107
        interpretation, 107
    staff privileges, 653-656
        adequate time to prepare defense, 654
        appearance before panel, 655
        assistance of legal counsel, 655
        cross-examination of witnesses, 655
        initial *versus* existing, 654
        notification of adverse recommendation, 654
        physician's interest in, 653-654
        physician's rights, 654-656
        prehearing discovery, 654
        presentation of witnesses and evidence in
          defense, 655
        private *versus* public hospitals, 653-654
        scope of judicial review, 656
        transcript of panel hearing, 655
        written decision from panel, 656
        written notice of charges, 654
Durable power of attorney, 411
Duress
    contract law, 51-52
    crime, 204
Duty to defend, insurance contract, 64
Duty to warn
    acquired immunodeficiency syndrome, 325-326
    blood bank, 326
    contagious disease, 325-328
    disclosure, 322-328
    human immunodeficiency virus, 325-326
    medical conditions, 324
    medication, 324-325
    patient-psychotherapist privilege, 323-324
    threats to others, 322-324
Duty to warn and control, 136-137
Dying, 404-422, 409-417
    changing patient population, 409-410
    double effect, 409
    ethical issues, 359-361
    good death, 424
    medical futility, 414-415
    patient without capacity, 410-413
        best interests standard, 412
        decision making by families, 412-413
        subjective standard, 411-412
        substituted judgment standard, 412
    technology, 409-410
    traditional physician role, 409

E

Echocardiography, 698
Economic credentialing, 111-113
    defined, 111
Education, right to be a physician, 93
Elder abuse and neglect, geriatric patient,
    490-492
Election, liability insurance, 222-223
Electrocardiogram, 696
Electroconvulsive therapy, 586
Electrocution, 564
Electroencephalography, 700-701
Electromyography, 699-700
Electrophysiologic testing, 699-700
Emancipation, minor, 460
Embryo, 364
    cryopreservation, 443-444
    frozen, 369-370
Emergency, minor, 459
Emergency care
    hospital liability, 643-644
    informed consent, 283-284
    physician-patient relationship, 267
Employee Retirement Security Act, malpractice,
    166
Employment contract, insurance contract, 66
Endoscopy, 702-703
English medical ethics, 7
Entitlement doctrine, 20
Entrapment, 204
Environmental law, defined, 4
Equal protection, 20
Estoppel, liability insurance, 222-223

Ethical issues, 351-361
  in advising patients, 353
  basis for ethical conduct, 351-353
  current trends, 11-13
  decisions near end of life, 418-419
  dying, 359-361
  euthanasia, 359-361
  experimentation, 711-726
    benefit *versus* risk rule, 717-718
    children as subjects, 714-715
    civil liability, 718-720
    criminal liability, 718-720
    fetal research, 715-716
    geriatric patient, 716-717
    historical background, 711-717
    radiation experiments, 721-722
  historical aspects, 6-17
  medical resources, 358-359
  rationing, 358-359
  research, 353-354, 355-358, 711-726
    benefit *versus* risk rule, 717-718
    children as subjects, 714-715
    civil liability, 718-720
    criminal liability, 718-720
    fetal research, 715-716
    geriatric patient, 716-717
    historical background, 711-717
    radiation experiments, 721-722
  scientific writing, 353-354, 355-358
  standards, 12
Euthanasia, 206, 415-417, 419, 425
  ethical issues, 359-361
Evidentiary privilege, privileged communication, 316-317
Evoked potential, 700
Ex parte discovery, 331-332
Exclusionary clause, insurance contract, 64
Exclusive dealing, antitrust law, 184-186
Exculpatory agreement, negligence, 127
Executory contract, 221
Experimental procedure, consent, 292
Experimentation
  Declaration of Helsinki, 714
  ethical issues, 711-726
    benefit *versus* risk rule, 717-718
    children as subjects, 714-715
    civil liability, 718-720
    criminal liability, 718-720
    fetal research, 715-716
    geriatric patient, 716-717
    historical background, 711-717
    radiation experiments, 721-722
  government-sponsored, 712-713
  LSD, 713
  Nuremberg Code, 713-714

Expert testimony, 141-153
  ethical issues, 152-153
  forensic medicine, 560-561
    court-appointed experts, 561
    opinion testimony, 561
  limitations, 148-149
  opinion discovery, 151
  opinion foundation, 146-148
  qualification, 143-146
  rules of admissibility, 142-149
  scientific evidence acceptance, 148-149
  subject matter of opinion, 142-143
Expressed consent, 275

F

Fact-finding, alternative dispute resolution, 80
Failure to mitigate, 57
Failure to protect, psychiatry, 601-604
Failure to warn, psychiatry, 601-604
False Claims Act, 674
False imprisonment, 131-132
  geriatric patient, 490
Family
  consent, 276-278
  disclosure, 333-334
Family planning, 433-434
Federal court, 26
Federal court of appeals, 25
Federal court system, 24-26
Federal physicians' immunity, 40-41
Federal Trade Commission, Antitrust law, 191
Federation of State Medical Boards, 102
Fetal protection policies, discrimination, 549-550
Fetal research, 715-716
Fetus, 364-370
  conscience clause, 369
  constitutional rights of the unborn, 365
  court-ordered obstetrical interventions, 452
  criminal law, 367-368
  ethical considerations, 364-365
  fetal rights under tort law, 365-367
  forced medical intervention on behalf of, 368
  meta-ethics, 365
  organ donation, 379-382
  parental tort liability, 367
  preconception tort liability, 366
  previable, 368
  protection by third parties, 368-369
  rights of conscience, 369
  viable, 368
  wrongful death, 366-367
Fire, 564
Food, Drug, and Cosmetic Act, 88, 169
Food and Drug Administration, 169
Forcible feeding, 206

Forensic anthropology, 570
Forensic biochemistry, defined, 4
Forensic dentistry, 570
Forensic medicine, 558-565
    adversarial process, 560
    defined, 4
    expert witness, 560-561
        court-appointed experts, 561
        opinion testimony, 561
    history, 558-560
Forensic orthopedic surgery, defined, 4
Forensic pathology, 567-584
    child abuse, 579-581
    defined, 4
    DNA, 582-583
    drug abuse, 581-582
    hospital pathology, compared, 568-575
    identifying deceased, 570
    manner of death, 573-575
    paternity, 578-579
    rape, 575-578
    time of death, 570-572
    time of injury, 572-573
Forensic psychiatry, 564-565, 585-613
    criminal law, 590-598
        competency to stand trial, 591-592
        defenses, 592-598
        diminished capacity, 596
        insanity defense, 592-598
    guilty but mentally ill, 598
    mental state, 585-586
Forensic psychologist, 564-565
Forensic toxicology, defined, 4
Fourteenth Amendment, 18-20
    equal protection, 20
    privileges and immunities clause, 18-19
    procedural due process, 19-20
    substantive due process, 19
Fraud, 672-679
    administrative hearing, 674
    contract law, 52
    liability insurance, 222
    limitations, 673
    Medicaid, 207, 673
    Medicare, 207, 673
        civil monetary penalties, 672-673
    preliminary investigation and negotiations, 673-674
    research, 353-354, 355-358
    scientific writing, 353-354, 355-358
    statute, 89
Freedom of Information Act, disclosure, 321-322
Full faith and credit, 22

G

Galan, 7

Gamete, cryopreservation, 443-444
Gender discrimination, 549-550
Genetic counseling, 432-433
Geriatric patient, 488-493
    Alzheimer's disease, 492
    case management, 492-493
    decision making, 492-493
    elder abuse and neglect, 490-492
    false imprisonment, 490
    psychological problems, 492
Good Samaritan statute, immunity, 33, 38-39
Governmental immunity, 39-40
Guardian, 32-33
    definition, 32
    determination of need for, 32-33
    general, 32, 33
    role of, 33
    selection of, 33
    specific, 32, 33
Guardian ad litem, 33
Gunshot wound, 573-574, 575

H

Hazard communication policies, 685-686
Hazard Communication Standard, 683-684
    occupational health law, 547
Hazard label, 684
Hazardous chemical, 683-684
Head injury
    alternative causes, 612
    anatomy, 610
    clinical findings, 611
    clinical presentation, 610-611
    dissimulation, 612-613
    epidemiology, 610
    pathology, 610
    permanent neuropsychiatric deficits, 611-612
    prognosis, 611
    secondary complications, 612
    testing, 612
Health care economics, 11-12
Health care proxy, 411
Health Care Quality Improvement Act, 37-38, 106, 107, 652
Health Care Quality Improvement Initiative, peer review organization, 680
Health care reform, antitrust law, 191
Health law, defined, 4
Health law study, 11
Health maintenance organization, 620-622
    contract warranty, 165-166
    corporate structure, 622
    cost containment, 662-663
    direct liability, 165
    group model, 621

independent practice association, 621
liability, 156, 164-165
mixed models, 621
models, 621-622
primary care model, 621
staff model, 621
statute, 88
Hepatitis B, bloodborne pathogen, 686
Hindu medical ethics, 7
Hippocratic oath, 6
physician-assisted suicide, 426
Historical development, 46-47
HIV; *see* Human immunodeficiency virus
Holter recording, 699
Homicide, 205
Hospital
apparent agency, 642
corporate liability, 644-645
expanding hospital legal duties, 163-164
legal basis for duty to patients, 157-159
quality assurance, evolution of legal responsibilities, 641-642
regulation, 88
risk management, 652-653
Hospital admission
hospital liability
emergency, 642-643
nonemergency, 642
medical staff physician liability
emergency, 642-643
nonemergency, 642
Hospital and medical staff bylaws, credentialing, 650
Hospital ethics committee, 12
Hospital law, defined, 4
Hospital liability
emergency room care, 643-644
hospital admission, 642-643
emergency, 642-643
nonemergency, 642
Hospital medical record, 297-298
Hospital pathology, forensic pathology, compared, 568-575
Hospital record, retention, 305
House officer, 96-97
House staff, physician-patient relationship, 267
Human cloning, 723
Human immunodeficiency virus (HIV), 516-530
duty to warn, 325-326
evaluation guidelines, 528-529
information sources, 522-523
legal responses, 518-520
management, 528-529
pathogenesis, 517
protection of individual rights, 520
reporting requirements, 530

Revised Classification System 1993, 523-528
societal concerns, 519-520
testing, 517-518
treatment, 517-518
Human subject research
consent, 291-292
informed consent, 291-292

I

Immunity, 33-42; *see also Specific type*
child abuse reporting, 41-42
Good Samaritan statute, 33, 38-39
peer review committee, 35
reportable condition, 41-42
Impairment, 531-533
defined, 532
determination, 532-533
Implied consent, 275-276
Impossibility, contract law, 52
In vitro fertilization, 439-440
Incident report, 242, 262, 301-302
Incompetent patient, disclosure, 335
Incontestability clause, liability insurance, 222
Indemnification
contract law, 62
negligence, 127
Independent contractor, 619
apparent agency, 642
coprovider, 639
Independent practice association
contract warranty, 165-166
direct liability, 165
health maintenance organization, 621
liability, 156, 164-165
Infanticide, 205-206
Informed consent, 137, 278-279, 425; *see also* Consent
assumption of risk, 286-287
causes of action, 284-285
competency, 31-32
defenses to action for lack of, 286-287
elements, 278-279
emergency care, 283-284
failure of, 121
human subject research, 291-292
minor, 456-461
consent tests, 458
parental consent exceptions, 458-461
surgery for benefit of another, 457-458
obtaining, 287
oncology patient, 495-496
phantom physician, 289
sterilization, 292-293
whether to disclose, 278
Informed refusal, 288-289
Innovative therapy, 720-721

Insanity defense, 592-598
    abolition, 596-598
Institutional practice, 641-659, 642
    historical origins, 641-642
Insurance, hospital-required malpractice insurance,
        656-659
Insurance contract, 63-66
    antitrust, 64
    bad faith, 64
    claims-made coverage, 65
    duty to defend, 64
    employment contract, 66
    exclusionary clause, 64
    getting in, 65
    getting out, 65
    intentional tort, 64
    payment provisions, 65-66
    public policy, 64
    punitive damages, 64
    unjust dismissal, 66
    vicarious liability, 65
Insurance fraud, 197-198
Intentional tort, 130-131
    insurance contract, 64
    physician countersuit, 217
Intimate therapy, 207-208
Intrauterine device, 434-435
Involuntary commitment
    minor, 474-475
        institutional conditions, 475
    psychiatric patient, 588-590
        commitment procedures, 588-589
        commitment standards, 588
        least restrictive alternative, 589
        patient rights, 587, 589-590
Involuntary sterilization, 435-436
    minor, 468-470
        courts' power, 468
        judicial immunity, 468-469
        procedure, 469-470

J

Jewish medical ethics, 7
Joint and successive tortfeasors, 137
Joint Commission on Accreditation of Healthcare
        Organizations
    medical record, 304
    risk management, 258-259
Joint venture, 624-626
    antitrust law, 631-632
    contractual alternative dispute resolution, 633
    contractual model, 626
    conventional financing, 627
    corporate model, 626

corporate practice of medicine, 630
debt offering, 627-628
defined, 625
equipment lease financing, 628
ethical considerations, 628
financing considerations, 627-628
franchise model, 627
franchising, 628
general partnership model, 626
hospital goals, 625
insurance regulations, 632
liability, 632-633
licensure, 629
limited partnership model, 626-627
limited partnership syndications, 628
management contracts, 628
Medicaid fraud and abuse, 630-631
MeSh model, 626
need for, 625
nonprofit corporate financing, 628
organizational structural models, 626
physician goals, 625
public and private equity, 627-628
Racketeering Influence Corruption Act, 630-631, 632
reasons for, 625
reimbursement, 629
securities regulation, 629-630
taxation, 629
tax-exempt bonds, 627
types, 625-626
unrelated business taxable income, 629
utilization review, 629
venture capital, 628
venture capital model, 627
voluntary accreditation, 629
Judgment, civil trial, 76
Judgment notwithstanding the verdict, 76
Judicial review, 113-116
    bias, 114-115
    sufficiency of evidence, 115-116
    violation of hospital bylaws, 115
Judicial system, 24-26
Judicial tenure, 26
Jury instruction, civil trial, 76
Jury selection, civil trial, 73-74
Jury trial, 210-211

L

Labeling, pharmaceutical product liability, 172
Laboratory requirements, statute, 88
Laboratory tests, 705
Law, conflict of, 22-23
Law school, 8
    health law, 11

medical school, jointly sponsored clinics, 10-11
Learning technique, 703-705
Legal medicine
    current trends, 11-13
    definition, 3
    journals, 6
    law school education, 8
    medical school education, 9
    nineteenth-century American scholars, 5-6
    standards, 12
Legal medicine consultant, 12-13
Legal psychiatry, defined, 4
Legal risk, sources, 238-240
Legal system, 17-23
    adversarial process, 560
Lesser included offense, 200
Liability
    health maintenance organization, 156, 164-165
    independent practice association, 156, 164-165
    joint venture, 632-633
    legal basis for duty to patients, 157-159
    managed care organization, 156, 164-165
    medical staff, 162-163
        monitoring, 162-163
        selection, 162-163
        supervision, 162-163
    nondelegable duty, 159
    physician liability for other health care providers,
        123-124
    preferred provider organization, 156, 164-165
    professional association, 156, 164-165, 166
    professional corporation, 156, 164-165, 166
    professional service corporation, 166
    standards to measure hospital conduct, 159-162
Liability insurance, 220-234
    accounting reports, 226-230
    bad faith, 223-224
    claims, 230-233
    contract, 220-224
    contract formation, 221-222
    differences between statutory and GAAP
        accounting, 228-229
    direct regulation, 225
    election, 222-223
    estoppel, 222-223
    fraud, 222
    glossary, 235-236
    incontestability clause, 222
    incurred but not reported claims, 228
    loss reserves, 227-228
    National Association of Insurance Commissioners
        blank, 228
    occurrence *versus* claims-made policy, 230-231
    policy provisions, 230-233

    pricing, 232-233
    prior knowledge of claim, 231
    problems, 227
    property-casualty company reports, 229-230
    rates, 224-226
    rating bureaus, 224
    regulation, 224-226
    reporting endorsements, 231-232
    reservation of rights, 223
    retroactive exclusion clause, 231
    risk retention group, 233-234
    state regulation, 225-226
    state *versus* federal regulation, 226
    statutory accounting, 228-229
    waiver, 222-223
Licensure
    appeal, 103
    attorney fees, 101
    board member recusal, 101
    commingling investigative and judicial functions, 100
    coprovider, 636
    defenses to disciplinary charges, 99-100
    disciplinary proceedings after formal charges are
        filed, 100-101
    disciplinary proceedings before formal charges are
        filed, 100
    disciplinary sanctions, 98-103
    disclosure, 337-338
    discovery, 101
    grounds for discipline, 98-99
    national collectors of disciplinary data, 102
    obtaining, 97-98
    Open Records Act, 102-103
    Opening Meetings Act, 102-103
    power of the state, 97
    requirements, 97-98
    restoration, 103
    sanctions, 101-102
    statute, by state, 91
    supervision, 98-103
    theory, 97-98
    types of, 97
Life-sustaining treatment, 425
Liquidated damages, 51
    contract law, 61
Living will, 411
Long arm statute, 22
Loss of chance, 134-136
Loss of consortium, 137-138
Loss of enjoyment of life, oncology patient, 500-501
Loss retention, 256

M

Malicious prosecution, physician countersuit, 214-216

Malpractice, 129-139
  allegations by average cost, 260
  allegations by cost, 260
  allegations by frequency, 260, 261
  allegations by location, 261
  allegations issues, 261
  allegations with highest indemnity, 260
  Employee Retirement Security Act, 166
  historical background, 129-130
  history of physician as defendant, 118
  hospital-required malpractice insurance, 656-659
  medical record, 305
  negotiation, 127-128
  occupational health care provider, 551-552
  plaintiff theories against physicians, 118-124
  psychiatrists, 598-606
  settlement, 127-128
  statute, by state, 92
  transplantation, 389-390
Managed care, cost containment, 663
Managed care organization
  contract warranty, 165-166
  direct liability, 165
  liability, 156, 164-165
Managed health care delivery system, 620-624
Market allocation, antitrust law, 187
Material safety data sheet, 684
MD/JD degree, 10
Mediation
  alternative dispute resolution, 80
  in health care, 80
Medicaid, 670-672
  abuse, 673
  beneficiaries, 670
  exclusion regulations, 671-672
  fee control, 670-671
  fraud, 197-198, 207, 673
  prospective payment system, 674-675
  scope of benefits, 670
Medical device
  statute, 88
  strict liability, 123
Medical evidence law and procedure, defined, 4
Medical examiner, 561
  organ donation, 375
Medical futility
  do-not-resuscitate order, 414-415
  dying, 414-415
Medical jurisprudence, 4-5
  defined, 4
Medical law, defined, 4
Medical literature, use as evidence, 149-150
Medical record, 297-308
  access, 302-304

access laws, 303
accuracy, 299
Age Discrimination in Employment Act, 304
AHA recommendations, 304
alcohol and drug abuse treatment records, 304
AMRA recommendations, 304
authorization, 301
autoauthentication, 307-408
  regulatory and accrediting issues, 307-408
clarity, 300-301
computerized, 306-307
confidentiality, 301
control of, 303-304
corrections and alterations, 299-300
custody, 303-304
destruction, 306
disclosure, 332-333
documentation, 301
employee, 305
function, 297-298
inappropriate entries, 300
information, 299
Joint Commission on Accreditation of Healthcare
    Organizations, 304
legal actions regarding access, 303
legibility, 300-301
loss, 303
malpractice, 305
Medicare, 306
ownership, 302-304
privacy, 301
purpose, 297-298
record keeping standards, 298-301
retention requirements, 304-306
spoilation of evidence, 303
statute of limitations, 304-305
storage, 303-304
transfer, 303
wrongful death, 305
Medical resources, ethical issues, 358-359
Medical school, 9
  academic dismissals, 94-95
  admissions criteria, 93-94
    Americans with Disabilities Act, 94
    Bakke decision, 94
    judicial review, 93
    reaction to *Bakke,* 94
  Americans with Disabilities Act, 96
  contractual relations, 96
  disciplinary dismissal, 95
  graduation, 94-97
  law school, jointly sponsored clinics, 10-11
  retention, 94-97
  substance of content of education, 96

substantive due process, 95-96
Medical staff
    liability, 162-163
        emergency, 642
        monitoring, 162-163
        nonemergency, 642
        selection, 162-163
        supervision, 162-163
    peer review, 651-652
Medical staff committee immunity, 35-38
Medical staff credentialing; *see* Credentialing
Medical technology, 691-709
Medical testimony, 141-153
    reasonable degree of medical certainty standard,
        150-151
Medicare
    abuse, 673
    administrative hearings, 668
    basis of denial, 666
    carrier fair hearing, 667-668
    carrier reconsideration, 667
    claims denial, 666
    conditions of participation, 664
    cost containment, 663-670
    court of appeals, 667
    diagnostic test billing, 665
    electronic billing, 675
    exclusion regulations, 671-672
    fraud, 197-198, 207, 673
        civil monetary penalties, 672-673
    judicial interpretation, 665
    judicial review, 668
    medical record, 306, 665
    Part B claims processing, 666
    participating provider, 664
    physician fee limits, 665
    physician's orders, 664-665
    prospective payment system, 674-675
    Provider Reimbursement Review Board, 669-670
    regulated fees, 665
    secondary payer, 670
    state statute, 665
    supplier or beneficiary procedural fairness, 667
    waiver of deductibles, 665
    waiver of liability provisions, 666-667
Medicolegal relations, defined, 4
Mental illness, crime, 203
Mental state, 585-586
Mental status examination, 609
Merger, antitrust law, 188
Microbiology, 705
Military physician, statute, 89
Minor, 456-479; *see also* Child abuse
    abortion, 446-447, 472-474

        bypass procedure, 472-473
        parental consent, 472
        parental notification, 473-474
    consent, 276
    contraception, 470-472
        parental consent, 471
        parental notification, 471-472
    contractual liability, 66-67
        health care, 67
        legal services, 67
        necessaries, 66-67
    disclosure, 334-335
    emancipation, 460
    emergency, 459
    informed consent, 456-461
        consent tests, 458
        parental consent exceptions, 458-461
        surgery for benefit of another, 457-458
    involuntary commitment, 474-475
        institutional conditions, 475
    involuntary sterilization, 468-470
        courts' power, 468
        judicial immunity, 468-469
        procedure, 469-470
    mature, 459-460
    parens patriae, 463-465
    police power, 465-466
    public health measures, 465-466
    religious convictions, 461, 466-468
    remote parents, 460
    rights, 461-462
    standard of care applicable to parents, 462
    state intervention, 462-468
    sterilization, 468-470
        hospital's refusal, 470
        institutionalized developmentally disabled,
            470
    transfusion, 466-468
    treatment against parental wishes, 461
    voluntary sterilization, 468
Miranda warning, crime, 209
Misrepresentation, contract law, 52
Mistake, contract law, 52
Monopolization, antitrust law, 187-188
Motion, civil trial, 71-72
Motion in limine, civil trial, 73
Mutuality of obligation, contract law, 49-50

N

National Committee on Quality Assurance, risk
    management, 258
National Health Service Corps, statute, 89
National Organ Transplant Act, 384, 397-403
National Practitioner Data Bank, 102, 106

Negligence, 118, 119-120, 132-133
   absence of duty, 124-125
   breach of duty, 119
   causation, 119-120
   compliance with the standard of care, 125-126
   corporate liability, 156-167
   damages, 120
   duty, 119
   exculpatory agreement, 127
   indemnification contract, 127
   lack of causation, 126
   no breach of duty, 125-126
   no damages, 126
   other defenses, 126-127
   physicians' defense theories against plaintiffs'
      claims, 124-127
   statute of limitations, 127
Negligent infliction of emotional distress, 134
Nerve conduction, 700
Neuropsychiatry, 608-613
New York
   do-not-resuscitate law, 420-421
   health care agents and proxies law, 421-422
No code order, 289
Noerr-Pennington doctrine, antitrust law, 190
No-fault compensation option, alternative dispute
     resolution, 80-81
No-fault plan, alternative dispute resolution, 80
Noncompetition clause, 51
   contract law, 61-62
Nondelegable duty, 643
   liability, 159
Notification, 326
Nuclear magnetic resonance imaging, 693-694

O

Occupational disease, disclosure, 322
Occupational health care provider
   legal liability, 551-552
   malpractice, 551-552
   risk management, 552
Occupational health law, 545-552
   Hazard Communication Standard, 547
   worker information, 547-548
Occupational Safety and Health Act, 545-547
   coverage, 545-546
   enforcement, 546-547
   penalties, 546
   record access, 548
   recording, 547-548
   reporting, 547-548
   standard setting, 546
   violations, 546
Occurrence screening, 242-243

Offer, contract law, 48-49
Oncology patient, 494-506
   causation, 499-500
   chemotherapy, 503-504
   comparative negligence, 500
   contributory negligence, 500
   damages, 499-500
   delay in diagnosis, 496-503
   disclosure, 496, 497-498
   informed consent, 495-496
   loss of enjoyment of life, 500-501
   misdiagnosis, 496-503
   radiation therapy, 503
   standard of care, 494-495
   unorthodox treatments, 504-506
Open Records Act, licensure, 102-103
Opening Meetings Act, licensure, 102-103
Opening statement, civil trial, 74
Oral contraceptive, 434
Organ donation, 372-390
   acceptance, 374-375
   anencephalic, 379-382
   cadaver organs, 379
   confidentiality, 383
   decedent gift, 373
   determination of death, 379
   donor consent, 382
   donor screening, 384
   execution, 374
   federal legislation, 384-386
   fetus, 379-382
   Food and Drug Administration, 385-386
   immunity, 375
   incompetent donor, 382-383
   living related donor, 382
   medical examiner, 375
   next-of-kin gift, 373-374
   organ sale, 385
   presumed/implied consent, 376
   required request, 375-376, 377-378
   routine inquiry, 375-376, 377-378
   state anatomical gift acts, 373-375
   Uniform Anatomical Gift Act, 373, 375
Ostensible agency, coprovider, 639-640

P

Package insert, pharmaceutical product liability, 172
Pain, 534-544, 701
   behavioral medicine, 541-542
   defined, 536
   diagnostic processes, 537-539
   disability, 531-532
   epidemiology, 536
   functional capacity assessment, 539

incidence, 536
medication, 540-541
medicolegal issues, 538-539
medicolegal/political issues, 542-544
multidisciplinary treatment, 539-542
physiotherapy, 542
sociolegal economic principles, 542-544
treatment processes, 539-542
types, 536-537
vocational rehabilitation, 542
Pain medicine, 534-535, 540-541
concepts, 535-536
Parens patriae, minor, 463-465
Parole evidence rule, 53
Partnership, 618-619
Part-time faculty, physician-patient relationship, 267
Passive euthanasia, 206, 415-416, 425
Paternity suit, 447-448
forensic pathology, 578-579
Patient control and supervision, psychiatry, 605-606
Patient-psychotherapist privilege, duty to warn, 323-324
Peer review, 105-111
appeal, 110
application limits, 110-111
California law overview, 107-108
confidentiality, 110
conflict of interest, 106-107
coprovider, 636-638
disciplinary actions, 638
normative *versus* actual standards of care, 637-638
quality assurance program, 637
standards of care, 637
due process, 107
definition, 107
interpretation, 107
immunities, 109-110
Judicial Review Committee bias, 109
legal representation, 106-107
medical staff, 651-652
modification and expansion, 107-111
notice requirements, 109
overlap of investigatory, prosecutorial, and adjudicatory functions, 110
preliminary investigation, 108-109
reportable sanctions, 109
right to representation, 106
rights of discovery of evidence, 109
statute, 90
Peer review committee, immunity, 35
Peer review organization, 679-680
case review, 680
Health Care Quality Improvement Initiative, 680
profiling, 679

quality intervention plan, 679-680
sanctions, 680
Penile plethysmography, 702
Per se rule, antitrust law, 181-188
Peritoneal lavage, 703
Persian medical ethics, 7
Personal protective equipment, 685
Pharmaceutical industry
government regulation, 169-170
history, 169
history, 168-169
Pharmaceutical product liability, 168-175
adverse reaction reporting, 169-170
advertising, 172-173
assumption of risk, 174
causation, 173
comparative fault, 174
damages, 174
defenses, 174
detail person, 173
drug testing, 169
labeling, 172
package insert, 172
pharmacist liability, 173-174
physician liability, 173-174
product misuse, 174
strict liability, 170-174
design defects, 170-171
manufacturing defects, 170
types of defects, 170-171
warning, 171-173
Pharmacist liability, pharmaceutical product liability, 173-174
Phonocardiography, 698-699
Photon imaging, 693-696
Physician
as employee, 619-620
as employer, 683-690
Physician aid-in-dying, 415-417
Physician countersuit, 213-218
abuse of process, 216
appeals results, 218
constitutional mandate, 217-218
defamation, 216-217
intentional tort, 217
malicious prosecution, 214-216
negligence, 217
policy considerations, 213-214
prima facie tort, 218
Physician immunity, 33-34
federal physicians, 40-41
Physician liability, pharmaceutical product liability, 173-174
Physician office record, 298

Physician Payment Review Commission, statute, 90
Physician-assisted suicide, 416, 419, 424-430
    common law, 426
    current positions of proponents, 429-430
    defined, 425
    definition of terms, 425
    Hippocratic oath, 426
    legal aspects, 426-427
    practical problems, 429
    request for assistance, 427-429
    state interests, 426
Physician-patient contract, 62-63
Physician-patient relationship, 248, 265-271
    abandonment, 270
    breach of contract, 267
    clinical faculty, 267
    covering physician, 267
    creation of, 265-266
    curbstone consultation, 267
    emergency room physician, 267
    house staff, 267
    indirect relationships with physicians, 269
    liability for injury to third parties, 268-269
    limiting, 266
    nature, 265-266
    nonpatient relationships with physicians, 268-269
    part-time faculty, 267
    patient autonomy, 425-426
    physician authority, 425-426
    problems, 270-271
    relationships formed by contract with others, 269-270
    second opinion program, 267
    sexual contact, 268
    sidewalk consultation, 267
    telephone contact, 268
    termination of, 270
    volunteer faculty, 267
Physiotherapy, pain, 542
Plea bargaining, crime, 210
Pleading, civil trial, 71
Pneumatic antishock garment, 696
Polygraph, coroner's case, 563
Positron emission tomography, 695
Postmortem examination, 567-568
Practice organization, 617-618
    among physicians, 618-620
Preconception issues, 432-437
Preconception tort liability, 366
Preembryo, protection under criminal law, 370
Preemployment physical, 335
Preemption clause, 20
Preferred provider organization, 621-622
    contract warranty, 165-166

corporate structure, 622
cost containment, 663
direct liability, 165
liability, 156, 164-165
Pregnancy, discrimination, 448, 549-550
Pregnancy Discrimination Act, 448
Prenatal injury issues, 444-445
President's Commission for the Study of Ethical
    Problems in Medicine and Biomedical and
    Behavioral Research, death, 406
Price-fixing, antitrust law, 183-184
Prima facie tort, physician countersuit, 218
Prison system, statute, 89
Privacy, 312-313
    educational use of patient information, 313-314
    erosion of patients' rights, 313
    health care team responsibility, 313
    medical record, 301
Privacy tort, 336-337
Privileged communication, 314-320
    evidentiary privilege, 316-317
Privileged conduct, crime, 204
Problem-oriented medical record, 307
Procedural due process, 19-20
    credentialing, 651
Product Liability Risk Retention Act, 233
Product misuse, pharmaceutical product liability, 174
Professional association
    contract warranty, 165-166
    direct liability, 165
    liability, 156, 164-165, 166
Professional corporation
    contract warranty, 165-166
    direct liability, 165
    liability, 156, 164-165, 166
Professional service corporation, liability, 166
Prospective payment system
    cost containment, 663
    Medicaid, 674-675
    Medicare, 674-675
Proton radiography, 693
Provider Reimbursement Review Board
    cost containment, 669-670
    Medicare, 669-670
Pseudodementia, 608-609
Psychiatric history, 609
Psychiatric malpractice, 598-606
Psychiatric patient, 585-613
    civil rights, 586-590
    criminal law, 590-598
        competency to stand trial, 591-592
        defenses, 592-598
        diminished capacity, 596
        insanity defense, 592-598

guilty but mentally ill, 598
  involuntary hospitalization, 588-590
    commitment procedures, 588-589
    commitment standards, 588
    least restrictive alternative, 589
    patient rights, 587, 589-590
  mental state, 585-586
  therapeutic methods, 586
  voluntary hospitalization, 586-587
Psychiatry
  abandonment, 604-605
  breach of confidentiality, 600-601
  failure to protect, 601-604
  failure to warn, 601-604
  informed consent, 599-600
  patient control and supervision, 605-606
  refusal of medication, 606-608
  sexual exploitation, 604
  suicide, 605-606
  treatment refusal, 599-600
  unusual and experimental therapies, 606
Psychosurgery, 586
Psychotherapy, 586
Psychotropic medication, 586
Public health law, defined, 4
Public health record, retention, 305-306
Public (medicolegal) death investigation program,
    defined, 4
Public policy, insurance contract, 64
Punitive damages, insurance contract, 64

Q

Quality assurance
  Clinical Laboratory Improvement Amendments,
    689-690
  Frederick II, 7
  hospital, evolution of legal responsibilities, 641-642
Quality assurance program, 637
Quality intervention plan, peer review organization,
    679-680
Quasi contract, 60

R

Racketeering Influence Corruption Act, joint venture,
    630-631, 632
Radiation therapy, oncology patient, 503
Radionuclide imaging, 695
Rape
  consent, 576-577
  forensic pathology, 575-578
Rationing, ethical issues, 358-359
Reasonable degree of medical certainty standard,
    150-151
Referral, disclosure, 280

Referring physician, coprovider, 640
Refusal of medication, psychiatry, 606-608
Reimbursement, 662-680
Reliance theory, 642
Religious convictions, minor, 461, 466-468
Relocation effect, 489-490
  legal implications, 489-490
Reportable condition, immunity, 41-42
Reporting statute, 137
Reproduction, 432-452, 722-724
Res ipsa loquitur, 133-134
Research
  Declaration of Helsinki, 714
  ethical issues, 353-354, 355-358, 711-726
    benefit *versus* risk rule, 717-718
    children as subjects, 714-715
    civil liability, 718-720
    criminal liability, 718-720
    fetal research, 715-716
    geriatric patient, 716-717
    historical background, 711-717
    radiation experiments, 721-722
  fraud, 353-354, 355-358
  LSD, 713
  Nuremberg Code, 713-714
  statute, 89-90
Reservation of rights, liability insurance, 223
Respiratory impedance pneumography, 699
Respondeat superior, 123-124, 156, 157, 268
  charitable immunity, 34, 35
Restitution, 57
Right of confidentiality, 312-313
Right of privacy, 312-313
Right to know, 326-328
Right to refuse treatment, 287-289, 410
  exceptions to, 287-288
Right to sue, 23
Rights of conscience, fetus, 369
Risk administrator, 237
Risk management, 237-259
  assessing risk exposure, 253-254
  assisting defense counsel, 249-251
  conducting investigations, 248-249
  continuous risk reduction cycle, 255-256
  defense counsel selection, 249
  defining performance expectations, 254-255
  external risk management requirements,
    257-259
  federal requirements, 257
  hospital, 652-653
  initial investigation, 246-248
  insurance carrier notification, 249
  Joint Commission on Accreditation of Healthcare
    Organizations, 258-259

Risk management—cont'd
National Committee on Quality Assurance, 258
occupational health care provider, 552
origin, 237-240
potential plaintiff prediction, 248
principles, 652-653
retaining risk, 256
risk avoidance strategies, 255
risk control, 246-251
risk financing, 256
risk identification, 240-245
case evaluation, 243-244
data-based performance monitoring, 244-245
external case identification, 241
internal case identification, 242-243
limitations, 244
methods, 241
strengths, 244
risk prevention, 251-256
risk prioritization, 245-246
scope, 237-240
state requirements, 257-258
transferring risk, 256-257
Robinson-Patman Act, 190-191
Roentgenography, 692-693

S

Scientific evidence, general acceptance, 148-149
Scientific literature
ethical issues, 353-354, 355-358
fraud, 353-354, 355-358
use as evidence, 149-150
Second opinion program, physician-patient
relationship, 267
Sexual exploitation, psychiatry, 604
Sharing arrangement, 618
Sherman Act, 180-181, 622, 623
Sidewalk consultation, physician-patient relationship,
267
Single-photon emission computerized tomography,
695
Skilled listening, 705
Social Security Act, 88-89
Solo practice, sole proprietor, 618
Sovereign immunity, 39-40
Spermicidal jelly, 435
Sports medicine, 554-557
definition, 554, 555, 556
equipment industry liability, 555
legal issues, 554
nonlicensed providers, 556
Spouse, consent, 276-278
Stab, 563
Staff privileges, 645-651

due process, 653-656
adequate time to prepare defense, 654
appearance before panel, 655
assistance of legal counsel, 655
cross-examination of witnesses, 655
initial *versus* existing, 654
notification of adverse recommendation,
654
physician's interest in, 653-654
physician's rights, 654-656
prehearing discovery, 654
presentation of witnesses and evidence in
defense, 655
private *versus* public hospitals, 653-654
scope of judicial review, 656
transcript of panel hearing, 655
written decision from panel, 656
written notice of charges, 654
Standard medical practice, 720
Standard of care, 12, 125-126
Stare decisis, 35
State court, 26
State jurisdiction, 89
Statute, 20
advanced health care directive, by state, 90
alternative medicine, 89
antitrust, 87
contract law, 55-56
controlled substance, by state, 91
fraud, 89
health maintenance organization, 88
laboratory requirements, 88
licensure, by state, 91
malpractice, by state, 92
medical device, 88
military physician, 89
National Health Service Corps, 89
peer review, 90
Physician Payment Review Commission, 90
prison system, 89
reporting, 137
research, 89-90
special types of patient employment, 89
Statute of limitations, 138
medical record, 304-305
negligence, 127
Statutory malpractice arbitration, alternative dispute
resolution, 79
Sterilization, 435-437
failure, 448-449
informed consent, 292-293
minor, 468-470
hospital's refusal, 470
institutionalized developmentally disabled, 470

Strict liability, 133
  drug, 123
  medical device, 123
  pharmaceutical product liability, 170-174
    design defects, 170-171
    manufacturing defects, 170
    types of defects, 170-171
    warning, 171-173
Subdermal implant, 435
Subpoena, 330-331
Substance abuse
  disclosure, 329
  treatment records, 304
Substantive due process, 19
  credentialing, 651
  medical school, 95-96
Sudden infant death syndrome, 564
Suicide, 360
  assisted, 200-201
  psychiatry, 605-606
Supervisory liability, coprovider, 638-639
Supreme Court, 25-26
Surface electromyography, 700
Surrogate motherhood, 440-443
Survival acts, 138

T

Tax Equity and Fiscal Responsibility Act, 675-679
Team physician, 554
Telephone management
  coverage, 346
  delegation of responsibility, 345
  development, 343-344
  documentation, 346
  evaluation, 346
  impact on medical practice, 343
  legal implications, 347-349
  medical implications, 347-349
  medication, 347-348
  physician-patient relationship, 268
  principles, 344-346
  recording phone calls, 347
  supervision, 346
  telephone assessment protocols, 345
  telephone assessment training, 345-346
  telephone call anatomy, 346-347
Testamentary capacity, competency, 29-31
  legal requirements, 30
  undue influence, 30-31
Testimonial disclosure, 317-320
  committee reports, 317-318
  exceptions, 318-319
  patient names, 317
  waivers, 319-320

Thermography, 691-692
Tort, 129; *see also* Intentional tort
  disclosure, 336-337
  historical background, 129-130
Tort liability, workers' compensation, 551
Transfer trauma, 489-490
  legal implications, 489-490
Transfusion, minor, 466-468
Transplantation, 372-390
  animal transplant, 383-384
  artificial transplant, 383-384
  cost, 387-389
  malpractice, 389-390
  organs used in, 392-393
  selection of organ recipients, 386-387
Transplantation shock, 489-490
  legal implications, 489-490
Traumatic brain impairment, 513-514
Traumatic encephalopathy, 610
Treatment
  proportionality/disproportionality, 419-420
  refusal, 287-289
    psychiatry, 599-600
  withdrawing, 410-413, 417
  withholding, 410-413, 417
Tying, antitrust law, 184-186

U

Ultrasound, 695-696
Ultrasound compression technique, 696
Undue influence, 30
  contract law, 51-52
Unemployment compensation, 687
  federal provisions, 687
  state provisions, 687
Uniform Anatomical Gift Act, 373, 375, 393-397
  consent, 293
Uniform Commercial Code, 55
Universal precautions, 685
Unjust dismissal, insurance contract, 66
Urine, 705
U.S. Constitution, 17-20
  constitutional supremacy clause, 18
  Fourteenth Amendment, 18-20
    privileges and immunities clause, 18-19

V

Vectorcardiogram, 696
Verbal contract, 58
Verbal order, 298
Vicarious liability, 638
  insurance contract, 65
Vital statistics, disclosure, 320-321
Vocational rehabilitation, pain, 542

Voluntary active euthanasia, physician-committed, 416
Voluntary hospitalization, psychiatric patient, 586-587
Voluntary sterilization, 435-436
  minor, 468
Volunteer faculty, physician-patient relationship, 267

W

Waiver, liability insurance, 222-223
Warrant, crime, 209
Warranty to cure, 122-123
Will, competency, 29-31
  undue influence, 30-31
Workers' compensation, 550-551, 686-687
  appeals, 687
  claim types, 686
  confidentiality, 551

disclosure, 321
records, 686-687
tort liability, 551
types, 686
World Medical Association, 7
Wrongful birth, 449-450
Wrongful conception, 448-449
Wrongful death, 138
Wrongful life, 433, 450-451
  fetus, 366-367
  medical record, 305
Wrongful pregnancy, 448-449

X

Xeroradiography, 692
X-ray, 692-693